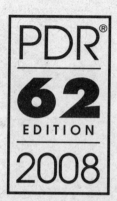

PHYSICIANS' DESK REFERENCE®

Supplement A

www.PDR.net
Web | PDA | Print

IMPORTANT NOTICE

Supplements to *Physicians' Desk Reference* are published twice yearly to provide readers with significant revisions of existing product listings as well as comprehensive information on new drugs and other products not included in the current annual edition. Before prescribing or administering any product described in *Physicians' Desk Reference*, be sure to consult this supplement to determine whether revisions have occurred since the 2008 edition of *PDR* went to press.

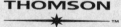

Officers of Thomson Healthcare: *President & Chief Executive Officer:* Mike Boswood; *Chief Medical Officer:* Alan Ying, MD; *Senior Vice President & Chief Technology Officer:* Frank Licata; *Chief Strategy Officer:* Courtney Morris; *Executive Vice President, Payer Decision Support:* Jon Newpol; *Executive Vice President, Provider Markets:* Terry Cameron; *Executive Vice President, Marketing & Innovation:* Doug Schneider; *Senior Vice President, Finance:* Phil Buckingham; *Vice President, Human Resources:* Pamela M. Bilash; *General Counsel:* Darren Pocsik

NEW AND REVISED PRODUCT LISTINGS INDEX

Listed below are new *PDR* listings first appearing in 2008 *PDR Supplement A,* as well as listings that have been revised since the publication of the main 2008 edition. New listings are in **bold type** and include comprehensive descriptions of new pharmaceutical products, new dosage forms of previously described products, and existing products not described in the main 2008 edition. Revised listings are in light type and may include new research data or clinical findings of importance.

ERRATA

PDR 2008

Mylan Pharmaceuticals

Page 7, third column, under "Direct Inquiries to:": The phone number is incorrectly listed as (804) 599-2595. It should be (304) 599-2595.

PBM Pharmaceuticals

Page 2468, top of first column: The product "Donnatel" is misspelled in the Continued Line. It is correctly spelled "Donnatal".

NEW PRODUCT LISTINGS

This section contains comprehensive descriptions of new pharmaceutical products introduced since publication of the 2008 *PDR*, new dosage forms of products already described, and existing pharmaceutical products not described in the 2008 *PDR*.

Allergan, Inc.
2525 DUPONT DRIVE
P.O. BOX 19534
IRVINE, CA 92623-9534

Direct Inquiries to:
1(800)433-8871

COMBIGAN™   ℞
(brimonidine tartrate/timolol maleate ophthalmic solution)

HIGHLIGHTS OF PRESCRIBING INFORMATION
These highlights do not include all the information needed to use COMBIGAN™ safely and effectively. See full prescribing information for COMBIGAN™.
COMBIGAN™ (brimonidine tartrate/timolol maleate ophthalmic solution) 0.2%/0.5%
Initial U.S. Approval: 2007

--------------INDICATIONS AND USAGE---------------
COMBIGAN™ is an alpha adrenergic receptor agonist with a beta adrenergic receptor inhibitor indicated for the reduction of elevated intraocular pressure (IOP) in patients with glaucoma or ocular hypertension who require adjunctive or replacement therapy due to inadequately controlled IOP; the IOP-lowering of COMBIGAN™ dosed twice a day was slightly less than that seen with the concomitant administration of timolol maleate ophthalmic solution, 0.5% dosed twice a day and brimonidine tartrate ophthalmic solution, 0.2% dosed three times per day. (1)

-----------DOSAGE AND ADMINISTRATION-----------
• One drop in the affected eye(s), twice daily approximately 12 hours apart. (2)

---------DOSAGE FORMS AND STRENGTHS----------
• Solution containing 2 mg/mL brimonidine tartrate and 5 mg/mL timolol. (3)

-----------------CONTRAINDICATIONS-----------------
• Bronchial asthma, a history of bronchial asthma, severe chronic obstructive pulmonary disease. (4, 5.1, 5.3)
• Sinus bradycardia, second or third degree atrioventricular block, overt cardiac failure, cardiogenic shock. (4, 5.2)
• Hypersensitivity to any component of this product. (4)

------------WARNINGS AND PRECAUTIONS------------
• Potentiation of respiratory reactions including asthma (5.1)
• Cardiac Failure (5.2)
• Obstructive Pulmonary Disease (5.3)
• Potentiation of vascular insufficiency (5.4)
• Increased reactivity to allergens (5.5)
• Potentiation of muscle weakness (5.6)
• Masking of hypoglycemic symptoms in patients with diabetes mellitus (5.7)
• Masking of thyrotoxicosis (5.8)

-------------------ADVERSE REACTIONS-----------------
Most common adverse reactions occurring in approximately 5 to 15% of patients included allergic conjunctivitis, conjunctival folliculosis, conjunctival hyperemia, eye pruritus, ocular burning, and stinging. (6.1)
To report SUSPECTED ADVERSE REACTIONS, contact Allergan at 800-433-8871 or the FDA at 800-FDA-1088 or www.fda.gov/medwatch.

-----------------DRUG INTERACTIONS-----------------
• Antihypertensives/cardiac glycosides may lower blood pressure. (7.1)
• Concomitant use with systemic beta-blockers may potentiate systemic beta-blockade. (7.2)
• Oral or intravenous calcium antagonists may cause atrioventricular conduction disturbances, left ventricular failure, and hypotension. (7.3)

• Catecholamine-depleting drugs may have additive effects and produce hypotension and/or marked bradycardia. (7.4)
• Use with CNS depressants may result in an additive or potentiating effect. (7.5)
• Digitalis and calcium antagonists may have additive effects in prolonging atrioventricular conduction time. (7.6)
• CYP2D6 inhibitors may potentiate systemic beta-blockade. (7.7)
• Tricyclic antidepressants may potentially blunt the hypotensive effect of systemic clonidine. (7.8)
• Monoamine oxidase inhibitors may result in increased hypotension. (7.9)

-------------USE IN SPECIFIC POPULATIONS-------------
• Not for use in children below the age of 2 years. (8.4)
See 17 for Patient Counseling Information
Revised: 01/2008

FULL PRESCRIBING INFORMATION

1   INDICATIONS AND USAGE
COMBIGAN™ (brimonidine tartrate/timolol maleate ophthalmic solution) 0.2%/0.5% is an alpha adrenergic receptor agonist with a beta adrenergic receptor inhibitor indicated for the reduction of elevated intraocular pressure (IOP) in patients with glaucoma or ocular hypertension who require adjunctive or replacement therapy due to inadequately controlled IOP; the IOP-lowering of COMBIGAN™ dosed twice a day was slightly less than that seen with the concomitant administration of 0.5% timolol maleate ophthalmic solution dosed twice a day and 0.2% brimonidine tartrate ophthalmic solution dosed three times per day.

2   DOSAGE AND ADMINISTRATION
The recommended dose is one drop of COMBIGAN™ in the affected eye(s) twice daily approximately 12 hours apart. If more than one topical ophthalmic product is to be used, the different products should be instilled at least 5 minutes apart.

3   DOSAGE FORMS AND STRENGTHS
Solution containing 2 mg/mL brimonidine tartrate and 5 mg/mL timolol (6.8 mg/mL timolol maleate).

4   CONTRAINDICATIONS
Asthma, COPD
COMBIGAN™ is contraindicated in patients with bronchial asthma; a history of bronchial asthma; severe chronic obstructive pulmonary disease (see **Warnings and Precautions**, 5.1, 5.3).

Sinus bradycardia, AV block, Cardiac failure, Cardiogenic shock
COMBIGAN™ is contraindicated in patients with sinus bradycardia; second or third degree atrioventricular block; overt cardiac failure (see **Warnings and Precautions**, 5.2); cardiogenic shock.

Hypersensitivity reactions
Local hypersensitivity reactions have occurred following the use of different components of COMBIGAN™. COMBIGAN™ is contraindicated in patients who have exhibited a hypersensitivity reaction to any component of this medication in the past.

5   WARNINGS AND PRECAUTIONS
5.1   Potentiation of respiratory reactions including asthma
COMBIGAN™ contains timolol maleate; and although administered topically can be absorbed systemically. Therefore, the same types of adverse reactions found with systemic administration of beta-adrenergic blocking agents may occur with topical administration. For example, severe respiratory reactions including death due to bronchospasm in patients with asthma have been reported following systemic or ophthalmic administration of timolol maleate (see **Contraindications**, 4).

5.2   Cardiac Failure
Sympathetic stimulation may be essential for support of the circulation in individuals with diminished myocardial contractility, and its inhibition by beta-adrenergic receptor blockade may precipitate more severe failure.
In patients without a history of cardiac failure, continued depression of the myocardium with beta-blocking agents over a period of time can, in some cases, lead to cardiac failure. At the first sign or symptom of cardiac failure, COMBIGAN™ should be discontinued (see also **Contraindications**, 4).

5.3   Obstructive Pulmonary Disease
Patients with chronic obstructive pulmonary disease (e.g., chronic bronchitis, emphysema) of mild or moderate severity, bronchospastic disease, or a history of bronchospastic disease (other than bronchial asthma or a history of bronchial asthma, in which COMBIGAN™ is contraindicated (see **Contraindications**, 4)) should, in general, not receive beta-blocking agents, including COMBIGAN™.

Continued on next page

Combigan—Cont.

5.4 Potentiation of vascular insufficiency

COMBIGAN™ may potentiate syndromes associated with vascular insufficiency. **COMBIGAN™** should be used with caution in patients with depression, cerebral or coronary insufficiency, Raynaud's phenomenon, orthostatic hypotension, or thromboangiitis obliterans.

5.5 Increased reactivity to allergens

While taking beta-blockers, patients with a history of atopy or a history of severe anaphylactic reactions to a variety of allergens may be more reactive to repeated accidental, diagnostic, or therapeutic challenge with such allergens. Such patients may be unresponsive to the usual doses of epinephrine used to treat anaphylactic reactions.

5.6 Potentiation of muscle weakness

Beta-adrenergic blockade has been reported to potentiate muscle weakness consistent with certain myasthenic symptoms (e.g., diplopia, ptosis, and generalized weakness). Timolol has been reported rarely to increase muscle weakness in some patients with myasthenia gravis or myasthenic symptoms.

5.7 Masking of hypoglycemic symptoms in patients with diabetes mellitus

Beta-adrenergic blocking agents should be administered with caution in patients subject to spontaneous hypoglycemia or to diabetic patients (especially those with labile diabetes) who are receiving insulin or oral hypoglycemic agents. Beta-adrenergic receptor blocking agents may mask the signs and symptoms of acute hypoglycemia.

5.8 Masking of thyrotoxicosis

Beta-adrenergic blocking agents may mask certain clinical signs (e.g., tachycardia) of hyperthyroidism. Patients suspected of developing thyrotoxicosis should be managed carefully to avoid abrupt withdrawal of beta-adrenergic blocking agents that might precipitate a thyroid storm.

5.9 Contamination of topical ophthalmic products after use

There have been reports of bacterial keratitis associated with the use of multiple dose containers of topical ophthalmic products. These containers had been inadvertently contaminated by patients who, in most cases, had a concurrent corneal disease or a disruption of the ocular epithelial surface (see **Patient Counseling Information**, 17).

5.10 Impairment of beta-adrenergically mediated reflexes during surgery

The necessity or desirability of withdrawal of beta-adrenergic blocking agents prior to major surgery is controversial. Beta-adrenergic receptor blockade impairs the ability of the heart to respond to beta-adrenergically mediated reflex stimuli. This may augment the risk of general anesthesia in surgical procedures. Some patients receiving beta-adrenergic receptor blocking agents have experienced protracted severe hypotension during anesthesia. Difficulty in restarting and maintaining the heartbeat has also been reported. For these reasons, in patients undergoing elective surgery, some authorities recommend gradual withdrawal of beta-adrenergic receptor blocking agents.

If necessary during surgery, the effects of beta-adrenergic blocking agents may be reversed by sufficient doses of adrenergic agonists.

6 ADVERSE REACTIONS

6.1 Clinical Studies Experience

Because clinical studies are conducted under widely varying conditions, adverse reaction rates observed in the clinical studies of a drug cannot be directly compared to rates in the clinical studies of another drug and may not reflect the rates observed in practice.

COMBIGAN™

In clinical trials of 12 months duration with **COMBIGAN™**, the most frequent reactions associated with its use occurring in approximately 5% to 15% of the patients included: allergic conjunctivitis, conjunctival folliculosis, conjunctival hyperemia, eye pruritus, ocular burning, and stinging. The following adverse reactions were reported in 1% to 5% of patients: asthenia, blepharitis, corneal erosion, depression, epiphora, eye discharge, eye dryness, eye irritation, eye pain, eyelid edema, eyelid erythema, eyelid pruritus, foreign body sensation, headache, hypertension, oral dryness, somnolence, superficial punctate keratitis, and visual disturbance.

Other adverse reactions that have been reported with the individual components are listed below.

Brimonidine Tartrate (0.1%-0.2%)

Abnormal taste, allergic reaction, blepharoconjunctivitis, blurred vision, bronchitis, cataract, conjunctival edema, conjunctival hemorrhage, conjunctivitis, cough, dizziness, dyspepsia, dyspnea, fatigue, flu syndrome, follicular conjunctivitis, gastrointestinal disorder, hypercholesterolemia, hypotension, infection (primarily colds and respiratory infections), hordeolum, insomnia, keratitis, lid disorder, nasal dryness, ocular allergic reaction, pharyngitis, photophobia, rash, rhinitis, sinus infection, sinusitis, taste perversion, tearing, visual field defect, vitreous detachment, vitreous disorder, vitreous floaters, and worsened visual acuity.

Timolol (Ocular Administration)

Body as a whole: chest pain; *Cardiovascular*: Arrhythmia, bradycardia, cardiac arrest, cardiac failure, cerebral ischemia, cerebral vascular accident, claudication, cold hands and feet, edema, heart block, palpitation, pulmonary edema, Raynaud's phenomenon, syncope, and worsening of angina pectoris; *Digestive*: Anorexia, diarrhea, nausea; *Immunologic*: Systemic lupus erythematosus; *Nervous System/Psychiatric*: Increase in signs and symptoms of myasthenia gravis, insomnia, nightmares, paresthesia, behavioral changes and psychic disturbances including confusion, hallucinations, anxiety, disorientation, nervousness, and memory loss; *Skin*: Alopecia, psoriasiform rash or exacerbation of psoriasis; *Hypersensitivity*: Signs and symptoms of systemic allergic reactions, including anaphylaxis, angioedema, urticaria, and generalized and localized rash; *Respiratory*: Bronchospasm (predominantly in patients with pre-existing bronchospastic disease), dyspnea, nasal congestion, respiratory failure; *Endocrine*: Masked symptoms of hypoglycemia in diabetes patients (see **Warnings and Precautions**, 5.7); *Special Senses*: diplopia, choroidal detachment following filtration surgery, cystoid macular edema, decreased corneal sensitivity, pseudopemphigoid, ptosis, refractive changes, tinnitus; *Urogenital*: Decreased libido, impotence, Peyronie's disease, retroperitoneal fibrosis.

6.2 Postmarketing Experience

Brimonidine

The following reactions have been identified during postmarketing use of brimonidine tartrate ophthalmic solutions in clinical practice. Because they are reported voluntarily from a population of unknown size, estimates of frequency cannot be made. The reactions, which have been chosen for inclusion due to either their seriousness, frequency of reporting, possible causal connection to brimonidine tartrate ophthalmic solutions, or a combination of these factors, include: bradycardia, depression, iritis, keratoconjunctivitis sicca, miosis, nausea, skin reactions (including erythema, eyelid pruritus, rash, and vasodilation), and tachycardia. Apnea, bradycardia, hypotension, hypothermia, hypotonia, and somnolence have been reported in infants receiving brimonidine tartrate ophthalmic solutions.

Oral Timolol/Oral Beta-blockers

The following additional adverse reactions have been reported in clinical experience with ORAL timolol maleate or other ORAL beta-blocking agents and may be considered potential effects of ophthalmic timolol maleate: *Allergic*: Erythematous rash, fever combined with aching and sore throat, laryngospasm with respiratory distress; *Body as a whole*: Decreased exercise tolerance, extremity pain, weight loss; *Cardiovascular*: Vasodilatation, worsening of arterial insufficiency; *Digestive*: Gastrointestinal pain, hepatomegaly, ischemic colitis, mesenteric arterial thrombosis, vomiting; *Hematologic*: Agranulocytosis, nonthrombocytopenic purpura, thrombocytopenic purpura; *Endocrine*: Hyperglycemia, hypoglycemia; *Skin*: Increased pigmentation, pruritus, skin irritation, sweating; *Musculoskeletal*: Arthralgia; *Nervous System/Psychiatric*: An acute reversible syndrome characterized by disorientation for time and place, decreased performance on neuropsychometrics, diminished concentration, emotional lability, local weakness, reversible mental depression progressing to catatonia, slightly clouded sensorium, vertigo; *Respiratory*: Bronchial obstruction, rales; *Urogenital*: Urination difficulties.

7 DRUG INTERACTIONS

7.1 Antihypertensives/Cardiac Glycosides

Because **COMBIGAN™** may reduce blood pressure, caution in using drugs such as antihypertensives and/or cardiac glycosides with **COMBIGAN™** is advised.

7.2 Beta-adrenergic Blocking Agents

Patients who are receiving a beta-adrenergic blocking agent orally and **COMBIGAN™** should be observed for potential additive effects of beta-blockade, both systemic and on intraocular pressure. The concomitant use of two topical beta-adrenergic blocking agents is not recommended.

7.3 Calcium Antagonists

Caution should be used in the co-administration of beta-adrenergic blocking agents, such as **COMBIGAN™**, and oral or intravenous calcium antagonists because of possible atrioventricular conduction disturbances, left ventricular failure, and hypotension. In patients with impaired cardiac function, co-administration should be avoided.

7.4 Catecholamine-depleting Drugs

Close observation of the patient is recommended when a beta blocker is administered to patients receiving catecholamine-depleting drugs such as reserpine, because of possible additive effects and the production of hypotension and/or marked bradycardia, which may result in vertigo, syncope, or postural hypotension.

7.5 CNS Depressants

Although specific drug interaction studies have not been conducted with **COMBIGAN™**, the possibility of an additive or potentiating effect with CNS depressants (alcohol, barbiturates, opiates, sedatives, or anesthetics) should be considered.

7.6 Digitalis and Calcium Antagonists

The concomitant use of beta-adrenergic blocking agents with digitalis and calcium antagonists may have additive effects in prolonging atrioventricular conduction time.

7.7 CYP2D6 Inhibitors

Potentiated systemic beta-blockade (e.g., decreased heart rate, depression) has been reported during combined treatment with CYP2D6 inhibitors (e.g., quinidine, SSRIs) and timolol.

7.8 Tricyclic Antidepressants

Tricyclic antidepressants have been reported to blunt the hypotensive effect of systemic clonidine. It is not known whether the concurrent use of these agents with **COMBIGAN™** in humans can lead to resulting interference with the IOP lowering effect. Caution, however, is advised in patients taking tricyclic antidepressants which can affect the metabolism and uptake of circulating amines.

7.9 Monoamine oxidase inhibitors

Monoamine oxidase (MAO) inhibitors may theoretically interfere with the metabolism of brimonidine and potentially result in an increased systemic side-effect such as hypotension. Caution is advised in patients taking MAO inhibitors which can affect the metabolism and uptake of circulating amines.

8 USE IN SPECIFIC POPULATIONS

8.1 Pregnancy

Pregnancy Category C: Teratogenicity studies have been performed in animals.

Brimonidine tartrate was not teratogenic when given orally during gestation days 6 through 15 in rats and days 6 through 18 in rabbits. The highest doses of brimonidine tartrate in rats (1.65 mg/kg/day) and rabbits (3.33 mg/kg/day) achieved AUC exposure values 580 and 37-fold higher, respectively, than similar values estimated in humans treated with **COMBIGAN™**, 1 drop in both eyes twice daily.

Teratogenicity studies with timolol in mice, rats, and rabbits at oral doses up to 50 mg/ kg/day [4,200 times the maximum recommended human ocular dose of 0.012 mg/kg/day on a mg/kg basis (MRHOD)] demonstrated no evidence of fetal malformations. Although delayed fetal ossification was observed at this dose in rats, there were no adverse effects on postnatal development of offspring. Doses of 1,000 mg/kg/day (83,000 times the MRHOD) were maternotoxic in mice and resulted in an increased number of fetal resorptions. Increased fetal resorptions were also seen in rabbits at doses 8,300 times the MRHOD without apparent maternotoxicity.

There are no adequate and well-controlled studies in pregnant women; however, in animal studies, brimonidine crossed the placenta and entered into the fetal circulation to a limited extent. Because animal reproduction studies are not always predictive of human response, **COMBIGAN™** should be used during pregnancy only if the potential benefit to the mother justifies the potential risk to the fetus.

8.3 Nursing Mothers

Timolol has been detected in human milk following oral and ophthalmic drug administration. It is not known whether brimonidine tartrate is excreted in human milk, although in animal studies, brimonidine tartrate has been shown to be excreted in breast milk. Because of the potential for serious adverse reactions from **COMBIGAN™** in nursing infants, a decision should be made whether to discontinue nursing or to discontinue the drug, taking into account the importance of the drug to the mother.

8.4 Pediatric Use

COMBIGAN™ is not recommended for use in children under the age of 2 years. During post-marketing surveillance, apnea, bradycardia, hypotension, hypothermia, hypotonia, and somnolence have been reported in infants receiving brimonidine. The safety and effectiveness of brimonidine tartrate and timolol maleate have not been studied in children below the age of two years.

The safety and effectiveness of **COMBIGAN™** have been established in the age groups 2–16 years of age. Use of **COMBIGAN™** in these age groups is supported by evidence from adequate and well-controlled studies of **COMBIGAN™** in adults with additional data from a study of the concomitant use of brimonidine tartrate ophthalmic solution 0.2% and timolol maleate ophthalmic solution in pediatric glaucoma patients (ages 2 to 7 years). In this study, brimonidine tartrate ophthalmic solution 0.2% was dosed three times a day as adjunctive therapy to beta-blockers. The most commonly observed adverse reactions were somnolence (50%-83% in patients 2 to 6 years) and decreased alertness. In pediatric patients 7 years of age or older (>20 kg), somnolence appears to occur less frequently (25%). Approximately 16% of patients on brimonidine tartrate ophthalmic solution discontinued from the study due to somnolence.

8.5 Geriatric Use

No overall differences in safety or effectiveness have been observed between elderly and other adult patients.

10 OVERDOSAGE

No information is available on overdosage with **COMBIGAN™** in humans. There have been reports of inadvertent overdosage with timolol ophthalmic solution resulting in systemic effects similar to those seen with systemic beta-adrenergic blocking agents such as dizziness, headache, shortness of breath, bradycardia, bronchospasm, and cardiac arrest. Treatment of an oral overdose includes supportive and symptomatic therapy; a patent airway should be maintained.

11 DESCRIPTION

COMBIGAN™ (brimonidine tartrate/timolol maleate ophthalmic solution) 0.2%/0.5%, sterile, is a relatively selective alpha-2 adrenergic receptor agonist with a non-selective beta-adrenergic receptor inhibitor (topical intraocular pressure lowering agent).

The structural formulae are:

Brimonidine tartrate:

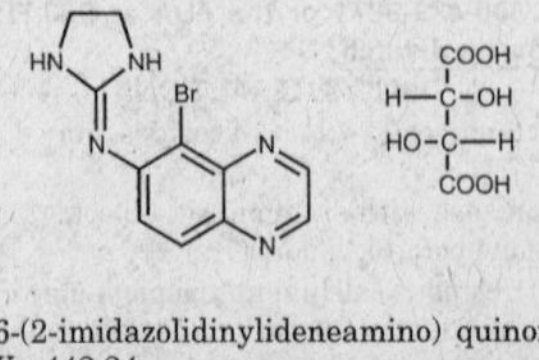

5-bromo-6-(2-imidazolidinylideneamino) quinoxaline L-tartrate; MW= 442.24

Timolol maleate:

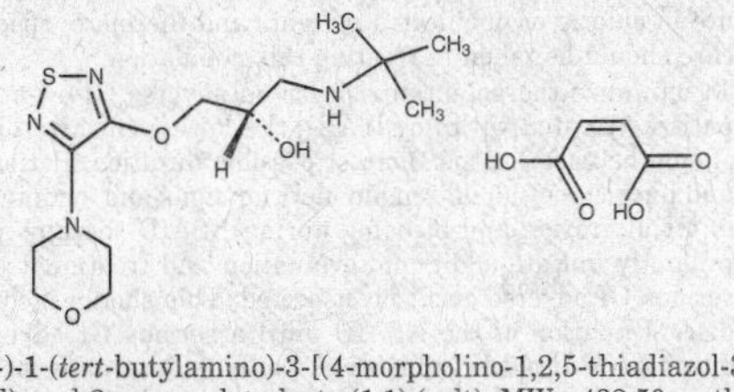

(-)-1-(*tert*-butylamino)-3-[(4-morpholino-1,2,5-thiadiazol-3-yl)-oxy]-2-propanol maleate (1:1) (salt); MW= 432.50 as the maleate salt

In solution, **COMBIGAN™** (brimonidine tartrate/timolol maleate ophthalmic solution) 0.2%/0.5% has a clear, greenish-yellow color. It has an osmolality of 260-330 mOsmol/kg and a pH during its shelf life of 6.5-7.3. Brimonidine tartrate appears as an off-white, or white to pale-yellow powder and is soluble in both water (1.5 mg/mL) and in the product vehicle (3.0 mg/mL) at pH 7.2. Timolol maleate appears as a white, odorless, crystalline powder and is soluble in water, methanol, and alcohol.

Each mL of **COMBIGAN™** contains the active ingredients brimonidine tartrate 0.2% and timolol 0.5% with the inactive ingredients benzalkonium chloride 0.005%; sodium phosphate, monobasic; sodium phosphate, dibasic; purified water; and hydrochloric acid and/or sodium hydroxide to adjust pH.

12 CLINICAL PHARMACOLOGY

12.1 Mechanism of Action

COMBIGAN™ is comprised of two components: brimonidine tartrate and timolol. Each of these two components decreases elevated intraocular pressure, whether or not associated with glaucoma. Elevated intraocular pressure is a major risk factor in the pathogenesis of optic nerve damage and glaucomatous visual field loss. The higher the level of intraocular pressure, the greater the likelihood of glaucomatous field loss and optic nerve damage.

COMBIGAN™ is a selective alpha-2 adrenergic receptor agonist with a non-selective beta-adrenergic receptor inhibitor. Both brimonidine and timolol have a rapid onset of action, with peak ocular hypotensive effect seen at two hours post-dosing for brimonidine and one to two hours for timolol.

Fluorophotometric studies in animals and humans suggest that brimonidine tartrate has a dual mechanism of action by reducing aqueous humor production and increasing non-pressure dependent uveoscleral outflow.

Timolol maleate is a beta$_1$ and beta$_2$ adrenergic receptor inhibitor that does not have significant intrinsic sympathomimetic, direct myocardial depressant, or local anesthetic (membrane-stabilizing) activity.

12.3 Pharmacokinetics

Absorption

Systemic absorption of brimonidine and timolol was assessed in healthy volunteers and patients following topical dosing with **COMBIGAN™**. Normal volunteers dosed with one drop of **COMBIGAN™** twice daily in both eyes for seven days showed peak plasma brimonidine and timolol concentrations of 30 pg/mL and 400 pg/mL, respectively. Plasma concentrations of brimonidine peaked at 1 to 4 hours after ocular dosing. Peak plasma concentrations of timolol occurred approximately 1 to 3 hours post-dose. In a crossover study of **COMBIGAN™**, brimonidine tartrate 0.2%, and timolol 0.5% administered twice daily for 7 days in healthy volunteers, the mean brimonidine area-under-the-plasma-concentration-time curve (AUC) for **COMBIGAN™** was 128 ± 61 pg•hr/mL versus 141 ± 106 pg•hr/mL for the respective monotherapy treatments; mean C_{max} values of brimonidine were comparable following **COMBIGAN™** treatment versus monotherapy (32.7 ± 15.0 pg/mL versus 34.7 ± 22.6 pg/mL, respectively). Mean timolol AUC for **COMBIGAN™** was similar to that of the respective monotherapy treatment (2919 ± 1679 pg•hr/mL versus 2909 ± 1231 pg•hr/mL, respectively); mean C_{max} of timolol was approximately 20% lower following **COMBIGAN™** treatment versus monotherapy.

In a parallel study in patients dosed twice daily with **COMBIGAN™**, twice daily with timolol 0.5%, or three times daily with brimonidine tartrate 0.2%, one-hour post dose plasma concentrations of timolol and brimonidine were approximately 30-40% lower with **COMBIGAN™** than their respective monotherapy values. The lower plasma brimonidine concentrations with **COMBIGAN™** appears to be due to twice-daily dosing for **COMBIGAN™** versus three-times dosing with brimonidine tartrate 0.2%.

Distribution

The protein binding of timolol is approximately 60%. The protein binding of brimonidine has not been studied.

Metabolism

In humans, brimonidine is extensively metabolized by the liver. Timolol is partially metabolized by the liver.

Excretion

In the crossover study in healthy volunteers, the plasma concentration of brimonidine declined with a systemic half-life of approximately 3 hours. The apparent systemic half-life of timolol was about 7 hours after ocular administration. Urinary excretion is the major route of elimination of brimonidine and its metabolites. Approximately 87% of an orally-administered radioactive dose of brimonidine was eliminated within 120 hours, with 74% found in the urine. Unchanged timolol and its metabolites are excreted by the kidney.

Special Populations

COMBIGAN™ has not been studied in patients with hepatic impairment.

COMBIGAN™ has not been studied in patients with renal impairment.

A study of patients with renal failure showed that timolol was not readily removed by dialysis. The effect of dialysis on brimonidine pharmacokinetics in patients with renal failure is not known.

Following oral administration of timolol maleate, the plasma half-life of timolol is essentially unchanged in patients with moderate renal insufficiency.

13 NONCLINICAL TOXICOLOGY

13.1 Carcinogenesis, Mutagenesis, and Impairment of Fertility

With brimonidine tartrate, no compound-related carcinogenic effects were observed in either mice or rats following a 21-month and 24-month study, respectively. In these studies, dietary administration of brimonidine tartrate at doses up to 2.5 mg/kg/day in mice and 1 mg/kg/day in rats achieved 150 and 210 times, respectively, the plasma C_{max} drug concentration in humans treated with one drop **COMBIGAN™** into both eyes twice daily, the recommended daily human dose.

In a two-year study of timolol maleate administered orally to rats, there was a statistically significant increase in the incidence of adrenal pheochromocytomas in male rats administered 300 mg/kg/day [approximately 25,000 times the maximum recommended human ocular dose of 0.012 mg/kg/day on a mg/kg basis (MRHOD)]. Similar differences were not observed in rats administered oral doses equivalent to approximately 8,300 times the daily dose of **COMBIGAN™** in humans.

In a lifetime oral study of timolol maleate in mice, there were statistically significant increases in the incidence of benign and malignant pulmonary tumors, benign uterine polyps and mammary adenocarcinomas in female mice at 500 mg/kg/day, (approximately 42,000 times the MRHOD), but not at 5 or 50 mg/kg/day (approximately 420 to 4,200 times higher, respectively, than the MRHOD). In a subsequent study in female mice, in which post-mortem examinations were limited to the uterus and the lungs, a statistically significant increase in the incidence of pulmonary tumors was again observed at 500 mg/kg/day.

The increased occurrence of mammary adenocarcinomas was associated with elevations in serum prolactin which occurred in female mice administered oral timolol at 500 mg/kg/day, but not at doses of 5 or 50 mg/kg/day. An increased incidence of mammary adenocarcinomas in rodents has been associated with administration of several other therapeutic agents that elevate serum prolactin, but no correlation between serum prolactin levels and mammary tumors has been established in humans. Furthermore, in adult human female subjects who received oral dosages of up to 60 mg of timolol maleate (the maximum recommended human oral dosage), there were no clinically meaningful changes in serum prolactin.

Brimonidine tartrate was not mutagenic or clastogenic in a series of in vitro and in vivo studies including the Ames bacterial reversion test, chromosomal aberration assay in Chinese Hamster Ovary (CHO) cells, and three in vivo studies in CD-1 mice: a host-mediated assay, cytogenetic study, and dominant lethal assay.

Timolol maleate was devoid of mutagenic potential when tested in vivo (mouse) in the micronucleus test and cytogenetic assay (doses up to 800 mg/kg) and in vitro in a neoplastic cell transformation assay (up to 100 mcg/mL). In Ames tests the highest concentrations of timolol employed, 5,000 or 10,000 mcg/plate, were associated with statistically significant elevations of revertants observed with tester strain TA100 (in seven replicate assays), but not in the remaining three strains. In the assays with tester strain TA100, no consistent dose response relationship was observed, and the ratio of test to control revertants did not reach 2. A ratio of 2 is usually considered the criterion for a positive Ames test.

Reproduction and fertility studies in rats with timolol maleate and in rats with brimonidine tartrate demonstrated no adverse effect on male or female fertility at doses up to approximately 100 times the systemic exposure following the maximum recommended human ophthalmic dose of **COMBIGAN™**.

14 CLINICAL STUDIES

Clinical studies were conducted to compare the IOP-lowering effect over the course of the day of **COMBIGAN™** administered twice a day (BID) to individually-administered brimonidine tartrate ophthalmic solution, 0.2% administered three times per day (TID) and timolol maleate ophthalmic solution, 0.5% BID in patients with glaucoma or ocular hypertension. **COMBIGAN™** BID provided an additional 1 to 3 mm Hg decrease in IOP over brimonidine treatment TID and an additional 1 to 2 mm Hg decrease over timolol treatment BID during the first 7 hours post dosing. However, the IOP-lowering of **COMBIGAN™** BID was less (approximately 1-2 mm Hg) than that seen with the concomitant administration of 0.5% timolol BID and 0.2% brimonidine tartrate TID.

COMBIGAN™ administered BID had a favorable safety profile versus concurrently administered brimonidine TID and timolol BID in the self-reported level of severity of sleepiness for patients over age 40.

16 HOW SUPPLIED/STORAGE AND HANDLING

COMBIGAN™ is supplied sterile, in white opaque plastic LDPE bottles and tips, with blue high impact polystyrene (HIPS) caps as follows:

5 mL in 10 mL bottle NDC 0023-9211-05
10 mL in 10 mL bottle NDC 0023-9211-10

Storage: Store between 15° to 25°C (59° to 77°F). Protect from light.

17 PATIENT COUNSELING INFORMATION

Patients with bronchial asthma, a history of bronchial asthma, severe chronic obstructive pulmonary disease, sinus bradycardia, second or third degree atrioventricular block, or cardiac failure should be advised not to take this product (see **Contraindications**, 4).

Patients should be instructed that ocular solutions, if handled improperly or if the tip of the dispensing container contacts the eye or surrounding structures, can become contaminated by common bacteria known to cause ocular infections. Serious damage to the eye and subsequent loss of vision may result from using contaminated solutions (see **Warnings and Precautions**, 5.9).

Patients also should be advised that if they have ocular surgery or develop an intercurrent ocular condition (e.g., trauma or infection), they should immediately seek their physician's advice concerning the continued use of the present multidose container.

If more than one topical ophthalmic drug is being used, the drugs should be administered at least five minutes apart.

Patients should be advised that **COMBIGAN™** contains benzalkonium chloride which may be absorbed by soft contact lenses. Contact lenses should be removed prior to administration of the solution. Lenses may be reinserted 15 minutes following administration of **COMBIGAN™**.

As with other similar medications, **COMBIGAN™** may cause fatigue and/or drowsiness in some patients. Patients who engage in hazardous activities should be cautioned of the potential for a decrease in mental alertness.

Irvine, CA 92612, U.S.A.
™ mark owned by Allergan, Inc.
U.S. Patents 6,248,741; 6,194,415; 6,465,464; and 7,030,149
71969US11U

Alpharma Pharmaceuticals LLC

ONE NEW ENGLAND AVENUE
PISCATAWAY, NJ 08854

Direct Inquiries to:
Medical Affairs
888-840-8884

FLECTOR® PATCH ℞

(diclofenac epolamine topical patch) 1.3%
Rx Only

Cardiovascular Risk

- NSAIDs may cause an increased risk of serious cardiovascular thrombotic events, myocardial infarction, and stroke, which can be fatal. This risk may increase with duration of use. Patients with cardiovascular disease or risk factors for cardiovascular disease may be at greater risk. (See **WARNINGS** and **CLINICAL TRIALS**).
- Flector® Patch is contraindicated for the treatment of peri-operative pain in the setting of coronary artery bypass graft (CABG) surgery (see **WARNINGS**).

Gastrointestinal Risk

- NSAIDs cause an increased risk of serious gastrointestinal adverse events including bleeding, ulceration, and perforation of the stomach or intestines, which can be fatal. These events can occur at any time during use and without warning symptoms. Elderly patients are at greater risk for serious gastrointestinal events. (See **WARNINGS**).

DESCRIPTION

Flector® Patch (10 cm × 14 cm) is comprised of an adhesive material containing 1.3% diclofenac epolamine which is applied to a non-woven polyester felt backing and covered with a polypropylene film release liner. The release liner is removed prior to topical application to the skin.

Diclofenac epolamine is a non-opioid analgesic chemically designated as 2-[(2,6-dichlorophenyl) amino]benzeneacetic acid, (2-(pyrrolidin-1-yl) ethanol salt, with a molecular formula of $C_{20}H_{24}Cl_2N_2O_3$ (molecular weight 411.3), an n-octanol/water partition coefficient of 8 at pH 8.5, and the following structure:

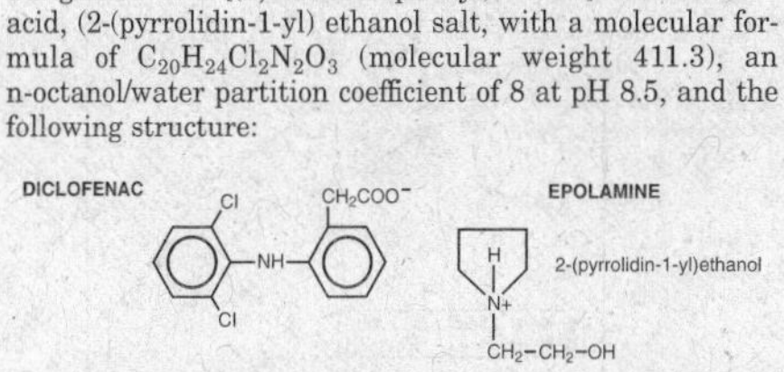

Each adhesive patch contains 180 mg of diclofenac epolamine (13 mg per gram adhesive) in an aqueous base. It also contains the following inactive ingredients: 1,3-butylene glycol, dihydroxyaluminum aminoacetate, diso-

Continued on next page

Flector Patch—Cont.

dium edetate, D-sorbitol, fragrance (Dalin PH), gelatin, kaolin, methylparaben, polysorbate 80, povidone, propylene glycol, propylparaben, sodium carboxymethylcellulose, sodium polyacrylate, tartaric acid, titanium dioxide, and purified water.

CLINICAL PHARMACOLOGY

Pharmacodynamics

Flector® Patch applied to intact skin provides local analgesia by releasing diclofenac epolamine from the patch into the skin. Diclofenac is a nonsteroidal anti-inflammatory drug (NSAID). In pharmacologic studies, diclofenac has shown anti-inflammatory, analgesic, and antipyretic activity. As with other NSAIDs, its mode of action is not known; its ability to inhibit prostaglandin synthesis, however, may be involved in its anti-inflammatory activity, as well as contribute to its efficacy in relieving pain associated with inflammation.

Pharmacokinetics

Absorption

Following a single application of the Flector® Patch on the upper inner arm, peak plasma concentrations of diclofenac (range 0.7 – 6 ng/mL) were noted between 10 – 20 hours of application. Plasma concentrations of diclofenac in the range of 1.3 – 8.8 ng/mL were noted after five days with twice-a-day Flector® Patch application.

Distribution

Diclofenac has a very high affinity (>99%) for human serum albumin.

Metabolism and Excretion

The plasma elimination half-life of diclofenac after application of Flector® Patch is approximately 12 hours. Diclofenac is eliminated through metabolism and subsequent urinary and biliary excretion of the glucuronide and the sulfate conjugates of the metabolites.

CLINICAL STUDIES

Efficacy of Flector® Patch was demonstrated in two of four studies of patients with minor sprains, strains, and contusions. Patients were randomly assigned to treatment with the Flector® Patch, or a placebo patch identical to the Flector® Patch minus the active ingredient. In the first of these two studies, patients with ankle sprains were treated once daily for a week. In the second study, patients with sprains, strains and contusions were treated twice daily for up to two weeks. Pain was assessed over the period of treatment. Patients treated with the Flector® Patch experienced a greater reduction in pain as compared to patients randomized to placebo patch as evidenced by the responder curves presented below.

Figure 1: Patients Achieving Various Levels of Pain Relief at Day 3; 14-Day Study

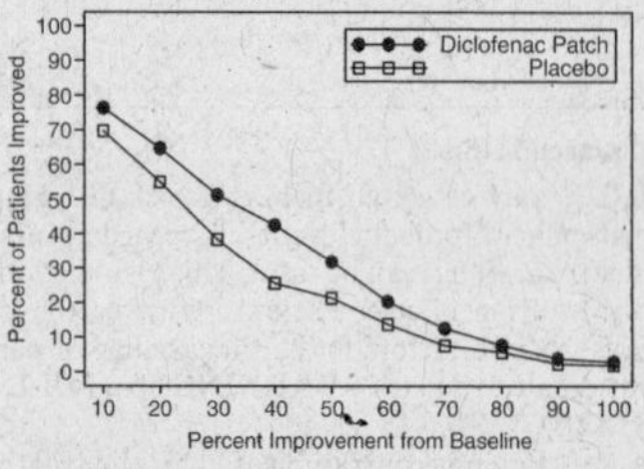

Figure 2: Patients Achieving Various Levels of Pain Relief at End of Study; 14-Day Study

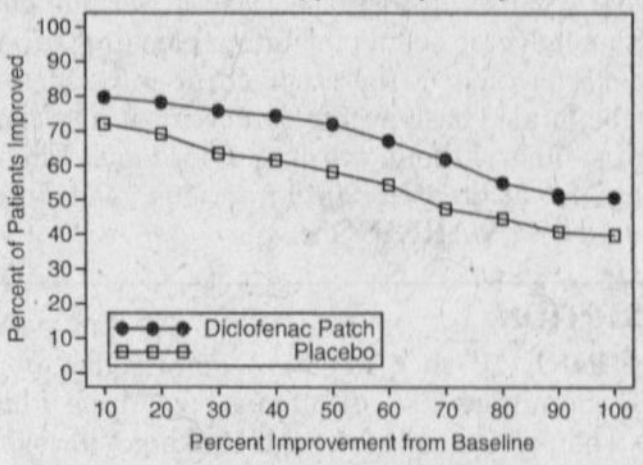

Figure 3: Patients Achieving Various Levels of Pain Relief at Day 3; 7-Day Study

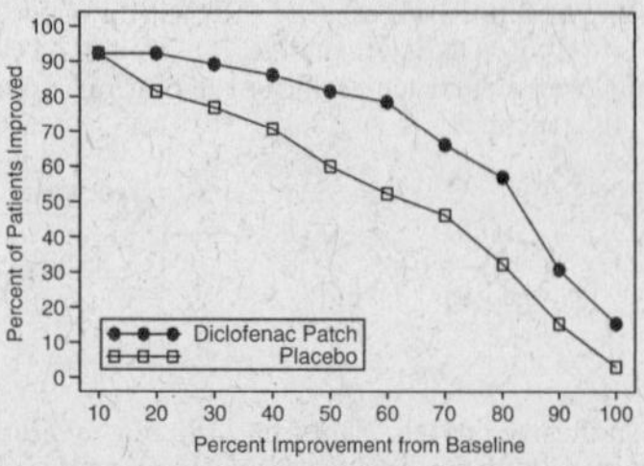

[See figure 4 at top of next column]

INDICATION AND USAGE

Carefully consider the potential benefits and risks of Flector® Patch and other treatment options before deciding to use Flector® Patch. Use the lowest effective dose for the shortest duration consistent with individual patient treatment goals (see **WARNINGS**).

Figure 4: Patients Achieving Various Levels of Pain Relief at End of Study; 7-Day Study

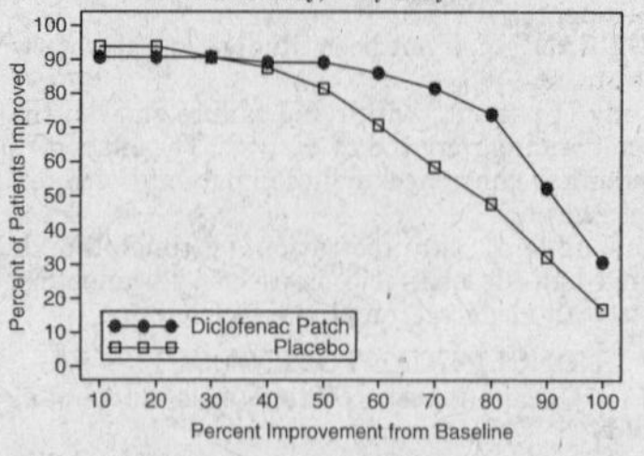

Flector® Patch is indicated for the topical treatment of acute pain due to minor strains, sprains, and contusions.

CONTRAINDICATIONS

Flector® Patch is contraindicated in patients with known hypersensitivity to diclofenac.

Flector® Patch should not be given to patients who have experienced asthma, urticaria, or allergic-type reactions after taking aspirin or other NSAIDs. Severe, rarely fatal, anaphylactic-like reactions to NSAIDs have been reported in such patients (see **WARNINGS - Anaphylactoid Reactions**, and **PRECAUTIONS - Preexisting Asthma**).

Flector® Patch is contraindicated for the treatment of perioperative pain in the setting of coronary artery bypass graft (CABG) surgery (see **WARNINGS**).

Flector® Patch should not be applied to non-intact or damaged skin resulting from any etiology e.g. exudative dermatitis, eczema, infected lesion, burns or wounds.

WARNINGS

CARDIOVASCULAR EFFECTS

Cardiovascular Thrombotic Events

Clinical trials of several COX-2 selective and nonselective NSAIDs of up to three years duration have shown an increased risk of serious cardiovascular (CV) thrombotic events, myocardial infarction, and stroke, which can be fatal. All NSAIDs, both COX-2 selective and nonselective, may have a similar risk. Patients with known CV disease or risk factors for CV disease may be at greater risk. To minimize the potential risk for an adverse CV event in patients treated with an NSAID, the lowest effective dose should be used for the shortest duration possible. Physicians and patients should remain alert for the development of such events, even in the absence of previous CV symptoms. Patients should be informed about the signs and/or symptoms of serious CV events and the steps to take if they occur.

There is no consistent evidence that concurrent use of aspirin mitigates the increased risk of serious CV thrombotic events associated with NSAID use. The concurrent use of aspirin and an NSAID does increase the risk of serious GI events (see **GI WARNINGS**).

Two large, controlled, clinical trials of a COX-2 selective NSAID for the treatment of pain in the first 10-14 days following CABG surgery found an increased incidence of myocardial infarction and stroke (see **CONTRAINDICATIONS**).

Hypertension

NSAIDs, including Flector® Patch, can lead to onset of new hypertension or worsening of pre-existing hypertension, either of which may contribute to the increased incidence of CV events. Patients taking thiazides or loop diuretics may have impaired response to these therapies when taking NSAIDs. NSAIDs, including Flector® Patch, should be used with caution in patients with hypertension. Blood pressure (BP) should be monitored closely during the initiation of NSAID treatment and throughout the course of therapy.

Congestive Heart Failure and Edema

Fluid retention and edema have been observed in some patients taking NSAIDs. Flector® Patch should be used with caution in patients with fluid retention or heart failure.

Gastrointestinal Effects- Risk of Ulceration, Bleeding, and Perforation

NSAIDs, including Flector® Patch, can cause serious gastrointestinal (GI) adverse events including inflammation, bleeding, ulceration, and perforation of the stomach, small intestine, or large intestine, which can be fatal. These serious adverse events can occur at any time, with or without warning symptoms, in patients treated with NSAIDs. Only one in five patients, who develop a serious upper GI adverse event on NSAID therapy, is symptomatic. Upper GI ulcers, gross bleeding, or perforation caused by NSAIDs occur in approximately 1% of patients treated for 3-6 months, and in about 2-4% of patients treated for one year. These trends continue with longer duration of use, increasing the likelihood of developing a serious GI event at some time during the course of therapy. However, even short-term therapy is not without risk.

NSAIDs should be prescribed with extreme caution in those with a prior history of ulcer disease or gastrointestinal bleeding. Patients with a *prior history of peptic ulcer disease and/or gastrointestinal bleeding* who use NSAIDs have a greater than 10-fold increased risk for developing a GI bleed compared to patients with neither of these risk factors. Other factors that increase the risk for GI bleeding in patients treated with NSAIDs include concomitant use of oral corticosteroids or anticoagulants, longer duration of NSAID therapy, smoking, use of alcohol, older age, and poor general health status. Most spontaneous reports of fatal GI events are in elderly or debilitated patients and therefore, special care should be taken in treating this population.

To minimize the potential risk for an adverse GI event in patients treated with an NSAID, the lowest effective dose should be used for the shortest possible duration. Patients and physicians should remain alert for signs and symptoms of GI ulceration and bleeding during NSAID therapy and promptly initiate additional evaluation and treatment if a serious GI adverse event is suspected. This should include discontinuation of the NSAID until a serious GI adverse event is ruled out. For high risk patients, alternate therapies that do not involve NSAIDs should be considered.

Renal Effects

Long-term administration of NSAIDs has resulted in renal papillary necrosis and other renal injury. Renal toxicity has also been seen in patients in whom renal prostaglandins have a compensatory role in the maintenance of renal perfusion. In these patients, administration of a nonsteroidal anti-inflammatory drug may cause a dose-dependent reduction in prostaglandin formation and, secondarily, in renal blood flow, which may precipitate overt renal decompensation. Patients at greatest risk of this reaction are those with impaired renal function, heart failure, liver dysfunction, those taking diuretics and ACE inhibitors, and the elderly. Discontinuation of NSAID therapy is usually followed by recovery to the pretreatment state.

Advanced Renal Disease

No information is available from controlled clinical studies regarding the use of Flector® Patch in patients with advanced renal disease. Therefore, treatment with Flector® Patch is not recommended in these patients with advanced renal disease. If Flector® Patch therapy is initiated, close monitoring of the patient's renal function is advisable.

Anaphylactoid Reactions

As with other NSAIDs, anaphylactoid reactions may occur in patients without known prior exposure to Flector® Patch. Flector® Patch should not be given to patients with the aspirin triad. This symptom complex typically occurs in asthmatic patients who experience rhinitis with or without nasal polyps, or who exhibit severe, potentially fatal bronchospasm after taking aspirin or other NSAIDs (see **CONTRAINDICATIONS** and **PRECAUTIONS - Preexisting Asthma**). Emergency help should be sought in cases where an anaphylactoid reaction occurs.

Skin Reactions

NSAIDs, including Flector® Patch, can cause serious skin adverse events such as exfoliative dermatitis, Stevens-Johnson Syndrome (SJS), and toxic epidermal necrolysis (TEN), which can be fatal. These serious events may occur without warning. Patients should be informed about the signs and symptoms of serious skin manifestations and use of the drug should be discontinued at the first appearance of skin rash or any other sign of hypersensitivity.

Pregnancy

In late pregnancy, as with other NSAIDs, Flector® Patch should be avoided because it may cause premature closure of the ductus arteriosus.

PRECAUTIONS

General

Flector® Patch cannot be expected to substitute for corticosteroids or to treat corticosteroid insufficiency. Abrupt discontinuation of corticosteroids may lead to disease exacerbation. Patients on prolonged corticosteroid therapy should have their therapy tapered slowly if a decision is made to discontinue corticosteroids.

The pharmacological activity of Flector® Patch in reducing inflammation may diminish the utility of these diagnostic signs in detecting complications of presumed noninfectious, painful conditions.

Hepatic Effects

Borderline elevations of one or more liver tests may occur in up to 15% of patients taking NSAIDs including Flector® Patch. These laboratory abnormalities may progress, may remain unchanged, or may be transient with continuing therapy. Notable elevations of ALT or AST (approximately three or more times the upper limit of normal) have been reported in approximately 1% of patients in clinical trials with NSAIDs. In addition, rare cases of severe hepatic reactions, including jaundice and fatal fulminant hepatitis, liver necrosis and hepatic failure, some of them with fatal outcomes have been reported.

A patient with symptoms and/or signs suggesting liver dysfunction, or in whom an abnormal liver test has occurred, should be evaluated for evidence of the development of a more severe hepatic reaction while on therapy with Flector® Patch. If clinical signs and symptoms consistent with liver disease develop, or if systemic manifestations occur (e.g., eosinophilia, rash, etc.), Flector® Patch should be discontinued.

Hematological Effects

Anemia is sometimes seen in patients receiving NSAIDs. This may be due to fluid retention, occult or gross GI blood loss, or an incompletely described effect upon erythropoiesis. Patients on long-term treatment with NSAIDs, including Flector® Patch, should have their hemoglobin or hematocrit checked if they exhibit any signs or symptoms of anemia.

NSAIDs inhibit platelet aggregation and have been shown to prolong bleeding time in some patients. Unlike aspirin, their effect on platelet function is quantitatively less, of shorter duration, and reversible. Patients receiving Flector® Patch who may be adversely affected by alterations in platelet function, such as those with coagulation disorders or patients receiving anticoagulants, should be carefully monitored.

Preexisting Asthma

Patients with asthma may have aspirin-sensitive asthma. The use of aspirin in patients with aspirin-sensitive asthma has been associated with severe bronchospasm which can be fatal. Since cross reactivity, including bronchospasm, between aspirin and other nonsteroidal anti-inflammatory drugs has been reported in such aspirin-sensitive patients, Flector® Patch should not be administered to patients with this form of aspirin sensitivity and should be used with caution in patients with preexisting asthma.

Eye Exposure

Contact of Flector® Patch with eyes and mucosa, although not studied, should be avoided. If eye contact occurs, immediately wash out the eye with water or saline. Consult a physician if irritation persists for more than an hour.

Accidental Exposure in Children

Even a used Flector® Patch contains a large amount of diclofenac epolamine (as much as 170 mg). The potential therefore exists for a small child or pet to suffer serious adverse effects from chewing or ingesting a new or used Flector® Patch. It is important for patients to store and dispose of Flector® Patch out of the reach of children and pets.

Information for Patients

Patients should be informed of the following information before initiating therapy with an NSAID and periodically during the course of ongoing therapy. Patients should also be encouraged to read the NSAID Medication Guide that accompanies each prescription dispensed.

1. Flector® Patch, like other NSAIDs, may cause serious CV side effects, such as MI or stroke, which may result in hospitalization and even death. Although serious CV events can occur without warning symptoms, patients should be alert for the signs and symptoms of chest pain, shortness of breath, weakness, slurring of speech, and should ask for medical advice when observing any indicative sign or symptoms. Patients should be apprised of the importance of this follow-up (see **WARNINGS, Cardiovascular Effects**).
2. Flector® Patch, like other NSAIDs, may cause GI discomfort and, rarely, serious GI side effects, such as ulcers and bleeding, which may result in hospitalization and even death. Although serious GI tract ulcerations and bleeding can occur without warning symptoms, patients should be alert for the signs and symptoms of ulcerations and bleeding, and should ask for medical advice when observing any indicative sign or symptoms including epigastric pain, dyspepsia, melena, and hematemesis. Patients should be apprised of the importance of this follow-up (see **WARNINGS, Gastrointestinal Effects: Risk of Ulceration, Bleeding, and Perforation**).
3. Flector® Patch, like other NSAIDs, may cause serious skin side effects such as exfoliative dermatitis, SJS, and TEN, which may result in hospitalizations and even death. Although serious skin reactions may occur without warning, patients should be alert for the signs and symptoms of skin rash and blisters, fever, or other signs of hypersensitivity such as itching, and should ask for medical advice when observing any indicative signs or symptoms. Patients should be advised to stop the drug immediately if they develop any type of rash and contact their physicians as soon as possible.
4. Patients should be instructed to promptly report signs or symptoms of unexplained weight gain or edema to their physicians (see **WARNINGS, Cardiovascular Effects**).
5. Patients should be informed of the warning signs and symptoms of hepatotoxicity (e.g., nausea, fatigue, lethargy, pruritus, jaundice, right upper quadrant tenderness, and "flu like" symptoms). If these occur, patients should be instructed to stop therapy and seek immediate medical therapy.
6. Patients should be informed of the signs of an anaphylactoid reaction (e.g. difficulty breathing, swelling of the face or throat). If these occur, patients should be instructed to seek immediate emergency help (see **WARNINGS**).
7. In late pregnancy, as with other NSAIDs, Flector® Patch should be avoided because it may cause premature closure of the ductus arteriosus.
8. Patients should be advised not to use Flector® Patch if they have an aspirin-sensitive asthma. Flector® Patch, like other NSAIDs, could cause severe and even fatal bronchospasm in these patients (see **PRECAUTIONS, Preexisting asthma**). Patients should discontinue use of Flector® Patch and should immediately seek emergency help if they experience wheezing or shortness of breath.
9. Patients should be informed that Flector® Patch should be used only on intact skin.
10. Patients should be advised to avoid contact of Flector® Patch with eyes and mucosa. Patients should be instructed that if eye contact occurs, they should immediately wash out the eye with water or saline, and consult a physician if irritation persists for more than an hour.
11. Patients and caregivers should be instructed to wash their hands after applying, handling or removing the patch.
12. Patients should be informed that, if Flector® Patch begins to peel off, the edges of the patch may be taped down.
13. Patients should be instructed not to wear Flector® Patch during bathing or showering. Bathing should take place in between scheduled patch removal and application (see **DOSAGE AND ADMINISTRATION**).
14. Patients should be advised to store Flector® Patch and to discard used patches out of the reach of children and pets. If a child or pet accidentally ingests Flector® Patch, medical help should be sought immediately (see **PRECAUTIONS, Accidental Exposure in Children**).

Table 1. Common Adverse Events (by body system and preferred term) in ≥1% of Patients treated with Flector® Patch or Placebo Patch[1]

	Diclofenac N=572		Placebo N=564	
	N	Percent	N	Percent
Application Site Conditions	64	11	70	12
Pruritus	31	5	44	8
Dermatitis	9	2	3	< 1
Burning	2	<1	8	1
Other[2]	22	4	15	3
Gastrointestinal Disorders	49	9	33	6
Nausea	17	3	11	2
Dysgeusia	10	2	3	< 1
Dyspepsia	7	1	8	1
Other[3]	15	3	11	2
Nervous System Disorders	13	2	18	3
Headache	7	1	10	2
Paresthesia	6	1	8	1
Somnolence	4	1	6	1
Other[4]	4	1	3	< 1

[1] The table lists adverse events occurring in placebo-treated patients because the placebo-patch was comprised of the same ingredients as Flector® Patch except for diclofenac. Adverse events in the placebo group may therefore reflect effects of the non-active ingredients.
[2] Includes: application site dryness, irritation, erythema, atrophy, discoloration, hyperhidriosis, and vesicles.
[3] Includes: gastritis, vomiting, diarrhea, constipation, upper abdominal pain, and dry mouth.
[4] Includes: hypoaesthesia, dizziness, and hyperkinesias.

Laboratory Tests

Because serious GI tract ulcerations and bleeding can occur without warning symptoms, physicians should monitor for signs or symptoms of GI bleeding. Patients on long-term treatment with NSAIDs, should have their CBC and a chemistry profile checked periodically. If clinical signs and symptoms consistent with liver or renal disease develop, systemic manifestations occur (e.g., eosinophilia, rash, etc.) or if abnormal liver tests persist or worsen, Flector® Patch should be discontinued.

Drug Interactions

ACE-inhibitors

Reports suggest that NSAIDs may diminish the antihypertensive effect of ACE-inhibitors. This interaction should be given consideration in patients taking NSAIDs concomitantly with ACE- inhibitors.

Aspirin

When Flector® Patch is administered with aspirin, the binding of diclofenac to protein is reduced, although the clearance of free diclofenac is not altered. The clinical significance of this interaction is not known; however, as with other NSAIDs, concomitant administration of diclofenac and aspirin is not generally recommended because of the potential of increased adverse effects.

Diuretics

Clinical studies, as well as post marketing observations, have shown that Flector® Patch may reduce the natriuretic effect of furosemide and thiazides in some patients. This response has been attributed to inhibition of renal prostaglandin synthesis. During concomitant therapy with NSAIDs, the patient should be observed closely for signs of renal failure (see **WARNINGS, Renal Effects**), as well as to assure diuretic efficacy.

Lithium

NSAIDs have produced an elevation of plasma lithium levels and a reduction in renal lithium clearance. The mean minimum lithium concentration increased 15% and the renal clearance was decreased by approximately 20%. These effects have been attributed to inhibition of renal prostaglandin synthesis by the NSAID. Thus, when NSAIDs and lithium are administered concurrently, subjects should be observed carefully for signs of lithium toxicity.

Methotrexate

NSAIDs have been reported to competitively inhibit methotrexate accumulation in rabbit kidney slices. This may indicate that they could enhance the toxicity of methotrexate. Caution should be used when NSAIDs are administered concomitantly with methotrexate.

Warfarin

The effects of warfarin and NSAIDs on GI bleeding are synergistic, such that users of both drugs together have a risk of serious GI bleeding higher than users of either drug alone.

Carcinogenesis, Mutagenesis, Impairment of Fertility

Carcinogenesis

Long-term studies in animals have not been performed to evaluate the carcinogenic potential of either diclofenac epolamine or Flector® Patch.

Mutagenesis

Diclofenac epolamine is not mutagenic in *Salmonella Typhimurium* strains, nor does it induce an increase in metabolic aberrations in cultured human lymphocytes, or the frequency of micronucleated cells in the bone marrow micronucleus test performed in rats.

Impairment of Fertility

Male and female Sprague Dawley rats were administered 1, 3, or 6 mg/kg/day diclofenac epolamine via oral gavage (males treated for 60 days prior to conception and during mating period, females treated for 14 days prior to mating through day 19 of gestation). Diclofenac epolamine treatment with 6 mg/kg/day resulted in increased early resorptions and postimplantation losses; however, no effects on the mating and fertility indices were found. The 6 mg/kg/day dose corresponds to 3-times the maximum recommended daily exposure in humans based on a body surface area comparison.

Pregnancy

Teratogenic Effects. Pregnancy Category C.

Pregnant Sprague Dawley rats were administered 1, 3, or 6 mg/kg diclofenac epolamine via oral gavage daily from gestation days 6-15. Maternal toxicity, embryotoxicity, and increased incidence of skeletal anomalies were noted with 6 mg/kg/day diclofenac epolamine, which corresponds to 3-times the maximum recommended daily exposure in humans based on a body surface area comparison. Pregnant New Zealand White rabbits were administered 1, 3, or 6 mg/kg diclofenac epolamine via oral gavage daily from gestation days 6-18. No maternal toxicity was noted; however, embryotoxicity was evident at 6 mg/kg/day group which corresponds to 6.5-times the maximum recommended daily exposure in humans based on a body surface area comparison.

There are no adequate and well-controlled studies in pregnant women. Flector® Patch should be used during pregnancy only if the potential benefit justifies the potential risk to the fetus.

Nonteratogenic Effects

Because of the known effects of nonsteroidal anti-inflammatory drugs on the fetal cardiovascular system (closure of ductus arteriosus), use during pregnancy (particularly late pregnancy) should be avoided.

Male rats were orally administered diclofenac epolamine (1, 3, 6 mg/kg) for 60 days prior to mating and throughout the mating period, and females were given the same doses 14 days prior to mating and through mating, gestation, and lactation. Embryotoxicity was observed at 6 mg/kg diclofenac epolamine (3-times the maximum recommended daily exposure in humans based on a body surface area comparison), and was manifested as an increase in early resorptions, post-implantation losses, and a decrease in live fetuses. The number of live born and total born were also

Continued on next page

Flector Patch—Cont.

reduced as was F1 postnatal survival, but the physical and behavioral development of surviving F1 pups in all groups was the same as the deionized water control, nor was reproductive performance adversely affected despite a slight treatment-related reduction in body weight.

Labor and Delivery
In rat studies with NSAIDs, as with other drugs known to inhibit prostaglandin synthesis, an increased incidence of dystocia, delayed parturition, and decreased pup survival occurred. The effects of Flector® Patch on labor and delivery in pregnant women are unknown.

Nursing Mothers
It is not known whether this drug is excreted in human milk. Because many drugs are excreted in human milk and because of the potential for serious adverse reactions in nursing infants from Flector® Patch, a decision should be made whether to discontinue nursing or to discontinue the drug, taking into account the importance of the drug to the mother.

Pediatric Use
Safety and effectiveness in pediatric patients have not been established.

Geriatric Use
Clinical studies of Flector® Patch did not include sufficient numbers of subjects aged 65 and over to determine whether they respond differently from younger subjects. Other reported clinical experience has not identified differences in responses between the elderly and younger patients.
Diclofenac, as with any NSAID, is known to be substantially excreted by the kidney, and the risk of toxic reactions to Flector® Patch may be greater in patients with impaired renal function. Because elderly patients are more likely to have decreased renal function, care should be taken when using Flector® Patch in the elderly, and it may be useful to monitor renal function.

ADVERSE REACTIONS
In controlled trials during the premarketing development of Flector® Patch, approximately 600 patients with minor sprains, strains, and contusions have been treated with Flector® Patch for up to two weeks.

Adverse Events Leading to Discontinuation of Treatment
In the controlled trials, 3% of patients in both the Flector® Patch and placebo patch groups discontinued treatment due to an adverse event. The most common adverse events leading to discontinuation were application site reactions, occurring in 2% of both the Flector® Patch and placebo patch groups. Application site reactions leading to dropout included pruritus, dermatitis, and burning.

Common Adverse Events
Localized Reactions
Overall, the most common adverse events associated with Flector® Patch treatment were skin reactions at the site of treatment.
Table 1 lists all adverse events, regardless of causality, occurring in ≥ 1% of patients in controlled trials of Flector® Patch. A majority of patients treated with Flector® Patch had adverse events with a maximum intensity of "mild" or "moderate."
[See table 1 at top of previous page]
Foreign labeling describes that dermal allergic reactions may occur with Flector® Patch treatment. Additionally, the treated area may become irritated or develop itching, erythema, edema, vesicles, or abnormal sensation.

DRUG ABUSE AND DEPENDENCE
Controlled Substance Class
Flector® Patch is not a controlled substance.
Physical and Psychological Dependence
Diclofenac, the active ingredient in Flector® Patch, is an NSAID that does not lead to physical or psychological dependence.

OVERDOSAGE
There is limited experience with overdose of Flector® Patch. In clinical studies, the maximum single dose administered was one Flector® Patch containing 180 mg of diclofenac epolamine. There were no serious adverse events.
Should systemic side effects occur due to incorrect use or accidental overdose of this product, the general measures recommended for intoxication with non-steroidal anti-inflammatory drugs should be taken.

DOSAGE AND ADMINISTRATION
Carefully consider the potential benefits and risks of Flector® Patch and other treatment options before deciding to use Flector® Patch. Use the lowest effective dose for the shortest duration consistent with individual patient treatment goals (see WARNINGS).
The recommended dose of Flector® Patch is one (1) patch to the most painful area twice a day.
Flector® patch should not be applied to damaged or non-intact skin.
Flector® patch should not be worn when bathing or showering.

HANDLING AND DISPOSAL
Patients and caregivers should wash their hands after applying, handling or removing the patch. Eye contact should be avoided.

HOW SUPPLIED
The Flector® Patch is supplied in resealable envelopes, each containing 5 patches (10 cm × 14 cm), with six envelopes per box (NDC 63857-111-33). Each individual patch is embossed with "FLECTOR PATCH <DICLOFENAC EPOLAMINE TOPICAL PATCH> 1.3%".

- Each patch contains 180 mg of diclofenac epolamine in an aqueous base (13 mg of active per gram of adhesive or 1.3%).
- The product is intended for topical use only.
- Keep out of reach of children and pets.
- The ENVELOPES SHOULD BE SEALED AT ALL TIMES WHEN NOT IN USE.
- Store at 25°C (77°F); excursions permitted to 15°-30°C (59°-86°F). [See USP Controlled Room Temperature].

Distributed by: Alpharma Pharmaceuticals LLC
One New England Avenue, Piscataway, NJ 08854 USA
(Telephone: 1-888-840-8884) • www.FlectorPatch.com
Manufactured for: IBSA Institut Biochimique SA,
CH-6903 Lugano, Switzerland
Manufactured by: Teikoku Seiyaku Co., Ltd.,
Sanbonmatsu, Kagawa 769-2695 Japan
Version March 2008
8283

Bristol-Myers Squibb Company
P.O. BOX 4500
PRINCETON, NJ 08543-4500

NOUS08AB00401

For Medical Information Contact:
Generally:
Bristol-Myers Squibb Medical Information Department
P.O. Box 4500
Princeton, NJ 08543-4500
(800) 321-1335
To report SUSPECTED ADVERSE REACTIONS, contact Bristol-Myers Squibb at 1-800-721-5072 between 8:00 AM–5:00 PM EST
Sales and Ordering:
Orders may be placed by:
1. Calling your purchase orders in toll-free between 8:30 AM–6:00 PM EST:
(800) 631-5244
2. Mailing your purchase orders to:
Bristol-Myers Squibb U.S. Pharmaceuticals
Attn: Customer Service
P.O. Box 4500
Princeton, NJ 08543-4500
3. Faxing your purchase orders to:
(800) 523-2965
4. Transmitting computer-to-computer on the NWDA and UCS formats through Ordernet Services use:
DEA#PE0048579
NOUS08AB00402

IXEMPRA™ KIT FOR INJECTION   ℞
[Ĭk-ˈsĕm-prǎ]
(ixabepilone)
for intravenous infusion only

HIGHLIGHTS OF PRESCRIBING INFORMATION
These highlights do not include all the information needed to use IXEMPRA™ safely and effectively. See full prescribing information for IXEMPRA™.
IXEMPRA™ Kit (ixabepilone) For Injection, for intravenous infusion only
Initial U.S. Approval: 2007

> **WARNING: TOXICITY IN HEPATIC IMPAIRMENT**
> *See full prescribing information for complete boxed warning.*
> IXEMPRA™ in combination with capecitabine must not be given to patients with AST or ALT >2.5 × ULN or bilirubin >1 × ULN due to increased risk of toxicity and neutropenia-related death. (4, 5.3)

INDICATIONS AND USAGE
IXEMPRA (ixabepilone), a microtubule inhibitor, in combination with capecitabine is indicated for the treatment of metastatic or locally advanced breast cancer in patients after failure of an anthracycline and a taxane (1).
IXEMPRA as monotherapy is indicated for the treatment of metastatic or locally advanced breast cancer in patients after failure of an anthracycline, a taxane, and capecitabine (1).

DOSAGE AND ADMINISTRATION
- The recommended dose of IXEMPRA is 40 mg/m² infused intravenously over 3 hours every 3 weeks (2.1).
- Dose reduction is required in certain patients with elevated AST, ALT, or bilirubin (2.2, 8.6).
IXEMPRA (ixabepilone) for Injection must be constituted with supplied DILUENT. The ixabepilone concentration in constituted solution is 2 mg/mL.
Constituted solution must be diluted with Lactated Ringer's Injection, USP, to a final ixabepilone concentration of 0.2 mg/mL to 0.6 mg/mL. The final solution must be used within 6 hours of preparation (2.4).

DOSAGE FORMS AND STRENGTHS
- IXEMPRA for Injection, 15 mg supplied with DILUENT for IXEMPRA, 8 mL (3)
- IXEMPRA (ixabepilone) for Injection, 45 mg supplied with DILUENT for IXEMPRA, 23.5 mL (3)

CONTRAINDICATIONS
- Hypersensitivity to drugs formulated with Cremophor® EL (4).
- Baseline neutrophil count <1500 cells/mm³ or a platelet count <100,000 cells/mm³ (4).
- Patients with AST or ALT >2.5 × ULN or bilirubin >1 × ULN must not be treated with IXEMPRA (ixabepilone) in combination with capecitabine (4).

WARNINGS AND PRECAUTIONS
- Peripheral Neuropathy: Monitor for symptoms of neuropathy, primarily sensory. Neuropathy is cumulative, generally reversible and should be managed by dose adjustment and delays (2.2, 5.1).
- Myelosuppression: Primarily neutropenia. Monitor with peripheral blood cell counts and adjust dose as appropriate (2.2, 5.2).
- Hypersensitivity reactions: Must premedicate all patients with an H₁ antagonist and an H₂ antagonist before treatment (2.3, 5.4).
- Fetal harm can occur when administered to a pregnant woman. Women should be advised not to become pregnant when taking IXEMPRA (5.5, 8.1).

ADVERSE REACTIONS
- The most common adverse reactions (≥20%) are peripheral sensory neuropathy, fatigue/asthenia, myalgia/arthralgia, alopecia, nausea, vomiting, stomatitis/mucositis, diarrhea, and musculoskeletal pain. Additional reactions occurred in ≥20% in combination treatment: palmar-plantar erythrodysesthesia syndrome, anorexia, abdominal pain, nail disorder, and constipation (6).
- Drug-associated hematologic abnormalities (>40%) include neutropenia, leukopenia, anemia, and thrombocytopenia (6).

To report SUSPECTED ADVERSE REACTIONS, contact Bristol-Myers Squibb at 1-800-721-5072 or FDA at 1-800-FDA-1088 or www.fda.gov/medwatch

DRUG INTERACTIONS
- Inhibitors of CYP3A4 may increase plasma concentrations of ixabepilone; dose of IXEMPRA (ixabepilone) must be reduced with strong CYP3A4 inhibitors (7.1).
- Inducers of CYP3A4 may decrease plasma concentrations of ixabepilone; alternative therapeutic agents with low enzyme induction potential should be considered (7.1).

See 17 for PATIENT COUNSELING INFORMATION and FDA-Approved Patient Labeling.

Revised: 10/2007

FULL PRESCRIBING INFORMATION

WARNING: TOXICITY IN HEPATIC IMPAIRMENT
IXEMPRA in combination with capecitabine is contraindicated in patients with AST or ALT >2.5 × ULN or bilirubin >1 × ULN due to increased risk of toxicity and neutropenia-related death [see *Contraindications (4)* and *Warnings and Precautions (5.3)*].

1 INDICATIONS AND USAGE

IXEMPRA (ixabepilone) is indicated in combination with capecitabine for the treatment of patients with metastatic or locally advanced breast cancer resistant to treatment with an anthracycline and a taxane, or whose cancer is taxane resistant and for whom further anthracycline therapy is contraindicated. Anthracycline resistance is defined as progression while on therapy or within 6 months in the adjuvant setting or 3 months in the metastatic setting. Taxane resistance is defined as progression while on therapy or within 12 months in the adjuvant setting or 4 months in the metastatic setting.

IXEMPRA is indicated as monotherapy for the treatment of metastatic or locally advanced breast cancer in patients whose tumors are resistant or refractory to anthracyclines, taxanes, and capecitabine.

2 DOSAGE AND ADMINISTRATION

2.1 General Dosing Information

The recommended dosage of IXEMPRA is 40 mg/m^2 administered intravenously over 3 hours every 3 weeks. Doses for patients with body surface area (BSA) greater than 2.2 m^2 should be calculated based on 2.2 m^2.

2.2 Dose Modification

Dose Adjustments During Treatment

Patients should be evaluated during treatment by periodic clinical observation and laboratory tests including complete blood cell counts. If toxicities are present, treatment should be delayed to allow recovery. Dosing adjustment guidelines for monotherapy and combination therapy are shown in Table 1. If toxicities recur, an additional 20% dose reduction should be made.

[See table 1 above]

Table 1: Dose Adjustment Guidelines[a]

IXEMPRA (Monotherapy or Combination Therapy)	IXEMPRA Dose Modification
Nonhematologic:	
Grade 2 neuropathy (moderate) lasting ≥7 days	Decrease the dose by 20%
Grade 3 neuropathy (severe) lasting <7 days	Decrease the dose by 20%
Grade 3 neuropathy (severe) lasting ≥7 days or disabling neuropathy	Discontinue treatment
Any grade 3 toxicity (severe) other than neuropathy	Decrease the dose by 20%
Transient grade 3 arthralgia/myalgia or fatigue	No change in dose of IXEMPRA
Grade 3 hand-foot syndrome (palmar-plantar erythrodysesthesia)	
Any grade 4 toxicity (disabling)	Discontinue treatment
Hematologic:	
Neutrophil <500 cells/mm^3 for ≥7 days	Decrease the dose by 20%
Febrile neutropenia	Decrease the dose by 20%
Platelets <25,000/mm^3 or platelets <50,000/mm^3 with bleeding	Decrease the dose by 20%
CAPECITABINE (when used in combination with IXEMPRA)	**Capecitabine Dose Modification**
Nonhematologic:	Follow Capecitabine Label
Hematologic:	
Platelets <25,000/mm^3 or <50,000/mm^3 with bleeding	Hold for concurrent diarrhea or stomatitis until platelet count >50,000/mm^3, then continue at same dose.
Neutrophils <500 cells/mm^3 for ≥7 days or febrile neutropenia	Hold for concurrent diarrhea or stomatitis until neutrophil count >1,000 cells/mm^3, then continue at same dose.

[a] Toxicities graded in accordance with National Cancer Institute (NCI) Common Terminology Criteria for Adverse Events (CTCAE v3.0).

Re-treatment Criteria: Dose adjustments at the start of a cycle should be based on nonhematologic toxicity or blood counts from the preceding cycle following the guidelines in Table 1. Patients should not begin a new cycle of treatment unless the neutrophil count is at least 1500 cells/mm^3, the platelet count is at least 100,000 cells/mm^3, and nonhematologic toxicities have improved to grade 1 (mild) or resolved.

Dose Adjustments in Special Populations - Hepatic Impairment

Combination Therapy:

IXEMPRA (ixabepilone) in combination with capecitabine is contraindicated in patients with AST or ALT >2.5 × ULN or bilirubin >1 × ULN. Patients receiving combination treatment who have AST and ALT ≤2.5 × ULN and bilirubin ≤1 × ULN may receive the standard dose of ixabepilone (40 mg/m^2). [See *Boxed Warning*, *Contraindications (4)*, *Warnings and Precautions (5.3)* and *Use in Specific Populations (8.6)*.]

Monotherapy:

Patients with hepatic impairment should be dosed with IXEMPRA based on the guidelines in Table 2. Patients with moderate hepatic impairment should be started at 20 mg/m^2, the dosage in subsequent cycles may be escalated up to, but not exceeding, 30 mg/m^2 if tolerated. Use in patients with AST or ALT >10 × ULN or bilirubin >3 × ULN is not recommended. Limited data are available for patients with baseline AST or ALT >5 × ULN. Caution should be used when treating these patients. [See *Warnings and Precautions (5.3)* and *Use in Specific Populations (8.6)*.]

[See table 2 above]

Table 2: Dose Adjustments for IXEMPRA as Monotherapy in Patients with Hepatic Impairment

	Transaminase Levels		Bilirubin Levels[a]	IXEMPRA[b] (mg/m^2)
Mild	AST and ALT ≤2.5 × ULN	and	≤1 × ULN	40
	AST or ALT ≤10 × ULN	and	≤1.5 × ULN	32
Moderate	AST and ALT ≤10 × ULN	and	>1.5 × ULN - ≤3 × ULN	20-30

[a] Excluding patients whose total bilirubin is elevated due to Gilbert's disease.
[b] Dosage recommendations are for first course of therapy; further decreases in subsequent courses should be based on individual tolerance.

Strong CYP3A4 Inhibitors

The use of concomitant strong CYP3A4 inhibitors should be avoided (eg, ketoconazole, itraconazole, clarithromycin, atazanavir, nefazodone, saquinavir, telithromycin, ritonavir, amprenavir, indinavir, nelfinavir, delavirdine, or voriconazole). Grapefruit juice may also increase plasma concentrations of IXEMPRA and should be avoided. Based on pharmacokinetic studies, if a strong CYP3A4 inhibitor must be coadministered, a dose reduction to 20 mg/m^2 is predicted to adjust the ixabepilone AUC to the range observed without inhibitors and should be considered. If the strong inhibitor is discontinued, a washout period of approximately 1 week should be allowed before the IXEMPRA dose is adjusted upward to the indicated dose. [See *Drug Interactions (7.1)*.]

2.3 Premedication

To minimize the chance of occurrence of a hypersensitivity reaction, all patients must be premedicated approximately 1 hour before the infusion of IXEMPRA with:

- An H_1 antagonist (eg, diphenhydramine 50 mg orally or equivalent) and
- An H_2 antagonist (eg, ranitidine 150 - 300 mg orally or equivalent).

Patients who experienced a hypersensitivity reaction to IXEMPRA require premedication with corticosteroids (eg, dexamethasone 20 mg intravenously, 30 minutes before infusion or orally, 60 minutes before infusion) in addition to pretreatment with H_1 and H_2 antagonists.

2.4 Instructions for Preparation and IV Administration

IXEMPRA *Kit* contains two vials, a vial labeled IXEMPRA (ixabepilone) for Injection which contains ixabepilone powder and a vial containing DILUENT for IXEMPRA. Only supplied DILUENT must be used for constituting IXEMPRA (ixabepilone) for Injection. IXEMPRA *Kit* must be stored in a refrigerator at 2° C - 8° C (36° F - 46° F) in the original package to protect from light. Prior to constituting IXEMPRA for Injection, the *Kit* should be removed from the refrigerator and allowed to stand at room temperature for approximately 30 minutes. When the vials are first removed from the refrigerator, a white precipitate may be observed in the DILUENT vial. This precipitate will dissolve to form a clear solution once the DILUENT warms to room temperature. To allow for withdrawal losses, the vial labeled as 15 mg IXEMPRA for Injection contains 16 mg of ixabepilone and the vial labeled as 45 mg IXEMPRA for Injection contains 47 mg of ixabepilone. The 15-mg IXEMPRA *Kit* is supplied with a vial providing 8 mL of the DILUENT and the 45-mg IXEMPRA *Kit* is supplied with a vial providing 23.5 mL of the DILUENT. After constituting with the DILUENT, the concentration of ixabepilone is 2 mg/mL.

Please refer to Preparation and Handling Precautions [see Dosage and Administration (2.5)] before preparation.

A. To constitute:

1. With a suitable syringe, aseptically withdraw the DILUENT and slowly inject it into the IXEMPRA (ixabepilone) for Injection vial. The 15-mg IXEMPRA is constituted with 8 mL of DILUENT and the 45-mg IXEMPRA is constituted with 23.5 mL of DILUENT.
2. Gently swirl and invert the vial until the powder in IXEMPRA is completely dissolved.

B. To dilute:

Before administration, the constituted solution must be further diluted only with Lactated Ringer's Injection, USP (LRI) supplied in DEHP [di-(2-ethylhexyl)phthalate] free bags. For most doses, a 250 mL bag of Lactated Ringer's Injection is sufficient. However, it is necessary to check the final infusion concentration of each dose based on the volume of Lactated Ringer's Injection to be used. The final concentration for infusion must be between 0.2 mg/mL and 0.6 mg/mL. To calculate the final infusion concentration, use the following formulas:

Total Infusion Volume = mL of Constituted Solution + mL of LRI

Final Infusion Concentration = Dose of IXEMPRA (mg)/ Total Infusion Volume (mL)

1. Aseptically, withdraw the appropriate volume of constituted solution containing 2 mg of ixabepilone per mL.
2. Aseptically, transfer to an intravenous (IV) bag containing an appropriate volume of Lactated Ringer's Injection, USP to achieve the final desired concentration of ixabepilone.
3. Thoroughly mix the infusion bag by manual rotation.

The infusion solution must be administered through an appropriate in-line filter with a microporous membrane of 0.2 to 1.2 microns. DEHP-free infusion containers and administration sets must be used. Any remaining solution should be discarded according to institutional procedures for antineoplastics.

Stability

After constituting ixabepilone for injection, the constituted solution should be further diluted with Lactated Ringer's Injection as soon as possible, but may be stored in the vial (not the syringe) for a maximum of 1 hour at room temperature and room light. Once diluted with Lactated Ringer's Injection, USP the solution is stable at room temperature and room light for a maximum of 6 hours. Administration of diluted IXEMPRA (ixabepilone) must be completed within this 6-hour period. Lactated Ringer's Injection, USP is specified because it has a pH range of 6 to 7.5, which is required to maintain IXEMPRA stability. Other diluents should not be used with IXEMPRA.

2.5 Preparation and Handling Precautions

Procedures for proper handling and disposal of antineoplastic drugs [see *References (15)*] should be followed. To minimize the risk of dermal exposure, impervious gloves should be worn when handling vials containing IXEMPRA, regardless of the setting, including unpacking and inspection, transport within a facility, and dose preparation and administration.

3 DOSAGE FORMS AND STRENGTHS

IXEMPRA, for Injection 15 mg supplied with DILUENT for IXEMPRA, 8 mL.

IXEMPRA, for Injection 45 mg supplied with DILUENT for IXEMPRA, 23.5 mL.

4 CONTRAINDICATIONS

IXEMPRA is contraindicated in patients with a history of a severe (CTC grade 3/4) hypersensitivity reaction to agents containing Cremophor® EL or its derivatives (eg, polyoxyethylated castor oil) [see *Warnings and Precautions (5.4)*].

IXEMPRA is contraindicated in patients who have a neutrophil count <1500 cells/mm^3 or a platelet count <100,000 cells/mm^3 [see *Warnings and Precautions (5.2)*].

IXEMPRA in combination with capecitabine is contraindicated in patients with AST or ALT >2.5 × ULN or bilirubin >1 × ULN [see *Boxed Warning* and *Warnings and Precautions (5.3)*].

5 WARNINGS AND PRECAUTIONS

5.1 Peripheral Neuropathy

Peripheral neuropathy was common (see Table 3). Patients treated with IXEMPRA should be monitored for symptoms

Continued on next page

Product information on these pages reflects product labeling on June 1, 2007. Current information on products of Bristol-Myers Squibb may be obtained at 1-800-321-1335 or www.bms.com.
NOUS08AB00403

Ixempra—Cont.

of neuropathy, such as burning sensation, hyperesthesia, hypoesthesia, paresthesia, discomfort, or neuropathic pain. Neuropathy occurred early during treatment; ~75% of new onset or worsening neuropathy occurred during the first 3 cycles. Patients experiencing new or worsening symptoms may require a reduction or delay in the dose of IXEMPRA (ixabepilone) [see *Dosage and Administration (2.2)*]. In clinical studies, peripheral neuropathy was managed through dose reductions, dose delays and treatment discontinuation. Neuropathy was the most frequent cause of treatment discontinuation due to drug toxicity. In Studies 046 and 081, 80% and 87%, respectively, of patients with peripheral neuropathy who received IXEMPRA had improvement or no worsening of their neuropathy following dose reduction. For patients with grade 3/4 neuropathy in Studies 046 and 081, 76% and 79%, respectively, had documented improvement to baseline or grade 1, twelve weeks after onset.

Table 3: Treatment-related Peripheral Neuropathy

	IXEMPRA with capecitabine Study 046	IXEMPRA as monotherapy Study 081
Peripheral neuropathy (all grades)[a,b]	67%	63%
Peripheral neuropathy (grades 3/4)[a,b]	23%	14%
Discontinuation due to neuropathy	21%	6%
Median number of cycles to onset of grade 3/4 neuropathy	4	4
Median time to improvement of grade 3/4 neuropathy to baseline or to grade 1	6.0 weeks	4.6 weeks

[a] Sensory and motor neuropathy combined.
[b] 24% and 27% of patients in 046 and 081, respectively, had preexisting neuropathy (grade 1).

A pooled analysis of 945 cancer patients treated with IXEMPRA (ixabepilone) indicated that patients with diabetes mellitus may be at increased risk of severe neuropathy. The presence of grade 1 neuropathy and prior therapy with neurotoxic chemotherapy agents did not predict either the development or worsening of neuropathy. Patients with moderate to severe neuropathy (grade 2 or greater) were excluded from studies with IXEMPRA. Caution should be used when treating patients with diabetes mellitus or existing moderate to severe neuropathy.

5.2 Myelosuppression

Myelosuppression is dose-dependent and primarily manifested as neutropenia. In clinical studies, grade 4 neutropenia (<500 cells/mm³) occurred in 36% of patients treated with IXEMPRA in combination with capecitabine and 23% of patients treated with IXEMPRA monotherapy. Febrile neutropenia and infection with neutropenia were reported in 5% and 6% of patients treated with IXEMPRA in combination with capecitabine, respectively, and 3% and 5% of patients treated with IXEMPRA as monotherapy, respectively. Neutropenia-related death occurred in 1.9% of 414 patients with normal hepatic function or mild hepatic impairment treated with IXEMPRA in combination with capecitabine. The rate of neutropenia-related deaths was higher (29%, 5 out of 17) in patients with AST or ALT >2.5 × ULN or bilirubin >1.5 × ULN. [See *Boxed Warning, Contraindications (4), and Warnings and Precautions (5.3)*.] Neutropenia-related death occurred in 0.4% of 240 patients treated with IXEMPRA as monotherapy. No neutropenia-related deaths were reported in 24 patients with AST or ALT >2.5 × ULN or bilirubin >1.5 × ULN treated with IXEMPRA monotherapy. IXEMPRA must not be administered to patients with a neutrophil count <1500 cells/mm³. To monitor for myelosuppression, frequent peripheral blood cell counts are recommended for all patients receiving IXEMPRA. Patients who experience severe neutropenia or thrombocytopenia should have their dose reduced [see *Dosage and Administration (2.2)*].

5.3 Hepatic Impairment

Patients with baseline AST or ALT >2.5 × ULN or bilirubin >1.5 × ULN experienced greater toxicity than patients with baseline AST or ALT ≤2.5 × ULN or bilirubin ≤1.5 × ULN when treated with IXEMPRA at 40 mg/m² in combination with capecitabine or as monotherapy in breast cancer studies. In combination with capecitabine, the overall frequency of grade 3/4 adverse reactions, febrile neutropenia, serious adverse reactions, and toxicity related deaths was greater [see *Warnings and Precautions (5.2)*]. With monotherapy, grade 4 neutropenia, febrile neutropenia, and serious adverse reactions were more frequent. The safety and pharmacokinetics of IXEMPRA as monotherapy were evaluated in a dose escalation study in 56 patients with varying degrees of hepatic impairment. Exposure was increased in patients with elevated AST or bilirubin [see *Use in Specific Populations (8.6)*].

IXEMPRA in combination with capecitabine is contraindicated in patients with AST or ALT >2.5 × ULN or bilirubin >1 × ULN due to increased risk of toxicity and neutropenia-related death [see *Boxed Warning, Contraindications (4), and Warnings and Precautions (5.2)*]. Patients who are treated with IXEMPRA as monotherapy should receive a reduced dose depending on the degree of hepatic impairment [see *Dosage and Administration (2.2)*]. Use in patients with AST or ALT >10 × ULN or bilirubin >3 × ULN is not recommended. Limited data are available for patients with AST or ALT >5 × ULN. Caution should be used when treating these patients [see *Dosage and Administration (2.2)*].

5.4 Hypersensitivity Reactions

Patients with a history of a severe hypersensitivity reaction to agents containing Cremophor® EL or its derivatives (eg, polyoxyethylated castor oil) should not be treated with IXEMPRA (ixabepilone). All patients should be premedicated with an H₁ and an H₂ antagonist approximately 1 hour before IXEMPRA infusion and be observed for hypersensitivity reactions (eg, flushing, rash, dyspnea and bronchospasm). In case of severe hypersensitivity reactions, infusion of IXEMPRA should be stopped and aggressive supportive treatment (eg, epinephrine, corticosteroids) started. Of the 1323 patients treated with IXEMPRA (ixabepilone) in clinical studies, 9 patients (1%) had experienced severe hypersensitivity reactions (including anaphylaxis). Three of the 9 patients were able to be retreated. Patients who experience a hypersensitivity reaction in one cycle of IXEMPRA must be premedicated in subsequent cycles with a corticosteroid in addition to the H₁ and H₂ antagonists, and extension of the infusion time should be considered [see *Dosage and Administration (2.3) and Contraindications (4)*].

5.5 Pregnancy

Pregnancy Category D.
IXEMPRA (ixabepilone) may cause fetal harm when administered to pregnant women. There are no adequate and well-controlled studies with IXEMPRA in pregnant women. Women should be advised not to become pregnant when taking IXEMPRA. If this drug is used during pregnancy, or if the patient becomes pregnant while taking this drug, the patient should be apprised of the potential hazard to the fetus.

Table 4: Nonhematologic Drug-related Adverse Reactions Occurring in at Least 5% of Patients with Metastatic or Locally Advanced Breast Cancer Treated with IXEMPRA

	Study 046				Study 081	
	IXEMPRA with capecitabine n=369		Capecitabine n=368		IXEMPRA monotherapy n=126	
System Organ Class[a]/ Preferred Term	Total (%)	Grade 3/4 (%)	Total (%)	Grade 3/4 (%)	Total (%)	Grade 3/4 (%)
Infections and Infestations						
Upper respiratory tract infection[b]	4	0	3	0	6	0
Blood and Lymphatic System Disorders						
Febrile neutropenia	5	4[c]	1	1[d]	3	3[d]
Immune System Disorders						
Hypersensitivity[b]		1[d]	0	0	5	1[d]
Metabolism and Nutrition Disorders						
Anorexia[b]	34	3[d]	15	1[d]	19	2[d]
Dehydration[b]	5	2	2	<1[d]	2	1[d]
Psychiatric						
Insomnia[b]	9	<1[d]	2	0	5	0
Nervous System Disorders						
Peripheral neuropathy						
Sensory neuropathy[b,e]	65	21	16	0	62	14
Motor neuropathy[b]	16	5[d]	<1	0	10	1[d]
Headache	8	<1[d]	3	0	11	0
Taste disorder[b]	12	0	4	0	6	0
Dizziness	8	1[d]	5	1[d]	7	0
Eye Disorders						
Lacrimation increased	5	0	4	<1[d]	4	0
Vascular Disorders						
Hot flush[b]	5	0	2	0	6	0
Respiratory, Thoracic, and Mediastinal Disorders						
Dyspnea[b]	7	1	4	1	9	1[d]
Cough[b]	6	0	2	0	2	0
Gastrointestinal Disorders						
Nausea	53	3[d]	40	2[d]	42	2[d]
Vomiting[b]	39	4[d]	24	2	29	1[d]
Stomatitis/mucositis[b]	31	4	20	3[d]	29	6
Diarrhea[b]	44	6[d]	39	9	22	1[d]
Constipation	22	0	6	<1[d]	16	2[d]
Abdominal pain[b]	24	2[d]	14	1[d]	13	2[d]
Gastroesophageal reflux disease[b]	7	1[d]	8	0	6	0
Skin and Subcutaneous Tissue Disorders						
Alopecia[b]	31	0	3	0	48	0
Skin rash[b]	17	1[d]	7	0	9	2[d]
Nail disorder[b]	24	2[d]	10	<1[d]	9	0
Palmar-plantar erythrodysesthesia syndrome[b,f]	64	18[d]	63	17[d]	8	2[d]
Pruritus	5	0	2	0	6	1[d]
Skin exfoliation[b]	5	<1[d]	3	0	2	0
Skin hyperpigmentation[b]	11	0	14	0	2	0
Musculoskeletal, Connective Tissue, and Bone Disorders						
Myalgia/arthralgia[b]	39	8[d]	5	<1[d]	49	8[d]
Musculoskeletal pain[b]	23	2[d]	5	0	20	3[d]
General Disorders and Administrative Site Conditions						
Fatigue/asthenia[b]	60	16	29	4	56	13
Edema[b]	8	0	5	<1[d]	9	1[d]
Pyrexia	10	1[d]	4	0	8	1[d]
Pain[b]	9	1[d]	2	0	8	3[d]
Chest pain[b]	4	1[d]	<1	0	5	1[d]
Investigations						
Weight decreased	11	0	3	0	6	0

[a] System organ class presented as outlined in Guidelines for Preparing Core Clinical Safety Information on Drugs by the Council for International Organizations of Medical Sciences (CIOMS).
[b] A composite of multiple MedDRA Preferred Terms.
[c] NCI CTC grading for febrile neutropenia ranges from Grade 3 to 5. Three patients (1%) experienced Grade 5 (fatal) febrile neutropenia. Other neutropenia-related deaths (9) occurred in the absence of reported febrile neutropenia [see *Warnings and Precautions (5.2)*].
[d] No grade 4 reports.
[e] Peripheral sensory neuropathy (graded with the NCI CTC scale) was defined as the occurrence of any of the following: areflexia, burning sensation, dysesthesia, hyperesthesia, hypoesthesia, hyporeflexia, neuralgia, neuritis, neuropathy, neuropathy peripheral, neurotoxicity, painful response to normal stimuli, paresthesia, pallanesthesia, peripheral sensory neuropathy, polyneuropathy, polyneuropathy toxic and sensorimotor disorder.
Peripheral motor neuropathy was defined as the occurrence of any of the following: multifocal motor neuropathy, neuromuscular toxicity, peripheral motor neuropathy, and peripheral sensorimotor neuropathy.
[f] Palmar-plantar erythrodysesthesia (hand-foot syndrome) was graded on a 1-3 severity scale in Study 046.

Ixabepilone was studied for effects on embryo-fetal development in pregnant rats and rabbits given IV doses of 0.02, 0.08, and 0.3 mg/kg/day and 0.01, 0.03, 0.11 and 0.3 mg/kg/day, respectively. There were no teratogenic effects. In rats, an increase in resorptions and post-implantation loss and a decrease in the number of live fetuses and fetal weight was observed at the maternally toxic dose of 0.3 mg/kg/day (approximately one-tenth the human clinical exposure based on AUC). Abnormalities included a reduced ossification of caudal vertebrae, sternebrae, and metacarpals. In rabbits, ixabepilone caused maternal toxicity (death) and embryo-fetal toxicity (resorptions) at 0.3 mg/kg/day (approximately one-tenth the human clinical dose based on body surface area). No fetuses were available at this dose for evaluation.

5.6   Cardiac Adverse Reactions
The frequency of cardiac adverse reactions (myocardial ischemia and ventricular dysfunction) was higher in the IXEMPRA (ixabepilone) in combination with capecitabine (1.9%) than in the capecitabine alone (0.3%) treatment group. Supraventricular arrhythmias were observed in the combination arm (0.5%) and not in the capecitabine alone arm. Caution should be exercised in patients with a history of cardiac disease. Discontinuation of IXEMPRA should be considered in patients who develop cardiac ischemia or impaired cardiac function.

5.7   Potential for Cognitive Impairment from Excipients
Since IXEMPRA contains dehydrated alcohol USP, consideration should be given to the possibility of central nervous system and other effects of alcohol [see *Description (11)*].

6   ADVERSE REACTIONS
The following adverse reactions are discussed in greater detail in other sections.
- Peripheral neuropathy [see *Warnings and Precautions (5.1)*]
- Myelosuppression [see *Warnings and Precautions (5.2)*]
- Hypersensitivity reactions [see *Warnings and Precautions (5.4)*]

Because clinical trials are conducted under widely varying conditions, the adverse reaction rates observed in the clinical trials of a drug cannot be directly compared to rates in other clinical trials and may not reflect the rates observed in clinical practice.

Unless otherwise specified, assessment of adverse reactions is based on one randomized study (Study 046) and one single-arm study (Study 081). In Study 046, 369 patients with metastatic breast cancer were treated with IXEMPRA 40 mg/m^2 administered intravenously over 3 hours every 21 days, combined with capecitabine 1000 mg/m^2 twice daily for 2 weeks followed by a 1-week rest period. Patients treated with capecitabine as monotherapy (n=368) in this study received 1250 mg/m^2 twice daily for 2 weeks every 21 days. In Study 081, 126 patients with metastatic or locally advanced breast cancer were treated with IXEMPRA 40 mg/m^2 administered intravenously over 3 hours every 3 weeks.

The most common adverse reactions (≥20%) reported by patients receiving IXEMPRA were peripheral sensory neuropathy, fatigue/asthenia, myalgia/arthralgia, alopecia, nausea, vomiting, stomatitis/mucositis, diarrhea, and musculoskeletal pain. The following additional reactions occurred in ≥20% in combination treatment: palmar-plantar erythrodysesthesia (hand-foot) syndrome, anorexia, abdominal pain, nail disorder, and constipation. The most common hematologic abnormalities (>40%) include neutropenia, leukopenia, anemia, and thrombocytopenia.

Table 4 presents nonhematologic adverse reactions reported in 5% or more of patients. Hematologic abnormalities are presented separately in Table 5.

[See table 4 at top of previous page]
[See table 5 above]

The following serious adverse reactions were also reported in 1323 patients treated with IXEMPRA as monotherapy or in combination with other therapies in Phase 2 and 3 studies.

Infections and Infestations: sepsis, pneumonia, infection, neutropenic infection, urinary tract infection, bacterial infection, enterocolitis, laryngitis, lower respiratory tract infection

Blood and Lymphatic System Disorders: coagulopathy, lymphopenia

Metabolism and Nutrition Disorders: hyponatremia, metabolic acidosis, hypokalemia, hypovolemia

Nervous System Disorders: cognitive disorder, syncope, cerebral hemorrhage, abnormal coordination, lethargy

Cardiac Disorders: myocardial infarction, supraventricular arrhythmia, left ventricular dysfunction, angina pectoris, atrial flutter, cardiomyopathy, myocardial ischemia

Vascular Disorders: hypotension, thrombosis, embolism, hemorrhage, hypovolemic shock, vasculitis

Respiratory, Thoracic, and Mediastinal Disorders: pneumonitis, hypoxia, respiratory failure, acute pulmonary edema, dysphonia, pharyngolaryngeal pain

Gastrointestinal Disorders: ileus, colitis, impaired gastric emptying, esophagitis, dysphagia, gastritis, gastrointestinal hemorrhage

Hepatobiliary Disorders: acute hepatic failure, jaundice

Skin and Subcutaneous Tissue Disorders: erythema multiforme

Musculoskeletal, Connective Tissue Disorders, and Bone Disorders: muscular weakness, muscle spasms, trismus

Renal and Urinary Disorders: nephrolithiasis, renal failure

General Disorders and Administration Site Conditions: chills

Investigations: increased transaminases, increased blood alkaline phosphatase, increased gamma-glutamyltransferase.

7   DRUG INTERACTIONS
7.1   Effect of Other Drugs on Ixabepilone
Drugs That May Increase Ixabepilone Plasma Concentrations

CYP3A4 Inhibitors: Co-administration of ixabepilone with ketoconazole, a potent CYP3A4 inhibitor, increased ixabepilone AUC by 79% compared to ixabepilone treatment alone. If alternative treatment cannot be administered, a dose adjustment should be considered. The effect of mild or moderate inhibitors (eg, erythromycin, fluconazole, or verapamil) on exposure to ixabepilone has not been studied. Therefore, caution should be used when administering mild or moderate CYP3A4 inhibitors during treatment with IXEMPRA (ixabepilone), and alternative therapeutic agents that do not inhibit CYP3A4 should be considered. Patients receiving CYP3A4 inhibitors during treatment with IXEMPRA should be monitored closely for acute toxicities (eg, frequent monitoring of peripheral blood counts between cycles of IXEMPRA). [See *Dosage and Administration (2.2)*.]

Drugs That May Decrease Ixabepilone Plasma Concentrations

CYP3A4 Inducers: IXEMPRA is a CYP3A4 substrate. Strong CYP3A4 inducers (eg, dexamethasone, phenytoin, carbamazepine, rifampin, rifampicin, rifabutin, and phenobarbital) may decrease ixabepilone concentrations leading to subtherapeutic levels. Therefore, therapeutic agents with low enzyme induction potential should be considered for co-administration with IXEMPRA. St. John's wort may decrease ixabepilone plasma concentrations unpredictably and should be avoided.

7.2   Effect of Ixabepilone on Other Drugs
Ixabepilone does not inhibit CYP enzymes at relevant clinical concentrations and is not expected to alter the plasma concentrations of other drugs [see *Clinical Pharmacology (12.3)*].

7.3   Capecitabine
In patients with cancer who received ixabepilone (40 mg/m^2) in combination with capecitabine (1000 mg/m^2), ixabepilone C_{max} decreased by 19%, capecitabine C_{max} decreased by 27%, and 5-fluorouracil AUC increased by 14%, as compared to ixabepilone or capecitabine administered separately. The interaction is not clinically significant given that the combination treatment is supported by efficacy data.

8   USE IN SPECIFIC POPULATIONS
8.1   Pregnancy
Pregnancy Category D [See *Warnings and Precautions (5.5)*.]

8.3   Nursing Mothers
It is not known whether ixabepilone is excreted into human milk. Following intravenous administration of radiolabeled ixabepilone to rats on days 7 to 9 postpartum, concentrations of radioactivity in milk were comparable with those in plasma and declined in parallel with the plasma concentrations. Because many drugs are excreted in human milk and because of the potential for serious adverse reactions in nursing infants from ixabepilone, a decision must be made whether to discontinue nursing or to discontinue IXEMPRA (ixabepilone) taking into account the importance of the drug to the mother.

8.4   Pediatric Use
The safety and effectiveness of IXEMPRA in pediatric patients have not been established.

8.5   Geriatric Use
Clinical studies of IXEMPRA did not include sufficient numbers of subjects aged sixty five and over to determine whether they respond differently from younger subjects.

Forty-five of 431 patients treated with IXEMPRA in combination with capecitabine were ≥65 years of age and 3 patients were ≥75. Overall, the incidence of grade 3/4 adverse reactions were higher in patients ≥65 years of age versus those <65 years of age (82% versus 68%) including grade 3/4 stomatitis (9% versus 1%), diarrhea (9% versus 6%), palmar-plantar erythrodysesthesia syndrome (27% versus 20%), peripheral neuropathy (24% versus 22%), febrile neutropenia (9% versus 3%), fatigue (16% versus 12%), and asthenia (11% versus 6%). Toxicity-related deaths occurred in

2 (4.7%) of 43 patients ≥65 years with normal baseline hepatic function or mild impairment.

Thirty-two of 240 breast cancer patients treated with IXEMPRA (ixabepilone) as monotherapy were ≥65 years of age and 6 patients were ≥75. No overall differences in safety were observed in these patients compared to those <65 years of age.

8.6   Hepatic Impairment
IXEMPRA was evaluated in 56 patients with mild to severe hepatic impairment defined by bilirubin levels and AST levels. Compared to patients with normal hepatic function (n=17), the area under the curve ($AUC_{0-infinity}$) of ixabepilone increased by:
- 22% in patients with a) bilirubin >1 – 1.5 × ULN or b) AST >ULN but bilirubin <1.5 × ULN;
- 30% in patients with bilirubin >1.5 – 3 × ULN and any AST level; and
- 81% in patients with bilirubin >3 × ULN and any AST level.

Doses of 10 and 20 mg/m^2 as monotherapy were tolerated in 17 patients with severe hepatic impairment (bilirubin >3 × ULN).

IXEMPRA in combination with capecitabine must not be given to patients with AST or ALT >2.5 × ULN or bilirubin >1 × ULN [see *Boxed Warning, Contraindications (4)*, and *Warnings and Precautions (5.3)*]. Dose reduction is recommended when administering IXEMPRA as monotherapy to patients with hepatic impairment [see *Dosage and Administration (2.3)*]. Because there is a need for dosage adjustment based upon hepatic function, assessment of hepatic function is recommended before initiation of IXEMPRA and periodically thereafter.

8.7   Renal Impairment
Ixabepilone is minimally excreted via the kidney. No controlled pharmacokinetic studies were conducted with IXEMPRA in patients with renal impairment. IXEMPRA in combination with capecitabine has not been evaluated in patients with calculated creatinine clearance of <50 mL/min. IXEMPRA as monotherapy has not been evaluated in patients with creatinine >1.5 times ULN. In a population pharmacokinetic analysis of IXEMPRA as monotherapy, there was no meaningful effect of mild and moderate renal insufficiency (CrCL >30 mL/min) on the pharmacokinetics of ixabepilone.

10   OVERDOSAGE
One case of overdose of IXEMPRA has been reported. The patient mistakenly received 100 mg/m^2 (total dose 185 mg) and was admitted to the hospital for observation. The patient experienced myalgia (grade 1) and fatigue (grade 1) one day after infusion and was treated with a centrally acting analgesic. The patient recovered and was discharged without incident.

There is no known antidote for overdosage of IXEMPRA. In case of overdosage, the patient should be closely monitored, and supportive treatment should be administered. Management of overdose should include supportive medical interventions to treat the presenting clinical manifestations.

11   DESCRIPTION
IXEMPRA (ixabepilone) is a microtubule inhibitor belonging to a class of antineoplastic agents, the epothilones and their analogs. The epothilones are isolated from the myxobacterium *Sorangium cellulosum*. Ixabepilone is a semisynthetic analog of epothilone B, a 16-membered polyketide macrolide, with a chemically modified lactam substitution for the naturally existing lactone.

The chemical name for ixabepilone is (1S,3S,7S,10R, 11S,12S,16R)-7,11-dihydroxy-8,8,10,12,16-pentamethyl-3-[(1E)-1-methyl-2-(2-methyl-4-thiazolyl)ethenyl]-17-oxa-4-azabicyclo[14.1.0] heptadecane-5,9-dione, and it has a mo-

Continued on next page

Product information on these pages reflects product labeling on June 1, 2007. Current information on products of Bristol-Myers Squibb may be obtained at 1-800-321-1335 or www.bms.com.
NOUS08AB00403

Table 5:   Hematologic Abnormalities in Patients with Metastatic or Locally Advanced Breast Cancer Treated with IXEMPRA (ixabepilone)

Hematology Parameter	Study 046				Study 081	
	IXEMPRA with capecitabine n=369		Capecitabine n=368		IXEMPRA monotherapy n=126	
	Grade 3 (%)	Grade 4 (%)	Grade 3 (%)	Grade 4 (%)	Grade 3 (%)	Grade 4 (%)
Neutropenia[a]	32	36	9	2	31	23
Leukopenia (WBC)	41	16	5	1	36	13
Anemia (Hgb)	8	2	4	1	6	2
Thrombocytopenia	5	3	2	2	5	2

[a] G-CSF (granulocyte colony stimulating factor) or GM-CSF (granulocyte macrophage stimulating factor) was used in 20% and 17% of patients who received IXEMPRA in Study 046 and Study 081, respectively.

Ixempra—Cont.

lecular weight of 506.7. Ixabepilone has the following structural formula:

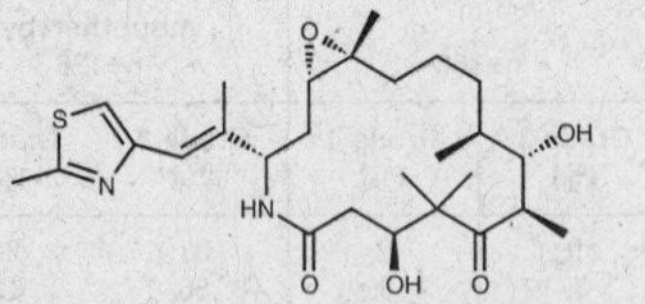

IXEMPRA (ixabepilone) for Injection is intended for intravenous infusion only after constitution with the supplied DILUENT and after further dilution with Lactated Ringer's Injection, USP. IXEMPRA (ixabepilone) for Injection is supplied as a sterile, non-pyrogenic single-use vial containing 15 mg or 45 mg ixabepilone as lyophilized white powder. The DILUENT for IXEMPRA is a sterile, non-pyrogenic solution of 52.8% (w/v) purified polyoxyethylated castor oil and 39.8% (w/v) dehydrated alcohol, USP. The IXEMPRA (ixabepilone) for Injection and the DILUENT for IXEMPRA are co-packaged and supplied as IXEMPRA *Kit*.

12 CLINICAL PHARMACOLOGY

12.1 Mechanism of Action

Ixabepilone is a semi-synthetic analog of epothilone B. Ixabepilone binds directly to β-tubulin subunits on microtubules, leading to suppression of microtubule dynamics. Ixabepilone suppresses the dynamic instability of αβ-II and αβ-III microtubules. Ixabepilone possesses low *in vitro* susceptibility to multiple tumor resistance mechanisms including efflux transporters, such as MRP-1 and P-glycoprotein (P-gp). Ixabepilone blocks cells in the mitotic phase of the cell division cycle, leading to cell death.

12.2 Pharmacodynamics

In cancer patients, ixabepilone has a plasma concentration-dependent effect on tubulin dynamics in peripheral blood mononuclear cells that is observed as the formation of microtubule bundles. Ixabepilone has antitumor activity *in vivo* against multiple human tumor xenografts, including drug-resistant types that overexpress P-gp, MRP-1, and βIII tubulin isoforms, or harbor tubulin mutations. Ixabepilone is active in xenografts that are resistant to multiple agents including taxanes, anthracyclines, and vinca alkaloids. Ixabepilone demonstrated synergistic antitumor activity in combination with capecitabine *in vivo*. In addition to direct antitumor activity, ixabepilone has antiangiogenic activity.

12.3 Pharmacokinetics

Absorption

Following administration of a single 40 mg/m^2 dose of IXEMPRA in patients with cancer, the mean C_{max} was 252 ng/mL (coefficient of variation, CV 56%) and the mean AUC was 2143 ng•hr/mL (CV 48%).Typically C_{max} occurred at the end of the 3 hour infusion. In cancer patients, the pharmacokinetics of ixabepilone were linear at doses of 15 to 57 mg/m^2.

Distribution

The mean volume of distribution of 40 mg/m^2 ixabepilone at steady-state was in excess of 1000 L. *In vitro*, the binding of ixabepilone to human serum proteins ranged from 67 to 77%, and the blood-to-plasma concentration ratios in human blood ranged from 0.65 to 0.85 over a concentration range of 50 to 5000 ng/mL.

Metabolism

Ixabepilone is extensively metabolized in the liver. *In vitro* studies indicated that the main route of oxidative metabolism of ixabepilone is via CYP3A4. More than 30 metabolites of ixabepilone are excreted into human urine and feces. No single metabolite accounted for more than 6% of the administered dose. The biotransformation products generated from ixabepilone by human liver microsomes were not active when tested for *in vitro* cytotoxicity against a human tumor cell line.

In vitro studies using human liver microsomes indicate that clinically relevant concentrations of ixabepilone do not inhibit CYP3A4, CYP1A2, CYP2A6, CYP2B6, CYP2C8, CYP2C9, CYP2C19, or CYP2D6. Ixabepilone does not induce the activity or the corresponding mRNA levels of CYP1A2, CYP2B6, CYP2C9, or CYP3A4 in cultured human hepatocytes at clinically relevant concentrations. Therefore, it is unlikely that ixabepilone will affect the plasma levels of drugs that are substrates of CYP enzymes.

Elimination

Ixabepilone is eliminated primarily as metabolized drug. After an intravenous ^{14}[C]-ixabepilone dose to patients, approximately 86% of the dose was eliminated within 7 days in feces (65% of the dose) and in urine (21% of the dose). Unchanged ixabepilone accounted for approximately 1.6% and 5.6% of the dose in feces and urine, respectively. Ixabepilone has a terminal elimination half-life of approximately 52 hours. No accumulation in plasma is expected for ixabepilone administered every 3 weeks.

Effects of Age, Gender, and Race

Based upon a population pharmacokinetic analysis in 676 cancer patients, gender, race, and age do not have meaningful effects on the pharmacokinetics of ixabepilone.

13 NONCLINICAL TOXICOLOGY

13.1 Carcinogenesis, Mutagenesis, Impairment of Fertility

Carcinogenicity studies with ixabepilone have not been conducted. Ixabepilone did not induce mutations in the microbial mutagenesis (Ames) assay and was not clastogenic in an *in vitro* cytogenetic assay using primary human lymphocytes. Ixabepilone was clastogenic (induction of micronuclei) in the *in vivo* rat micronucleus assay at doses ≥0.625 mg/kg/day.

There were no effects on male or female rat mating or fertility at doses up to 0.2 mg/kg/day in both males and females (approximately one-fifteenth the expected human clinical exposure based on AUC). The effect of ixabepilone on human fertility is unknown. However, when rats were given an IV infusion of ixabepilone during breeding and through the first 7 days of gestation, a significant increase in resorptions and pre- and post-implantation loss and a decrease in the number of corpora lutea was observed at 0.2 mg/kg/day. Testicular atrophy or degeneration was observed in 6-month rat and 9-month dog studies when ixabepilone was given every 21 days at intravenous doses of 6.7 mg/kg (40 mg/m^2) in rats (approximately 2.1 times the expected clinical exposure based on AUC) and 0.5 and 0.75 mg/kg (10 and 15 mg/m^2) in dogs (approximately 0.2 and 0.4 times the expected clinical exposure based on AUC).

13.2 Animal Toxicology

Overdose

In rats, single intravenous doses of ixabepilone from 60 to 180 mg/m^2 (mean AUC values ≥8156 ng•h/mL) were associated with mortality occurring between 5 and 14 days after dosing, and toxicity was principally manifested in the gastrointestinal, hematopoietic (bone-marrow), lymphatic, peripheral-nervous, and male-reproductive systems. In dogs, a single intravenous dose of 100 mg/m^2 (mean AUC value of 6925 ng•h/mL) was markedly toxic, inducing severe gastrointestinal toxicity and death 3 days after dosing.

14 CLINICAL STUDIES

Combination Therapy

In an open-label, multicenter, multinational, randomized trial of 752 patients with metastatic or locally advanced breast cancer, the efficacy and safety of IXEMPRA (ixabepilone) (40 mg/m^2 every 3 weeks) in combination with capecitabine (at 1000 mg/m^2 twice daily for 2 weeks followed by 1 week rest) were assessed in comparison with capecitabine as monotherapy (at 1250 mg/m^2 twice daily for 2 weeks followed by 1 week rest). Patients were previously treated with anthracyclines and taxanes. Patients were required to have demonstrated tumor progression or resistance to taxanes and anthracyclines as follows:

- tumor progression within 3 months of the last anthracycline dose in the metastatic setting or recurrence within 6 months in the adjuvant or neoadjuvant setting, and
- tumor progression within 4 months of the last taxane dose in the metastatic setting or recurrence within 12 months in the adjuvant or neoadjuvant setting.

For anthracyclines, patients who received a minimum cumulative dose of 240 mg/m^2 of doxorubicin or 360 mg/m^2 of epirubicin were also eligible.

Sixty-seven percent of patients were White, 23% were Asian and 3% were Black. Both arms were evenly matched with regards to race, age (median 53 years), baseline performance status (Karnofsky 70-100%), and receipt of prior adjuvant or neo-adjuvant chemotherapy (75%). Tumors were ER-positive in 47% of patients, ER-negative in 43%, HER2-positive in 15%, HER2-negative in 61%, and ER-negative, PR-negative, HER2-negative in 25%. The baseline disease characteristics and previous therapies for all patients (n=752) are shown in Table 6.

Table 6: Baseline Disease Characteristics and Previous Therapies

	IXEMPRA with capecitabine n=375	Capecitabine n=377
Site of disease		
Visceral disease (liver or lung)	316 (84%)	315 (84%)
Liver	245 (65%)	228 (61%)
Lung	180 (48%)	174 (46%)
Lymph node	250 (67%)	249 (66%)
Bone	168 (45%)	162 (43%)
Skin/soft tissue	60 (16%)	62 (16%)
Number of prior chemotherapy regimens in metastatic setting[a]		
0	27 (7%)	33 (9%)
1	179 (48%)	184 (49%)
2	152 (41%)	138 (37%)
≥3	17 (5%)	22 (6%)
Anthracycline resistance[b]	164 (44%)	165 (44%)
Taxane Resistance[c]		
Neoadjuvant/adjuvant setting	40 (11%)	44 (12%)
Metastatic setting	327 (87%)	319 (85%)

[a] For IXEMPRA plus capecitabine versus capecitabine only, prior treatment in the metastatic setting included cyclophosphamide (25% vs. 23%), fluorouracil (22% vs. 16%), vinorelbine (11% vs. 12%), gemcitabine (9% each arm), carboplatin (9% vs. 7%), liposomal doxorubicin (3% each arm), and cisplatin (2% vs. 3%).

[b] Tumor progression within 3 months in the metastatic setting or recurrence within 6 months in the adjuvant or neoadjuvant setting.

[c] 24% and 21% of patients had received 2 or more taxane-containing regimens in the combination and single agent treatment groups, respectively.

The patients in the combination treatment group received a median of 5 cycles of treatment and patients in the capecitabine monotherapy treatment group received a median of 4 cycles of treatment.

The primary endpoint of the study was progression-free survival (PFS) defined as time from randomization to radiologic progression as determined by Independent Radiologic Review (IRR), clinical progression of measurable skin lesions or death from any cause. Other study endpoints included objective tumor response based on Response Evaluation Criteria in Solid Tumors (RECIST), time to response, response duration, and overall survival. The data for overall survival analysis are not mature.

IXEMPRA (ixabepilone) in combination with capecitabine resulted in a statistically significant improvement in PFS compared to capecitabine. The results of the study are presented in Table 7 and Figure 1.

Table 7: Efficacy of IXEMPRA in Combination with Capecitabine vs Capecitabine Alone – Intent-to-Treat Analysis

Efficacy Parameter	IXEMPRA with capecitabine n=375	Capecitabine n=377
PFS		
Number of events[a]	242	256
Median	5.7 months	4.1 months
(95% CI)	(4.8-6.7)	(3.1-4.3)
Hazard Ratio[b] (95% CI)	0.69 (0.58-0.83)	
p-value[c] (Log rank)	<0.0001	
Objective Tumor Response Rate (95% CI)	34.7% (29.9-39.7)	14.3% (10.9-18.3)
p-value[c] (CMH)[d]	<0.0001	
Duration of Response, Median (95% CI)	6.4 months (5.6-7.1)	5.6 months (4.2-7.5)

[a] Patients were censored for PFS at the last date of tumor assessment prior to the start of subsequent therapy. In patients where independent review was not available PFS was censored at the randomization date.

[b] For the hazard ratio, a value less than 1.00 favors combination treatment, CI adjusted for interim analysis.

[c] Stratified by visceral metastasis in liver/lung, prior chemotherapy in metastatic setting, and anthracycline resistance.

[d] Cochran-Mantel-Haenszel test.

Figure 1: Progression-free Survival Kaplan Meier Curves

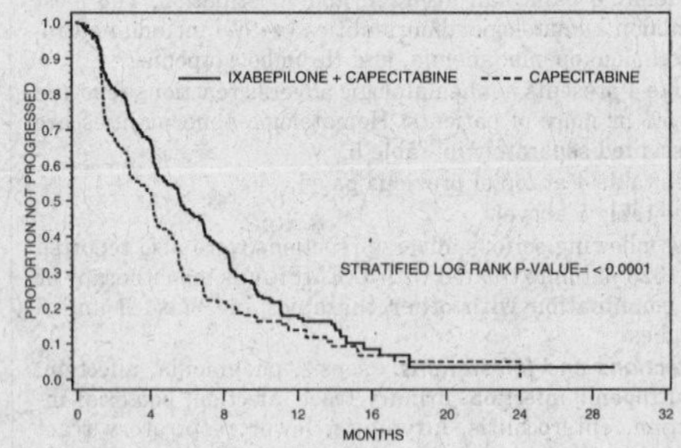

Monotherapy

IXEMPRA was evaluated as a single agent in a multicenter single-arm study in 126 women with metastatic or locally advanced breast cancer. The study enrolled patients whose tumors had recurred or had progressed following two or more chemotherapy regimens including an anthracycline, a taxane, and capecitabine. Patients who had received a minimum cumulative dose of 240 mg/m^2 of doxorubicin or 360 mg/m^2 of epirubicin were also eligible. Tumor progression or recurrence were prospectively defined as follows:

- Disease progression while on therapy in the metastatic setting (defined as progression while on treatment or within 8 weeks of last dose),
- Recurrence within 6 months of the last dose in the adjuvant or neoadjuvant setting (only for anthracycline and taxane),
- HER2-positive patients must also have progressed during or after discontinuation of trastuzumab.

In this study, the median age was 51 years (range, 30-78), and 79% were White, 5% Black, and 2% Asian, Karnofsky performance status was 70-100%, 88% had received two or more prior chemotherapy regimens for metastatic disease, and 86% had liver and/or lung metastases. Tumors were ER-positive in 48% of patients, ER-negative in 44%, HER2-positive in 7%, HER2-negative in 72%, and ER-negative, PR-negative, HER2-negative in 33%.

- IXEMPRA (ixabepilone) was administered at a dose of 40 mg/m^2 intravenously over 3 hours every 3 weeks. Patients received a median of 4 cycles (range 1 to 18) of IXEMPRA therapy.

Objective tumor response was determined by independent radiologic and investigator review using RECIST. Efficacy results are presented in Table 8.

Table 8: Efficacy of IXEMPRA (ixabepilone) in Metastatic and Locally Advanced Breast Cancer

Endpoint	Result
Objective tumor response rate (95% CI)	
IRR Assessment[a] (n = 113)	12.4% (6.9-19.9)
Investigator Assessment (n = 126)	18.3% (11.9-26.1)
Time to response[b] (n = 14)	
Median, weeks (min - max)	6.1 (5-54.4)
Duration of response[b] (n = 14)	
Median, months (95% CI)	6.0 (5.0-7.6)

[a] All responses were partial.
[b] As assessed by IRR.

15 REFERENCES

1. Preventing Occupational Exposures to Antineoplastic and Other Hazardous Drugs in Health Care Settings. NIOSH Alert 2004-165.
2. OSHA Technical Manual, TED 1-0.15A, Section VI: Chapter 2. Controlling Occupational Exposure to Hazardous Drugs. OSHA, 1999. http://www.osha.gov/dts/osta/otm/otm_vi/otm_vi_2.html.
3. American Society of Health-System Pharmacists. ASHP guidelines on handling hazardous drugs. *Am J Health-Syst Pharm.* 2006;63:1172-1193.
4. Polovich, M., White, J.M., & Kelleher, L.O. (eds.) 2005. Chemotherapy and biotherapy guidelines and recommendations for practice (2nd. ed.) Pittsburgh, PA: Oncology Nursing Society.

16 HOW SUPPLIED/STORAGE AND HANDLING

IXEMPRA is supplied as a *Kit* containing one vial of IXEMPRA™ (ixabepilone) for Injection and one vial of DILUENT for IXEMPRA.

NDC 0015-1910-12	IXEMPRA™ *Kit* containing one vial of IXEMPRA™ (ixabepilone) for Injection, 15 mg and one vial of DILUENT for IXEMPRA, 8 mL
NDC 0015-1911-13	IXEMPRA™ *Kit* containing one vial of IXEMPRA™ (ixabepilone) for Injection, 45 mg and one vial of DILUENT for IXEMPRA, 23.5 mL

IXEMPRA *Kit* must be stored in a refrigerator at 2° C to 8° C (36° F to 46° F). Retain in original package until time of use to protect from light.

Procedures for proper handling and disposal of antineoplastic drugs [see *References (15)*] should be followed. To minimize the risk of dermal exposure, impervious gloves should be worn when handling vials containing IXEMPRA, regardless of the setting, including unpacking and inspection, transport within a facility, and dose preparation and administration.

17 PATIENT COUNSELING INFORMATION

See *FDA-Approved Patient Labeling (17.6)*

17.1 Peripheral Neuropathy

Patients should be advised to report to their physician any numbness and tingling of the hands or feet [see *Warnings and Precautions (5.1)*].

17.2 Fever/Neutropenia

Patients should be instructed to call their physician if a fever of 100.5° F or greater or other evidence of potential infection such as chills, cough, or burning or pain on urination develops [see *Warnings and Precautions (5.2)*].

17.3 Hypersensitivity Reactions

Patients should be advised to call their physician if they experience urticaria, pruritus, rash, flushing, swelling, dyspnea, chest tightness or other hypersensitivity related symptoms following an infusion of IXEMPRA [see *Warnings and Precautions (5.4)*].

17.4 Pregnancy

Patients should be advised to use effective contraceptive measures to prevent pregnancy and to avoid nursing during treatment with IXEMPRA [see *Warnings and Precautions (5.5)* and *Use in Specific Populations (8.1, 8.3)*].

17.5 Cardiac Adverse Reactions

Patients should be advised to report to their physician chest pain, difficulty breathing, palpitations or unusual weight gain [see *Warnings and Precautions (5.6)*].

17.6 FDA-Approved Patient Labeling

Patient Information

IXEMPRA™ *Kit* (pronounced as ĭk-'sĕm-prä)
(ixabepilone)
for Injection, for intravenous infusion only

Read the Patient Information that comes with IXEMPRA (ixabepilone) before you start receiving it and before each injection. There may be new information. This leaflet does not take the place of talking with your healthcare provider about your medical condition or your treatment.

What is the most important information I should know about IXEMPRA (ixabepilone)?

Your healthcare provider should do blood tests to check your liver function:
- before you begin receiving IXEMPRA
- as needed while you are receiving IXEMPRA

If blood tests show that you have liver problems, do not receive injections of IXEMPRA (ixabepilone) along with the medicine capecitabine. Taking these two medicines together if you have liver problems increases your chance of serious problems. These include: serious infection and death due to a very low white blood cell count (neutropenia).

What is IXEMPRA?

IXEMPRA is a cancer medicine. IXEMPRA is used alone or with another cancer medicine called capecitabine. IXEMPRA is used to treat breast cancer, when certain other medicines have not worked or no longer work.

Who should not take IXEMPRA?

Do not receive injections of IXEMPRA if you:
- are allergic to a medicine, such as TAXOL®, that contains Cremophor® EL or polyoxyethylated castor oil
- have low white blood cell or platelet counts. Your healthcare provider will check your blood counts.
- are also taking a cancer medicine called capecitabine and you have liver problems. **See "What is the most important information I should know about IXEMPRA?"**

What should I tell my healthcare provider before receiving IXEMPRA?

IXEMPRA may not be right for you. Before you receive IXEMPRA, tell your healthcare provider about all of your medical conditions, including if you:
- have liver problems
- have heart problems or a history of heart problems
- have had an allergic reaction to IXEMPRA. You will receive medicines before each injection of IXEMPRA to decrease the chance of an allergic reaction. **See "How will I receive IXEMPRA?"**
- are pregnant or plan to become pregnant. You should not receive IXEMPRA during pregnancy because it may harm your unborn baby. Talk with your healthcare provider about how to prevent pregnancy while receiving IXEMPRA. Tell your healthcare provider right away if you become pregnant or think you are pregnant while receiving IXEMPRA.
- are breast-feeding. It is not known if IXEMPRA passes into breast milk. You and your healthcare provider should decide if you will take IXEMPRA or breast-feed. You should not do both.

Tell your healthcare provider about all the medicines you take, including prescription and non-prescription medicines, vitamins and herbal supplements.

IXEMPRA and certain other medicines may affect each other causing side effects. IXEMPRA may affect the way other medicines work, and other medicines may affect how IXEMPRA works. Know the medicines you take. Keep a list of your medicines with you to show your healthcare provider.

How will I receive IXEMPRA?

IXEMPRA is given by an injection directly into your vein (intravenous infusion). IXEMPRA is usually given once every three weeks. Each treatment with IXEMPRA will take about 3 hours.

Your healthcare provider will decide how much IXEMPRA you will receive and how often you will receive it.

To lower the chance of allergic reaction, you will receive other medicines about 1 hour before each treatment with IXEMPRA. (**See "What are the possible side effects of IXEMPRA?"**)

If you have an allergic reaction to IXEMPRA, you will receive a steroid medicine before future doses of IXEMPRA.You may also need to receive your doses of IXEMPRA more slowly.

What should I avoid while receiving IXEMPRA?

IXEMPRA contains alcohol. If you are dizzy or drowsy, avoid activities that may be dangerous, such as driving or operating machinery.

Do not drink grapefruit juice while receiving IXEMPRA. Drinking grapefruit juice may cause you to have too much IXEMPRA in your blood and lead to side effects.

What are the possible side effects of IXEMPRA?

IXEMPRA may cause serious side effects including:
- **Numbness, tingling, or burning in the hands or feet can occur while taking IXEMPRA (neuropathy).** These symptoms may be new or get worse while you are receiving IXEMPRA. These symptoms often occur early during treatment with IXEMPRA. Tell your healthcare provider if you have any of these symptoms.
  Your dose of IXEMPRA (ixabepilone) may need to be decreased, stopped until your symptoms get better, or totally stopped.
- **Low white blood cell count (neutropenia).** White blood cells help protect the body from infections caused by bacteria. If you get a fever or infection when your white blood cells are very low, you can become seriously ill and die. You may need treatment in the hospital with antibiotic medicines. Your healthcare provider will monitor your white blood cell count often with blood tests. Tell your healthcare provider right away or go to the nearest hospital emergency room if you have a fever (temperature above 100.5° F) or other sign of infection, such as chills, cough, burning or pain when you urinate, any time between treatments with IXEMPRA.
- **Allergic Reactions.** Severe allergic reactions can occur with IXEMPRA and may cause death in rare cases. Allergic reactions are most likely to occur while IXEMPRA is being injected into your vein. Tell your healthcare provider right away if you get any of the following signs and symptoms of an allergic reaction:
  - itching, hives (raised itchy welts), rash
  - flushed face
  - sudden swelling of face, throat or tongue
  - chest tightness, trouble breathing
  - feel dizzy or faint
  - feel your heart beating (palpitations)
- **Harm to an unborn child.** See "What should I tell my healthcare provider before taking IXEMPRA (ixabepilone)?"
- **Heart problems.** IXEMPRA might cause decreased blood flow to the heart, problems with heart function, and abnormal heart beat. This is seen more often in patients who also take capecitabine. **Tell your healthcare provider right away if you have any of the following symptoms:**
  - chest pain,
  - difficulty breathing,
  - feel your heart beating (palpitations), or
  - unusual weight gain.

The most common side effects with IXEMPRA used alone or with capecitabine may include:
- tiredness
- loss of appetite
- disorders of toenails and fingernails
- hair loss
- fever
- decreased red blood cells (anemia)
- joint and muscle pain
- headache
- decreased platelets (thrombocytopenia)
- nausea, vomiting, diarrhea, constipation, and abdominal pain
- sores on the lip, in the mouth and esophagus
- tender, red palms and soles of feet (hand-foot syndrome) that looks like a sunburn; the skin may become dry and peel. There may also be numbness and tingling.

Tell your healthcare provider about any side effect that bothers you or that does not go away.

These are not all of the side effects of IXEMPRA. Ask your healthcare provider or pharmacist for more information if you have questions or concerns.

General information about IXEMPRA?

This patient information leaflet summarizes the most important information about IXEMPRA. Medicines are sometimes prescribed for purposes other than those listed in a Patient Information Leaflet. If you would like more information about IXEMPRA, talk with your healthcare provider. You can ask your healthcare provider or pharmacist for information about IXEMPRA that is written for health professionals. For more information about IXEMPRA, call 1-888-IXEMPRA.

IXEMPRA™ (ixabepilone) for Injection Manufactured by: Baxter Oncology GmbH, 33790 Halle/Westfalen, Germany
DILUENT for IXEMPRA Manufactured by: Baxter Oncology GmbH, 33790 Halle/Westfalen, Germany
Distributed by Bristol-Myers Squibb Company, Princeton, NJ 08543 USA

Bristol-Myers Squibb Company
Princeton, NJ 08543 USA

1234735 Iss October 2007 XG-B0001-01-08
691US08LC08001

Daiichi Sankyo, Inc.

2 HILTON COURT
PARSIPPANY, NJ 07054

Direct Inquiries to:
1-877-4DS-PROD (1-877-437-7763)
www.daiichisankyo-us.com

AZOR™ ℞

[*AY-sawr*]
(amlodipine and olmesartan medoxomil)

HIGHLIGHTS OF PRESCRIBING INFORMATION
These highlights do not include all the information needed to use AZOR™ safely and effectively. See full prescribing information for AZOR™
AZOR™
(amlodipine and olmesartan medoxomil) tablets
Initial U.S. Approval: 2007

USE IN PREGNANCY
See full prescribing information for complete boxed warning.
When used in pregnancy during the second and third trimesters, drugs that act directly on the renin-angiotensin system can cause injury and even death to the developing fetus. When pregnancy is detected, AZOR™ should be discontinued as soon as possible (5.1).

--------------INDICATIONS AND USAGE--------------
- AZOR™ is a dihydropyridine calcium channel blocker and angiotensin II receptor blocker combination product indicated for the treatment of hypertension, alone or with other antihypertensive agents (1).

Continued on next page

Azor—Cont.

··········DOSAGE AND ADMINISTRATION ··········

• AZOR™ may be substituted for its individually titrated components for patients on amlodipine and olmesartan medoxomil. AZOR™ may also be given with increased amounts of amlodipine, olmesartan medoxomil, or both, as needed (2).

• AZOR™ may be used as add-on therapy for patients not adequately controlled on amlodipine or olmesartan medoxomil (2).

• Dosage may be increased after 2 weeks to a maximum dose of 10/40 mg once daily, usually by increasing one component at a time but both components can be raised to achieve more rapid control (2).

• Maximum antihypertensive effects are attained within 2 weeks after a change in dose (2).

········DOSAGE FORMS AND STRENGTHS ········

Tablets: (amlodipine/olmesartan medoxomil content) 5/20 mg; 10/20 mg; 5/40 mg; and 10/40 mg (3).

··············CONTRAINDICATIONS ··············

None (4).

··········WARNINGS AND PRECAUTIONS··········

• Hypotension in volume- or salt-depleted patients with treatment initiation may occur. Start treatment under close supervision (5.2).

• Increased angina or myocardial infarction with calcium channel blockers may occur upon dosage initiation or increase (5.4).

• Impaired renal function: changes in renal function may be anticipated in susceptible individuals (5.6).

···············ADVERSE REACTIONS ···············

Most common adverse reaction (incidence ≥3%) is edema (6.1).

To report SUSPECTED ADVERSE REACTIONS, contact Daiichi Sankyo, Inc. at 1-877-437-7763 or FDA at 1-800-332-1088 or www.fda.gov/medwatch.

··········USE IN SPECIFIC POPULATIONS ··········

• In patients with an activated renin-angiotensin system, such as volume- or salt-depletion, renin-angiotensin-aldosterone system (RAAS) blockers such as olmesartan medoxomil can cause excessive hypotension. In susceptible patients, e.g., with renal artery stenosis, RAAS blockers can cause renal failure (5.2, 5.6).

• When starting or adding amlodipine in patients ≥75 years old or hepatically impaired patients, starting it at 2.5 mg is recommended. Elderly and patients with hepatic impairment have decreased clearance of amlodipine. (8.5, 8.6).

See 17 for PATIENT COUNSELING INFORMATION

Revised 09/2007

FULL PRESCRIBING INFORMATION: CONTENTS*

*Sections or subsections omitted from the full prescribing information are not listed.

FULL PRESCRIBING INFORMATION

AZOR™

(amlodipine and olmesartan medoxomil) tablets

> **USE IN PREGNANCY**
>
> When used in pregnancy during the second and third trimesters, drugs that act directly on the renin-angiotensin system can cause injury and even death to the developing fetus. When pregnancy is detected, AZOR™ should be discontinued as soon as possible *[see Warnings and Precautions (5.1)].*

1　INDICATIONS AND USAGE

AZOR™ is indicated for the treatment of hypertension, alone or with other anti-hypertensive agents.

This fixed combination drug is not indicated for the initial therapy of hypertension (see DOSAGE AND ADMINISTRATION).

2　DOSAGE AND ADMINISTRATION

General Considerations

The side effects of olmesartan medoxomil are generally rare and apparently independent of dose. Those of amlodipine are generally dose-dependent (mostly edema).

Maximum antihypertensive effects are attained within 2 weeks after a change in dose.

AZOR™ may be taken with or without food.

AZOR™ may be administered with other antihypertensive agents.

Dosage may be increased after 2 weeks. The maximum recommended dose of AZOR™ is 10/40 mg.

Replacement Therapy

AZOR™ may be substituted for its individually titrated components.

When substituting for individual components, the dose of one or both of the components can be increased if blood pressure control has not been satisfactory.

Add-on Therapy for Patients with Hypertension Not Adequately Controlled on Amlodipine or Olmesartan Medoxomil Alone.

AZOR™ may be used as add-on therapy for patients not adequately controlled on amlodipine or olmesartan medoxomil.

3　DOSAGE FORMS AND STRENGTHS

AZOR™ tablets are formulated for oral administration in the following strength combinations:

	5/20	5/40	10/20	10/40
amlodipine equivalent (mg)	5	5	10	10
olmesartan medoxomil (mg)	20	40	20	40

4　CONTRAINDICATIONS

None.

5　WARNINGS AND PRECAUTIONS

The adverse reactions of AZOR™ are generally related to those of each of its components.

5.1　Fetal/Neonatal Morbidity and Mortality

Olmesartan medoxomil. Drugs that act directly on the renin-angiotensin system can cause fetal and neonatal morbidity and death when administered to pregnant women. There have been several dozen cases reported in the world literature of patients who were taking angiotensin converting enzyme inhibitors. When pregnancy is detected, AZOR™ should be discontinued as soon as possible.

During the second and third trimesters of pregnancy, these drugs have been associated with fetal injury that includes hypotension, neonatal skull hypoplasia, anuria, reversible or irreversible renal failure, and death. Oligohydramnios has also been reported, presumably resulting from decreased fetal renal function; oligohydramnios in this setting has been associated with fetal limb contractures, craniofacial deformation, and hypoplastic lung development. Prematurity, intrauterine growth retardation, and patent ductus arteriosus have also been reported, although it is not clear whether these occurrences were due to exposure to the drug.

These adverse effects do not appear to have resulted from intrauterine drug exposure that has been limited to the first trimester. Mothers whose embryos and fetuses are exposed to an angiotensin II receptor antagonist only during the first trimester should be so informed. Nonetheless, when patients become pregnant, physicians should have the patient discontinue the use of AZOR™ as soon as possible.

Rarely (probably less often than once in every thousand pregnancies), no alternative to a drug acting on the renin-angiotensin system will be found. In these rare cases, the mothers should be apprised of the potential hazards to their fetuses and serial ultrasound examinations should be performed to assess the intra-amniotic environment.

If oligohydramnios is observed, AZOR™ should be discontinued unless it is considered life-saving for the mother. Contraction stress testing (CST), a non-stress test (NST), or biophysical profiling (BPP) may be appropriate, depending upon the week of pregnancy. Patients and physicians should be aware, however, that oligohydramnios may not appear until after the fetus has sustained irreversible injury.

Infants with histories of *in utero* exposure to an angiotensin II receptor antagonist should be closely observed for hypotension, oliguria, and hyperkalemia. If oliguria occurs, attention should be directed toward support of blood pressure and renal perfusion. Exchange transfusion or dialysis may be required as means of reversing hypotension and/or substituting for disordered renal function.

No teratogenic effects were observed when olmesartan medoxomil was administered to pregnant rats at oral doses up to 1000 mg/kg/day (240 times the maximum recommended human dose (MRHD) on a mg/m² basis) or pregnant rabbits at oral doses up to 1 mg/kg/day (half the MRHD on a mg/m² basis; higher doses could not be evaluated for effects on fetal development as they were lethal to the does). In rats, significant decreases in pup birth weight and weight gain were observed at doses ≥1.6 mg/kg/day, and delays in developmental milestones (delayed separation of ear auricular, eruption of lower incisors, appearance of abdominal hair, descent of testes, and separation of eyelids) and dose-dependent increases in the incidence of dilation of the renal pelvis were observed at doses ≥8 mg/kg/day. The no observed effect dose for developmental toxicity in rats is 0.3 mg/kg/day, about one-tenth the MRHD of 40 mg/day.

5.2　Hypotension in Volume- or Salt-Depleted Patients

Olmesartan medoxomil. Symptomatic hypotension may occur after initiation of treatment with olmesartan medoxomil. Patients with an activated renin-angiotensin system, such as volume- and/or salt-depleted patients (e.g., those being treated with high doses of diuretics) may be particularly vulnerable. Treatment with AZOR™ should start under close medical supervision. If hypotension does occur, the patient should be placed in the supine position and, if necessary, given an intravenous infusion of normal saline. A transient hypotensive response is not a contraindication to further treatment, which usually can be continued without difficulty once the blood pressure has stabilized.

5.3　Vasodilation

Amlodipine. Since the vasodilation attributable to amlodipine in AZOR™ is gradual in onset, acute hypotension has rarely been reported after oral administration. Nonetheless, caution, as with any other peripheral vasodilator, should be exercised when administering AZOR™, particularly in patients with severe aortic stenosis.

5.4　Patients with Severe Obstructive Coronary Artery Disease

Patients, particularly those with severe obstructive coronary artery disease, may develop increased frequency, duration, or severity of angina or acute myocardial infarction on starting calcium channel blocker therapy or at the time of dosage increase. The mechanism of this effect has not been elucidated.

5.5　Patients with Congestive Heart Failure

Amlodipine. In general, calcium channel blockers should be used with caution in patients with heart failure. Amlodipine (5-10 mg per day) has been studied in a placebo-controlled trial of 1153 patients with NYHA Class III or IV heart failure on stable doses of ACE inhibitor, digoxin, and diuretics. Follow-up was at least 6 months, with a mean of about 14 months. There was no overall adverse effect on survival or cardiac morbidity (as defined by life-threatening arrhythmia, acute myocardial infarction, or hospitalization for worsened heart failure). Amlodipine has been compared to placebo in four 8-12 week studies of patients with NYHA class II/III heart failure, involving a total of 697 patients. In these studies, there was no evidence of worsening of heart failure based on measures of exercise tolerance, NYHA classification, symptoms, or LVEF.

5.6　Patients with Impaired Renal Function

Olmesartan medoxomil. Changes in renal function may be anticipated in susceptible individuals treated with olmesartan medoxomil as a consequence of inhibiting the renin-angiotensin-aldosterone system. In patients whose renal function may depend upon the activity of the renin-angiotensin-aldosterone system (e.g., patients with severe congestive heart failure), treatment with angiotensin converting enzyme inhibitors and angiotensin receptor antagonists has been associated with oliguria or progressive azotemia and (rarely) with acute renal failure and/or death. Similar effects may occur in patients treated with AZOR™ due to the olmesartan medoxomil component *[See Clinical Pharmacology (12.3)].*

In studies of ACE inhibitors in patients with unilateral or bilateral renal artery stenosis, increases in serum creatinine or blood urea nitrogen (BUN) have been reported. There has been no long-term use of olmesartan medoxomil in patients with unilateral or bilateral renal artery stenosis, but similar effects would be expected with AZOR™ because of the olmesartan medoxomil component.

5.7　Patients with Hepatic Impairment

Amlodipine. Since amlodipine is extensively metabolized by the liver and the plasma elimination half-life ($t_{1/2}$) is 56 hours in patients with severely impaired hepatic function, caution should be exercised when administering AZOR™ to patients with severe hepatic impairment.

5.8　Laboratory Tests

AZOR™. There was a greater decrease in hemoglobin and hematocrit in the combination product compared to either component. Other laboratory changes can usually be attributed to either monotherapy component.

Amlodipine. In post-marketing experience, hepatic enzyme elevations have been reported (6.2).

Olmesartan medoxomil. In post-marketing experience, increased blood creatinine levels and hyperkalemia have been reported.

6 ADVERSE REACTIONS

6.1 Clinical Trials Experience

Because clinical studies are conducted under widely varying conditions, adverse reaction rates observed in the clinical studies of a drug cannot be directly compared to rates in the clinical studies of another drug and may not reflect the rates observed in practice.

AZOR™

The data described below reflect exposure to AZOR™ in more than 1600 patients including more than 1000 exposed for at least 6 months and more than 700 exposed for 1 year. AZOR™ was studied in one placebo-controlled factorial trial (see Section 14.1). The population had a mean age of 54 years and included approximately 55% males. Seventy-one percent were Caucasian and 25% were Black. Patients received doses ranging from 5/20 mg to 10/40 mg orally once daily.

The overall incidence of adverse reactions on therapy with AZOR™ was similar to that seen with corresponding doses of the individual components of AZOR™, and to placebo. The reported adverse reactions were generally mild and seldom led to discontinuation of treatment (2.6% for AZOR™ and 6.8% for placebo).

Edema

Edema is a known, dose-dependent adverse effect of amlodipine but not of olmesartan medoxomil.

The placebo-subtracted incidence of edema during the 8-week, randomized, double-blind treatment period was highest with amlodipine 10 mg monotherapy. The incidence was significantly reduced when 20 mg or 40 mg of olmesartan medoxomil was added to the 10 mg amlodipine dose.

Placebo-Subtracted Incidence of Edema during the Double-Blind Treatment Period

		Olmesartam Medoxomil		
		Placebo	**20 mg**	**40 mg**
Amiodipine	**Placebo**	0%*	(-2.4%)	6.2%
	5 mg	0.7%	5.7%	6.2%
	10 mg	24.5%	13.3%	11.2%

*12.3%=actual placebo incidence

Across all treatment groups, the frequency of edema was generally higher in women than men, as has been observed in previous studies of amlodipine.

Adverse reactions seen at lower rates during the double-blind period also occurred in the patients treated with AZOR™ at about the same or greater incidence as in patients receiving placebo. These included hypotension, orthostatic hypotension, rash, pruritus, palpitation, urinary frequency, and nocturia.

The adverse event profile obtained from 44 weeks of open-label combination therapy with amlodipine plus olmesartan medoxomil was similar to that observed during the 8-week, double-blind, placebo-controlled period.

Amlodipine

Amlodipine has been evaluated for safety in more than 11,000 patients in U.S. and foreign clinical trials. Most adverse reactions reported during therapy with amlodipine were of mild or moderate severity. In controlled clinical trials directly comparing amlodipine (N=1730) in doses up to 10 mg to placebo (N=1250), discontinuation of amlodipine due to adverse reactions was required in only about 1.5% of amlodipine-treated patients and about 1% of placebo-treated patients. The most common side effects were headache and edema. The incidence (%) of dose-related side effects was as follows:

Adverse Event	Placebo N=520	2.5 mg N=275	5.0 mg N=296	10.0 mg N=268
Edema	0.6	1.8	3.0	10.8
Dizziness	1.5	1.1	3.4	3.4
Flushing	0.0	0.7	1.4	2.6
Palpitation	0.6	0.7	1.4	4.5

For several adverse experiences that appear to be drug- and dose-related, there was a greater incidence in women than men associated with amlodipine treatment as shown in the following table:

Adverse Event	Placebo		Amlodipine	
	Male=% (N=914)	Female=% (N=336)	Male=% (N=1218)	Female=% (N=512)
Edema	1.4	5.1	5.6	14.6
Flushing	0.3	0.9	1.5	4.5
Palpitation	0.9	0.9	1.4	3.3
Somnolence	0.8	0.3	1.3	1.6

Olmesartan medoxomil

Olmesartan medoxomil has been evaluated for safety in more than 3825 patients/subjects, including more than 3275 patients treated for hypertension in controlled trials. This experience included about 900 patients treated for at least 6 months and more than 525 for at least 1 year. Treatment with olmesartan medoxomil was well tolerated, with an incidence of adverse events similar to that seen with placebo. Events were generally mild, transient, and without relationship to the dose of olmesartan medoxomil.

The overall frequency of adverse events was not dose-related. Analysis of gender, age, and race groups demonstrated no differences between olmesartan medoxomil- and placebo-treated patients. The rate of withdrawals due to adverse events in all trials of hypertensive patients was 2.4% (i.e., 79/3278) of patients treated with olmesartan medoxomil and 2.7% (i.e., 32/1179) of control patients. In placebo-controlled trials, the only adverse event that occurred in more than 1% of patients treated with olmesartan medoxomil and at a higher incidence in olmesartan medoxomil treated patients vs. placebo was dizziness (3% vs 1%).

6.2 Post-Marketing Experience

The following adverse reactions have been identified during post-approval use of the individual components of AZOR™. Because these reactions are reported voluntarily from a population of uncertain size, it is not always possible to reliably estimate their frequency or establish a causal relationship to drug exposure.

Amlodipine. The following post-marketing event has been reported infrequently where a causal relationship is uncertain: gynecomastia. In post-marketing experience, jaundice and hepatic enzyme elevations (mostly consistent with cholestasis or hepatitis), in some cases severe enough to require hospitalization, have been reported in association with use of amlodipine.

Olmesartan medoxomil. The following adverse reactions have been reported in post-marketing experience:

Body as a Whole: asthenia, angioedema
Gastrointestinal: vomiting
Musculoskeletal: rhabdomyolysis
Urogenital System: acute renal failure
Skin and Appendages: alopecia, pruritus, urticaria

7 DRUG INTERACTIONS

7.1 Drug Interactions with AZOR™

The pharmacokinetics of amlodipine and olmesartan medoxomil are not altered when the drugs are co-administered.

No drug interaction studies have been conducted with AZOR™ and other drugs, although studies have been conducted with the individual amlodipine and olmesartan medoxomil components of AZOR™, as described below, and no significant drug interactions have been observed.

7.2 Drug Interactions with Amlodipine

In vitro data indicate that amlodipine has no effect on the human plasma protein binding of digoxin, phenytoin, warfarin, and indomethacin.

Effect of Other Agents on Amlodipine

Cimetidine: Co-administration of amlodipine with cimetidine did not alter the pharmacokinetics of amlodipine.

Grapefruit juice: Co-administration of 240 mL of grapefruit juice with a single oral dose of amlodipine 10 mg in 20 healthy volunteers had no significant effect on the pharmacokinetics of amlodipine.

Maalox® (antacid): Co-administration of the antacid Maalox® with a single dose of amlodipine had no significant effect on the pharmacokinetics of amlodipine.

Sildenafil: A single 100 mg dose of sildenafil in subjects with essential hypertension had no effect on the pharmacokinetic parameters of amlodipine. When amlodipine and sildenafil were used in combination, each agent independently exerted its own blood pressure lowering effect.

Effect of Amlodipine on Other Agents

Atorvastatin: Co-administration of multiple 10 mg doses of amlodipine with 80 mg of atorvastatin resulted in no significant change in the steady state pharmacokinetic parameters of atorvastatin.

Digoxin: Co-administration of amlodipine with digoxin did not change serum digoxin levels or digoxin renal clearance in normal volunteers.

Ethanol (alcohol): Single and multiple 10 mg doses of amlodipine had no significant effect on the pharmacokinetics of ethanol.

Warfarin: Co-administration of amlodipine with warfarin did not change the warfarin prothrombin response time.

In clinical trials, amlodipine has been safely administered with thiazide diuretics, beta-blockers, angiotensin-converting enzyme inhibitors, long-acting nitrates, sublingual nitroglycerin, digoxin, warfarin, non-steroidal anti-inflammatory drugs, antibiotics, and oral hypoglycemic drugs.

7.3 Drug Interactions with Olmesartan Medoxomil

No significant drug interactions were reported in studies in which olmesartan medoxomil was co-administered with digoxin or warfarin in healthy volunteers.

The bioavailability of olmesartan medoxomil was not significantly altered by the co-administration of antacids [$Al(OH)_3/Mg(OH)_2$].

Olmesartan medoxomil is not metabolized by the cytochrome P450 system and has no effects on P450 enzymes; thus, interactions with drugs that inhibit, induce, or are metabolized by those enzymes are not expected.

8 USE IN SPECIFIC POPULATIONS

8.1 Pregnancy

Olmesartan medoxomil. Pregnancy Categories C (first trimester) and D (second and third trimesters). *[See Warnings and Precautions (5.1)]*

Amlodipine. No evidence of teratogenicity or other embryo/fetal toxicity was found when pregnant rats and rabbits were treated orally with amlodipine maleate at doses of up to 10 mg amlodipine/kg/day (respectively about 10 and 20 times the maximum recommended human dose of 10 mg amlodipine on a mg/m^2 basis) during their respective periods of major organogenesis. (Calculations based on a patient weight of 60 kg). However, litter size was significantly decreased (by about 50%) and the number of intrauterine deaths was significantly increased (about 5-fold) in rats receiving amlodipine maleate at a dose equivalent to 10 mg amlodipine/kg/day for 14 days before mating and throughout mating and gestation. Amlodipine maleate has been shown to prolong both the gestational period and the duration of labor in rats at this dose. There are no adequate and well-controlled studies in pregnant women. Amlodipine should be used during pregnancy only if the potential benefit justifies the potential risk to the fetus.

8.3 Nursing Mothers

It is not known whether the amlodipine or olmesartan medoxomil components of AZOR™ are excreted in human milk, but olmesartan is secreted at low concentration in the milk of lactating rats. Because of the potential for adverse effects on the nursing infant, a decision should be made whether to discontinue nursing or discontinue the drug, taking into account the importance of the drug to the mother.

8.4 Pediatric Use

The safety and effectiveness of AZOR™ in pediatric patients have not been established.

Amlodipine. The effect of amlodipine on blood pressure in patients less than 6 years of age is not known.

Olmesartan medoxomil. Safety and effectiveness of olmesartan medoxomil in pediatric patients have not been established.

8.5 Geriatric Use

Of the total number of subjects in the double-blind clinical study of AZOR™, 20% (384/1940) were 65 years of age or older and 3% (62/1940) were 75 years or older. No overall differences in safety or effectiveness were observed between subjects 65 years of age or older and younger subjects.

Amlodipine. Reported clinical experience has not identified differences in responses between the elderly and younger patients. In general, dose selection for an elderly patient should be cautious, usually starting at the low end of the dosing range, reflecting the greater frequency of decreased hepatic, renal, or cardiac function, and of concomitant disease or other drug therapy. Elderly patients have decreased clearance of amlodipine with a resulting increase of AUC of approximately 40% to 60%, and a lower initial dose may be required.

Olmesartan medoxomil. Of the total number of hypertensive patients receiving olmesartan medoxomil in clinical studies, more than 20% were 65 years of age and over, while more than 5% were 75 years of age and older. No overall differences in effectiveness or safety were observed between elderly patients and younger patients. Other reported clinical experience has not identified differences in responses between the elderly and younger patients, but greater sensitivity of some older individuals cannot be ruled out.

8.6 Hepatic Impairment

There are no studies of AZOR™ in patients with hepatic insufficiency, but both amlodipine and olmesartan medoxomil show moderate increases in exposure in patients with hepatic impairment. Use caution when administering AZOR™ to patients with severe hepatic impairment.

8.7 Renal Impairment

There are no studies of AZOR™ in patients with renal impairment.

Amlodipine. The pharmacokinetics of amlodipine are not significantly influenced by renal impairment. Patients with renal failure may therefore receive the usual initial dose.

Olmesartan medoxomil. Patients with renal insufficiency have elevated serum concentrations of olmesartan compared with patients with normal renal function. After repeated dosing, AUC was approximately tripled in patients with severe renal impairment (creatinine clearance <20 mL/min). No initial dosage adjustment is recommended for patients with moderate to marked renal impairment (creatinine clearance <40 mL/min).

8.8 Black Patients

Of the total number of subjects in the double-blind clinical study of AZOR™, 25% (481/1940) were black patients. AZOR™ was effective in treating black patients (usually a low-renin population), and the magnitude of blood pressure reduction in black patients approached that observed for non-black patients.

10 OVERDOSAGE

There is no information on overdosage with AZOR™ in humans.

Amlodipine. Single oral doses of amlodipine maleate equivalent to 40 mg amlodipine/kg and 100 mg amlodipine/kg in mice and rats, respectively, caused deaths. Single oral

Continued on next page

Azor—Cont.

amlodipine maleate doses equivalent to 4 or more mg amlodipine/kg or higher in dogs (11 or more times the maximum recommended human dose on a mg/m^2 basis) caused a marked peripheral vasodilation and hypotension.

Overdosage might be expected to cause excessive peripheral vasodilation with marked hypotension and possibly a reflex tachycardia. In humans, experience with intentional overdosage of amlodipine is limited.

If massive overdose should occur, active cardiac and respiratory monitoring should be instituted. Frequent blood pressure measurements are essential. Should hypotension occur, cardiovascular support including elevation of the extremities and the judicious administration of fluids should be initiated. If hypotension remains unresponsive to these conservative measures, administration of vasopressors (such as phenylephrine) should be considered with attention to circulating volume and urine output. Intravenous calcium gluconate may help to reverse the effects of calcium entry blockade. As amlodipine is highly protein bound, hemodialysis is not likely to be of benefit.

Olmesartan medoxomil. Limited data are available related to overdosage in humans. The most likely manifestations of overdosage would be hypotension and tachycardia; bradycardia could be encountered if parasympathetic (vagal) stimulation occurs. If symptomatic hypotension should occur, supportive treatment should be initiated. The dialyzability of olmesartan is unknown.

11 DESCRIPTION

AZOR™ is a combination of the calcium channel receptor blocker (CCB) amlodipine besylate and the angiotensin II receptor blocker (ARB) olmesartan medoxomil.

The amlodipine besylate component of AZOR™ is chemically described as 3-ethyl-5-methyl (±)-2-[(2-aminoethoxy)methyl]-4-(2-chlorophenyl)-1,4-dihydro-6-methyl-3,5-pyridinedicarboxylate, monobenzenesulphonate. Its empirical formula is $C_{20}H_{25}ClN_2O_5 \bullet C_6H_6O_3S$.

Olmesartan medoxomil, a prodrug, is hydrolyzed to olmesartan during absorption from the gastrointestinal tract.

The olmesartan medoxomil component of AZOR™ is chemically described as 2,3-dihydroxy-2-butenyl 4-(1-hydroxy-1-methylethyl)-2-propyl-1-[p-(o-1*H*-tetrazol-5-ylphenyl)benzyl]imidazole-5-carboxylate, cyclic 2,3-carbonate. Its empirical formula is $C_{29}H_{30}N_6O_6$.

The structural formula for amlodipine besylate is:

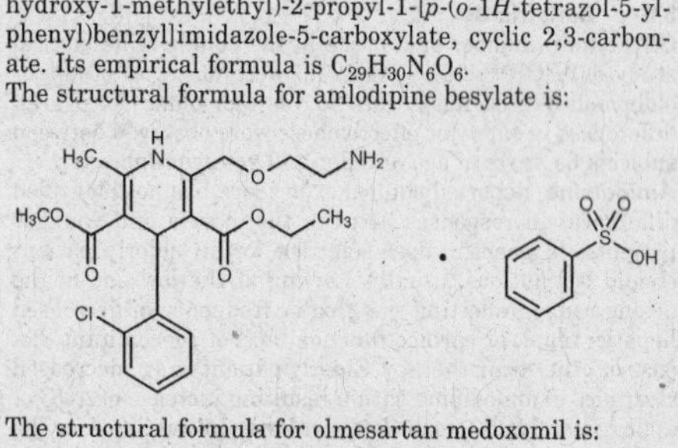

The structural formula for olmesartan medoxomil is:

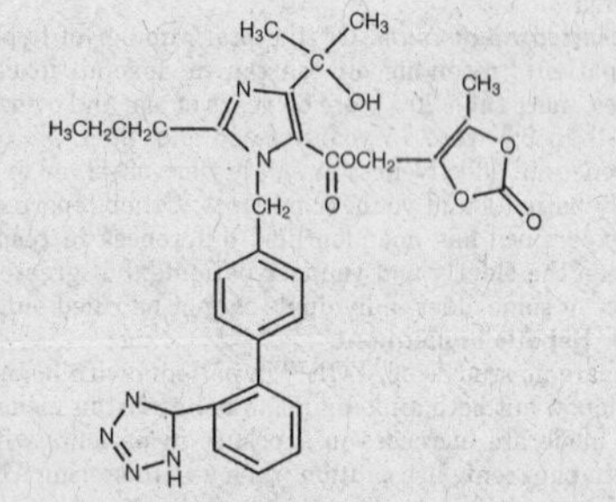

AZOR™ contains amlodipine besylate, a white to off-white crystalline powder, and olmesartan medoxomil, a white to light yellowish-white powder or crystalline powder. The molecular weights of amlodipine besylate and olmesartan medoxomil are 567.1 and 558.59, respectively. Amlodipine besylate is slightly soluble in water and sparingly soluble in ethanol. Olmesartan medoxomil is practically insoluble in water and sparingly soluble in methanol.

Each tablet of AZOR™ also contains the following inactive ingredients: silicified microcrystalline cellulose, pregelatinized starch, croscarmellose sodium, and magnesium stearate. The color coatings contain polyvinyl alcohol, macrogol/polyethylene glycol 3350, titanium dioxide, talc, iron oxide yellow (5/40 mg, 10/20 mg, 10/40 mg tablets), iron oxide red (10/20 mg and 10/40 mg tablets), and iron oxide black (10/20 mg tablets).

12 CLINICAL PHARMACOLOGY

12.1 Mechanism of Action

AZOR™. AZOR™ is a combination of two antihypertensive drugs: a dihydropyridine calcium antagonist (calcium ion antagonist or slow-channel blocker), amlodipine besylate, and an angiotensin II receptor blocker, olmesartan medoxomil. The amlodipine component of AZOR™ inhibits the transmembrane influx of calcium ions into vascular smooth muscle and cardiac muscle, and the olmesartan medoxomil component of AZOR™ blocks the vasoconstrictor effects of angiotensin II.

Amlodipine. Experimental data suggests that amlodipine binds to both dihydropyridine and nonhydropyridine binding sites. The contractile processes of cardiac muscle and vascular smooth muscle are dependent upon the movement of extracellular calcium ions into these cells through specific ion channels. Amlodipine inhibits calcium ion influx across cell membranes selectively, with a greater effect on vascular smooth muscle cells than on cardiac muscle cells. Negative inotropic effects can be detected *in vitro* but such effects have not been seen in intact animals at therapeutic doses. Serum calcium concentration is not affected by amlodipine. Within the physiologic pH range, amlodipine is an ionized compound (pKa=8.6), and its kinetic interaction with the calcium channel receptor is characterized by a gradual rate of association and dissociation with the receptor binding site, resulting in a gradual onset of effect.

Amlodipine is a peripheral arterial vasodilator that acts directly on vascular smooth muscle to cause a reduction in peripheral vascular resistance and reduction in blood pressure.

Olmesartan medoxomil. Angiotensin II is formed from angiotensin I in a reaction catalyzed by angiotensin converting enzyme (ACE, kininase II). Angiotensin II is the principal pressor agent of the renin-angiotensin system, with effects that include vasoconstriction, stimulation of synthesis and release of aldosterone, cardiac stimulation and renal reabsorption of sodium. Olmesartan blocks the vasoconstrictor effects of angiotensin II by selectively blocking the binding of angiotensin II to the AT_1 receptor in vascular smooth muscle. Its action is, therefore, independent of the pathways for angiotensin II synthesis.

An AT_2 receptor is found also in many tissues, but this receptor is not known to be associated with cardiovascular homeostasis. Olmesartan has more than a 12,500-fold greater affinity for the AT_1 receptor than for the AT_2 receptor.

Blockade of the renin-angiotensin system with ACE inhibitors, which inhibit the biosynthesis of angiotensin II from angiotensin I, is a mechanism of many drugs used to treat hypertension. ACE inhibitors also inhibit the degradation of bradykinin, a reaction also catalyzed by ACE. Because olmesartan does not inhibit ACE (kininase II), it does not affect the response to bradykinin. Whether this difference has clinical relevance is not yet known.

Blockade of the angiotensin II receptor inhibits the negative regulatory feedback of angiotensin II on renin secretion, but the resulting increased plasma renin activity and circulating angiotensin II levels do not overcome the effect of olmesartan on blood pressure.

12.2 Pharmacodynamics

Amlodipine. Following administration of therapeutic doses to patients with hypertension, amlodipine produces vasodilation resulting in a reduction of supine and standing blood pressures. These decreases in blood pressure are not accompanied by a significant change in heart rate or plasma catecholamine levels with chronic dosing.

With chronic once daily oral administration, antihypertensive effectiveness is maintained for at least 24 hours. Plasma concentrations correlate with effect in both young and elderly patients. The magnitude of reduction in blood pressure with amlodipine is also correlated with the height of pretreatment elevation; thus, individuals with moderate hypertension (diastolic pressure 105-114 mmHg) had about a 50% greater response than patients with mild hypertension (diastolic pressure 90-104 mmHg). Normotensive subjects experienced no clinically significant change in blood pressures (+1/-2 mmHg).

In hypertensive patients with normal renal function, therapeutic doses of amlodipine resulted in a decrease in renal vascular resistance and an increase in glomerular filtration rate and effective renal plasma flow without change in filtration fraction or proteinuria.

As with other calcium channel blockers, hemodynamic measurements of cardiac function at rest and during exercise (or pacing) in patients with normal ventricular function treated with amlodipine have generally demonstrated a small increase in cardiac index without significant influence on dP/dt or on left ventricular end diastolic pressure or volume. In hemodynamic studies, amlodipine has not been associated with a negative inotropic effect when administered in the therapeutic dose range to intact animals and man, even when co-administered with beta-blockers to man. Similar findings, however, have been observed in normal or well-compensated patients with heart failure with agents possessing significant negative inotropic effects.

Amlodipine does not change sinoatrial nodal function or atrioventricular conduction in intact animals or man. In clinical studies in which amlodipine was administered in combination with beta-blockers to patients with either hypertension or angina, no adverse effects on electrocardiographic parameters were observed.

Olmesartan medoxomil. Olmesartan medoxomil doses of 2.5 mg to 40 mg inhibit the pressor effects of angiotensin I infusion. The duration of the inhibitory effect was related to dose, with doses of olmesartan medoxomil >40 mg giving >90% inhibition at 24 hours.

Plasma concentrations of angiotensin I and angiotensin II and plasma renin activity (PRA) increase after single and repeated administration of olmesartan medoxomil to healthy subjects and hypertensive patients. Repeated administration of up to 80 mg olmesartan medoxomil had minimal influence on aldosterone levels and no effect on serum potassium.

12.3 Pharmacokinetics

The pharmacokinetics of amlodipine and olmesartan medoxomil from AZOR™ are equivalent to the pharmacokinetics of amlodipine and olmesartan medoxomil when administered separately. The bioavailability of both components is well below 100%, but neither component is affected by food. The effective half-lives of amlodipine (45±11 hours) and olmesartan (7±1 hours) result in a 2- to 3-fold accumulation for amlodipine and negligible accumulation for olmesartan with once-daily dosing.

Amlodipine. After oral administration of therapeutic doses of amlodipine, absorption produces peak plasma concentrations between 6 and 12 hours. Absolute bioavailability is estimated as between 64% and 90%.

Olmesartan medoxomil. Olmesartan medoxomil is rapidly and completely bioactivated by ester hydrolysis to olmesartan during absorption from the gastrointestinal tract. The absolute bioavailability of olmesartan medoxomil is approximately 26%. After oral administration, the peak plasma concentration (C_{max}) of olmesartan is reached after 1 to 2 hours. Food does not affect the bioavailability of olmesartan medoxomil.

Distribution

Amlodipine. *Ex vivo* studies have shown that approximately 93% of the circulating drug is bound to plasma proteins in hypertensive patients. Steady-state plasma levels of amlodipine are reached after 7 to 8 days of consecutive daily dosing.

Olmesartan medoxomil. The volume of distribution of olmesartan is approximately 17 L. Olmesartan is highly bound to plasma proteins (99%) and does not penetrate red blood cells. The protein binding is constant at plasma olmesartan concentrations well above the range achieved with recommended doses.

In rats, olmesartan crossed the blood-brain barrier poorly, if at all. Olmesartan passed across the placental barrier in rats and was distributed to the fetus. Olmesartan was distributed to milk at low levels in rats.

Metabolism and Excretion

Amlodipine. Amlodipine is extensively (about 90%) converted to inactive metabolites via hepatic metabolism. Elimination from the plasma is biphasic with a terminal elimination half-life of about 30 to 50 hours. Ten percent of the parent compound and 60% of the metabolites are excreted in the urine.

Olmesartan medoxomil. Following the rapid and complete conversion of olmesartan medoxomil to olmesartan during absorption, there is virtually no further metabolism of olmesartan. Total plasma clearance of olmesartan is 1.3 L/h, with a renal clearance of 0.6 L/h. Approximately 35% to 50% of the absorbed dose is recovered in urine while the remainder is eliminated in feces via the bile.

Olmesartan appears to be eliminated in a biphasic manner with a terminal elimination half-life of approximately 13 hours. Olmesartan shows linear pharmacokinetics following single oral doses of up to 320 mg and multiple oral doses of up to 80 mg. Steady-state levels of olmesartan are achieved within 3 to 5 days and no accumulation in plasma occurs with once-daily dosing.

Geriatric

The pharmacokinetic properties of AZOR™ in the elderly are similar to those of the individual components.

Amlodipine. Elderly patients have decreased clearance of amlodipine with a resulting increase in AUC of approximately 40% to 60%, and a lower initial dose may be required.

Olmesartan medoxomil. The pharmacokinetics of olmesartan medoxomil were studied in the elderly (≥65 years). Overall, maximum plasma concentrations of olmesartan were similar in young adults and the elderly. Modest accumulation of olmesartan was observed in the elderly with repeated dosing; $AUC_{ss,\tau}$ was 33% higher in elderly patients, corresponding to an approximate 30% reduction in CL_R.

Pediatric

Amlodipine. Sixty-two hypertensive patients aged 6 to 17 years received doses of amlodipine between 1.25 mg and 20 mg. Weight-adjusted clearance and volume of distribution were similar to values in adults.

Olmesartan medoxomil. The pharmacokinetics of olmesartan medoxomil have not been investigated in patients <18 years of age.

Gender

Population pharmacokinetic analysis indicated that female patients had approximately 15% smaller clearances of olmesartan than male patients. Gender had no effect on the clearance of amlodipine.

Olmesartan medoxomil. Minor differences were observed in the pharmacokinetics of olmesartan medoxomil in women compared to men. AUC and C_{max} were 10% to 15% higher in women than in men.

Renal Insufficiency

Amlodipine. The pharmacokinetics of amlodipine are not significantly influenced by renal impairment. Patients with renal failure may therefore receive the usual initial dose.

Olmesartan medoxomil. In patients with renal insufficiency, serum concentrations of olmesartan were elevated compared to subjects with normal renal function. After repeated dosing, the AUC was approximately tripled in patients with severe renal impairment (creatinine clearance <20 mL/min). The pharmacokinetics of olmesartan medoxomil in patients undergoing hemodialysis has not been studied.

Hepatic Insufficiency

Amlodipine. Patients with hepatic insufficiency have decreased clearance of amlodipine with a resulting increase in AUC of approximately 40% to 60%.

Olmesartan medoxomil. Increases in $AUC_{0-\infty}$ and C_{max} were observed in patients with moderate hepatic impairment

**Reduction in Seated Systolic/Diastolic Blood Pressure (mmHg):
Combination Therapy vs. Monotherapy Components (Double-Blind Treatment Period)**

			Olmesartan Medoxomil			
		(mmHg)	Placebo	10 mg	20 mg	40 mg
Amlodipine	Placebo	Mean Change	-5/-3	-12/-8	-14/-9	-16/-10
		Placebo-Adjusted Mean Change	-	-8/-5	-10/-6	-13/-7
	5 mg	Mean Change	-15/-9	-24/-14	-24/-14	-25/-16
		Placebo-Adjusted Mean Change	-12/-7	-20/-11	-20/-11	-22/-13
	10 mg	Mean Change	-20/-13	-25/-16	-29/-17	-30/-19
		Placebo-Adjusted Mean Change	-16/-10	-22/-13	-25/-14	-26/-16

Tablet Strength (amlodipine equivalent/olmesartan medoxomil) mg	Package Configuration	NDC#	Product Code	Tablet Color
5/20 mg	Bottle of 30 Bottle of 90 10 blisters of 10 Bottle of 1000	65597-110-30 65597-110-90 65597-110-10 65597-110-11	C73	White
10/20 mg	Bottle of 30 Bottle of 90 10 blisters of 10 Bottle of 1000	65597-111-30 65597-111-90 65597-111-10 65597-111-11	C74	Grayish Orange
5/40 mg	Bottle of 30 Bottle of 90 10 blisters of 10 Bottle of 1000	65597-112-30 65597-112-90 65597-112-10 65597-112-11	C75	Cream
10/40 mg	Bottle of 30 Bottle of 90 10 blisters of 10 Bottle of 1000	65597-113-30 65597-113-90 65597-113-10 65597-113-11	C77	Brownish Red

compared to those in matched controls, with an increase in AUC of about 60%.

Heart Failure

Amlodipine. Patients with heart failure have decreased clearance of amlodipine with a resulting increase in AUC of approximately 40% to 60%.

13 NONCLINICAL TOXICOLOGY

13.1 Carcinogenesis, Mutagenesis, Impairment of Fertility

Amlodipine. Rats and mice treated with amlodipine maleate in the diet for up to two years, at concentrations calculated to provide daily dosage levels of amlodipine 0.5, 1.25, and 2.5 mg/kg/day showed no evidence of a carcinogenic effect of the drug. For the mouse, the highest dose was, on a mg/m^2 basis, similar to the maximum recommended human dose (MRHD) of amlodipine 10 mg/day. For the rat, the highest dose was, on a mg/m^2 basis, about two and a half times the MRHD. (Calculations based on á 60 kg patient.) Mutagenicity studies conducted with amlodipine maleate revealed no drug related effects at either the gene or chromosome level.

There was no effect on the fertility of rats treated orally with amlodipine maleate (males for 64 days and females for 14 days prior to mating) at doses of amlodipine up to 10 mg/kg/day (about 10 times the MRHD of 10 mg/day on a mg/m^2 basis).

Olmesartan medoxomil. Olmesartan was not carcinogenic when administered by dietary administration to rats for up to 2 years. The highest dose tested (2000 mg/kg/day) was, on a mg/m^2 basis, about 480 times the maximum recommended human dose (MRHD) of 40 mg/day. Two carcinogenicity studies conducted in mice, a 6-month gavage study in the p53 knockout mouse and a 6-month dietary administration study in the Hras2 transgenic mouse, at doses of up to 1000 mg/kg/day (about 120 times the MRHD), revealed no evidence of a carcinogenic effect of olmesartan. Both olmesartan medoxomil and olmesartan tested negative in the in vitro Syrian hamster embryo cell transformation assay and showed no evidence of genetic toxicity in the Ames (bacterial mutagenicity) test. However, both were shown to induce chromosomal aberrations in cultured cells in vitro (Chinese hamster lung) and tested positive for thymidine kinase mutations in the in vitro mouse lymphoma assay. Olmesartan medoxomil tested negative in vivo for mutations in the MutaMouse intestine and kidney and for clastogenicity in mouse bone marrow (micronucleus test) at oral doses of up to 2000 mg/kg (olmesartan not tested).

Fertility of rats was unaffected by administration of olmesartan at dose levels as high as 1000 mg/kg/day (240 times the MRHD) in a study in which dosing was begun 2 (female) or 9 (male) weeks prior to mating.

14 CLINICAL STUDIES

14.1 AZOR™

An 8-week multicenter, randomized, double-blind, placebo controlled, parallel group factorial study in patients with mild to severe hypertension was conducted to determine if treatment with AZOR™ was associated with clinically significant reduction in blood pressure compared to the respective monotherapies. The study randomized 1940 patients equally to one of the following 12 treatment arms: placebo, monotherapy treatment with amlodipine 5 mg or 10 mg, monotherapy treatment with olmesartan medoxomil 10 mg, 20 mg, or 40 mg, or combination therapy with amlodipine/olmesartan medoxomil at doses of 5/10 mg, 5/20 mg, 5/40 mg, 10/10 mg, 10/20 mg, and 10/40 mg.

Treatment with AZOR™ resulted in significantly greater reductions in diastolic and systolic blood pressure compared to the respective monotherapy components.

The following table presents the results for mean reduction in seated systolic and diastolic blood pressure following 8 weeks of treatment with AZOR™. Placebo-adjusted reductions from baseline in blood pressure were progressively greater with increases in dose of both amlodipine and olmesartan medoxomil components of AZOR™.

[See first table above]

The antihypertensive effect of AZOR™ was similar in patients with and without prior antihypertensive medication use, in patients with and without diabetes, in patients ≥65 years of age and <65 years of age, and in women and men. AZOR™ was effective in treating black patients (usually a low-renin population), and the magnitude of blood pressure reduction in black patients approached that observed for non-black patients. This effect in black patients has been seen with ACE inhibitors, angiotensin receptor blockers, and beta-blockers.

The blood pressure lowering effect was maintained throughout the 24-hour period with AZOR™ once daily, with trough-to-peak ratios for systolic and diastolic response between 71% and 82%.

Upon completing the 8-week, double-blind, placebo-controlled study, 1684 patients entered a 44-week open-label extension and received combination therapy with amlodipine 5 mg plus olmesartan medoxomil 40 mg. During the open-label extension, patients whose blood pressure was not adequately controlled (i.e., did not achieve a blood pressure goal of <140/90 mmHg, or <130/80 mmHg for those patients with diabetes) on amlodipine/olmesartan medoxomil 5/40 mg were titrated to amlodipine/olmesartan medoxomil 10/40 mg. Patients whose blood pressure was still not adequately controlled were offered additional hydrochlorothiazide 12.5 mg and subsequently 25 mg as required to achieve adequate blood pressure goal.

14.2 Amlodipine

The antihypertensive efficacy of amlodipine has been demonstrated in a total of 15 double-blind, placebo-controlled, randomized studies involving 800 patients on amlodipine and 538 on placebo. Once daily administration produced statistically significant placebo-corrected reductions in supine and standing blood pressures at 24 hours postdose, averaging about 12/6 mmHg in the standing position and 13/7 mmHg in the supine position in patients with mild to moderate hypertension. Maintenance of the blood pressure effect over the 24-hour dosing interval was observed, with little difference in peak and trough effect.

14.3 Olmesartan medoxomil

The antihypertensive effects of olmesartan medoxomil have been demonstrated in seven placebo-controlled studies at doses ranging from 2.5 mg to 80 mg for 6 to 12 weeks, each showing statistically significant reductions in peak and trough blood pressure. A total of 2693 patients (2145 olmesartan medoxomil; 548 placebo) with essential hypertension were studied. The blood pressure lowering effect was maintained throughout the 24-hour period with olmesartan medoxomil once daily, with trough-to-peak ratios for systolic and diastolic response between 60% and 80%.

16 HOW SUPPLIED/STORAGE AND HANDLING

AZOR™ tablets contain amlodipine besylate at a dose equivalent to 5 or 10 mg amlodipine and olmesartan medoxomil in the strengths described below.

AZOR™ tablets are differentiated by tablet color/size and are debossed with an individual product tablet code on one side. AZOR™ tablets are supplied for oral administration in the following strength and package configurations:

[See second table above]

Store at 25°C (77°F); excursions permitted to 15-30°C (59-86°F) [see USP Controlled Room Temperature].

17 PATIENT COUNSELING INFORMATION

Physicians should instruct female patients of childbearing age about the consequences of second and third trimester exposure to drugs that act on the renin-angiotensin system and they should be told that these consequences do not appear to have resulted from intrauterine drug exposure that has been limited to the first trimester. These patients should be informed to report pregnancies to their physicians as soon as possible. *[See Warnings and Precautions (5.1)].*

Manufactured for Daiichi Sankyo, Inc., Parsippany, New Jersey 07054

Manufactured by Daiichi Sankyo Pharma GmbH, Germany
Copyright © Daiichi Sankyo, Inc. 2007. All rights reserved.

P1801701

Forest Pharmaceuticals, Inc. (Subsidiary of Forest Laboratories, Inc.)

13600 SHORELINE DRIVE
ST. LOUIS, MO 63045

Direct Inquiries to:
Professional Affairs Department
13600 Shoreline Drive
St. Louis, MO 63045
(800) 678-1605

BYSTOLIC™   ℞
(nebivolol) Tablets
2.5 mg, 5 mg and 10 mg
Rx Only

DESCRIPTION

The chemical name for the active ingredient in BYSTOLIC (nebivolol) tablets is (1RS,1'RS)-1,1'-[(2RS,2'SR)-bis (6-fluoro-3,4-dihydro-2H-1-benzopyran-2-yl)]-2,2'-iminodiethanol hydrochloride. Nebivolol is a racemate composed of d-nebivolol and l-nebivolol with the stereochemical designations of [SRRR]-nebivolol and [RSSS]-nebivolol, respectively. Nebivolol's molecular formula is $(C_{22}H_{25}F_2NO_4 \bullet HCl)$ with the following structural formula:

SRRR – or d-nebivolol hydrochloride

RSSS – or l-nebivolol hydrochloride

MW: 441.90 g/mol

Nebivolol hydrochloride is a white to almost white powder that is soluble in methanol, dimethylsulfoxide, and N,N-dimethylformamide, sparingly soluble in ethanol, propylene glycol, and polyethylene glycol, and very slightly soluble in hexane, dichloromethane, and methylbenzene.

BYSTOLIC as tablets for oral administration contains nebivolol hydrochloride equivalent to 2.5, 5, and 10 mg of nebivolol base. In addition, BYSTOLIC contains the following inactive ingredients: colloidal silicon dioxide, croscarmellose sodium, D&C Red #27 Lake, FD&C Blue #2 Lake, FD&C Yellow #6 Lake, hypromellose, lactose monohydrate, magnesium stearate, microcrystalline cellulose, pregelatinized starch, polysorbate 80, and sodium lauryl sulfate.

Continued on next page

Bystolic—Cont.

CLINICAL PHARMACOLOGY

General

Nebivolol is a β-adrenergic receptor blocking agent. In extensive metabolizers (most of the population) and at doses less than or equal to 10 mg, nebivolol is preferentially β_1 selective. In poor metabolizers and at higher doses, nebivolol inhibits both β_1 and β_2-adrenergic receptors. Nebivolol lacks intrinsic sympathomimetic and membrane stabilizing activity at therapeutically relevant concentrations. At clinically relevant doses, BYSTOLIC does not demonstrate α_1-adrenergic receptor blockade activity. Various metabolites, including glucuronides, contribute to β-blocking activity.

Pharmacodynamics

The mechanism of action of the antihypertensive response of BYSTOLIC has not been definitively established. Possible factors that may be involved include: (1) decreased heart rate, (2) decreased myocardial contractility, (3) diminution of tonic sympathetic outflow to the periphery from cerebral vasomotor centers, (4) suppression of renin activity and (5) vasodilation and decreased peripheral vascular resistance.

Pharmacokinetics

Nebivolol is metabolized by a number of routes, including glucuronidation and hydroxylation by CYP2D6. The active isomer (d-nebivolol) has an effective half-life of about 12 hours in CYP2D6 extensive metabolizers (most people), and 19 hours in poor metabolizers and exposure to d-nebivolol is substantially increased in poor metabolizers. This has less importance than usual, however, because the metabolites, including the hydroxyl metabolite and glucuronides (the predominant circulating metabolites), contribute to β-blocking activity.

Plasma levels of d–nebivolol increase in proportion to dose in EMs and PMs for doses up to 20 mg. Exposure to l-nebivolol is higher than to d-nebivolol but l-nebivolol contributes little to the drug's activity as d-nebivolol's beta receptor affinity is >1000-fold higher than l-nebivolol. For the same dose, PMs attain a 5-fold higher Cmax and 10-fold higher AUC of d-nebivolol than do EMs. d-Nebivolol accumulates about 1.5-fold with repeated once-daily dosing in EMs.

Absorption and Distribution

Absorption of BYSTOLIC is similar to an oral solution. The absolute bioavailability has not been determined.

Mean peak plasma nebivolol concentrations occur approximately 1.5 to 4 hours post-dosing in EMs and PMs.

Food does not alter the pharmacokinetics of nebivolol. Under fed conditions, nebivolol glucuronides are slightly reduced. BYSTOLIC may be administered without regard to meals.

The *in vitro* human plasma protein binding of nebivolol is approximately 98%, mostly to albumin, and is independent of nebivolol concentrations.

Metabolism and Excretion

Nebivolol is predominantly metabolized via direct glucuronidation of parent and to a lesser extent via N-dealkylation and oxidation via cytochrome P450 2D6. Its stereospecific metabolites contribute to the pharmacologic activity. (see **Drug Interactions**).

After a single oral administration of ^{14}C-nebivolol, 38% of the dose was recovered in urine and 44% in feces for EMs and 67% in urine and 13% in feces for PMs. Essentially all nebivolol was excreted as multiple oxidative metabolites or their corresponding glucuronide conjugates.

Drug Interactions

Drugs that inhibit CYP2D6 can be expected to increase plasma levels of nebivolol. When BYSTOLIC is co-administered with an inhibitor or an inducer of this enzyme, patients should be closely monitored and the nebivolol dose adjusted according to blood pressure response. *In vitro* studies have demonstrated that at therapeutically relevant concentrations, d- and l-nebivolol do not inhibit any cytochrome P450 pathways.

Digoxin: Concomitant administration of BYSTOLIC (10 mg once daily) and digoxin (0.25 mg once daily) for 10 days in 14 healthy adult individuals resulted in no significant changes in the pharmacokinetics of digoxin or nebivolol (see **PRECAUTIONS, Drug Interactions**).

Warfarin: Administration of BYSTOLIC (10 mg once daily for 10 days) led to no significant changes in the pharmacokinetics of nebivolol or R- or S-warfarin following a single 10 mg dose of warfarin. Similarly, nebivolol has no significant effects on the anticoagulant activity of warfarin, as assessed by Prothrombin time and INR profiles from 0 to 144 hours after a single 10 mg warfarin dose in 12 healthy adult volunteers.

Diuretics: No pharmacokinetic interactions were observed in healthy adults between nebivolol (10 mg daily for 10 days) and furosemide (40 mg single dose), hydrochlorothiazide (25 mg once daily for 10 days), or spironolactone (25 mg once daily for 10 days).

Ramipril: Concomitant administration of BYSTOLIC (10 mg once daily) and ramipril (5 mg once daily) for 10 days in 15 healthy adult volunteers produced no pharmacokinetic interactions.

Losartan: Concomitant administration of BYSTOLIC (10 mg single dose) and losartan (50 mg single dose) in 20 healthy adult volunteers did not result in pharmacokinetic interactions.

Fluoxetine: Fluoxetine, a CYP2D6 inhibitor, administered at 20 mg per day for 21 days prior to a single 10 mg dose of nebivolol to 10 healthy adults, led to an 8-fold increase in the AUC and 3-fold increase in Cmax for d-nebivolol (see **PRECAUTIONS, Drug Interactions**).

Histamine-2 Receptor Antagonists: The pharmacokinetics of nebivolol (5 mg single dose) were not affected by the co-administration of ranitidine (150 mg twice daily). Cimetidine (400 mg twice daily) causes a 23% increase in the plasma levels of d-nebivolol.

Charcoal: The pharmacokinetics of nebivolol (10 mg single dose) were not affected by repeated co-administration (4, 8, 12, 16, 22, 28, 36, and 48 hours after nebivolol administration) of activated charcoal (Actidose-Aqua®).

Sildenafil: The co-administration of nebivolol and sildenafil decreased AUC and Cmax of sildenafil by 21 and 23% respectively. The effect on the Cmax and AUC for d -nebivolol was also small (<20%). The effect on vital signs (e.g., pulse and blood pressure) was approximately the sum of the effects of sildenafil and nebivolol.

Other Concomitant Medications: Utilizing population pharmacokinetic analyses, derived from hypertensive patients, the following drugs were observed not to have an effect on the pharmacokinetics of nebivolol: acetaminophen, acetylsalicylic acid, atorvastatin, esomeprazole, ibuprofen, levothyroxine sodium, metformin, sildenafil, simvastatin, or tocopherol.

Protein Binding: No meaningful changes in the extent of *in vitro* binding of nebivolol to human plasma proteins were noted in the presence of high concentrations of diazepam, digoxin, diphenylhydantoin, enalapril, hydrochlorothiazide, imipramine, indomethacin, propranolol, sulfamethazine, tolbutamide, or warfarin. Additionally, nebivolol did not significantly alter the protein binding of the following drugs: diazepam, digoxin, diphenylhydantoin, hydrochlorothiazide, imipramine, or warfarin at their therapeutic concentrations.

Special Populations

Renal Disease: The apparent clearance of nebivolol was unchanged following a single 5 mg dose of BYSTOLIC in patients with mild renal impairment (ClCr 50 to 80 mL/min, n=7), and it was reduced negligibly in patients with moderate (ClCr 30 to 50 mL/min, n=9), but by 53% in patients with severe renal impairment (ClCr <30 mL/min, n=5). The dose of BYSTOLIC should be adjusted in patients with severe renal impairment. BYSTOLIC should be used with caution in patients receiving dialysis, since no formal studies have been conducted in this population (see **DOSAGE AND ADMINISTRATION**).

Hepatic Disease: d-Nebivolol peak plasma concentration increased 3-fold, exposure (AUC) increased 10-fold, and the apparent clearance decreased by 86% in patients with moderate hepatic impairment (Child-Pugh Class B). The starting dose should be reduced in patients with moderate hepatic impairment. No formal studies have been performed in patients with severe hepatic impairment and nebivolol should be contraindicated for these patients (see **DOSAGE AND ADMINISTRATION**).

Clinical Studies

The antihypertensive effectiveness of BYSTOLIC as monotherapy has been demonstrated in three randomized, double-blind, multi-center, placebo-controlled trials at doses ranging from 1.25 to 40 mg for 12 weeks (Studies 1, 2, and 3). A fourth placebo-controlled trial demonstrated additional antihypertensive effects of BYSTOLIC at doses ranging from 5 to 20 mg when administered concomitantly with up to two other antihypertensive agents (ACE inhibitors, angiotensin II receptor antagonists, and thiazide diuretics) in patients with inadequate blood pressure control.

The three monotherapy trials included a total of 2016 patients (1811 BYSTOLIC, 205 placebo) with mild to moderate hypertension who had baseline diastolic blood pressures (DBP) of 95 to 109 mmHg. Patients received either BYSTOLIC or placebo once daily for twelve weeks. Two of these monotherapy trials (Studies 1 and 2) studied 1716 patients in the general hypertensive population with a mean age of 54 years, 55% males, 26% non-Caucasians, 7% diabetics and 6% genotyped as PMs. The third monotherapy trial (Study 3) studied 300 Black patients with a mean age of 51 years, 45% males, 14% diabetics, and 3% as PMs.

Placebo-subtracted blood pressure reductions by dose for each study are presented in **Table 1**. Most studies showed increasing response to doses above 5 mg.

[See table 1 below]

Table 1. Placebo-Subtracted Least-Square Mean Reductions in Trough Sitting Systolic/Diastolic Blood Pressure (SiSBP/SiDBP mmHg) by Dose in Studies with Once-Daily BYSTOLIC

	Nebivolol dose (mg)					
	1.25	2.5	5.0	10	20	30-40
Study 1	-6.6*/-5.1*	-8.5*/-5.6*	-8.1*/-5.5*	-9.2*/-6.3*	-8.7*/-6.9*	-11.7*/-8.3*
Study 2			-3.8/-3.2*	-3.1/-3.9*	-6.3*/-4.5*	
Study 3¶		-1.5/-2.9	-2.6/-4.9*	-6.0*/-6.1*	-7.2*/-6.1*	-6.8*/-5.5*
Study 4^			-5.7*/-3.3*	-3.7*/-3.5*	-6.2*/-4.6*	

* p<0.05 based on pair-wise comparison vs placebo
¶ Study enrolled only African Americans.
^ Study on top of one or two other antihypertensive medications.

Study 4 enrolled 669 patients with a mean age of 54 years, 55% males, 54% Caucasians, 29% Blacks, 15% Hispanics, 1% Asians, 14% diabetics, and 5% PMs. BYSTOLIC, 5 mg to 20 mg, administered once daily concomitantly with stable doses of up to two other antihypertensive agents (ACE inhibitors, angiotensin II receptor antagonists, and thiazide diuretics) resulted in significant additional antihypertensive effects over placebo compared to baseline blood pressure.

Effectiveness was similar in subgroups analyzed by age and sex. Effectiveness was established in Blacks, but as monotherapy the magnitude of effect was somewhat less than in Caucasians.

The blood pressure lowering effect of BYSTOLIC was seen within two weeks of treatment and was maintained over the 24-hour dosing interval.

INDICATIONS AND USAGE

BYSTOLIC is indicated for the treatment of hypertension. BYSTOLIC may be used alone or in combination with other antihypertensive agents.

CONTRAINDICATIONS

BYSTOLIC is contraindicated in patients with severe bradycardia, heart block greater than first degree, cardiogenic shock, decompensated cardiac failure, sick sinus syndrome (unless a permanent pacemaker is in place), or severe hepatic impairment (Child-Pugh >B), and in patients who are hypersensitive to any component of this product.

WARNINGS

Abrupt Cessation of Therapy

Patients with coronary artery disease treated with BYSTOLIC should be advised against abrupt discontinuation of therapy. Severe exacerbation of angina and the occurrence of myocardial infarction and ventricular arrhythmias have been reported in patients with coronary artery disease following the abrupt discontinuation of therapy with β-blockers. Myocardial infarction and ventricular arrhythmias may occur with or without preceding exacerbation of the angina pectoris. Even patients without overt coronary artery disease should be cautioned against interruption or abrupt discontinuation of therapy. As with other β-blockers, when discontinuation of BYSTOLIC is planned, patients should be carefully observed and advised to minimize physical activity. BYSTOLIC should be tapered over 1 to 2 weeks when possible. If the angina worsens or acute coronary insufficiency develops, it is recommended that BYSTOLIC be promptly reinstituted, at least temporarily.

Cardiac Failure

Sympathetic stimulation is a vital component supporting circulatory function in the setting of congestive heart failure, and β-blockade may result in further depression of myocardial contractility and precipitate more severe failure. In patients who have compensated congestive heart failure, BYSTOLIC should be administered cautiously. If heart failure worsens, discontinuation of BYSTOLIC should be considered.

Angina and Acute Myocardial Infarction

BYSTOLIC was not studied in patients with angina pectoris or who had a recent MI.

Bronchospastic Diseases

In general, patients with bronchospastic diseases should not receive β-blockers.

Anesthesia and Major Surgery

If BYSTOLIC is to be continued perioperatively, patients should be closely monitored when anesthetic agents which depress myocardial function, such as ether, cyclopropane, and trichloroethylene, are used. If β-blocking therapy is withdrawn prior to major surgery, the impaired ability of the heart to respond to reflex adrenergic stimuli may augment the risks of general anesthesia and surgical procedures.

The β-blocking effects of BYSTOLIC can be reversed by β-agonists, e.g., dobutamine or isoproterenol. However, such patients may be subject to protracted severe hypotension. Additionally, difficulty in restarting and maintaining the heartbeat has been reported with β-blockers.

Diabetes and Hypoglycemia

β-blockers may mask some of the manifestations of hypoglycemia, particularly tachycardia. Nonselective β-blockers may potentiate insulin-induced hypoglycemia and delay recovery of serum glucose levels. It is not known whether nebivolol has these effects. Patients subject to spontaneous hypoglycemia, or diabetic patients receiving insulin or oral hypoglycemic agents, should be advised about these possibilities and nebivolol should be used with caution.

Thyrotoxicosis

β-blockers may mask clinical signs of hyperthyroidism, such as tachycardia. Abrupt withdrawal of β-blockers may be followed by an exacerbation of the symptoms of hyperthyroidism or may precipitate a thyroid storm.

Peripheral Vascular Disease

β-blockers can precipitate or aggravate symptoms of arterial insufficiency in patients with peripheral vascular disease. Caution should be exercised in these patients.

Non-dihydropyridine Calcium Channel Blockers

Because of significant negative inotropic and chronotropic effects in patients treated with β-blockers and calcium channel blockers of the verapamil and diltiazem type, caution should be used in patients treated concomitantly with these agents and ECG and blood pressure should be monitored.

PRECAUTIONS

Use with CYP2D6 inhibitors

Nebivolol exposure increases with inhibition of CYP2D6 (see **Drug Interactions**). The dose of BYSTOLIC may need to be reduced.

Impaired Renal Function

BYSTOLIC should be used with caution in patients with severe renal impairment because of decreased renal clearance. BYSTOLIC has not been studied in patients receiving dialysis.

Impaired Hepatic Function

BYSTOLIC should be used with caution in patients with moderate hepatic impairment because of decreased metabolism. Since BYSTOLIC has not been studied in patients with severe hepatic impairment, BYSTOLIC is contraindicated in this population (see **CLINICAL PHARMACOLOGY, Special Populations** and **DOSAGE AND ADMINISTRATION**).

Risk of Anaphylactic Reactions

While taking β-blockers, patients with a history of severe anaphylactic reactions to a variety of allergens may be more reactive to repeated challenge either accidental, diagnostic, or therapeutic. Such patients may be unresponsive to the usual doses of epinephrine used to treat allergic reactions. In patients with known or suspected pheochromocytoma, an alpha-blocker should be initiated prior to the use of any β-blocker.

Information for Patients

Patients should be advised to take BYSTOLIC regularly and continuously, as directed. BYSTOLIC can be taken with or without food. If a dose is missed, the patient should take the next scheduled dose only (without doubling it). Patients should not interrupt or discontinue BYSTOLIC without consulting the physician.

Patients should know how they react to this medicine before they operate automobiles, use machinery, or engage in other tasks requiring alertness.

Patients should be advised to consult a physician if any difficulty in breathing occurs, or if they develop signs or symptoms of worsening congestive heart failure such as weight gain or increasing shortness of breath, or excessive bradycardia.

Patients subject to spontaneous hypoglycemia, or diabetic patients receiving insulin or oral hypoglycemic agents, should be cautioned that β-blockers may mask some of the manifestations of hypoglycemia, particularly tachycardia. Nebivolol should be used with caution in these patients.

Drug Interactions

BYSTOLIC should be used with care when myocardial depressants or inhibitors of AV conduction, such as certain calcium antagonists (particularly of the phenylalkylamine [verapamil] and benzothiazepine [diltiazem] classes), or antiarrhythmic agents, such as disopyramide, are used concurrently. Both digitalis glycosides and β-blockers slow atrioventricular conduction and decrease heart rate. Concomitant use can increase the risk of bradycardia.

BYSTOLIC should not be combined with other β-blockers. Patients receiving catecholamine-depleting drugs, such as reserpine or guanethidine, should be closely monitored, because the added β-blocking action of BYSTOLIC may produce excessive reduction of sympathetic activity. In patients who are receiving BYSTOLIC and clonidine, BYSTOLIC should be discontinued for several days before the gradual tapering of clonidine.

CYP2D6 Inhibitors: Use caution when BYSTOLIC is co-administered with CYP2D6 inhibitors (quinidine, propafenone, fluoxetine, paroxetine, etc.) (see **CLINICAL PHARMACOLOGY, Drug Interactions**).

Carcinogenesis, Mutagenesis, Impairment of Fertility

In a two-year study of nebivolol in mice, a statistically significant increase in the incidence of testicular Leydig cell hyperplasia and adenomas was observed at 40 mg/kg/day (5 times the maximally recommended human dose of 40 mg on a mg/m^2 basis). Similar findings were not reported in mice administered doses equal to approximately 0.3 or 1.2 times the maximum recommended human dose. No evidence of a tumorigenic effect was observed in a 24-month study in Wistar rats receiving doses of nebivolol of 2.5, 10 and 40 mg/kg/day (equivalent to 0.6, 2.4, and 10 times the maximally recommended human dose). Co-administration of dihydrotestosterone reduced blood LH levels and prevented the Leydig cell hyperplasia, consistent with an indirect LH-mediated effect of nebivolol in mice and not thought to be clinically relevant in man.

A randomized, double-blind, placebo- and active-controlled, parallel-group study in healthy male volunteers was conducted to determine the effects of nebivolol on adrenal function, luteinizing hormone, and testosterone levels. This study demonstrated that 6 weeks of daily dosing with 10 mg of nebivolol had no significant effect on ACTH-stimulated mean serum cortisol $AUC_{0-120\ min}$, serum LH, or serum total testosterone.

Effects on spermatogenesis were seen in male rats and mice at ≥40 mg/kg/day (10 and 5 times the MRHD, respectively). For rats, the effects on spermatogenesis were not reversed and may have worsened during a four week recovery period. The effects of nebivolol on sperm in mice, however, were partially reversible.

Mutagenesis: Nebivolol was not genotoxic when tested in a battery of assays (Ames, *in vitro* mouse lymphoma TK$^{+/-}$, *in vitro* human peripheral lymphocyte chromosome aberration, *in vivo* Drosophila melanogaster sex-linked recessive lethal, and *in vivo* mouse bone marrow micronucleus tests).

Pregnancy: Teratogenic Effects. Pregnancy Category C: Decreased pup body weights occurred at 1.25 and 2.5 mg/kg in rats, when exposed during the perinatal period (late gestation, parturition and lactation). At 5 mg/kg and higher doses (1.2 times the MRHD), prolonged gestation, dystocia and reduced maternal care were produced with corresponding increases in late fetal deaths and stillbirths and decreased birth weight, live litter size and pup survival. Insufficient numbers of pups survived at 5 mg/kg to evaluate the offspring for reproductive performance.

In studies in which pregnant rats were given nebivolol during organogenesis, reduced fetal body weights were observed at maternally toxic doses of 20 and 40 mg/kg/day (5 and 10 times the MRHD), and small reversible delays in sternal and thoracic ossification associated with the reduced fetal body weights and a small increase in resorption occurred at 40 mg/kg/day (10 times the MRHD). No adverse effects on embryo-fetal viability, sex, weight or morphology were observed in studies in which nebivolol was given to pregnant rabbits at doses as high as 20 mg/kg/day (10 times the MRHD).

Labor and Delivery

Nebivolol caused prolonged gestation and dystocia at doses ≥5 mg/kg in rats (1.2 times the MRHD). These effects were associated with increased fetal deaths and stillborn pups, and decreased birth weight, live litter size and pup survival rate, events that occurred only when nebivolol was given during the perinatal period (late gestation, parturition and lactation).

No studies of nebivolol were conducted in pregnant women. BYSTOLIC should be used during pregnancy only if the potential benefit justifies the potential risk to the fetus.

Nursing Mothers

Studies in rats have shown that nebivolol or its metabolites cross the placental barrier and are excreted in breast milk. It is not known whether this drug is excreted in human milk.

Because of the potential for β-blockers to produce serious adverse reactions in nursing infants, especially bradycardia, BYSTOLIC is not recommended during nursing.

Geriatric Use

Of the 2800 patients in the U.S. sponsored placebo-controlled clinical hypertension studies, 478 patients were 65 years of age or older. No overall differences in efficacy or in the incidence of adverse events were observed between older and younger patients.

Pediatric Use

Safety and effectiveness in pediatric patients have not been established. Pediatric studies in ages newborn to 18 years old have not been conducted because of incomplete characterization of developmental toxicity and possible adverse effects on long-term fertility (see **Carcinogenesis, Mutagenesis and Impairment of Infertility**).

ADVERSE REACTIONS

The data described below reflect worldwide clinical trial exposure to BYSTOLIC in 6545 patients, including 5038 patients treated for hypertension and the remaining 1507 subjects treated for other cardiovascular diseases. Doses ranged from 0.5 mg to 40 mg. Patients received BYSTOLIC for up to 24 months, with over 1900 patients treated for at least 6 months, and approximately 1300 patients for more than one year. In placebo-controlled clinical trials comparing BYSTOLIC with placebo, discontinuation of therapy due to adverse events was reported in 2.8% of patients treated with nebivolol and 2.2% of patients given placebo. The most common adverse events that led to discontinuation of BYSTOLIC were headache (0.4%), nausea (0.2%) and bradycardia (0.2%).

Adverse Reactions in Controlled Trials

Table 2 lists treatment-emergent signs and symptoms that were reported in three 12-week, placebo-controlled monotherapy trials involving 1597 hypertensive patients treated with either 5 mg, 10 mg or 20-40 mg of BYSTOLIC and 205 patients given placebo and for which the rate of occurrence was at least 1% of patients treated with nebivolol and greater than the rate for those treated with placebo in at least one dose group.

Table 2. Treatment-Emergent Adverse Events with an Incidence (over 6 weeks) ≥1% in BYSTOLIC-treated Patients and at a Higher Frequency than Placebo-treated Patients

	Placebo (n = 205) (%)	Nebivolol 5 mg (n = 459) (%)	Nebivolol 10 mg (n = 461) (%)	Nebivolol 20-40 mg (n = 677) (%)
Headache	6	9	6	7
Fatigue	1	2	2	5
Dizziness	2	2	3	4
Diarrhea	2	2	2	3
Nausea	0	1	3	2
Insomnia	0	1	1	1
Chest pain	0	0	1	1
Bradycardia	0	0	0	1
Dyspnea	0	0	1	1
Rash	0	0	1	1
Peripheral edema	0	1	1	1

Other Adverse Events Observed During Worldwide Clinical Trials

Listed below are other reported adverse events with an incidence of at least 1% in the more than 5300 patients treated with BYSTOLIC in controlled or open-label trials, whether or not attributed to treatment, except for those already appearing in **Table 2**, terms too general to be informative, minor symptoms, or events unlikely to be attributable to drug because they are common in the population. These adverse events were in most cases observed at a similar frequency in placebo-treated patients in the controlled studies.

Body as a whole: asthenia.

Gastrointestinal System Disorders: abdominal pain

Metabolic and Nutritional Disorders: hypercholesterolemia and hyperuricemia

Nervous System Disorders: paraesthesia

Laboratory

In controlled monotherapy trials, BYSTOLIC was associated with an increase in BUN, uric acid, triglycerides and a decrease in HDL cholesterol and platelet count.

Events Identified from Spontaneous Reports of BYSTOLIC Received Worldwide.

The following adverse events have been identified from spontaneous reports of BYSTOLIC received worldwide and have not been listed elsewhere. These adverse events have been chosen for inclusion due to a combination of seriousness, frequency of reporting or potential causal connection to BYSTOLIC. Events common in the population have generally been omitted. Because these events were reported voluntarily from a population of uncertain size, it is not possible to estimate their frequency or establish a causal relationship to BYSTOLIC exposure: abnormal hepatic function (including increased AST, ALT and bilirubin), acute pulmonary edema, acute renal failure, atrioventricular block (both second and third degree), bronchospasm, erectile dysfunction, hypersensitivity (including urticaria, allergic vasculitis and rare reports of angioedema), myocardial infarction, pruritus, psoriasis, Raynaud's phenomenon, peripheral ischemia/claudication, somnolence, syncope, thrombocytopenia, various rashes and skin disorders, vertigo, and vomiting.

OVERDOSAGE

In clinical trials and worldwide postmarketing experience there were reports of BYSTOLIC overdose. The most common signs and symptoms associated with BYSTOLIC overdosage are bradycardia and hypotension. Other important adverse events reported with BYSTOLIC overdose include cardiac failure, dizziness, hypoglycemia, fatigue and vomiting. Other adverse events associated with β-blocker overdose include bronchospasm and heart block.

The largest known ingestion of BYSTOLIC worldwide involved a patient who ingested up to 500 mg of BYSTOLIC along with several 100 mg tablets of acetylsalicylic acid in a suicide attempt. The patient experienced hyperhidrosis, pallor, depressed level of consciousness, hypokinesia, hypotension, sinus bradycardia, hypoglycemia, hypokalemia, respiratory failure and vomiting. The patient recovered.

Due to extensive drug binding to plasma proteins, hemodialysis is not expected to enhance nebivolol clearance.

If overdose occurs, BYSTOLIC should be stopped and general supportive and specific symptomatic treatment should be provided. Based on expected pharmacologic actions and recommendations for other β-blockers, the following general measures should be considered when clinically warranted:

Bradycardia: Administer IV atropine. If the response is inadequate, isoproterenol or another agent with positive chronotropic properties may be given cautiously. Under some circumstances, transthoracic or transvenous pacemaker placement may be necessary.

Hypotension: Administer IV fluids and vasopressors. Intravenous glucagon may be useful.

Heart Block (second or third degree): Patients should be carefully monitored and treated with isoproterenol infusion. Under some circumstances, transthoracic or transvenous pacemaker placement may be necessary.

Congestive Heart Failure: Initiate therapy with digitalis glycoside and diuretics. In certain cases, consideration should be given to the use of inotropic and vasodilating agents.

Continued on next page

BYSTOLIC

Tablet Strength	Package Configuration	NDC #	Tablet Color
2.5 mg	Bottle of 30	0456-1402-30	Light Blue
	Bottle of 100	0456-1402-01	
5 mg	Bottle of 30	0456-1405-30	Beige
	Bottle of 100	0456-1405-01	
	10 × 10 Unit Dose	0456-1405-63	
10 mg	Bottle of 30	0456-1410-30	Pinkish-Purple
	Bottle of 100	0456-1410-01	
	10 × 10 Unit Dose	0456-1410-63	

Bystolic—Cont.

Bronchospasm: Administer bronchodilator therapy such as a short acting inhaled β_2-agonist and/or aminophylline.
Hypoglycemia: Administer IV glucose. Repeated doses of IV glucose or possibly glucagon may be required.
In the event of intoxication where there are symptoms of shock, treatment must be continued for a sufficiently long period consistent with the 12-19 hour effective half-life of BYSTOLIC. Supportive measures should continue until clinical stability is achieved.
Call the National Poison Control Center (800-222-1222) for the most current information on β-blocker overdose treatment.

DOSAGE AND ADMINISTRATION

The dose of BYSTOLIC should be individualized to the needs of the patient. For most patients, the recommended starting dose is 5 mg once daily, with or without food, as monotherapy or in combination with other agents. For patients requiring further reduction in blood pressure, the dose can be increased at 2-week intervals up to 40 mg. A more frequent dosing regimen is unlikely to be beneficial.

Renal Impairment
In patients with severe renal impairment (ClCr less than 30 mL/min) the recommended initial dose is 2.5 mg once daily; upward titration should be performed cautiously if needed. BYSTOLIC has not been studied in patients receiving dialysis (see **CLINICAL PHARMACOLOGY, Special Populations**).

Hepatic Impairment
In patients with moderate hepatic impairment, the recommended initial dose is 2.5 mg once daily; upward titration should be performed cautiously if needed. BYSTOLIC has not been studied in patients with severe hepatic impairment and therefore it is not recommended in that population (see **PRECAUTIONS** and **CLINICAL PHARMACOLOGY, Special Populations**).

Geriatric Patients
It is not necessary to adjust the dose in the elderly (see above and **PRECAUTIONS, Geriatric Use**).

CYP2D6 Polymorphism (see **CLINICAL PHARMACOLOGY, Pharmacokinetics**)
No dose adjustments are necessary for patients who are CYP2D6 poor metabolizers. The clinical effect and safety profiles observed in poor metabolizers were similar to those of extensive metabolizers.

HOW SUPPLIED

BYSTOLIC is available as tablets for oral administration containing nebivolol hydrochloride equivalent to 2.5, 5, and 10 mg of nebivolol.
BYSTOLIC tablets are triangular-shaped, biconvex, unscored, differentiated by color and are engraved with "FL" on one side and the number of mg (2 ½, 5, or 10) on the other side. BYSTOLIC tablets are supplied in the following strengths and package configurations:
[See table above]

Store at 20° to 25°C (68° to 77°F). [See USP for Controlled Room Temperature.]
Dispense in a tight, light-resistant container as defined in the USP using a child-resistant closure.
Forest Pharmaceuticals, Inc.
Subsidiary of Forest Laboratories, Inc.
St. Louis, MO 63045, USA
Licensed from Mylan Laboratories, Inc.
Under license from Janssen Pharmaceutica N.V., Beerse, Belgium
Actidose-Aqua® is a registered trademark of Paddock Laboratories, Inc.
Rev. 12/07
© 2007 Forest Laboratories, Inc.

To keep your **PDR** up to date throughout the year, note these revisions on the corresponding pages of the annual volume. Simply write **"See Supplement A"** next to the product heading.

Inspire Pharmaceuticals, Inc.
4222 EMPEROR BOULEVARD
SUITE 200
DURHAM, NC 27703

Direct Inquiries to:
Telephone: 919-941-9777
Fax: 919-941-9797
E-mail: info@inspirepharm.com

AZASITE™
[ah-zuh-site]
(azithromycin ophthalmic solution)

R

HIGHLIGHTS OF PRESCRIBING INFORMATION
These highlights do not include all the information needed to use AzaSite safely and effectively. See full prescribing information for AzaSite.
AZASITE™ (azithromycin ophthalmic solution) 1%
Sterile topical ophthalmic drops
Initial U.S. Approval: 2007
----------------**INDICATIONS AND USAGE**----------------
AzaSite™ is a macrolide antibiotic indicated for the treatment of bacterial conjunctivitis caused by susceptible isolates of the following microorganisms: CDC coryneform group G, *Haemophilus influenzae*, *Staphylococcus aureus*, *Streptococcus mitis* group, and *Streptococcus pneumoniae*. (1)
------------**DOSAGE AND ADMINISTRATION**------------
Instill 1 drop in the affected eye (s) twice daily, eight to twelve hours apart for the first two days and then instill 1 drop in the affected eye (s) once daily for the next five days. (2)
----------**DOSAGE FORMS AND STRENGTHS**----------
5 mL size bottle filled with 2.5 mL of 1% sterile topical ophthalmic solution. (3)
FULL PRESCRIBING INFORMATION: CONTENTS*
1 INDICATIONS AND USAGE
2 DOSAGE AND ADMINISTRATION
3 DOSAGE FORMS AND STRENGTHS
4 CONTRAINDICATIONS
5 WARNINGS AND PRECAUTIONS
5.1 Topical Ophthalmic Use Only
5.2 Anaphylaxis and Hypersensitivity with Systemic Use of Azithromycin
5.3 Growth of Resistant Organisms with Prolonged Use
5.4 Avoidance of Contact Lenses
6 ADVERSE REACTIONS
7 DRUG INTERACTIONS
8 USE IN SPECIFIC POPULATIONS
8.1 Pregnancy
8.3 Nursing Mothers
8.4 Pediatric Use
8.5 Geriatric Use
----------------------**CONTRAINDICATIONS**----------------------
None (4)
--------------**WARNING AND PRECAUTIONS**--------------
• For topical ophthalmic use only. (5.1)
• Anaphylaxis and hypersensitivity have been reported with systemic use of azithromycin. (5.2)
• Growth of resistant organisms may occur with prolonged use. (5.3)
• Patients should not wear contact lenses if they have signs or symptoms of bacterial conjunctivitis. (5.4)
----------------------**ADVERSE REACTIONS**----------------------
Most common adverse reaction reported in patients was eye irritation (1–2% of patients). (6)
To report SUSPECTED ADVERSE REACTIONS, contact Inspire Pharmaceuticals, Inc. at 1-888-881-4696 or FDA at 1-800-FDA-1088 or www.fda.gov/medwatch.
See 17 for PATIENT COUNSELING INFORMATION.
Revised: 5/2007
11 DESCRIPTION
12 CLINICAL PHARMACOLOGY
12.1 Mechanism of Action
12.3 Pharmacokinetics
12.4 Microbiology
13 NONCLINICAL TOXICOLOGY
13.1 Carcinogenesis, Mutagenesis, Impairment of Fertility
13.2 Animal Toxicology and/or Pharmacology
14 CLINICAL STUDIES

---

16 HOW SUPPLIED/STORAGE AND HANDLING
17 PATIENT COUNSELING INFORMATION
* Sections or subsections omitted from the full prescribing information are not listed
FULL PRESCRIBING INFORMATION

1 INDICATIONS AND USAGE

AzaSite is indicated for the treatment of bacterial conjunctivitis caused by susceptible isolates of the following microorganisms:
CDC coryneform group G*
Haemophilus influenzae
Staphylococcus aureus
Streptococcus mitis group
Streptococcus pneumoniae
*Efficacy for this organism was studied in fewer than 10 infections.

2 DOSAGE AND ADMINISTRATION

The recommended dosage regimen for the treatment of bacterial conjunctivitis is: Instill 1 drop in the affected eye(s) twice daily, eight to twelve hours apart for the first two days and then instill 1 drop in the affected eye(s) once daily for the next five days.

3 DOSAGE FORMS AND STRENGTHS

5 mL bottle containing 2.5 mL of a 1% sterile topical ophthalmic solution.

4 CONTRAINDICATIONS

None

5 WARNINGS AND PRECAUTIONS

5.1 Topical Ophthalmic Use Only
NOT FOR INJECTION. AzaSite is indicated for topical ophthalmic use only, and should not be administered systemically, injected subconjunctivally, or introduced directly into the anterior chamber of the eye.

5.2 Anaphylaxis and Hypersensitivity with Systemic Use of Azithromycin
In patients receiving systemically administered azithromycin, serious allergic reactions, including angioedema, anaphylaxis, and dermatologic reactions including Stevens Johnson Syndrome and toxic epidermal necrolysis have been reported rarely in patients on azithromycin therapy. Although rare, fatalities have been reported. While these reactions have not been observed with topical ophthalmic use of AzaSite, the potential for anaphylaxis or other hypersensitivity reactions should be considered since patients with a known hypersensitivity to azithromycin or erythromycin were excluded from study.

5.3 Growth of Resistant Organisms with Prolonged Use
As with other anti-infectives, prolonged use may result in overgrowth of non-susceptible organisms, including fungi. If super-infection occurs, discontinue use and institute alternative therapy. Whenever clinical judgment dictates, the patient should be examined with the aid of magnification, such as slit-lamp biomicroscopy, and where appropriate, fluorescein staining.

5.4 Avoidance of Contact Lenses
Patients should be advised not to wear contact lenses if they have signs or symptoms of bacterial conjunctivitis.

6 ADVERSE REACTIONS

Because clinical trials are conducted under widely varying conditions, adverse reaction rates observed in one clinical trial of a drug cannot be directly compared with the rates in the clinical trials of the same or another drug and may not reflect the rates observed in practice.
The data described below reflect exposure to AzaSite in 698 patients. The population was between 1 and 87 years old with clinical signs and symptoms of bacterial conjunctivitis. The most frequently reported ocular adverse reaction reported in patients receiving AzaSite was eye irritation. This reaction occurred in approximately 1–2% of patients. Other adverse reactions associated with the use of AzaSite were reported in less than 1% of patients and included: burning, stinging and irritation upon instillation, contact dermatitis, corneal erosion, dry eye, dysgeusia, nasal congestion, ocular discharge, punctate keratitis, and sinusitis.

7 DRUG INTERACTIONS

Drug interaction studies have not been conducted with AzaSite ophthalmic solution.

8 USE IN SPECIFIC POPULATIONS

8.1 Pregnancy
Pregnancy Category B. Reproduction studies have been performed in rats and mice at doses up to 200 mg/kg/d. The highest dose was associated with moderate maternal toxicity. These doses are estimated to be approximately 5000 times, the maximum human ocular daily dose of 2 mg. In the animal studies, no evidence of harm to the fetus due to azithromycin was found. There are, however, no adequate and well-controlled studies in pregnant women. Because animal reproduction studies are not always predictive of human response, azithromycin should be used during pregnancy only if clearly needed.

8.3 Nursing Mothers
It is not known whether azithromycin is excreted in human milk. Because many drugs are excreted in human milk, caution should be exercised when azithromycin is administered to a nursing woman.

8.4 Pediatric Use
The safety and effectiveness of AzaSite solution in pediatric patients below 1 year of age have not been established. The efficacy of AzaSite in treating bacterial conjunctivitis in pediatric patients one year or older has been demonstrated in controlled clinical trials [see Clinical Studies (14)].

8.5 Geriatric Use
No overall differences in safety or effectiveness have been observed between elderly and younger patients.

11 DESCRIPTION

AzaSite (azithromycin ophthalmic solution) is a 1% sterile aqueous topical ophthalmic solution of azithromycin formulated in DuraSite® (polycarbophil, edetate disodium, sodium chloride). AzaSite is an off-white, viscous liquid with an osmolality of approximately 290 mOsm/kg.

Preservative: 0.003% benzalkonium chloride.

Inactives: mannitol, citric acid, sodium citrate, poloxamer 407, polycarbophil, edetate disodium (EDTA), sodium chloride, water for injection, and sodium hydroxide to adjust pH to 6.3.

Azithromycin is a macrolide antibiotic with a 15-membered ring. Its chemical name is (2R,3S, 4R,5R,8R,10R, 11R,12S,13S,14R)-13-[(2,6-dideoxy-3-C-methyl-3-O-methyl-α-L-ribohexopyranosyl)oxy]-2-ethyl-3,4,10-trihydroxy-3,5, 6,8,10,12,14-heptamethyl-11-[[3,4,6-trideoxy-3-(dimethylamino)-ß-D-xylohexopyranosyl] oxy]-1-oxa-6-aza-cyclopentadecan-15-one, and the structural formula is:

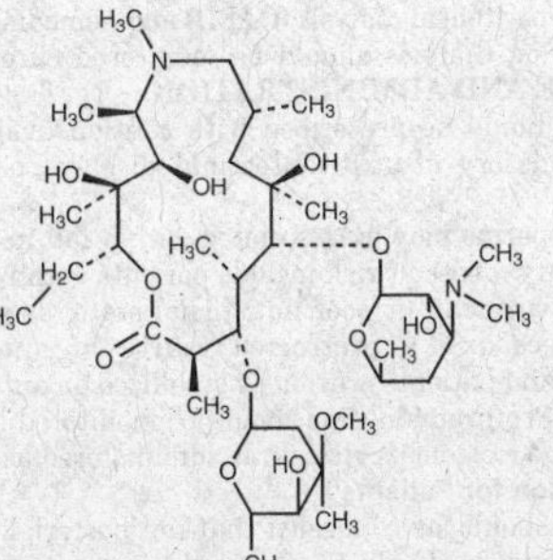

Azithromycin has a molecular weight of 749, and its empirical formula is $C_{38}H_{72}N_2O_{12}$.

12 CLINICAL PHARMACOLOGY

12.1 Mechanism of Action
Azithromycin is a macrolide antibiotic *[see Clinical Pharmacology, Microbiology (12.4)]*.

12.3 Pharmacokinetics
The plasma concentration of azithromycin following ocular administration of AzaSite (azithromycin ophthalmic solution) in humans is unknown. Based on the proposed dose of one drop to each eye (total dose of 100 mcL or 1 mg) and exposure information from systemic administration, the systemic concentration of azithromycin following ocular administration is estimated to be below quantifiable limits (δ10 ng/mL) at steady-state in humans, assuming 100% systemic availability.

12.4 Microbiology
Azithromycin acts by binding to the 50S ribosomal subunit of susceptible microorganisms and interfering with microbial protein synthesis.

Azithromycin has been shown to be active against most isolates of the following microorganisms, both *in vitro* and clinically in conjunctival infections as described in the INDICATIONS AND USAGE section:

CDC coryneform group G*
Haemophilus influenzae
Staphylococcus aureus
Streptococcus mitis group
Streptococcus pneumoniae

The following *in vitro* data are also available, **but their clinical significance in ophthalmic infections is unknown**. The safety and effectiveness of AzaSite in treating ophthalmological infections due to these microorganisms have not been established.

The following microorganisms are considered susceptible when evaluated using systemic breakpoints. However, a correlation between the *in vitro* systemic breakpoint and ophthalmological efficacy has not been established. This list of microorganisms is provided as an aid only in assessing the potential treatment of conjunctival infections. Azithromycin exhibits *in vitro* minimal inhibitory concentrations (MICs) of equal or less (systemic susceptible breakpoint) against most (є90%) of isolates of the following ocular pathogens:

Chlamydia pneumoniae
Chlamydia trachomatis
Legionella pneumophila
Moraxella catarrhalis
Mycoplasma hominis
Mycoplasma pneumoniae
Neisseria gonorrhoeae
Peptostreptococcus species
Streptococci (Groups C, F, G)
Streptococcus pyogenes
Streptococcus agalactiae
Ureaplasma urealyticum
Viridans group streptococci

**Efficacy for this organism was studied in fewer than 10 infections.*

13 NONCLINICAL TOXICOLOGY

13.1 Carcinogenesis, Mutagenesis, Impairment of Fertility
Long term studies in animals have not been performed to evaluate carcinogenic potential. Azithromycin has shown no mutagenic potential in standard laboratory tests: mouse lymphoma assay, human lymphocyte clastogenic assay, and mouse bone marrow clastogenic assay. No evidence of impaired fertility due to azithromycin was found in mice or rats that received oral doses of up to 200 mg/kg/day.

13.2 Animal Toxicology and/or Pharmacology
Phospholipidosis (intracellular phospholipid accumulation) has been observed in some tissues of mice, rats, and dogs given multiple systemic doses of azithromycin. Cytoplasmic microvacuolation, which is likely a manifestation of phospholipidosis, has been observed in the corneas of rabbits given multiple ocular doses of AzaSite. This effect was reversible upon cessation of AzaSite treatment. The significance of this toxicological finding for animals and for humans is unknown.

14 CLINICAL STUDIES

In a randomized, vehicle-controlled, double-blind, multicenter clinical study in which patients were dosed twice daily for the first two days, then once daily on days 3, 4, and 5, AzaSite solution was superior to vehicle on days 6–7 in patients who had a confirmed clinical diagnosis of bacterial conjunctivitis. Clinical resolution was achieved in 63% (82/130) of patients treated with AzaSite versus 50% (74/149) of patients treated with vehicle. The p value for the comparison was 0.03 and the 95% confidence interval around the 13% (63%–50%) difference was 2% to 25%. The microbiological success rate for the eradication of the baseline pathogens was approximately 88% compared to 66% of patients treated with vehicle (p<.001, confidence interval around the 22% difference was 13% to 31%). Microbiologic eradication does not always correlate with clinical outcome in anti-infective trials.

16 HOW SUPPLIED/STORAGE AND HANDLING

AzaSite is a sterile aqueous topical ophthalmic formulation of 1% azithromycin in a white, round, low-density polyethylene (LDPE) bottle, with a natural LDPE dropper tip, and a tan colored high-density polyethylene (HDPE) eyedropper cap. A white tamper evident overcap is provided.
2.5 mL in 5 mL bottle containing a total of 25 mg of azithromycin
(NDC 31357-040-25)

Storage and Handling:
Store unopened bottle under refrigeration at 2°C to 8°C (36°F to 46°F). Once the bottle is opened, store at 2°C to 25°C (36°F to 77°F) for up to 14 days. Discard after the 14 days.

17 PATIENT COUNSELING INFORMATION

Patients should be advised to avoid contaminating the applicator tip by allowing it to touch the eye, fingers or other sources.

Patients should be directed to discontinue use and contact a physician if any signs of an allergic reaction occur.

Patients should be told that although it is common to feel better early in the course of the therapy, the medication should be taken exactly as directed. Skipping doses or not completing the full course of therapy may (1) decrease the effectiveness of the immediate treatment and (2) increase the likelihood that bacteria will develop resistance and will not be treatable by AzaSite (azithromycin ophthalmic solution) or other antibacterial drugs in the future.

Patients should be advised not to wear contact lenses if they have signs or symptoms of bacterial conjunctivitis.

Patients are advised to thoroughly wash hands prior to using AzaSite.

Invert closed bottle (upside down) and shake once before each use. Remove cap with bottle still in the inverted position. Tilt head back, and with bottle inverted, gently squeeze bottle to instill one drop into the affected eye (s).

Inspire Pharmaceuticals Inc.
Licensee of InSite Vision Incorporated
Manufactured by Cardinal Health
U.S. PAT NO. 5,225,196; 5,192,535;
6,239,113; 6,569,443; 6,861,411;
7,056,893; and Patents Pending
AZA-0000

Lupin Pharmaceuticals, Inc.

HARBOR PLACE TOWER
111 SOUTH CALVERT STREET, 21ST FLOOR
BALTIMORE, MD 21202

Direct Inquiries to:
Phone (410) 576-2000

SUPRAX® ℞

CEFIXIME TABLETS USP, 400 mg
Rx only

To reduce the development of drug-resistant bacteria and maintain the effectiveness of Suprax (cefixime) Tablets and other antibacterial drugs, Suprax should be used only to treat or prevent infections that are proven or strongly suspected to be caused by bacteria.

DESCRIPTION

Suprax (cefixime) Tablets is a semisynthetic, cephalosporin antibiotic for oral administration. Chemically, it is (6*R*,7*R*)-7-[2-(2-Amino-4-thiazolyl)glyoxylamido]-8-oxo-3-vinyl-5-thia-1-azabicyclo[4.2.0] oct-2-ene-2-carboxylic-acid, 7^2-(*Z*)-[*O*-(carboxymethyl) oxime] trihydrate.

Molecular weight = 507.50 as the trihydrate. Chemical Formula is $C_{16}H_{15}N_5O_7S_2.3H_2O$

The structural formula for cefixime is:

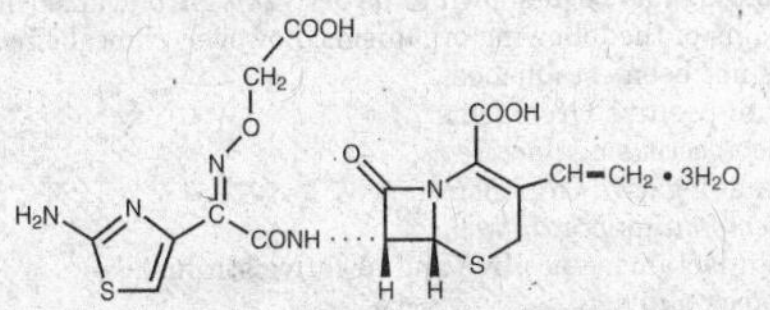

Each film coated tablet for oral administration contains 400 mg of cefixime as the trihydrate. In addition, each tablet contains the following inactive ingredients: dibasic calcium phosphate, hypromellose, titanium dioxide, lactose monohydrate, polyethylene glycol, triacetin, magnesium stearate, microcrystalline cellulose and pregelatinized starch.

CLINICAL PHARMACOLOGY

Suprax, given orally, is about 40%-50% absorbed whether administered with or without food; however, time to maximal absorption is increased approximately 0.8 hours when administered with food. A single 200 mg tablet of cefixime produces an average peak serum concentration of approximately 2 mcg/mL (range 1 to 4 mcg/mL); a single 400 mg tablet produces an average peak concentration of approximately 3.7 mcg/mL (range 1.3 to 7.7 mcg/mL). The oral suspension produces average peak concentrations approximately 25%-50% higher than the tablets, when tested in normal adult volunteers. The area under the time versus concentration curve is greater by approximately 10%-25% with the oral suspension than with the tablet after doses of 100 to 400 mg, when tested in normal adult volunteers. This increased absorption should be taken into consideration if the oral suspension is to be substituted for the tablet. Because of the lack of bioequivalence, tablets should not be substituted for oral suspension in the treatment of otitis media. (See **DOSAGE AND ADMINISTRATION**). Crossover studies of tablet versus suspension have not been performed in children.

Peak serum concentrations occur between 2 and 6 hours following oral administration of a single 200 mg tablet or a single 400 mg tablet.
[See table below]

Approximately 50% of the absorbed dose is excreted unchanged in the urine in 24 hours. In animal studies, it was noted that cefixime is also excreted in the bile in excess of 10% of the administered dose. Serum protein binding is concentration independent with a bound fraction of approximately 65%. In a multiple dose study conducted with a research formulation which is less bioavailable than the tablet or suspension, there was little accumulation of drug in serum or urine after dosing for 14 days. The serum half-life of cefixime in healthy subjects is independent of dosage form and averages 3-4 hours but may range up to 9 hours in some normal volunteers. Average AUCs at steady state in elderly patients are approximately 40% higher than average AUCs in other healthy adults.

In subjects with moderate impairment of renal function (20 to 40 mL/min creatinine clearance), the average serum half-life of cefixime is prolonged to 6.4 hours. In severe renal impairment (5 to 20 mL/min creatinine clearance), the half-life increased to an average of 11.5 hours. The drug is not cleared significantly from the blood by hemodialysis or peritoneal dialysis. However, a study indicated that with doses of 400 mg, patients undergoing hemodialysis have similar blood profiles as subjects with creatinine clearances of 21-60 mL/min. There is no evidence of metabolism of cefixime *in vivo*.

Adequate data on CSF levels of cefixime are not available.

Microbiology
As with other cephalosporins, bactericidal action of cefixime results from inhibition of cell-wall synthesis. Cefixime is highly stable in the presence of beta-lactamase enzymes. As a result, many organisms resistant to penicillins and some cephalosporins due to the presence of beta-lactamases, may be susceptible to cefixime. Cefixime has been shown to be active against most strains of the following organisms both *in vitro* and in clinical infections (see **INDICATIONS AND USAGE**):

Gram-positive Organisms.
Streptococcus pneumoniae,
Streptococcus pyogenes.
Gram-negative Organisms.
Haemophilus influenzae
(beta-lactamase positive and negative strains),
Moraxella (Branhamella) catarrhalis
(most of which are beta-lactamase positive),
Escherichia coli,
Proteus mirabilis,

Continued on next page

TABLE

Serum Levels of Cefixime after Administration of Tablets (mcg/mL)

DOSE	1h	2h	4h	6h	8h	12h	24h
100 mg	0.3	0.8	1	0.7	0.4	0.2	0.02
200 mg	0.7	1.4	2	1.5	1	0.4	0.03
400 mg	1.2	2.5	3.5	2.7	1.7	0.6	0.04

Suprax—Cont.

Neisseria gonorrhoeae
(including penicillinase- and non-penicillinase-producing strains).
Cefixime has been shown to be active *in vitro* against most strains of the following organisms; however, clinical efficacy has not been established.
Gram-positive Organisms.
Streptococcus agalactiae.
Gram-negative Organisms.
Haemophilus parainfluenzae
(beta-lactamase positive and negative strains),
Proteus vulgaris,
Klebsiella pneumoniae,
Klebsiella oxytoca,
Pasteurella multocida,
Providencia species,
Salmonella species,
Shigella species,
Citrobacter amalonaticus,
Citrobacter diversus,
Serratia marcescens.
Note: *Pseudomonas* species, strains of group D streptococci (including enterococci), *Listeria monocytogenes*, most strains of staphylococci (including methicillin-resistant strains) and most strains of *Enterobacter* are resistant to cefixime. In addition, most strains of *Bacteroides fragilis* and *Clostridia* are resistant to cefixime.

Susceptibility Testing
Susceptibility Tests:
Diffusion Techniques

Quantitative methods that require measurement of zone diameters give an estimate of antibiotic susceptibility. One such procedure[1-3] has been recommended for use with disks to test susceptibility to cefixime. Interpretation involves correlation of the diameters obtained in the disk test with minimum inhibitory concentration (MIC) for cefixime.
Reports from the laboratory giving results of the standard single-disk susceptibility test with a 5-mcg cefixime disk should be interpreted according to the following criteria:
[See first table above]
A report of "Susceptible" indicates that the pathogen is likely to be inhibited by generally achievable blood levels. A report of "Moderately Susceptible" indicates that inhibitory concentrations of the antibiotic may well be achieved if high dosage is used or if the infection is confined to tissues and fluids (e.g., urine) in which high antibiotic levels are attained. A report of "Resistant" indicates that achievable concentrations of the antibiotic are unlikely to be inhibitory and other therapy should be selected.
Standardized procedures require the use of laboratory control organisms. The 5-mcg disk should give the following zone diameter:

Organism	Zone diameter (mm)
E. coli ATCC 25922	23-27
N. gonorrhoeae ATCC 49226[a]	37-45

[a] Using GC Agar Base with a defined 1% supplement without cysteine.

The class disk for cephalosporin susceptibility testing (the cephalothin disk) is not appropriate because of spectrum differences with cefixime. The 5-mcg cefixime disk should be used for all *in vitro* testing of isolates.

Dilution Techniques

Broth or agar dilution methods can be used to determine the minimum inhibitory concentration (MIC) value for susceptibility of bacterial isolates to cefixime. The recommended susceptibility breakpoints are as follows:
[See second table above]
As with standard diffusion methods, dilution procedures require the use of laboratory control organisms. Standard cefixime powder should give the following MIC ranges in daily testing of quality control organisms:

Organism	MIC range (mcg/mL)
E. coli ATCC 25922	0.25-1
S. aureus ATCC 29213	8-32
N. gonorrhoeae ATCC 49226[a]	0.008-0.03

[a] Using GC Agar Base with a defined 1% supplement without cysteine.

INDICATIONS AND USAGE

To reduce the development of drug resistant bacteria and maintain the effectiveness of Suprax (cefixime) Tablets and other antibacterial drugs, Suprax should be used only to treat or prevent infections that are proven or strongly suspected to be caused by susceptible bacteria. When culture and susceptibility information are available, they should be considered in selecting or modifying antimicrobial therapy. In the absence of such data, local epidemiology and susceptibility patterns may contribute to the empiric selection of therapy.
Suprax is indicated in the treatment of the following infections when caused by susceptible strains of the designated microorganisms:
Uncomplicated Urinary Tract Infections caused by *Escherichia coli* and *Proteus mirabilis*.
Pharyngitis and *Tonsillitis*, caused by *S. pyogenes*.

Recommended Susceptibility Ranges: Agar Disk Diffusion

Organisms	Resistant	Moderately Susceptible	Susceptible
Neisseria gonorrhoeae[a]	—	—	≥ 31 mm
All other organisms	≤ 15 mm	16-18 mm	≥ 19 mm

[a] Using GC Agar Base with a defined 1% supplement without cysteine.

MIC Interpretive Standards (mcg/mL)

Organisms	Resistant	Moderately Susceptible	Susceptible
Neisseria gonorrhoeae[a]	—	—	≤ 0.25
All other organisms	≥ 4	2	≤ 1

Note: Penicillin is the usual drug of choice in the treatment of *S. pyogenes* infections, including the prophylaxis of rheumatic fever. Suprax is generally effective in the eradication of *S. pyogenes* from the nasopharynx; however, data establishing the efficacy of Suprax in the subsequent prevention of rheumatic fever are not available.
Acute Bronchitis and *Acute Exacerbations of Chronic Bronchitis*, caused by *Streptococcus pneumoniae* and *Haemophilus influenzae* (beta-lactamase positive and negative strains).
Uncomplicated gonorrhea (cervical/urethral), caused by *Neisseria gonorrhoeae* (penicillinase-and non-penicillinase-producing strains).
Appropriate cultures and susceptibility studies should be performed to determine the causative organism and its susceptibility to cefixime; however, therapy may be started while awaiting the results of these studies. Therapy should be adjusted, if necessary, once these results are known.

CONTRAINDICATIONS

Suprax is contraindicated in patients with known allergy to the cephalosporin group of antibiotics.

WARNINGS

BEFORE THERAPY WITH SUPRAX IS INSTITUTED, CAREFUL INQUIRY SHOULD BE MADE TO DETERMINE WHETHER THE PATIENT HAS HAD PREVIOUS HYPERSENSITIVITY REACTIONS TO CEPHALOSPORINS, PENICILLINS, OR OTHER DRUGS. IF THIS PRODUCT IS TO BE GIVEN TO PENICILLIN-SENSITIVE PATIENTS, CAUTION SHOULD BE EXERCISED BECAUSE CROSS HYPERSENSITIVITY AMONG BETA-LACTAM ANTIBIOTICS HAS BEEN CLEARLY DOCUMENTED AND MAY OCCUR IN UP TO 10% OF PATIENTS WITH A HISTORY OF PENICILLIN ALLERGY. IF AN ALLERGIC REACTION TO SUPRAX OCCURS, DISCONTINUE THE DRUG. SERIOUS ACUTE HYPERSENSITIVITY REACTIONS MAY REQUIRE TREATMENT WITH EPINEPHRINE AND OTHER EMERGENCY MEASURES, INCLUDING OXYGEN, INTRAVENOUS FLUIDS, INTRAVENOUS ANTIHISTAMINES, CORTICOSTEROIDS, PRESSOR AMINES AND AIRWAY MANAGEMENT, AS CLINICALLY INDICATED.
Anaphylactic/anaphylactoid reactions (including shock and fatalities) have been reported with the use of cefixime.
Antibiotics, including Suprax, should be administered cautiously to any patient who has demonstrated some form of allergy, particularly to drugs.
Treatment with broad spectrum antibiotics, including Suprax, alters the normal flora of the colon and may permit overgrowth of clostridia. Studies indicate that a toxin produced by *Clostridium difficile* is a primary cause of severe antibiotic-associated diarrhea including pseudomembranous colitis.
Pseudomembranous colitis has been reported with the use of Suprax and other broad-spectrum antibiotics (including macrolides, semisynthetic penicillins, and cephalosporins); therefore, it is important to consider this diagnosis in patients who develop diarrhea in association with the use of antibiotics. Symptoms of pseudomembranous colitis may occur during or after antibiotic treatment and may range in severity from mild to life-threatening. Mild cases of pseudomembranous colitis usually respond to drug discontinuation alone. In moderate to severe cases, management should include fluids, electrolytes, and protein supplementation. If the colitis does not improve after the drug has been discontinued, or if the symptoms are severe, oral vancomycin is the drug of choice for antibiotic-associated pseudomembranous colitis produced by *C. difficile*. Other causes of colitis should be excluded.

PRECAUTIONS

General

Prescribing Suprax (Cefixime) Tablets in the absence of a proven or strongly suspected bacterial infection of a prophylactic indication is unlikely to provide benefit to the patient and increases the risk of the development of drug-resistant bacteria.
The possibility of the emergence of resistant organisms which might result in overgrowth should be kept in mind, particularly during prolonged treatment. In such use, careful observation of the patient is essential. If superinfection occurs during therapy, appropriate measures should be taken.
The dose of Suprax should be adjusted in patients with renal impairment as well as those undergoing continuous ambulatory peritoneal dialysis (CAPD) and hemodialysis (HD). Patients on dialysis should be monitored carefully. (See **DOSAGE AND ADMINISTRATION**.)
Suprax should be prescribed with caution in individuals with a history of gastrointestinal disease, particularly colitis.
Cephalosporins may be associated with a fall in prothrombin activity. Those at risk include patients with renal or hepatic impairment, or poor nutritional state, as well as patients receiving a protracted course of antimicrobial therapy, and patients previously stabilized on anticoagulant therapy. Prothrombin time should be monitored in patients at risk and exogenous vitamin K administered as indicated.

Information for Patients

Patients should be counseled that antibacterial drugs, including Suprax, should only be used to treat bacterial infections. They do not treat viral infections (e.g., the common cold). When Suprax is prescribed to treat a bacterial infection, patients should be told that although it is common to feel better early in the course of therapy, the medication should be taken exactly as directed. Skipping doses or not completing the full course of therapy may: (1) decrease the effectiveness of the immediate treatment and (2) increase the likelihood that bacteria will develop resistance and will not be treatable by Suprax or other antibacterial drugs in the future.

Drug Interactions

Carbamazepine: Elevated carbamazepine levels have been reported in postmarketing experience when cefixime is administered concomitantly. Drug monitoring may be of assistance in detecting alterations in carbamazepine plasma concentrations.
Warfarin and Anticoagulants: Increased prothrombin time, with or without clinical bleeding, has been reported when cefixime is administered concomitantly.

Drug/Laboratory Test Interactions

A false-positive reaction for ketones in the urine may occur with tests using nitroprusside but not with those using nitroferricyanide.
The administration of cefixime may result in a false-positive reaction for glucose in the urine using Clinitest®**, Benedict's solution, or Fehling's solution. It is recommended that glucose tests based on enzymatic glucose oxidase reactions (such as Clinistix®** or TesTape®**) be used. A false-positive direct Coombs test has been reported during treatment with other cephalosporin antibiotics; therefore, it should be recognized that a positive Coombs test may be due to the drug.

Carcinogenesis, Mutagenesis, Impairment of Fertility

Lifetime studies in animals to evaluate carcinogenic potential have not been conducted. Cefixime did not cause point mutations in bacteria or mammalian cells, DNA damage, or chromosome damage *in vitro* and did not exhibit clastogenic potential *in vivo* in the mouse micronucleus test. In rats, fertility and reproductive performance were not affected by cefixime at doses up to 125 times the adult therapeutic dose.

Usage in Pregnancy

Pregnancy Category B. Reproduction studies have been performed in mice and rats at doses up to 400 times the human dose and have revealed no evidence of harm to the fetus due to cefixime. There are no adequate and well-controlled studies in pregnant women. Because animal reproduction studies are not always predictive of human response, this drug should be used during pregnancy only if clearly needed.

Labor and Delivery

Cefixime has not been studied for use during labor and delivery. Treatment should only be given if clearly needed.

Nursing Mothers

It is not known whether cefixime is excreted in human milk. Consideration should be given to discontinuing nursing temporarily during treatment with this drug.

Pediatric Use

Safety and effectiveness of cefixime in children aged less than six months old have not been established.
The incidence of gastrointestinal adverse reactions, including diarrhea and loose stools, in the pediatric patients receiving the suspension, was comparable to the incidence seen in adult patients receiving tablets.

ADVERSE REACTIONS

Most of adverse reactions observed in clinical trials were of a mild and transient nature. Five percent (5%) of patients in the U.S. trials discontinued therapy because of drug-related adverse reactions. The most commonly seen adverse reac-

PEDIATRIC DOSAGE CHART 200 mg/5 mL

Patient Weight (kg)	Dose/Day mg	Dose/Day mL	Dose/Day tsp of Suspension
6.25	50	1.25	¼
12.5	100	2.5	½
18.75	150	3.75	¾
25	200	5	1
31.25	250	6.25	1¼
37.5	300	7.5	1½

tions in U.S. trials of the tablet formulation were gastrointestinal events, which were reported in 30% of adult patients on either the BID or the QD regimen. Clinically mild gastrointestinal side effects occurred in 20% of all patients, moderate events occurred in 9% of all patients and severe adverse reactions occurred in 2% of all patients. Individual event rates included diarrhea 16%, loose or frequent stools 6%, abdominal pain 3%, nausea 7%, dyspepsia 3%, and flatulence 4%. The incidence of gastrointestinal adverse reactions, including diarrhea and loose stools, in pediatric patients receiving the suspension was comparable to the incidence seen in adult patients receiving tablets.

These symptoms usually responded to symptomatic therapy or ceased when cefixime was discontinued.

Several patients developed severe diarrhea and/or documented pseudomembranous colitis, and a few required hospitalization.

The following adverse reactions have been reported following the use of cefixime. Incidence rates were less than 1 in 50 (less than 2%), except as noted above for gastrointestinal events.

Gastrointestinal (see above): Diarrhea, loose stools, abdominal pain, dyspepsia, nausea, and vomiting. Several cases of documented pseudomembranous colitis were identified during the studies. The onset of pseudomembranous colitis symptoms may occur during or after therapy.

Hypersensitivity Reactions: Anaphylactic/anaphylactoid reactions (including shock and fatalities), skin rashes, urticaria, drug fever, pruritus, angioedema, and facial edema. Erythema multiforme, Stevens-Johnson syndrome, and serum sickness-like reactions have been reported.

Hepatic: Transient elevations in SGPT, SGOT, alkaline phosphatase, hepatitis, jaundice.

Renal: Transient elevations in BUN or creatinine, acute renal failure.

Central Nervous System: Headaches, dizziness, seizures.

Hemic and Lymphatic Systems: Transient thrombocytopenia, leukopenia, neutropenia, and eosinophilia. Prolongation in prothrombin time was seen rarely.

Abnormal Laboratory Tests: Hyperbilirubinemia.

Other: Genital pruritus, vaginitis, candidiasis, toxic epidermal necrolysis.

In addition to the adverse reactions listed above which have been observed in patients treated with cefixime, the following adverse reactions and altered laboratory tests have been reported for cephalosporin-class antibiotics:

Adverse reactions: Allergic reactions, superinfection, renal dysfunction, toxic nephropathy, hepatic dysfunction including cholestasis, aplastic anemia, hemolytic anemia, hemorrhage, and colitis.

Several cephalosporins have been implicated in triggering seizures, particularly in patients with renal impairment when the dosage was not reduced. (See **DOSAGE AND ADMINISTRATION** and **OVERDOSAGE**.) If seizures associated with drug therapy occur, the drug should be discontinued. Anticonvulsant therapy can be given if clinically indicated.

Abnormal Laboratory Tests: Positive direct Coombs test, elevated LDH, pancytopenia, agranulocytosis.

OVERDOSAGE

Gastric lavage may be indicated; otherwise, no specific antidote exists. Cefixime is not removed in significant quantities from the circulation by hemodialysis or peritoneal dialysis. Adverse reactions in small numbers of healthy adult volunteers receiving single doses up to 2 g of cefixime did not differ from the profile seen in patients treated at the recommended doses.

DOSAGE AND ADMINISTRATION

Adults: The recommended dose of cefixime is 400 mg daily. This may be given as a 400 mg tablet daily or as 200 mg tablet every 12 hours. For the treatment of uncomplicated cervical/urethral gonococcal infections, a single oral dose of 400 mg is recommended.

Children: The recommended dose is 8 mg/kg/day of the suspension. This may be administered as a single daily dose or may be given in two divided doses, as 4 mg/kg every 12 hours.

[See table above]

Children weighing more than 50 kg or older than 12 years should be treated with the recommended adult dose.

Otitis media should be treated with the suspension. Clinical studies of otitis media were conducted with the suspension, and the suspension results in higher peak blood levels than the tablet when administered at the same dose. Therefore, the tablet should not be substituted for the suspension in the treatment of otitis media. (See **CLINICAL PHARMACOLOGY**.)

Efficacy and safety in infants aged less than six months have not been established.

In the treatment of infections due to *S. pyogenes*, a therapeutic dosage of Suprax should be administered for at least 10 days.

Renal Impairment

Suprax may be administered in the presence of impaired renal function. Normal dose and schedule may be employed in patients with creatinine clearances of 60 mL/min or greater. Patients whose clearance is between 21 and 60 mL/min or patients who are on renal hemodialysis may be given 75% of the standard dosage at the standard dosing interval (i.e., 300 mg daily). Patients whose clearance is < 20 mL/min, or patients who are on continuous ambulatory peritoneal dialysis may be given half the standard dosage at the standard dosing interval (i.e., 200 mg daily). Neither hemodialysis nor peritoneal dialysis remove significant amounts of drug from the body.

HOW SUPPLIED

Each film coated tablet contains 400 mg of cefixime as the trihydrate. Suprax® (cefixime) Tablets, 400 mg, are white to off-white film coated capsule shaped tablets with beveled edges and a divided score line on each side, debossed with "SUPRAX" across one side and "LUPIN" across other side, supplied as follows:

NDC 27437-201-01—Bottle of 100 tablets
NDC 27437-201-08—Bottle of 50 tablets
NDC 27437-201-10—Bottle of 10 tablets with CRC

Store at 20°-25°C (68°-77°F) [See USP Controlled Room Temperature].

REFERENCES

1. Bauer AW, Kirby WMM, Sherris JC, et al.: Antibiotic susceptibility testing by a standard single disk method. *Am J Clin Pathol* 1966; 45:493.
2. National Committee for Clinical Laboratory Standards, Approved Standard: Performance Standards for Antimicrobial Disk Susceptibility Tests (M2-A3), December 1984.
3. Standardized disk susceptibility test. Federal Register 1974; 39 (May 30): 19182-19184.
**Clinitest® and Clinistix® are registered trademarks of Ames Division, Miles Laboratories, Inc. Tes-Tape® is a registered trademark of Eli Lilly and Company.

Manufactured for: Lupin Pharma
                     Baltimore, Maryland 21202
                     United States
Manufactured by: Lupin Limited
                     Mumbai 400 098
                     INDIA

Revised: October, 2007   ID: 212954

MedImmune Vaccines, Inc.
A subsidiary of MedImmune, Inc.

ONE MEDIMMUNE WAY
GAITHERSBURG, MD 20878

For all inquiries including emergencies (24 hours), medical information, adverse drug experiences, product sales and ordering, and customer service, please contact:
(877) FLUMIST (358-6478)
www.medimmune.com

FLUMIST®   ℞
Influenza Virus Vaccine Live, Intranasal
Intranasal Spray

HIGHLIGHTS OF PRESCRIBING INFORMATION
These highlights do not include all the information needed to use FluMist safely and effectively. See full prescribing information for FluMist.

FluMist® Influenza Virus Vaccine Live, Intranasal Intranasal Spray
2007-2008 Formula
Initial U.S. Approval: 2003

RECENT MAJOR CHANGES

Indications and Usage (1)	9/2007
Dosage and Administration, Dosing Information (2.1)	9/2007
Warnings and Precautions (5)	9/2007

INDICATIONS AND USAGE

FluMist is a live attenuated influenza virus vaccine indicated for the active immunization of individuals 2-49 years of age against influenza disease caused by influenza virus subtypes A and type B contained in the vaccine. (1)

DOSAGE AND ADMINISTRATION

For intranasal administration by a health care provider.

Age Group	Vaccination Status	Dosage Schedule
Children (2-8 years)	Not previously vaccinated with influenza vaccine	2 doses (0.2 mL* each, at least 1 month apart) (2.1)
Children (2-8 years)	Previously vaccinated with influenza vaccine	1 dose (0.2 mL*) (2.1)
Children, adolescents and adults (9-49 years)	Not applicable	1 dose (0.2 mL*) (2.1)

* Administer as 0.1 mL per nostril.

DOSAGE FORMS AND STRENGTHS

0.2 mL pre-filled, single-use intranasal spray (3)
Each 0.2 mL dose contains $10^{6.5-7.5}$ FFU (fluorescent focus units) of live attenuated influenza virus reassortants of each of the three strains for the 2007-2008 season: A/Solomon Islands/3/2006 (H1N1), A/Wisconsin/67/2005 (H3N2), and B/Malaysia/2506/2004. (3)

CONTRAINDICATIONS

- Hypersensitivity to eggs, egg proteins, gentamicin, gelatin or arginine or life threatening reactions to previous influenza vaccination. (4.1)
- Concomitant aspirin therapy in children and adolescents. (4.2)

WARNINGS AND PRECAUTIONS

- Do not administer FluMist to children <24 months because of increased risk of hospitalization and wheezing observed in clinical trials. (5.1)
- FluMist should not be administered to any individuals with asthma and children < 5 years of age with recurrent wheezing because of the potential for increased risk of wheezing post vaccination. (5.2)
- If Guillain-Barré syndrome has occurred within 6 weeks of any prior influenza vaccination, the decision to give FluMist should be based on careful consideration of the potential benefits and risks. (5.3)
- Administration of FluMist, a live virus vaccine, to immunocompromised persons should be based on careful consideration of potential benefits and risks. (5.4)
- Safety has not been established in individuals with underlying medical conditions predisposing them to wild-type influenza infection complications. (5.5)

ADVERSE REACTIONS

Most common adverse reactions (≥ 10% in FluMist and at least 5% greater than in control) are runny nose or nasal congestion in all ages, fever >100°F in children 2-6 years of age, and sore throat in adults. (6.1)

To report SUSPECTED ADVERSE REACTIONS, contact MedImmune at 1-877-633-4411 or VAERS at 1-800-822-7967 and *http://vaers.hhs.gov.*

DRUG INTERACTIONS

- Antiviral agents active against influenza A and/or B: Do not administer FluMist until 48 hours after antiviral cessation. Antiviral agents should not be administered until 2 weeks after FluMist administration unless medically necessary. (7.2)

USE IN SPECIFIC POPULATIONS

- Safety and effectiveness of FluMist have not been studied in pregnant women or nursing mothers. (8.1, 8.3)
- FluMist is not indicated for use in children <2 years of age. (8.4)
- FluMist is not indicated for use in individuals ≥50 years of age. (8.5, 8.6)

See 17 for PATIENT COUNSELING INFORMATION.

Revised: 09/2007

FULL PRESCRIBING INFORMATION: CONTENTS*

Continued on next page

FluMist—Cont.

FULL PRESCRIBING INFORMATION

1 INDICATIONS AND USAGE

FluMist is a live attenuated influenza virus vaccine indicated for the active immunization of individuals 2-49 years of age against influenza disease caused by influenza virus subtypes A and type B contained in the vaccine.

2 DOSAGE AND ADMINISTRATION

FOR INTRANASAL ADMINISTRATION BY A HEALTH CARE PROVIDER.

2.1 Dosing Information

FluMist should be administered according to the following schedule:

Age Group	Vaccination Status	Dosage Schedule
Children age 2 years through 8 years	Not previously vaccinated with influenza vaccine	2 doses (0.2 mL* each, at least 1 month apart)
Children age 2 years through 8 years	Previously vaccinated with influenza vaccine	1 dose (0.2 mL*)
Children, adolescents and adults age 9 through 49 years	Not applicable	1 dose (0.2 mL*)

* Administer as 0.1 mL per nostril.

For children age 2 years through 8 years who have not previously received influenza vaccine, the recommended dosage schedule for nasal administration is one 0.2 mL dose (0.1 mL per nostril) followed by a second 0.2 mL dose (0.1 mL per nostril) given at least 1 month later.
For all other individuals, including children age 2-8 years who have previously received influenza vaccine, the recommended schedule is one 0.2 mL dose (0.1 mL per nostril).
FluMist should be administered prior to exposure to influenza. Annual revaccination with influenza vaccine is recommended.

2.2 Administration Instructions

Each sprayer contains a single dose of FluMist; approximately one-half of the contents should be administered into each nostril. 0.1 mL (i.e., half of the dose from a single FluMist sprayer) is administered into each nostril while the recipient is in an upright position. Insert the tip of the sprayer just inside the nose and rapidly depress the plunger until the dose-divider clip stops the plunger. The dose-divider clip is removed from the sprayer to administer the second half of the dose (0.1 mL) into the other nostril. Once FluMist has been administered, the sprayer should be disposed of according to the standard procedures for medical waste (e.g., sharps container or biohazard container).

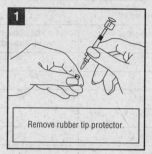

Remove rubber tip protector.

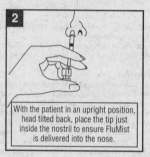

With the patient in an upright position, head tilted back, place the tip just inside the nostril to ensure FluMist is delivered into the nose.

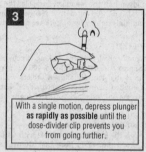

With a single motion, depress plunger **as rapidly as possible** until the dose-divider clip prevents you from going further.

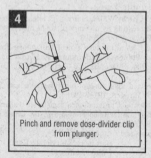

Pinch and remove dose-divider clip from plunger.

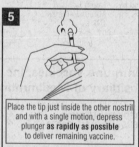

Place the tip just inside the other nostril and with a single motion, depress plunger **as rapidly as possible** to deliver remaining vaccine.

3 DOSAGE FORMS AND STRENGTHS

0.2 mL pre-filled, single-use intranasal spray.
Each 0.2 mL dose of FluMist is formulated to contain $10^{6.5-7.5}$ FFU (fluorescent focus units) of each of three live attenuated influenza virus reassortants: A/Solomon Islands/3/2006 (H1N1), A/Wisconsin/67/2005 (H3N2), and B/Malaysia/2506/2004 [1].

4 CONTRAINDICATIONS

4.1 Hypersensitivity

FluMist is contraindicated in individuals with a history of hypersensitivity, especially anaphylactic reactions, to eggs, egg proteins, gentamicin, gelatin, or arginine or with life-threatening reactions to previous influenza vaccinations.

4.2 Concomitant Pediatric and Adolescent Aspirin Therapy and Reye's Syndrome

FluMist is contraindicated in children and adolescents (2-17 years of age) receiving aspirin therapy or aspirin-containing therapy, because of the association of Reye's syndrome with aspirin and wild-type influenza infection.

5 WARNINGS AND PRECAUTIONS

5.1 Risks in Children <24 Months of Age

Do not administer FluMist to children <24 months of age. In clinical trials, an increased risk of wheezing post-vaccination was observed in FluMist recipients <24 months of age. An increase in hospitalizations was observed in children <24 months of age after vaccination with FluMist. [See *Adverse Reactions (6.1)*.]

5.2 Asthma/Recurrent Wheezing

FluMist should not be administered to any individuals with asthma and children < 5 years of age with recurrent wheezing because of the potential for increased risk of wheezing post vaccination unless the potential benefit outweighs the potential risk.
Do not administer FluMist to individuals with severe asthma or active wheezing because these individuals have not been studied in clinical trials.

5.3 Guillain-Barré Syndrome

If Guillain-Barré syndrome has occurred within 6 weeks of any prior influenza vaccination, the decision to give FluMist should be based on careful consideration of the potential benefits and potential risks [see also *Adverse Reactions (6.2)*].

5.4 Altered Immunocompetence

Administration of FluMist, a live virus vaccine, to immunocompromised persons should be based on careful consideration of potential benefits and risks. Although FluMist was studied in 57 asymptomatic or mildly symptomatic adults with HIV infection [see *Clinical Studies (14.3)*], data supporting the safety and effectiveness of FluMist administration in immunocompromised individuals are limited.

5.5 Medical Conditions Predisposing to Influenza Complications

The safety of FluMist in individuals with underlying medical conditions that may predispose them to complications following wild-type influenza infection has not been established. FluMist should not be administered unless the potential benefit outweighs the potential risk.

5.6 Preventing and Managing Allergic Vaccine Reactions

Prior to vaccination, review the individual's medical history for possible sensitivity to influenza vaccine or vaccine components. Treatment must be readily available in the event of an acute anaphylactic reaction following vaccination [see *Contraindications (4.1)*].

5.7 Limitations of Vaccine Effectiveness

FluMist may not protect all individuals receiving the vaccine.

6 ADVERSE REACTIONS

FluMist is not indicated in children <24 months of age. In a clinical trial, among children 6-23 months of age, wheezing requiring bronchodilator therapy or with significant respiratory symptoms occurred in 5.9% of FluMist recipients compared to 3.8% of active control recipients (Relative Risk 1.5, 95% CI: 1.2, 2.1). Wheezing was not increased in children ≥24 months of age.
Hypersensitivity, including anaphylactic reaction, has been reported post-marketing.
[See *Warnings and Precautions (5.1)* and *Adverse Reactions (6.1, 6.2)*.]

6.1 Adverse Reactions in Clinical Trials

Because clinical trials are conducted under widely varying conditions, adverse reaction rates observed in the clinical trials of a drug cannot be directly compared to rates in the clinical trials of another drug and may not reflect the rates observed in practice.
A total of 9537 children and adolescents 1-17 years of age and 3041 adults 18-64 years of age received FluMist in randomized, placebo-controlled Studies D153-P501, AV006, D153-P526, AV019 and AV009 described below. In addition, 4179 children 6-59 months of age received FluMist in Study MI-CP111, a randomized, active-controlled trial. Among pediatric FluMist recipients 6 months-17 years of age, 50% were female; in the study of adults, 55% were female. In MI-CP111, AV006, D153-P526, AV019 and AV009, subjects were White (71%), Hispanic (11%), Asian (7%), Black (6%), and Other (5%), while in D153-P501, 99% of subjects were Asian.

Adverse Reactions in Children and Adolescents

In a placebo-controlled safety study (AV019) conducted in a large Health Maintenance Organization (HMO) in children 1-17 years of age (n = 9689), an increase in asthma events, captured by review of diagnostic codes, was observed in children <5 years of age (Relative Risk 3.53, 90% CI: 1.1, 15.7). This observation was prospectively evaluated in Study MI-CP111.
In MI-CP111, an active-controlled study, increases in wheezing and hospitalization (for any cause) were observed in children <24 months of age, as shown in Table 1.

Table 1
Percentages of Children with Hospitalizations and Wheezing from MI-CP111

Adverse Reaction	Age Group	FluMist	Active Control[a]
Hospitalizations[b]	6-23 months (n = 3967)	4.2 %	3.2 %
	24-59 months (n = 4385)	2.1 %	2.5 %
Wheezing[c]	6-23 months (n = 3967)	5.9 %	3.8 %
	24-59 months (n = 4385)	2.1 %	2.5 %

[a] Injectable influenza vaccine

[b] From randomization through 180 days post last vaccination.

[c] Wheezing requiring bronchodilator therapy or with significant respiratory symptoms evaluated from randomization through 42 days post last vaccination.

Most hospitalizations observed were gastrointestinal and respiratory tract infections and occurred more than 6 weeks post vaccination. In post hoc analysis, rates of hospitalization in children 6-11 months of age (n = 1376) were 6.1% in FluMist recipients and 2.6% in active control recipients.

Table 2 shows an analysis of pooled solicited events, occurring in at least 1% of FluMist recipients and at a higher rate compared to placebo, post Dose 1 for Study D153-P501 and AV006 and solicited events post Dose 1 for Study MI-CP111. Solicited events were those about which parents/guardians were specifically queried after vaccination with FluMist. In these studies, solicited events were documented for 10 days post vaccination. Solicited events post Dose 2 for FluMist were similar to those post Dose 1 and were generally observed at a lower frequency.

[See table 2 above]

Table 2
Summary of Solicited Events Observed within 10 Days after Dose 1 for Vaccine[a] and either Placebo or Active Control Recipients; Children 2-6 Years of Age

	D153-P501 & AV006		MI-CP111	
	FluMist N=876-1764[c]	Placebo N=424-1036[c]	FluMist N=2170[c]	Active Control[b] N=2165[c]
Event	%	%	%	%
Runny Nose/Nasal Congestion	58	50	51	42
Decreased Appetite	21	17	13	12
Irritability	21	19	12	11
Decreased Activity (Lethargy)	14	11	7	6
Sore Throat	11	9	5	6
Headache	9	7	3	3
Muscle Aches	6	3	2	2
Chills	4	3	2	2
Fever				
100-101°F Oral	9	6	6	4
101-102°F Oral	4	3	4	3

[a] Frozen formulation used in AV006; Refrigerated formulation used in D153-P501 and MI-CP111.

[b] Injectable influenza vaccine

[c] Number of evaluable subjects (those who returned diary cards) for each event. Range reflects differences in data collection between the 2 pooled studies.

In clinical studies D153-P501 and AV006, other adverse reactions in children occurring in at least 1% of FluMist recipients and at a higher rate compared to placebo were: abdominal pain (2% FluMist vs. 0% placebo) and otitis media (3% FluMist vs. 1% placebo).

An additional adverse reaction identified in the active-controlled trial, MI-CP111, occurring in at least 1% of FluMist recipients and at a higher rate compared to active control was sneezing (2% FluMist vs. 1% active control).

In a separate trial (MI-CP112) that compared the refrigerated and frozen formulations of FluMist in children and adults ages 5-49 years of age, the solicited events and other adverse events were consistent with observations from previous trials. Fever of >103°F was observed in 1 to 2% of children 5-8 years of age.

In a separate placebo-controlled trial (D153-P526) using the refrigerated formulation in a subset of older children and adolescents 9-17 years of age who received one dose of FluMist, the solicited events and other adverse events were generally consistent with observations from previous trials. Abdominal pain was reported in 12% of FluMist recipients compared to 4% of placebo recipients and decreased activity was reported in 6% of FluMist recipients compared to 0% of placebo recipients.

Adverse Reactions in Adults

In adults 18-49 years of age in Study AV009, summary of solicited adverse events occurring in at least 1% of FluMist recipients and at a higher rate compared to placebo include runny nose (44% FluMist vs. 27% placebo), headache (40% FluMist vs. 38% placebo), sore throat (28% FluMist vs. 17% placebo), tiredness/weakness (26% FluMist vs. 22% placebo), muscle aches (17% FluMist vs. 15% placebo), cough (14% FluMist vs. 11% placebo), and chills (9% FluMist vs. 6% placebo).

In addition to the solicited events, other adverse reactions from Study AV009 occurring in at least 1% of FluMist recipients and at a higher rate compared to placebo were: nasal congestion (9% FluMist vs. 2% placebo) and sinusitis (4% FluMist vs. 2% placebo).

6.2 Postmarketing Experience

The following adverse reactions have been identified during postapproval use of FluMist. Because these reactions are reported voluntarily from a population of uncertain size, it is not always possible to reliably estimate their frequency or establish a causal relationship to vaccine exposure.

Gastrointestinal disorders: Nausea, vomiting, diarrhea

Immune system disorders: Hypersensitivity reactions (including anaphylactic reaction, facial edema and urticaria)

Nervous system disorders: Guillain-Barré syndrome, Bell's Palsy

Respiratory, thoracic and mediastinal disorders: Epistaxis

Skin and subcutaneous tissue disorders: Rash

7 DRUG INTERACTIONS

7.1 Aspirin Therapy

Do not administer FluMist to children or adolescents who are receiving aspirin therapy or aspirin-containing therapy *[see Contraindications (4.2)]*.

7.2 Antiviral Agents Against Influenza A and/or B

The concurrent use of FluMist with antiviral agents that are active against influenza A and/or B viruses has not been evaluated. However, based upon the potential for antiviral agents to reduce the effectiveness of FluMist, do not administer FluMist until 48 hours after the cessation of antiviral therapy and antiviral agents should not be administered until two weeks after administration of FluMist unless medically indicated. If antiviral agents and FluMist are administered concomitantly, revaccination should be considered when appropriate.

7.3 Concomitant Inactivated Vaccines

The safety and immunogenicity of FluMist when administered concurrently with inactivated vaccines have not been determined. Studies of FluMist excluded subjects who received any inactivated or subunit vaccine within two weeks of enrollment. Therefore, healthcare providers should consider the risks and benefits of concurrent administration of FluMist with inactivated vaccines.

7.4 Concomitant Live Vaccines

Concurrent administration of FluMist with the measles, mumps and rubella vaccine and the varicella vaccine was studied in 1245 children 12-15 months of age. Adverse events were similar to those seen in other clinical trials with FluMist [see *Adverse Reactions* (6.1)]. No evidence of interference with immune responses to measles, mumps, rubella, varicella and FluMist vaccines was observed. The safety and immunogenicity in children >15 months of age have not been studied.

7.5 Intranasal Products

There are no data regarding co-administration of FluMist with other intranasal preparations.

8 USE IN SPECIFIC POPULATIONS

8.1 Pregnancy

Pregnancy Category C

Animal reproduction studies have not been conducted with FluMist. It is not known whether FluMist can cause fetal harm when administered to a pregnant woman or can affect reproduction capacity. FluMist should be given to a pregnant woman only if clearly needed.

The effect of the vaccine on embryo-fetal and pre-weaning development was evaluated in a developmental toxicity study using pregnant rats receiving the frozen formulation. Groups of animals were administered the vaccine either once (during the period of organogenesis on gestation day 6) or twice (prior to gestation and during the period of organogenesis on gestation day 6), 250mcL/rat/occasion (approximately 110-140 human dose equivalents based on $TCID_{50}$), by intranasal instillation. No adverse effects on pregnancy, parturition, lactation, embryo-fetal or pre-weaning development were observed. There were no vaccine related fetal malformations or other evidence of teratogenesis noted in this study.

8.3 Nursing Mothers

It is not known whether FluMist is excreted in human milk. Therefore, as some viruses are excreted in human milk and additionally, because of the possibility of shedding of vaccine virus and the close proximity of a nursing infant and mother, caution should be exercised if FluMist is administered to nursing mothers.

8.4 Pediatric Use

FluMist is not indicated for use in children <24 months of age. FluMist use in children <24 months has been associated with increased risk of hospitalization and wheezing in clinical trials *[see Warnings and Precautions (5.1)* and *Adverse Reactions (6.1)]*.

8.5 Geriatric Use

FluMist is not indicated for use in individuals ≥65 years of age. Subjects with underlying high-risk medical conditions (n=200) were studied for safety. Compared to controls, FluMist recipients had a higher rate of sore throat.

8.6 Use in Individuals 50-64 Years of Age

FluMist is not indicated for use in individuals 50-64 years of age. In Study AV009, effectiveness was not demonstrated in individuals 50-64 years of age (n=641). Solicited adverse events were similar in type and frequency to those reported in younger adults.

11 DESCRIPTION

FluMist (Influenza Virus Vaccine Live, Intranasal) is a live trivalent vaccine for administration by intranasal spray. The influenza virus strains in FluMist are (a) *cold-adapted (ca)* (i.e., they replicate efficiently at 25°C, a temperature that is restrictive for replication of many wild-type influenza viruses); (b) *temperature-sensitive (ts)* (i.e., they are restricted in replication at 37°C (Type B strains) or 39°C (Type A strains), temperatures at which many wild-type influenza viruses grow efficiently); and (c) *attenuated (att)* (they do not produce classic influenza-like illness in the ferret model of human influenza infection). The cumulative effect of the antigenic properties and the *ca, ts,* and *att* phenotypes is that the attenuated vaccine viruses replicate in the nasopharynx to induce protective immunity.

No evidence of reversion has been observed in the recovered vaccine strains that have been tested (135 of possible 250 recovered isolates) *[see Clinical Studies (14.5)]*. For each of the three reassortant strains in FluMist, the six internal gene segments responsible for *ca, ts,* and *att* phenotypes are derived from a master donor virus (MDV), and the two segments that encode the two surface glycoproteins, hemagglutinin (HA) and neuraminidase (NA), are derived from the corresponding antigenically relevant wild-type influenza viruses that have been recommended by the USPHS for inclusion in the annual vaccine formulation. Thus, the three viruses contained in FluMist maintain the replication characteristics and phenotypic properties of the MDV and express the HA and NA of wild-type viruses that are related to strains expected to circulate during the 2007-2008 influenza season. For the Type A MDV, at least five genetic loci in three different internal gene segments contribute to the *ts* and *att* phenotypes. For the Type B MDV, at least three genetic loci in two different internal gene segments contribute to both the *ts* and *att* properties; five genetic loci in three gene segments control the *ca* property.

Specific pathogen-free (SPF) eggs are inoculated with each of the reassortant strains and incubated to allow vaccine virus replication. The allantoic fluid of these eggs is harvested, pooled and then clarified by filtration. The virus is concentrated by ultracentrifugation and diluted with stabilizing buffer to obtain the final sucrose and potassium phosphate concentrations. In addition, ethylene diamine tetracetic acid (EDTA) is added to the dilution buffer for H3N2 strains. The viral harvests are then sterile filtered to produce the monovalent bulks. Each lot is tested for *ca, ts,* and *att* phenotypes and is also tested extensively by *in vitro* and *in vivo* methods to detect adventitious agents. Monovalent bulks from the three strains are subsequently blended and diluted as required to attain the desired potency with stabilizing buffers to produce the trivalent bulk vaccine. The bulk vaccine is then filled directly into individual sprayers for nasal administration.

Each pre-filled refrigerated FluMist sprayer contains a single 0.2 mL dose. Each 0.2 mL dose contains $10^{6.5-7.5}$ FFU of live attenuated influenza virus reassortants of each of the three strains: A/Solomon Islands/3/2006 (H1N1), A/Wisconsin/67/2005 (H3N2), and B/Malaysia/2506/2004 [1]. Each 0.2 mL dose also contains 0.188 mg/dose monosodium glutamate, 2.00 mg/dose hydrolyzed porcine gelatin, 2.42 mg/dose arginine, 13.68 mg/dose sucrose, 2.26 mg/dose dibasic potassium phosphate, 0.96 mg/dose monosodium phosphate, and <0.015 mcg/mL gentamicin sulfate. FluMist contains no preservatives.

The tip attached to the sprayer is equipped with a nozzle that produces a fine mist that is primarily deposited in the nose and nasopharynx. FluMist is a colorless to pale yellow liquid and is clear to slightly cloudy.

12 CLINICAL PHARMACOLOGY

12.1 Mechanism of Action

Immune mechanisms conferring protection against influenza following receipt of FluMist vaccine are not fully understood. Likewise, naturally acquired immunity to wild-type influenza has not been completely elucidated. Serum antibodies, mucosal antibodies and influenza-specific T cells may play a role in prevention and recovery from infection.

Influenza illness and its complications follow infection with influenza viruses. Global surveillance of influenza identifies yearly antigenic variants. For example, since 1977, antigenic variants of influenza A (H1N1 and H3N2) viruses and influenza B viruses have been in global circulation. Antibody against one influenza virus type or subtype confers limited or no protection against another. Furthermore, antibody to one antigenic variant of influenza virus might not protect against a new antigenic variant of the same type or subtype. Frequent development of antigenic variants through antigenic drift is the virologic basis for seasonal epidemics and the reason for the usual change of one or more new strains in each year's influenza vaccine. Therefore, influenza vaccines are standardized to contain the strains (i.e., typically two type A and one type B), representing the influenza viruses likely to be circulating in the United States in the upcoming winter.

Annual revaccination with the current vaccine is recommended because immunity declines during the year after vaccination, and because circulating strains of influenza virus change from year to year.

Continued on next page

FluMist—Cont.

12.2 Biodistribution

A biodistribution study of intranasally administered radio-labeled placebo was conducted in 7 healthy adult volunteers. The mean percentage of the delivered doses detected were as follows: nasal cavity 89.7%, stomach 2.6%, brain 2.4%, and lung 0.4%. The clinical significance of these findings is unknown.

13 NONCLINICAL TOXICOLOGY

13.1 Carcinogenesis, Mutagenesis, Impairment of Fertility

FluMist has not been evaluated for its carcinogenic or mutagenic potential or its potential to impair fertility.

14 CLINICAL STUDIES

FluMist, in refrigerated and frozen formulations, was administered to approximately 35,000 subjects in controlled clinical studies. FluMist has been studied in placebo-controlled trials over multiple years, using different vaccine strains. Comparative efficacy has been studied where FluMist was compared to an inactivated influenza vaccine.

14.1 Studies in Children and Adolescents

Study MI-CP111: Pediatric Comparative Study

A multinational, randomized, double-blind, active-controlled trial (MI-CP111) was performed to assess the efficacy and safety of FluMist compared to an injectable influenza vaccine (active control) in children <5 years of age, using the refrigerated formulation. During the 2004-2005 influenza season, a total number of 3916 children <5 years of age and without severe asthma, without use of bronchodilator or steroids and without wheezing within the prior 6 weeks were randomized to FluMist and 3936 were randomized to active control. Participants were then followed through the influenza season to identify illness caused by influenza virus. As the primary endpoint, culture-confirmed modified CDC-ILI (CDC-defined influenza-like illness) was defined as a positive culture for a wild-type influenza virus associated within ±7 days of modified CDC-ILI. Modified CDC-ILI was defined as fever (temperature ≥100°F oral or equivalent) plus cough, sore throat, or runny nose/nasal congestion on the same or consecutive days.

In the primary efficacy analysis, FluMist demonstrated a 44.5% (95%CI: 22.4, 60.6) reduction in influenza rate compared to active control as measured by culture-confirmed modified CDC-ILI caused by wild-type strains antigenically similar to those contained in the vaccine. See Table 3 for a description of the results by strain and antigenic similarity. [See table 3 above]

Study D153-P501: Pediatric Study

A randomized, double-blind, placebo-controlled trial (D153-P501) was performed to evaluate the efficacy of FluMist in children 12 to 35 months of age without high-risk medical conditions against culture-confirmed influenza illness, using the refrigerated formulation. A total of 3174 children were randomized 3:2 (vaccine:placebo) to receive 2 doses of study vaccine or placebo at least 28 days apart in Year 1. See Table 4 for a description of the results.

Study AV006: Pediatric Study

AV006 was a multi-center, randomized, double-blind, placebo-controlled trial performed in U.S. children without high-risk medical conditions to evaluate the efficacy of FluMist against culture-confirmed influenza over two successive seasons using the frozen formulation. The primary endpoint of the trial was the prevention of culture-confirmed influenza illness due to antigenically matched wild-type influenza in children, who received two doses of vaccine in the first year and a single revaccination dose in the second year. During the first year of the study 1602 children 15-71 months of age were randomized 2:1 (vaccine:placebo). Approximately 85% of the participants in the first year returned for the second year of the study. In Year 2, children remained in the same treatment group as in year one and received a single dose of FluMist or placebo. See Table 4 for a description of the results. [See table 4 above]

During the second year of Study AV006, the primary circulating strain was the A/Sydney/05/97 H3N2 strain, which was antigenically dissimilar from the H3N2 strain represented in the vaccine, A/Wuhan/359/95; FluMist demonstrated 87.0% (95% CI: 77.0, 92.6) efficacy against culture-confirmed influenza illness.

14.2 Study in Adults

AV009 was a multi-center, randomized, double-blind, placebo-controlled trial to evaluate effectiveness in adults 18-64 years of age without high-risk medical conditions. Participants were randomized 2:1, vaccine:placebo. Cultures for influenza virus were not obtained from subjects in the trial, so that the efficacy against culture-confirmed influenza was not assessed. The A/Wuhan/359/95 (H3N2) strain, which was contained in FluMist, was antigenically distinct from the predominant circulating strain of influenza virus during the trial period, A/Sydney/05/97 (H3N2). Type A/Wuhan (H3N2) and Type B strains also circulated in the U.S. during the study period. The primary endpoint of the trial was the reduction in the proportion of participants with one or more episodes of any febrile illness and prospective secondary endpoints were severe febrile illness, and febrile upper respiratory illness. Effectiveness for any of the three endpoints was not demonstrated in a subgroup of adults 50-64 years of age. Primary and secondary effectiveness endpoints from the age group 18-49 years of age are presented in Table 5. Effectiveness was not demonstrated for the primary endpoint in adults 18-49 years of age. [See table 5 above]

Effectiveness was shown in a post-hoc analysis using CDC-ILI in the age group 18-49 years.

14.3 Study in Adults with Human Immunodeficiency Virus (HIV) Infection

Safety and shedding of vaccine virus following FluMist administration were evaluated in 57 HIV-infected [median CD4 cell count of 541 cells/mm³] and 54 HIV-negative adults 18-58 years of age in a randomized, double-blind, placebo controlled trial using the frozen formulation. No serious adverse events were reported during the one-month follow-up period. Vaccine strain (type B) virus was detected in 1 of 28 HIV-infected subjects on Day 5 only and none of the HIV-negative FluMist recipients. No adverse effects on HIV viral load or CD4 counts were identified following FluMist. The effectiveness of FluMist in preventing influenza illness in HIV-infected individuals has not been evaluated.

14.4 Refrigerated Formulation Study

A double-blind, randomized multi-center trial was conducted to evaluate the comparative immunogenicity and safety of refrigerated and frozen formulations of FluMist in individuals 5 to 49 years of age without high risk medical conditions. Nine hundred and eighty-one subjects were randomized at a 1:1 ratio to receive either vaccine formulation. Subjects 5-8 years of age received two doses of study vaccine 46-60 days apart; subjects 9-49 years of age received one dose of study vaccine. The study met its primary endpoint. The GMT ratios of refrigerated and frozen formulations (adjusted for baseline serostatus) for H1N1, H3N2 and B strains, respectively, were 1.24, 1.02 and 1.00 in the two dose group and 1.14, 1.12 and 0.96 in the one dose group.

14.5 Transmission Study

FluMist contains live attenuated influenza viruses that must infect and replicate in cells lining the nasopharynx of the recipient to induce immunity. Vaccine viruses capable of infection and replication can be cultured from nasal secretions obtained from vaccine recipients. The relationship of viral replication in a vaccine recipient and transmission of vaccine viruses to other individuals has not been established.

Using the frozen formulation, a prospective, randomized, double-blind, placebo-controlled trial was performed in a daycare setting in children <3 years of age to assess the transmission of vaccine viruses from a vaccinated individual to a non-vaccinated individual. A total of 197 children 8-36 months of age were randomized to receive one dose of FluMist (n=98) or placebo (n=99). Virus shedding was eval-

---

Table 3
Comparative Efficacy against Culture-Confirmed Modified CDC-ILI[a] Caused by Wild-Type Strains in Children <5 Years of Age

	FluMist			Active Control[b]			% Reduction in Rate for FluMist[c]	95% CI
	N	# of Cases	Rate (cases/N)	N	# of Cases	Rate (cases/N)		
Matched Strains								
All strains	3916	53	1.4%	3936	93	2.4%	44.5%	22.4, 60.6
A/H1N1	3916	3	0.1%	3936	27	0.7%	89.2%	67.7, 97.4
A/H3N2	3916	0	0.0%	3936	0	0.0%	—	
B	3916	50	1.3%	3936	67	1.7%	27.3%	-4.8, 49.9
Mismatched Strains								
All strains	3916	102	2.6%	3936	245	6.2%	58.2%	47.4, 67.0
A/H1N1	3916	0	0.0%	3936	0	0.0%	—	
A/H3N2	3916	37	0.9%	3936	178	4.5%	79.2%	70.6, 85.7
B	3916	66	1.7%	3936	71	1.8%	6.3%	-31.6, 33.3
Regardless of Match								
All strains	3916	153	3.9%	3936	338	8.6%	54.9%	45.4, 62.9
A/H1N1	3916	3	0.1%	3936	27	0.7%	89.2%	67.7, 97.4
A/H3N2	3916	37	0.9%	3936	178	4.5%	79.2%	70.6, 85.7
B	3916	115	2.9%	3936	136	3.5%	16.1%	-7.7, 34.7

ATP Population.
[a] Modified CDC-ILI was defined as fever (temperature ≥100°F oral or equivalent) plus cough, sore throat, or runny nose/nasal congestion on the same or consecutive days.
[b] Injectable influenza vaccine.
[c] Reduction in rate was adjusted for country, age, prior influenza vaccination status, and wheezing history status.

Table 4
D153-P501 & AV006, Years 1[a]: Efficacy of FluMist vs. Placebo against Culture-Confirmed Influenza Illness due to Wild-Type Strains

	D153-P501			AV006		
	FluMist n[b] (%)	Placebo n[b] (%)	% Efficacy (95% CI)	FluMist n[b] (%)	Placebo n[b] (%)	% Efficacy (95% CI)
	N[c]=1653	N[c]=1111		N[c]=849	N[c]=410	
Any strain	56 (3.4%)	139 (12.5%)	72.9%[d] (62.8, 80.5)	10 (1%)	73 (18%)	93.4% (87.5, 96.5)
A/H1N1	23 (1.4%)	81 (7.3%)	80.9% (69.4, 88.5)[e]	0	0	—
A/H3N2	4 (0.2%)	27 (2.4%)	90.0% (71.4, 97.5)	4 (0.5%)	48 (12%)	96.0% (89.4, 98.5)
B	29 (1.8%)	35 (3.2%)	44.3% (6.2, 67.2)	6 (0.7%)	31 (7%)	90.5% (78.0, 95.9)

[a] D153-P501 and AV006 data are for subjects who received two doses of study vaccine.
[b] Number and percent of subjects in per-protocol efficacy analysis population with culture-confirmed influenza illness.
[c] Number of subjects in per-protocol efficacy analysis population of each treatment group of each study for the "any strain" analysis.
[d] For D153-P501, influenza circulated through 12 months following vaccination.
[e] Estimate includes A/H1N1 and A/H1N2 strains. Both were considered antigenically similar to the vaccine.

Table 5
Effectiveness of FluMist[a] in Adults 18-49 Years of Age During the 7-week Site-Specific Outbreak Period

Endpoint	FluMist N=2411[b] n (%)	Placebo N=1226[b] n (%)	Percent Reduction	(95% CI)
Participants with one or more events of:[c]				
Primary Endpoint:				
Any febrile illness	331 (13.73)	189 (15.42)	10.9	(-5.1, 24.4)
Secondary Endpoints:				
Severe febrile illness	250 (10.37)	158 (12.89)	19.5	(3.0, 33.2)
Febrile upper respiratory illness	213 (8.83)	142 (11.58)	23.7	(6.7, 37.5)

[a] Frozen formulation used.
[b] Number of evaluable subjects (92.7% and 93.0% of FluMist and placebo recipients, respectively).
[c] The predominantly circulating virus during the trial period was A/Sydney/05/97 (H3N2), an antigenic variant not included in the vaccine.

uated for 21 days by culture of nasal swab specimens. Wild-type A (H3N2) influenza virus was documented to have circulated in the community and in the study population during the trial, whereas Type A (H1N1) and Type B strains did not.

At least one vaccine strain was isolated from 80% of FluMist recipients; strains were recovered from 1-21 days post vaccination (mean duration of 7.6 days ± 3.4 days). The cold-adapted *(ca)* and temperature-sensitive *(ts)* phenotypes were preserved in 135 tested of 250 strains isolated at the local laboratory. Ten influenza isolates (9 influenza A, 1 influenza B) were cultured from a total of seven placebo subjects. One placebo subject had mild symptomatic Type B virus infection confirmed as a transmitted vaccine virus by a FluMist recipient in the same playgroup. This Type B isolate retained the *ca*, *ts*, and *att* phenotypes of the vaccine strain, and had the same genetic sequence when compared to a Type B virus cultured from a vaccine recipient within the same playgroup. Four of the influenza Type A isolates were confirmed as wild-type A/Panama (H3N2). The remaining isolates could not be further characterized.
Assuming a single transmission event (isolation of the Type B vaccine strain), the probability of a young child acquiring vaccine virus following close contact with a single FluMist vaccinee in this daycare setting was 0.58% (95% CI: 0, 1.7) based on the Reed-Frost model. With documented transmission of one Type B in one placebo subject and possible transmission of Type A viruses in four placebo subjects, the probability of acquiring a transmitted vaccine virus was estimated to be 2.4% (95% CI: 0.13, 4.6), using the Reed-Frost model.
The duration of FluMist vaccine virus replication and shedding have not been established.

15 REFERENCES
1. Centers for Disease Control and Prevention. Prevention and Control of Influenza: Recommendations of the Advisory Committee on Immunization Practices (ACIP). *MMWR* 2006;55(RR-10):1-42.

16 HOW SUPPLIED/STORAGE AND HANDLING
FluMist is supplied for intranasal delivery in a package of 10 pre-filled, single-use sprayers. NDC 66019-105-01
Storage and Handling
Once FluMist has been administered, the sprayer should be disposed of according to the standard procedures for medical waste (e.g., sharps container or biohazard container).
FLUMIST SHOULD BE STORED IN A REFRIGERATOR BETWEEN 2-8°C (35-46°F) UPON RECEIPT AND UNTIL USE BEFORE THE EXPIRATION DATE ON THE SPRAYER LABEL. DO NOT FREEZE.
The cold chain (2 to 8°C) must be maintained when transporting FluMist.

17 PATIENT COUNSELING INFORMATION
Vaccine recipients or their parents/guardians should be informed by the health care provider of the potential benefits and risks of FluMist, and the need for two doses at least 1 month apart in children 2-8 years old who have not previously received influenza vaccine.
17.1 Asthma and Recurrent Wheezing
Ask the vaccinee or their parent/guardian if the vaccinee has asthma. For children <5 years of age, also ask if the vaccinee has recurrent wheezing since this may be an asthma equivalent in this age group.
17.2 Vaccination with a Live Virus Vaccine
Vaccine recipients or their parents/guardians should be informed by the health care provider that FluMist is an attenuated live virus vaccine and has the potential for transmission to immunocompromised household contacts.
17.3 Adverse Event Reporting
The vaccine recipient or the parent/guardian accompanying the vaccine recipient should be told to report any suspected adverse events to the physician or clinic where the vaccine was administered.
FluMist® is a registered trademark of MedImmune Vaccines, Inc.
Manufactured by:
MedImmune Vaccines, Inc.
Gaithersburg, MD 20878
For other product information regarding FluMist, call 1-877-FLUMIST (358-6478).
Issue Date: September 2007   RAL-FLUV7
U.S. Government License No. 1652

To keep your **PDR** up to date
throughout the year, note these revisions
on the corresponding pages of the annual
volume. Simply write **"See Supplement A"**
next to the product heading.

Merck & Co., Inc.
PO BOX 4 WP39-206
WEST POINT, PA 19486-0004

For Medical Information Contact:
Generally:
Product and service information:
Call the Merck National Service Center, 8:00 AM to 7:00 PM (ET), Monday through Friday:
(800) NSC-MERCK
(800) 672-6372
FAX: (800) MERCK-68
FAX: (800) 637-2568
Adverse Drug Experiences:
Call the Merck National Service Center, 8:00 AM to 7:00 PM (ET), Monday through Friday:
(800) NSC-MERCK
(800) 672-6372
Pregnancy Registries
(800) 986-8999
In Emergencies:
24-hour emergency information for healthcare professionals:
(800) NSC-MERCK
(800) 672-6372
Sales and Ordering:
For product orders and direct account inquiries only, call the Order Management Center,
8:00 AM to 7:00 PM (ET), Monday through Friday:
(800) MERCK RX
(800) 637-2579

EMEND®   ℞
[ē'mĕnd]
(fosaprepitant dimeglumine)
for Injection

DESCRIPTION
EMEND[1] (fosaprepitant dimeglumine) for Injection is a sterile, lyophilized prodrug of aprepitant and is chemically described as 1-Deoxy-1-(methylamino)-D-glucitol [3-[[(2R,3S)-2-[(1R)-1-[3,5-bis(trifluoromethyl)phenyl]ethoxy]-3-(4-fluorophenyl)-4-morpholinyl]methyl]-2,5-dihydro-5-oxo-1H-1,2,4-triazol-1-yl]phosphonate (2:1) (salt).
Its empirical formula is $C_{23}H_{22}F_7N_4O_6P \cdot 2(C_7H_{17}NO_5)$ and its structural formula is:

Fosaprepitant dimeglumine is a white to off-white amorphous powder with a molecular weight of 1004.83. It is freely soluble in water.
EMEND for Injection is a lyophilized prodrug of aprepitant containing polysorbate 80 (PS80), to be administered intravenously as an infusion.
Each vial of EMEND for Injection for intravenous administration contains 188 mg of fosaprepitant dimeglumine equivalent to 115 mg of fosaprepitant and the following inactive ingredients: edetate disodium (14.4 mg), polysorbate 80 (57.5 mg), lactose anhydrous (287.5 mg), sodium hydroxide and/or hydrochloric acid (for pH adjustment). Fosaprepitant dimeglumine hereafter will be referred to as fosaprepitant.
Aprepitant is a substance P/neurokinin 1 (NK₁) receptor antagonist, chemically described as 5-[[(2R,3S)-2-[(1R)-1-[3,5-bis(trifluoromethyl)phenyl]ethoxy]-3-(4-fluorophenyl)-4-morpholinyl]methyl]-1,2-dihydro-3H-1,2,4-triazol-3-one.
Its empirical formula is $C_{23}H_{21}F_7N_4O_3$, and its structural formula is:

CLINICAL PHARMACOLOGY
Fosaprepitant, a prodrug of aprepitant, when administered intravenously is rapidly converted to aprepitant, a substance P/neurokinin 1 (NK1) receptor antagonist. Plasma concentrations of fosaprepitant are below the limits of quantification (10 ng/mL) within 30 minutes of the completion of infusion (see CLINICAL PHARMACOLOGY, *Pharmacokinetics*). Upon conversion of 115 mg of fosaprepitant to aprepitant, 18.3 mg of phosphate and 73 mg of meglumine are liberated from fosaprepitant.

Mechanism of Action
Fosaprepitant is a prodrug of aprepitant and accordingly, its antiemetic effects are attributable to aprepitant.
Aprepitant is a selective high-affinity antagonist of human substance P/neurokinin 1 (NK₁) receptors. Aprepitant has little or no affinity for serotonin (5-HT₃), dopamine, and corticosteroid receptors, the targets of existing therapies for chemotherapy-induced nausea and vomiting (CINV). Aprepitant has been shown in animal models to inhibit emesis induced by cytotoxic chemotherapeutic agents, such as cisplatin, via central actions. Animal and human Positron Emission Tomography (PET) studies with aprepitant have shown that it crosses the blood brain barrier and occupies brain NK₁ receptors. Animal and human studies show that aprepitant augments the antiemetic activity of the 5-HT₃-receptor antagonist ondansetron and the corticosteroid dexamethasone and inhibits both the acute and delayed phases of cisplatin-induced emesis.
Pharmacokinetics
Aprepitant after Fosaprepitant Administration
Following a single intravenous dose of fosaprepitant administered as a 15-minute infusion to healthy volunteers the mean AUC₀₋∞ of aprepitant was 31.7 (± 14.3) mcg•hr/mL and the mean maximal aprepitant concentration (Cₘₐₓ) was 3.27 (± 1.16) mcg/mL. The mean aprepitant plasma concentration at 24 hours postdose was similar between the 125-mg oral aprepitant dose and the 115-mg intravenous fosaprepitant dose (See Figure 1).

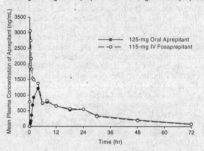

Figure 1: Mean Plasma Concentration of Aprepitant Following 125-mg Oral Aprepitant and 115-mg I.V. Fosaprepitant

Distribution
Fosaprepitant is rapidly converted to aprepitant. Aprepitant is greater than 95% bound to plasma proteins. The mean apparent volume of distribution at steady state (Vd₍ss₎) is approximately 70 L in humans.
Aprepitant crosses the placenta in rats and rabbits and crosses the blood brain barrier in humans (see CLINICAL PHARMACOLOGY, *Mechanism of Action*).
Metabolism
Fosaprepitant was rapidly converted to aprepitant in *in vitro* incubations with liver preparations from nonclinical species (rat and dog) and humans. Furthermore, fosaprepitant underwent rapid and nearly complete conversion to aprepitant in S9 preparations from multiple other human tissues including kidney, lung and ileum. Thus, it appears that the conversion of fosaprepitant to aprepitant can occur in multiple extrahepatic tissues in addition to the liver. In humans, fosaprepitant administered intravenously was rapidly converted to aprepitant within 30 minutes following the end of infusion.
Aprepitant undergoes extensive metabolism. *In vitro* studies using human liver microsomes indicate that aprepitant is metabolized primarily by CYP3A4 with minor metabolism by CYP1A2 and CYP2C19. Metabolism is largely via oxidation at the morpholine ring and its side chains. No metabolism by CYP2D6, CYP2C9, or CYP2E1 was detected. In healthy young adults, aprepitant accounts for approximately 24% of the radioactivity in plasma over 72 hours following a single oral 300-mg dose of [¹⁴C]-aprepitant, indicating a substantial presence of metabolites in the plasma. Seven metabolites of aprepitant, which are only weakly active, have been identified in human plasma.
Excretion
Following administration of a single I.V. 100-mg dose of [¹⁴C]-fosaprepitant to healthy subjects, 57% of the radioactivity was recovered in urine and 45% in feces.
Aprepitant is eliminated primarily by metabolism; aprepitant is not renally excreted. The apparent terminal half-life of aprepitant ranged from approximately 9 to 13 hours.
Special Populations
Fosaprepitant, a prodrug of aprepitant, when administered intravenously is rapidly converted to aprepitant.
Gender
Following oral administration of a single 125-mg dose of aprepitant, no difference in AUC₀₋₂₄ₕᵣ was observed between males and females. The Cₘₐₓ for aprepitant is 16% higher in females as compared with males. The half-life of aprepitant is 25% lower in females as compared with males and Tₘₐₓ occurs at approximately the same time. These differences are not considered clinically meaningful. No dosage adjustment is necessary based on gender.

Continued on next page

Emend Injection—Cont.

Geriatric

Following oral administration of a single 125-mg dose of aprepitant on Day 1 and 80 mg once daily on Days 2 through 5, the AUC_{0-24hr} of aprepitant was 21% higher on Day 1 and 36% higher on Day 5 in elderly ($\geq$65 years) relative to younger adults. The C_{max} was 10% higher on Day 1 and 24% higher on Day 5 in elderly relative to younger adults. These differences are not considered clinically meaningful. No dosage adjustment is necessary in elderly patients.

Pediatric

Fosaprepitant has not been evaluated in patients below 18 years of age.

Race

Following oral administration of a single 125-mg dose of aprepitant, the AUC_{0-24hr} is approximately 25% and 29% higher in Hispanics as compared with Whites and Blacks, respectively. The C_{max} is 22% and 31% higher in Hispanics as compared with Whites and Blacks, respectively. These differences are not considered clinically meaningful. There was no difference in AUC_{0-24hr} or C_{max} between Whites and Blacks. No dosage adjustment is necessary based on race.

Hepatic Insufficiency

Fosaprepitant is metabolized in various extrahepatic tissues; therefore hepatic insufficiency is not expected to alter the conversion of fosaprepitant to aprepitant.

Oral aprepitant was well tolerated in patients with mild to moderate hepatic insufficiency. Following administration of a single 125-mg dose of oral aprepitant on Day 1 and 80 mg once daily on Days 2 and 3 to patients with mild hepatic insufficiency (Child-Pugh score 5 to 6), the AUC_{0-24hr} of aprepitant was 11% lower on Day 1 and 36% lower on Day 3, as compared with healthy subjects given the same regimen. In patients with moderate hepatic insufficiency (Child-Pugh score 7 to 9), the AUC_{0-24hr} of aprepitant was 10% higher on Day 1 and 18% higher on Day 3, as compared with healthy subjects given the same regimen. These differences in AUC_{0-24hr} are not considered clinically meaningful; therefore, no dosage adjustment is necessary in patients with mild to moderate hepatic insufficiency.

There are no clinical or pharmacokinetic data in patients with severe hepatic insufficiency (Child-Pugh score >9) (see PRECAUTIONS).

Renal Insufficiency

A single 240-mg dose of oral aprepitant was administered to patients with severe renal insufficiency (CrCl<30 mL/min) and to patients with end stage renal disease (ESRD) requiring hemodialysis.

In patients with severe renal insufficiency, the $AUC_{0-\infty}$ of total aprepitant (unbound and protein bound) decreased by 21% and C_{max} decreased by 32%, relative to healthy subjects. In patients with ESRD undergoing hemodialysis, the $AUC_{0-\infty}$ of total aprepitant decreased by 42% and C_{max} decreased by 32%. Due to modest decreases in protein binding of aprepitant in patients with renal disease, the AUC of pharmacologically active unbound drug was not significantly affected in patients with renal insufficiency compared with healthy subjects. Hemodialysis conducted 4 or 48 hours after dosing had no significant effect on the pharmacokinetics of aprepitant; less than 0.2% of the dose was recovered in the dialysate.

No dosage adjustment is necessary for patients with renal insufficiency or for patients with ESRD undergoing hemodialysis.

Pharmacodynamics

Cardiac Electrophysiology

In a randomized, double-blind, positive-controlled, thorough QTc study, a single 200-mg dose of fosaprepitant had no effect on the QTc interval.

Clinical Studies

Fosaprepitant, a prodrug of aprepitant, when administered intravenously is rapidly converted to aprepitant. Fosaprepitant 115 mg I.V. infused over 15 minutes can be substituted for 125 mg oral aprepitant on Day 1 (see DOSAGE AND ADMINISTRATION). Pivotal efficacy studies were conducted with oral aprepitant.

Oral administration of aprepitant in combination with ondansetron and dexamethasone (aprepitant regimen) has been shown to prevent acute and delayed nausea and vomiting associated with highly emetogenic chemotherapy including high-dose cisplatin, and nausea and vomiting associated with moderately emetogenic chemotherapy.

Highly Emetogenic Chemotherapy

In 2 multicenter, randomized, parallel, double-blind, controlled clinical studies, the aprepitant regimen (see table below) was compared with standard therapy in patients receiving a chemotherapy regimen that included cisplatin >50 mg/m^2 (mean cisplatin dose = 80.2 mg/m^2). Of the 550 patients who were randomized to receive the aprepitant regimen, 42% were women, 58% men, 59% White, 5% Asian, 5% Black, 12% Hispanic American, and 21% Multi-Racial. The aprepitant-treated patients in these clinical studies ranged from 14 to 84 years of age, with a mean age of 56 years. 170 patients were 65 years or older, with 29 patients being 75 years or older.

Patients (N = 1105) were randomized to either the aprepitant regimen (N = 550) or standard therapy (N = 555). The treatment regimens are defined in the table below.

[See first table above]

During these studies 95% of the patients in the aprepitant group received a concomitant chemotherapeutic agent in addition to protocol-mandated cisplatin. The most common chemotherapeutic agents and the number of aprepitant patients exposed follow: etoposide (106), fluorouracil (100), gemcitabine (89), vinorelbine (82), paclitaxel (52), cyclophosphamide (50), doxorubicin (38), docetaxel (11).

The antiemetic activity of oral aprepitant was evaluated during the acute phase (0 to 24 hours post-cisplatin treatment), the delayed phase (25 to 120 hours post-cisplatin treatment) and overall (0 to 120 hours post-cisplatin treatment) in Cycle 1. Efficacy was based on evaluation of the following endpoints:

Primary endpoint:

- complete response (defined as no emetic episodes and no use of rescue therapy)

Other prespecified endpoints:

- complete protection (defined as no emetic episodes, no use of rescue therapy, and a maximum nausea visual analogue scale [VAS] score <25 mm on a 0 to 100 mm scale)
- no emesis (defined as no emetic episodes regardless of use of rescue therapy)
- no nausea (maximum VAS <5 mm on a 0 to 100 mm scale)
- no significant nausea (maximum VAS <25 mm on a 0 to 100 mm scale)

A summary of the key study results from each individual study analysis is shown in Table 1 and in Table 2.

[See table 1 above]

[See table 2 at top of next page]

In both studies, a statistically significantly higher proportion of patients receiving the aprepitant regimen in Cycle 1 had a complete response (primary endpoint), compared with patients receiving standard therapy. A statistically significant difference in complete response in favor of the aprepitant regimen was also observed when the acute phase and the delayed phase were analyzed separately.

In both studies, the estimated time to first emesis after initiation of cisplatin treatment was longer with the aprepitant regimen, and the incidence of first emesis was reduced in the aprepitant regimen group compared with standard therapy group as depicted in the Kaplan-Meier curves in Figure 2.

Treatment Regimens Highly Emetogenic Chemotherapy Trials

Treatment Regimen	Day 1	Days 2 to 4
Aprepitant	Aprepitant 125 mg PO Dexamethasone 12 mg PO Ondansetron 32 mg I.V.	Aprepitant 80 mg PO Daily (Days 2 and 3 only) Dexamethasone 8 mg PO Daily (morning)
Standard Therapy	Dexamethasone 20 mg PO Ondansetron 32 mg I.V.	Dexamethasone 8 mg PO Daily (morning) Dexamethasone 8 mg PO Daily (evening)

Aprepitant placebo and dexamethasone placebo were used to maintain blinding.

Table 1
Percent of Patients Receiving Highly Emetogenic Chemotherapy Responding by Treatment Group and Phase for Study 1 — Cycle 1

ENDPOINTS	Aprepitant Regimen (N = 260)[†] %	Standard Therapy (N = 261)[†] %	p-Value
PRIMARY ENDPOINT			
Complete Response			
Overall[‡]	73	52	<0.001
OTHER PRESPECIFIED ENDPOINTS			
Complete Response			
Acute phase[§]	89	78	<0.001
Delayed phase[‖]	75	56	<0.001
Complete Protection			
Overall	63	49	0.001
Acute phase	85	75	NS*
Delayed phase	66	52	<0.001
No Emesis			
Overall	78	55	<0.001
Acute phase	90	79	0.001
Delayed phase	81	59	<0.001
No Nausea			
Overall	48	44	NS**
Delayed phase	51	48	NS**
No Significant Nausea			
Overall	73	66	NS**
Delayed phase	75	69	NS**

[†]N: Number of patients (older than 18 years of age) who received cisplatin, study drug, and had at least one post-treatment efficacy evaluation.
[‡]Overall: 0 to 120 hours post-cisplatin treatment.
[§]Acute phase: 0 to 24 hours post-cisplatin treatment.
[‖]Delayed phase: 25 to 120 hours post-cisplatin treatment.
*Not statistically significant when adjusted for multiple comparisons.
**Not statistically significant.
Visual analogue scale (VAS) score range: 0 mm = no nausea; 100 mm = nausea as bad as it could be.

Figure 2: Percent of Patients Receiving Highly Emetogenic Chemotherapy Who Remain Emesis Free Over Time – Cycle 1

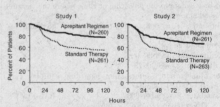

p-Value <0.001 based on a log rank test for Study 1 and Study 2; nominal p-values not adjusted for multiplicity.

Patient-Reported Outcomes: The impact of nausea and vomiting on patients' daily lives was assessed in Cycle 1 of both Phase III studies using the Functional Living Index–Emesis (FLIE), a validated nausea- and vomiting-specific patient-reported outcome measure. Minimal or no impact of nausea and vomiting on patients' daily lives is defined as a FLIE total score >108. In each of the 2 studies, a higher proportion of patients receiving the aprepitant regimen reported minimal or no impact of nausea and vomiting on daily life (Study 1: 74% versus 64%; Study 2: 75% versus 64%).

Multiple-Cycle Extension: In the same 2 clinical studies, patients continued into the Multiple-Cycle extension for up to 5 additional cycles of chemotherapy. The proportion of patients with no emesis and no significant nausea by treatment group at each cycle is depicted in Figure 3. Antiemetic effectiveness for the patients receiving the aprepitant regimen is maintained throughout repeat cycles for those patients continuing in each of the multiple cycles.

Figure 3: Proportion of Patients Receiving Highly Emetogenic Chemotherapy With No Emesis and No Significant Nausea by Treatment Group and Cycle

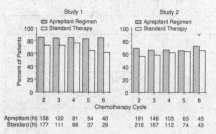

| Aprepitant (N) | 158 | 122 | 81 | 54 | 40 | | 191 | 148 | 103 | 63 | 43 |
| Standard (N) | 177 | 111 | 68 | 37 | 29 | | 216 | 167 | 112 | 74 | 43 |

Moderately Emetogenic Chemotherapy

In a multicenter, randomized, double-blind, parallel-group, clinical study in breast cancer patients, the aprepitant regimen (see table that follows) was compared with a standard of care therapy in patients receiving a moderately emetogenic chemotherapy regimen that included cyclophosphamide 750-1500 mg/m^2; or cyclophosphamide 500-1500 mg/m^2 and doxorubicin ($\leq$60 mg/m^2) or epirubicin ($\leq$100 mg/m^2).

In this study, the most common combinations were cyclophosphamide + doxorubicin (60.6%); and cyclophosphamide + epirubicin + fluorouracil (21.6%).

Of the 438 patients who were randomized to receive the aprepitant regimen, 99.5% were women. Of these, approximately 80% were White, 8% Black, 8% Asian, 4% Hispanic, and <1% Other. The aprepitant-treated patients in this clinical study ranged from 25 to 78 years of age, with a mean age of 53 years; 70 patients were 65 years or older, with 12 patients being over 74 years.

Patients (N = 866) were randomized to either the aprepitant regimen (N = 438) or standard therapy (N = 428). The treatment regimens are defined in the table that follows.

[See second table above]

The antiemetic activity of oral aprepitant was evaluated based on the following endpoints:

Primary endpoint:

Complete response (defined as no emetic episodes and no use of rescue therapy) in the overall phase (0 to 120 hours post-chemotherapy)

Other prespecified endpoints:

- no emesis (defined as no emetic episodes regardless of use of rescue therapy)
- no nausea (maximum VAS <5 mm on a 0 to 100 mm scale)
- no significant nausea (maximum VAS <25 mm on a 0 to 100 mm scale)
- complete protection (defined as no emetic episodes, no use of rescue therapy, and a maximum nausea visual analogue scale [VAS] score <25 mm on a 0 to 100 mm scale)
- complete response during the acute and delayed phases.

A summary of the key results from this study is shown in Table 3.

[See table 3 at top of next page]

In this study, a statistically significantly (p=0.015) higher proportion of patients receiving the aprepitant regimen (51%) in Cycle 1 had a complete response (primary endpoint) during the overall phase compared with patients receiving standard therapy (42%). The difference between treatment groups was primarily driven by the "No Emesis Endpoint", a principal component of this composite primary endpoint. In addition, a higher proportion of patients receiving the aprepitant regimen in Cycle 1 had a complete response during the acute (0-24 hours) and delayed (25-120 hours) phases compared with patients receiving standard therapy; however, the treatment group differences failed to reach statistical significance, after multiplicity adjustments.

Patient-Reported Outcomes: In a phase III study in patients receiving moderately emetogenic chemotherapy, the impact of nausea and vomiting on patients' daily lives was assessed in Cycle 1 using the FLIE. A higher proportion of patients receiving the aprepitant regimen reported minimal or no impact on daily life (64% versus 56%). This difference between treatment groups was primarily driven by the "No Vomiting Domain" of this composite endpoint.

Multiple-Cycle Extension: Patients receiving moderately emetogenic chemotherapy were permitted to continue into the Multiple-Cycle extension of the study for up to 3 additional cycles of chemotherapy. Antiemetic effect for patients receiving the aprepitant regimen is maintained during all cycles.

INDICATIONS AND USAGE

EMEND for Injection, in combination with other antiemetic agents, is indicated for the:

- prevention of acute and delayed nausea and vomiting associated with initial and repeat courses of highly emetogenic cancer chemotherapy including high-dose cisplatin
- prevention of nausea and vomiting associated with initial and repeat courses of moderately emetogenic cancer chemotherapy (see DOSAGE AND ADMINISTRATION).

Table 2
Percent of Patients Receiving Highly Emetogenic Chemotherapy Responding by Treatment Group and Phase for Study 2 — Cycle 1

ENDPOINTS	Aprepitant Regimen (N = 261)[†] %	Standard Therapy (N = 263)[†] %	p-Value
PRIMARY ENDPOINT			
Complete Response			
Overall[‡]	63	43	<0.001
OTHER PRESPECIFIED ENDPOINTS			
Complete Response			
Acute phase[§]	83	68	<0.001
Delayed phase[||]	68	47	<0.001
Complete Protection			
Overall	56	41	<0.001
Acute phase	80	65	<0.001
Delayed phase	61	44	<0.001
No Emesis			
Overall	66	44	<0.001
Acute phase	84	69	<0.001
Delayed phase	72	48	<0.001
No Nausea			
Overall	49	39	NS*
Delayed phase	53	40	NS*
No Significant Nausea			
Overall	71	64	NS**
Delayed phase	73	65	NS**

[†]N: Number of patients (older than 18 years of age) who received cisplatin, study drug, and had at least one post-treatment efficacy evaluation.
[‡]Overall: 0 to 120 hours post-cisplatin treatment.
[§]Acute phase: 0 to 24 hours post-cisplatin treatment.
[||]Delayed phase: 25 to 120 hours post-cisplatin treatment.
*Not statistically significant when adjusted for multiple comparisons.
**Not statistically significant.
Visual analogue scale (VAS) score range: 0 mm = no nausea; 100 mm = nausea as bad as it could be.

Treatment Regimens Moderately Emetogenic Chemotherapy Trial

Treatment Regimen	Day 1	Days 2 to 3
Aprepitant	Aprepitant 125 mg PO[†] Dexamethasone 12 mg PO[‡] Ondansetron 8 mg PO × 2 doses[§]	Aprepitant 80 mg PO Daily
Standard Therapy	Dexamethasone 20 mg PO Ondansetron 8 mg PO × 2 doses	Ondansetron 8 mg PO Daily (every 12 hours)

Aprepitant placebo and dexamethasone placebo were used to maintain blinding.
[†]1 hour prior to chemotherapy.
[‡]30 minutes prior to chemotherapy.
[§]30 to 60 minutes prior to chemotherapy and 8 hours after first ondansetron dose.

CONTRAINDICATIONS

EMEND for Injection is contraindicated in patients who are hypersensitive to EMEND for Injection, aprepitant, polysorbate 80 or any other components of the product.

Aprepitant, when administered orally, is a moderate cytochrome P450 isoenzyme 3A4 (CYP3A4) inhibitor following the 3-day antiemetic dosing regimen for CINV. Since fosaprepitant is rapidly converted to aprepitant, fosaprepitant should not be used concurrently with pimozide, terfenadine, astemizole, or cisapride. Inhibition of CYP3A4 by aprepitant could result in elevated plasma concentrations of these drugs, potentially causing serious or life-threatening reactions (see PRECAUTIONS, *Drug Interactions*).

PRECAUTIONS

General

Fosaprepitant is rapidly converted to aprepitant, which is a moderate inhibitor of CYP3A4 when administered as a 3-day antiemetic dosing regimen for CINV. Fosaprepitant should be used with caution in patients receiving concomitant medications that are primarily metabolized through CYP3A4. Inhibition of CYP3A4 by aprepitant could result in elevated plasma concentrations of these concomitant medications. When fosaprepitant is used concomitantly with another CYP3A4 inhibitor, aprepitant plasma concentrations could be elevated. (See PRECAUTIONS; *Drug Interactions*.)

Chemotherapy agents that are known to be metabolized by CYP3A4 include docetaxel, paclitaxel, etoposide, irinotecan, ifosfamide, imatinib, vinorelbine, vinblastine and vincristine. In clinical studies, the oral aprepitant regimen was administered commonly with etoposide, vinorelbine, or paclitaxel. The doses of these agents were not adjusted to account for potential drug interactions.

In separate pharmacokinetic studies no clinically significant change in docetaxel or vinorelbine pharmacokinetics was observed when the oral aprepitant regimen was co-administered.

Due to the small number of patients in clinical studies who received the CYP3A4 substrates vinblastine, vincristine, or ifosfamide, particular caution and careful monitoring are advised in patients receiving these agents or other chemotherapy agents metabolized primarily by CYP3A4 that were not studied (see PRECAUTIONS, *Drug Interactions*).

Chronic continuous use of EMEND for Injection for prevention of nausea and vomiting is not recommended because it has not been studied and because the drug interaction profile may change during chronic continuous use.

Coadministration of aprepitant with warfarin may result in a clinically significant decrease in International Normalized Ratio (INR) of prothrombin time. In patients on chronic warfarin therapy, the INR should be closely monitored in the 2-week period, particularly at 7 to 10 days, following initiation of the 3-day regimen of fosaprepitant followed by oral aprepitant with each chemotherapy cycle (see PRECAUTIONS, *Drug Interactions*).

Upon coadministration with aprepitant, the efficacy of hormonal contraceptives during and for 28 days following the last dose of aprepitant may be reduced. Alternative or back-up methods of contraception should be used during

Continued on next page

Information on the Merck & Co., Inc., products listed on these pages is from the full prescribing information in use March 1, 2008. For information, please call 1-800-NSC-MERCK [1-800-672-6372].

Emend Injection—Cont.

treatment with aprepitant and for 1 month following the last dose of aprepitant (see PRECAUTIONS, *Drug Interactions*).
There are no clinical or pharmacokinetic data in patients with severe hepatic insufficiency (Child-Pugh score >9). Therefore, caution should be exercised when fosaprepitant or aprepitant is administered in these patients (see CLINICAL PHARMACOLOGY, *Special Populations, Hepatic Insufficiency* and DOSAGE AND ADMINISTRATION).

Information for Patients

Physicians should instruct their patients to read the patient package insert before starting therapy with EMEND for Injection and to reread it each time the prescription is renewed.
Patients should follow the physician's instructions for the EMEND for Injection regimen.
For the prevention of CINV, patients should be given their dose of EMEND for Injection as an infusion over 15 minutes, 30 minutes prior to chemotherapy on Day 1.
EMEND for Injection may interact with some drugs including chemotherapy; therefore, patients should be advised to report to their doctor the use of any other prescription, nonprescription medication or herbal products.
Patients on chronic warfarin therapy should be instructed to have their clotting status closely monitored in the 2-week period, particularly at 7 to 10 days, following initiation of the 3-day regimen of fosaprepitant followed by aprepitant, with each chemotherapy cycle.
Administration of EMEND for Injection may reduce the efficacy of hormonal contraceptives. Patients should be advised to use alternative or back-up methods of contraception during treatment with EMEND for Injection and for 1 month following the last dose of the 3-day aprepitant regimen.

Drug Interactions

Drug interactions following administration of fosaprepitant are likely to occur with drugs that interact with oral aprepitant. The following information was derived from data with oral aprepitant and one study conducted with fosaprepitant and oral midazolam.
Aprepitant is a substrate, a moderate inhibitor, and an inducer of CYP3A4 when administered as a 3-day antiemetic dosing regimen for CINV. Aprepitant is also an inducer of CYP2C9.

Effect of aprepitant on the pharmacokinetics of other agents

As a moderate inhibitor of CYP3A4, aprepitant can increase plasma concentrations of orally coadministered medicinal products that are metabolized through CYP3A4 (see CONTRAINDICATIONS).
Aprepitant has been shown to induce the metabolism of S(-) warfarin and tolbutamide, which are metabolized through CYP2C9. Coadministration of fosaprepitant or oral aprepitant with these drugs or other drugs that are known to be metabolized by CYP2C9, such as phenytoin, may result in lower plasma concentrations of these drugs.
Fosaprepitant or aprepitant is unlikely to interact with drugs that are substrates for the P-glycoprotein transporter, as demonstrated by the lack of interaction of oral aprepitant with digoxin in a clinical drug interaction study.
5-HT$_3$ antagonists: In clinical drug interaction studies, aprepitant did not have clinically important effects on the pharmacokinetics of ondansetron, granisetron, or hydrodolasetron (the active metabolite of dolasetron).
Corticosteroids:
Dexamethasone: Oral aprepitant, when given as a regimen of 125 mg with dexamethasone coadministered orally as 20 mg on Day 1, and oral aprepitant when given as 80 mg/day with dexamethasone coadministered orally as 8 mg on Days 2 through 5, increased the AUC of dexamethasone, a CYP3A4 substrate, by 2.2-fold on Days 1 and 5. The oral dexamethasone doses should be reduced by approximately 50% when coadministered with a regimen of fosaprepitant followed by aprepitant, to achieve exposures of dexamethasone similar to those obtained when dexamethasone is given without aprepitant. The daily dose of dexamethasone administered in clinical CINV studies with oral aprepitant reflects an approximate 50% reduction of the dose of dexamethasone (see DOSAGE AND ADMINISTRATION).
Methylprednisolone: Oral aprepitant, when given as a regimen of 125 mg on Day 1 and 80 mg/day on Days 2 and 3, increased the AUC of methylprednisolone, a CYP3A4 substrate, by 1.34-fold on Day 1 and by 2.5-fold on Day 3, when methylprednisolone was coadministered intravenously as 125 mg on Day 1 and orally as 40 mg on Days 2 and 3. The I.V. methylprednisolone dose should be reduced by approximately 25%, and the oral methylprednisolone dose should be reduced by approximately 50% when coadministered with a regimen of fosaprepitant followed by aprepitant to achieve exposures of methylprednisolone similar to those obtained when it is given without aprepitant.
Chemotherapeutic agents: See PRECAUTIONS, *General*.
Docetaxel: In a pharmacokinetic study, oral aprepitant (CINV regimen) did not influence the pharmacokinetics of docetaxel.
Vinorelbine: In a pharmacokinetic study, oral aprepitant (CINV regimen) did not influence the pharmacokinetics of vinorelbine to a clinically significant degree.
Warfarin: A single 125-mg dose of oral aprepitant was administered on Day 1 and 80 mg/day on Days 2 and 3 to healthy subjects who were stabilized on chronic warfarin therapy. Although there was no effect of oral aprepitant on the plasma AUC of R(+) or S(-) warfarin determined on Day 3, there was a 34% decrease in S(−) warfarin (a CYP2C9 substrate) trough concentration accompanied by a 14% decrease in the prothrombin time (reported as International Normalized Ratio or INR) 5 days after completion of dosing with oral aprepitant. In patients on chronic warfarin therapy, the prothrombin time (INR) should be closely monitored in the 2-week period, particularly at 7 to 10 days, following initiation of the 3-day regimen of fosaprepitant followed by aprepitant with each chemotherapy cycle.
Tolbutamide: Oral aprepitant, when given as 125 mg on Day 1 and 80 mg/day on Days 2 and 3, decreased the AUC of tolbutamide (a CYP2C9 substrate) by 23% on Day 4, 28% on Day 8, and 15% on Day 15, when a single dose of tolbutamide 500 mg was administered orally prior to the administration of the 3-day regimen of oral aprepitant and on Days 4, 8, and 15.
Oral contraceptives: Aprepitant, when given once daily for 14 days as a 100-mg capsule with an oral contraceptive containing 35 mcg of ethinyl estradiol and 1 mg of norethindrone, decreased the AUC of ethinyl estradiol by 43%, and decreased the AUC of norethindrone by 8%.
In another study, a daily dose of an oral contraceptive containing ethinyl estradiol and norethindrone was administered on Days 1 through 21, and oral aprepitant was given as a 3-day regimen of 125 mg on Day 8 and 80 mg/day on Days 9 and 10 with ondansetron 32 mg I.V. on Day 8 and oral dexamethasone given as 12 mg on Day 8 and 8 mg/day on Days 9, 10, and 11. In the study, the AUC of ethinyl estradiol decreased by 19% on Day 10 and there was as much as a 64% decrease in ethinyl estradiol trough concentrations during Days 9 through 21. While there was no effect of oral aprepitant on the AUC of norethindrone on Day 10, there was as much as a 60% decrease in norethindrone trough concentrations during Days 9 through 21. The coadministration of fosaprepitant or aprepitant may reduce the efficacy of hormonal contraceptives during and for 28 days after administration of the last dose of either. Alternative or back-up methods of contraception should be used during treatment with fosaprepitant or aprepitant and for 1 month following the last dose.
Midazolam: A study was completed with fosaprepitant and oral midazolam. Fosaprepitant was given at a dose of 100 mg over 15 minutes along with a single dose of midazolam 2 mg. The plasma AUC of midazolam was increased by 1.6-fold. This effect was not considered clinically important. Oral aprepitant increased the AUC of midazolam by 2.3-fold on Day 1 and 3.3-fold on Day 5, when a single oral dose of midazolam 2 mg was coadministered on Day 1 and Day 5 of a regimen of oral aprepitant 125 mg on Day 1 and 80 mg/day on Days 2 through 5. The potential effects of increased plasma concentrations of midazolam or other benzodiazepines metabolized via CYP3A4 (alprazolam, triazolam) should be considered when coadministering these agents with a 3-day regimen of fosaprepitant followed by aprepitant. In another study with intravenous administration of midazolam, oral aprepitant was given as 125 mg on Day 1 and 80 mg/day on Days 2 and 3, and midazolam 2 mg I.V. was given prior to the administration of the 3-day regimen of oral aprepitant and on Days 4, 8, and 15. Oral aprepitant increased the AUC of midazolam by 25% on Day 4 and decreased the AUC of midazolam by 19% on Day 8 relative to the dosing of oral aprepitant on Days 1 through 3. These effects were not considered clinically important. The AUC of midazolam on Day 15 was similar to that observed at baseline.
An additional study was completed with intravenous administration of midazolam and oral aprepitant. Intravenous midazolam 2 mg was given 1 hour after oral administration of a single dose of oral aprepitant 125 mg. The plasma AUC of midazolam was increased by 1.5-fold.

Effect of other agents on the pharmacokinetics of aprepitant

Aprepitant is a substrate for CYP3A4; therefore, coadministration of fosaprepitant or aprepitant with drugs that inhibit CYP3A4 activity may result in increased plasma concentrations of aprepitant. Consequently, concomitant administration of fosaprepitant or aprepitant with strong CYP3A4 inhibitors (e.g., ketoconazole, itraconazole, nefazodone, troleandomycin, clarithromycin, ritonavir, nelfinavir) should be approached with caution. Because moderate CYP3A4 inhibitors (e.g., diltiazem) result in a 2-fold increase in plasma concentrations of aprepitant, concomitant administration should also be approached with caution.
Aprepitant is a substrate for CYP3A4; therefore, coadministration of fosaprepitant or aprepitant with drugs that strongly induce CYP3A4 activity (e.g., rifampin, carbamazepine, phenytoin) may result in reduced plasma concentrations and decreased efficacy.
Ketoconazole: When a single 125-mg dose of oral aprepitant was administered on Day 5 of a 10-day regimen of 400 mg/day of ketoconazole, a strong CYP3A4 inhibitor, the AUC of aprepitant increased approximately 5-fold and the mean terminal half-life of aprepitant increased approximately 3-fold. Concomitant administration of fosaprepitant or aprepitant with strong CYP3A4 inhibitors should be approached cautiously.
Rifampin: When a single 375-mg dose of oral aprepitant was administered on Day 9 of a 14-day regimen of 600 mg/day of rifampin, a strong CYP3A4 inducer, the AUC of aprepitant decreased approximately 11-fold and the mean terminal half-life decreased approximately 3-fold.
Coadministration of fosaprepitant or aprepitant with drugs that induce CYP3A4 activity may result in reduced plasma concentrations and decreased efficacy.

Additional interactions

Diltiazem: In a study in 10 patients with mild to moderate hypertension, intravenous infusion of 100 mg fosaprepitant over 15 minutes with diltiazem 120 mg 3 times daily, resulted in a 1.5-fold increase of aprepitant AUC and a 1.4-fold increase in diltiazem AUC. It also resulted in a small but clinically meaningful further maximum decrease in diastolic blood pressure [mean (SD) of 24.3 (± 10.2) mm Hg with fosaprepitant versus 15.6 (± 4.1) mm Hg without fosaprepitant] and resulted in a small further maximum decrease in systolic blood pressure [mean (SD) of 29.5 (± 7.9) mm Hg with fosaprepitant versus 23.8 (± 4.8) mm Hg without fosaprepitant], which may be clinically meaningful, but did not result in a clinically meaningful further change in heart rate or PR interval, beyond those changes induced by diltiazem alone.
In the same study, administration of aprepitant once daily, as a tablet formulation comparable to 230 mg of the capsule formulation, with diltiazem 120 mg 3 times daily for 5 days, resulted in a 2-fold increase of aprepitant AUC and a simultaneous 1.7-fold increase of diltiazem AUC. These pharmacokinetic effects did not result in clinically meaningful changes in ECG, heart rate or blood pressure beyond those changes induced by diltiazem alone.
Paroxetine: Coadministration of once daily doses of aprepitant, as a tablet formulation comparable to 85 mg or 170 mg of the capsule formulation, with paroxetine 20 mg once daily, resulted in a decrease in AUC by approximately 25% and C_{max} by approximately 20% of both aprepitant and paroxetine.

Carcinogenesis, Mutagenesis, Impairment of Fertility

Carcinogenicity studies were conducted in Sprague-Dawley rats and in CD-1 mice for 2 years. In the rat carcinogenicity studies, animals were treated with oral doses ranging from 0.05 to 1000 mg/kg twice daily. The highest dose produced a systemic exposure to aprepitant (plasma $AUC_{0\text{-}24hr}$) of 0.7 to 1.6 times the human exposure ($AUC_{0\text{-}24hr}$ = 19.6 mcg•hr/mL) at the recommended dose of 125 mg/day. Treatment with aprepitant at doses of 5 to 1000 mg/kg twice daily caused an increase in the incidences of thyroid follicular cell adenomas and carcinomas in male rats. In female rats, it produced hepatocellular adenomas at 5 to 1000 mg/kg twice daily and hepatocellular carcinomas and thyroid follicular cell adenomas at 125 to 1000 mg/kg twice daily. In the mouse carcinogenicity studies, the animals were treated with oral doses ranging from 2.5 to 2000 mg/kg/day. The highest dose produced a systemic exposure of about 2.8 to 3.6 times the human exposure at the recommended dose.

Table 3
Percent of Patients Receiving Moderately Emetogenic Chemotherapy Responding by Treatment Group and Phase — Cycle 1

ENDPOINTS	Aprepitant Regimen (N = 433)[†] %	Standard Therapy (N = 424)[†] %	p-Value
PRIMARY ENDPOINT			
Complete Response[‡]	51	42	0.015
OTHER PRESPECIFIED ENDPOINTS			
No Emesis	76	59	NS*
No Nausea	33	33	NS
No Significant Nausea	61	56	NS
No Rescue Therapy	59	56	NS
Complete Protection	43	37	NS

†N: Number of patients included in the primary analysis of complete response.
‡Overall: 0 to 120 hours post-chemotherapy treatment.
*NS when adjusted for prespecified multiple comparisons rule; unadjusted p-value <0.001.

Treatment with aprepitant produced skin fibrosarcomas at 125 and 500 mg/kg/day doses in male mice. Carcinogenicity studies were not conducted with fosaprepitant.

Aprepitant and fosaprepitant were not genotoxic in the Ames test, the human lymphoblastoid cell (TK6) mutagenesis test, the rat hepatocyte DNA strand break test, the Chinese hamster ovary (CHO) cell chromosome aberration test and the mouse micronucleus test.

Fosaprepitant, when administered intravenously, is rapidly converted to aprepitant. In the fertility studies conducted with fosaprepitant and aprepitant, the highest systemic exposures to aprepitant were obtained following oral administration of aprepitant. Oral aprepitant did not affect the fertility or general reproductive performance of male or female rats at doses up to the maximum feasible dose of 1000 mg/kg twice daily (providing exposure in male rats lower than the exposure at the recommended human dose and exposure in female rats at about 1.6 times the human exposure).

Pregnancy. Teratogenic Effects: Category B. In the teratology studies conducted with fosaprepitant and aprepitant, the highest systemic exposures to aprepitant were obtained following oral administration of aprepitant. Teratology studies performed in rats at oral doses of aprepitant up to 1000 mg/kg twice daily (plasma AUC_{0-24hr} of 31.3 mcg•hr/mL, about 1.6 times the human exposure at the recommended dose) and in rabbits at oral doses up to 25 mg/kg/day (plasma AUC_{0-24hr} of 26.9 mcg•hr/mL, about 1.4 times the human exposure at the recommended dose) revealed no evidence of impaired fertility or harm to the fetus due to aprepitant. There are, however, no adequate and well-controlled studies in pregnant women. Because animal reproduction studies are not always predictive of human response, this drug should be used during pregnancy only if clearly needed.

Nursing Mothers

Aprepitant is excreted in the milk of rats. It is not known whether this drug is excreted in human milk. Because many drugs are excreted in human milk and because of the potential for possible serious adverse reactions in nursing infants from aprepitant and because of the potential for tumorigenicity shown for aprepitant in rodent carcinogenicity studies, a decision should be made whether to discontinue nursing or to discontinue the drug, taking into account the importance of the drug to the mother.

Pediatric Use

Safety and effectiveness in pediatric patients have not been established.

Geriatric Use

In 2 well-controlled chemotherapy-induced nausea and vomiting clinical studies, of the total number of patients (N=544) treated with oral aprepitant, 31% were 65 and over, while 5% were 75 and over. No overall differences in safety or effectiveness were observed between these subjects and younger subjects. Greater sensitivity of some older individuals cannot be ruled out. Dosage adjustment in the elderly is not necessary.

ADVERSE REACTIONS

The overall safety of aprepitant was evaluated in approximately 4900 individuals.

Since EMEND for Injection is converted to aprepitant, those adverse experiences associated with aprepitant might also be expected to occur with EMEND for Injection.

Fosaprepitant (intravenous formulation)

In a randomized, open-label, incomplete crossover, bioequivalence study, 66 subjects were dosed with 115 mg of EMEND for Injection intravenously and 72 subjects received 125 mg of aprepitant orally. Systemic exposure of 115 mg of intravenous EMEND for Injection is equivalent to 125 mg oral aprepitant. The following clinical adverse experiences, regardless of causality, were reported in subjects dosed with EMEND for Injection: infusion site pain, 5 (7.6%); infusion site induration, 1(1.5%); headache, 2(3%).

Oral Aprepitant

Highly Emetogenic Chemotherapy

In 2 well-controlled clinical trials in patients receiving highly emetogenic cancer chemotherapy, 544 patients were treated with aprepitant during Cycle 1 of chemotherapy and 413 of these patients continued into the Multiple-Cycle extension for up to 6 cycles of chemotherapy. Oral aprepitant was given in combination with ondansetron and dexamethasone and was generally well tolerated. Most adverse experiences reported in these clinical studies were described as mild to moderate in intensity.

In Cycle 1, clinical adverse experiences were reported in approximately 69% of patients treated with the aprepitant regimen compared with approximately 68% of patients treated with standard therapy. Table 4 shows the percent of patients with clinical adverse experiences reported at an incidence ≥3%.

Table 4
Percent of Patients Receiving Highly Emetogenic Chemotherapy With Clinical Adverse Experiences (Incidence ≥3%) - Cycle 1

	Aprepitant Regimen (N = 544)	Standard Therapy (N = 550)
Body as a Whole/Site Unspecified		
Abdominal Pain	4.6	3.3
Asthenia/Fatigue	17.8	11.8
Dehydration	5.9	5.1
Dizziness	6.6	4.4
Fever	2.9	3.5
Mucous Membrane Disorder	2.6	3.1
Digestive System		
Constipation	10.3	12.2
Diarrhea	10.3	7.5
Epigastric Discomfort	4.0	3.1
Gastritis	4.2	3.1
Heartburn	5.3	4.9
Nausea	12.7	11.8
Vomiting	7.5	7.6
Eyes, Ears, Nose, and Throat		
Tinnitus	3.7	3.8
Hemic and Lymphatic System		
Neutropenia	3.1	2.9
Metabolism and Nutrition		
Anorexia	10.1	9.5
Nervous System		
Headache	8.5	8.7
Insomnia	2.9	3.1
Respiratory System		
Hiccups	10.8	5.6

In addition, isolated cases of serious adverse experiences, regardless of causality, of bradycardia, disorientation, and perforating duodenal ulcer were reported in highly emetogenic CINV clinical studies.

Moderately Emetogenic Chemotherapy

During Cycle 1 of a moderately emetogenic chemotherapy study, 438 patients were treated with the aprepitant regimen and 385 of these patients continued into the Multiple-Cycle extension for up to 4 cycles of chemotherapy. In Cycle 1, clinical adverse experiences were reported in approximately 73% of patients treated with the aprepitant regimen compared with approximately 75% of patients treated with standard therapy.

The adverse experience profile in the moderately emetogenic chemotherapy study was generally comparable to the highly emetogenic chemotherapy studies. Table 5 shows the percent of patients with clinical adverse experiences reported at an incidence ≥3%.

Table 5
Percent of Patients Receiving Moderately Emetogenic Chemotherapy With Clinical Adverse Experiences (Incidence ≥3%) — Cycle 1

	Aprepitant Regimen (N = 438)	Standard Therapy (N = 428)
Blood and Lymphatic System Disorders		
Neutropenia	8.9	8.4
Metabolism and Nutrition Disorders		
Anorexia	4.3	5.8
Psychiatric Disorders		
Insomnia	4.1	5.6
Nervous System Disorders		
Dizziness	3.4	4.2
Headache	16.4	16.4
Vascular Disorders		
Hot Flush	3.0	1.4
Respiratory, Thoracic and Mediastinal Disorders		
Pharyngolaryngeal pain	3.0	2.3
Gastrointestinal Disorders		
Constipation	12.3	18.0
Diarrhea	5.5	6.3
Dyspepsia	8.4	4.9
Nausea	7.1	7.5
Stomatitis	5.3	4.4
Skin and Subcutaneous Tissue Disorders		
Alopecia	24.0	22.2
General Disorders and General Administration Site Conditions		
Asthenia	3.4	3.7
Fatigue	21.9	21.5
Mucosal inflammation	2.5	3.5

Isolated cases of serious adverse experiences, regardless of causality, of dehydration, enterocolitis, febrile neutropenia, hypertension, hypoesthesia, neutropenic sepsis, pneumonia, and sinus tachycardia were reported in the moderately emetogenic CINV clinical study.

Highly and Moderately Emetogenic Chemotherapy

The following additional clinical adverse experiences (incidence >0.5% and greater than standard therapy), regardless of causality, were reported in patients treated with aprepitant regimen:

Infections and infestations: candidiasis, herpes simplex, lower respiratory infection, pharyngitis, septic shock, upper respiratory infection, urinary tract infection.

Neoplasms benign, malignant and unspecified (including cysts and polyps): malignant neoplasm, non-small cell lung carcinoma.

Blood and lymphatic system disorders: anemia, febrile neutropenia, thrombocytopenia.

Metabolism and nutrition disorders: appetite decreased, diabetes mellitus, hypokalemia.

Psychiatric disorders: anxiety disorder, confusion, depression.

Nervous system: peripheral neuropathy, sensory neuropathy, taste disturbance, tremor.

Eye disorders: conjunctivitis.

Cardiac disorders: myocardial infarction, palpitations, tachycardia.

Vascular disorders: deep venous thrombosis, flushing, hypertension, hypotension.

Respiratory, thoracic and mediastinal disorders: cough, dyspnea, nasal secretion, pneumonitis, pulmonary embolism, respiratory insufficiency, vocal disturbance.

Gastrointestinal disorders: acid reflux, deglutition disorder, dry mouth, dysgeusia, dysphagia, eructation, flatulence, obstipation, salivation increased.

Skin and subcutaneous tissue disorders: acne, diaphoresis, rash.

Musculoskeletal and connective tissue disorders: arthralgia, back pain, muscular weakness, musculoskeletal pain, myalgia.

Renal and urinary disorders: dysuria, renal insufficiency.

Reproductive system and breast disorders: pelvic pain.

General disorders and administrative site conditions: edema, malaise, rigors.

Investigations: weight loss.

Laboratory Adverse Experiences

Table 6 shows the percent of patients with laboratory adverse experiences reported at an incidence ≥3% in patients receiving highly emetogenic chemotherapy.

Table 6
Percent of Patients Receiving Highly Emetogenic Chemotherapy With Laboratory Adverse Experiences (Incidence ≥3%) - Cycle 1

	Aprepitant Regimen (N = 544)	Standard Therapy (N = 550)
ALT Increased	6.0	4.3
AST Increased	3.0	1.3
Blood Urea Nitrogen Increased	4.7	3.5
Serum Creatinine Increased	3.7	4.3
Proteinuria	6.8	5.3

The following additional laboratory adverse experiences (incidence >0.5% and greater than standard therapy), regardless of causality, were reported in patients treated with aprepitant regimen: alkaline phosphatase increased, hyperglycemia, hyponatremia, leukocytes increased, erythrocyturia, leukocyturia.

The adverse experiences of increased AST and ALT were generally mild and transient.

The following laboratory adverse experiences were reported at an incidence ≥3% during Cycle 1 of the moderately emetogenic chemotherapy study in patients treated with the aprepitant regimen or standard therapy, respectively: decreased hemoglobin (2.3%, 4.7%) and decreased white blood cell count (9.3%, 9.0%).

The adverse experience profiles in the Multiple-Cycle extensions for up to 6 cycles of chemotherapy were generally similar to that observed in Cycle 1.

Stevens-Johnson syndrome was reported as a serious adverse experience in a patient receiving aprepitant with cancer chemotherapy in another CINV study.

Other Studies with Postoperative Nausea and Vomiting

In well-controlled clinical studies in patients receiving general anesthesia, 564 patients were administered 40 mg aprepitant orally and 538 patients were administered 4 mg ondansetron I.V. EMEND was generally well tolerated. Most adverse experiences reported in these clinical studies were described as mild to moderate in intensity. Clinical adverse experiences were reported in approximately 60% of patients treated with 40 mg aprepitant compared with approximately 64% of patients treated with 4 mg ondansetron I.V.

Additional adverse experiences were observed in patients receiving general anesthesia. In the patients treated with aprepitant (40 mg) for postoperative nausea and vomiting, the following additional adverse experiences were reported, regardless of causality, at an incidence ≥3%: anemia, bradycardia, flatulence, hypotension, pruritus, pyrexia.

The following adverse experiences were reported, regardless of causality, in patients treated with aprepitant for postop-

Continued on next page

Information on the Merck & Co., Inc., products listed on these pages is from the full prescribing information in use March 1, 2008. For information, please call 1-800-NSC-MERCK [1-800-672-6372].

Emend Injection—Cont.

erative nausea and vomiting at an incidence of >0.5% and greater than with ondansetron: abdominal pain, abdominal pain upper, blood pressure decreased, dizziness, dyspepsia, hematoma, hypoesthesia, hypothermia, hypovolemia, hypoxia, operative hemorrhage, pain, postoperative infection, respiratory depression, syncope, urticaria, wound dehiscence.

Other adverse experiences (incidence ≤0.5%) reported, regardless of causality, in patients treated with aprepitant 40 mg for postoperative nausea and vomiting included: bowel sounds abnormal, dysarthria, miosis, sensory disturbance, stomach discomfort, visual acuity reduced, wheezing.

Laboratory Adverse Experiences with Postoperative Nausea and Vomiting

One laboratory adverse experience, hemoglobin decreased (40 mg aprepitant), was reported, regardless of causality, at an incidence ≥3% in a patient receiving general anesthesia.

The following additional laboratory adverse experiences (incidence >0.5% and greater than ondansetron), regardless of causality, were reported in patients treated with aprepitant 40 mg: blood albumin decreased, blood bilirubin increased, blood glucose increased, blood potassium decreased, glucose urine present.

The adverse experience of ALT increased occurred with similar incidence in patients treated with aprepitant as in patients treated with ondansetron.

Other Studies

In addition, two serious adverse experiences were reported in postoperative nausea and vomiting (PONV) clinical studies in patients taking a higher dose of aprepitant: one case of constipation, and one case of sub-ileus.

Angioedema and urticaria were reported as serious adverse experiences in a patient receiving aprepitant in a non-CINV/non-PONV study.

OVERDOSAGE

No specific information is available on the treatment of overdosage. Single doses up to 200 mg of fosaprepitant I.V. and 600 mg of oral aprepitant were generally well tolerated in healthy subjects.

Three out of 33 subjects receiving 200 mg of fosaprepitant experienced mild injection site thrombosis. Aprepitant was generally well tolerated when administered as 375 mg once daily for up to 42 days to patients in non-CINV studies. In 33 cancer patients, administration of a single 375-mg dose of aprepitant on Day 1 and 250 mg once daily on Days 2 to 5 was generally well tolerated.

Drowsiness and headache were reported in one patient who ingested 1440 mg of aprepitant.

In the event of overdose, oral aprepitant should be discontinued and general supportive treatment and monitoring should be provided. Because of the antiemetic activity of aprepitant, drug-induced emesis may not be effective.

Aprepitant cannot be removed by hemodialysis.

DOSAGE AND ADMINISTRATION

EMEND for Injection is a sterile, lyophilized prodrug of aprepitant containing polysorbate 80 (PS80), to be administered intravenously as an infusion. Aprepitant is available as capsules (EMEND[2]) for oral administration.

EMEND for Injection (115 mg) may be substituted for EMEND (125 mg) 30 minutes prior to chemotherapy, on Day 1 only of the CINV regimen as an infusion administered over 15 minutes.

EMEND for Injection should not be mixed or reconstituted with solutions for which physical and chemical compatibility have not been established. EMEND for Injection is incompatible with any solutions containing divalent cations (e.g., Ca^{2+}, Mg^{2+}), including Lactated Ringer's Solution and Hartmann's Solution.

The 3-day CINV regimen includes EMEND for Injection (115 mg) or EMEND (125 mg orally) on Day 1; EMEND (80 mg orally) on Days 2 and 3; in addition to a corticosteroid and a 5-HT_3 antagonist as specified in the tables below.

In clinical studies with EMEND, the following regimen was used for the prevention of nausea and vomiting associated with highly emetogenic cancer chemotherapy:

[See first table above]

	Day 1	Day 2	Day 3	Day 4
EMEND*	125 mg orally	80 mg orally	80 mg orally	none
Dexamethasone**	12 mg orally	8 mg orally	8 mg orally	8 mg orally
Ondansetron†	32 mg I.V.	none	none	none

*EMEND was administered orally 1 hour prior to chemotherapy treatment on Day 1 and in the morning on Days 2 and 3.
**Dexamethasone was administered 30 minutes prior to chemotherapy treatment on Day 1 and in the morning on Days 2 through 4. The dose of dexamethasone was chosen to account for drug interactions.
† Ondansetron was administered 30 minutes prior to chemotherapy treatment on Day 1.

In a clinical study with EMEND, the following regimen was used for the prevention of nausea and vomiting associated with moderately emetogenic cancer chemotherapy:

[See second table above]

	Day 1	Day 2	Day 3
EMEND*	125 mg orally	80 mg orally	80 mg orally
Dexamethasone**	12 mg orally	none	none
Ondansetron†	2 × 8 mg orally	none	none

*EMEND was administered orally 1 hour prior to chemotherapy treatment on Day 1 and in the morning on Days 2 and 3.
**Dexamethasone was administered 30 minutes prior to chemotherapy treatment on Day 1. The dose of dexamethasone was chosen to account for drug interactions.
† Ondansetron 8-mg capsule was administered 30 to 60 minutes prior to chemotherapy treatment and one 8-mg capsule was administered 8 hours after the first dose on Day 1.

Preparation of EMEND for Injection

1. Aseptically inject 5 mL 0.9% Sodium Chloride for Injection (saline) into the vial. Assure that saline is added to the vial along the vial wall in order to prevent foaming. Swirl the vial gently. Avoid shaking and jetting saline into the vial.
2. Aseptically prepare an infusion bag filled with 110 mL of saline.
3. Aseptically withdraw the entire volume from the vial and transfer it into the infusion bag containing 110 mL of saline to yield a total volume of 115 mL and a final concentration of 1 mg/1 mL.
4. Gently invert the bag 2-3 times.

The reconstituted final drug solution is stable for 24 hours at ambient room temperature (at or below 25°C).

Parenteral drug products should be inspected visually for particulate matter and discoloration before administration whenever solution and container permit.

Caution: EMEND for Injection should not be mixed or reconstituted with solutions for which physical and chemical compatibility have not been established. EMEND for Injection is incompatible with any solutions containing divalent cations (e.g., Ca^{2+}, Mg^{2+}), including Lactated Ringer's Solution and Hartmann's Solution.

General Information

EMEND for Injection has not been studied for the treatment of established nausea and vomiting.

Chronic continuous administration is not recommended (see PRECAUTIONS).

See PRECAUTIONS, *Drug Interactions* for additional information on dose adjustment for corticosteroids when coadministered with EMEND for Injection.

Refer to the full prescribing information for coadministered antiemetic agents.

EMEND for Injection may be administered with or without food.

No dosage adjustment is necessary for the elderly.

No dosage adjustment is necessary for patients with renal insufficiency or for patients with end stage renal disease undergoing hemodialysis.

No dosage adjustment is necessary for patients with mild to moderate hepatic insufficiency (Child-Pugh score 5 to 9). There are no clinical data in patients with severe hepatic insufficiency (Child-Pugh score >9).

[2] Registered trademark of MERCK & CO., Inc.

HOW SUPPLIED

No. 3884 — One 115 mg single dose per 10 mL glass vial: White to off-white lyophilized solid. Supplied as follows:
NDC 0006-3884-32 1 vial per carton.

Storage

Vials: Store at 2-8°C (36-46°F).

Sterile lyophilized powder for intravenous use only after reconstitution and dilution

Rx only

Manufactured for:
MERCK & CO., INC., Whitehouse Station, NJ 08889, USA
Manufactured by:
DSM Pharmaceuticals, Inc., 5900 Martin Luther King Jr. Highway, Greenville, NC 27834
U.S. Patent Nos.: 5,512,570; 5,691,336
9840000 Issued January 2008
Printed in USA

Patient Information

EMEND®
(fosaprepitant dimeglumine)
for Injection

You should read this information before you start taking EMEND[1] (fosaprepitant dimeglumine) for Injection. Also, read the leaflet each time you refill your prescription, in case any information has changed. This leaflet provides only a summary of certain information about EMEND for Injection. Your doctor or pharmacist can give you an additional leaflet that is written for health professionals that contains more complete information. This leaflet does not take the place of careful discussions with your doctor. You and your doctor should discuss EMEND for Injection when you start taking your medicine.

What is EMEND for Injection?

EMEND for Injection is an antiemetic medicine for use in adult patients, to be given intravenously by your doctor. An antiemetic is a medicine used to prevent and control nausea and vomiting. EMEND for Injection is always used WITH OTHER MEDICINES to prevent and control nausea and vomiting caused by your chemotherapy treatment. EMEND for Injection is not used to treat nausea and vomiting that you already have.

Who should not take EMEND for Injection?

Do not take EMEND for Injection if you:

- are taking any of the following medicines[2]:
  - ORAP® (pimozide)
  - SELDANE® (terfenadine)
  - HISMANAL® (astemizole)
  - PROPULSID® (cisapride)

Taking EMEND for Injection with these medicines could cause serious or life-threatening problems.

- are allergic to fosaprepitant or any of the ingredients in EMEND for Injection. The active ingredient is fosaprepitant. See the end of this leaflet for a list of all the ingredients in EMEND for Injection.

What should I tell my doctor before and during treatment with EMEND for Injection?

Tell your doctor:

- if you are pregnant or plan to become pregnant. It is not known if EMEND for Injection can harm your unborn baby.
- if you are breast-feeding. It is not known if EMEND for Injection passes into your milk and if it can harm your baby.
- if you have liver problems.
- about all your medical problems.
- about all the medicines that you are taking or plan to take, prescription and nonprescription medicines, vitamins, and herbal supplements. EMEND for Injection may cause **serious life-threatening reactions** if used with certain medicines (see the section **Who should not take EMEND for Injection?**). Some medicines can affect EMEND for Injection. EMEND for Injection may also affect some medicines, including chemotherapy, causing them to work differently in your body.

[1] Trademark of MERCK & CO., Inc.
COPYRIGHT © 2008 MERCK & CO., Inc.
All rights reserved.
[2] The brands listed are the registered trademarks of their respective owners and are not trademarks of Merck & Co., Inc.

Your doctor may check to make sure your other medicines are working, while you are taking EMEND for Injection. Patients who take COUMADIN® (warfarin) may need to have blood tests after each 3-day treatment to check their blood clotting.

Women who use birth control medicines during treatment with EMEND for Injection and for up to 1 month after using EMEND for Injection should also use a back-up method of contraception to avoid pregnancy.

How should I take EMEND for Injection?

- EMEND for Injection is given intravenously on Day 1 only of a 3-day regimen.

The recommended dose of EMEND for Injection is:

- 115 mg given intravenously 30 minutes before you start your chemotherapy treatment;

AND

- One 80-mg capsule of EMEND[3] (aprepitant) each morning for the 2 days following your chemotherapy treatment.
- EMEND for Injection may be administered with or without food.
- Tell your doctor if you already have nausea and vomiting before you are given EMEND for Injection.

What are the possible side effects of EMEND for Injection?

The most common side effects of EMEND for Injection are:

- tiredness
- nausea
- hiccups
- constipation
- diarrhea
- loss of appetite
- headache
- hair loss
- injection site pain
- hardening of site of injection

These are not all of the possible side effects of EMEND for Injection. For further information ask your doctor or pharmacist. Talk to your doctor about any side effect that bothers you.

General information about the use of EMEND for Injection
This leaflet summarizes the most important information about EMEND for Injection. If you would like to know more information, talk with your doctor. You can ask your doctor or pharmacist for information about EMEND for Injection that is written for health professionals.
What are the ingredients in EMEND for Injection?
Active ingredient: fosaprepitant
Inactive ingredients: edetate disodium, polysorbate 80, lactose anhydrous, sodium hydroxide and/or hydrochloric acid (for pH adjustment).

[3] Registered trademark of MERCK & CO., Inc.
U.S. Patent Nos.: 5,512,570; 5,691,336
9840000 Issued January 2008
Manufactured for:
MERCK & CO., INC., Whitehouse Station, NJ 08889, USA
Manufactured by:
DSM Pharmaceuticals, Inc., 5900 Martin Luther King Jr. Highway, Greenville, NC 27834

ISENTRESS ℞
[eye sén tris]
(raltegravir)
Tablets
Initial U.S. Approval: 2007

HIGHLIGHTS OF PRESCRIBING INFORMATION
These highlights do not include all the information needed to use ISENTRESS safely and effectively. See full prescribing information for ISENTRESS.
INDICATIONS AND USAGE
ISENTRESS™ is a human immunodeficiency virus integrase strand transfer inhibitor (HIV-1 INSTI) indicated:
• In combination with other antiretroviral agents for the treatment of HIV-1 infection in treatment-experienced adult patients who have evidence of viral replication and HIV-1 strains resistant to multiple antiretroviral agents (1).
The safety and efficacy of ISENTRESS have not been established in treatment-naïve adult patients or pediatric patients (1).
DOSAGE AND ADMINISTRATION
• 400 mg administered orally, twice daily with or without food (2.1).
DOSAGE FORMS AND STRENGTHS
Tablets: 400 mg (3).
CONTRAINDICATIONS
None
WARNINGS AND PRECAUTIONS
Monitor for Immune Reconstitution Syndrome (5.1)
Drug Interactions
• Caution should be used when coadministering ISENTRESS with strong inducers of uridine diphosphate glucuronosyltransferase (UGT) 1A1 (e.g., rifampin) due to reduced plasma concentrations of raltegravir (5.2).
ADVERSE REACTIONS
• The most common adverse reactions (>10%) of all intensities, reported in subjects in either the ISENTRESS or the placebo treatment group, regardless of causality were: nausea, headache, diarrhea and pyrexia (6.1).
• Creatine kinase elevations were observed in subjects who received ISENTRESS. Myopathy and rhabdomyolysis have been reported; however, the relationship of ISENTRESS to these events is not known. Use with caution in patients at increased risk of myopathy or rhabdomyolysis, such as patients receiving concomitant medications known to cause these conditions (6.1).
To report SUSPECTED ADVERSE REACTIONS, contact Merck & Co., Inc. at 1-877-888-4231 or FDA at 1-800-FDA-1088 or www.fda.gov/medwatch.
USE IN SPECIFIC POPULATIONS
Pregnancy:
• ISENTRESS should be used during pregnancy only if the potential benefit justifies the potential risk to the fetus. Physicians are encouraged to register pregnant women exposed to ISENTRESS by calling 1-800-258-4263 so that Merck can monitor maternal and fetal outcomes (8.1).
Nursing Mothers:
• Breast-feeding is not recommended while taking ISENTRESS (8.3).
See 17 for PATIENT COUNSELING INFORMATION and FDA-approved patient labeling.

Revised: 10/2007

FULL PRESCRIBING INFORMATION: CONTENTS*

FULL PRESCRIBING INFORMATION

1 INDICATIONS AND USAGE
ISENTRESS[1] in combination with other antiretroviral agents is indicated for the treatment of HIV-1 infection in treatment-experienced adult patients who have evidence of viral replication and HIV-1 strains resistant to multiple antiretroviral agents.
This indication is based on analyses of plasma HIV-1 RNA levels up through 24 weeks in two controlled studies of ISENTRESS. These studies were conducted in clinically advanced, 3-class antiretroviral (NNRTI, NRTI, PI) treatment-experienced adults.
The use of other active agents with ISENTRESS is associated with a greater likelihood of treatment response [see Clinical Studies (14)].
The safety and efficacy of ISENTRESS have not been established in treatment-naïve adult patients or pediatric patients.
There are no study results demonstrating the effect of ISENTRESS on clinical progression of HIV-1 infection.

[1] Trademark of MERCK & CO., Inc.
  COPYRIGHT © 2007 MERCK & CO., Inc.
  All rights reserved

2 DOSAGE AND ADMINISTRATION
2.1 Dosing Information
For the treatment of patients with HIV-1 infection, the dosage of ISENTRESS is 400 mg administered orally, twice daily with or without food.

3 DOSAGE FORMS AND STRENGTHS
400 mg pink, oval-shaped, film-coated tablets with "227" on one side.

4 CONTRAINDICATIONS
None

5 WARNINGS AND PRECAUTIONS
5.1 Immune Reconstitution Syndrome
During the initial phase of treatment, patients responding to antiretroviral therapy may develop an inflammatory response to indolent or residual opportunistic infections (such as *Mycobacterium avium* complex, cytomegalovirus, *Pneumocystis jiroveci* pneumonia, *Mycobacterium* tuberculosis, or reactivation of varicella zoster virus), which may necessitate further evaluation and treatment.
5.2 Drug Interactions
Caution should be used when coadministering ISENTRESS with strong inducers of uridine diphosphate glucuronosyltransferase (UGT) 1A1 (e.g., rifampin) due to reduced plasma concentrations of raltegravir [see Drug Interactions (7)].

6 ADVERSE REACTIONS
6.1 Clinical Trials Experience
Because clinical trials are conducted under widely varying conditions, adverse reaction rates observed in the clinical trials of a drug cannot be directly compared to rates in the clinical trials of another drug and may not reflect the rates observed in practice.
Treatment-Experienced Studies
The safety assessment of ISENTRESS in treatment-experienced subjects is based on the pooled safety data from the randomized, double-blind, placebo-controlled trials, BENCHMRK 1 and BENCHMRK 2 (Protocols 018 and 019), and the randomized, double-blind, placebo-controlled, dose-ranging trial (Protocol 005) in antiretroviral treatment-experienced HIV-1 infected adult subjects reported using the recommended dose of ISENTRESS 400 mg twice daily in combination with optimized background therapy (OBT) in 507 subjects, in comparison to 282 subjects taking placebo in combination with OBT. During double-blind treatment, the total follow-up was 332.2 patient-years in the ISENTRESS 400 mg twice daily group and 150.2 patient-years in the placebo group.
The most commonly (>10%) reported adverse reactions, of all intensities, regardless of causality in subjects treated with ISENTRESS and OBT versus placebo and OBT are presented in Table 1.

Table 1: Percentage of Subjects with the Most Commonly Reported (>10%) Adverse Reactions of All Intensities* and Regardless of Causality Occurring in Treatment-Experienced Adult Subjects

System Organ Class, Adverse Reactions	Randomized Studies P005, P018 and P019	
	ISENTRESS 400 mg twice daily + OBT (n=507)[†] %	Placebo + OBT (n=282)[†] %
Gastrointestinal Disorders		
Diarrhea	16.6	19.5
Nausea	9.9	14.2
Nervous System Disorders		
Headache	9.7	11.7
General Disorders and Administration Site Conditions		
Pyrexia	4.9	10.3

* Intensities are defined as follows: Mild (awareness of sign or symptom, but easily tolerated); Moderate (discomfort enough to cause interference with usual activity); Severe (incapacitating with inability to work or do usual activity).
[†] n=total number of subjects per treatment group.

The clinical adverse reactions listed below were considered by investigators to be of moderate to severe intensity and causally related to any drug in the combination regimen (ISENTRESS/placebo alone or in combination with OBT, or OBT alone):
Common Adverse Reactions
Drug-related clinical adverse reactions of moderate to severe intensity occurring in ≥2% of subjects treated with ISENTRESS + OBT are presented in Table 2.

Table 2: Percentage of Subjects with Drug-Related* Adverse Reactions of Moderate to Severe Intensity[†] Occurring in ≥2% of Treatment-Experienced Adult Subjects

System Organ Class, Adverse Reactions	Randomized Studies P005, P018 and P019	
	ISENTRESS 400 mg Twice Daily + OBT (n = 507)[‡] %	Placebo + OBT (n = 282)[‡] %
Gastrointestinal Disorders		
Diarrhea	3.7	4.6
Nausea	2.2	3.2
Nervous System Disorders		
Headache	2.4	1.4

* Includes adverse reactions at least possibly, probably, or very likely related to the drug.
[†] Intensities are defined as follows: Moderate (discomfort enough to cause interference with usual activity); Severe (incapacitating with inability to work or do usual activity).
[‡] n=total number of subjects per treatment group.

Less Common Adverse Reactions
Drug-related adverse reactions occurring in at least 1% but less than 2% of treatment-experienced subjects (n=507) receiving ISENTRESS + OBT and of moderate (discomfort enough to cause interference with usual activity) to severe (incapacitating with inability to work or do usual activity) intensity are listed below by system organ class:
Gastrointestinal Disorders: abdominal pain, vomiting
General Disorders and Administration Site Conditions: asthenia, fatigue
Nervous System Disorders: dizziness
Skin and Subcutaneous Tissue Disorders: lipodystrophy acquired
Discontinuations
In the pooled analyses for studies P005, P018 and P019, the rates of discontinuation of therapy due to adverse reactions were 2.0% in subjects receiving ISENTRESS + OBT and 1.4% in subjects receiving placebo + OBT.
Serious Events
Drug Related
The following serious drug-related reactions were reported in the clinical studies, P005, P018 and P019: hypersensitiv-

Continued on next page

Isentress—Cont.

ity (hypersensitivity was seen in 2 subjects with ISENTRESS; therapy was interrupted and upon rechallenge the subjects were able to resume drug), anemia, neutropenia, myocardial infarction, gastritis, hepatitis, herpes simplex, toxic nephropathy, renal failure, chronic renal failure and renal tubular necrosis.

Regardless of Drug Relationship
Cancers were reported in treatment-experienced subjects who initiated ISENTRESS with OBT; several were recurrent. The types and rates of specific cancers were those expected in a highly immunodeficient population (many had CD4+ cell counts below 50 cells/mm³ and most had prior AIDS diagnoses). The cancers included Kaposi's sarcoma, lymphoma, squamous cell carcinoma, hepatocellular carcinoma and anal cancer. Most subjects had other risk factors for cancer including tobacco use, papillomavirus and active hepatitis B virus infection. It is unknown if these cancer diagnoses were related to ISENTRESS use.

Grade 2-4 creatine kinase laboratory abnormalities were observed in subjects treated with ISENTRESS (see Table 3). Myopathy and rhabdomyolysis have been reported; however, the relationship of ISENTRESS to these events is not known. Use with caution in patients at increased risk of myopathy or rhabdomyolysis, such as patients receiving concomitant medications known to cause these conditions.

Patients with Co-existing Conditions
Patients Co-infected with Hepatitis B and/or Hepatitis C Virus
In the clinical studies, P018 and P019, subjects with chronic (but not acute) active hepatitis B and/or hepatitis C virus

co-infection (N = 113/699 or 16.2%) were permitted to enroll provided that baseline liver function tests did not exceed 5 times the upper limit of normal (ULN). The rates of AST and ALT abnormalities were somewhat higher in the subgroup of subjects with hepatitis B and/or hepatitis C virus co-infection for both treatment groups. In general the safety profile of ISENTRESS in subjects with hepatitis B and/or hepatitis C virus co-infection was similar to subjects without hepatitis B and/or hepatitis C virus co-infection. Grade 2 or higher laboratory abnormalities that represent a worsening from baseline of AST, ALT or total bilirubin occurred in 26%, 27% and 12%, respectively, of raltegravir-treated coinfected subjects as compared to 9%, 8% and 7% of all other raltegravir-treated subjects.

Laboratory Abnormalities
The percentages of adult subjects treated with ISENTRESS 400 mg twice daily in P005, P018 and P019 with selected Grades 2 to 4 laboratory abnormalities that represent a worsening from baseline are presented in Table 3.
[See table 3 below]

7   DRUG INTERACTIONS
7.1   Effect of Raltegravir on the Pharmacokinetics of Other Agents
Raltegravir does not inhibit (IC$_{50}$>100 µM) CYP1A2, CYP2B6, CYP2C8, CYP2C9, CYP2C19, CYP2D6 or CYP3A *in vitro*. Moreover, *in vitro*, raltegravir did not induce CYP3A4. A midazolam drug interaction study confirmed the low propensity of raltegravir to alter the pharmacokinetics of agents metabolized by CYP3A4 *in vivo* by demonstrating a lack of effect of raltegravir on the pharmacokinetics of midazolam, a sensitive CYP3A4 substrate. Similarly, raltegravir is not an inhibitor (IC$_{50}$>50 µM) of the UDP-glucuronosyltransferases (UGT) tested (UGT1A1,

UGT2B7), and raltegravir does not inhibit P-glycoprotein-mediated transport. Based on these data, ISENTRESS is not expected to affect the pharmacokinetics of drugs that are substrates of these enzymes or P-glycoprotein (e.g., protease inhibitors, NNRTIs, methadone, opioid analgesics, statins, azole antifungals, proton pump inhibitors, oral contraceptives, and anti-erectile dysfunction agents).

In drug interaction studies, raltegravir did not have a clinically meaningful effect on the pharmacokinetics of the following: lamivudine, tenofovir.

7.2   Effect of Other Agents on the Pharmacokinetics of Raltegravir
Raltegravir is not a substrate of cytochrome P450 (CYP) enzymes. Based on *in vivo* and *in vitro* studies, raltegravir is eliminated mainly by metabolism via a UGT1A1-mediated glucuronidation pathway.

Rifampin, a strong inducer of UGT1A1, reduces plasma concentrations of ISENTRESS. Therefore, caution should be used when coadministering ISENTRESS with rifampin or other strong inducers of UGT1A1 *[see Warnings and Precautions (5.2)]*. The impact of other inducers of drug metabolizing enzymes, such as phenytoin and phenobarbital, on UGT1A1 is unknown. Other less strong inducers (e.g., efavirenz, nevirapine, rifabutin, St. John's wort) may be used with the recommended dose of ISENTRESS.

Similar to rifampin, tipranavir/ritonavir reduces plasma concentrations of ISENTRESS. However, approximately 100 subjects received raltegravir in combination with tipranavir/ritonavir in Protocols 018 and 019. Comparable efficacy was observed in this subgroup relative to subjects not receiving tipranavir/ritonavir. Based on these data, tipranavir/ritonavir may be coadministered with ISENTRESS without dose adjustment of ISENTRESS.

Atazanavir, a strong inhibitor of UGT1A1, and atazanavir/ritonavir increase plasma concentrations of raltegravir. However, concomitant use of ISENTRESS and atazanavir/ritonavir did not result in a unique safety signal in Protocol 005 and Protocols 018 and 019. Based on these data, atazanavir/ritonavir may be coadministered with ISENTRESS without dose adjustment of ISENTRESS.

Coadministration of ISENTRESS with other drugs that inhibit UGT1A1 may increase plasma levels of raltegravir.

8   USE IN SPECIFIC POPULATIONS
8.1   Pregnancy
Pregnancy Category C
ISENTRESS should be used during pregnancy only if the potential benefit justifies the potential risk to the fetus. There are no adequate and well-controlled studies in pregnant women. In addition, there have been no pharmacokinetic studies conducted in pregnant patients.

Developmental toxicity studies were performed in rabbits (at oral doses up to 1000 mg/kg/day) and rats (at oral doses up to 600 mg/kg/day). The reproductive toxicity study in rats was performed with pre-, peri-, and postnatal evaluation. The highest doses in these studies produced systemic exposures in these species approximately 3- to 4-fold the exposure at the recommended human dose. In both rabbits and rats, no treatment-related effects on embryonic/fetal survival or fetal weights were observed. In addition, no treatment-related external, visceral, or skeletal changes were observed in rabbits. However, treatment-related increases over controls in the incidence of supernumerary ribs were seen in rats at 600 mg/kg/day (exposures 3-fold the exposure at the recommended human dose).

Placenta transfer of drug was demonstrated in both rats and rabbits. At a maternal dose of 600 mg/kg/day in rats, mean drug concentrations in fetal plasma were approximately 1.5- to 2.5-fold greater than in maternal plasma at 1 hour and 24 hours postdose, respectively. Mean drug concentrations in fetal plasma were approximately 2% of the mean maternal concentration at both 1 and 24 hours postdose at a maternal dose of 1000 mg/kg/day in rabbits.

Antiretroviral Pregnancy Registry
To monitor maternal-fetal outcomes of pregnant patients exposed to ISENTRESS, an Antiretroviral Pregnancy Registry has been established. Physicians are encouraged to register patients by calling 1-800-258-4263.

8.3   Nursing Mothers
Breast-feeding is not recommended while taking ISENTRESS. In addition, it is recommended that HIV-infected mothers not breast-feed their infants to avoid risking postnatal transmission of HIV.

It is not known whether raltegravir is secreted in human milk. However, raltegravir is secreted in the milk of lactating rats. Mean drug concentrations in milk were approximately 3-fold greater than those in maternal plasma at a maternal dose of 600 mg/kg/day in rats. There were no effects in rat offspring attributable to exposure of ISENTRESS through the milk.

8.4   Pediatric Use
Safety and effectiveness of ISENTRESS in pediatric patients less than 16 years of age have not been established.

8.5   Geriatric Use
Clinical studies of ISENTRESS did not include sufficient numbers of subjects aged 65 and over to determine whether they respond differently from younger subjects. Other reported clinical experience has not identified differences in responses between the elderly and younger subjects. In general, dose selection for an elderly patient should be cautious, reflecting the greater frequency of decreased hepatic, renal, or cardiac function, and of concomitant disease or other drug therapy.

Table 3: Selected Grade 2 to 4 Laboratory Abnormalities Reported in Treatment-Experienced Subjects

Laboratory Parameter Preferred Term (Unit)	Limit	Randomized Studies P005, P018 and P019	
		ISENTRESS 400 mg Twice Daily + OBT (N = 507)	Placebo + OBT (N = 282)
Hematology			
Absolute neutrophil count (10³/µL)			
Grade 2	0.75–0.999	3.7%	7.4%
Grade 3	0.50–0.749	2.4%	2.5%
Grade 4	<0.50	1.0%	1.1%
Hemoglobin (gm/dL)			
Grade 2	7.5–8.4	1.0%	2.8%
Grade 3	6.5–7.4	1.0%	0.4%
Grade 4	<6.5	0.0%	0.0%
Platelet count (10³/µL)			
Grade 2	50–99.999	3.7%	5.7%
Grade 3	25–49.999	0.4%	0.4%
Grade 4	<25	0.8%	0.4%
Blood chemistry			
Fasting (non-random) serum glucose test (mg/dL)			
Grade 2	126–250	9.3%	6.8%
Grade 3	251–500	1.4%	1.4%
Grade 4	>500	0.0%	0.0%
Total serum bilirubin			
Grade 2	1.6–2.5 × ULN	5.3%	6.7%
Grade 3	2.6–5.0 × ULN	3.2%	2.5%
Grade 4	>5.0 × ULN	0.8%	0.0%
Serum aspartate aminotransferase			
Grade 2	2.6–5.0 × ULN	9.1%	5.7%
Grade 3	5.1–10.0 × ULN	2.2%	2.1%
Grade 4	>10.0 × ULN	0.4%	0.7%
Serum alanine aminotransferase			
Grade 2	2.6–5.0 × ULN	6.9%	7.8%
Grade 3	5.1–10.0 × ULN	3.0%	1.4%
Grade 4	>10.0 × ULN	0.6%	1.1%
Serum alkaline phosphatase			
Grade 2	2.6–5.0 × ULN	2.0%	0.4%
Grade 3	5.1–10.0 × ULN	0.4%	1.1%
Grade 4	>10.0 × ULN	0.4%	0.4%
Serum pancreatic amylase test			
Grade 2	1.6–2.0 × ULN	1.4%	0.7%
Grade 3	2.1–5.0 × ULN	3.6%	2.1%
Grade 4	>5.0 × ULN	0.2%	0.0%
Serum lipase test			
Grade 2	1.6–3.0 × ULN	3.4%	1.8%
Grade 3	3.1–5.0 × ULN	0.6%	0.4%
Grade 4	>5.0 × ULN	0.2%	0.0%
Serum creatine kinase			
Grade 2	6.0–9.9 × ULN	2.2%	1.4%
Grade 3	10.0–19.9 × ULN	2.4%	1.8%
Grade 4	≥20.0 × ULN	2.2%	0.7%

ULN = Upper limit of normal range

Table 4: Effect of Other Agents on the Pharmacokinetics of Raltegravir

Coadministered Drug	Coadministered Drug Dose/Schedule	Raltegravir Dose/Schedule	Ratio (90% Confidence Interval) of Raltegravir Pharmacokinetic Parameters with/without Coadministered Drug; No Effect = 1.00			
			n	C_{max}	AUC	C_{min}
atazanavir	400 mg daily	100 mg single dose	10	1.53 (1.11, 2.12)	1.72 (1.47, 2.02)	1.95 (1.30, 2.92)
atazanavir/ritonavir	300 mg/100 mg daily	400 mg twice daily	10	1.24 (0.87, 1.77)	1.41 (1.12, 1.78)	1.77 (1.39, 2.25)
efavirenz	600 mg daily	400 mg single dose	9	0.64 (0.41, 0.98)	0.64 (0.52, 0.80)	0.79 (0.49, 1.28)
rifampin	600 mg daily	400 mg single dose	9	0.62 (0.37, 1.04)	0.60 (0.39, 0.91)	0.39 (0.30, 0.51)
ritonavir	100 mg twice daily	400 mg single dose	10	0.76 (0.55, 1.04)	0.84 (0.70, 1.01)	0.99 (0.70, 1.40)
tenofovir	300 mg daily	400 mg twice daily	9	1.64 (1.16, 2.32)	1.49 (1.15, 1.94)	1.03 (0.73, 1.45)
tipranavir/ritonavir	500 mg/200 mg twice daily	400 mg twice daily	15 (14 for C_{min})	0.82 (0.46, 1.46)	0.76 (0.49, 1.19)	0.45 (0.31, 0.66)

8.6 Use in Patients with Hepatic Impairment

No clinically important pharmacokinetic differences between subjects with moderate hepatic impairment and healthy subjects were observed. No dosage adjustment is necessary for patients with mild to moderate hepatic impairment. The effect of severe hepatic impairment on the pharmacokinetics of raltegravir has not been studied *[see Clinical Pharmacology (12.3)]*.

8.7 Use in Patients with Renal Impairment

No clinically important pharmacokinetic differences between subjects with severe renal impairment and healthy subjects were observed. No dosage adjustment is necessary *[see Clinical Pharmacology (12.3)]*.

10 OVERDOSAGE

No specific information is available on the treatment of overdosage with ISENTRESS. Doses as high as 1600-mg single dose and 800-mg twice-daily multiple doses were studied in healthy volunteers without evidence of toxicity. Occasional doses of up to 1800 mg per day were taken in the P005/P018 & P019 studies without evidence of toxicity.

In the event of an overdose, it is reasonable to employ the standard supportive measures, e.g., remove unabsorbed material from the gastrointestinal tract, employ clinical monitoring (including obtaining an electrocardiogram), and institute supportive therapy if required. The extent to which ISENTRESS may be dialyzable is unknown.

11 DESCRIPTION

ISENTRESS contains raltegravir potassium, a human immunodeficiency virus integrase strand transfer inhibitor. The chemical name for raltegravir potassium is *N*-[(4-Fluorophenyl)methyl]-1,6-dihydro-5-hydroxy-1-methyl-2-[1-methyl-1-[[(5-methyl-1,3,4-oxadiazol-2-yl)carbonyl]amino]ethyl]-6-oxo-4-pyrimidinecarboxamide monopotassium salt. The empirical formula is $C_{20}H_{20}FKN_6O_5$ and the molecular weight is 482.51. The structural formula is:

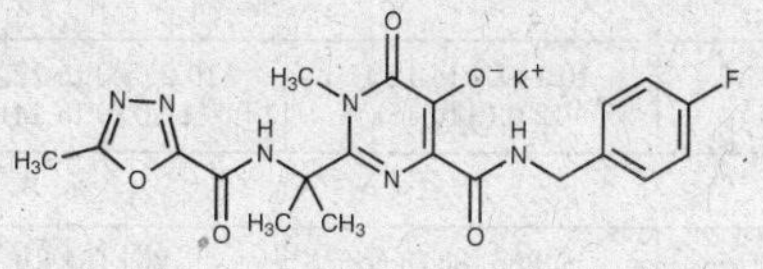

Raltegravir potassium is a white to off-white powder. It is soluble in water, slightly soluble in methanol, very slightly soluble in ethanol and acetonitrile and insoluble in isopropanol.

Each film-coated tablet of ISENTRESS for oral administration contains 434.4 mg of raltegravir potassium (as salt), equivalent to 400 mg of raltegravir (free phenol) and the following inactive ingredients: microcrystalline cellulose, lactose monohydrate, calcium phosphate dibasic anhydrous, hypromellose 2208, poloxamer 407 (contains 0.01% butylated hydroxytoluene as antioxidant), sodium stearyl fumarate, magnesium stearate. In addition, the film coating contains the following inactive ingredients: polyvinyl alcohol, titanium dioxide, polyethylene glycol 3350, talc, red iron oxide and black iron oxide.

12 CLINICAL PHARMACOLOGY

12.1 Mechanism of Action

Raltegravir is an HIV-1 antiviral drug *[see Clinical Pharmacology (12.4)]*.

12.2 Pharmacodynamics

In a monotherapy study raltegravir (400 mg twice daily) demonstrated rapid antiviral activity with mean viral load reduction of 1.66 log_{10} copies/mL by Day 10.

In Protocol 005 and Protocols 018 and 019, antiviral responses were similar among subjects regardless of dose.

Effects on Electrocardiogram

In a randomized, placebo-controlled, crossover study, 31 healthy subjects were administered a single oral supratherapeutic dose of raltegravir 1600 mg and placebo. Peak raltegravir plasma concentrations were approximately 4-fold higher than the peak concentrations following a 400 mg dose. ISENTRESS did not appear to prolong the QTc interval for 12 hours postdose. After baseline and placebo adjustment, the maximum mean QTc change was -0.4 msec (1-sided 95% upper Cl: 3.1 msec).

12.3 Pharmacokinetics

Absorption

Raltegravir is absorbed with a T_{max} of approximately 3 hours postdose in the fasted state. Raltegravir AUC and C_{max} increase dose proportionally over the dose range 100 mg to 1600 mg. Raltegravir C_{12hr} increases dose proportionally over the dose range of 100 to 800 mg and increases slightly less than dose proportionally over the dose range 100 mg to 1600 mg. With twice-daily dosing, pharmacokinetic steady state is achieved within approximately the first 2 days of dosing. There is little to no accumulation in AUC and C_{max}. The average accumulation ratio for C_{12hr} ranged from approximately 1.2 to 1.6.

The absolute bioavailability of raltegravir has not been established.

In subjects who received 400 mg twice daily alone, raltegravir drug exposures were characterized by a geometric mean $AUC_{0\text{-}12hr}$ of 14.3 μM•hr and C_{12hr} of 142 nM.

Considerable variability was observed in the pharmacokinetics of raltegravir. For observed C_{12hr} in Protocols 018 and 019, the coefficient of variation (CV) for inter-subject variability = 212% and the CV for intra-subject variability = 122%.

Effect of Food on Oral Absorption

ISENTRESS may be administered without regard to food. Administration of raltegravir following a high-fat meal increased raltegravir AUC by approximately 19%. A high-fat meal slowed the rate of absorption resulting in an approximately 34% decrease in C_{max}, an 8.5-fold increase in C_{12hr}, and a delay in T_{max} following a single 400 mg dose. The effect of consumption of a range of food types on steady-state pharmacokinetics is not known. Raltegravir was administered without regard to food in the pivotal safety and efficacy studies in HIV-1 positive subjects.

Distribution

Raltegravir is approximately 83% bound to human plasma protein over the concentration range of 2 to 10 μM.

Metabolism and Excretion

The apparent terminal half-life of raltegravir is approximately 9 hours, with a shorter α-phase half-life (~1 hour) accounting for much of the AUC. Following administration of an oral dose of radiolabeled raltegravir, approximately 51 and 32% of the dose was excreted in feces and urine, respectively. In feces, only raltegravir was present, most of which is likely derived from hydrolysis of raltegravir-glucuronide secreted in bile as observed in preclinical species. Two components, namely raltegravir and raltegravir-glucuronide, were detected in urine and accounted for approximately 9 and 23% of the dose, respectively. The major circulating entity was raltegravir and represented approximately 70% of the total radioactivity; the remaining radioactivity in plasma was accounted for by raltegravir-glucuronide. Studies using isoform-selective chemical inhibitors and cDNA-expressed UDP-glucuronosyltransferases (UGT) show that UGT1A1 is the main enzyme responsible for the formation of raltegravir-glucuronide. Thus, the data indicate that the major mechanism of clearance of raltegravir in humans is UGT1A1-mediated glucuronidation.

Special Populations

Pediatric

The pharmacokinetics of raltegravir in pediatric patients has not been established.

Age

The effect of age on the pharmacokinetics of raltegravir was evaluated in the composite analysis. No dosage adjustment is necessary.

Race

The effect of race on the pharmacokinetics of raltegravir was evaluated in the composite analysis. No dosage adjustment is necessary.

Gender

A study of the pharmacokinetics of raltegravir was performed in young healthy males and females. Additionally, the effect of gender was evaluated in a composite analysis of pharmacokinetic data from 103 healthy subjects and 28 HIV-1 infected subjects receiving raltegravir monotherapy with fasted administration. No dosage adjustment is necessary.

Hepatic Impairment

Raltegravir is eliminated primarily by glucuronidation in the liver. A study of the pharmacokinetics of raltegravir was performed in subjects with moderate hepatic impairment. Additionally, hepatic impairment was evaluated in the composite pharmacokinetic analysis. There were no clinically important pharmacokinetic differences between subjects with moderate hepatic impairment and healthy subjects. No dosage adjustment is necessary for patients with mild to moderate hepatic impairment. The effect of severe hepatic impairment on the pharmacokinetics of raltegravir has not been studied.

Renal Impairment

Renal clearance of unchanged drug is a minor pathway of elimination. A study of the pharmacokinetics of raltegravir was performed in subjects with severe renal impairment. Additionally, renal impairment was evaluated in the composite pharmacokinetic analysis. There were no clinically important pharmacokinetic differences between subjects with severe renal impairment and healthy subjects. No dosage adjustment is necessary. Because the extent to which ISENTRESS may be dialyzable is unknown, dosing before a dialysis session should be avoided.

UGT1A1 Polymorphism

Data currently available are not sufficient to determine the impact of UGT1A1 polymorphism on raltegravir pharmacokinetics.

Drug Interactions *[see Drug Interactions (7)]*.

[See table 4 above]

12.4 Microbiology

Mechanism of Action

Raltegravir inhibits the catalytic activity of HIV-1 integrase, an HIV-1 encoded enzyme that is required for viral replication. Inhibition of integrase prevents the covalent insertion, or integration, of unintegrated linear HIV-1 DNA into the host cell genome preventing the formation of the HIV-1 provirus. The provirus is required to direct the production of progeny virus, so inhibiting integration prevents propagation of the viral infection. Raltegravir did not significantly inhibit human phosphoryltransferases including DNA polymerases α, β, and γ.

Antiviral Activity in Cell Culture

Raltegravir at concentrations of 31 ± 20 nM resulted in 95% inhibition (EC_{95}) of viral spread (relative to an untreated virus-infected culture) in human T-lymphoid cell cultures infected with the cell-line adapted HIV-1 variant H9IIIB. In addition, raltegravir at concentrations of 6 to 50 nM resulted in 95% inhibition of viral spread in cultures of mitogen-activated human peripheral blood mononuclear cells infected with diverse, primary clinical isolates of HIV-1, including isolates resistant to reverse transcriptase inhibitors and protease inhibitors. Raltegravir also inhibited replication of an HIV-2 isolate when tested in CEMx174 cells (EC_{95} value = 6 nM). Additive to synergistic antiretroviral activity was observed when human T-lymphoid cells infected with the H9IIIB variant of HIV-1 were incubated with raltegravir in combination with non-nucleoside reverse transcriptase inhibitors (delavirdine, efavirenz, or nevirapine); nucleoside analog reverse transcriptase inhibitors (abacavir, didanosine, lamivudine, stavudine, tenofovir, zalcitabine, or zidovudine); protease inhibitors (amprenavir, atazanavir, indinavir, lopinavir, nelfinavir, ritonavir, or saquinavir); or the entry inhibitor enfuvirtide.

Continued on next page

Information on the Merck & Co., Inc., products listed on these pages is from the full prescribing information in use March 1, 2008. For information, please call 1-800-NSC-MERCK [1-800-672-6372].

Isentress—Cont.

Resistance

The mutations observed in the HIV-1 integrase coding sequence that contributed to raltegravir resistance (evolved either in cell culture or in subjects treated with raltegravir) generally included an amino acid substitution at either Q148 (changed to H, K, or R) or N155 (changed to H) plus one or more additional substitutions (i.e., L74M/R, E92Q, T97A, E138A/K, G140A/S, V151I, G163R, H183P, Y226D/F/H, S230R and D232N). Amino acid substitution at Y143C/H/R is another pathway to raltegravir resistance.

13   NONCLINICAL TOXICOLOGY

13.1   Carcinogenesis, Mutagenesis, Impairment of Fertility

Long-term (2-year) carcinogenicity studies of raltegravir in rodents are ongoing.

No evidence of mutagenicity or genotoxicity was observed in *in vitro* microbial mutagenesis (Ames) tests, *in vitro* alkaline elution assays for DNA breakage and *in vitro* and *in vivo* chromosomal aberration studies.

No effect on fertility was seen in male and female rats at doses up to 600 mg/kg/day which resulted in a 3-fold exposure above the exposure at the recommended human dose.

14   CLINICAL STUDIES

Description of Clinical Studies

The evidence of efficacy of ISENTRESS is based on the analyses of 24-week data from 2 ongoing, randomized, double-blind, placebo-controlled trials, BENCHMRK 1 and BENCHMRK 2 (Protocols 018 and 019), in antiretroviral treatment-experienced HIV-1 infected adult subjects. These efficacy results were supported by the 48-week analysis of a randomized, double-blind, controlled, dose-ranging trial, Protocol 005, in antiretroviral treatment-experienced HIV-1 infected adult subjects.

Treatment-Experienced Subjects

BENCHMRK 1 and BENCHMRK 2 are Phase III studies to evaluate the safety and antiretroviral activity of ISENTRESS 400 mg twice daily in combination with an optimized background therapy (OBT), versus OBT alone, in HIV-infected subjects, 16 years or older, with documented resistance to at least 1 drug in each of 3 Classes (NNRTIs, NRTIs, PIs) of antiretroviral therapies. Randomization was stratified by degree of resistance to PI (1PI vs. >1PI) and use of enfuvirtide in the OBT. Prior to randomization, OBT was selected by the investigator based on genotypic/phenotypic resistance testing and prior ART history.

Table 5 shows the demographic characteristics of subjects in the ISENTRESS 400 mg twice daily arm and subjects in the placebo arm.

[See table 5 above]

Table 6 compares the characteristics of optimized background therapy at baseline in the ISENTRESS 400 mg twice daily arm and subjects in the control arm.

[See table 6 above]

Week 24 outcomes for subjects on the recommended dose of ISENTRESS 400 mg twice daily from the pooled studies BENCHMRK 1 and 2 are shown in Table 7. The efficacy responses were evaluated based upon the 436 subjects from the pooled studies BENCHMRK 1 and 2 who had completed 24 weeks of treatment or discontinued earlier. All other outcomes were based upon the total 699 subjects who were randomized and treated.

[See table 7 at top of next page]

The mean changes in plasma HIV-1 RNA from baseline were -1.85 $\log_{10}$ copies/mL in the ISENTRESS 400 mg twice daily arm and -0.84 $\log_{10}$ copies/mL for the control arm. The mean increase from baseline in CD4+ cell counts was higher in the arm receiving ISENTRESS 400 mg twice daily (89 cells/mm^3) than in the control arm (35 cells/mm^3).

Virologic responses at Week 24 by baseline genotypic and phenotypic sensitivity score are shown in Table 8.

[See table 8 at top of next page]

16   HOW SUPPLIED/STORAGE AND HANDLING

ISENTRESS tablets 400 mg are pink, oval-shaped, film-coated tablets with "227" on one side. They are supplied as follows:

NDC 0006-0227-61 unit-of-use bottles of 60.

No. 3894

Storage and Handling

Store at 20-25°C (68-77°F); excursions permitted to 15-30°C (59-86°F). See USP Controlled Room Temperature.

17   PATIENT COUNSELING INFORMATION

[See FDA-Approved Patient Labeling].

Patients should be informed that ISENTRESS is not a cure for HIV infection or AIDS. They should also be told that people taking ISENTRESS may still get infections or other conditions common in people with HIV (opportunistic infections). In addition, patients should be told that the long-term effects of ISENTRESS are not known at this time. Patients should also be told that it is very important that they stay under a physician's care during treatment with ISENTRESS.

Patients should be informed that ISENTRESS does not reduce the chance of passing HIV to others through sexual contact, sharing needles, or being exposed to blood. Patients should be advised to continue to practice safer sex and to use latex or polyurethane condoms or other barrier methods to lower the chance of sexual contact with any body fluids such as semen, vaginal secretions or blood. Patients should also be advised to never re-use or share needles.

Table 5: Baseline Characteristics

BENCHMRK 1 and 2 Pooled	ISENTRESS 400 mg Twice Daily + OBT (N = 462)	Placebo + OBT (N = 237)
Gender n (%)		
Male	405 (87.7)	210 (88.6)
Female	57 (12.3)	27 (11.4)
Race n (%)		
White	301 (65.2)	173 (73.0)
Black	66 (14.3)	26 (11.0)
Asian	16 (3.5)	6 (2.5)
Hispanic	53 (11.5)	19 (8.0)
Others	26 (5.6)	13 (5.5)
Age (years)		
Median (min, max)	45.0 (16 to 74)	45.0 (17 to 70)
CD4+ Cell Count		
Median (min, max), cells/mm^3	119 (1 to 792)	123 (0 to 759)
≤50 cells/mm^3, n (%)	146 (31.6)	78 (32.9)
>50 and ≤200 cells/mm^3, n (%)	173 (37.4)	85 (35.9)
Plasma HIV-1 RNA		
Median (min, max), $\log_{10}$ copies/mL	4.8 (2 to 6)	4.7 (2 to 6)
>100,000 copies/mL, n (%)	164 (35.5)	78 (32.9)
History of AIDS n (%)		
Yes	426 (92.2)	216 (91.1)
Prior Use of ART, Median (1st Quartile, 3rd Quartile)		
Years of ART Use	10.1 (7.4 to 12.1)	10.2 (7.9 to 12.4)
Number of ART	12.0 (9 to 15)	12.0 (9 to 14)
Hepatitis Co-infection* n (%)		
No Hepatitis B or C virus	385 (83.3)	201 (84.8)
Hepatitis B virus only	36 (7.8)	7 (3.0)
Hepatitis C virus only	37 (8.0)	27 (11.4)
Co-infection of Hepatitis B and C virus	4 (0.9)	2 (0.8)
Stratum n (%)		
Enfuvirtide in OBT	175 (37.9)	89 (37.6)
Resistant to ≥2 PI	447 (96.8)	226 (95.4)

* Hepatitis B virus surface antigen positive or hepatitis C virus antibody positive.

Table 6: Characteristics of Optimized Background Therapy at Baseline

BENCHMRK 1 and 2 Pooled	ISENTRESS 400 mg Twice Daily + OBT (N = 462)	Placebo + OBT (N = 237)
Number of ARTs in OBT		
Median (min, max)	4.0 (1 to 7)	4.0 (2 to 7)
Number of Active PI in OBT by Phenotypic Resistance Test*		
0	166 (35.9)	97 (40.9)
1 or more	278 (60.2)	137 (57.8)
Phenotypic Sensitivity Score (PSS)[†]		
0	67 (14.5)	44 (18.6)
1	145 (31.4)	71 (30.0)
2	142 (30.7)	66 (27.8)
3 or more	85 (18.4)	48 (20.3)
Genotypic Sensitivity Score (GSS)[†]		
0	115 (24.9)	65 (27.4)
1	178 (38.5)	96 (40.5)
2	111 (24.0)	49 (20.7)
3 or more	51 (11.0)	23 (9.7)

* Darunavir use in OBT in darunavir naïve subjects was counted as one active PI.
† The Phenotypic Sensitivity Score (PSS) and the Genotypic Sensitivity Score (GSS) were defined as the total oral ARTs in OBT to which a subject's viral isolate showed phenotypic sensitivity and genotypic sensitivity, respectively, based upon phenotypic and genotypic resistance tests. Enfuvirtide use in OBT in enfuvirtide-naïve subjects was counted as one active drug in OBT in the GSS and PSS. Similarly, darunavir use in OBT in darunavir-naïve subjects was counted as one active drug in OBT.

Physicians should instruct their patients that if they miss a dose, they should take it as soon as they remember. If they do not remember until it is time for the next dose, they should be instructed to skip the missed dose and go back to the regular schedule. Patients should not take two tablets of ISENTRESS at the same time.

Physicians should instruct their patients to read the Patient Package Insert before starting ISENTRESS therapy and to reread each time the prescription is renewed. Patients should be instructed to inform their physician or pharmacist if they develop any unusual symptom, or if any known symptom persists or worsens.

Manufactured and Distributed by:
MERCK & CO., INC., Whitehouse Station, NJ 08889, USA
Printed in USA

9795100
U.S. Patent Nos. US 7,169,780

Patient Information

ISENTRESS™ (eye **sen** tris)
(raltegravir)
Tablets

Read the patient information that comes with ISENTRESS[1] before you start taking it and each time you get a refill. There may be new information. This leaflet is a summary of the information for patients. Your doctor or pharmacist can give you additional information. This leaflet does not take the place of talking with your doctor about your medical condition or your treatment.

[1] Trademark of MERCK & CO., Inc.

What is ISENTRESS?
- ISENTRESS is an anti-HIV (antiretroviral) medicine that helps to control HIV infection. The term HIV stands for Human Immunodeficiency Virus. It is the virus that causes AIDS (Acquired Immune Deficiency Syndrome). ISENTRESS is used along with other anti-HIV medicines in patients who are already taking or have taken anti-HIV medicines and the medicines are not controlling their HIV infection. ISENTRESS will NOT cure HIV infection.
- People taking ISENTRESS may still develop infections, including opportunistic infections or other conditions that happen with HIV infection.
- Stay under the care of your doctor during treatment with ISENTRESS.
- The long-term effects of ISENTRESS are not known at this time.
- The safety and effectiveness of ISENTRESS in children less than 16 years of age has not been studied.

ISENTRESS must be used with other anti-HIV medicines.

How does ISENTRESS work?
- ISENTRESS blocks an enzyme which the virus (HIV) needs in order to make more virus. The enzyme that ISENTRESS blocks is called HIV integrase.
- When used with other anti-HIV medicines, ISENTRESS may do two things:
  1. It may reduce the amount of HIV in your blood. This is called your "viral load".
  2. It may also increase the number of white blood cells called CD4 (T) cells that help fight off other infections.
- ISENTRESS may not have these effects in all patients.

Does ISENTRESS lower the chance of passing HIV to other people?
No. ISENTRESS does not reduce the chance of passing HIV to others through sexual contact, sharing needles, or being exposed to your blood.
- Continue to practice safer sex.
- Use latex or polyurethane condoms or other barrier methods to lower the chance of sexual contact with any body fluids. This includes semen from a man, vaginal secretions from a woman, or blood.
- Never re-use or share needles.

Ask your doctor if you have any questions about safer sex or how to prevent passing HIV to other people.

What should I tell my doctor before and during treatment with ISENTRESS?
Tell your doctor about all of your medical conditions. Include any of the following that applies to you:
- You have any allergies.
- You are pregnant or plan to become pregnant.
  - ISENTRESS is not recommended for use during pregnancy. ISENTRESS has not been studied in pregnant women. If you take ISENTRESS while you are pregnant, talk to your doctor about how you can be included in the Antiretroviral Pregnancy Registry.
- You are breast-feeding or plan to breast-feed.
  - It is recommended that HIV-infected women should not breast-feed their infants. This is because their babies could be infected with HIV through their breast milk.
  - Talk with your doctor about the best way to feed your baby.

Tell your doctor about all the medicines you take. Include the following:
- prescription medicines
- non-prescription medicines
- vitamins
- herbal supplements

Know the medicines you take.
- Keep a list of your medicines. Show the list to your doctor and pharmacist when you get a new medicine.

How should I take ISENTRESS?
Take ISENTRESS <u>exactly</u> as your doctor has prescribed.
The recommended dose is as follows:
- Take only one 400 mg tablet at a time.
- Take it twice a day.
- Take it by mouth.
- Take it with or without food.

Do not change your dose or stop taking ISENTRESS or your other anti-HIV medicines without first talking with your doctor.
IMPORTANT: Take ISENTRESS exactly as your doctor prescribed and at the right times of day because if you don't:
- The amount of virus (HIV) in your blood may increase if the medicine is stopped for even a short period of time.
- The virus may develop resistance to ISENTRESS and become harder to treat.
- Your medicines may stop working to fight HIV.
- The activity of ISENTRESS may be reduced (due to resistance).

If you fail to take ISENTRESS the way you should, here's what to do:
- If you miss a dose, take it as soon as you remember. If you do not remember until it is time for your next dose, skip the missed dose and go back to your regular schedule. Do NOT take two tablets of ISENTRESS at the same time. In other words, do NOT take a double dose.
- If you take too much ISENTRESS, call your doctor or local Poison Control Center.

Be sure to keep a supply of your anti-HIV medicines.
- When your ISENTRESS supply starts to run low, get more from your doctor or pharmacy.
- Do not wait until your medicine runs out to get more.

What are the possible side effects of ISENTRESS?
When ISENTRESS has been given with other anti-HIV drugs, the most common side effects included:
- diarrhea
- nausea
- headache

A condition called Immune Reconstitution Syndrome can happen in some patients with advanced HIV infection (AIDS) when combination antiretroviral treatment is started. Signs and symptoms of inflammation from opportunistic infections that a person has or had may occur as the medicines work to control the HIV infection and strengthen the immune system. Call your doctor right away if you notice any signs or symptoms of an infection after starting ISENTRESS with other anti-HIV medicines.

Contact your doctor promptly if you experience unexplained muscle pain, tenderness, or weakness while taking ISENTRESS.

Tell your doctor if you have any side effect that bothers you or that does not go away.

These are not all the side effects of ISENTRESS. For more information, ask your doctor or pharmacist.

How should I store ISENTRESS?
- Store ISENTRESS at room temperature (68 to 77°F).
- **Keep ISENTRESS and all medicines out of the reach of children.**

General information about the use of ISENTRESS
Medicines are sometimes prescribed for conditions that are not mentioned in patient information leaflets.
- Do not use ISENTRESS for a condition for which it was not prescribed.
- Do not give ISENTRESS to other people, even if they have the same symptoms you have. It may harm them.

This leaflet gives you the most important information about ISENTRESS.
- If you would like to know more, talk with your doctor.
- You can ask your doctor or pharmacist for additional information about ISENTRESS that is written for health professionals.
- For more information go to www.ISENTRESS.com or call 1-800-622-4477.

What are the ingredients in ISENTRESS?
Active ingredient: Each film-coated tablet contains 400 mg of raltegravir.
Inactive ingredients: Microcrystalline cellulose, lactose monohydrate, calcium phosphate dibasic anhydrous, hypromellose 2208, poloxamer 407 (contains 0.01% butylated hydroxytoluene as antioxidant), sodium stearyl fumarate, magnesium stearate. In addition, the film coating contains the following inactive ingredients: polyvinyl alcohol, titanium dioxide, polyethylene glycol 3350, talc, red iron oxide and black iron oxide.

Manufactured and Distributed by:
MERCK & CO., Inc.
Whitehouse Station, NJ 08889, USA
Revised October 2007
9795100
U.S. Patent Nos. US 7,169,780

Information on the Merck & Co., Inc., products listed on these pages is from the full prescribing information in use March 1, 2008. For information, please call 1-800-NSC-MERCK [1-800-672-6372].

Table 7: Outcomes by Treatment Group through Week 24

BENCHMRK 1 and 2 Pooled n (%)	ISENTRESS 400 mg Twice Daily + OBT (N = 462)	Placebo + OBT (N = 237)
Outcome at Week 24	n (%)	n (%)
Subjects with Week 24 data	286	150
Subjects with HIV-1 RNA less than 400 copies/mL*	216 (75.5)	59 (39.3)
Subjects with HIV-1 RNA less than 50 copies/mL*	179 (62.6)	50 (33.3)
Virologic Failure (confirmed)[†,‡]	74 (16.0)	121 (51.1)
Non-responder[†,‡]	13 (2.8)	78 (32.9)
Rebound[†,‡]	61 (13.2)	43 (18.1)
Death[‡,§]	6 (1.3)	3 (1.3)
Discontinuation due to adverse experiences[‡,§]	9 (1.9)	5 (2.1)
Discontinuation due to other reasons[‡,§,¶]	6 (1.3)	1 (0.4)

* Based upon the 436 subjects with Week 24 data
[†] Virologic failure: defined as non-responders who did not achieve >1.0 $\log_{10}$ HIV-1 RNA reduction and <400 HIV-1 RNA copies/mL by Week 16, or viral rebound, which was defined as: (a) HIV-1 RNA >400 copies/mL (on 2 consecutive measurements at least 1 week apart) after initial response with HIV-1 RNA <400 copies/mL, or (b) >1.0 $\log_{10}$ increase in HIV-1 RNA above nadir level (on 2 consecutive measurements at least 1 week apart).
[‡] Based upon the total 699 subjects randomized and treated, not all subjects complete to Week 24
[§] Includes available data beyond Week 24
[¶] Includes loss to follow-up, subjects withdrew consent, noncompliance, protocol violation and other reasons.

Table 8: Virologic Response at Week 24 by Baseline Genotypic/Phenotypic Sensitivity Score

BENCHMRK 1 and 2 Pooled (Noncompleters as failures approach)	Percent with HIV RNA <400 copies/mL at Week 24				Percent with HIV RNA <50 copies/mL at Week 24			
	n	ISENTRESS 400 mg Twice Daily + OBT (N = 286)	n	Placebo + OBT (N = 150)	n	ISENTRESS 400 mg Twice Daily + OBT (N = 286)	n	Placebo + OBT (N = 150)
Phenotypic Sensitivity Score (PSS)*								
0	44	50	26	4	44	41	26	4
1	89	75	50	34	89	66	50	30
2	95	86	36	42	95	70	36	36
3 or more	48	73	33	67	48	56	33	55
Genotypic Sensitivity Score (GSS)*								
0	69	54	40	8	69	41	40	5
1	115	82	64	36	115	70	64	33
2	67	88	27	78	67	75	27	63
3 or more	30	70	18	61	30	53	18	50

* The Phenotypic Sensitivity Score (PSS) and the Genotypic Sensitivity Score (GSS) were defined as the total oral ARTs in OBT to which a subject's viral isolate showed phenotypic sensitivity and genotypic sensitivity, respectively, based upon phenotypic and genotypic resistance tests. Enfuvirtide use in OBT in enfuvirtide-naïve subjects was counted as one active drug in OBT in the GSS and PSS. Similarly, darunavir use in OBT in darunavir-naïve subjects was counted as one active drug in OBT.

Novo Nordisk Inc.
100 COLLEGE ROAD WEST
PRINCETON, NJ 08540

Direct Inquiries to:
Novo Nordisk Inc.
(800) 727-6500
8:00am - 7:00pm EST M–F
In Emergencies after hours and weekends:
609-987-5800
Novo Nordisk Diabetes Care® Hotline
1-800-727-6500
Norditropin Hotline
1-888-NOVO-444
NovoSeven® Hotline
1-877-NOVO-777
Activella Hotline
866-668-6336
Vagifem Hotline
(888) VAGIFEM

ACTIVELLA® ℞
(estradiol/norethindrone acetate) tablets
1.0 mg/0.5 mg
0.5 mg/0.1 mg
Rx Only

CARDIOVASCULAR AND OTHER RISKS

Estrogens with or without progestins should not be used for the prevention of cardiovascular disease or dementia. (See **CLINICAL STUDIES** and **WARNINGS, Cardiovascular disorders** and **Dementia**.)

The estrogen plus progestin substudy of the Women's Health Initiative (WHI) reported increased risks of myocardial infarction, stroke, invasive breast cancer, pulmonary emboli, and deep vein thrombosis in postmenopausal women (50 to 79 years of age) during 5.6 years of treatment with oral conjugated estrogens (CE 0.625 mg) combined with medroxyprogesterone acetate (MPA 2.5 mg) per day, relative to placebo. (See **CLINICAL STUDIES** and **WARNINGS, Cardiovascular disorders** and **Malignant neoplasms, *Breast cancer*.**)

The estrogen-alone substudy of the WHI reported increased risks of stroke and deep vein thrombosis (DVT) in postmenopausal women (50 to 79 years of age) during 6.8 years and 7.1 years, respectively, of treatment with oral conjugated estrogens (CE 0.625 mg) per day, relative to placebo. (See **CLINICAL STUDIES** and **WARNINGS, Cardiovascular disorders.**)

The Women's Health Initiative Memory Study (WHIMS), a substudy of the WHI study, reported increased risk of developing probable dementia in postmenopausal women 65 years of age or older during 4 years of treatment with CE 0.625 mg combined with MPA 2.5 mg and during 5.2 years of treatment with CE 0.625 mg alone, relative to placebo. It is unknown whether this finding applies to younger postmenopausal women. (See **CLINICAL STUDIES, WARNINGS, Dementia**, and **PRECAUTIONS, Geriatric Use.**)

Other doses of oral conjugated estrogens with medroxyprogesterone acetate, and other combinations and dosage forms of estrogens and progestins were not studied in the WHI clinical trials and, in the absence of comparable data, these risks should be assumed to be similar. Because of these trials, estrogens with or without progestins should be prescribed at the lowest effective doses and for the shortest duration consistent with treatment goals and risks for the individual woman.

DESCRIPTION

Activella 1.0 mg/0.5 mg is a single tablet for oral administration containing 1 mg of estradiol and 0.5 mg of norethindrone acetate and the following excipients: lactose monohydrate, starch (corn), copovidone, talc, magnesium stearate, hypromellose and triacetin.

Activella 0.5 mg/0.1 mg is a single tablet for oral administration containing 0.5 mg of estradiol and 0.1 mg of norethindrone acetate and the following excipients: lactose monohydrate, starch (corn), hydroxypropylcellulose, talc, magnesium stearate, hypromellose and triacetin.

Estradiol (E_2) is a white or almost white crystalline powder. Its chemical name is estra-1, 3, 5 (10)-triene-3, 17β-diol hemihydrate with the empirical formula of $C_{18}H_{24}O_2$, 1/2 H_2O and a molecular weight of 281.4. The structural formula of E_2 is as follows:

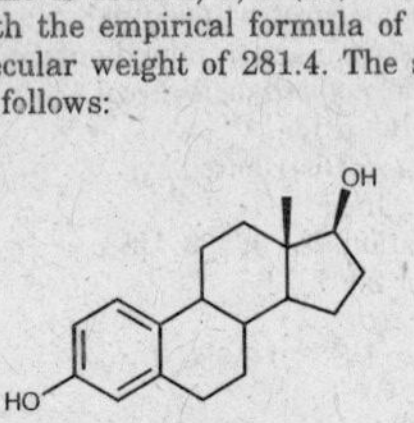

Estradiol

Norethindrone acetate (NETA) is a white or yellowish-white crystalline powder. Its chemical name is 17β-acetoxy-19-nor-17α-pregn-4-en-20-yn-3-one with the empirical formula of $C_{22}H_{28}O_3$ and molecular weight of 340.5. The structural formula of NETA is as follows:

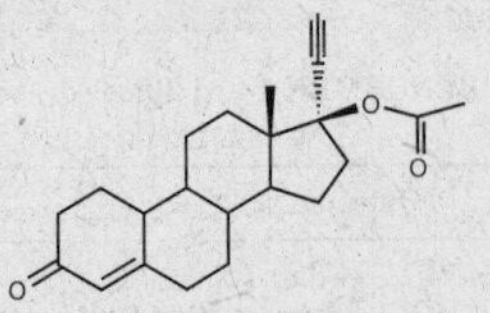

Norethindrone Acetate

CLINICAL PHARMACOLOGY

Endogenous estrogens are largely responsible for the development and maintenance of the female reproductive system and secondary sexual characteristics. Although circulating estrogens exist in a dynamic equilibrium of metabolic interconversions, estradiol is the principal intracellular human estrogen and is substantially more potent than its metabolites, estrone and estriol, at the receptor level.

The primary source of estrogen in normally cycling adult women is the ovarian follicle, which secretes 70 to 500 mcg of estradiol daily, depending on the phase of the menstrual cycle. After menopause, most endogenous estrogen is produced by conversion of androstenedione, secreted by the adrenal cortex, to estrone by peripheral tissues. Thus, estrone and the sulfate conjugated form, estrone sulfate, are the most abundant circulating estrogens in postmenopausal women.

Estrogens act through binding to nuclear receptors in estrogen-responsive tissues. To date, two estrogen receptors have been identified. These vary in proportion from tissue to tissue.

Circulating estrogens modulate the pituitary secretion of the gonadotropins, luteinizing hormone (LH), and follicle-stimulating hormone (FSH) through a negative feedback mechanism. Estrogens act to reduce the elevated levels of these hormones seen in postmenopausal women.

Progestin compounds enhance cellular differentiation and generally oppose the actions of estrogens by decreasing estrogen receptor levels, increasing local metabolism of estrogens to less active metabolites, or inducing gene products that blunt cellular responses to estrogen. Progestins exert their effects in target cells by binding to specific progesterone receptors that interact with progesterone response elements in target genes. Progesterone receptors have been identified in the female reproductive tract, breast, pituitary, hypothalamus, and central nervous system. Progestins produce similar endometrial changes to those of the naturally occurring hormone progesterone.

PHARMACOKINETICS

A. Absorption - Estradiol is well absorbed through the gastrointestinal tract. Following oral administration of Activella tablets, peak plasma estradiol concentrations are reached slowly within 5–8 hours. When given orally, estradiol is extensively metabolized (first-pass effect) to estrone sulfate, with smaller amounts of other conjugated and unconjugated estrogens. After oral administration, norethindrone acetate is rapidly absorbed and transformed to norethindrone. It undergoes first-pass metabolism in the liver and other enteric organs, and reaches a peak plasma concentration within 0.5-1.5 hours after the administration of Activella tablets. The oral bioavailability of estradiol and norethindrone following administration of Activella 1.0 mg/0.5 mg when compared to a combination oral solution is 53% and 100%, respectively. Administration of Activella 1.0 mg/0.5 mg with food did not modify the bioavailability of estradiol, although increases in AUC_{0-72} of 19% and decreases in C_{max} of 36% for norethindrone were seen.

The pharmacokinetic parameters of estradiol (E_2), estrone (E_1), and norethindrone (NET) following oral administration of 1 Activella 1.0 mg/0.5 mg or 2 Activella 0.5 mg/0.1 mg tablet(s) to healthy postmenopausal women are summarized in Table 1.

TABLE 1. PHARMACOKINETIC PARAMETERS AFTER ADMINISTRATION OF 1 TABLET OF ACTIVELLA 1.0 MG/0.5 MG OR 2 TABLETS OF ACTIVELLA 0.5 MG/0.1 MG TO HEALTHY POSTMENOPAUSAL WOMEN

	1x Activella 1.0 mg/0.5 mg (n=24) Mean[a] (%CV)[b]	2x Activella 0.5 mg/0.1 mg (n=24) Mean[a] (%CV)[b]
Estradiol[c] (E_2)		
AUC_{0-t} (pg/mL*h)	766.5 (48)	697.3 (53)
C_{max} (pg/mL)	26.8 (36)	26.5 (37)
t_{max} (h): median (range)	6.0 (0.5-16.0)	6.5 (0.5-16.0)
$t_{1/2}$ (h)[d]	14.0[e] (29)	14.5[f] (27)
Estrone[c] (E_1)		
AUC_{0-t} (pg/mL*h)	4469.1 (48)	4506.4 (44)
C_{max} (pg/mL)	195.5 (37)	199.5 (30)
t_{max} (h): median (range)	6.0 (1.0-9.0)	6.0 (2.0-9.0)
$t_{1/2}$ (h)[d]	10.7 (44)[g]	11.8 (25)[g]
Norethindrone (NET)		
AUC_{0-t} (pg/mL*h)	21043 (41)	8407.2 (43)
C_{max} (pg/mL)	5249.5 (47)	2375.4 (41)
t_{max} (h): median (range)	0.7 (0.7-1.25)	0.8 (0.7-1.3)
$t_{1/2}$ (h)	9.8 (32)[h]	11.4 (36)[i]

AUC = area under the curve, 0 – last quantifiable sample
C_{max} = maximum plasma concentration,
t_{max} = time at maximum plasma concentration,
$t_{1/2}$ = half-life,
[a] geometric mean; [b] geometric % coefficient of variation; [c] baseline unadjusted data; [d] baseline unadjusted data; [e] n=18; [f] n=16; [g] n=13; [h] n=22; [i] n=21

Following continuous dosing with once-daily administration of Activella 1.0 mg/0.5 mg, serum levels of estradiol, estrone, and norethindrone reached steady-state within two weeks with an accumulation of 33-47% above levels following single dose administration. Unadjusted circulating levels of E_2, E_1, and NET during Activella 1.0 mg/0.5 mg treatment at steady state (dosing at time 0) are provided in Figures 1a and 1b.

Figure 1a. Levels of Estradiol and Estrone at Steady State During Continuous Dosing with Activella 1.0 mg/0.5 mg (n=24)

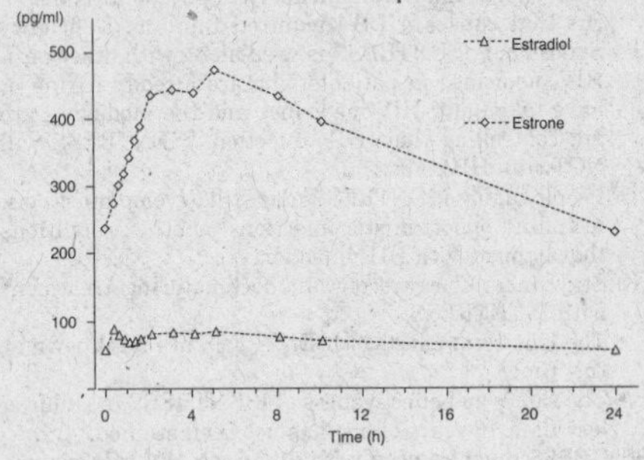

Figure 1b. Levels of Norethindrone at Steady State During Continuous Dosing with Activella 1.0 mg/0.5 mg (n=24)

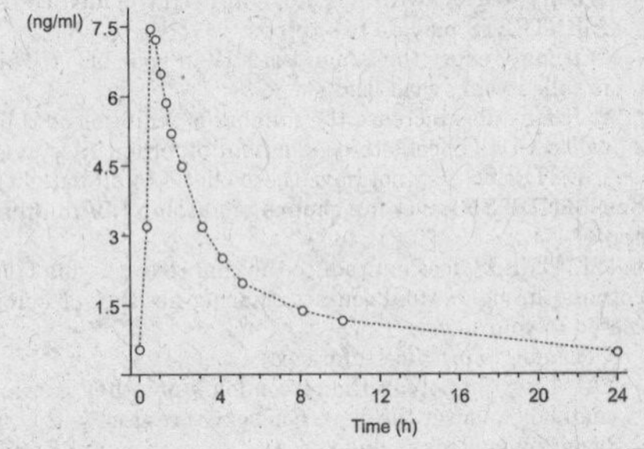

B. Distribution - The distribution of exogenous estrogens is similar to that of endogenous estrogens. Estrogens are widely distributed in the body and are generally found in higher concentrations in the sex hormone target organs. Estradiol circulates in the blood bound to sex-hormone-binding globulin (SHBG) (37%) and to albumin (61%), while only approximately 1–2% is unbound. Norethindrone also binds to a similar extent to SHBG (36%) and to albumin (61%).

C. Metabolism - Estradiol: Exogenous estrogens are metabolized in the same manner as endogenous estrogens. Circulating estrogens exist in a dynamic equilibrium of metabolic interconversions. These transformations take place mainly in the liver. Estradiol is converted reversibly to estrone, and both can be converted to estriol, which is the major urinary metabolite. Estrogens also undergo enterohepatic recirculation via sulfate and glucuronide conjugation in the liver, biliary secretion of conjugates into the intestine, and hydrolysis in the intestine followed by reabsorption. In postmenopausal women, a significant proportion of the circulating estrogens exist as sulfate conjugates, especially estrone sulfate, which serves as a circulating reservoir for the formation of more active estrogens.

Norethindrone Acetate: The most important metabolites of norethindrone are isomers of 5α-dihydro-norethindrone and tetrahydro-norethindrone, which are excreted mainly in the urine as sulfate or glucuronide conjugates.

D. Excretion - Estradiol, estrone, and estriol are excreted in the urine along with glucuronide and sulfate conjugates. The half-life of estradiol following single dose administration of Activella 1.0 mg/0.5 mg is 12-14 hours. The terminal half-life of norethindrone is about 8-11 hours.

E. Special Populations - No pharmacokinetic studies were conducted in special populations, including patients with renal or hepatic impairment.

F. Drug Interactions - Coadministration of estradiol with norethindrone acetate did not elicit any apparent influence on the pharmacokinetics of norethindrone. Similarly, no relevant interaction of norethindrone on the pharmacokinetics of estradiol was found within the NETA dose range investigated in a single dose study.

In-vitro and in-vivo studies have shown that estrogens are metabolized partially by cytochrome P450 3A4 (CYP3A4). Therefore, inducers or inhibitors of CYP3A4 may affect estrogen drug metabolism. Inducers of CYP3A4 such as St. John's Wort preparations (Hypericum perforatum), phenobarbital, carbamazepine, and rifampin may reduce plasma concentrations of estrogens, possibly resulting in a decrease in therapeutic effects and/or changes in the uterine bleeding profile. Inhibitors of CYP3A4 such as erythromycin, clarithromycin, ketoconazole, itraconazole, ritonavir and grapefruit juice may increase plasma concentrations of estrogens and result in side effects.

CLINICAL STUDIES

Effects on Vasomotor Symptoms

In a 12-week randomized clinical trial involving 92 subjects, Activella 1.0 mg/0.5 mg was compared to 1 mg of estradiol and to placebo. The mean number and intensity of hot flushes were significantly reduced from baseline to week 4 and 12 in both the Activella 1.0 mg/0.5 mg and the 1 mg estradiol group compared to placebo (see Figure 2).

Figure 2. Mean Weekly Number of Moderate and Severe Hot Flushes in a 12-Week Study

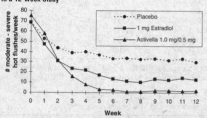

In a study conducted in Europe a total of 577 postmenopausal women were randomly assigned to either Activella 0.5 mg/0.1 mg, 0.5 mg E$_2$/0.25 mg NETA, or placebo for 24 weeks of treatment. The mean number and severity of hot flushes were significantly reduced at week 4 and week 12 in the Activella 0.5 mg/0.1 mg (see Figure 3) and 0.5 mg E$_2$/0.25 mg NETA groups compared to placebo.

Figure 3. Mean Number of Moderate to Severe Hot Flushes for Weeks 0 Through 12

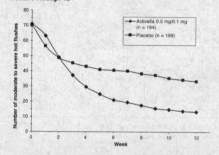

Effects on the Endometrium

Activella 1.0 mg/0.5 mg reduced the incidence of estrogen-induced endometrial hyperplasia at 1 year in a randomized, controlled clinical trial. This trial enrolled 1,176 subjects who were randomized to one of 4 arms: 1 mg estradiol unopposed (n=296), 1 mg E$_2$ + 0.1 mg NETA (n=294), 1 mg E$_2$ + 0.25 mg NETA (n=291), and Activella 1.0 mg/0.5 mg (n=295). At the end of the study, endometrial biopsy results were available for 988 subjects. The results of the 1 mg estradiol unopposed arm compared to Activella 1.0 mg/0.5 mg are shown in Table 2.
[See table 2 above]

Effects on Uterine Bleeding or Spotting

During the initial months of therapy, irregular bleeding or spotting occurred with Activella 1.0 mg/0.5 mg treatment. However, bleeding tended to decrease over time, and after 12 months of treatment with Activella 1.0 mg/0.5 mg, about 86% of women were amenorrheic (see Figure 4).

Figure 4. Patients Treated with Activella 1.0 mg/0.5 mg with Cumulative Amenorrhea over Time Percentage of Women with no Bleeding or Spotting at any Cycle Through Cycle 13, Intent to Treat Population, LOCF

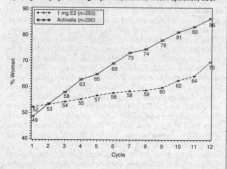

Note: the percentage of patients who were amenorrheic in a given cycle and through cycle 13 is shown. If data were missing, the bleeding value from the last reported day was carried forward (LOCF).

TABLE 2. INCIDENCE OF ENDOMETRIAL HYPERPLASIA WITH UNOPPOSED ESTRADIOL AND ACTIVELLA 1.0 MG/0.5 MG IN A 12-MONTH STUDY

	1 mg E$_2$ (n=296)	Activella 1 mg E$_2$/0.50 mg NETA (n=295)	1 mg E$_2$/ 0.25 mg NETA (n=291)	1 mg E$_2$/ 0.1 mg NETA (n=294)
No. of subjects with histological evaluation at the end of the study	247	241	251	249
No. (%) of subjects with endometrial hyperplasia at the end of the study	36 (14.6%)	1 (0.4%)	1 (0.4%)	2 (0.8%)

TABLE 3. PERCENTAGE CHANGE (MEAN ± SD) IN BONE MINERAL DENSITY (BMD) FOR ACTIVELLA 1.0 MG/0.5 MG AND 0.5 MG E$_2$[†] (Intent to Treat Analysis, Last Observation Carried Forward)

	US Trial			EU Trial	
	Placebo (n=37)	0.5 mg E$_2$[†] (n=31)	Activella 1.0 mg/0.5 mg (n=37)	Placebo (n=40)	Activella 1.0 mg/0.5 mg (n=38)
Lumbar spine	-2.1 ± 2.9	2.3 ± 2.8*	3.8 ± 3.0*	-0.9 ± 4.0	5.4 ± 4.8*
Femoral neck	-2.3 ± 3.4	0.3 ± 2.9**	1.8 ± 4.1*	-1.0 ± 4.6	0.7 ± 6.1
Femoral trochanter	-2.0 ± 4.3	1.7 ± 4.1***	3.7 ± 4.3*	0.8 ± 6.9	6.3 ± 7.6*

US=United States, EU=European
[†] While Activella 0.5 mg/0.1 mg was not directly studied in these trials, the US trial showed that addition of NETA to estradiol enhances the effect on BMD, therefore the BMD changes expected from treatment with Activella 0.5 mg/0.1 mg should be at least as great as observed with estradiol 0.5 mg.
* Significantly (p<0.001) different from placebo
** Significantly (p<0.007) different from placebo
*** Significantly (p<0.002) different from placebo

In the clinical trial with Activella 0.5 mg/0.1 mg, 88% of women were amenorrheic after 6 months of treatment (See Figure 5).

Figure 5. Patients Treated with Activella 0.5 mg/0.1 mg with Cumulative Amenorrhea over Time Percentage of Women with no Bleeding or Spotting at any Cycle Through Cycle 6, Intent to Treat Population, LOCF

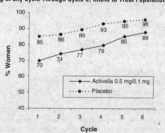

Effects on Bone Mineral Density

The results of two randomized, multicenter, calcium-supplemented (500-1000 mg/day), placebo-controlled, 2 year clinical trials have shown that Activella 1.0 mg/0.5 mg and estradiol 0.5 mg are effective in preventing bone loss in postmenopausal women. While Activella 0.5 mg/0.1 mg was not directly studied in these trials, the US trial showed that addition of NETA to estradiol enhances the effect on BMD, therefore the BMD changes expected from treatment with Activella 0.5 mg/0.1 mg should be at least as great as observed with estradiol 0.5 mg. A total of 462 postmenopausal women with intact uteri and baseline BMD values for lumbar spine within 2 standard deviations of the mean in healthy young women were enrolled. In a US trial, 327 postmenopausal women (mean time from menopause 2.5 to 3.1 years) with a mean age of 53 years were randomized to 7 groups (0.25 mg, 0.5 mg, and 1 mg of estradiol alone, 1 mg estradiol with 0.25 mg norethindrone acetate, 1 mg estradiol with 0.5 mg norethindrone acetate, and 2 mg estradiol with 1 mg norethindrone acetate, and placebo.) In a European trial (EU trial), 135 postmenopausal women (mean time from menopause 8.4 to 9.3 years) with a mean age of 58 years were randomized to 1 mg estradiol with 0.25 mg norethindrone acetate, 1 mg estradiol with 0.5 mg norethindrone acetate, and placebo. Approximately 58% and 67% of the randomized subjects in the two clinical trials, respectively, completed the two clinical trials. BMD was measured using dual-energy x-ray absorptiometry (DEXA). A summary of the results comparing Activella 1.0 mg/0.5 mg and estradiol 0.5 mg to placebo from the two prevention trials is shown in Table 3.
[See table 3 above]
The overall difference in mean percentage change in BMD at the lumbar spine in the US trial (1000 mg/day calcium) between Activella 1.0 mg/0.5 mg and placebo was 5.9% and between estradiol 0.5 mg and placebo was 4.4%. In the European trial (500 mg/day calcium), the overall difference in mean percentage change in BMD at the lumbar spine was 6.3%. Activella 1.0 mg/0.5 mg and estradiol 0.5 mg also increased BMD at the femoral neck and femoral trochanter compared to placebo. The increase in lumbar spine BMD in the US and European clinical trials for Activella 1.0 mg/ 0.5 mg and estradiol 0.5 mg is displayed in Figure 6.
[See figure 6 at top of next column]

Effect on Bone Turnover

Activella 1.0 mg/0.5 mg reduced serum and urine markers of bone turnover with a marked decrease in bone resorption markers (e.g., urinary pyridinoline crosslinks Type 1 colla-

Figure 6. Percentage Change in Bone Mineral Density (BMD) ± SEM of the Lumbar Spine (L1-L4) for Activella 1.0 mg/0.5 mg and Estradiol 0.5 mg[†] (Intent to Treat Analysis with Last Observation Carried Forward)

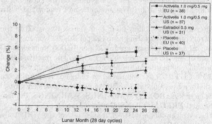

[†] While Activella 0.5 mg/0.1 mg was not directly studied in these trials, the US trial showed that addition of NETA to estradiol enhances the effect on BMD, therefore the BMD changes expected from treatment with Activella 0.5 mg/0.1 mg should be at least as great as observed with estradiol 0.5 mg.

gen C-telopeptide, pyridinoline, deoxypyridinoline) and to a lesser extent in bone formation markers (e.g., serum osteocalcin, bone-specific alkaline phosphatase, C-terminal propetide of type 1 collagen). The suppression of bone turnover markers was evident by 3 months and persisted throughout the 24-month treatment period.

Treatment with 0.5 mg estradiol decreased biochemical markers of bone resorption (urinary pyridinoline, urinary deoxypyridinoline) and bone formation (bone-specific alkaline phosphatase) compared to placebo. These decreases occurred by 6 months of treatment after which the levels were maintained throughout the 24 months.

Women's Health Initiative Studies

The WHI enrolled a total of 27,000 predominantly healthy postmenopausal women in two substudies to assess the risks and benefits of either the use of oral conjugated estrogens (CE 0.625 mg per day) alone or the use of oral conjugated estrogens (CE 0.625 mg) plus medroxyprogesterone acetate (MPA 2.5 mg per day) compared to placebo in the prevention of certain chronic diseases. The primary endpoint was the incidence of coronary heart disease (CHD) (nonfatal myocardial infarction (MI), silent MI and CHD death), with invasive breast cancer as the primary adverse outcome studied. A "global index" included the earliest occurrence of CHD, invasive breast cancer, stroke, pulmonary embolism (PE), endometrial cancer, colorectal cancer, hip fracture, or death due to other cause. The study did not evaluate the effects of CE or CE/MPA on menopausal symptoms.

The estrogen-plus-progestin substudy was stopped early. According to the predefined stopping rule, after an average follow-up of 5.2 years of treatment, the increased risk of breast cancer and cardiovascular events exceeded the specified benefits included in the "global index." The absolute excess risk of events included in the "global index" was 19 per 10,000 women-years (RR 1.15, 95% nCI 1.03-1.28).

For those outcomes included in the WHI "global index," that reached statistical significance after 5.6 years of follow-up, the absolute excess risks per 10,000 women-years in the group treated with CE/MPA were six more CHD events, seven more strokes, ten more PEs, and eight more invasive breast cancers, while the absolute risk reductions per 10,000 women-years were seven fewer colorectal cancers and five fewer hip fractures. (See **BOXED WARNINGS, WARNINGS**, and **PRECAUTIONS**.)

Continued on next page

Activella—Cont.

Results of the estrogen-plus-progestin substudy, which included 16,608 women (average age of 63 years, range 50 to 79; 83.9% White, 6.8% Black, 5.4% Hispanic, 3.9% Other) are presented in Table 4 below:
[See table 4 above]
The estrogen-alone substudy was also stopped early because an increased risk of stroke was observed, and it was deemed that no further information would be obtained regarding the risks and benefits of estrogen alone in predetermined primary endpoints. Results of the estrogen-alone substudy, which included 10,739 women (average age of 63 years, range 50 to 79; 75.3% White, 15.1% Black, 6.1% Hispanic, 3.6% Other), after an average follow-up of 6.8 years are presented in Table 5 below.
[See table 5 above]
For those outcomes included in the WHI "global index" that reached statistical significance, the absolute excess risk per 10,000 women-years in the group treated with estrogen-alone was 12 more strokes, while the absolute risk reduction per 10,000 women-years was six fewer hip fractures. The absolute excess risk of events included in the "global index" was a nonsignificant two events per 10,000 women-years. There was no difference between the groups in terms of all-cause mortality. (See **BOXED WARNINGS, WARNINGS,** and **PRECAUTIONS.**)
Final adjudicated results for CHD events from the estrogen-alone substudy, after an average follow-up of 7.1 years, reported no overall difference for primary CHD events (non-fatal MI, silent MI and CHD death) in women receiving CE alone compared with placebo (see Table 5).

Women's Health Initiative Memory Study

The estrogen plus progestin Women's Health Initiative Memory Study (WHIMS) substudy of WHI enrolled 4,532 predominantly healthy postmenopausal women 65 years of age and older (47%, age 65 to 69 years, 35%, age 70 to 74 years, 18%, 75 years of age and older) to evaluate the effects of CE 0.625 mg plus MPA 2.5 mg daily on the incidence of probable dementia (primary outcome) compared with placebo.
After an average follow-up of four years, 40 women in the estrogen-plus-progestin group (45 per 10,000 women-years) and 21 in the placebo group (22 per 10,000 women-years) were diagnosed with probable dementia. The relative risk of probable dementia in the hormone therapy group was 2.05 (95% CI 1.21-3.48) compared to placebo. It is unknown whether these findings apply to younger postmenopausal women. (See **BOXED WARNINGS, WARNINGS, Dementia**, and **PRECAUTIONS, Geriatric Use.**)
The estrogen-alone WHIMS, a substudy of the WHI study, enrolled 2,947 predominantly healthy postmenopausal women 65 years of age and older (45%, age 65 to 69 years, 36%, age 70 to 74 years, 19%, 75 years of age and older) to evaluate the effects of conjugated estrogens (CE 0.625 mg) on the incidence of probable dementia (primary outcome) compared with placebo.
After an average follow-up of 5.2 years, 28 women in the estrogen-alone group (37 per 10,000 women-years) and 19 in the placebo group (25 per 10,000 women-years) were diagnosed with probable dementia. The relative risk of probable dementia in the estrogen-alone group was 1.49 (95% CI 0.83-2.66) compared to placebo.
When data from the two populations were pooled as planned in the WHIMS protocol, the reported overall relative risk for probable dementia was 1.76 (95% CI 1.19-2.60). Differences between groups became apparent in the first year of treatment. It is unknown whether these findings apply to younger postmenopausal women. (See **BOXED WARNINGS, WARNINGS, Dementia**, and **PRECAUTIONS, Geriatric Use.**)

INDICATIONS AND USAGE

Activella 1.0 mg/0.5 mg and 0.5 mg/0.1 mg are indicated in women who have a uterus for the:
1. Treatment of moderate to severe vasomotor symptoms associated with menopause.
2. Prevention of postmenopausal osteoporosis. When prescribing solely for the prevention of postmenopausal osteoporosis, therapy should only be considered for women at significant risk of osteoporosis and non-estrogen medications should be carefully considered.

The mainstays for decreasing the risk of postmenopausal osteoporosis are weight bearing exercise, adequate calcium and vitamin D intake, and when indicated, pharmacologic therapy.
Postmenopausal women require an average of 1500 mg/day of elemental calcium. Therefore, when not contraindicated, calcium supplementation may be helpful for women with suboptimal dietary intake. Vitamin D supplementation of 400-800 IU/day may also be required to ensure adequate daily intake in postmenopausal women.
Activella 1.0 mg/0.5 mg is also indicated in women who have a uterus for the:
3. Treatment of moderate to severe symptoms of vulvar and vaginal atrophy associated with menopause. When used solely for the treatment of symptoms of vulvar and vaginal atrophy, topical vaginal products should be considered.

CONTRAINDICATIONS

Activella should not be used in women with any of the following conditions:
1. Undiagnosed abnormal genital bleeding.
2. Known, suspected, or history of cancer of the breast.
3. Known or suspected estrogen-dependent neoplasia.
4. Active deep vein thrombosis, pulmonary embolism, or history of these conditions.
5. Active or recent (e.g., within the past year) arterial thromboembolic disease (e.g., stroke, myocardial infarction).
6. Liver dysfunction or disease.
7. Known hypersensitivity to the ingredients of Activella 1.0 mg/0.5 mg or Activella 0.5 mg/0.1 mg.
8. Known or suspected pregnancy. There is no indication for Activella in pregnancy. There appears to be little or no increased risk of birth defects in children born to women who have used estrogens and progestins from oral contraceptives inadvertently during early pregnancy. (See **PRECAUTIONS.**)

WARNINGS

See **BOXED WARNINGS.**

1. Cardiovascular disorders

Estrogen-plus-progestin therapy has been associated with an increased risk of myocardial infarction as well as stroke, venous thrombosis and pulmonary embolism.
Estrogen-alone therapy has been associated with an increased risk of stroke and deep vein thrombosis (DVT). Should any of these events occur or be suspected, estrogens should be discontinued immediately.
Risk factors for arterial vascular disease (e.g., hypertension, diabetes mellitus, tobacco use, hypercholesterolemia, and obesity) and/or venous thromboembolism (e.g., personal history or family history of VTE, obesity, and systemic lupus erythematosus) should be managed appropriately.
a. Stroke - In the estrogen plus progestin substudy of the Women's Health Initiative (WHI), a statistically significant increased risk of stroke was reported in women receiving CE/MPA 0.625 mg/2.5 mg daily compared to woman receiving placebo (31 vs. 24 per 10,000 women-years). The increase in risk was demonstrated after the first year and persisted. (See **CLINICAL STUDIES.**)
In the estrogen-alone substudy of the WHI, a statistically significant increased risk of stroke was reported in women receiving CE 0.625 mg daily compared to women receiving placebo (44 vs. 32 per 10,000 women-years). The increase in risk was demonstrated in year one and persisted.
b. Coronary heart disease - In the estrogen-plus progestin sub-study of WHI, no statistically significant increase in CHD events (defined as non-fatal, MI, silent MI, or death, due to CHD) was reported in women receiving CE/MPA compared to women receiving placebo (39 vs. 33 per 10,000 women-years). An increase in relative risk was demonstrated in year one, and a trend toward decreasing relative risk was reported in years 2 through 5. (See **CLINICAL STUDIES.**)
In the estrogen-alone substudy of WHI, no overall effect on coronary disease (CHD) events was reported in women receiving estrogen alone compared to placebo. (See **CLINICAL STUDIES.**)
In postmenopausal women with documented heart disease (n=2,763, average age 66.7 years), a controlled clinical trial of secondary prevention of cardiovascular disease (Heart and Estrogen/Progestin Replacement Study (HERS)) treatment with CE/MPA (0.625 mg/2.5 mg per day) demonstrated no cardiovascular benefit. During an average follow-up of 4.1 years, treatment with CE/MPA did not reduce the overall rate of CHD events in postmenopausal women with established coronary heart disease. There were more CHD events in the CE/MPA treated group than in the placebo group in year 1, but not during the subsequent years. Participation in an open-label extension of the original HERS trial (HERS II) was agreed to by 2,321 women. Average follow-up in HERS II was an additional 2.7 years, for a total of 6.8 years overall. Rates of CHD events were comparable among women in the CE/MPA group and the placebo group in HERS, HERS II, and overall.
Large doses of estrogen (5 mg conjugated estrogens per day), comparable to those used to treat cancer of the prostate and breast, have been shown in a large prospective clinical trial in men to increase the risk of nonfatal myocardial infarction, pulmonary embolism, and thrombophlebitis.
c. Venous thromboembolism - In the estrogen-plus-progestin substudy of the Women's Health Initiative (WHI), a statis-

TABLE 4. RELATIVE AND ABSOLUTE RISK SEEN IN THE ESTROGEN-PLUS-PROGESTIN SUBSTUDY OF WHI AT AN AVERAGE OF 5.6 YEARS[a]

Event	Relative Risk CE/MPA vs. Placebo (95% nCI[b])	CE/MPA n = 8,506	Placebo n = 8,102
		Absolute Risk per 10,000 Women-years	
CHD events	1.24 (1.00-1.54)	39	33
Non-fatal MI	*1.28 (1.00-1.63)*	*31*	*25*
CHD death	*1.10 (0.70-1.75)*	*8*	*8*
All strokes	1.31 (1.02-1.68)	31	24
Ischemic stroke	*1.44 (1.09-1.90)*	*26*	*18*
Deep vein thrombosis	1.95 (1.43-2.67)	26	13
Pulmonary embolism	2.13 (1.45-3.11)	18	8
Invasive breast cancer[c]	1.24 (1.01-1.54)	41	33
Invasive colorectal cancer	0.56 (0.38-0.81)	9	16
Endometrial cancer	0.81 (0.48-1.36)	6	7
Cervical cancer	1.44 (0.47-4.42)	2	1
Hip fracture	0.67 (0.47-0.96)	11	16
Vertebral fractures	0.65 (0.46-0.92)	11	17
Lower arm/wrist fractures	0.71 (0.59-0.85)	44	62
Total fractures	0.76 (0.69-0.83)	152	199

[a] Results are based on centrally adjudicated data. Mortality data was not part of the adjudicated data; however, data at 5.2 years of follow-up showed no difference between the groups in terms of all-cause mortality (RR 0.98, 95% nCI 0.82-1.18).
[b] Nominal confidence intervals unadjusted for multiple looks and multiple comparisons.
[c] Includes metastatic and non-metastatic breast cancer, with the exception of in situ breast cancer.

TABLE 5. RELATIVE AND ABSOLUTE RISK SEEN IN THE ESTROGEN-ALONE SUBSTUDY OF WHI[a]

Event	Relative Risk CE vs. Placebo (95% nCI[a])	CE n = 5,310	Placebo n = 5,429
		Absolute Risk per 10,000 Women-years	
CHD events[b]	0.95 (0.79-1.16)	53	56
Non-fatal MI[b]	*0.91 (0.73-1.14)*	*40*	*43*
CHD death[b]	*1.01 (0.71-1.43)*	*16*	*16*
Stroke[c]	1.39 (1.10-1.77)	44	32
Deep vein thrombosis[b,d]	1.47 (1.06-2.06)	23	15
Pulmonary embolism[b]	1.37 (0.90-2.07)	14	10
Invasive breast cancer[b]	0.80 (0.62-1.04)	28	34
Colorectal cancer[c]	1.08 (0.75-1.55)	17	16
Hip fracture[c]	0.61 (0.41-0.91)	11	17
Vertebral fractures[c,d]	0.62 (0.42-0.93)	11	17
Total fractures[c,d]	0.70 (0.63-0.79)	139	195
Death due to other causes[c,e]	1.08 (0.88-1.32)	53	50
Overall mortality[c,d]	1.04 (0.88-1.22)	81	78
Global index[c,f]	1.01 (0.91-1.12)	192	190

[a] Nominal confidence intervals unadjusted for multiple looks and multiple comparisons.
[b] Results are based on centrally adjudicated data for an average follow-up of 7.1 years.
[c] Results are based on an average follow-up of 6.8 years.
[d] Not included in Global Index.
[e] All deaths, except from breast or colorectal cancer, definite/probable CHD, PE or cerebrovascular disease.
[f] A subset of the events was combined in a "global index," defined as the earliest occurrence of CHD events, invasive breast cancer, stroke, pulmonary embolism, colorectal cancer, hip fracture, or death due to other causes.

tically significant 2-fold greater rate of VTE (DVT and pulmonary embolism [PE]), was reported in women receiving CE/MPA compared to women receiving placebo (35 vs. 17 per 10,000 women-years). Statistically significant increases in risk for both DVT (26 vs. 13 per 10,000 women-years) and PE (18 vs. 8 per 10,000 women-years) were also demonstrated. The increase in VTE risk was demonstrated during the first year and persisted. (See **CLINICAL STUDIES**.) In the estrogen-alone substudy of WHI, the risk of VTE was reported to be increased for women taking conjugated estrogens (30 vs. 22 per 10,000 women-years), although only the increased risk of DVT reached statistical significance (23 vs. 15 per 10,000 women-years). The increase in VTE risk was demonstrated during the first two years.

If feasible, estrogens should be discontinued at least 4 to 6 weeks before surgery of the type associated with an increased risk of thromboembolism, or during periods of prolonged immobilization.

2. Malignant neoplasms

a. Breast cancer - In some studies, the use of estrogens and progestins by postmenopausal women has been reported to increase the risk of breast cancer. The most important randomized clinical trial providing information about this issue is the CE/MPA substudy of the WHI study (see **CLINICAL STUDIES**). The results from observational studies are generally consistent with those of the WHI clinical trial.

Observational studies have also reported an increased risk of breast cancer for estrogen-plus-progestin combination therapy, and a smaller increased risk for estrogen-alone therapy, after several years of use. For both findings, the excess risk increased with duration of use, and appeared to return to baseline over about five years after stopping treatment (only the observational studies have substantial data on risk after stopping). In these studies, the risk of breast cancer was greater, and became apparent earlier, with estrogen-plus-progestin combination therapy as compared to estrogen-alone therapy. However, these studies have not found significant variation in the risk of breast cancer among different estrogens or among different estrogen-plus-progestin combinations, doses, or routes of administration.

In the estrogen-plus-progestin substudy, after a mean follow-up of 5.6 years, the WHI substudy reported an increased risk of breast cancer. In this substudy, prior use of estrogen alone or estrogen-plus-progestin combination hormone therapy was reported by 26% of the women. The relative risk of invasive breast cancer was 1.24 (95% nCI 1.01-1.54), and the absolute risk was 41 vs. 33 cases per 10,000 women-years, for estrogen plus progestin compared with placebo, respectively. Among women who reported prior use of hormone therapy, the relative risk of invasive breast cancer was 1.86, and the absolute risk was 46 vs. 25 cases per 10,000 women-years, for estrogen plus progestin compared with placebo. Among women who reported no prior use of hormone therapy, the relative risk of invasive breast cancer was 1.09, and the absolute risk was 40 vs. 36 cases per 10,000 women-years of estrogen plus progestin compared with placebo. In the WHI trial, invasive breast cancers were larger and diagnosed at a more advanced stage in the estrogen-plus-progestin group compared with the placebo group. Metastatic disease was rare, with no apparent difference between the two groups. Other prognostic factors, such as histologic subtype, grade and hormone receptor status did not differ between the groups.

In the estrogen-alone substudy of WHI, after an average of 7.1 years of follow-up, CE (0.625 mg daily) was not associated with an increased risk of invasive breast cancer (RR 0.80, 95% nCI 0.62-1.04).

In a one-year trial among 1,176 women who received either unopposed 1 mg estradiol or a combination of 1 mg estradiol plus one of three different doses of NETA (0.1, 0.25, and 0.5 mg), seven new cases of breast cancer were diagnosed, two of which occurred among the group of 295 women treated with Activella 1.0 mg/0.5 mg and two of which occurred among the group of 294 women treated with 1 mg estradiol/0.1 mg NETA.

The use of estrogen alone and estrogen plus progestin has been reported to result in an increase in abnormal mammograms requiring further evaluation. All women should receive yearly breast examinations by a health care provider and perform monthly breast self-examinations. In addition, mammography examinations should be scheduled based on patient age, risk factors, and prior mammogram results.

b. Endometrial cancer - The use of unopposed estrogens in women with intact uteri has been associated with an increased risk of endometrial cancer. The reported endometrial cancer risk among unopposed estrogen users is about 2 to 12 fold greater than in nonusers, and appears dependent on duration of treatment and on estrogen dose. Most studies show no significant increased risk associated with use of estrogens for less than one year. The greatest risk appears associated with prolonged use, with an increased risk of 15- to 24-fold for five to ten years or more. This risk has been shown to persist for at least 8 to 15 years after estrogen therapy is discontinued.

Clinical surveillance of all women taking estrogen/progestin combinations is important. Adequate diagnostic measures, including endometrial sampling when indicated, should be undertaken to rule out malignancy in all cases of undiagnosed persistent or recurring abnormal vaginal bleeding. There is no evidence that the use of natural estrogens results in a different endometrial risk profile than synthetic estrogens of equivalent estrogen dose. Adding a progestin to estrogen therapy has been shown to reduce the risk of endometrial hyperplasia, which may be a precursor to endometrial cancer.

TABLE 6. ALL TREATMENT-EMERGENT ADVERSE EVENTS REGARDLESS OF RELATIONSHIP REPORTED AT A FREQUENCY OF ≥5% WITH ACTIVELLA 1.0 MG/0.5 MG

	Endometrial Hyperplasia Study (12-months)		Vasomotor Symptoms Study (3-months)		Osteoporosis Study (2 years)	
	Activella 1.0 mg/ 0.5 mg (n=295)	1 mg E_2 (n=296)	Activella 1.0 mg/ 0.5 mg (n=29)	Placebo (n=34)	Activella 1.0 mg/ 0.5 mg (n=47)	Placebo (n=48)
Body as a Whole						
Back Pain	6%	5%	3%	3%	6%	4%
Headache	16%	16%	17%	18%	11%	6%
Digestive System						
Nausea	3%	5%	10%	0%	11%	0%
Gastroenteritis	2%	2%	0%	0%	6%	4%
Nervous System						
Insomnia	6%	4%	3%	3%	0%	8%
Emotional Lability	1%	1%	0%	0%	6%	0%
Respiratory System						
Upper Respiratory Tract Infection	18%	15%	10%	6%	15%	19%
Sinusitis	7%	11%	7%	0%	15%	10%
Metabolic and Nutritional						
Weight Increase	0%	0%	0%	0%	9%	6%
Urogenital System						
Breast Pain	24%	10%	21%	0%	17%	8%
Post-Menopausal Bleeding	5%	15%	10%	3%	11%	0%
Uterine Fibroid	5%	4%	0%	0%	4%	8%
Ovarian Cyst	3%	2%	7%	0%	0%	8%
Resistance Mechanism						
Infection Viral	4%	6%	0%	3%	6%	6%
Moniliasis Genital	4%	7%	0%	0%	6%	0%
Secondary Terms						
Injury Accidental	4%	3%	3%	0%	17%*	4%*
Other Events	2%	3%	3%	0%	6%	4%

*including one upper extremity fracture in each group

Endometrial hyperplasia (a possible precursor of endometrial cancer) has been reported to occur in approximately 1% or less with Activella in one large clinical trial.

3. Dementia

In the estrogen-plus-progestin Women's Health Initiative Memory Study (WHIMS), a substudy of WHI, a population of 4,532 postmenopausal women aged 65 to 79 years was randomized to CE/MPA (0.625 mg/2.5 mg daily) or placebo.

In the estrogen-alone WHIMS substudy, a population of 2,947 hysterectomized women, aged 65 to 79 years, was randomized to CE (0.625 mg daily) or placebo.

In the estrogen-plus-progestin substudy, after an average follow-up of four years, 40 women in the estrogen-plus-progestin group and 21 women in the placebo group were diagnosed with probable dementia. The relative risk of probable dementia for estrogen plus progestin vs. placebo was 2.05 (95% CI 1.21-3.48). The absolute risk of probable dementia for CE/MPA vs. placebo was 45 vs. 22 cases per 10,000 women-years.

In the estrogen-alone substudy, after an average follow-up of 5.2 years, 28 women in the estrogen-alone group and 19 women in the placebo group were diagnosed with probable dementia. The relative risk of probable dementia for CE alone vs. placebo was 1.49 (95% CI 0.83-2.66). The absolute risk of probable dementia for CE alone vs. placebo was 37 vs. 25 cases per 10,000 women-years.

When data from the two populations were pooled as planned in the WHIMS protocol, the reported overall relative risk of probable dementia was 1.76 (95% CI 1.19-2.60). Since both substudies were conducted in women ages 65 to 79, it is unknown whether these findings apply to younger postmenopausal women. (See **BOXED WARNINGS** and **PRECAUTIONS, Geriatric Use.**)

4. Gallbladder disease

A two-to four fold increase in the risk of gallbladder disease requiring surgery in postmenopausal women receiving estrogens has been reported.

5. Hypercalcemia

Estrogen administration may lead to severe hypercalcemia in patients with breast cancer and bone metastases. If hypercalcemia occurs, use of the drug should be stopped and appropriate measures taken to reduce the serum calcium level.

6. Visual abnormalities

Retinal vascular thrombosis has been reported in patients receiving estrogens. Discontinue medication pending examination if there is a sudden partial or complete loss of vision, or a sudden onset of proptosis, diplopia, or migraine. If examination reveals papilledema or retinal vascular lesions, estrogens should be permanently discontinued.

PRECAUTIONS

A. General

1. Addition of a progestin when a woman has not had a hysterectomy

Studies of the addition of a progestin for 10 or more days of a cycle of estrogen administration, or daily with estrogen in a continuous regimen, have reported a lowered incidence of endometrial hyperplasia than would be induced by estrogen treatment alone. Endometrial hyperplasia may be a precursor to endometrial cancer.

There are, however, possible risks that may be associated with the use of progestins with estrogens compared to estrogen-alone treatment. These include a possible increased risk of breast cancer.

2. Elevated blood pressure

In a small number of case reports, substantial increases in blood pressure have been attributed to idiosyncratic reactions to estrogens. In a large, randomized, placebo-controlled clinical trial, a generalized effect of estrogens on blood pressure was not seen. Blood pressure should be monitored at regular intervals with estrogen use.

3. Hypertriglyceridemia

In patients with preexisting hypertriglyceridemia, estrogen therapy may be associated with elevations of plasma triglycerides leading to pancreatitis and other complications.

4. Impaired liver function and past history of cholestatic jaundice

Estrogens may be poorly metabolized in patients with impaired liver function. For patients with a history of cholestatic jaundice associated with past estrogen use or with pregnancy, caution should be exercised, and in the case of recurrence, medication should be discontinued.

5. Hypothyroidism

Estrogen administration leads to increased thyroid-binding globulin (TBG) levels. Patients with normal thyroid function can compensate for the increased TBG by making more thyroid hormone, thus maintaining free T_4 and T_3 serum concentrations in the normal range. Patients dependent on thyroid hormone replacement therapy who are also receiving estrogen may require increased doses of their thyroid replacement therapy. These patients should have their thyroid function monitored to maintain their free thyroid hormone levels in an acceptable range.

6. Fluid retention

Estrogens may cause some degree of fluid retention. Because of this, patients who have conditions that might be influenced by this factor, such as a cardiac or renal dysfunction, warrant careful observation when estrogens are prescribed.

7. Hypocalcemia

Estrogens should be used with caution in individuals with severe hypocalcemia.

8. Ovarian cancer

The estrogen-plus-progestin substudy of WHI reported that after an average follow-up of 5.6 years, the relative risk for ovarian cancer for estrogen plus progestin vs. placebo was 1.58 (95% CI 0.77-3.24), but was not statistically significant. The absolute risk for estrogen plus progestin vs. placebo was 4.2 vs. 2.7 cases per 10,000 women-years. In some epidemiologic studies, the use of estrogen-only products, in particular for 10 or more years, has been associated with an increased risk of ovarian cancer. Other epidemiologic studies have not found these associations.

9. Exacerbation of endometriosis

Endometriosis may be exacerbated with administration of estrogens.

Malignant transformation of residual endometrial implants has been reported in women treated post-hysterectomy with estrogen-alone therapy. For patients known to have residual endometriosis post-hysterectomy, the addition of progestin should be considered.

10. Exacerbation of other conditions

Estrogens may cause an exacerbation of asthma, diabetes mellitus, epilepsy, migraine or porphyria, systemic lupus erythematosus, and hepatic hemangiomas and should be used with caution in women with these conditions.

Continued on next page

Activella—Cont.

B. Patient Information
Physicians are advised to discuss the contents of the Patient Information leaflet with patients for whom they prescribe Activella 1.0 mg/0.5 mg or Activella 0.5 mg/0.1 mg.

C. Laboratory Tests
Estrogen administration should be initiated at the lowest dose approved for the indication and then guided by clinical response, rather than by serum hormone levels (e.g., estradiol, FSH).

D. Drug/Laboratory Test Interactions
1. Accelerated prothrombin time, partial thromboplastin time, and platelet aggregation time; increased platelet count; increased factors II, VII antigen, VIII coagulant activity, IX, X, XII, VII-X complex, and beta-thromboglobulin; decreased levels of anti-factor Xa and antithrombin III, decreased antithrombin III activity, increased levels of fibrinogen and fibrinogen activity; increased plasminogen antigen and activity.
2. Increased thyroid-binding globulin (TBG) levels leading to increased circulating total thyroid hormone levels as measured by protein-bound iodine (PBI), T_4 levels (by column or by radioimmunoassay), or T_3 levels by radioimmunoassay. T_3 resin uptake is decreased, reflecting the elevated TBG. Free T_4 and free T_3 concentrations are unaltered. Patients on thyroid replacement therapy may require higher doses of thyroid hormone.
3. Other binding proteins may be elevated in serum (i.e., corticosteroid binding globulin (CBG), SHBG) leading to increased total circulating corticosteroids and sex steroids, respectively. Free hormone concentrations may be decreased. Other plasma proteins may be increased (angiotensinogen/rennin substrate, alpha-1 antitrypsin, ceruloplasmin).
4. Increased plasma HDL and HDL_2 cholesterol subfraction concentration, reduced LDL cholesterol concentration, increased triglyceride levels.
5. Impaired glucose tolerance.
6. Reduced response to metyrapone test.

E. Carcinogenesis, Mutagenesis, Impairment of Fertility
Long-term continuous administration of estrogen, with or without progestin, in women with or without a uterus, has shown an increased risk of endometrial cancer, breast cancer, and ovarian cancer. (See **BOXED WARNINGS**, **WARNINGS**, and **PRECAUTIONS**.)

Long-term continuous administration of natural and synthetic estrogens in certain animal species increases the frequency of carcinomas of the breast, uterus, cervix, vagina, testis, and liver.

F. Pregnancy
Activella should not be used during pregnancy. (See **CONTRAINDICATIONS**.)

G. Nursing Mothers
Estrogen administration to nursing mothers has been shown to decrease the quantity and quality of breast milk. Detectable amounts of estrogens have been identified in the milk of mothers receiving this drug. Caution should be exercised when Activella is administered to a nursing mother.

H. Pediatric Use
Activella is not indicated in children.

I. Geriatric Use
Clinical studies of Activella did not include sufficient number of subjects aged 65 and over to determine if they responded differently from younger subjects.

Of the total number of subjects in the estrogen-plus-progestin substudy of the Women's Health Initiative (WHI) study, 44% (n=7,320) were 65–74 years of age, while 6.6% (n=1,095) were 75 years and over. There was a higher relative risk (CE/MPA vs. placebo) of non-fatal stroke and invasive breast cancer in women 75 and over compared to women less than 75 years of age. In women greater than 75, the increased risk of non-fatal stroke and invasive breast cancer observed in the estrogen-plus-progestin combination group compared to the placebo group was 75 vs. 24 per 10,000 women-years and 52 vs. 12 per 10,000 women-years, respectively.

In the estrogen-plus-progestin Women's Health Initiative Memory Study (WHIMS), a substudy of WHI, a population of 4,532 hysterectomized women, aged 65 to 79 years, was randomized to CE/MPA (0.625 mg/2.5 mg daily) or placebo. In the estrogen-plus-progestin group, after an average follow-up of four years, the relative risk (CE/MPA vs. placebo) of probable dementia was 2.05 (95% CI 1.21-3.48). The absolute risk of developing probable dementia with CE/MPA was 45 vs. 22 cases per 10,000 women-years with placebo. Of the total number of subjects in the estrogen-alone substudy of WHI, 46% (n=4,943) were 65 years and over, while 7.1% (n=767) were 75 years and over. There was a higher relative risk (CE vs. placebo) of stroke in women less than 75 years of age compared to women 75 years and over. In the estrogen-alone WHIMS substudy, a population of 2,947 hysterectomized women, aged 65 to 79 years, was randomized to CE (0.625 mg daily) or placebo. After an average follow-up of 5.2 years, the relative risk (CE vs. placebo) of probable dementia was 1.49 (95% CI 0.83-2.66). The absolute risk of developing probable dementia with estrogen alone was 37 vs. 25 cases per 10,000 women-years with placebo.

Seventy-nine percent of the cases of probable dementia occurred in women that were older than 70 for the CE-alone group, and 82 percent of the cases of probable dementia occurred in women who were older than 70 in the CE/MPA group. The most common classification of probable dementia in both the treatment groups and placebo groups was Alzheimer's disease.

When data from the two populations were pooled as planned in the WHIMS protocol, the reported overall relative risk for probable dementia was 1.76 (95% CI 1.19-2.60). Since both substudies were conducted in women aged 65 to 79 years, it is unknown whether these findings apply to younger postmenopausal women. (See **BOXED WARNINGS** and **WARNINGS, Dementia**.)

ADVERSE REACTIONS
See **BOXED WARNINGS**, **WARNINGS**, and **PRECAUTIONS**.

Because clinical trials are conducted under widely varying conditions, adverse reaction rates observed in the clinical trials of a drug cannot be directly compared to rates in the clinical trials of another drug and may not reflect the rates observed in practice. The adverse reaction information from clinical trials does, however, provide a basis for identifying the adverse events that appear to be related to drug use and for approximating rates.

Adverse events reported with Activella 1.0 mg/0.5 mg by investigators in the Phase 3 studies regardless of causality assessment are shown in Table 6.

[See table 6 at top of previous page]

Adverse events reported with Activella 0.5 mg/0.1 mg by investigators during the Phase 3 study regardless of causality assessment are shown in Table 7.

TABLE 7. ALL TREATMENT-EMERGENT ADVERSE EVENTS REGARDLESS OF RELATIONSHIP REPORTED AT A FREQUENCY OF ≥5% WITH ACTIVELLA 0.5 MG/0.1 MG

	Activella 0.5 mg/0.1 mg (n=194)	Placebo (n=200)
Body as a Whole		
Back Pain	10%	4%
Headache	22%	19%
Pain in extremity	5%	4%
Digestive System		
Nausea	5%	4%
Diarrhea	6%	6%
Respiratory System		
Nasopharyngitis	21%	18%
Urogenital System		
Endometrial thickening	10%	4%
Vaginal hemorrhage	26%	12%

The following adverse reactions have been reported with estrogen and/or progestin therapy:

1. Genitourinary system
Changes in vaginal bleeding pattern and abnormal withdrawal bleeding or flow; breakthrough bleeding; spotting; dysmenorrhea, increase in size of uterine leiomyomata; vaginitis, including vaginal candidiasis; change in amount of cervical secretion; changes in cervical ectropion; premenstrual-like syndrome; cystitis-like syndrome; ovarian cancer; endometrial hyperplasia; endometrial cancer.

2. Breasts
Tenderness, enlargement, pain, nipple discharge, galactorrhea; fibrocystic breast changes; breast cancer.

3. Cardiovascular
Deep and superficial venous thrombosis; pulmonary embolism; thrombophlebitis; myocardial infarction, stroke; increase in blood pressure.

4. Gastrointestinal
Nausea, vomiting; changes in appetite; cholestatic jaundice; abdominal pain/cramps, flatulence, bloating; increased incidence of gallbladder disease; pancreatitis; enlargement of hepatic hemangiomas.

5. Skin
Chloasma or melasma that may persist when drug is discontinued; erythema multiforme; erythema nodosum; hemorrhagic eruption; loss of scalp hair; seborrhea; hirsutism; itching; skin rash; pruritus.

6. Eyes
Retinal vascular thrombosis, intolerance to contact lenses.

7. Central nervous system
Headache; migraine; dizziness; mental depression; chorea; insomnia; nervousness; mood disturbances; irritability; exacerbation of epilepsy; probable dementia.

8. Miscellaneous
Increase or decrease in weight; aggravation of porphyria; edema; leg cramps; changes in libido; fatigue; reduced carbohydrate tolerance; anaphylactoid/anaphylactic reactions; hypocalcemia; exacerbation of asthma; increased triglycerides; back pain; arthralgia; myalgia.

OVERDOSAGE
Serious ill effects have not been reported following acute ingestion of large doses of estrogen-containing drug products by young children. Overdosage of estrogen may cause nausea and vomiting, and withdrawal bleeding may occur in females.

DOSAGE AND ADMINISTRATION
Use of estrogen, alone or in combination with a progestin, should be with the lowest effective dose and for the shortest duration consistent with treatment goals and risks for the individual woman. Patients should be re-evaluated periodically as clinically appropriate (e.g., 3 to 6 month intervals) to determine if treatment is still necessary (See **BOXED WARNINGS** and **WARNINGS**). For women who have a uterus, adequate diagnostic measures, such as endometrial sampling, when indicated, should be undertaken to rule out malignancy in cases of undiagnosed persistent or recurring abnormal vaginal bleeding.

Activella therapy consists of a single tablet to be taken once daily.

1. For the treatment of moderate to severe vasomotor symptoms associated with menopause, and the prevention of postmenopausal osteoporosis. When prescribing solely for the prevention of postmenopausal osteoporosis, therapy should only be considered for women at significant risk of osteoporosis and non-estrogen medications should be carefully considered.
   - Activella 1.0 mg/0.5 mg
   - Activella 0.5 mg/0.1 mg
2. For the treatment of moderate to severe symptoms of vulvar and vaginal atrophy. When used solely for the treatment of symptoms of vulvar and vaginal atrophy, topical vaginal products should be considered.
   - Activella 1.0 mg/0.5 mg

Patients should be started at the lowest dose.

HOW SUPPLIED
Activella 1.0 mg/0.5 mg is a white, film-coated tablet, engraved with NOVO 288 on one side and the APIS bull on the other. It is round, 6mm in diameter and bi-convex. (NDC 0169-5174-02). It is supplied as 28 tablets in a calendar dial pack dispenser. Store in a dry place protected from light.

Activella 0.5 mg/0.1 mg is a white, film-coated tablet, engraved with NOVO 291 on one side and the APIS bull on the other. It is round, 6mm in diameter and bi-convex. (NDC 0169-5175-10). It is supplied as 28 tablets in a calendar dial pack dispenser. Keep the container in the outer carton. Store at 25°C (77°F), excursions permitted to 15-30°C (59-86°F).

[See USP Controlled Room Temperature.]

Rx Only

Activella® is a trademark owned by Novo Nordisk FemCare AG

Revised December 2006
Version 7
Novo Nordisk Inc.
Princeton, NJ 08540
1-866-668-6336
www.novonordisk-us.com
Manufactured by
Novo Nordisk A/S
2880 Bagsvaerd, Denmark
© 2000-2006 Novo Nordisk Inc.
131688R   04/07

Ortho-McNeil, Inc.
RARITAN, NJ 08869-0602

www.ortho-mcneil.com
For Medical Information Contact:
(800) 682-6532
In Emergencies:
(908) 218-7325
For Patient Education Materials Contact:
877-323-2200
For Customer Service (Sales and Ordering):
800-631-5273

DORIBAX™
[dor-ebaks]
(doripenem for injection)
for Intravenous Infusion

℞

HIGHLIGHTS OF PRESCRIBING INFORMATION
These highlights do not include all the information needed to use DORIBAX™ safely and effectively. See full prescribing information for DORIBAX™.
Initial U.S. Approval: 2007

To reduce the development of drug-resistant bacteria and maintain the effectiveness of DORIBAX™ and other antibacterial drugs, DORIBAX™ should be used only to treat or prevent infections that are proven or strongly suspected to be caused by bacteria.

INDICATIONS AND USAGE
DORIBAX™ is a penem antibacterial indicated in the treatment of the following infections caused by designated susceptible bacteria:
- Complicated intra-abdominal infections (1.1)
- Complicated urinary tract infections, including pyelonephritis (1.2)

DOSAGE AND ADMINISTRATION
- 500 mg every 8 hours by intravenous infusion administered over one hour for patients ≥18 years of age. (2.1)
- Dosage in patients with impaired renal function (2.2):

CrCl (mL/min)	Recommended Dose of DORIBAX™
>50	No dosage adjustment necessary
≥30 to ≤50	250 mg IV (over 1 hour) every 8 hours
>10 to < 30	250 mg IV (over 1 hour) every 12 hours

DOSAGE FORMS AND STRENGTHS

500 mg single-use vial (3)

CONTRAINDICATIONS

Patients with known serious hypersensitivity to doripenem or to other drugs in the same class or patients who have demonstrated anaphylactic reactions to beta-lactams (4)

WARNINGS AND PRECAUTIONS

- Serious hypersensitivity (anaphylactic) reactions have been reported with carbapenems and other beta-lactams (5.1)
- Loss of seizure control due to lower serum valproic acid levels may result from interaction with sodium valproate (5.2)
- *Clostridium difficile*-associated diarrhea (ranging from mild diarrhea to fatal colitis): Evaluate if diarrhea occurs (5.3)

ADVERSE REACTIONS

Most common adverse reactions (≥5%) are headache, nausea, diarrhea, rash and phlebitis.

To report SUSPECTED ADVERSE REACTIONS, contact Ortho-McNeil Pharmaceutical, Inc. at 1-800-526-7736 or FDA at 1-800-FDA-1088 or *www.fda.gov/medwatch*.

DRUG INTERACTIONS

Interacting Drug	Interaction
Valproic acid	Carbapenems may reduce serum valproic acid levels (7.1)
Probenecid	Reduces renal clearance of doripenem, resulting in increased doripenem concentrations (7.2, 12.3)
Drugs metabolized by cytochrome P450 enzymes	Doripenem neither inhibits nor induces major cytochrome P450 enzymes (12.3)

USE IN SPECIFIC POPULATIONS

- Dosage adjustment is required in patients with moderately or severely impaired renal function (2.2, 12.3)
- DORIBAX™ has not been studied in pediatric patients. (8.4)

See 17 for PATIENT COUNSELING INFORMATION

Revised: 10/2007

FULL PRESCRIBING INFORMATION:

CONTENTS*

1 INDICATIONS AND USAGE

To reduce the development of drug-resistant bacteria and maintain the effectiveness of DORIBAX™ and other antibacterial drugs, DORIBAX™ should be used only to treat infections that are proven or strongly suspected to be caused by susceptible bacteria. When culture and suscepti-

Table 1: Dosage of DORIBAX™ by Infection

Infection	Dosage	Frequency	Infusion Time (hours)	Duration
Complicated intra-abdominal infection	500 mg	q8h	1	5-14 days*
Complicated UTI, including pyelonephritis	500 mg	q8h	1	10 days*§

* Duration includes a possible switch to an appropriate oral therapy, after at least 3 days of parenteral therapy, once clinical improvement has been demonstrated.
§ Duration can be extended up to 14 days for patients with concurrent bacteremia.

Males: Creatinine clearance (mL/min) = $\dfrac{\text{weight (kg)} \times (140 - \text{age in years})}{72 \times \text{serum creatinine (mg/dL)}}$

Females: Creatinine clearance (mL/min) = $0.85 \times$ value calculated for males

---

bility information are available, they should be considered in selecting and modifying antibacterial therapy. In the absence of such data, local epidemiology and susceptibility patterns may contribute to the empiric selection of therapy.

1.1 Complicated Intra-Abdominal Infections

DORIBAX™ (doripenem for injection) is indicated as a single agent for the treatment of complicated intra-abdominal infections caused by *Escherichia coli*, *Klebsiella pneumoniae*, *Pseudomonas aeruginosa*, *Bacteroides caccae*, *Bacteroides fragilis*, *Bacteroides thetaiotaomicron*, *Bacteroides uniformis*, *Bacteroides vulgatus*, *Streptococcus intermedius*, *Streptococcus constellatus* and *Peptostreptococcus micros*.

1.2 Complicated Urinary Tract Infections, Including Pyelonephritis

DORIBAX™ (doripenem for injection) is indicated as a single agent for the treatment of complicated urinary tract infections, including pyelonephritis caused by *Escherichia coli* including cases with concurrent bacteremia, *Klebsiella pneumoniae*, *Proteus mirabilis*, *Pseudomonas aeruginosa*, and *Acinetobacter baumannii*.

2 DOSAGE AND ADMINISTRATION

2.1 Recommended Dosage

The recommended dosage of DORIBAX™ is 500 mg administered every 8 hours by intravenous infusion over one hour in patients ≥18 years of age. The recommended dosage and administration by infection is described in Table 1:
[See table 1 above]

2.2 Patients with Renal Impairment

Table 2: Dosage of DORIBAX™ in Patients with Renal Impairment

Estimated CrCl (mL/min)	Recommended Dosage Regimen of DORIBAX™
> 50	No dosage adjustment necessary
≥ 30 to ≤50	250 mg intravenously (over 1 hour) every 8 hours
> 10 to < 30	250 mg intravenously (over 1 hour) every 12 hours

The following formula may be used to estimate CrCl. The serum creatinine used in the formula should represent a steady state of renal function.
[See second table above]
DORIBAX™ is hemodialyzable; however, there is insufficient information to make dose adjustment recommendations in patients on hemodialysis.

2.3 Preparation of Solutions

DORIBAX™ does not contain a bacteriostatic preservative. Aseptic technique must be followed in preparation of the infusion solution.
Preparation of 500 mg dose:
- Constitute the vial with 10 mL of sterile water for injection or 0.9% sodium chloride injection (normal saline) and gently shake to form a suspension. The resultant concentration is 50 mg/mL. **CAUTION: THE CONSTITUTED SUSPENSION IS NOT FOR DIRECT INJECTION.**
- Withdraw the suspension using a syringe with a 21 gauge needle and add it to an infusion bag containing 100 mL of normal saline or 5% dextrose; gently shake until clear. The final infusion solution concentration is 4.5 mg/mL.

Preparation of 250 mg dose for patients with moderate or severe renal impairment:
- Constitute the vial with 10 mL of sterile water for injection or 0.9% sodium chloride injection (normal saline) and gently shake to form a suspension. The resultant concentration is 50 mg/mL. **CAUTION: THE CONSTITUTED SUSPENSION IS NOT FOR DIRECT INJECTION.**
- Withdraw the suspension using a syringe with a 21 gauge needle and add it to an infusion bag containing 100 mL of normal saline or 5% dextrose; gently shake until clear. Remove 55 mL of this solution from the bag and discard. Infuse the remaining solution, which contains 250 mg (4.5 mg/mL).

To prepare DORIBAX infusions in Baxter Minibag Plus™ infusion bags consult the infusion bag manufacturer's instructions.
Parenteral drug products should be inspected visually for particulate matter and discoloration prior to use whenever solution and container permit. DORIBAX infusions range

from clear, colorless solutions to solutions that are clear and slightly yellow. Variations in color within this range do not affect the potency of the product.

2.4 Compatibility

The compatibility of DORIBAX™ with other drugs has not been established. DORIBAX™ should not be mixed with or physically added to solutions containing other drugs.

2.5 Storage of Constituted Solutions

Upon constitution with sterile water for injection or 0.9% sodium chloride (normal saline) injection, DORIBAX suspension in the vial may be held for 1-hour prior to transfer and dilution in the infusion bag.
Following dilution of the suspension with normal saline or 5% dextrose, DORIBAX infusions stored at controlled room temperature or under refrigeration should be completed according to the times in Table 3.

Table 3: Storage and Stability Times of Infusion Solutions Prepared in Normal Saline or 5% Dextrose

Infusion prepared in	Stability Time at Room Temp. (includes room temperature storage and infusion time)	Stability time at 2-8°C (Refrigeration) (includes refrigerator storage and infusion time)
Normal saline	8 hours	24 hours
5% Dextrose	4 hours	24 hours

Constituted DORIBAX suspension or DORIBAX infusion should not be frozen. This storage information applies also to DORIBAX™ diluted in Baxter Minibag Plus™.

3 DOSAGE FORMS AND STRENGTHS

Single use clear glass vials containing 500 mg (on an anhydrous basis) of sterile doripenem powder.

4 CONTRAINDICATIONS

DORIBAX™ is contraindicated in patients with known serious hypersensitivity to doripenem or to other drugs in the same class or in patients who have demonstrated anaphylactic reactions to beta-lactams.

5 WARNINGS AND PRECAUTIONS

5.1 Hypersensitivity Reactions

Serious and occasionally fatal hypersensitivity (anaphylactic) and serious skin reactions have been reported in patients receiving beta-lactam antibiotics. These reactions are more likely to occur in individuals with a history of sensitivity to multiple allergens. Before therapy with DORIBAX™ is instituted, careful inquiry should be made to determine whether the patient has had a previous hypersensitivity reaction to other carbapenems, cephalosporins, penicillins or other allergens. If this product is to be given to a penicillin- or other beta-lactam-allergic patient, caution should be exercised because cross-hyperreactivity among beta-lactam antibiotics has been clearly documented.
If an allergic reaction to DORIBAX™ occurs, discontinue the drug. Serious acute hypersensitivity (anaphylactic) reactions require emergency treatment with epinephrine and other emergency measures, including oxygen, IV fluids, IV antihistamines, corticosteroids, pressor amines and airway management, as clinically indicated.

5.2 Interaction with Sodium Valproate

Carbapenems may reduce serum valproic acid concentrations to subtherapeutic levels, resulting in loss of seizure control. Serum valproic acid concentrations should be monitored frequently after initiating carbapenem therapy. Alternative antibacterial or anticonvulsant therapy should be considered if serum valproic acid concentrations cannot be maintained in the therapeutic range or seizures occur. [see *Drug Interactions (7.1)*]

5.3 *Clostridium difficile*-Associated Diarrhea

Clostridium difficile-associated diarrhea (CDAD) has been reported with nearly all antibacterial agents and may range in severity from mild diarrhea to fatal colitis.
Treatment with antibacterial agents alters the normal flora of the colon and may permit overgrowth of *C. difficile*.
C. difficile produces toxins A and B which contribute to the development of CDAD. Hypertoxin producing strains of *C. difficile* cause increased morbidity and mortality, as these

Continued on next page

Doribax—Cont.

infections can be refractory to antimicrobial therapy and may require colectomy. CDAD must be considered in all patients who present with diarrhea following antibiotic use. Careful medical history is necessary since CDAD has been reported to occur over two months after the administration of antibacterial agents.

If CDAD is suspected or confirmed, ongoing antibiotic use not directed against *C. difficile* may need to be discontinued. Appropriate fluid and electrolyte management, protein supplementation, antibiotic treatment of *C. difficile*, and surgical evaluation should be instituted as clinically indicated. *[see Adverse Reactions (6.1)]*

5.4 Development of Drug-Resistant Bacteria

Prescribing DORIBAX™ in the absence of a proven or strongly suspected bacterial infection is unlikely to provide benefit to the patient and increases the risk of the development of drug-resistant bacteria.

5.5 Pneumonitis with Inhalational Use

When DORIBAX™ has been used investigationally via inhalation, pneumonitis has occurred. DORIBAX™ should not be administered by this route.

6 ADVERSE REACTIONS

The following adverse reactions are discussed in greater detail in other sections of labeling:

- Anaphylaxis and serious hypersensitivity reactions *[see Warnings and Precautions (5.1)]*
- Interaction with sodium valproate *[see Warnings and Precautions (5.2)* and *Drug Interactions (7.1)]*
- *Clostridium difficile*-associated diarrhea *[see Warnings and Precautions (5.3)]*
- Development of drug-resistant bacteria *[see Warnings and Precautions (5.4)]*
- Pneumonitis with inhalational use *[see Warnings and Precautions (5.5)]*

6.1 Adverse Reactions from Clinical Trials

Because clinical trials are conducted under widely varying conditions, adverse reaction rates observed in clinical trials of a drug cannot be compared directly to rates from clinical trials of another drug and may not reflect rates observed in practice.

During clinical investigations, 853 adult patients were treated with DORIBAX™ IV (500 mg administered over 1 hour q8h) in the three comparative phase 3 clinical studies; in some patients, parenteral therapy was followed by a switch to an oral antimicrobial. *[see Clinical Studies (14)]* The median age of patients treated with DORIBAX™ was 54 years (range 18-90) in the comparative cUTI study and 46 years (range 18-94) in the pooled comparative cIAI studies. There was a female predominance (62%) in the comparative cUTI study and a male predominance (63%) in the pooled cIAI studies. The patients treated with DORIBAX™ were predominantly Caucasian (77%) in the three pooled phase 3 studies.

The most common adverse reactions (≥5%) observed in the DORIBAX™ phase 3 clinical trials were headache, nausea, diarrhea, rash and phlebitis. During clinical trials, adverse drug reactions that led to DORIBAX™ discontinuation were nausea (0.2%), vulvomycotic infection (0.1%) and rash (0.1%).

Adverse reactions due to DORIBAX™ 500 mg q8h that occurred at a rate ≥1 % in either indication are listed in Table 4. Hypersensitivity reactions related to intravenous study drug and *C. difficile* colitis occurred at a rate of less than 1% in the three controlled phase 3 clinical trials.

[See table 4 above]

6.2 Postmarketing Experience

The following adverse reaction has been identified during post-approval use of doripenem outside of the U.S. Because this reaction was reported voluntarily from a population of uncertain size, it is not possible to reliably estimate its frequency or establish a causal relationship to drug exposure.

Anaphylaxis

The following treatment-emergent adverse events (known to occur with beta-lactams including carbapenems) have been reported voluntarily during post-approval use of DORIBAX™ outside of the U.S. They are included due to their seriousness, although it is not possible to estimate their frequency and causality has not been established:

Stevens Johnson Syndrome
Toxic epidermal necrolysis
Interstitial pneumonia
Seizure

7 DRUG INTERACTIONS

7.1 Valproic Acid

A clinically significant reduction in serum valproic acid concentrations has been reported in patients receiving carbapenem antibiotics and may result in loss of seizure control. Although the mechanism of this interaction is not fully understood, data from *in vitro* and animal studies suggest that carbapenem antibiotics may inhibit valproic acid glucuronide hydrolysis. Serum valproic acid concentrations should be monitored frequently after initiating carbapenem therapy. Alternative antibacterial or anticonvulsant therapy should be considered if serum valproic acid concentrations cannot be maintained in the therapeutic range or a seizure occurs. *[see Warnings and Precautions (5.2)]*

7.2 Probenecid

Probenecid interferes with the active tubular secretion of doripenem, resulting in increased plasma concentrations of

doripenem. *[see Clinical Pharmacology (12.3)]* Coadministration of probenecid with DORIBAX™ is not recommended.

8 USE IN SPECIFIC POPULATIONS

8.1 Pregnancy

Category B: Doripenem was not teratogenic and did not produce effects on ossification, developmental delays or fetal weight following intravenous administration during organogenesis at doses as high as 1 g/kg/day in rats and 50 mg/kg/day in rabbits (based on AUC, at least 2.4 and 0.8 times the exposure to humans dosed at 500 mg q8h, respectively). There are no adequate and well-controlled studies in pregnant women. Because animal reproduction studies are not always predictive of human response, this drug should be used during pregnancy only if clearly needed.

8.3 Nursing Mothers

It is not known whether this drug is excreted in human milk. Because many drugs are excreted in human milk, caution should be exercised when DORIBAX™ is administered to a nursing woman.

8.4 Pediatric Use

Safety and effectiveness in pediatric patients have not been established.

8.5 Geriatric Use

Of the total number of subjects in clinical studies of DORIBAX™, 28% were 65 and over, while 12% were 75 and over. Clinical cure rates in complicated intra-abdominal and complicated urinary tract infections were slightly lower in patients ≥65 years of age and also in the subgroup of patients ≥75 years of age versus patients <65. These results were similar between doripenem and comparator treatment groups.

No overall differences in safety were observed between older and younger subjects, but greater sensitivity of some older individuals cannot be ruled out.

Elderly subjects had greater doripenem exposure relative to non-elderly subjects; however, this increase in exposure was mainly attributed to age-related changes in renal function. *[see Clinical Pharmacology (12.3)]*

This drug is known to be excreted substantially by the kidney, and the risk of adverse reactions to this drug may be greater in patients with impaired renal function or pre-renal azotemia. Because elderly patients are more likely to have decreased renal function or pre-renal azotemia, care should be taken in dose selection, and it may be useful to monitor renal function.

8.6 Patients with Renal Impairment

Dosage adjustment is required in patients with moderately or severely impaired renal function. *[see Dosage and Administration (2.2)* and *Clinical Pharmacology (12.3)]* In such patients, renal function should be monitored.

10 OVERDOSAGE

In the event of overdose, DORIBAX™ should be discontinued and general supportive treatment given.

Doripenem can be removed by hemodialysis. In subjects with end-stage renal disease administered DORIBAX™

500 mg, the mean total recovery of doripenem and doripenem-M1 in the dialysate following a 4-hour hemodialysis session was 259 mg (52% of the dose). However, no information is available on the use of hemodialysis to treat overdosage. *[see Clinical Pharmacology (12.3)]*

11 DESCRIPTION

DORIBAX™, doripenem monohydrate for injection vials contain 500 mg of doripenem on an anhydrous basis, a white to slightly-yellowish off-white sterile crystalline powder. All references to doripenem activity are expressed in terms of the active doripenem moiety. The powder is constituted for intravenous infusion. The pH of the infusion solution is between 4.5 and 5.5.

DORIBAX™ is not formulated with any inactive ingredients.

DORIBAX™ (doripenem monohydrate) is a synthetic broad-spectrum carbapenem antibiotic structurally related to beta-lactam antibiotics. The chemical name for doripenem monohydrate is $(4R,5S,6S)$-3-$[((3S,5S)$-5-$[[(aminosulfonyl)amino]$ methyl]-3-pyrrolidinyl)thio]-6-$[(1R)$-1-hydroxyethyl]-4-methyl-7-oxo-1-azabicyclo[3.2.0] hept-2-ene-2-carboxylic acid monohydrate.

Its molecular weight is 438.52, and its chemical structure is:

12 CLINICAL PHARMACOLOGY

Doripenem is a carbapenem with *in vitro* antibacterial activity against aerobic and anaerobic Gram-positive and Gram-negative bacteria.

12.1 Mechanism of Action

Doripenem is an antibacterial drug. *[see Clinical Pharmacology (12.4)]*

12.2 Pharmacodynamics

Similar to other beta-lactam antimicrobial agents, the time that unbound plasma concentration of doripenem exceeds the MIC of the infecting organism has been shown to best correlate with efficacy in animal models of infection. However, the pharmacokinetic/pharmacodynamic relationship for doripenem has not been evaluated in patients.

In a randomized, positive- and placebo-controlled crossover QT study, 60 healthy subjects were administered DORIBAX™ 500 mg IV every 8 hours × 4 doses and DORIBAX™ 1g IV every 8 hours × 4 doses, placebo, and a single oral dose of positive control. At both the 500 mg and 1g DORIBAX™ doses, no significant effect on QTc interval was detected at peak plasma concentration or at any other time.

Table 4: Adverse Reactions[†] with Incidence Rates (%) of ≥1% and Adverse Events[††] Having Clinically Important Differences in Frequency by Indication in the Three Controlled, Comparative DORIBAX™ Phase 3 Clinical Trials

System organ class	Complicated Urinary Tract Infections (one trial)		Complicated Intra-Abdominal Infections (two trials)	
	DORIBAX™ 500 mg q8h (n =376)	Levofloxacin 250 mg IV q24h (n = 372)	DORIBAX™ 500 mg q8h (n = 477)	Meropenem 1 g q8h (n = 469)
Nervous system disorders				
Headache	16	15	4	5
Vascular disorders				
Phlebitis	4	4	8	6
Gastro-intestinal disorders				
Nausea	4	6	12	9
Diarrhea	6	10	11	11
Blood and Lymphatic System Disorders				
Anemia[††]	2	1	10	5
Renal and Urinary Disorders				
Renal impairment/Renal failure[††]	<1	0	1	<1
Skin and subcutaneous disorders				
Pruritus	<1	1	3	2
Rash*	1	1	5	2
Investigations				
Hepatic enzyme elevation**	2	3	1	3
Infection and Infestations				
Oral candidiasis	1	0	1	2
Vulvomycotic infection	2	1	1	<1

* includes reactions reported as allergic and bullous dermatitis, erythema, macular/papular eruptions, urticaria and erythema multiforme

**includes reactions reported as alanine aminotransferase increased, aspartate aminotransferase increased, hepatic enzyme increased, and transaminases increased

[†] An adverse drug reaction was defined as an undesirable effect, reasonably associated with the use of DORIBAX™ that may occur as part of its pharmacological action or may be unpredictable in its occurrence.

[††] An adverse event refers to any untoward medical event associated with the use of the drug in humans, whether or not considered drug-related.

12.3 Pharmacokinetics
Plasma Concentrations
Mean plasma concentrations of doripenem following a single 1-hour intravenous infusion of a 500 mg dose of DORIBAX™ to 24 healthy subjects are shown below in Figure 1. The mean (SD) plasma C_{max} and $AUC_{0-\infty}$ values were 23.0 (6.6) µg/mL and 36.3 (8.8) µg•hr/mL, respectively.

Figure 1. Average Doripenem Plasma Concentrations Versus Time Following a Single 1-Hour Intravenous Infusion of DORIBAX™ 500 mg in Healthy Subjects (N=24)

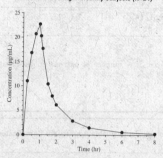

The pharmacokinetics of doripenem (C_{max} and AUC) are linear over a dose range of 500 mg to 1g when intravenously infused over 1 hour. There is no accumulation of doripenem following multiple intravenous infusions of either 500 mg or 1g administered every 8 hours for 7 to 10 days in subjects with normal renal function.

Distribution
The average binding of doripenem to plasma proteins is approximately 8.1% and is independent of plasma drug concentrations. The median (range) volume of distribution at steady state in healthy subjects is 16.8 L (8.09-55.5 L), similar to extracellular fluid volume (18.2 L).

Doripenem penetrates into several body fluids and tissues, including those at the site of infection for the approved indications. Doripenem concentrations in peritoneal and retroperitoneal fluid either match or exceed those required to inhibit most susceptible bacteria; however, the clinical relevance of this finding has not been established. Concentrations achieved in selected tissues and fluids following administration of DORIBAX™ are shown in Table 5:
[See table 5 above]

Metabolism
Metabolism of doripenem to a microbiologically inactive ring-opened metabolite (doripenem-M1) occurs primarily via dehydropeptidase-I. The mean (SD) plasma doripenem-M1-to-doripenem AUC ratio following single 500 mg and 1 g doses in healthy subjects is 18% (7.2%).

In pooled human liver microsomes, no *in vitro* metabolism of doripenem could be detected, indicating that doripenem is not a substrate for hepatic CYP450 enzymes.

Excretion
Doripenem is primarily eliminated unchanged by the kidneys. The mean plasma terminal elimination half-life of doripenem in healthy non-elderly adults is approximately 1 hour and mean (SD) plasma clearance is 15.9 (5.3) L/hour. Mean (SD) renal clearance is 10.8 (3.5) L/hour. The magnitude of this value, coupled with the significant decrease in the elimination of doripenem with concomitant probenecid administration, suggests that doripenem undergoes both glomerular filtration and active tubular secretion. In healthy adults given a single 500 mg dose of DORIBAX™, a mean of 70% and 15% of the dose was recovered in urine as unchanged drug and the ring-opened metabolite, respectively, within 48 hours. Following the administration of a single 500 mg dose of radiolabeled doripenem to healthy adults, less than 1% of the total radioactivity was recovered in feces after one week.

Special Populations
Patients with Renal Impairment
Following a single 500 mg dose of DORIBAX™, the mean AUC of doripenem in subjects with mild (CrCl 50-79 mL/min), moderate (CrCl 31-50 mL/min), and severe renal impairment (CrCl ≤ 30 mL/min) was 1.6-, 2.8-, and 5.1-times that of age-matched healthy subjects with normal renal function (CrCl ≥ 80 mL/min), respectively. Dosage adjustment is necessary in patients with moderate and severe renal impairment. *[see Dosage and Administration (2.2)]*

A single 500 mg dose of DORIBAX™ was administered to subjects with end stage renal disease (ESRD) either one hour prior to or one hour after hemodialysis (HD). The mean doripenem AUC following the post-HD infusion was 7.8-times that of healthy subjects with normal renal function. The mean total recovery of doripenem and doripenem-M1 in the dialysate following a 4-hour HD session was 231 mg and 28 mg, respectively, or a total of 259 mg (52% of the dose). There is insufficient information to make dose adjustment recommendations in patients on hemodialysis.

Patients with Hepatic Impairment
The pharmacokinetics of doripenem in patients with hepatic impairment have not been established. As doripenem does not appear to undergo hepatic metabolism, the pharmacokinetics of doripenem are not expected to be affected by hepatic impairment.

Geriatric Patients
The impact of age on the pharmacokinetics of doripenem was evaluated in healthy male (n=6) and female (n=6) subjects ≥ 66 years of age. Mean doripenem $AUC_{0-\infty}$ was 49% higher in elderly adults relative to non-elderly adults. This difference in exposure was mainly attributed to age-related changes in creatinine clearance. No dosage adjustment is recommended for elderly patients with normal (for their age) renal function.

Gender
The effect of gender on the pharmacokinetics of doripenem was evaluated in healthy male (n=12) and female (n=12) subjects. Doripenem C_{max} and AUC were similar between males and females. No dose adjustment is recommended based on gender.

Race
The effect of race on doripenem pharmacokinetics was examined using a population pharmacokinetic analysis of data from phase 1 and 2 studies. Compared to Caucasians, mean doripenem clearance was 14% greater in Hispanic/Latino subjects whereas no difference in clearance was observed for African Americans. Doripenem clearance in Japanese studies is similar to what has been observed in Western populations. No dosage adjustment is recommended based on race.

Drug Interactions
Probenecid interferes with the active tubular secretion of doripenem, resulting in increased plasma concentrations. Probenecid increased doripenem AUC by 75% and prolonged the plasma elimination half-life by 53%. *[see also Drug Interactions (7.2)]*

In vitro studies in human liver microsomes and hepatocytes indicate that doripenem does not inhibit the major cytochrome P450 isoenzymes (CYP1A2, CYP2A6, CYP2B6, CYP2C8, CYP2C9, CYP2C19, CYP2D6, CYP2E1, CYP3A4/5, and CYP4A11). Therefore, DORIBAX™ is not expected to inhibit the clearance of drugs that are metabolized by these metabolic pathways in a clinically relevant manner.

DORIBAX™ is also not expected to have CYP1A2, CYP2B6, CYP2C9, CYP2C19, CYP3A4/5, or UGT1A1 enzyme-inducing properties based on *in vitro* studies in cultured human hepatocytes.

12.4 Microbiology
Mechanism of Action
Doripenem belongs to the carbapenem class of antimicrobials. Doripenem exerts its bactericidal activity by inhibiting bacterial cell wall biosynthesis. Doripenem inactivates multiple essential penicillin-binding proteins (PBPs) resulting in inhibition of cell wall synthesis with subsequent cell death. In *E. coli* and *P. aeruginosa*, doripenem binds to PBP 2, which is involved in the maintenance of cell shape, as well as to PBPs 3 and 4.

Mechanism(s) of Resistance
Bacterial resistance mechanisms that affect doripenem include drug inactivation by carbapenem-hydrolyzing enzymes, mutant or acquired PBPs, decreased outer membrane permeability and active efflux. Doripenem is stable to hydrolysis by most beta-lactamases, including penicillinases and cephalosporinases produced by Gram-positive and Gram-negative bacteria, with the exception of carbapenem hydrolyzing beta-lactamases. Although cross-resistance may occur, some isolates resistant to other carbapenems may be susceptible to doripenem.

Interaction with Other Antimicrobials
In vitro synergy tests with doripenem show doripenem has little potential to antagonize or be antagonized by other antibiotics (e.g., levofloxacin, amikacin, trimethoprim-sulfamethoxazole, daptomycin, linezolid, and vancomycin).

Doripenem has been shown to be active against most isolates of the following microorganisms, both *in vitro* and in clinical infections. *[see Indications and Usage (1)]*

Facultative Gram-negative microorganisms
Acinetobacter baumannii
Escherichia coli
Klebsiella pneumoniae
Proteus mirabilis
Pseudomonas aeruginosa

Facultative Gram-positive microorganisms
Streptococcus constellatus
Streptococcus intermedius

Anaerobic microorganisms
Bacteroides caccae
Bacteroides fragilis
Bacteroides thetaiotaomicron
Bacteroides uniformis
Bacteroides vulgatus
Peptostreptococcus micros

At least 90 percent of the following microorganisms exhibit an *in vitro* minimal inhibitory concentration (MIC) less than or equal to the susceptible breakpoint for doripenem of

Continued on next page

Table 5: Doripenem Concentrations in Selected Tissues and Fluids

Tissue or Fluid	Dose (mg)	Infusion Duration (h)	Number of Samples or Subjects[a]	Sampling Period[b]	Concentration Range (µg/mL or µg/g)	Tissue- or Fluid-To-Plasma Concentration Ratio (%) Mean (Range)
Retroperitoneal fluid	250	0.5	9[c]	30-90 min[d]	3.15-52.4	Range: 4.1 (0.5-9.7) at 0.25 h to 990 (173-2609) at 2.5 h
	500	0.5	4[c]	90 min[d]	9.53-13.9	Range: 3.3 (0.0-8.1) at 0.25 h to 516 (311-842) at 6.5 h
Peritoneal exudate	250	0.5	5[c]	30-150 min[d]	2.36-5.17	Range: 19.7 (0.00-47.3) at 0.5 h to 160 (32.2-322) at 4.5 h
Gallbladder	250	0.5	10	20-215 min	BQL-1.87[e]	8.02 (0.00-44.4)
Bile	250	0.5	10	20-215 min	BQL-15.4[f]	117 (0.00-611)
Urine	500	1	110	0-4 hr	601 (BQL[f]-3360)[g]	–
	500	1	110	4-8 hr	49.7 (BQL[f]-635)[g]	–

[a] Unless stated otherwise, only one sample was collected per subject; [b] Time from start of infusion; [c] Serial samples were collected; maximum concentrations reported; [d] t_{max} range; [e] BQL (Below Quantifiable Limits) in 6 subjects; [f] BQL in 1 subject; [g] Median (range)

Table 6: Susceptibility Test Result Interpretive Criteria for Doripenem

Pathogen	Minimum Inhibitory Concentrations (µg/mL) Susceptible[a]	Disk Diffusion (zone diameters in mm) Susceptible
Enterobacteriaceae	≤0.5	≥23
Pseudomonas aeruginosa	≤2	≥24
Acinetobacter baumannii	≤1	≥17
Streptococcus anginosus group (*S. constellatus* and *S. intermedius*)	≤0.12	≥24
Anaerobes	≤1	n/a[b]

[a] The current absence of resistant isolates precludes defining any results other than "Susceptible". Isolates yielding MIC or disk diffusion results suggestive of "Nonsusceptible" should be subjected to additional testing.
[b] n/a = not applicable

Table 7: Acceptable Quality Control Ranges for Susceptibility Testing

QC Organism	Minimum Inhibitory Concentrations (µg/mL)	Disk Diffusion (zone diameters in mm)
Escherichia coli ATCC 25922	0.015-0.06	28-35
Pseudomonas aeruginosa ATCC 27853	0.12-0.5	29-35
Streptococcus pneumoniae ATCC 49619[a]	0.03-0.12	30-38
Bacteroides fragilis ATCC 25285	0.12-0.5	n/a
Bacteroides thetaiotaomicron ATCC 29741	0.12-1	n/a

[a] This organism may be used for validation of susceptibility test results when testing organisms of the *Streptococcus anginosus* group

Doribax—Cont.

organisms of the same type shown in Table 6. The safety and efficacy of doripenem in treating clinical infections due to these microorganisms has not been established in adequate and well-controlled clinical trials.

Facultative Gram-positive microorganisms
Staphylococcus aureus (methicillin-susceptible isolates only)
Streptococcus agalactiae
Streptococcus pyogenes

Facultative Gram-negative microorganisms
Citrobacter freundii
Enterobacter cloacae
Enterobacter aerogenes
Klebsiella oxytoca
Morganella morganii
Serratia marcescens

- **Susceptibility Test Methods**

When available, the clinical microbiology laboratory should provide the results of *in vitro* susceptibility test results for antimicrobial drugs used in local hospitals and practice areas to the physician as periodic reports that describe the susceptibility profile of nosocomial and community-acquired pathogens. These reports should aid the physician in selecting the most effective antimicrobial.

Dilution Techniques
Quantitative methods are used to determine antimicrobial minimum inhibitory concentrations (MICs). These MICs provide estimates of the susceptibility of bacteria to antimicrobial compounds. The MICs should be determined using a standardized procedure. Standardized procedures are based on a dilution method [1,3] (broth or agar) or equivalent with standardized inoculum concentrations and standardized concentrations of doripenem powder. The MIC values should be interpreted according to the criteria provided in Table 6.

Diffusion Techniques
Quantitative methods that require measurement of zone diameters provide reproducible estimates of the susceptibility of bacteria to antimicrobial compounds. One such standardized procedure [2,3] requires the use of standardized inoculum concentrations. This procedure uses paper disks impregnated with 10 µg of doripenem to test the susceptibility of microorganisms to doripenem. Results should be interpreted according to the criteria in Table 6.

Anaerobic Techniques
For anaerobic bacteria, the susceptibility to doripenem as MICs should be determined by standardized test methods [4]. The MIC values obtained should be interpreted according to the criteria in Table 6.
[See table 6 at top of previous page]
A report of *Susceptible* indicates that the antimicrobial is likely to inhibit growth of the pathogen if the antimicrobial compound in the blood reaches the concentrations usually achievable.

Quality Control
Standardized susceptibility test procedures require the use of laboratory control microorganisms to monitor the performance of the supplies and reagents used in the assay, and the techniques of the individuals performing the test. Standard doripenem powder should provide the MIC values provided in Table 7. For the diffusion techniques using a 10 µg doripenem disk, the criteria noted in Table 7 should be achieved.
[See table 7 at top of previous page]

13 NON-CLINICAL TOXICOLOGY

13.1 Carcinogenesis, Mutagenesis, and Impairment of Fertility
Because of the short duration of treatment and intermittent clinical use, long-term carcinogenicity studies have not been conducted with doripenem.

Doripenem did not show evidence of mutagenic activity in standard tests that included bacterial reverse mutation assay, chromosomal aberration assay with Chinese hamster lung fibroblast cells, and mouse bone marrow micronucleus assay.

Intravenous injection of doripenem had no adverse effects on general fertility of treated male and female rats or on postnatal development and reproductive performance of the offspring at doses as high as 1g/kg/day (based on AUC, greater than 1.5 times the exposure to humans at the dose of 500 mg q8h).

14 CLINICAL STUDIES

14.1 Complicated Intra-Abdominal Infections
A total of 946 adults with complicated intra-abdominal infections were randomized and received study medications in two identical multinational, multi-center, double-blind studies comparing DORIBAX™ (500 mg administered over 1 hour q8h) to meropenem (1 g administered over 3-5 minutes q8h). Both regimens allowed the option to switch to oral amoxicillin/clavulanate (875 mg/125 mg twice daily) after a minimum of 3 days of intravenous therapy for a total of 5-14 days of intravenous and oral treatment. Patients with complicated appendicitis, or other complicated intra-abdominal infections, including bowel perforation, cholecystitis, intra-abdominal or solid organ abscess and generalized peritonitis were enrolled.

DORIBAX™ was non-inferior to meropenem with regard to clinical cure rates in microbiologically evaluable (ME) patients, i.e., in patients with susceptible pathogens isolated at baseline and no major protocol deviations at test of cure (TOC) visit, 25-45 days after completing therapy.

Table 8: Clinical Cure Rates in Two Phase 3 Studies of Adults with Complicated Intra-Abdominal Infections

Analysis Populations	DORIBAX™[a] n/N (%)[c]	Meropenem[b] n/N (%)[c]	Treatment Difference (2-sided 95% CI[f])
Study 1:			
ME[d]	130/157 (82.8)	128/149 (85.9)	-3.1 (-11.3; 5.2)
mMITT[e]	143/194 (73.7)	149/191 (78.0)	-4.3 (-12.8; 4.3)
Study 2:			
ME[d]	128/158 (81.0)	119/145 (82.1)	-1.1 (-9.8; 7.8)
mMITT[e]	143/199 (71.9)	138/186 (74.2)	-2.3 (-11.2; 6.6)

[a] 500 mg administered over 1 hour q8h
[b] 1 g administered over 3 - 5 minutes q8h
[c] n = number of patients in the designated population who were cured; N = number of patients in the designated population
[d] ME = microbiologically evaluable patients
[e] mMITT = microbiological modified intent-to-treat patients
[f] CI = confidence interval

Table 9: Microbiological Cure Rates by Infecting Pathogen in Microbiologically Evaluable Adults with Complicated Intra-abdominal Infections

Pathogen	DORIBAX™ N[a]	DORIBAX™ n[b]	DORIBAX™ %	Meropenem N[a]	Meropenem n[b]	Meropenem %
Gram-positive, aerobic						
Streptococcus constellatus	10	9	90.0	7	5	71.4
Streptococcus intermedius	36	30	83.3	29	21	72.4
Gram-positive, anaerobic						
Peptostreptococcus micros	13	11	84.6	14	11	78.6
Gram-negative, aerobic						
Enterobacteriaceae	315	271	86.0	274	234	85.4
Escherichia coli	216	189	87.5	199	168	84.4
Klebsiella pneumoniae	32	25	78.1	20	19	95.0
Non-fermenters	51	44	86.3	39	28	71.8
Pseudomonas aeruginosa	40	34	85.0	32	24	75.0
Gram-negative, anaerobic						
Bacteroides fragilis group	173	152	87.9	181	152	84.0
Bacteroides caccae	25	23	92.0	19	18	94.7
Bacteroides fragilis	67	56	83.6	68	54	79.4
Bacteroides thetaiotaomicron	34	30	88.2	36	32	88.9
Bacteroides uniformis	22	19	86.4	18	15	83.3
Non-fragilis Bacteroides	14	13	92.9	13	9	69.2
Bacteroides vulgatus	11	11	100.0	8	6	75.0

[a] N = number of unique baseline isolates
[b] n = number of pathogens assessed as cured

Table 10: Microbiological Eradication Rates from the Phase 3 Comparative Study of Adults with Complicated Urinary Tract Infections, Including Pyelonephritis

Analysis populations	DORIBAX™[a] n/N (%)[c]	Levofloxacin[b] n/N (%)[c]	Treatment Difference (2-sided 95% CI[f])
ME[d]	230/280 (82.1)	221/265 (83.4)	-1.3 (-8.0, 5.5)
mMITT[e]	259/327 (79.2)	251/321 (78.2)	1.0 (-5.6, 7.6)

[a] 500 mg administered over 1 hour q8h
[b] 250 mg administered intravenously q24h
[c] n = number of patients in the designated population who were cured; N = number of patients in the designated population
[d] ME = microbiologically evaluable patients
[e] mMITT = microbiological modified intent-to-treat patients
[f] CI= confidence interval

Table 11: Microbiological Eradication Rates By Infecting Pathogen in Microbiologically Evaluable Adults with Complicated Urinary Tract Infections, Including Pyelonephritis

Pathogen	DORIBAX™[a] N[b]	DORIBAX™[a] n[c]	DORIBAX™[a] %	Levofloxacin N[b]	Levofloxacin n[c]	Levofloxacin %
Gram-negative, aerobic						
Escherichia coli	357	313	87.7	211	184	87.2
Klebsiella pneumoniae	33	26	78.8	8	5	62.5
Proteus mirabilis	30	22	73.3	15	13	86.7
Non-fermenters	38	27	71.1	8	5	62.5
Acinetobacter baumannii	10	8	80.0	1	0	0.0
Pseudomonas aeruginosa	27	19	70.4	7	5	71.4

[a] data from comparative and non-comparative studies
[b] N = number of unique baseline isolates
[c] n = number of pathogens with a favorable outcome (eradication)

DORIBAX™ was also non-inferior to meropenem in microbiological modified intent-to-treat (mMITT) patients, i.e., patients with baseline pathogens isolated regardless of susceptibility. Clinical cure rates at TOC are displayed by patient populations in Table 8. Microbiological cure rates at TOC by pathogen in ME patients are presented in Table 9.
[See table 8 above]
[See table 9 above]

14.2 Complicated Urinary Tract Infections, Including Pyelonephritis
A total of 1171 adults with complicated urinary tract infections, including pyelonephritis (49 percent of microbiologi-cally evaluable patients) were randomized and received study medications in two multi-center, multinational studies. Complicated pyelonephritis, i.e., pyelonephritis associated with predisposing anatomical or functional abnormality, comprised 17% of patients with pyelonephritis. One study was double-blind and compared DORIBAX™ (500 mg administered over 1 hour q8h) to IV levofloxacin (250 mg q24h). The second study was a non-comparative study but of otherwise similar design. Both studies permitted the option of switching to oral levofloxacin (250 mg every q24h) after a minimum of 3 days of IV therapy for a total of 10 days of treatment. Patients with confirmed concurrent bacteremia

were allowed to receive 500 mg of IV levofloxacin (either IV or oral as appropriate) for a total of 10 to 14 days of treatment.

DORIBAX™ was non-inferior to levofloxacin with regard to the microbiological eradication rates in microbiologically evaluable (ME) patients, i.e., patients with baseline uropathogens isolated, no major protocol deviations and urine cultures at test of cure (TOC) visit 5-11 days after completing therapy. DORIBAX™ was also non-inferior to levofloxacin in microbiological modified intent-to-treat (mMITT) patients, i.e., patients with pretreatment urine cultures. Overall microbiological eradication rates at TOC and the 95% CIs for the comparative study are displayed in Table 10. Microbiological eradication rates at TOC by pathogen in ME patients are presented in Table 11.

[See table 10 at top of previous page]
[See table 11 at top of previous page]

15 REFERENCES

1. Clinical and Laboratory Standards Institute (CLSI). Methods for Dilution Antimicrobial Susceptibility Tests for Bacteria that Grow Aerobically; Approved Standard – 7th ed. CLSI Document M7-A7. CLSI, 940 West Valley Rd., Suite 1400, Wayne, PA 19087, 2006.
2. CLSI. Performance Standards for Antimicrobial Disk Susceptibility Tests; Approved Standard – 9th ed. CLSI Document M2-A9. CLSI, Wayne, PA 19087, 2006.
3. CLSI. Performance Standards for Antimicrobial Susceptibility Testing; 17th Informational Supplement. CLSI document M100-S17. CLSI, Wayne, PA 19087, 2007.
4. CLSI. Methods for Antimicrobial Susceptibility Testing of Anaerobic Bacteria; Approved Standard – 7th ed. CLSI document M11-A7. CLSI, Wayne, PA 19087, 2007.

16 HOW SUPPLIED/STORAGE AND HANDLING

• DORIBAX™ is supplied as single use type 1 clear glass vials containing 500 mg (on an anhydrous basis) of sterile doripenem powder. Vials are packaged individually (NDC: 0062-4010-01) in cartons containing 10 vials (NDC: 0062-4010-02).

• Storage of DORIBAX vials: DORIBAX™ should be stored at 25°C (77°F); excursions permitted to 15°-30°C (59° to 86°F) [refer to USP controlled room temperature].

17 PATIENT COUNSELING INFORMATION

• Patients should be advised that allergic reactions, including serious allergic reactions, could occur and that serious reactions require immediate treatment. They should report any previous hypersensitivity reactions to DORIBAX™, other carbapenems, beta-lactams or other allergens.

• Patients should be counseled that anti-bacterial drugs including DORIBAX™ should only be used to treat bacterial infections. They do not treat viral infections (e.g., the common cold). When DORIBAX™ is prescribed to treat a bacterial infection, patients should be told that although it is common to feel better early in the course of therapy, the medication should be taken exactly as directed. Skipping doses or not completing the full course of therapy may (1) decrease the effectiveness of the immediate treatment and (2) increase the likelihood that bacteria will develop resistance and will not be treatable by DORIBAX™ or other antibacterial drugs in the future.

• Keep out of the reach of children.

MINI-BAG Plus is a trademark of Baxter International Inc.
Manufactured by:
Shionogi & Co. Ltd.
Osaka 541-0045, Japan
Distributed by:
Ortho-McNeil Pharmaceutical, Inc.
Raritan, NJ 08869
10157600   10/2007

Otsuka America Pharmaceutical, Inc.

**2440 RESEARCH BOULEVARD
ROCKVILLE, MD 20850**

For Medical Information about products marketed by Otsuka America Pharmaceutical, Inc., or to report an adverse event, please contact: 1-800-562-3974

BUSULFEX®   ℞
(busulfan) Injection
Caution: Must be diluted prior to use.
Rx only

WARNING

BUSULFEX® (busulfan) Injection is a potent cytotoxic drug that causes profound myelosuppression at the recommended dosage. It should be administered under the supervision of a qualified physician who is experienced in allogeneic hematopoietic stem cell transplantation, the use of cancer chemotherapeutic drugs and the management of patients with severe pancytopenia. Appropriate management of therapy and complications is only possible when adequate diagnostic and treatment facilities are readily available. SEE "WARNINGS"

SECTION FOR INFORMATION REGARDING BUSULFAN-INDUCED PANCYTOPENIA IN HUMANS.

DESCRIPTION

Busulfan is a bifunctional alkylating agent known chemically as 1,4-butanediol, dimethanesulfonate. BUSULFEX® (busulfan) Injection is intended for intravenous administration. It is supplied as a clear, colorless, sterile, solution in 10 mL single use vials. Each vial of BUSULFEX contains 60 mg (6 mg/mL) of busulfan, the active ingredient, a white crystalline powder with a molecular formula of $CH_3SO_2O(CH_2)_4OSO_2CH_3$ and a molecular weight of 246 g/mole. Busulfan is dissolved in N,N-dimethylacetamide (DMA) 33% vol/vol and Polyethylene Glycol 400, 67% vol/vol. The solubility of busulfan in water is 0.1 g/L and the pH of BUSULFEX diluted to approximately 0.5 mg/mL busulfan in 0.9% Sodium Chloride Injection, USP or 5% Dextrose Injection, USP as recommended for infusion reflects the pH of the diluent used and ranges from 3.4 to 3.9.

BUSULFEX is intended for dilution with 0.9% Sodium Chloride Injection, USP or 5% Dextrose Injection, USP prior to intravenous infusion.

CLINICAL PHARMACOLOGY
Mechanism of Action:
Busulfan is a bifunctional alkylating agent in which two labile methanesulfonate groups are attached to opposite ends of a four-carbon alkyl chain. In aqueous media, busulfan hydrolyzes to release the methanesulfonate groups. This produces reactive carbonium ions that can alkylate DNA. DNA damage is thought to be responsible for much of the cytotoxicity of busulfan.

Pharmacokinetics:
The pharmacokinetics of BUSULFEX were studied in 59 patients participating in a prospective trial of a BUSULFEX-cyclophosphamide preparatory regimen prior to allogeneic hematopoietic progenitor stem cell transplantation. Patients received 0.8 mg/kg BUSULFEX every six hours, for a total of 16 doses over four days. Fifty-five of fifty-nine patients (93%) administered BUSULFEX maintained AUC values below the target value (<1500 µM•min).

Table 1
Steady State Pharmacokinetic Parameters Following Busulfex® (busulfan) Infusion (0.8 mg/kg; N=59)

	Mean	CV (%)	Range
C_{max} (ng/mL)	1222	18	496-1684
AUC (µM•min)	1167	20	556-1673
CL (mL/min/kg)*	2.52	25	1.49-4.31

*Clearance normalized to actual body weight for all patients.

BUSULFEX pharmacokinetics showed consistency between dose 9 and dose 13 as demonstrated by reproducibility of steady state C_{max} and a low coefficient of variation for this parameter.

In a pharmacokinetic study of BUSULFEX in 24 pediatric patients, the population pharmacokinetic (PPK) estimates of BUSULFEX for clearance (CL) and volume of distribution (V) were determined. For actual body weight, PPK estimates of CL and V were 4.04 L/hr/20 kg (3.37 mL/min/kg; interpatient variability 23%); and 12.8 L/20 kg (0.64 L/kg; interpatient variability 11%).

Distribution, Metabolism, Excretion:
Studies of distribution, metabolism, and elimination of BUSULFEX have not been done; however, the literature on oral busulfan is relevant. Additionally, for modulating effects on pharmacodynamic parameters see **Drug Interactions**.

Distribution: Busulfan achieves concentrations in the cerebrospinal fluid approximately equal to those in plasma. Irreversible binding to plasma elements, primarily albumin, has been estimated to be 32.4 ± 2.2% which is consistent with the reactive electrophilic properties of busulfan.

Metabolism: Busulfan is predominantly metabolized by conjugation with glutathione, both spontaneously and by glutathione S-transferase (GST) catalysis. This conjugate undergoes further extensive oxidative metabolism in the liver.

Excretion: Following administration of ^{14}C-labeled busulfan to humans, approximately 30% of the radioactivity was excreted into the urine over 48 hours; negligible amounts were recovered in feces. The incomplete recovery of radioactivity may be due to the formation of long-lived metabolites or due to nonspecific alkylation of macromolecules.

CLINICAL STUDIES
Documentation of the safety and efficacy of busulfan as a component of a conditioning regimen prior to allogeneic hematopoietic progenitor cell reconstitution is derived from two sources: i) analysis of a prospective clinical trial of BUSULFEX that involved 61 patients diagnosed with various hematologic malignancies, and ii) the published reports of randomized, controlled trials that employed high-dose oral busulfan as a component of a conditioning regimen for transplantation, which were identified in a literature review of five established commercial databases.

The prospective trial was a single-arm, open-label study in 61 patients who received BUSULFEX as part of a conditioning regimen for allogeneic hematopoietic stem cell transplantation. The study included patients with acute leukemia past first remission (first or subsequent relapse), with high-risk first remission, or with induction failure; chronic myelogenous leukemia (CML) in chronic phase, accelerated phase, or blast crisis; primary refractory or resistant relapsed Hodgkin's disease or non-Hodgkin's lymphoma; and myelodysplastic syndrome. Forty-eight percent of patients (29/61) were heavily pretreated, defined as having at least one of the following: prior radiation, ≥3 prior chemotherapeutic regimens, or prior hematopoietic stem cell transplant. Seventy-five percent of patients (46/61) were transplanted with active disease.

Patients received 16 BUSULFEX doses of 0.8 mg/kg every 6 hours as a two-hour infusion for 4 days, followed by cyclophosphamide 60 mg/kg once per day for two days (BuCy2 regimen). All patients received 100% of their scheduled BUSULFEX regimen. No dose adjustments were made. After one rest day, allogeneic hematopoietic progenitor cells were infused. The efficacy parameters in this study were myeloablation (defined as one or more of the following: absolute neutrophil count [ANC] less than 0.5×10^9/L, absolute lymphocyte count [ALC] less than 0.1×10^9/L, thrombocytopenia defined as a platelet count less than 20,000/mm³ or a platelet transfusion requirement) and engraftment (ANC ≥0.5×10^9/L).

All patients (61/61) experienced myeloablation. The median time to neutropenia was 4 days. All evaluable patients (60/60) engrafted at a median of 13 days post-transplant (range 9 to 29 days); one patient was considered non-evaluable because he died of a fungal pneumonia 20 days after BMT and before engraftment occurred. All but 13 of the patients were treated with prophylactic G-CSF. Evidence of donor cell engraftment and chimerism was documented in all patients who had a chromosomal sex marker or leukemic marker (43/43), and no patient with chimeric evidence of allogeneic engraftment suffered a later loss of the allogeneic graft. There were no reports of graft failure in the overall study population. The median number of platelet transfusions per patient was 6, and the median number of red blood cell transfusions per patient was 4.

Twenty-three patients (38%) relapsed at a median of 183 days post-transplant (range 36 to 406 days). Sixty-two percent of patients (38/61) were free from disease with a median follow-up of 269 days post-transplant (range 20 to 583 days). Forty-three patients (70%) were alive with a median follow up of 288 days post-transplant (range 51 to 583 days). There were two deaths before BMT Day +28 and six additional patients died by BMT Day +100. Ten patients (16%) died after BMT Day +100, at a median of 199 days post-transplant (range 113 to 275 days).

Oral Busulfan Literature Review. Four publications of randomized, controlled trials that evaluated a high-dose oral busulfan-containing conditioning regimen (busulfan 4 mg/kg/d × 4 days + cyclophosphamide 60 mg/kg/d × 2 days) for allogeneic transplantation in the setting of CML were identified. Two of the studies (Clift and Devergie) had populations confined to CML in chronic phase that were randomized between conditioning with busulfan/cyclophosphamide (BU/CY) and cyclophosphamide/total body irradiation (CY/TBI). A total of 138 patients were treated with BU/CY in these studies. The populations of the two remaining studies (Ringden and Blume) included patients with CML, acute lymphoblastic leukemia (ALL), and acute myelogenous leukemia (AML). In the Nordic BMT Group study published by Ringden, et al., 57 patients had CML, and of those, 30 were treated with BU/CY. Patients with CML in chronic phase, accelerated phase, and blast crisis were eligible for this study. The participants with CML (34/122 patients) in a SWOG study published by Blume, et al., had disease beyond first chronic phase. Twenty of those CML patients were treated with BU/CY, and the TBI comparator arm utilized etoposide instead of cyclophosphamide.

Table 2 below summarizes the efficacy analyses reported from these 4 studies.

[See table 2 at top of next page]

INDICATIONS AND USAGE

BUSULFEX® (busulfan) Injection is indicated for use in combination with cyclophosphamide as a conditioning regimen prior to allogeneic hematopoietic progenitor cell transplantation for chronic myelogenous leukemia.

CONTRAINDICATIONS

BUSULFEX is contraindicated in patients with a history of hypersensitivity to any of its components.

WARNINGS

BUSULFEX should be administered under the supervision of a qualified physician experienced in hematopoietic stem cell transplantation. Appropriate management of complications arising from its administration is possible only when adequate diagnostic and treatment facilities are readily available.

The following warnings pertain to different physiologic effects of BUSULFEX in the setting of allogeneic transplantation.

Hematologic: The most frequent serious consequence of treatment with BUSULFEX at the recommended dose and schedule is profound myelosuppression, occurring in all patients. Severe granulocytopenia, thrombocytopenia, anemia, or any combination thereof may develop. Frequent complete

Continued on next page

Busulfex—Cont.

blood counts, including white blood cell differentials, and quantitative platelet counts should be monitored during treatment and until recovery is achieved. Absolute neutrophil counts dropped below 0.5×10^9/L at a median of 4 days post-transplant in 100% of patients treated in the BUSULFEX clinical trial. The absolute neutrophil count recovered at a median of 13 days following allogeneic transplantation when prophylactic G-CSF was used in the majority of patients. Thrombocytopenia (<25,000/mm^3 or requiring platelet transfusion) occurred at a median of 5-6 days in 98% of patients. Anemia (hemoglobin <8.0 g/dL) occurred in 69% of patients. Antibiotic therapy and platelet and red blood cell support should be used when medically indicated.

Neurological: Seizures have been reported in patients receiving high-dose oral busulfan at doses producing plasma drug levels similar to those achieved following the recommended dosage of BUSULFEX. Despite prophylactic therapy with phenytoin, one seizure (1/42 patients) was reported during an autologous transplantation clinical trial of BUSULFEX. This episode occurred during the cyclophosphamide portion of the conditioning regimen, 36 hours after the last BUSULFEX dose. Anti-convulsant prophylactic therapy should be initiated prior to BUSULFEX treatment. Caution should be exercised when administering the recommended dose of BUSULFEX to patients with a history of a seizure disorder or head trauma or who are receiving other potentially epileptogenic drugs.

Hepatic: Current literature suggests that high busulfan area under the plasma concentration verses time curve (AUC) values (>1,500 µM•min) may be associated with an increased risk of developing hepatic veno-occlusive disease (HVOD). Patients who have received prior radiation therapy, greater than or equal to three cycles of chemotherapy, or a prior progenitor cell transplant may be at an increased risk of developing HVOD with the recommended BUSULFEX dose and regimen. Based on clinical examination and laboratory findings, hepatic veno-occlusive disease was diagnosed in 8% (5/61) of patients treated with BUSULFEX in the setting of allogeneic transplantation, was fatal in 2/5 cases (40%), and yielded an overall mortality from HVOD in the entire study population of 2/61 (3%). Three of the five patients diagnosed with HVOD were retrospectively found to meet the Jones' criteria. The incidence of HVOD reported in the literature from the randomized, controlled trials (see CLINICAL STUDIES) was 7.7%-12%.

Cardiac: Cardiac tamponade has been reported in pediatric patients with thalassemia (8/400 or 2% in one series) who received high doses of oral busulfan and cyclophosphamide as the preparatory regimen for hematopoietic progenitor cell transplantation. Six of the eight children died and two were saved by rapid pericardiocentesis. Abdominal pain and vomiting preceded the tamponade in most patients. No patients treated in the BUSULFEX (busulfan) Injection clinical trials experienced cardiac tamponade.

Pulmonary: Bronchopulmonary dysplasia with pulmonary fibrosis is a rare but serious complication following chronic busulfan therapy. The average onset of symptoms is 4 years after therapy (range 4 months to 10 years).

Carcinogenicity, Mutagenicity, Impairment of Fertility:

Busulfan is a mutagen and a clastogen. In *in vitro* tests it caused mutations in ***Salmonella typhimurium*** and ***Drosophila melanogaster***. Chromosomal aberrations induced by busulfan have been reported *in vivo* (rats, mice, hamsters, and humans) and *in vitro* (rodent and human cells). The intravenous administration of busulfan (48 mg/kg given as biweekly doses of 12 mg/kg, or 30% of the total BUSULFEX dose on a mg/m^2 basis) has been shown to increase the incidence of thymic and ovarian tumors in mice. Four cases of acute leukemia occurred among 19 patients who became pancytopenic in a 243 patient study incorporating busulfan as adjuvant therapy following surgical resection of bronchogenic carcinoma. Clinical appearance of leukemia was observed 5-8 years following oral busulfan treatment. Busulfan is a presumed human carcinogen.

Ovarian suppression and amenorrhea commonly occur in premenopausal women undergoing chronic, low-dose busulfan therapy for chronic myelogenous leukemia. Busulfan depleted oocytes of female rats. Busulfan induced sterility in male rats and hamsters. Sterility, azoospermia and testicular atrophy have been reported in male patients. The solvent DMA may also impair fertility. A DMA daily dose of 0.45 g/kg/d given to rats for nine days (equivalent to 44% of the daily dose of DMA contained in the recommended dose of BUSULFEX on a mg/m^2 basis) significantly decreased spermatogenesis in rats. A single sc dose of 2.2 g/kg (27% of the total DMA dose contained in BUSULFEX on a mg/m^2 basis) four days after insemination terminated pregnancy in 100% of tested hamsters.

Pregnancy: Busulfan may cause fetal harm when administered to a pregnant woman. Busulfan produced teratogenic changes in the offspring of mice, rats and rabbits when given during gestation. Malformations and anomalies included significant alterations in the musculoskeletal system, body weight gain, and size. In pregnant rats, busulfan produced sterility in both male and female offspring due to the absence of germinal cells in the testes and ovaries. The solvent, DMA, may also cause fetal harm when administered to a pregnant woman. In rats, DMA doses of 400 mg/kg/d (about 40% of the daily dose of DMA in the BUSULFEX dose on a mg/m^2 basis) given during organogenesis caused significant developmental anomalies. The most striking abnormalities included anasarca, cleft palate, vertebral anomalies, rib anomalies, and serious anomalies of the vessels of the heart. There are no adequate and well-controlled studies of either busulfan or DMA in pregnant women. If BUSULFEX is used during pregnancy, or if the patient becomes pregnant while receiving BUSULFEX, the patient should be apprised of the potential hazard to the fetus. Women of childbearing potential should be advised to avoid becoming pregnant.

Table 2
Summary of efficacy analyses from the randomized, controlled trials utilizing a high dose oral busulfan-containing conditioning regimen identified in a literature review

Clift, 1994 CML Chronic Phase;							
3 year Overall Survival		3 year DFS (p=0.43)		Relapse		Time to Engraftment (ANC≥500)	
BU/CY	CY/TBI	BU/CY	CY/TBI	BU/CY	CY/TBI	BU/CY	CY/TBI
80%	80%	71%	68%	13%	13%	22.6 days	22.3 days
Devergie, 1995 CML Chronic Phase;							
5 year Overall Survival (p=0.5)		5 year DFS (p=0.75)		Relapse (Relative Risk analysis BU/CY:CY/TBI) (p=0.04)		Time to Engraftment (ANC≥500)	
BU/CY	CY/TBI	BU/CY	CY/TBI	BU/CY	CY/TBI	BU/CY	CY/TBI
60.6% ±11.7%	65.8% ±12.5%	59.1% ±11.8%	51.0% ±14%	4.10 (95% CI =1.00-20.28)		None Given	None Given
Ringden, 1994 CML, AML, ALL;							
3 year Overall Survival (p<0.03)		3 year Relapse Free Survival (p=0.065)		Relapse (p=0.9)		Time to Engraftment (ANC>500)	
BU/CY	CY/TBI	BU/CY	CY/TBI	BU/CY	CY/TBI	BU/CY	CY/TBI
62%	76%	56%	67%	22%	26%	20 days	20 days
Blume, 1993* CML, AML, ALL; Relative Risk Analysis BU/CY: Etoposide/TBI							
RR of Mortality		DFS		RR of Relapse (Relative Risk analysis BU/CY:CY/TBI)		Time to Engraftment	
BU/CY	Eto/TBI	BU/CY	Eto/TBI	BU/CY	Eto/TBI	BU/CY	Eto/TBI
0.97 (95% CI=0.64-1.48)		Not Given		1.02 (95% CI=0.56-1.86)		Not Given	

*Eto = etoposide. TBI was combined with etoposide in the comparator arm of this study.
BU = Busulfan
CY = Cyclophosphamide
TBI = Total Body Irradiation
DFS = Disease Free Survival
ANC = Absolute Neutrophil Count

PRECAUTIONS

Hematologic: At the recommended dosage of BUSULFEX (busulfan) Injection, profound myelosuppression is universal, and can manifest as neutropenia, thrombocytopenia, anemia, or a combination thereof. Patients should be monitored for signs of local or systemic infection or bleeding. Their hematologic status should be evaluated frequently.

Information for Patients: The increased risk of a second malignancy should be explained to the patient.

Laboratory Tests: Patients receiving BUSULFEX should be monitored daily with a complete blood count, including differential count and quantitative platelet count, until engraftment has been demonstrated.

To detect hepatotoxicity, which may herald the onset of hepatic veno-occlusive disease, serum transaminases, alkaline phosphatase, and bilirubin should be evaluated daily through BMT Day +28.

Drug Interactions: Itraconazole decreases busulfan clearance by up to 25%, and may produce an AUC > 1500 µM•min in some patients. Fluconazole, and the 5-HT3 antiemetics odansetron (Zofran®) and granisetron (Kytril®) have all been used with BUSULFEX.

Phenytoin increases the clearance of busulfan by 15% or more, possibly due to the induction of glutathione-S-transferase. Since the pharmacokinetics of BUSULFEX were studied in patients treated with phenytoin, the clearance of BUSULFEX at the recommended dose may be lower and exposure (AUC) higher in patients not treated with phenytoin. Because busulfan is eliminated from the body via conjugation with glutathione, use of acetaminophen prior to (<72 hours) or concurrent with BUSULFEX may result in reduced busulfan clearance based upon the known property of acetaminophen to decrease glutathione levels in the blood and tissues.

Pregnancy: Pregnancy Category D. See **WARNINGS**.

Nursing Mothers: It is not known whether this drug is excreted in human milk. Because many drugs are excreted in human milk and because of the potential for tumorgenicity shown for busulfan in human and animal studies, a decision should be made whether to discontinue nursing or to discontinue the drug, taking into account the importance of the drug to the mother.

Special Populations

Pediatric: The effectiveness of BUSULFEX in the treatment of CML has not been specifically studied in pediatric patients. An open-label, uncontrolled study evaluated the pharmacokinetics of BUSULFEX in 24 pediatric patients receiving BUSULFEX as part of a conditioning regimen administered prior to hematopoietic progenitor cell transplantation for a variety of malignant hematologic (N=15) or non-malignant diseases (N=9). Patients ranged in age from 5 months to 16 years (median 3 years). BUSULFEX dosing was targeted to achieve an area under the plasma concentration curve (AUC) of 900-1350 µM•min with an initial dose of 0.8 mg/kg or 1.0 mg/kg (based on ABW) if the patient was >4 or ≤4 years, respectively. The dose was adjusted based on plasma concentration after completion of dose 1.

Patients received BUSULFEX doses every six hours as a two-hour infusion over four days for a total of 16 doses, followed by cyclophosphamide 50 mg/kg once daily for four days. After one rest day, hematopoietic progenitor cells were infused. All patients received phenytoin as seizure prophylaxis. The target AUC (900-1350 ± 5% µM•min) for BUSULFEX was achieved at dose 1 in 71% (17/24) of patients. Steady state pharmacokinetic testing was performed at dose 9 and 13. BUSULFEX levels were within the target range for 21 of 23 evaluable patients.

All 24 patients experienced neutropenia (absolute neutrophil count <0.5×10^9/L) and thrombocytopenia (platelet transfusions or platelet count <20,000/mm^3). Seventy-nine percent (19/24) of patients experienced lymphopenia (absolute lymphocyte count <0.1×10^9). In 23 patients, the ANC recovered to >0.5×10^9/L (median time to recovery = BMT day +13; range = BMT day +9 to +22). One patient who died on day +20 had not recovered to an ANC > 0.5×10^9/L.

Four (17%) patients died during the study. Two patients died within 28 days of transplant; one with pneumonia and capillary leak syndrome, and the other with pneumonia and veno-occlusive disease. Two patients died prior to day 100; one due to progressive disease and one due to multi-organ failure.

Adverse events were reported in all 24 patients during the study period (BMT day -10 through BMT day +28) or post-study surveillance period (day +29 through +100). These included vomiting (100%), nausea (83%), stomatitis (79%), hepatic veno-occlusive disease (HVOD) (21%), graft-versus host disease (GVHD) (25%), and pneumonia (21%).

Based on the results of this 24-patient clinical trial, a suggested dosing regimen of BUSULFEX in pediatric patients is shown in the following dosing nomogram:

BUSULFEX Dosing Nomogram

Patient's Actual Body Weight (ABW)	BUSULFEX Dosage
≤12 kgs	1.1 (mg/kg)
>12 kgs	0.8 (mg/kg)

Simulations based on a pediatric population pharmacokinetic model indicate that approximately 60% of pediatric patients will achieve a target BUSULFEX exposure (AUC) between 900 to 1350 µM•min with the first dose of BUSULFEX using this dosing nomogram. Therapeutic drug monitoring and dose adjustment following the first dose of BUSULFEX is recommended.

Dose Adjustment Based on Therapeutic Drug Monitoring
Instructions for measuring the AUC of busulfan at dose 1 (see **Blood Sample Collection for AUC Determination**), and the formula for adjustment of subsequent doses to achieve the desired target AUC (1125 µM•min), are provided below.
Adjusted dose (mg) = Actual Dose (mg) × Target AUC (µM•min)/Actual AUC (µM•min)
For example, if a patient received a dose of 11 mg busulfan and if the corresponding AUC measured was 800 µM•min, for a target AUC of 1125 µM•min, the target mg dose would be:
Mg dose = 11 mg × 1125 µM•min / 800 µM•min = 15.5 mg
Busulfex dose adjustment may be made using this formula and instructions below.

Blood Sample Collection for AUC Determination:
Calculate the AUC (µM•min) based on blood samples collected at the following time points:
For dose 1: 2 hr (end of infusion), 4 hr and 6 hr (immediately prior to the next scheduled BUSULFEX administration). Actual sampling times should be recorded.
For doses other than dose 1: Pre-infusion (baseline), 2 hr (end of infusion), 4 hr and 6 hr (immediately prior to the next scheduled BUSULFEX administration).
AUC calculations based on fewer than the three specified samples may result in inaccurate AUC determinations.
For each scheduled blood sample, collect one to three mL of blood into heparinized (Na or Li heparin) Vacutainer® tubes. The blood samples should be placed on wet ice immediately after collection and should be centrifuged (at 4°C) within one hour. The plasma, harvested into appropriate cryovial storage tubes, is to be frozen immediately at -20°C. All plasma samples are to be sent in a frozen state (i.e., on dry ice) to the assay laboratory for the determination of plasma busulfan concentrations.
Calculation of AUC:
BUSULFEX AUC calculations may be made using the following instructions and appropriate standard pharmacokinetic formula:
Dose 1 $AUC_{infinity}$ Calculation: $AUC_{infinity} = AUC_{0-6hr} + AUC_{extrapolated}$, where AUC_{0-6hr} is to be estimated using the linear trapezoidal rule and AUC extrapolated can be computed by taking the ratio of the busulfan concentration at Hour 6 and the terminal elimination rate constant, λ_z. The λ_z must be calculated from the terminal elimination phase of the busulfan concentration vs. time curve. A "0" pre-dose busulfan concentration should be assumed, and used in the calculation of AUC.
If the AUC is assessed subsequent to Dose 1, steady-state AUC_{ss} (AUC_{0-6hr}) is to be estimated from the trough, 2 hr, 4 hr and 6 hr concentrations using the linear trapezoidal rule.
Instructions for Drug Administration and Blood Sample Collection for Therapeutic Drug Monitoring:
An administration set with minimal residual hold up (priming) volume (1-3 mL) should be used for drug infusion to ensure accurate delivery of the entire prescribed dose and to ensure accurate collection of blood samples for therapeutic drug monitoring and dose adjustment.
Prime the administration set tubing with drug solution to allow accurate documentation of the start time of BUSULFEX infusion. Collect the blood sample from a peripheral IV line to avoid contamination with infusing drug. If the blood sample is taken directly from the existing central venous catheter (CVC), **DO NOT COLLECT THE BLOOD SAMPLE WHILE THE DRUG IS INFUSING** to ensure that the end of infusion sample is not contaminated with any residual drug. At the end of infusion (2 hr), disconnect the administration tubing and flush the CVC line with 5 cc of normal saline prior to the collection of the end of infusion sample from the CVC port. Collect the blood samples from a different port than that used for the BUSULFEX infusion. When recording the BUSULFEX infusion stop time, do not include the time required to flush the indwelling catheter line. Discard the administration tubing at the end of the two-hour infusion.
See Preparation for Intravenous Administration section for detailed instructions on drug preparation.
Geriatric: Five of sixty-one patients treated in the BUSULFEX clinical trial were over the age of 55 (range 57-64). All achieved myeloablation and engraftment.
Gender, Race: Adjusting BUSULFEX dosage based on gender or race has not been adequately studied.
Renal Insufficiency: BUSULFEX has not been studied in patients with renal impairment.

Hepatic Insufficiency: BUSULFEX has not been administered to patients with hepatic insufficiency.
Other: Busulfan may cause cellular dysplasia in many organs. Cytologic abnormalities characterized by giant, hyperchromatic nuclei have been reported in lymph nodes, pancreas, thyroid, adrenal glands, liver, lungs and bone marrow. This cytologic dysplasia may be severe enough to cause difficulty in the interpretation of exfoliative cytologic examinations of the lungs, bladder, breast and the uterine cervix.

ADVERSE REACTIONS

Dimethylacetamide (DMA), the solvent used in the BUSULFEX formulation, was studied in 1962 as a potential cancer chemotherapy drug. In a Phase 1 trial, the maximum tolerated dose (MTD) was 14.8 $g/m^2/d$ for four days. The daily recommended dose of BUSULFEX contains DMA equivalent to 42% of the MTD on a mg/m^2 basis. The dose-limiting toxicities in the Phase 1 study were hepatotoxicity as evidenced by increased liver transaminase (SGOT) levels and neurological symptoms as evidenced by hallucinations. The hallucinations had a pattern of onset at one day post completion of DMA administration and were associated with EEG changes. The lowest dose at which hallucinations were recognized was equivalent to 1.9 times that delivered in a conditioning regimen utilizing BUSULFEX 0.8 mg/kg every 6 hours × 16 doses. Other neurological toxicities included somnolence, lethargy, and confusion. The relative contribution of DMA and/or other concomitant medications to neurologic and hepatic toxicities observed with BUSULFEX is difficult to ascertain.
Treatment with BUSULFEX at the recommended dose and schedule will result in profound myelosuppression in 100% of patients, including granulocytopenia, thrombocytopenia, anemia, or a combined loss of formed elements of the blood. Adverse reaction information is primarily derived from the clinical study (N=61) of BUSULFEX and the data obtained for high-dose oral busulfan conditioning in the setting of randomized, controlled trials identified through a literature review.
BUSULFEX Clinical Trials: In the BUSULFEX (busulfan) Injection allogeneic stem cell transplantation clinical trial, all patients were treated with BUSULFEX 0.8 mg/kg as a two-hour infusion every six hours for 16 doses over four days, combined with cyclophosphamide 60 mg/kg × 2 days. Ninety-three percent (93%) of evaluable patients receiving this dose of BUSULFEX maintained an AUC less than 1,500 µM•min for dose 9, which has generally been considered the level that minimizes the risk of HVOD.

Table 3
Summary of the Incidence (≥20%) of Non-Hematologic Adverse Events through BMT Day +28 in Patients who Received BUSULFEX Prior to Allogeneic Hematopoietic Progenitor Cell Transplantation

Non-Hematological Adverse Events*	Percent Incidence
BODY AS A WHOLE	
Fever	80
Headache	69
Asthenia	51
Chills	46
Pain	44
Edema General	28
Allergic Reaction	26
Chest Pain	26
Inflammation at Injection Site	25
Pain Back	23
CARDIOVASCULAR SYSTEM	
Tachycardia	44
Hypertension	36
Thrombosis	33
Vasodilation	25
DIGESTIVE SYSTEM	
Nausea	98
Stomatitis (Mucositis)	97
Vomiting	95
Anorexia	85
Diarrhea	84
Abdominal Pain	72
Dyspepsia	44
Constipation	38
Dry Mouth	26
Rectal Disorder	25
Abdominal Enlargement	23
METABOLIC AND NUTRITIONAL SYSTEM	
Hypomagnesemia	77
Hyperglycemia	66
Hypokalemia	64
Hypocalcemia	49
Hyperbilirubinemia	49
Edema	36
SGPT Elevation	31
Creatinine Increased	21
NERVOUS SYSTEM	
Insomnia	84
Anxiety	72
Dizziness	30
Depression	23
RESPIRATORY SYSTEM	
Rhinitis	44
Lung Disorder	34
Cough	28
Epistaxis	25
Dyspnea	25
SKIN AND APPENDAGES	
Rash	57
Pruritus	28

*Includes all reported adverse events regardless of severity (toxicity grades 1-4)

The following sections describe clinically significant events occurring in the BUSULFEX clinical trials, regardless of drug attribution. For pediatric information, see Special Populations — Pediatric section.
Hematologic: At the indicated dose and schedule, BUSULFEX produced profound myelosuppression in 100% of patients. Following hematopoietic progenitor cell infusion, recovery of neutrophil counts to ≥500 cells/mm^3 occurred at median day 13 when prophylactic G-CSF was administered to the majority of participants on the study. The median number of platelet transfusions per patient on study was 6, and the median number of red blood cell transfusions on study was 4. Prolonged prothrombin time was reported in one patient (2%).
Gastrointestinal: Gastrointestinal toxicities were frequent and generally considered to be related to the drug. Few were categorized as serious. Mild or moderate nausea occurred in 92% of patients in the allogeneic clinical trial, and mild or moderate vomiting occurred in 95% through BMT Day +28; nausea was severe in 7%. The incidence of vomiting during BUSULFEX administration (BMT Day −7 to −4) was 43% in the allogeneic clinical trial. Grade 3-4 stomatitis developed in 26% of the participants, and Grade 3 esophagitis developed in 2%. Grade 3-4 diarrhea was reported in 5% of the allogeneic study participants, while mild or moderate diarrhea occurred in 75%. Mild or moderate constipation occurred in 38% of patients; ileus developed in 8% and was severe in 2%. Forty-four percent (44%) of patients reported mild or moderate dyspepsia. Two percent (2%) of patients experienced mild hematemesis. Pancreatitis developed in 2% of patients. Mild or moderate rectal discomfort occurred in 24% of patients. Severe anorexia occurred in 21% of patients and was mild/moderate in 64%.
Hepatic: Hyperbilirubinemia occurred in 49% of patients in the allogeneic BMT trial. Grade 3/4 hyperbilirubinemia occurred in 30% of patients within 28 days of transplantation and was considered life-threatening in 5% of these patients. Hyperbilirubinemia was associated with graft-versus-host disease in six patients and with hepatic veno-occlusive disease in 5 patients. Grade 3/4 SGPT elevations occurred in 7% of patients. Alkaline phosphatase increases were mild or moderate in 15% of patients. Mild or moderate jaundice developed in 12% of patients, and mild or moderate hepatomegaly developed in 6%.
Hepatic veno-occlusive disease: Hepatic veno-occlusive disease (HVOD) is a recognized potential complication of conditioning therapy prior to transplant. Based on clinical examination and laboratory findings, hepatic veno-occlusive disease was diagnosed in 8% (5/61) of patients treated with BUSULFEX in the setting of allogeneic transplantation, was fatal in 2/5 cases (40%), and yielded an overall mortality from HVOD in the entire study population of 2/61 (3%). Three of the five patients diagnosed with HVOD were retrospectively found to meet the Jones' criteria.
Graft-versus-host disease: Graft-versus-host disease developed in 18% of patients (11/61) receiving allogeneic transplants; it was severe in 3%, and mild or moderate in 15%. There were 3 deaths (5%) attributed to GVHD.
Edema: Patients receiving allogeneic transplant exhibited some form of edema (79%), hypervolemia, or documented weight increase (8%); all events were reported as mild or moderate.
Infection/Fever: Fifty-one percent (51%) of patients experienced one or more episodes of infection. Pneumonia was fatal in one patient (2%) and life-threatening in 3% of patients. Fever was reported in 80% of patients; it was mild or moderate in 78% and severe in 3%. Forty-six percent (46%) of patients experienced chills.
Cardiovascular: Mild or moderate tachycardia was reported in 44% of patients. In 7 patients (11%) it was first reported during BUSULFEX administration. Other rhythm abnormalities, which were all mild or moderate, included arrhythmia (5%), atrial fibrillation (2%), ventricular extrasystoles (2%), and third degree heart block (2%). Mild or moderate thrombosis occurred in 33% of patients, and all episodes were associated with the central venous catheter. Hypertension was reported in 36% of patients and was Grade 3/4 in 7%. Hypotension occurred in 11% of patients and was Grade 3/4 in 3%. Mild vasodilation (flushing and hot flashes) was reported in 25% of patients. Other cardiovascular events included cardiomegaly (5%), mild ECG abnormality (2%), Grade 3/4 left-sided heart failure in one patient (2%), and moderate pericardial effusion (2%). These events were reported primarily in the post-cyclophosphamide phase.
Pulmonary: Mild or moderate dyspnea occurred in 25% of patients and was severe in 2%. One patient (2%) experi-

Continued on next page

Busulfex—Cont.

enced severe hyperventilation; and in 2 (3%) additional patients it was mild or moderate. Mild rhinitis and mild or moderate cough were reported in 44% and 28% of patients, respectively. Mild epistaxis events were reported in 25%. Three patients (5%) on the allogeneic study developed documented alveolar hemorrhage. All required mechanical ventilatory support and all died. Non-specific interstitial fibrosis was found on wedge biopsies performed with video assisted thoracoscopy in one patient on the allogeneic study who subsequently died from respiratory failure on BMT Day +98. Other pulmonary events, reported as mild or moderate, included pharyngitis (18%), hiccup (18%), asthma (8%), atelectasis (2%), pleural effusion (3%), hypoxia (2%), hemoptysis (3%), and sinusitis (3%).

Neurologic: The most commonly reported adverse events of the central nervous system were insomnia (84%), anxiety (75%), dizziness (30%), and depression (23%). Severity was mild or moderate except for one patient (1%) who experienced severe insomnia. One patient (1%) developed a life-threatening cerebral hemorrhage and a coma as a terminal event following multi-organ failure after HVOD. Other events considered severe included delirium (2%), agitation (2%), and encephalopathy (2%). The overall incidence of confusion was 11%, and 5% of patients were reported to have experienced hallucinations. The patient who developed delirium and hallucination on the allogeneic study had onset of confusion at the completion of BUSULFEX (busulfan) Injection. The overall incidence of lethargy in the allogeneic BUSULFEX clinical trial was 7%, and somnolence was reported in 2%. One patient (2%) treated in an autologous transplantation study experienced a seizure while receiving cyclophosphamide, despite prophylactic treatment with phenytoin.

Renal: Creatinine was mildly or moderately elevated in 21% of patients. BUN was increased in 3% of patients and to a Grade 3/4 level in 2%. Seven percent of patients experienced dysuria, 15% oliguria, and 8% hematuria. There were 4 (7%) Grade 3/4 cases of hemorrhagic cystitis in the allogeneic clinical trial.

Skin: Rash (57%) and pruritus (28%) were reported; both conditions were predominantly mild. Alopecia was mild in 15% of patients and moderate in 2%. Mild vesicular rash was reported in 10% of patients and mild or moderate maculopapular rash in 8%. Vesiculo-bullous rash was reported in 10%, and exfoliative dermatitis in 5%. Erythema nodosum was reported in 2%, acne in 7%, and skin discoloration in 8%.

Metabolic: Hyperglycemia was observed in 67% of patients and Grade 3/4 hyperglycemia was reported in 15%. Hypomagnesemia was mild or moderate in 77% of patients; hypokalemia was mild or moderate in 62% and severe in 2%; hypocalcemia was mild or moderate in 46% and severe in 3%; hypophosphatemia was mild or moderate in 17%; and hyponatremia was reported in 2%.

Other: Other reported events included headache (mild or moderate 64%, severe 5%), abdominal pain (mild or moderate 69%, severe 3%), asthenia (mild or moderate 49%, severe 2%), unspecified pain (mild or moderate 43%, severe 2%), allergic reaction (mild or moderate 24%, severe 2%), injection site inflammation (mild or moderate 25%), injection site pain (mild or moderate 15%), chest pain (mild or moderate 26%), back pain (mild or moderate 23%), myalgia (mild or moderate 16%), arthralgia (mild or moderate 13%), and ear disorder in 3%.

Deaths: There were two deaths through BMT Day +28 in the allogeneic transplant setting. There were an additional six deaths BMT Day +29 through BMT Day +100 in the allogeneic transplant setting.

Oral Busulfan Literature Review. A literature review identified four randomized, controlled trials that evaluated a high-dose oral busulfan-containing conditioning regimen for allogeneic bone marrow transplantation in the setting of CML (see CLINICAL STUDIES). The safety outcomes reported in those trials are summarized in Table 4 below for a mixed population of hematological malignancies (AML, CML, and ALL).

[See table 4 below]

OVERDOSAGE

There is no known antidote to BUSULFEX other than hematopoietic progenitor cell transplantation. In the absence of hematopoietic progenitor cell transplantation, the recommended dosage for BUSULFEX would constitute an overdose of busulfan. The principal toxic effect is profound bone marrow hypoplasia/aplasia and pancytopenia, but the central nervous system, liver, lungs, and gastrointestinal tract may be affected. The hematologic status should be closely monitored and vigorous supportive measures instituted as medically indicated. Survival after a single 140 mg dose of Myleran® Tablets in an 18 kg, 4-year old child has been reported. Inadvertent administration of a greater than normal dose of oral busulfan (2.1 mg/kg; total dose of 23.3 mg/kg) occurred in a 2-year old child prior to a scheduled bone marrow transplant without sequelae. An acute dose of 2.4 g was fatal in a 10-year old boy. There is one report that busulfan is dialyzable, thus dialysis should be considered in the case of overdose. Busulfan is metabolized by conjugation with glutathione, thus administration of glutathione may be considered.

DOSAGE AND ADMINISTRATION

When BUSULFEX (busulfan) Injection is administered as a component of the BuCy conditioning regimen prior to bone marrow or peripheral blood progenitor cell replacement, the recommended doses are as follows:

Adults (BuCy2): The usual adult dose is 0.8 mg/kg of ideal body weight or actual body weight, whichever is lower, administered every six hours for four days (a total of 16 doses). For obese, or severely obese patients, BUSULFEX should be administered based on adjusted ideal body weight. Ideal body weight (IBW) should be calculated as follows (height in cm, and weight in kg): IBW (kg; men) = 50 + 0.91 × (height in cm -152); IBW (kg; women) = 45 + 0.91 × (height in cm - 152). Adjusted ideal body weight (AIBW) should be calculated as follows: AIBW = IBW + 0.25 × (actual weight -IBW). Cyclophosphamide is given on each of two days as a one-hour infusion at a dose of 60 mg/kg beginning on BMT day −3, no sooner than six hours following the 16th dose of BUSULFEX.

BUSULFEX clearance is best predicted when the BUSULFEX dose is administered based on adjusted ideal body weight. Dosing BUSULFEX based on actual body weight, ideal body weight or other factors can produce significant differences in BUSULFEX (busulfan) Injection clearance among lean, normal and obese patients.

BUSULFEX should be administered intravenously via a central venous catheter as a two-hour infusion every six hours for four consecutive days for a total of 16 doses. All patients should be premedicated with phenytoin as busulfan is known to cross the blood brain barrier and induce seizures. Phenytoin reduces busulfan plasma AUC by 15%. Use of other anticonvulsants may result in higher busulfan plasma AUCs, and an increased risk of VOD or seizures. In cases where other anticonvulsants must be used, plasma busulfan exposure should be monitored (See DRUG INTERACTIONS). Antiemetics should be administered prior to the first dose of BUSULFEX and continued on a fixed schedule through administration of BUSULFEX. Where available, pharmacokinetic monitoring may be considered to further optimize therapeutic targeting.

Pediatrics: The effectiveness of BUSULFEX in the treatment of CML has not been specifically studied in pediatric patients. For additional information see Special Populations -Pediatric section.

Preparation and Administration Precautions:
An administration set with minimal residual hold-up volume (2-5 cc) should be used for product administration.

As with other cytotoxic compounds, caution should be exercised in handling and preparing the solution of BUSULFEX. Skin reactions may occur with accidental exposure. The use of gloves is recommended. If BUSULFEX or diluted BUSULFEX solution contacts the skin or mucosa, wash the skin or mucosa thoroughly with water.

BUSULFEX is a clear, colorless solution. Parenteral drug products should be visually inspected for particulate matter and discoloration prior to administration whenever the solution and container permit. If particulate matter is seen in the BUSULFEX vial the drug should not be used.

Preparation for Intravenous Administration:
BUSULFEX must be diluted prior to use with either 0.9% Sodium Chloride Injection, USP (normal saline) or 5% Dextrose Injection, USP (D5W). The diluent quantity should be 10 times the volume of BUSULFEX, so that the final concentration of busulfan is approximately 0.5 mg/mL. Calculation of the dose for a 70 kg patient, would be performed as follows:

(70 kg patient) × (0.8 mg/kg) ÷ (6 mg/mL) = 9.3 mL BUSULFEX (56 mg total dose).

To prepare the final solution for infusion, add 9.3 mL of BUSULFEX to 93 mL of diluent (normal saline or D5W) as calculated below:

(9.3 mL BUSULFEX) × (10)=93 mL of either diluent plus the 9.3 mL of BUSULFEX to yield a final concentration of busulfan of 0.54 mg/mL (9.3 mL × 6 mg/mL ÷ 102.3 mL= 0.54 mg/mL).

All transfer procedures require strict adherence to aseptic techniques, preferably employing a vertical laminar flow safety hood while wearing gloves and protective clothing. DO NOT put the BUSULFEX into an intravenous bag or large-volume syringe that does not contain normal saline or D5W. Always add the BUSULFEX to the diluent, not the diluent to the BUSULFEX. Mix thoroughly by inverting several times. DO NOT USE POLYCARBONATE SYRINGES OR POLYCARBONATE FILTER NEEDLES WITH BUSULFEX.

Infusion pumps should be used to administer the diluted BUSULFEX solution. Set the flow rate of the pump to deliver the entire prescribed BUSULFEX dose over two hours. Prior to and following each infusion, flush the indwelling catheter line with approximately 5mL of 0.9% Sodium Chloride Injection, USP or 5% Dextrose Injection, USP. DO NOT infuse concomitantly with another intravenous solution of unknown compatibility. WARNING: RAPID INFUSION OF BUSULFEX HAS NOT BEEN TESTED AND IS NOT RECOMMENDED.

STABILITY
Unopened vials of BUSULFEX are stable until the date indicated on the package when stored under refrigeration at 2°-8°C (36°-46°F).

Table 4
Summary of safety analyses from the randomized, controlled trials utilizing a high dose oral busulfan-containing conditioning regimen that were identified in a literature review

Clift
CML Chronic Phase

TRM*	VOD**	GVHD***	Pulmonary	Hemorrhagic Cystitis	Seizure
Death ≤100d =4.1% (3/73)	No Report	Acute ≥Grade 2 =35% Chronic =41% (30/73)	1 death from Idiopathic Interstitial Pneumonitis And 1 death from Pulmonary Fibrosis	No Report	No Report

Devergie
CML Chronic Phase

TRM	VOD	GVHD	Pulmonary	Hemorrhagic Cystitis	Seizure
38%	7.7% (5/65) Deaths=4.6% (3/65)	Acute ≥Grade 2 =41% (24/59 at risk)	Interstitial Pneumonitis= 16.9% (11/65)	10.8% (7/65)	No report

Ringden
CML, AML, ALL

TRM	VOD	GVHD	Pulmonary	Hemorrhagic Cystitis	Seizure
28%	12%	Acute ≥Grade 2 GVHD=26% Chronic GVHD =45%	Interstitial Pneumonitis =14%	24%	6%

Blume
CML, AML, ALL

TRM	VOD	GVHD	Pulmonary	Hemorrhagic Cystitis	Seizure
No Report	Deaths =4.9%	Acute ≥Grade 2 GVHD=22% (13/58 at risk) Chronic GVHD =31% (14/45 at risk)	No Report	No Report	No Report

*TRM = Transplantation Related Mortality
**VOD = Veno-Occlusive Disease of the liver
***GVHD = Graft versus Host Disease

BUSULFEX diluted in 0.9% Sodium Chloride Injection, USP or 5% Dextrose Injection, USP is stable at room temperature (25°C) for up to 8 hours but the infusion must be completed within that time. BUSULFEX diluted in 0.9% Sodium Chloride Injection, USP is stable at refrigerated conditions (2°-8°C) for up to 12 hours but the infusion must be completed within that time.

HOW SUPPLIED

BUSULFEX is supplied as a sterile solution in 10 mL single-use clear glass vials each containing 60 mg of busulfan at a concentration of 6 mg/mL for intravenous use.

NDC 59148-070-90   10 mL (6mg/mL) in packages of eight vials

Unopened vials of BUSULFEX must be stored under refrigerated conditions between 2°-8°C (36°-46°F).

HANDLING AND DISPOSAL

Procedures for proper handling and disposal of anticancer drugs should be considered. Several guidelines on this subject have been published.[1,2,3,4,5,6] There is no general agreement that all of the procedures recommended in the guidelines are necessary or appropriate.

REFERENCES

1. Recommendations for the safe handling of parenteral antineoplastic drugs. Washington, DC: Division of Safety, National Institutes of Health; 1983. US Department of Health and Human Services, Public Health Service publication NIH 83-2621.
2. AMA Council on Scientific Affairs. Guidelines for handling parenteral antineoplastics. *JAMA* 1985; 253:1590-1591.
3. National Study Commission on Cytotoxic Exposure. Recommendations for handling cytotoxic agents. 1987. Available from Louis P. Jeffrey, Chairman, National Study Commission on Cytotoxic Exposure. Massachusetts College of Pharmacy and Allied Health Sciences, 179 Longwood Avenue, Boston, MA 02115.
4. Clinical Oncology Society of Australia. Guidelines and recommendations for safe handling of antineoplastic agents. *Med J Australia* 1983; 1:426-428.
5. Jones RB, Frank R, Mass T. Safe handling of chemotherapeutic agents: a report from the Mount Sinai Medical Center. *CA-A Cancer J for Clin* 1983; 33:258-263.
6. American Society of Hospital Pharmacists. ASHP technical assistance bulletin on handling cytotoxic and hazardous drugs. *Am J Hosp Pharm* 1990; 47:1033-1049.

Distributed and Marketed by:
Otsuka America Pharmaceutical, Inc.
Rockville, MD 20850
Manufactured by:
Ben Venue Labs, Inc.
Bedford, OH 44146
U.S. Patent Nos.: 5,430,057 and 5,559,148.
Canadian Patent No.: CA2171738.
European Union Patent No.: EP 0 725 637 B1.
Otsuka America Pharmaceutical, Inc.
Part No. 0608L-0001   Revised February 2008
© 2008, Otsuka Pharmaceutical Co., Ltd., Tokyo, 100-8535 Japan

---

Sepracor Inc.

84 WATERFORD DRIVE
MARLBOROUGH, MA 01752

For Medical Information
for Healthcare Professionals Contact:
1-800-739-0565
For Direct Inquiries to the
Customer Assistance Center (CAC) Contact:
1-888-394-7377
E-mail CAC@sepracor.com
or write to Sepracor CAC at the address above.
To report an Adverse Event contact
Sepracor's Drug Safety Department at:
1-877-737-7226

OMNARIS™   ℞

[ŏm-nĕ-rĭs]
(ciclesonide)
Nasal Spray, 50 mcg
For intranasal use only

DESCRIPTION

The active component of OMNARIS Nasal Spray is ciclesonide, a non-halogenated glucocorticoid having the chemical name pregna -1,4-diene-3,20-dione, 16,17-[[R-cyclohexylmethylene]bis(oxy)]-11-hydroxy-21-(2-methyl-1-oxopropoxy)-,(11b,16a)-. Ciclesonide is delivered as the R-epimer. The empirical formula is C32H44O7 and its molecular weight is 540.7. Its structural formula is as follows:
[See chemical structure at top of next column]

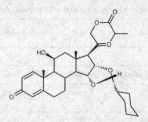

Ciclesonide is a white to yellow-white powder, practically insoluble in water and freely soluble in ethanol and acetone. OMNARIS Nasal Spray is a metered-dose, manual-pump spray formulation containing a hypotonic aqueous suspension of ciclesonide. OMNARIS Nasal Spray also contains microcrystalline cellulose, carboxymethylcellulose sodium, hypromellose, potassium sorbate and edetate sodium; and hydrochloric acid to adjust the pH to 4.5. The contents of one 12.5 gram bottle provide 120 actuations, after initial priming. Prior to initial use, OMNARIS Nasal Spray must be gently shaken and then the pump must be primed by actuating eight times. Once primed, each actuation of the pump delivers 50 mcg ciclesonide in a volume of 70 microliters from the nasal actuator. If the product is not used for four consecutive days, it should be gently shaken and re-primed with one spray or until a fine mist appears.

CLINICAL PHARMACOLOGY
Mechanism of Action

Ciclesonide is a pro-drug that is enzymatically hydrolyzed to a pharmacologically active metabolite, C21-desisobutyryl-ciclesonide (des-ciclesonide or RM1) following intranasal application. Des-ciclesonide has anti-inflammatory activity with affinity for the glucocorticoid receptor that is 120 times higher than the parent compound. The precise mechanism through which ciclesonide affects allergic rhinitis symptoms is not known. Corticosteroids have been shown to have a wide range of effects on multiple cell types (e.g., mast cells, eosinophils, neutrophils, macrophages, and lymphocytes) and mediators (e.g., histamine, eicosanoids, leukotrienes, and cytokines) involved in allergic inflammation.

Pharmacokinetics
Absorption

Ciclesonide and des-ciclesonide have negligible oral bioavailability (both less than 1%) due to low gastrointestinal absorption and high first-pass metabolism. The intranasal administration of ciclesonide at recommended doses results in negligible serum concentrations of ciclesonide. However, the known active metabolite (des-ciclesonide) is detected in the serum of some patients after nasal inhalation of ciclesonide. The bioanalytical assay used has a lower limit of quantification of 25 pg/mL and 10 pg/mL, for ciclesonide and des-ciclesonide, respectively.

In healthy adults treated for two weeks with 50 to 800 mcg of ciclesonide nasal spray daily (n=6 in each treatment group), the peak serum concentrations of des-ciclesonide in all subjects were found to be below 30 pg/mL. Of those treated with 800 mcg and 400 mcg daily, 100% and 67% had detectable levels of des-ciclesonide, respectively. With daily doses of 200 mcg or less, detectable serum levels of des-ciclesonide were not observed.

In pediatric subjects treated with 25 to 200 mcg of ciclesonide nasal spray daily, serum concentrations of des-ciclesonide were below 45 pg/mL, with the exception of one value of 64.5 pg/mL. In a 12-week study in children 6 to 11 years of age with perennial allergic rhinitis, des-ciclesonide was detected in 50% of the subjects treated with 200 mcg and in 5% of those treated with 100 mcg ciclesonide nasal spray daily. In a 6-week study in children 2 to 5 years of age with perennial allergic rhinitis, des-ciclesonide was detected in 41%, 22%, and 13% of the subjects treated with 200 mcg, 100 mcg, and 25 mcg ciclesonide nasal spray daily, respectively.

Distribution

Following intravenous administration of 800 mcg of ciclesonide, the volumes of distribution of ciclesonide and des-ciclesonide were approximately 2.9 L/kg and 12.1 L/kg, respectively. The percentage of ciclesonide and des-ciclesonide bound to human plasma proteins averaged ≥ 99% each, with ≤ 1% of unbound drug detected in the systemic circulation. Des-ciclesonide is not significantly bound to human transcortin.

Metabolism

Intranasal ciclesonide is hydrolyzed to a biologically active metabolite, des-ciclesonide, by esterases in the nasal mucosa. Des-ciclesonide undergoes further metabolism in the liver to additional metabolites mainly by the cytochrome P450 (CYP) 3A4 isozyme and to a lesser extent by CYP 2D6. The full range of potentially active metabolites of ciclesonide has not been characterized. After intravenous administration of 14C-ciclesonide, 19.3% of the resulting radioactivity in the plasma is accounted for by ciclesonide or des-ciclesonide; the remainder may be a result of other, as yet, unidentified multiple metabolites.

Elimination

Following intravenous administration of 800 mcg of ciclesonide, the clearance values of ciclesonide and des-ciclesonide were high (approximately 152 L/h and 228 L/h, respectively). 14C-labeled ciclesonide was predominantly excreted via the feces after intravenous administration (66%) indicating that excretion through bile is the major route of elimination. Approximately 20% or less of drug related radioactivity was excreted in the urine.

Special Populations

The pharmacokinetics of intranasally administered ciclesonide have not been assessed in patient subpopulations because the resulting blood levels of ciclesonide and des-ciclesonide are insufficient for pharmacokinetic calculations. However, population pharmacokinetic analysis showed that characteristics of des-ciclesonide after oral inhalation of ciclesonide were not appreciably influenced by a variety of subject characteristics such as body weight, age, race, and gender. Compared to healthy subjects, the systemic exposure (Cmax and AUC) in patients with liver impairment increased in the range of 1.4 to 2.7 fold after 1280 mcg ex-actuator ciclesonide by oral inhalation and dose adjustment in liver impairment is not necessary. Studies in renal impaired patients were not conducted.

Pharmacodynamics

In a 12-week study in children 6-11 years of age with perennial allergic rhinitis, daily doses of 200 mcg, 100 mcg, and 25 mcg of OMNARIS Nasal Spray were compared to placebo nasal spray. Adrenal function was assessed by measurement of 24-hour urinary free cortisol (in 32 to 44 patients per group) and morning plasma cortisol levels (in 45 to 61 patients per group) before and after 12 consecutive weeks of treatment. The ciclesonide-treated groups had a numerically greater decline in 24-hour urinary free cortisol compared to the placebo treated group. The differences (and 95% confidence intervals) from placebo in the mean change from baseline to 12 weeks were -0.81 (-4.0, 2.4), -0.08 (-3.1, 2.9), and -2.11 (-5.3, 1.1) mcg/day for 200 mcg, 100 mcg, and 25 mcg dose groups, respectively. The mean AM plasma cortisol value did not show any consistent treatment effect with differences (and 95% confidence intervals) from placebo in the mean change from baseline to 12 weeks of 0.35 (-1.4, 2.1), 0.12 (-1.5, 1.7), and -0.38 (-2.1, 1.3) mcg/dL for 200 mcg, 100 mcg, and 25 mcg dose groups respectively. In this study, serum was assayed for ciclesonide and des-ciclesonide (see CLINICAL PHARMACOLOGY: Pharmacokinetics: Absorption).

In a 6-week study in children 2 to 5 years of age with perennial allergic rhinitis, daily doses of 200 mcg, 100 mcg, and 25 mcg of OMNARIS Nasal Spray were compared to placebo nasal spray. Adrenal function was assessed by measurement of 24-hour urinary free cortisol (in 15 to 22 patients per group) and morning plasma cortisol levels (in 28 to 30 patients per group) before and after 6 consecutive weeks of treatment. The ciclesonide-treated groups had a numerically greater decline in 24-hour urinary free cortisol compared to the placebo treated group. The differences (and 95% confidence intervals) from placebo in the mean change from baseline to 6 weeks were -2.04 (-4.4, 0.3), -1.96 (-4.5, 0.6), and -1.76 (-4.3, 0.8) mcg/day for the 200 mcg, 100 mcg, and 25 mcg dose groups, respectively. The plasma cortisol also decreased numerically after treatment with ciclesonide. The differences (and 95% confidence intervals) from placebo in the mean change in plasma cortisol from baseline to 6 weeks were -1.04 (-2.7, 0.7), -0.36 (-2.1, 1.4), and -0.12 (-1.8, 1.6) mcg/dL for the 200 mcg, 100 mcg, and 25 mcg dose groups, respectively. In this study, serum was assayed for ciclesonide and des-ciclesonide (see CLINICAL PHARMACOLOGY: Pharmacokinetics: Absorption).

There are no adequately conducted studies in adults and adolescents that assess the effect of OMNARIS Nasal Spray on adrenal function.

CLINICAL TRIALS
Seasonal and Perennial Allergic Rhinitis
Adult and Adolescent Patients Aged 12 Years and Older:

The efficacy and safety of OMNARIS Nasal Spray were evaluated in 4 randomized, double-blind, parallel-group, multicenter, placebo-controlled clinical trials of 2 weeks to 1 year in duration conducted in the United States and Canada in adolescents and adults with allergic rhinitis. Three of these trials were 2 to 6 weeks in duration and primarily designed to assess efficacy. One of these trials was 1 year in duration and primarily designed to assess safety. The three trials of 2 to 6 weeks duration included a total of 1524 patients (495 males and 1029 females) of whom 79 were adolescents, ages 12 to 17 years. Of the 1524 patients, 546 patients received OMNARIS Nasal Spray 200 mcg once daily administered as 2 sprays in each nostril. Patients enrolled in the studies were 12 to 86 years of age with a history of seasonal or perennial allergic rhinitis, a positive skin test to at least one relevant allergen, and active symptoms of allergic rhinitis at study entry. Assessment of efficacy in these trials was based on patient recording of four nasal symptoms (runny nose, nasal itching, sneezing, and nasal congestion) on a 0-3 categorical severity scale (0=absent, 1=mild, 2=moderate, and 3=severe) as reflective or instantaneous scores. Reflective scoring required the patients to record symptom severity over the previous 12 hours; the instantaneous scoring required patients to record symptom severity at the time of recording. The results of these trials showed that patients treated with OMNARIS Nasal Spray 200 mcg once daily exhibited statistically significantly greater decreases in total nasal symptom scores than placebo treated patients. Secondary measures of efficacy were also generally supportive.

Of the three trials primarily designed to assess efficacy, one was a 2-week dose-ranging trial that evaluated efficacy of four doses of OMNARIS Nasal Spray in patients with seasonal allergic rhinitis. The primary efficacy endpoint was the difference from placebo in the change from baseline of the sum of morning and evening reflective total nasal symptom score averaged over the 2-week treatment period. Results of the primary efficacy endpoint are shown in Table 1. In this trial OMNARIS Nasal Spray 200 mcg once daily was statistically significantly different from placebo, but the lower doses were not statistically significantly different from placebo.

[See table 1 at top of next page]

Of the other trials primarily designed to assess efficacy, one was a 4-week single dose-level trial conducted in patients with seasonal allergic rhinitis and the other was a 6-week single dose-level trial conducted in patients with perennial allergic rhinitis. The primary efficacy endpoint in the seasonal allergic rhinitis trial was the difference from placebo in the change from baseline of the average of morning and evening reflective total nasal symptom score averaged over the first 2 weeks of treatment. The primary efficacy endpoint in the perennial allergic rhinitis trial was the difference from placebo in the change from baseline of the average of morning and evening reflective total nasal symptom

Continued on next page

Omnaris—Cont.

score averaged over the 6 weeks of treatment. Efficacy results of these two trials are shown in Table 2. In these trials, OMNARIS Nasal Spray 200 mcg once daily was statistically significantly different from placebo. Statistically significant differences in the morning pre-dose instantaneous total nasal symptom score indicate that the effect was maintained over the full 24-hour dosing interval.
[See table 2 above]
Onset of action was evaluated in two environmental exposure unit studies with a single dose of OMNARIS Nasal Spray 200 mcg. Results from these two studies did not demonstrate a replicate onset of action within the assessment period. Onset of action was also evaluated in the 4-week seasonal allergic rhinitis and in the 6-week perennial allergic rhinitis trial by frequent recording of instantaneous symptom score after the first dose. In these trials, onset of effect was seen within 24 to 48 hours with further symptomatic improvement observed over 1 to 2 weeks in seasonal allergic rhinitis and 5 weeks in perennial allergic rhinitis.
Pediatric Patients Aged 6 to 11 Years:
The efficacy of OMNARIS Nasal Spray was evaluated in two randomized, double-blind, parallel-group, multicenter, placebo-controlled clinical trials of 2 and 12 weeks in duration in 1282 patients 6 to 11 years of age with allergic rhinitis. Of the two trials, one was 2 weeks in duration conducted in patients with seasonal allergic rhinitis that evaluated efficacy of 200 mcg and 100 mcg of OMNARIS nasal spray once daily. The other trial was 12 weeks in duration conducted in patients with perennial allergic rhinitis that evaluated efficacy of 200 mcg, 100 mcg, and 25 mcg of OMNARIS nasal spray once daily. Of the total number of patients enrolled in the 2 studies, 380 were treated with 200 mcg of OMNARIS nasal spray once daily. The primary efficacy endpoint was the difference from placebo in the change from baseline of the average of morning and evening reflective total nasal symptom score averaged over 2 weeks of treatment in the seasonal allergic rhinitis trial and over the first 6 weeks of treatment in the perennial allergic rhinitis trial. In the 2-week trial in patients with seasonal allergic rhinitis, the OMNARIS Nasal Spray 200 mcg once daily dose was statistically significantly different from placebo, but the 100 mcg once daily dose was not statistically significantly different from placebo. The efficacy results for the seasonal allergic rhinitis trial are shown in Table 3.
[See table 3 above]
In the 12-week trial in patients with perennial allergic rhinitis, none of the ciclesonide doses were statistically significantly different from placebo. The means and 95% confidence intervals for the differences (OMNARIS Nasal Spray minus placebo) between OMNARIS Nasal Spray 200 mcg, 100 mcg, and 25 mcg treatment groups and placebo were -0.31 (-0.75, 0.13), 0.02 (-0.41, 0.46), and 0.09 (-0.35, 0.53), respectively.
Pediatric Patients Aged 2 to 5 Years:
Efficacy of OMNARIS Nasal Spray in patients 2 to 5 years of age has not been established (See PRECAUTIONS: Pediatric Use).

INDICATIONS AND USAGE
Seasonal Allergic Rhinitis
OMNARIS Nasal Spray is indicated for the treatment of nasal symptoms associated with seasonal allergic rhinitis in adults and children 6 years of age and older.
Perennial Allergic Rhinitis
OMNARIS Nasal Spray is indicated for the treatment of nasal symptoms associated with perennial allergic rhinitis in adults and adolescents 12 years of age and older.

CONTRAINDICATIONS
OMNARIS Nasal Spray is contraindicated in patients with a hypersensitivity to any of its ingredients.

WARNINGS
The replacement of a systemic corticosteroid with a topical corticosteroid can be accompanied by signs of adrenal insufficiency. In addition, some patients may experience symptoms of corticosteroid withdrawal, e.g., joint and/or muscular pain, lassitude, and depression. Patients previously treated for prolonged periods with systemic corticosteroids and transferred to topical corticosteroids should be carefully monitored for acute adrenal insufficiency in response to stress. In those patients who have asthma or other clinical conditions requiring long-term systemic corticosteroid treatment, rapid decreases in systemic corticosteroid dosages may cause a severe exacerbation of their symptoms.
Patients who are using drugs that suppress the immune system are more susceptible to infections than healthy individuals. Chickenpox and measles, for example, can have a more serious or even fatal course in children or adults using corticosteroids. In children or adults who have not had these diseases or been properly immunized, particular care should be taken to avoid exposure. How the dose, route, and duration of corticosteroid administration affect the risk of developing a disseminated infection is not known. The contribution of the underlying disease and/or prior corticosteroid treatment to the risk is also not known. If exposed to chickenpox, prophylaxis with varicella zoster immune globulin (VZIG) may be indicated. If exposed to measles, prophylaxis with pooled intramuscular immunoglobulin (IG) may be indicated. (See the respective package inserts for complete VZIG and IG prescribing information). If chickenpox develops, treatment with antiviral agents may be considered.

PRECAUTIONS
General
Intranasal corticosteroids may cause a reduction in growth velocity when administered to pediatric patients (see PRECAUTIONS: Pediatric Use). Rarely, immediate hypersensitivity reactions or contact dermatitis may occur after the administration of intranasal corticosteroids. Patients with a

known hypersensitivity reaction to other corticosteroid preparations should use caution when using ciclesonide nasal spray since cross reactivity to other corticosteroids including ciclesonide may also occur.
Because of the inhibitory effect of corticosteroids on wound healing, patients who have experienced recent nasal septal ulcers, nasal surgery, or nasal trauma should not use a nasal corticosteroid until healing has occurred. In clinical studies with OMNARIS Nasal Spray, the development of localized infections of the nose and pharynx with Candida albicans has rarely occurred. When such an infection develops, it may require treatment with appropriate local therapy and discontinuation of OMNARIS Nasal Spray. Therefore, patients using OMNARIS Nasal Spray over several months or longer should be examined periodically for evidence of Candida infection or other signs of adverse effects on the nasal mucosa. Intranasal corticosteroids should be used with caution, if at all, in patients with active or quiescent tuberculosis infections of the respiratory tract; or in patients with untreated local or systemic fungal or bacterial infections; systemic viral or parasitic infections; or ocular herpes simplex.

If recommended doses of intranasal corticosteroids are exceeded or if individuals are particularly sensitive or predisposed by virtue of recent systemic steroid therapy, symptoms of hypercorticism may occur, including very rare cases of menstrual irregularities, acneiform lesions, and cushingoid features. If such changes occur, topical corticosteroids should be discontinued slowly, consistent with accepted procedures for discontinuing oral steroid therapy.
The risk of glaucoma was evaluated by assessments of intraocular pressure in 3 studies including 943 patients. Of these, 390 adolescents or adults were treated for up to 52 weeks and 186 children ages 2 to 11 received treatment with OMNARIS Nasal Spray 200 mcg daily for up to 12 weeks. In these trials, no significant differences in intraocular pressure changes were observed between OMNARIS Nasal Spray 200 mcg and placebo-treated patients. Additionally, no significant differences between OMNARIS Nasal Spray 200 mcg and placebo-treated patients were noted during the 52-week study of adults and adolescent patients in whom thorough ophthalmologic assessments were performed including evaluation of cataract formation using slit lamp examinations. Rare instances of wheezing, nasal septum per-

Table 1 Mean change in reflective total nasal symptom score over 2 weeks in patients with seasonal allergic rhinitis

Treatment	N	Baseline*	Change from Baseline	Difference from Placebo		
				Estimate	95% CI	p-value
Seasonal Allergic Rhinitis Trial – Reflective total nasal symptom score						
Ciclesonide 200 mcg	144	18.8	-5.73	-1.35	(-2.43, -0.28)	0.014
Ciclesonide 100 mcg	145	18.7	-5.26	-0.88	(-1.96, 0.19)	0.11
Ciclesonide 50 mcg	143	18.4	-4.82	-0.44	(-1.52, 0.63)	0.42
Ciclesonide 25 mcg	146	18.7	-4.74	-0.35	(-1.42, 0.71)	0.51
Placebo	148	17.8	-4.38			

*Sum of AM and PM Scores; Maximum score = 24

Table 2 Mean changes in reflective total nasal symptom score and instantaneous total nasal symptom score in allergic rhinitis trials

Treatment	n	Baseline*	Change from Baseline	Difference from Placebo		
				Estimate	95% CI	p-value
Seasonal Allergic Rhinitis Trial – Reflective total nasal symptom score						
Ciclesonide 200 mcg	162	8.96	-2.40	-0.90	(-1.36, -0.45)	<0.001
Placebo	162	8.83	-1.50			
Seasonal Allergic Rhinitis Trial – Instantaneous total nasal symptom score						
Ciclesonide 200 mcg	162	8.45	-1.87	-0.84	(-1.30, -0.39)	<0.001
Placebo	162	8.33	-1.03			
Perennial Allergic Rhinitis Trial – Reflective total nasal symptom score						
Ciclesonide 200 mcg	232	7.59	-2.51	-0.62	(-0.97, -0.28)	<0.001
Placebo	229	7.72	-1.89			
Perennial Allergic Rhinitis Trial – Instantaneous total nasal symptom score						
Ciclesonide 200 mcg	232	7.05	-1.99	-0.53	(-0.90, -0.17)	0.004
Placebo	229	7.05	-1.46			

*Mean of AM and PM score from reflective total nasal symptom score; Mean of AM score for instantaneous total nasal symptom score; Maximum = 12

Table 3 Mean changes in reflective total nasal symptom score in 1 seasonal allergic rhinitis trial in children 6 to 11 years of age

Treatment	n	Baseline*	Change from Baseline	Difference from Placebo		
				Estimate	95% CI	p-value
Reflective total nasal symptom score						
Ciclesonide 200 mcg	215	8.25	-2.46	-0.39	(-0.76, -0.02)	0.040
Ciclesonide						
100 mcg	199	8.41	-2.38	-0.32	(-0.69, 0.06)	0.103
Placebo	204	8.41	-2.07			

*Mean of AM and PM score from reflective total nasal symptom score; Maximum = 12

foration, cataracts, glaucoma, and increased intraocular pressure have been reported following the intranasal application of corticosteroids. Close follow-up is warranted in patients with a change in vision and with a history of glaucoma and/or cataracts.

Information for Patients

Patients being treated with OMNARIS Nasal Spray should receive the following information and instructions. This information is intended to aid them in the safe and effective use of this medication. It is not a disclosure of all possible adverse or intended effects.

Patients who are on immunosuppressive doses of corticosteroids should be warned to avoid exposure to chickenpox or measles, and if exposed, to obtain medical advice. Patients should use OMNARIS Nasal Spray at regular intervals since its effectiveness depends on its regular use (See DOSAGE AND ADMINISTRATION).

In clinical trials, the onset of effect was seen within 24 to 48 hours with further symptomatic improvement observed over 1 to 2 weeks in seasonal allergic rhinitis and 5 weeks in perennial allergic rhinitis. Initial assessment of response should be made during this timeframe and periodically until the patients symptoms are stabilized.

The patient should take the medication as directed and should not exceed the prescribed dosage. The patient should contact the physician if symptoms do not improve by a reasonable time or if the condition worsens. For the proper use of this unit and to attain maximum improvement, the patients should read and follow the accompanying patient instructions carefully. Spraying OMNARIS Nasal Spray directly into the eyes or onto the nasal septum should be avoided. It is important that the bottle is gently shaken prior to use to ensure that a consistent amount is dispensed per actuation. The bottle should be discarded after 120 actuations following initial priming or after 4 months after the bottle is removed from the foil pouch, whichever occurs first.

Drug Interactions

Based on in vitro studies in human liver microsomes, des-ciclesonide appears to have no inhibitory or induction potential on the metabolism of other drugs metabolized by CYP 450 enzymes. The inhibitory potential of ciclesonide on CYP450 isoenzymes has not been studied. In vitro studies demonstrated that the plasma protein binding of des-ciclesonide was not affected by warfarin or salicylic acid, indicating no potential for protein binding-based drug interactions.

In a drug interaction study, co-administration of orally inhaled ciclesonide and oral erythromycin, an inhibitor of cytochrome P450 3A4, had no effect on the pharmacokinetics of either des-ciclesonide or erythromycin. In another drug interaction study, co-administration of orally inhaled ciclesonide and oral ketoconazole, a potent inhibitor of cytochrome P450 3A4, increased the exposure (AUC) of des-ciclesonide by approximately 3.6-fold at steady state, while levels of ciclesonide remained unchanged. Therefore, ketoconazole should be administered with caution with intranasal ciclesonide.

Carcinogenesis, Mutagenesis, Impairment of Fertility

Ciclesonide demonstrated no carcinogenic potential in a study of oral doses up to 900 mcg/kg (approximately 20 and 10 times the maximum human daily intranasal dose in adults and children, respectively, based on mcg/m2) in mice for 104 weeks and in a study of inhalation doses up to 193 mcg/kg (approximately 8 and 5 times the maximum human daily intranasal dose in adults and children, respectively, based on mcg/m2) in rats for 104 weeks. Ciclesonide was not mutagenic in an Ames test or in a forward mutation assay and was not clastogenic in a human lymphocyte assay or in an in vitro micronucleus test. However, ciclesonide was clastogenic in the in vivo mouse micronucleus test. The concurrent reference corticosteroid (dexamethasone) in this study showed similar findings. No evidence of impairment of fertility was observed in a reproductive study conducted in male and female rats both dosed orally up to 900 mcg/kg/day (approximately 35 times the maximum human daily intranasal dose in adults based on mcg/m2).

Pregnancy: Teratogenic Effects

Pregnancy Category C

Oral administration of ciclesonide in rats up to 900 mcg/kg (approximately 35 times the maximum human daily intranasal dose in adults based on mcg/m2) produced no teratogenicity or other fetal effects. However, subcutaneous administration of ciclesonide in rabbits at 5 mcg/kg (less than the maximum human daily intranasal dose in adults based on mcg/m2) or greater produced fetal toxicity. This included fetal loss, reduced fetal weight, cleft palate, skeletal abnormalities including incomplete ossifications, and skin effects. No toxicity was observed at 1 mcg/kg (less than the maximum human daily intranasal dose based on mcg/m2).

There are no adequate and well-controlled studies in pregnant women. OMNARIS Nasal Spray, like other corticosteroids, should be used during pregnancy only if the potential benefit justifies the potential risk to the fetus. Experience with oral corticosteroids since their introduction in pharmacologic, as opposed to physiologic, doses suggests that rodents are more prone to teratogenic effects from corticosteroids than humans. In addition, because there is a natural increase in corticosteroid production during pregnancy, most women will require a lower exogenous corticosteroid dose and many will not need corticosteroid treatment during pregnancy.

Nonteratogenic effects

Hypoadrenalism may occur in infants born of mothers receiving corticosteroids during pregnancy. Such infants should be carefully monitored.

Nursing Mothers

It is not known if ciclesonide is excreted in human milk. However, other corticosteroids are excreted in human milk. In a study with lactating rats, minimal but detectable levels of ciclesonide were recovered in milk. Caution should be used when OMNARIS Nasal Spray is administered to nursing women.

Pediatric Use

The safety and effectiveness for seasonal and perennial allergic rhinitis in children 12 years of age and older have been established. The efficacy of OMNARIS Nasal Spray in patients 6 to 11 years of age for treatment of the symptoms of seasonal allergic rhinitis is supported by evidence from four adequate and well-controlled studies in adults and adolescents 12 years of age and older with seasonal and perennial allergic rhinitis, and one study in patients 6 to 11 years of age with seasonal allergic rhinitis. The efficacy of OMNARIS Nasal Spray for the treatment of the symptoms of perennial allergic rhinitis in patients 6 to 11 years of age has not been established (see CLINICAL TRIALS: Pediatric Patients Aged 6 to 11 Years). The efficacy of OMNARIS Nasal Spray in children 2 to 5 years of age has not been established. The safety of OMNARIS Nasal Spray in children 2 to 11 years of age was evaluated in 4 controlled clinical studies of 2 to 12 weeks duration (See CLINICAL PHARMACOLOGY: Pharmacodynamics, CLINICAL TRIALS, ADVERSE REACTIONS: Pediatric Patients).

Clinical studies in children less than two years of age have not been conducted. Studies in children under 2 years of age are waived because of local and systemic safety concerns.

Controlled clinical studies have shown that intranasal corticosteroids may cause a reduction in growth velocity in pediatric patients. This effect has been observed in the absence of laboratory evidence of hypothalamic-pituitary-adrenal (HPA)-axis suppression, suggesting that growth velocity is a more sensitive indicator of systemic corticosteroid exposure in pediatric patients than some commonly used tests of HPA-axis function. The long-term effects of this reduction in growth velocity associated with intranasal corticosteroids, including the impact on final adult height, are unknown. The potential for "catch-up" growth following discontinuation of treatment with intranasal corticosteroids has not been adequately studied. The growth of pediatric patients receiving intranasal corticosteroids, including OMNARIS Nasal Spray, should be monitored routinely (e.g., via stadiometry). The potential growth effects of prolonged treatment should be weighed against clinical benefits obtained and the availability of safe and effective noncorticosteroid treatment alternatives. To minimize the systemic effects of intranasal corticosteroids, each patient should be titrated to the lowest dose that effectively controls his/her symptoms.

Geriatric Use

Clinical studies of OMNARIS Nasal Spray did not include sufficient numbers of subjects age 65 and over to determine whether they respond differently from younger subjects. Other reported clinical experience has not identified differences in responses between the elderly and younger patients. In general, dose selection for an elderly patient should be cautious, usually starting at the low end of the dosing range, reflecting the greater frequency of decreased hepatic, renal, or cardiac function, and of concomitant disease or other drug therapy.

ADVERSE REACTIONS

Adult and Adolescent Patients Aged 12 Years and Older:

In controlled clinical studies conducted in the US and Canada, a total of 1524 patients ages 12 years and older received treatment with ciclesonide administered intranasally. In studies of 2 to 6 weeks duration in patients 12 years and older, 546 patients were treated with OMNARIS Nasal Spray 200 mcg daily, and in a study of up to one year in duration, 441 patients were treated with OMNARIS Nasal Spray 200 mcg daily. The overall incidence of adverse events for patients treated with OMNARIS Nasal Spray was comparable to that in patients treated with placebo. Adverse events did not differ appreciably based on age, gender, or race. Approximately 2% of patients treated with OMNARIS Nasal Spray 200 mcg in clinical trials discontinued because of adverse events; this rate was similar for patients treated with placebo. Table 4 displays adverse events, irrespective of drug relationship, that occurred with an incidence of 2% or greater and more frequently with OMNARIS Nasal Spray 200 mcg than with placebo in clinical trials of 2 to 6 weeks in duration.

Table 4 Adverse Events from Controlled Clinical Trials 2 to 6 Weeks in Duration in Patients 12 Years of Age and Older with Seasonal or Perennial Allergic Rhinitis

Adverse Event	OMNARIS Nasal Spray 200 mcg Once Daily (N =546) %	Placebo (N = 544) %
Headache	6.0	4.6
Epistaxis	4.9	2.9
Nasopharyngitis	3.7	3.3
Ear Pain	2.2	0.6

In a 52-week long-term safety trial that included 663 adults and adolescent patients (441 treated with ciclesonide: 227 males and 436 females) with perennial allergic rhinitis, the adverse event profile over the treatment period was similar to the adverse event profile in trials of shorter duration. Adverse events considered likely or definitely related to OMNARIS Nasal Spray that were reported at an incidence of 1% or greater of patients and more commonly in OMNARIS Nasal Spray versus placebo were epistaxis, nasal discomfort, and headache. No patient experienced a nasal septal perforation or nasal ulcer during long-term use of OMNARIS Nasal Spray. While primarily designed to assess the long-term safety of OMNARIS Nasal Spray 200 mcg once daily, this 52-week trial demonstrated greater decreases in total nasal symptom scores with OMNARIS Nasal Spray versus placebo treated patients over the entire treatment period.

Pediatric Patients Aged 6 to 11 Years:

Two controlled clinical studies 2 and 12 weeks in duration were conducted in the US and Canada and included a total of 1282 patients with allergic rhinitis ages 6 to 11 years, of which 913 were treated with OMNARIS (ciclesonide) Nasal Spray 200 mcg, 100 mcg or 25 mcg daily. The overall incidence of adverse events for patients treated with OMNARIS Nasal Spray was comparable to that in patients treated with placebo. Adverse events did not differ appreciably based on age, gender, or race. In clinical trials, 1.6% and 2.7% of patients treated with OMNARIS Nasal Spray 200 mcg or 100 mcg, respectively, discontinued because of adverse events; these rates were lower than the rate in patients treated with placebo (2.8%). Table 5 displays adverse events, irrespective of drug relationship, that occurred with an incidence of 3% or greater and more frequently with OMNARIS Nasal Spray 200 mcg than with placebo.

Table 5 Adverse Events from Controlled Clinical Trials 2 to 12 Weeks in Duration in Patients 6 to 11 Years of Age and Older with Seasonal or Perennial Allergic Rhinitis

Adverse Event	OMNARIS Nasal Spray 200 mcg Once Daily (N =380) %	Placebo (N = 369) %
Headache	6.6	5.7
Nasopharyngitis	6.6	5.4
Pharyngolaryngeal pain	3.4	3.3

Pediatric Patients Aged 2 to 5 Years:

Two controlled clinical studies 6 and 12 weeks in duration were conducted in the US and included a total of 258 patients 2 to 5 years of age with perennial allergic rhinitis, of which 183 were treated with OMNARIS Nasal Spray 200 mcg, 100 mcg or 25 mcg daily. The distribution of adverse events was similar to that seen in the 6 to 11 year old children.

OVERDOSAGE

There are no data available on the effects of acute or chronic overdosage with OMNARIS Nasal Spray. Because of low systemic bioavailability, acute overdosage is unlikely to require any therapy other than observation. A single oral dose of up to 10 mg of ciclesonide in healthy volunteers was well tolerated and serum cortisol levels were virtually unchanged in comparison with placebo treatment. Chronic overdosage with any corticosteroid may result in signs or symptoms of hypercorticism (See PRECAUTIONS).

DOSAGE AND ADMINISTRATION

Seasonal Allergic Rhinitis

Adults and Children (6 Years of Age and Older): The recommended dose of OMNARIS Nasal Spray is 200 mcg per day administered as 2 sprays (50 mcg/spray) in each nostril once daily.

Perennial Allergic Rhinitis

Adults and Adolescents (12 Years of Age and Older): The recommended dose of OMNARIS Nasal Spray is 200 mcg per day administered as 2 sprays (50 mcg/spray) in each nostril once daily.

The maximum total daily dosage should not exceed 2 sprays in each nostril (200 mcg/day).

Prior to initial use, OMNARIS Nasal Spray must be gently shaken and then the pump must be primed by actuating eight times. If the product is not used for four consecutive days, it should be gently shaken and reprimed with one spray or until a fine mist appears.

Directions for Use

Illustrated patient's instructions for proper use accompany each package of OMNARIS Nasal Spray.

HOW SUPPLIED

OMNARIS is supplied in an amber glass bottle and provides for nasal delivery with a manual metered pump. OMNARIS Nasal Spray is supplied with an oxygen absorber sachet and enclosed in a foil pouch. OMNARIS Nasal Spray provides 120 metered sprays after initial priming. Each spray delivers 50 mcg of ciclesonide from the nasal actuator. The OMNARIS Nasal Spray bottle has been filled with an excess to accommodate the priming activity. The bottle should be discarded after removal from the foil pouch either after 120 sprays following initial priming (since the amount of ciclesonide delivered per spray thereafter may be substantially less than the labeled dose) or after 4 months. Patient instructions are also provided.

Store at 25°C (77°F); excursions permitted to 15-30°C (59-86°F) [See USP Controlled Room Temp]. Do not freeze. **Shake gently before use.** Do not spray in eyes. **Keep out of reach of children.**

OMNARIS Nasal Spray 50 mcg, 120 metered sprays; net fill weight 12.5 g. (NDC 63402-701-01)

Continued on next page

Omnaris—Cont.

Manufactured for:
Sepracor Inc.
Marlborough, MA 01752 USA
Made in Germany
For customer service, call 1-888-394-7377
To report adverse events, call 1-877-737-7226
For medical information, call 1-800-739-0565
November 2007
USA F.1/1207/3.5472.73

Vistakon® Pharmaceuticals, LLC

7500 CENTURION PARKWAY
JACKSONVILLE, FL 32256

Direct Inquiries to:
Phone (866) 427-6815

IQUIX® ℞

[*i-quiks*]
(levofloxacin ophthalmic solution) 1.5%

DESCRIPTION

IQUIX® (levofloxacin ophthalmic solution) 1.5% is a sterile topical ophthalmic solution. Levofloxacin is a fluoroquinolone antibacterial active against a broad spectrum of Gram-positive and Gram-negative ocular pathogens. Levofloxacin is a fluorinated 4-quinolone containing a six-member (pyridobenzoxazine) ring from positions 1 to 8 of the basic ring structure. Levofloxacin is the pure(-)-(*S*)-enantiomer of the racemic drug substance, ofloxacin. It is more soluble in water at neutral pH than ofloxacin.

Structural formula

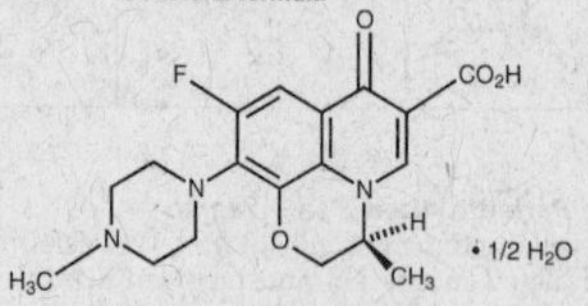

levofloxacin hemihydrate

$C_{18}H_{20}FN_3O_4 \cdot 1/2\ H_2O$ Mol Wt 370.38

Chemical Name: (-)-(*S*)-9-fluoro-2,3-dihydro-3-methyl-10-(4-methyl-1-piperazinyl)-7-oxo-7*H*-pyrido[1,2,3-de]-1,4 benzoxazine-6-carboxylic acid hemihydrate.
Levofloxacin (hemihydrate) is a yellowish-white crystalline powder.
Each mL of IQUIX® contains 15.36 mg of levofloxacin hemihydrate equivalent to 15 mg levofloxacin.

Contains:
Active: Levofloxacin 1.5% (15 mg/mL); **Inactives:** glycerin and water. May also contain hydrochloric acid and/or sodium hydroxide to adjust pH to approximately 6.5. IQUIX® solution is isotonic with an osmolality of approximately 290 mOsm/kg.

CLINICAL PHARMACOLOGY

Pharmacokinetics:
Levofloxacin concentration in plasma was measured in 14 healthy adult volunteers during a 16-day course of treatment with IQUIX® solution. The dosing schedule was 1-2 drops per eye once in the morning on Days 1 and 16; 1-2 drops per eye every two hours Days 2 through 8; and 1-2 drops per eye every four hours Days 9 through 15. The mean levofloxacin concentration in plasma 1 hour postdose ranged from 3.13 ng/mL on Day 1 to 10.4 ng/mL on Day 16. Maximum mean levofloxacin concentrations increased from 3.22 ng/mL on Day 1 to 10.9 ng/mL on Day 16, which is more than 400 times lower than those reported after standard oral doses of levofloxacin.
Levofloxacin concentration in tears was measured in 100 healthy adult volunteers at various time points following instillation of 2 drops of IQUIX® solution. Mean tear concentration measured 15 minutes after instillation was 757 µg/mL.

Microbiology:
Levofloxacin is the *L*-isomer of the racemate, ofloxacin, a quinolone antimicrobial agent. The antibacterial activity of ofloxacin resides primarily in the *L*-isomer. The mechanism of action of levofloxacin and other fluoroquinolone antimicrobials involves the inhibition of bacterial topoisomerase IV and DNA gyrase (both of which are type II topoisomerases), enzymes required for DNA replication, transcription, repair, and recombination.
Levofloxacin has *in vitro* activity against a wide range of Gram-negative and Gram-positive microorganisms and is often bactericidal at concentrations equal to or slightly greater than inhibitory concentrations.
Fluoroquinolones, including levofloxacin, differ in chemical structure and mode of action from β-lactam antibiotics and aminoglycosides, and therefore may be active against bacteria resistant to β-lactam antibiotics and aminoglycosides. Additionally, β-lactam antibiotics and aminoglycosides may be active against bacteria resistant to levofloxacin. Resistance to levofloxacin due to spontaneous mutation *in vitro* is a rare occurrence (range: 10^{-9} to 10^{-10}).
Levofloxacin has been shown to be active against most strains of the following microorganisms, both *in vitro* and in clinical infections as described in the INDICATIONS AND USAGE section:

AEROBIC GRAM-POSITIVE MICROORGANISMS:	**AEROBIC GRAM-NEGATIVE MICROORGANISMS:**
Corynebacterium species*	*Pseudomonas aeruginosa*
Staphylococcus aureus	*Serratia marcescens**
Staphylococcus epidermidis	
Streptococcus pneumoniae	
Viridans group streptococci*	

*Efficacy for this organism was studied in fewer than 10 infections.
The following *in vitro* data are also available, but their clinical significance in ophthalmic infections is unknown. The safety and effectiveness of levofloxacin in treating ophthalmological infections due to these microorganisms have not been established in adequate and well-controlled trials.
These organisms are considered susceptible when evaluated using systemic breakpoints. However, a correlation between the *in vitro* systemic breakpoint and ophthalmological efficacy has not been established. The list of organisms is provided as guidance only in assessing the potential treatment of corneal ulcer. Levofloxacin exhibits *in vitro* minimal inhibitory concentrations (MICs) of 2 µg/mL or less (systemic susceptible breakpoint) against most (≥90%) strains of the following ocular pathogens:

AEROBIC GRAM-POSITIVE MICROORGANISMS:
Enterococcus faecalis (many strains are only moderately susceptible)
Staphylococcus saprophyticus
Streptococcus agalactiae
Streptococcus pyogenes
Streptococcus (Group C/F)
Streptococcus (Group G)

AEROBIC GRAM-NEGATIVE MICROORGANISMS:

Acinetobacter baumannii	*Legionella pneumophila*
Acinetobacter lwoffii	*Moraxella catarrhalis*
Citrobacter koseri	*Morganella morganii*
Citrobacter freundii	*Neisseria gonorrhoeae*
Enterobacter aerogenes	*Pantoea agglomerans*
Enterobacter cloacae	*Proteus mirabilis*
Escherichia coli	*Proteus vulgaris*
Haemophilus influenzae	*Providencia rettgeri*
Haemophilus parainfluenzae	*Providencia stuartii*
Klebsiella oxytoca	*Pseudomonas fluorescens*
Klebsiella pneumoniae	

Clinical Studies:
In two randomized, double-masked, multicenter controlled clinical trials of 280 patients with positive cultures, subjects were dosed with IQUIX® or ofloxacin 0.3% ophthalmic solution. Dosing occurred on Days 1 through 3 every two hours while awake and 4 and 6 hours after retiring. Dosing occurred on Day 4 through treatment completion 4 times daily while awake. Clinical cure was defined as complete re-epithelialization and no progression of the infiltrate for two consecutive visits. The IQUIX® treated subjects had an approximately equal mean clinical cure rate of 80% (73% to 87%) compared to 84% (82% to 86%) for the subjects treated with ofloxacin 0.3% ophthalmic solution.

INDICATIONS AND USAGE

IQUIX® solution is indicated for the treatment of corneal ulcer caused by susceptible strains of the following bacteria:

GRAM-POSITIVE BACTERIA:	**GRAM-NEGATIVE BACTERIA:**
Corynebacterium species*	*Pseudomonas aeruginosa*
Staphylococcus aureus	*Serratia marcescens**
Staphylococcus epidermidis	
Streptococcus pneumoniae	
Viridans group streptococci*	

*Efficacy for this organism was studied in fewer than 10 infections.

CONTRAINDICATIONS

IQUIX® solution is contraindicated in patients with a history of hypersensitivity to levofloxacin, to other quinolones, or to any of the components in this medication.

WARNINGS

NOT FOR INJECTION.
IQUIX® solution should not be injected subconjunctivally, nor should it be introduced directly into the anterior chamber of the eye.
In patients receiving systemic quinolones, serious and occasionally fatal hypersensitivity (anaphylactic) reactions have been reported, some following the first dose. Some reactions were accompanied by cardiovascular collapse, loss of consciousness, angioedema (including laryngeal, pharyngeal or facial edema), airway obstruction, dyspnea, urticaria, and itching. If an allergic reaction to levofloxacin occurs, discontinue the drug. Serious acute hypersensitivity reactions may require immediate emergency treatment. Oxygen and airway management should be administered as clinically indicated.

PRECAUTIONS

General:
As with other anti-infectives, prolonged use may result in overgrowth of non-susceptible organisms, including fungi. If superinfection occurs, discontinue use and institute alternative therapy. Whenever clinical judgment dictates, the patient should be examined with the aid of magnification, such as slit-lamp biomicroscopy, and, where appropriate, fluorescein staining.
Patients should be advised not to wear contact lenses if they have signs and symptoms of corneal ulcer.

Information for Patients:
Avoid contaminating the applicator tip with material from the eye, fingers or other source.
Systemic quinolones have been associated with hypersensitivity reactions, even following a single dose. Discontinue use immediately and contact your physician at the first sign of a rash or allergic reaction.

Drug Interactions:
Specific drug interaction studies have not been conducted with IQUIX®. However, the systemic administration of some quinolones has been shown to elevate plasma concentrations of theophylline, interfere with the metabolism of caffeine, and enhance the effects of the oral anticoagulant warfarin and its derivatives, and has been associated with transient elevations in serum creatinine in patients receiving systemic cyclosporine concomitantly.

Carcinogenesis, Mutagenesis, Impairment of Fertility:
In a long term carcinogenicity study in rats, levofloxacin exhibited no carcinogenic or tumorigenic potential following daily dietary administration for 2 years; the highest dose (100 mg/kg/day) was 100 times the highest recommended human ophthalmic dose.
Levofloxacin was not mutagenic in the following assays: Ames bacterial mutation assay (*S. typhimurium* and *E. coli*), CHO/HGPRT forward mutation assay, mouse micronucleus test, mouse dominant lethal test, rat unscheduled DNA synthesis assay, and the *in vivo* mouse sister chromatid exchange assay. It was positive in the *in vitro* chromosomal aberration (CHL cell line) and *in vitro* sister chromatid exchange (CHL/IU cell line) assays.
Levofloxacin caused no impairment of fertility or reproduction in rats at oral doses as high as 360 mg/kg/day, corresponding to 400 times the highest recommended human ophthalmic dose.

Pregnancy: Teratogenic Effects. Pregnancy Category C:
Levofloxacin at oral doses of 810 mg/kg/day in rats, which corresponds to approximately 1000 times the highest recommended human ophthalmic dose, caused decreased fetal body weight and increased fetal mortality.
No teratogenic effect was observed when rabbits were dosed orally as high as 50 mg/kg/day, which corresponds to approximately 60 times the highest recommended maximum human ophthalmic dose, or when dosed intravenously as high as 25 mg/kg/day, corresponding to approximately 30 times the highest recommended human ophthalmic dose.
There are, however, no adequate and well-controlled studies in pregnant women. Levofloxacin should be used during pregnancy only if the potential benefit justifies the potential risk to the fetus.

Nursing Mothers:
Levofloxacin has not been measured in human milk. Based upon data from ofloxacin, it can be presumed that levofloxacin is excreted in human milk. Caution should be exercised when IQUIX® is administered to a nursing mother.

Pediatric Use:
Safety and effectiveness in children below the age of six years have not been established. Oral administration of systemic quinolones has been shown to cause arthropathy in immature animals. There is no evidence that the ophthalmic administration of levofloxacin has any effect on weight bearing joints.

Geriatric Use:
No overall differences in safety or effectiveness have been observed between elderly and other adult patients.

ADVERSE REACTIONS

The most frequently reported adverse events in the overall study population were headache and a taste disturbance following instillation. These events occurred in approximately 8–10% of patients.
Adverse events occurring in approximately 1–2% of patients included decreased/blurred vision, diarrhea, dyspepsia, fever, infection, instillation site irritation/discomfort, ocular infection, nausea, ocular pain/ discomfort, and throat irritation.
Other reported ocular reactions occurring in less than 1% of patients included chemosis, corneal erosion, corneal ulcer, diplopia, floaters, hyperemia, lid edema, and lid erythema.

DOSAGE AND ADMINISTRATION

Days 1 through 3:
Instill one to two drops in the affected eye(s) every 30 minutes to 2 hours while awake and approximately 4 and 6 hours after retiring.

Day 4 through treatment completion:
Instill one to two drops in the affected eye(s) every 1 to 4 hours while awake.

HOW SUPPLIED

IQUIX® (levofloxacin ophthalmic solution) 1.5% is supplied in a white, low density polyethylene bottle with a controlled dropper tip and a tan, high density polyethylene cap in the following size:
5 mL fill in 5 cc container–NDC 68669-145-05

Storage:
Store at 15°–25°C (59°–77°F).
Rx Only.

Manufactured by:
Santen Oy, P.O. Box 33, FIN-33721 Tampere, Finland
Santen®

Marketed by:
VISTAKON® Pharmaceuticals, LLC
Jacksonville, FL 32256 USA
Licensed from:
Daiichi Sankyo Co., Ltd.,
Tokyo, Japan
U.S. PAT. NO. 5,053,407
April 2007 Version

REVISED INFORMATION

As new research data and clinical findings become available, the product information in *PDR* is revised accordingly. Revisions submitted since the 2008 edition went to press can be found below. To remind yourself of a revision, write "See Supplement A" next to the product's heading in the book.

AstraZeneca Pharmaceuticals LP
WILMINGTON, DE 19850-5437

For Product Full Prescribing Information, Business Information, Medical Information, Adverse Drug Experiences, and Customer Service:
Information Center
1-800-236-9933
For Product Ordering:
Trade Customer Service
1-800-842-9920
For Product Full Prescribing Information:
Internet: www.astrazeneca-us.com

SEROQUEL XR™   ℞
(quetiapine fumarate)
extended-release tablets

HIGHLIGHTS OF PRESCRIBING INFORMATION

These highlights do not include all the information needed to use SEROQUEL XR safely and effectively. See full prescribing information for SEROQUEL XR.
SEROQUEL XR *(quetiapine fumarate) Extended-Release Tablets*
Initial U.S. Approval: 1997

WARNING: INCREASED MORTALITY IN ELDERLY PATIENTS WITH DEMENTIA *See full prescribing information for complete boxed warning.*

- Atypical antipsychotic drugs are associated with an increased risk of death (5.1)
- Quetiapine is not approved for elderly patients with Dementia-Related Psychoses (5.1)

WARNING: SUICIDALITY AND ANTIDEPRESSANT DRUGS *See full prescribing information for complete boxed warning.*
- Increased risk of suicidal thinking and behavior in children, adolescents and young adults taking antidepressants for major depressive disorder and other psychiatric disorders (5.2)
- SEROQUEL XR is not approved for the treatment of depression, however, an immediate release form of quetiapine (Seroquel) is approved for the treatment of bipolar depression. (5.2)

------------ RECENT MAJOR CHANGES --------------
WARNING: Suicidality and Antidepressant Drugs (see Boxed Warning) 06/2007
Warnings and Precautions, Suicidality and Antidepressant Drugs (5.2) 06/2007
Warnings: Hyperglycemia and Diabetes Mellitus (5.3), 06/2007
Warnings and Precautions, Leukopenia, Neutropenia, and Agranulocytosis (5.6) 11/2007

------------ INDICATIONS AND USAGE --------------
SEROQUEL XR is an atypical antipsychotic agent indicated for:
- The acute and maintenance treatment of schizophrenia (1)

------------ DOSAGE AND ADMINISTRATION --------------
Schizophrenia: SEROQUEL XR should be administered once daily, preferably in the evening. The recommended initial dose is 300 mg. The effective dose range for SEROQUEL XR is 400 – 800 mg per day depending on the response and tolerance of the individual patient. Dose increases can be made at intervals as short as 1 day and in increments of up to 300 mg/day. Individual dosage adjustments may be necessary. SEROQUEL XR Tablets should be swallowed whole and not split, chewed or crushed. SEROQUEL XR should be taken without food or with a light meal. (2)

------------ DOSAGE FORMS AND STRENGTHS --------------
Extended-Release Tablets: 200 mg, 300 mg, and 400 mg

------------ CONTRAINDICATIONS --------------
None

------------ WARNINGS AND PRECAUTIONS --------------
- **Increased Mortality in Elderly Patients with Dementia Related Psychoses:** Atypical antipsychotic drugs, including quetiapine, are associated with an increased risk of death; causes of death are variable. (5.1)
- **Suicidality and Antidepressant Drugs:** Seroquel XR is not approved for the treatment of depression, however, an immediate release form of quetiapine (Seroquel) is approved for the treatment of bipolar depression. (5.2)
- **Hyperglycemia and Diabetes Mellitus (DM):** Ketoacidosis, hyperosmolar coma and death have been reported in patients treated with atypical antipsychotics, including quetiapine. Any patient treated with atypical antipsychotics should be monitored for symptoms of hyperglycemia including polydipsia, polyuria, polyphagia, and weakness. When starting treatment, patients with DM risk factors should undergo blood glucose testing before and during treatment. (5.3)
- **Neuroleptic Malignant Syndrome (NMS):** Potentially fatal symptom complex has been reported with antipsychotic drugs, including quetiapine. (5.4)
- **Orthostatic Hypotension:** Associated dizziness, tachycardia and syncope especially during the initial dose titration period. (5.5)
- **Leukopenia, Neutropenia and Agranulocytosis:** have been reported with atypical antipsychotics including SEROQUEL XR. Patients with a pre-existing low white cell count (WBC) or a history of leukopenia/neutropenia should have complete blood count (CBC) monitored frequently during the first few months of treatment and should discontinue SEROQUEL XR at the first sign of a decline in WBC in absence of other causative factors. (5.6)
- **Tardive Dyskinesia** may develop acutely or chronically. (5.7)
- **Cataracts:** Lens changes have been observed in patients during long-term quetiapine treatment. Lens examination should be done when starting treatment and at 6 months intervals during chronic treatment. (5.8)
- **Hyperlipidemia** (5.11)
- The possibility of a suicide attempt is inherent in schizophrenia, and close supervision of high risk patients should accompany drug therapy. (5.18)
- See Full Prescribing Information for additional **WARNINGS and PRECAUTIONS**.

------------ ADVERSE REACTIONS --------------
Most common adverse reactions (incidence ≥5% and greater than placebo) are dry mouth, constipation, dyspepsia, sedation, somnolence, dizziness, and orthostatic hypotension. (6.1) **To report SUSPECTED ADVERSE REACTIONS, contact AstraZeneca at 1-800-236-9933 or FDA at 1-800-FDA-1088 or www.fda.gov/medwatch.**

------------ DRUG INTERACTIONS --------------
- **P450 3A Inhibitors:** May decrease the clearance of quetiapine. Lower doses of quetiapine may be required. (7.1)
- **Hepatic Enzyme Inducers:** May increase the clearance of quetiapine. Higher doses of quetiapine may be required with phenytoin or other inducers. (7.1)
- **Centrally Acting Drugs:** Caution should be used when quetiapine is used in combination with other CNS acting drugs. (7)
- **Antihypertensive Agents:** Quetiapine may add to the hypotensive effects of these agents. (7)
- **Levodopa and Dopamine Agents:** Quetiapine may antagonize the effect of these drugs. (7)

------------ USE IN SPECIFIC POPULATIONS --------------
- **Geriatric Use:** For the initial dosing in the elderly use the immediate release formulation of SEROQUEL instead of SEROQUEL XR. Consider a lower starting dose (25 mg/day immediate release formulation), slower titration, and careful monitoring during the initial dosing period in the elderly. (2.2, 8.5)
- **Hepatic Impairment:** For the initial dosing in patients with hepatic impairment, use the immediate release formulation of SEROQUEL instead of SEROQUEL XR. Lower starting doses (25 mg/day immediate release formulation) and slower titration may be needed. (2.2, 8.7, 12.3)
- **Pregnancy and Nursing Mothers:** Quetiapine should be used only if the potential benefit justifies the potential risk. (8.1) Breast feeding is not recommended. (8.3)
- **Pediatric Use:** Safety and effectiveness have not been established. (8.4)

SEE 17 FOR PATIENT COUNSELING INFORMATION
Revised 11/2007
*FULL PRESCRIBING INFORMATION: CONTENTS

Continued on next page

Seroquel XR—Cont.

* Sections or subsections omitted from the full prescribing information are not listed.

FULL PRESCRIBING INFORMATION

WARNING: INCREASED MORTALITY IN ELDERLY PATIENTS WITH DEMENTIA-RELATED PSYCHOSIS
Elderly patients with dementia-related psychosis treated with atypical antipsychotic drugs are at an increased risk of death compared to placebo. Analyses of seventeen placebo-controlled trials (modal duration of 10 weeks) in these patients revealed a risk of death in the drug-treated patients of between 1.6 to 1.7 times that seen in placebo-treated patients. Over the course of a typical 10-week controlled trial, the rate of death in drug-treated patients was about 4.5%, compared to a rate of about 2.6% in the placebo group. Although the causes of death were varied, most of the deaths appeared to be either cardiovascular (eg, heart failure, sudden death) or infectious (eg, pneumonia) in nature. SEROQUEL XR is not approved for the treatment of patients with Dementia-Related Psychosis.

SUICIDALITY AND ANTIDEPRESSANT DRUGS
Antidepressants increased the risk compared to placebo of suicidal thinking and behavior (suicidality) in children, adolescents, and young adults in short-term studies of major depressive disorder (MDD) and other psychiatric disorders. Anyone considering the use of SEROQUEL or any other antidepressant in a child, adolescent, or young adult must balance this risk with the clinical need. Short-term studies did not show an increase in the risk of suicidality with antidepressants compared to placebo in adults beyond age 24; there was a reduction in risk with antidepressants compared to placebo in adults aged 65 and older. Depression and certain other psychiatric disorders are themselves associated with increases in the risk of suicide. Patients of all ages who are started on antidepressant therapy should be monitored appropriately and observed closely for clinical worsening, suicidality, or unusual changes in behavior. Families and caregivers should be advised of the need for close observation and communication with the prescriber. SEROQUEL XR is not approved for use in pediatric patients. SEROQUEL XR is not approved for use in the treatment of depression, however, an immediate release form of quetiapine (SEROQUEL) is approved for the treatment of bipolar depression.

1 INDICATIONS AND USAGE

SEROQUEL XR is indicated for the acute and maintenance treatment of schizophrenia [see *Clinical Studies* (14.1)].
The efficacy of SEROQUEL XR in schizophrenia was established in part, on the basis of extrapolation from the established effectiveness of SEROQUEL. In addition, the efficacy of SEROQUEL XR was demonstrated in 1 short-term (6-week) controlled trial of schizophrenic inpatients and outpatients [see *Clinical Studies* (14.1)]. The longer-term benefit of maintaining patients on monotherapy with SEROQUEL XR after achieving a responder status for 16 weeks was demonstrated in a controlled trial [see *Clinical Studies* (14.1)].

2 DOSAGE AND ADMINISTRATION

2.1 Usual Dose
SEROQUEL XR should be administered once daily, preferably in the evening. The recommended initial dose is 300 mg/day. Patients should be titrated within a dose range of 400 – 800 mg/day depending on the response and tolerance of the individual patient [see *Clinical Studies* (14)]. Dose increases can be made at intervals as short as 1 day and in increments of up to 300 mg/day. The safety of doses above 800 mg/day has not been evaluated in clinical trials. SEROQUEL XR tablets should be swallowed whole and not split, chewed or crushed.
It is recommended that SEROQUEL XR be taken without food or with a light meal (approximately 300 calories) [see *Clinical Pharmacology* (12.3)].

2.2 Dosing in Special Populations
Consideration should be given to a slower rate of dose titration and a lower target dose in the elderly and in patients who are debilitated or who have a predisposition to hypotensive reactions [see *Use in Specific Populations* (8.5 and 8.7) and *Clinical Pharmacology* (12)]. When indicated, dose escalation should be performed with caution in these patients.
For those patients who require less than 200 mg per dose of SEROQUEL XR during the initial titration, use the immediate release formulation.
Elderly patients should be started on SEROQUEL immediate release formulation 25 mg/day and the dose can be increased in increments of 25-50 mg/day depending on the response and tolerance of the individual patient. When an effective dose has been reached, the patient may be switched to SEROQUEL XR at an equivalent total daily dose [see *Dosage and Administration* (2.5)].
Patients with hepatic impairment should be started on SEROQUEL immediate release formulation 25 mg/day. The dose can be increased daily in increments of 25-50 mg/day to an effective dose, depending on the clinical response and tolerance of the patient. When an effective dose has been reached, the patient may be switched to SEROQUEL XR at an equivalent total daily dose [see *Dosage and Administration* (2.5)].
The elimination of quetiapine was enhanced in the presence of phenytoin. Higher maintenance doses of quetiapine may be required when it is coadministered with phenytoin and other enzyme inducers such as carbamazepine and phenobarbital [see *Drug Interactions* (7.1)].

2.3 Maintenance Treatment
While there is no body of evidence available to specifically address how long the patient treated with SEROQUEL XR should remain on it, a longer-term study with SEROQUEL XR has shown this drug to be effective in delaying time to relapse in patients who were stabilized on SEROQUEL XR at doses of 400 to 800 mg/day for 16 weeks [see *Clinical Studies* (14.1)]. Patients should be periodically reassessed to determine the need for maintenance treatment and the appropriate dose for such treatment [see *Clinical Studies* (14.1)].

2.4 Re-initiation of Treatment in Patients Previously Discontinued
Although there are no data to specifically address reinitiation of treatment, it is recommended that when restarting therapy of patients who have been off SEROQUEL XR for more than one week, the initial dosing schedule should be followed. When restarting patients who have been off SEROQUEL XR for less than one week, gradual dose escalation may not be required and the maintenance dose may be reinitiated.

2.5 Switching Patients from SEROQUEL Tablets to SEROQUEL XR Tablets
Schizophrenic patients who are currently being treated with divided doses of SEROQUEL (immediate release formulation, eg, 2 to 3 times per day) may be switched to SEROQUEL XR at the equivalent total daily dose taken once daily. Individual dosage adjustments may be necessary.

2.6 Switching from Antipsychotics
There are no systematically collected data to specifically address switching patients with schizophrenia from other antipsychotics to SEROQUEL XR, or concerning concomitant administration with other antipsychotics. While immediate discontinuation of the previous antipsychotic treatment may be acceptable for some patients with schizophrenia, more gradual discontinuation may be most appropriate for others. In all cases, the period of overlapping antipsychotic administration should be minimized. When switching patients with schizophrenia from depot antipsychotics, if medically appropriate, initiate SEROQUEL XR therapy in place of the next scheduled injection. The need for continuing existing extrapyramidal syndrome medication should be re-evaluated periodically.

3 DOSAGE FORMS AND STRENGTHS

200 mg extended-release tablets
300 mg extended-release tablets
400 mg extended-release tablets

4 CONTRAINDICATIONS

None

5 WARNINGS AND PRECAUTIONS

5.1 Increased Mortality in Elderly Patients with Dementia-Related Psychosis
Elderly patients with dementia-related psychosis treated with atypical antipsychotic drugs are at an increased risk of death compared to placebo. SEROQUEL XR (quetiapine fumarate) is not approved for the treatment of patients with dementia-related psychosis (see Boxed Warning).

5.2 Clinical Worsening and Suicide Risk
Patients with major depressive disorder (MDD), both adult and pediatric, may experience worsening of their depression and/or the emergence of suicidal ideation and behavior (suicidality) or unusual changes in behavior, whether or not they are taking antidepressant medications, and this risk may persist until significant remission occurs. Suicide is a known risk of depression and certain other psychiatric disorders, and these disorders themselves are the strongest predictors of suicide. There has been a long-standing concern, however, that antidepressants may have a role in inducing worsening of depression and the emergence of suicidality in certain patients during the early phases of treatment. Pooled analyses of short-term placebo-controlled trials of antidepressant drugs (SSRIs and others) showed that these drugs increase the risk of suicidal thinking and behavior (suicidality) in children, adolescents, and young adults (ages 18-24) with major depressive disorder (MDD) and other psychiatric disorders. Short-term studies did not show an increase in the risk of suicidality with antidepressants compared to placebo in adults beyond age 24; there was a reduction with antidepressants compared to placebo in adults aged 65 and older.
The pooled analyses of placebo-controlled trials in children and adolescents with MDD, obsessive compulsive disorder (OCD), or other psychiatric disorders included a total of 24 short-term trials of 9 antidepressant drugs in over 4400 patients. The pooled analyses of placebo-controlled trials in adults with MDD or other psychiatric disorders included a total of 295 short-term trials (median duration of 2 months) of 11 antidepressant drugs in over 77,000 patients. There was considerable variation in risk of suicidality among drugs, but a tendency toward an increase in the younger patients for almost all drugs studied. There were differences in absolute risk of suicidality across the different indications, with the highest incidence in MDD. The risk differences (drug vs placebo), however, were relatively stable within age strata and across indications. These risk differences (drug-placebo difference in the number of cases of suicidality per 1000 patients treated) are provided in Table 1.

Table 1

Age Range	Drug-Placebo Difference in Number of Cases of Suicidality per 1000 Patients Treated
	Increases Compared to Placebo
<18	14 additional cases
18-24	5 additional cases
	Decreases Compared to Placebo
25-64	1 fewer case
≥65	6 fewer cases

No suicides occurred in any of the pediatric trials. There were suicides in the adult trials, but the number was not sufficient to reach any conclusion about drug effect on suicide.
It is unknown whether the suicidality risk extends to longer-term use, i.e., beyond several months. However, there is substantial evidence from placebo-controlled maintenance trials in adults with depression that the use of antidepressants can delay the recurrence of depression.
All patients being treated with antidepressants for any indication should be monitored appropriately and observed closely for clinical worsening, suicidality, and unusual changes in behavior, especially during the initial few months of a course of drug therapy, or at times of dose changes, either increases or decreases.
The following symptoms, anxiety, agitation, panic attacks, insomnia, irritability, hostility, aggressiveness, impulsivity, akathisia (psychomotor restlessness), hypomania, and mania, have been reported in adult and pediatric patients being treated with antidepressants for major depressive disorder as well as for other indications, both psychiatric and nonpsychiatric. Although a causal link between the emergence of such symptoms and either the worsening of depression and/or the emergence of suicidal impulses has not been established, there is concern that such symptoms may represent precursors to emerging suicidality.
Consideration should be given to changing the therapeutic regimen, including possibly discontinuing the medication, in patients whose depression is persistently worse, or who are experiencing emergent suicidality or symptoms that might be precursors to worsening depression or suicidality, especially if these symptoms are severe, abrupt in onset, or were not part of the patient's presenting symptoms.
Families and caregivers of patients being treated with antidepressants for major depressive disorder or other indications, both psychiatric and nonpsychiatric, should be alerted about the need to monitor patients for the emergence of agitation, irritability, unusual changes in behavior, and the other symptoms described above, as well as the emergence of suicidality, and to report such symptoms immediately to health care providers. Such monitoring should include daily observation by families and caregivers. Prescriptions for SEROQUEL should be written for the smallest quantity of tablets consistent with good patient management, in order to reduce the risk of overdose.
Screening Patients for Bipolar Disorder: A major depressive episode may be the initial presentation of bipolar disorder. It is generally believed (though not established in controlled trials) that treating such an episode with an antidepressant alone may increase the likelihood of precipitation of a mixed/manic episode in patients at risk for bipolar disorder. Whether any of the symptoms described above represent such a conversion is unknown. However, prior to initiating treatment with an antidepressant, patients with depressive symptoms should be adequately screened to determine if they are at risk for bipolar disorder; such screening should include a detailed psychiatric history, including a family history of suicide, bipolar disorder, and depression. It should be noted that SEROQUEL XR is not approved for use in treating depression, however, an

immediate release form of quetiapine (SEROQUEL) is approved for the treatment of bipolar depression.

5.3 Hyperglycemia and Diabetes Mellitus

Hyperglycemia, in some cases extreme and associated with ketoacidosis or hyperosmolar coma or death, has been reported in patients treated with atypical antipsychotics, including quetiapine [see *Adverse Reactions, Hyperglycemia* (6.2)]. Assessment of the relationship between atypical antipsychotic use and glucose abnormalities is complicated by the possibility of an increased background risk of diabetes mellitus in patients with schizophrenia and the increasing incidence of diabetes mellitus in the general population. Given these confounders, the relationship between atypical antipsychotic use and hyperglycemia-related adverse reactions is not completely understood. However, epidemiological studies suggest an increased risk of treatment-emergent hyperglycemia-related adverse reactions in patients treated with the atypical antipsychotics. Precise risk estimates for hyperglycemia-related adverse reactions in patients treated with atypical antipsychotics are not available.

Patients with an established diagnosis of diabetes mellitus who are started on atypical antipsychotics should be monitored regularly for worsening of glucose control. Patients with risk factors for diabetes mellitus (eg, obesity, family history of diabetes) who are starting treatment with atypical antipsychotics should undergo fasting blood glucose testing at the beginning of treatment and periodically during treatment. Any patient treated with atypical antipsychotics should be monitored for symptoms of hyperglycemia including polydipsia, polyuria, polyphagia, and weakness. Patients who develop symptoms of hyperglycemia during treatment with atypical antipsychotics should undergo fasting blood glucose testing. In some cases, hyperglycemia has resolved when the atypical antipsychotic was discontinued; however, some patients required continuation of anti-diabetic treatment despite discontinuation of the suspect drug.

5.4 Neuroleptic Malignant Syndrome (NMS)

A potentially fatal symptom complex sometimes referred to as Neuroleptic Malignant Syndrome (NMS) has been reported in association with administration of antipsychotic drugs, including quetiapine. Rare cases of NMS have been reported with quetiapine. Clinical manifestations of NMS are hyperpyrexia, muscle rigidity, altered mental status, and evidence of autonomic instability (irregular pulse or blood pressure, tachycardia, diaphoresis, and cardiac dysrhythmia). Additional signs may include elevated creatine phosphokinase, myoglobinuria (rhabdomyolysis) and acute renal failure.

The diagnostic evaluation of patients with this syndrome is complicated. In arriving at a diagnosis, it is important to exclude cases where the clinical presentation includes both serious medical illness (eg, pneumonia, systemic infection, etc.) and untreated or inadequately treated extrapyramidal signs and symptoms (EPS). Other important considerations in the differential diagnosis include central anticholinergic toxicity, heat stroke, drug fever and primary central nervous system (CNS) pathology.

The management of NMS should include: 1) immediate discontinuation of antipsychotic drugs and other drugs not essential to concurrent therapy; 2) intensive symptomatic treatment and medical monitoring; and 3) treatment of any concomitant serious medical problems for which specific treatments are available. There is no general agreement about specific pharmacological treatment regimens for NMS.

If a patient requires antipsychotic drug treatment after recovery from NMS, the potential reintroduction of drug therapy should be carefully considered. The patient should be carefully monitored since recurrences of NMS have been reported.

5.5 Orthostatic Hypotension

Quetiapine may induce orthostatic hypotension associated with dizziness, tachycardia and, in some patients, syncope, especially during the initial dose-titration period, probably reflecting its α1-adrenergic antagonist properties. Syncope was reported in 0.3% (3/951) of the patients treated with SEROQUEL XR, compared with 0.3% (1/319) on placebo. Syncope was reported in 1% (23/3265) of the patients treated with SEROQUEL, compared with 0.2% (2/527) on placebo.

Quetiapine should be used with particular caution in patients with known cardiovascular disease (history of myocardial infarction or ischemic heart disease, heart failure or conduction abnormalities), cerebrovascular disease or conditions which would predispose patients to hypotension (dehydration, hypovolemia and treatment with antihypertensive medications). If hypotension occurs during titration to the target dose, a return to the previous dose in the titration schedule is appropriate.

5.6 Leukopenia, Neutropenia and Agranulocytosis

In clinical trial and postmarketing experience, events of leukopenia/neutropenia have been reported temporally related to atypical antipsychotic agents, including quetiapine fumarate. Agranulocytosis (including fatal cases) has also been reported.

Possible risk factors for leukopenia/neutropenia include pre-existing low white cell count (WBC) and history of drug induced leukopenia/neutropenia. Patients with a pre-existing low WBC or a history of drug induced leukopenia/neutropenia should have their complete blood count (CBC) monitored frequently during the first few months of therapy and should discontinue SEROQUEL XR at the first sign of a decline in WBC in absence of other causative factors.

Patients with neutropenia should be carefully monitored for fever or other symptoms or signs of infection and treated promptly if such symptoms or signs occur. Patients with severe neutropenia (absolute neutrophil count <1000/mm^3) should discontinue SEROQUEL XR and have their WBC followed until recovery [see *Adverse Reactions* (6.2)].

5.7 Tardive Dyskinesia

A syndrome of potentially irreversible, involuntary, dyskinetic movements may develop in patients treated with antipsychotic drugs. Although the prevalence of the syndrome appears to be highest among the elderly, especially elderly women, it is impossible to rely upon prevalence estimates to predict, at the inception of antipsychotic treatment, which patients are likely to develop the syndrome. Whether antipsychotic drug products differ in their potential to cause tardive dyskinesia is unknown.

The risk of developing tardive dyskinesia and the likelihood that it will become irreversible are believed to increase as the duration of treatment and the total cumulative dose of antipsychotic drugs administered to the patient increase. However, the syndrome can develop, although much less commonly, after relatively brief treatment periods at low doses.

There is no known treatment for established cases of tardive dyskinesia, although the syndrome may remit, partially or completely, if antipsychotic treatment is withdrawn. Antipsychotic treatment, itself, however, may suppress (or partially suppress) the signs and symptoms of the syndrome and thereby may possibly mask the underlying process. The effect that symptomatic suppression has upon the long-term course of the syndrome is unknown.

Given these considerations, quetiapine should be prescribed in a manner that is most likely to minimize the occurrence of tardive dyskinesia. Chronic antipsychotic treatment should generally be reserved for patients who appear to suffer from a chronic illness that (1) is known to respond to antipsychotic drugs, and (2) for whom alternative, equally effective, but potentially less harmful treatments are not available or appropriate. In patients who do require chronic treatment, the smallest dose and the shortest duration of treatment producing a satisfactory clinical response should be sought. The need for continued treatment should be reassessed periodically.

If signs and symptoms of tardive dyskinesia appear in a patient on quetiapine, drug discontinuation should be considered. However, some patients may require treatment with quetiapine despite the presence of the syndrome.

5.8 Cataracts

The development of cataracts was observed in association with quetiapine treatment in chronic dog studies [see *Animal Toxicology* (13.2)]. Lens changes have also been observed in patients during long-term quetiapine treatment, but a causal relationship to quetiapine use has not been established. Nevertheless, the possibility of lenticular changes cannot be excluded at this time. Therefore, examination of the lens by methods adequate to detect cataract formation, such as slit lamp exam or other appropriately sensitive methods, is recommended at initiation of treatment or shortly thereafter, and at 6 month intervals during chronic treatment.

5.9 Seizures

During clinical trials with SEROQUEL XR, seizures occurred in 0.1% (1/951) of patients treated with SEROQUEL XR compared to 0.9% (3/319) on placebo. During clinical trials with SEROQUEL, seizures occurred in 0.5% (20/3490) patients treated with SEROQUEL compared to 0.2% (2/954) on placebo. As with other antipsychotics quetiapine should be used cautiously in patients with a history of seizures or with conditions that potentially lower the seizure threshold, eg, Alzheimer's dementia. Conditions that lower the seizure threshold may be more prevalent in a population of 65 years or older.

5.10 Hypothyroidism

In SEROQUEL XR clinical trials, 0.5% (4/806) of patients on SEROQUEL XR vs. 0% (0/262) on placebo experienced decreased free thyroxine and 2.7% (21/786) on SEROQUEL XR vs. 1.2% (3/256) on placebo experienced increased TSH; however, no patients experienced a combination of clinically significant decreased free thyroxine and increased TSH. No patients had reactions of hypothyroidism. Clinical trials with SEROQUEL demonstrated a dose-related decrease in total and free thyroxine (T4) of approximately 20% at the higher end of the therapeutic dose range and was maximal in the first two to four weeks of treatment and maintained without adaptation or progression during more chronic therapy. Generally, these changes were of no clinical significance and TSH was unchanged in most patients and levels of TBG were unchanged. In nearly all cases, cessation of quetiapine treatment was associated with a reversal of the effects on total and free T4, irrespective of the duration of treatment. About 0.4% (12/2791) of SEROQUEL patients did experience TSH increases in monotherapy studies. Six of these patients with TSH increases needed replacement thyroid treatment.

5.11 Cholesterol and Triglyceride Elevations

In schizophrenia clinical trials, SEROQUEL XR treated patients had increases from baseline in mean cholesterol and triglycerides of 4% and 15%, respectively compared to decreases from baseline in mean cholesterol and triglycerides of 2% and 6% for placebo treated patients. In schizophrenia clinical trials, SEROQUEL treated patients had increases from baseline in mean cholesterol and triglyceride of 11% and 17%, respectively, compared to slight decreases for placebo patients.

5.12 Hyperprolactinemia

An elevation of prolactin levels was not demonstrated in clinical trials with SEROQUEL XR as compared with placebo. Increased prolactin levels with quetiapine were observed in rat toxicity studies, and were associated with an increase in mammary gland neoplasia in rats [see *Carcinogenesis, Mutagenesis, Impairment of Fertility* (13.1)]. Tissue culture experiments indicate that approximately one-third of human breast cancers are prolactin dependent *in vitro*, a factor of potential importance if the prescription of these drugs is contemplated in a patient with previously detected breast cancer.

5.13 Transaminase Elevations

Asymptomatic, transient and reversible elevations in serum transaminases (primarily ALT) have been reported. The proportions of patients with transaminase elevations of >3 times the upper limits of the normal reference range in a pool of 6-week placebo controlled schizophrenia trials were approximately 1% for SEROQUEL XR compared to 2% for placebo. In schizophrenia trials, the proportions of patients with transaminase elevations of >3 times the upper limits of the normal reference range in a pool of 3- to 6-week placebo controlled trials were approximately 6% for SEROQUEL compared to 1% for placebo. These hepatic enzyme elevations usually occurred within the first 3 weeks of drug treatment and promptly returned to pre-study levels with ongoing treatment with SEROQUEL.

5.14 Potential for Cognitive and Motor Impairment

Somnolence was a commonly reported adverse event reported in patients treated with quetiapine especially during the 3-day period of initial dose titration. In schizophrenia trials, somnolence and sedation were reported in 12% and 13% of patients on SEROQUEL XR respectively compared to 4% and 7% of placebo patients. In schizophrenia trials, somnolence was reported in 18% of patients on SEROQUEL compared to 11% of placebo patients. Since quetiapine has the potential to impair judgment, thinking, or motor skills, patients should be cautioned about performing activities requiring mental alertness, such as operating a motor vehicle (including automobiles) or operating hazardous machinery until they are reasonably certain that quetiapine therapy does not affect them adversely.

5.15 Priapism

One case of priapism in a patient receiving quetiapine was reported prior to market introduction. While a causal relationship to use of quetiapine has not been established, other drugs with α-adrenergic blocking effects have been reported to induce priapism, and it is possible that quetiapine may share this capacity. Severe priapism may require surgical intervention.

5.16 Body Temperature Regulation

Disruption of the body's ability to reduce core body temperature has been attributed to antipsychotic agents. Appropriate care is advised when prescribing SEROQUEL XR for patients who will be experiencing conditions which may contribute to an elevation in core body temperature, eg, exercising strenuously, exposure to extreme heat, receiving concomitant medication with anticholinergic activity, or being subject to dehydration.

5.17 Dysphagia

Esophageal dysmotility and aspiration have been associated with antipsychotic drug use. Aspiration pneumonia is a common cause of morbidity and mortality in elderly patients, in particular those with advanced Alzheimer's dementia. SEROQUEL XR and other antipsychotic drugs should be used cautiously in patients at risk for aspiration pneumonia.

5.18 Suicide

The possibility of a suicide attempt is inherent in schizophrenia; close supervision of high risk patients should accompany drug therapy. Prescriptions for SEROQUEL XR should be written for the smallest quantity of tablets consistent with good patient management in order to reduce the risk of overdose.

In three, 6-week clinical studies in patients with schizophrenia (N=951) the incidence of treatment emergent suicidal ideation or suicide attempt, as measured by the Columbia Analysis of Suicidal Behavior, was low in SEROQUEL XR treated patients (0.6%) and similar to placebo (0.9%).

5.19 Use in Patients with Concomitant Illness

Clinical experience with SEROQUEL XR in patients with certain concomitant systemic illnesses [see *Pharmacokinetics* (12.3)] is limited.

SEROQUEL XR has not been evaluated or used to any appreciable extent in patients with a recent history of myocardial infarction or unstable heart disease. Patients with these diagnoses were excluded from premarketing clinical studies. Because of the risk of orthostatic hypotension with SEROQUEL XR, caution should be observed in cardiac patients [see *Warnings and Precautions* (5.5)].

5.20 Withdrawal

Acute withdrawal symptoms, such as nausea, vomiting, and insomnia have very rarely been described after abrupt cessation of atypical antipsychotic drugs, including quetiapine. Gradual withdrawal is advised.

6 ADVERSE REACTIONS

6.1. Clinical Studies Experience

Because clinical studies are conducted under widely varying conditions, adverse reaction rates observed in the clinical

Continued on next page

Seroquel XR—Cont.

studies of a drug cannot be directly compared to rates in the clinical studies of another drug and may not reflect the rates observed in practice.

The information below is derived from a clinical trial database for SEROQUEL XR consisting of 951 patients exposed to SEROQUEL XR for the treatment of schizophrenia in placebo controlled trials. This experience corresponds to approximately 82.9 patient-years. Adverse reactions were assessed by collecting adverse reactions, results of physical examinations, vital signs, body weights, laboratory analyses, and ECG results.

Adverse reactions during exposure were obtained by general inquiry and recorded by clinical investigators using terminology of their own choosing. Consequently, it is not possible to provide a meaningful estimate of the proportion of individuals experiencing adverse reactions without first grouping similar types of reactions into a smaller number of standardized event categories. In the tables and tabulations that follow, standard MedDRA terminology has been used to classify reported adverse reactions.

The stated frequencies of adverse reactions represent the proportion of individuals who experienced, at least once, a treatment-emergent adverse reaction of the type listed. An event was considered treatment-emergent if it occurred for the first time or worsened while receiving therapy following baseline evaluation.

Adverse Reactions Associated with Discontinuation of Treatment in Short-Term, Placebo-Controlled Trials
There was no difference in the incidence and type of adverse reactions associated with discontinuation (6.4% for SEROQUEL XR vs. 7.5% for placebo) in a pool of controlled trials.

Adverse Reactions Occurring at an Incidence of 5% or More Among SEROQUEL XR Treated Patients in Short-Term, Placebo-Controlled Trials
Table 2 enumerates the incidence, rounded to the nearest percent, of treatment-emergent adverse reactions that occurred during acute therapy of schizophrenia (up to 6 weeks) in ≥5% patients treated with SEROQUEL XR (doses ranging from 300 to 800 mg/day) where the incidence in patients treated with SEROQUEL XR was greater than the incidence in placebo-treated patients.

Table 2. Treatment-Emergent Adverse Reaction Incidence in 6-Week Placebo-Controlled Clinical Trials for the Treatment of Schizophrenia

Body System/ Preferred Term	SEROQUEL XR (n=951)	PLACEBO (n=319)
Gastrointestinal Disorders		
Dry mouth	12%	1%
Constipation	6%	5%
Dyspepsia	5%	2%
Nervous System Disorders		
Sedation	13%	7%
Somnolence	12%	4%
Dizziness	10%	4%
Vascular Disorders		
Orthostatic hypotension	7%	5%

[1] Reactions for which the SEROQUEL XR incidence was equal to or less than placebo are not listed in the table, but included the following: headache, insomnia, and nausea.

In these studies, the most commonly observed adverse reactions associated with the use of SEROQUEL XR (incidence of 5% or greater) and observed at a rate on SEROQUEL XR at least twice that of placebo were dry mouth (12%), somnolence (12%), dizziness (10%), and dyspepsia (5%).

Adverse Reactions Occurring at an Incidence of 5% or More Among SEROQUEL XR Treated Patients in Long-Term, Placebo-Controlled Trials
In a longer-term placebo-controlled trial, adult patients with schizophrenia who remained clinically stable on SEROQUEL XR during open label treatment for at least 4 months were randomized to placebo (n=103) or to continue on their current SEROQUEL XR (n=94) for up to 12 months of observation for possible relapse, the adverse reactions reported were generally consistent with those reported in the short-term, placebo-trials. Insomnia (8.5%) and headache (7.4%) were the only adverse events reported by 5% or more patients.

Adverse Reactions that occurred in <5% of patients and were considered drug-related (incidence greater than placebo and consistent with known pharmacology of drug class) in order of decreasing frequency:
heart rate increased, hypotension, weight increased, tremor, akathisia, increased appetite, blurred vision, postural dizziness, pyrexia, dysarthria, dystonia, drooling, syncope, tardive dyskinesia, dysphagia, leukopenia, and rash.

Adverse Reactions that have historically been associated with the use of SEROQUEL and not listed elsewhere in the label
The following adverse reactions have also been reported with SEROQUEL: anaphylactic reaction, peripheral edema, rhinitis, eosinophilia, hypersensitivity, elevations in gamma-GT levels and restless legs syndrome.
Extrapyramidal Symptoms:
Four methods were used to measure EPS: (1) Simpson-Angus total score (mean change from baseline) which evalu-

ates parkinsonism and akathisia, (2) Barnes Akathisia Rating Scale (BARS) Global Assessment Score (3) incidence of spontaneous complaints of EPS (akathisia, akinesia, cogwheel rigidity, extrapyramidal syndrome, hypertonia, hypokinesia, neck rigidity, and tremor), and (4) use of anticholinergic medications to treat emergent EPS.

In three-arm placebo-controlled clinical trials for the treatment of schizophrenia, utilizing doses between 300 mg and 800 mg of SEROQUEL XR, the incidence of any adverse reactions potentially related to EPS was 8% for SEROQUEL XR and 8% for SEROQUEL (without evidence of being dose related), and 5% in the placebo group. In these studies, the incidence of the individual adverse reactions (eg, akathisia, extrapyramidal disorder, tremor, dyskinesia, dystonia, restlessness, and muscle rigidity) was generally low and did not exceed 3% for any treatment group.

At the end of treatment, the mean change from baseline in SAS total score and BARS Global Assessment score was similar across the treatment groups. The use of concomitant anticholinergic medications was infrequent and similar across the treatment groups. The incidence of extrapyramidal symptoms was consistent with that seen with the profile of SEROQUEL in schizophrenia patients.

6.2   Vital Signs and Laboratory Studies
Vital Sign Changes:
Quetiapine is associated with orthostatic hypotension [see *Warnings and Precautions* (5.5)].
Weight Gain:
In schizophrenia trials with SEROQUEL XR, the proportions of patients meeting a weight gain criterion of ≥7% of body weight was 10% for SEROQUEL XR compared to 5% for placebo. In schizophrenia trials the proportions of patients meeting a weight gain criterion of ≥7% of body weight were compared in a pool of four 3- to 6-week placebo-controlled clinical trials, revealing a statistically significant greater incidence of weight gain for SEROQUEL (23%) compared to placebo (6%).
Laboratory Changes:
An assessment of the premarketing experience for SEROQUEL suggested that it is associated with asymptomatic increases in ALT and increases in both total cholesterol and triglycerides [see *Warnings and Precautions* (5.11; 5.13)]. In post-marketing clinical trials, elevations in total cholesterol (predominantly LDL cholesterol) have been observed.

In three-arm SEROQUEL XR placebo controlled monotherapy clinical trials, among patients with a baseline neutrophil count ≥1.5 × 10^9/L, the incidence of at least one occurrence of neutrophil count <1.5 × 10^9/L was 1.5% in patients treated with SEROQUEL XR and 1.5% for SEROQUEL, compared to 0.8% in placebo-treated patients. In placebo controlled monotherapy clinical trials involving 3368 patients on quetiapine fumarate and 1515 on placebo, the incidence of at least one occurrence of neutrophil count <1.0 × 10^9/L among patients with a normal baseline neutrophil count and at least one available follow up laboratory measurement was 0.3% (10/2967) in patients treated with quetiapine fumarate, compared to 0.1% (2/1349) in patients treated with placebo. Patients with a pre-existing low WBC or a history of drug induced leukopenia/neutropenia should have their complete blood count (CBC) monitored frequently during the first few months of therapy and should discontinue SEROQUEL XR at the first sign of a decline in WBC in absence of other causative factors [see *Warnings and Precautions* (5.6)].

Hyperglycemia:
In 2 long-term placebo-controlled clinical trials, mean exposure 213 days for SEROQUEL (646 patients) and 152 days for placebo (680 patients), the exposure-adjusted rate of any increased blood glucose level (≥126 mg/dL) for patients more than 8 hours since a meal was 18.0 per 100 patient years for SEROQUEL (10.7% of patients) and 9.5 for placebo per 100 patient years (4.6% of patients).
In short-term (12 weeks duration or less) placebo-controlled clinical trials (3342 patients treated with SEROQUEL and 1490 treated with placebo), the percent of patients who had a fasting blood glucose ≥126 mg/dL or a non fasting blood glucose ≥200 mg/dL was 3.5% for quetiapine fumarate and 2.1% for placebo.
In a 24 week trial (active-controlled, 115 patients treated with SEROQUEL) designed to evaluate glycemic status with oral glucose tolerance testing of all patients, at week 24 the incidence of a treatment-emergent post-glucose challenge glucose level ≥200 mg/dL was 1.7% and the incidence of a fasting treatment-emergent blood glucose level ≥126 mg/dL was 2.6%.
ECG Changes:
0.8% of SEROQUEL XR patients, and no placebo patients, had tachycardia (>120 bpm) at any time during the trials. SEROQUEL XR was associated with a mean increase in heart rate, assessed by ECG, of 7 beats per minute compared to a mean decrease of 1 beat per minute for placebo. This is consistent with the rates of SEROQUEL. The incidence of adverse reactions of tachycardia was 3% for SEROQUEL XR compared to 1% for placebo. SEROQUEL use was associated with a mean increase in heart rate, assessed by ECG, of 7 beats per minute compared to a mean increase of 1 beat per minute among placebo patients. The slight tendency for tachycardia may be related to quetiapine's potential for inducing orthostatic changes [see *Warnings and Precautions* (5)].

6.3   Post Marketing Experience:
The following adverse reactions were identified during post approval use of SEROQUEL. Because these reactions are

reported voluntarily from a population of uncertain size, it is not always possible to reliably estimate their frequency or establish a causal relationship to drug exposure.
Adverse reactions reported since market introduction which were temporally related to SEROQUEL therapy include: anaphylactic reaction, and restless legs.
Other adverse reactions reported since market introduction, which were temporally related to SEROQUEL therapy, but not necessarily causally related, include the following: agranulocytosis, cardiomyopathy hyponatremia, myocarditis rhabdomyolysis, syndrome of inappropriate antidiuretic hormone secretion (SIADH), and Stevens-Johnson syndrome (SJS).

7   DRUG INTERACTIONS

The risks of using SEROQUEL XR in combination with other drugs have not been extensively evaluated in systematic studies. Given the primary CNS effects of SEROQUEL XR, caution should be used when it is taken in combination with other centrally acting drugs. Quetiapine potentiated the cognitive and motor effects of alcohol in a clinical trial in subjects with selected psychotic disorders, and alcoholic beverages should be limited while taking quetiapine.
Because of its potential for inducing hypotension, SEROQUEL XR may enhance the effects of certain antihypertensive agents.
SEROQUEL XR may antagonize the effects of levodopa and dopamine agonists.

7.1   The Effect of Other Drugs on Quetiapine
Phenytoin
Coadministration of quetiapine (250 mg three times/day) and phenytoin (100 mg three times/day) increased the mean oral clearance of quetiapine by 5-fold. Increased doses of SEROQUEL XR may be required to maintain control of symptoms of schizophrenia in patients receiving quetiapine and phenytoin, or other hepatic enzyme inducers (eg, carbamazepine, barbiturates, rifampin, glucocorticoids). Caution should be taken if phenytoin is withdrawn and replaced with a non-inducer (eg, valproate) [see *Dosage and Administration* (2)].
Divalproex
Coadministration of quetiapine (150 mg bid) and divalproex (500 mg bid) increased the mean maximum plasma concentration of quetiapine at steady-state by 17% without affecting the extent of absorption or mean oral clearance.
Thioridazine
Thioridazine (200 mg bid) increased the oral clearance of quetiapine (300 mg bid) by 65%.
Cimetidine
Administration of multiple daily doses of cimetidine (400 mg tid for 4 days) resulted in a 20% decrease in the mean oral clearance of quetiapine (150 mg tid). Dosage adjustment for quetiapine is not required when it is given with cimetidine.
P450 3A Inhibitors
Coadministration of ketoconazole (200 mg once daily for 4 days), a potent inhibitor of cytochrome P450 3A, reduced oral clearance of quetiapine by 84%, resulting in a 335% increase in maximum plasma concentration of quetiapine. Caution (reduced dosage) is indicated when SEROQUEL XR is administered with ketoconazole and other inhibitors of cytochrome P450 3A (eg, itraconazole, fluconazole, erythromycin, protease inhibitors).
Fluoxetine, Imipramine, Haloperidol, and Risperidone
Coadministration of fluoxetine (60 mg once daily); imipramine (75 mg bid), haloperidol (7.5 mg bid), or risperidone (3 mg bid) with quetiapine (300 mg bid) did not alter the steady-state pharmacokinetics of quetiapine.
7.2.   Effect of Quetiapine on Other Drugs
Lorazepam
The mean oral clearance of lorazepam (2 mg, single dose) was reduced by 20% in the presence of quetiapine administered as 250 mg tid dosing.
Divalproex
The mean maximum concentration and extent of absorption of total and free valproic acid at steady-state were decreased by 10 to 12% when divalproex (500 mg bid) was administered with quetiapine (150 mg bid). The mean oral clearance of total valproic acid (administered as divalproex 500 mg bid) was increased by 11% in the presence of quetiapine (150 mg bid). The changes were not significant.
Lithium
Concomitant administration of quetiapine (250 mg tid) with lithium had no effect on any of the steady-state pharmacokinetic parameters of lithium.
Antipyrine
Administration of multiple daily doses up to 750 mg/day (on a tid schedule) of quetiapine to subjects with selected psychotic disorders had no clinically relevant effect on the clearance of antipyrine or urinary recovery of antipyrine metabolites. These results indicate that quetiapine does not significantly induce hepatic enzymes responsible for cytochrome P450 mediated metabolism of antipyrine.

8   USE IN SPECIFIC POPULATIONS
8.1   Pregnancy
Pregnancy Category C: The teratogenic potential of quetiapine was studied in Wistar rats and Dutch Belted rabbits dosed during the period of organogenesis. No evidence of a teratogenic effect was detected in rats at doses of 25 to 200 mg/kg or 0.3 to 2.4 times the maximum human dose on a mg/m² basis or in rabbits at 25 to 100 mg/kg or 0.6 to 2.4 times the maximum human dose on a mg/m² basis: There was, however, evidence of embryo/fetal toxicity. Delays in skeletal ossification were detected in rat fetuses at doses of 50 and 200 mg/kg (0.6 and 2.4 times the maximum

human dose on a mg/m^2 basis) and in rabbits at 50 and 100 mg/kg (1.2 and 2.4 times the maximum human dose on a mg/m^2 basis). Fetal body weight was reduced in rat fetuses at 200 mg/kg and rabbit fetuses at 100 mg/kg (2.4 times the maximum human dose on a mg/m^2 basis for both species). There was an increased incidence of a minor soft tissue anomaly (carpal/tarsal flexure) in rabbit fetuses at a dose of 100 mg/kg (2.4 times the maximum human dose on a mg/m^2 basis). Evidence of maternal toxicity (i.e., decreases in body weight gain and/or death) was observed at the high dose in the rat study and at all doses in the rabbit study. In a peri/postnatal reproductive study in rats, no drug-related effects were observed at doses of 1, 10, and 20 mg/kg or 0.01, 0.12, and 0.24 times the maximum human dose on a mg/m^2 basis. However, in a preliminary peri/postnatal study, there were increases in fetal and pup death, and decreases in mean litter weight at 150 mg/kg, or 3.0 times the maximum human dose on a mg/m^2 basis.

There are no adequate and well-controlled studies in pregnant women and quetiapine should be used during pregnancy only if the potential benefit justifies the potential risk to the fetus.

8.2 Labor and Delivery

The effect of SEROQUEL XR on labor and delivery in humans is unknown.

8.3 Nursing Mothers

SEROQUEL XR was excreted in milk of treated animals during lactation. It is not known if SEROQUEL XR is excreted in human milk. It is recommended that women receiving SEROQUEL XR should not breast feed.

8.4 Pediatric Use

The safety and effectiveness of SEROQUEL XR in pediatric patients have not been established.

8.5 Geriatric Use

Sixty-eight patients in clinical studies with SEROQUEL XR were 65 years of age or over. In general, there was no indication of any different tolerability of SEROQUEL XR in the elderly compared to younger adults. Nevertheless, the presence of factors that might decrease pharmacokinetic clearance, increase the pharmacodynamic response to SEROQUEL XR, or cause poorer tolerance or orthostasis, should lead to consideration of a lower starting dose, slower titration, and careful monitoring during the initial dosing period in the elderly. The mean plasma clearance of quetiapine was reduced by 30% to 50% in elderly patients when compared to younger patients [see *Use in Special Populations* (2.2) and *Pharmacokinetics* (12.3)].

8.6 Renal Impairment

Clinical experience with SEROQUEL XR in patients with renal impairment [see *Clinical Pharmacology* (12.3)] is limited.

8.7 Hepatic Impairment

Since quetiapine is extensively metabolized by the liver, higher plasma levels are expected in the hepatically impaired population, and dosage adjustment may be needed [see *Dosing and Administration* (2.2) and *Clinical Pharmacology* (12.3)].

9 DRUG ABUSE AND DEPENDENCE

9.1 Controlled Substance

SEROQUEL XR is not a controlled substance.

9.2 Abuse

SEROQUEL XR has not been systematically studied in animals or humans for its potential for abuse, tolerance or physical dependence. While the clinical trials did not reveal any tendency for any drug-seeking behavior, these observations were not systematic and it is not possible to predict on the basis of this limited experience the extent to which a CNS-active drug will be misused, diverted, and/or abused once marketed. Consequently, patients should be evaluated carefully for a history of drug abuse, and such patients should be observed closely for signs of misuse or abuse of SEROQUEL XR, (eg, development of tolerance, increases in dose, drug-seeking behaviour).

10 OVERDOSAGE

10.1 Human Experience

In clinical trials, survival has been reported in acute overdoses of up to 30 grams of quetiapine. Most patients who overdosed experienced no adverse events or recovered fully from the reported events. Death has been reported in a clinical trial following an overdose of 13.6 grams of quetiapine alone. In general, reported signs and symptoms were those resulting from an exaggeration of the drug's known pharmacological effects, ie, drowsiness and sedation, tachycardia and hypotension. Patients with pre-existing severe cardiovascular disease may be at an increased risk of the effects of overdose [see *Warnings and Precautions* (5.4)]. One case, involving an estimated overdose of 9600 mg, was associated with hypokalemia and first degree heart block. In post-marketing experience, there have been very rare reports of overdose of SEROQUEL alone resulting in death, coma, or QTc prolongation.

10.2 Management of Overdosage

In case of acute overdosage, establish and maintain an airway and ensure adequate oxygenation and ventilation. Gastric lavage (after intubation, if patient is unconscious) and administration of activated charcoal together with a laxative should be considered. The possibility of obtundation, seizure or dystonic reaction of the head and neck following overdose may create a risk of aspiration with induced emesis. Cardiovascular monitoring should commence immediately and should include continuous electrocardiographic monitoring to detect possible arrhythmias. If antiarrhythmic therapy is administered, disopyramide, procainamide and quinidine carry a theoretical hazard of additive QT-prolonging effects when administered in patients with acute overdosage of SEROQUEL XR. Similarly it is reasonable to expect that the α-adrenergic-blocking properties of bretylium might be additive to those of quetiapine, resulting in problematic hypotension.

There is no specific antidote to SEROQUEL XR. Therefore, appropriate supportive measures should be instituted. The possibility of multiple drug involvement should be considered. Hypotension and circulatory collapse should be treated with appropriate measures such as intravenous fluids and/or sympathomimetic agents (epinephrine and dopamine should not be used, since β stimulation may worsen hypotension in the setting of quetiapine-induced α blockade). In cases of severe extrapyramidal symptoms, anticholinergic medication should be administered. Close medical supervision and monitoring should continue until the patient recovers.

11 DESCRIPTION

SEROQUEL XR (quetiapine fumarate) is a psychotropic agent belonging to a chemical class, the dibenzothiazepine derivatives. The chemical designation is 2-[2-(4-dibenzo [*b,f*] [1,4]thiazepin-11-yl-1-piperazinyl)ethoxy]-ethanol fumarate (2:1) (salt). It is present in tablets as the fumarate salt. All doses and tablet strengths are expressed as milligrams of base, not as fumarate salt. Its molecular formula is $C_{42}H_{50}N_6O_4S_2 \bullet C_4H_4O_4$ and it has a molecular weight of 883.11 (fumarate salt). The structural formula is:

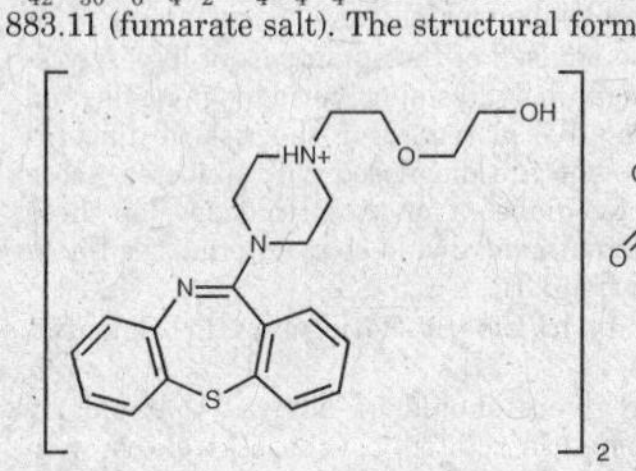

Quetiapine fumarate is a white to off-white crystalline powder which is moderately soluble in water.

SEROQUEL XR is supplied for oral administration as 200 mg (yellow), 300 mg (pale yellow), and 400 mg (white). All tablets are capsule shaped and film coated.

Inactive ingredients for SEROQUEL XR are, lactose monohydrate, microcrystalline cellulose, sodium citrate, hypromellose, and magnesium stearate. The film coating for all SEROQUEL XR tablets contain hypromellose, polyethylene glycol 400 and titanium dioxide. In addition yellow iron oxide (200 and 300 mg tablets) are included in the film coating of specific strengths.

Each 200 mg tablet contains 230 mg of quetiapine fumarate equivalent to 200 mg quetiapine. Each 300 mg tablet contains 345 mg of quetiapine fumarate equivalent to 300 mg quetiapine. Each 400 mg tablet contains 461 mg of quetiapine fumarate equivalent to 400 mg quetiapine.

12 CLINICAL PHARMACOLOGY

12.1 Mechanism of Action

The mechanism of action of quetiapine, as with other drugs having efficacy in the treatment of schizophrenia, is unknown. However, it is believed that this drug's efficacy in schizophrenia is mediated through a combination of dopamine type 2 (D_2) and serotonin type 2 ($5HT_2$) antagonism, by quetiapine and its active metabolite N-desalkyl quetiapine.

Antagonism at receptors other than dopamine D_2 and serotonin $5HT_2$ with similar or greater affinities may explain some of the other effects of quetiapine and N-desalkyl quetiapine; antagonism at histamine H_1 receptors may explain the somnolence and antagonism at adrenergic α_1 receptors may explain the orthostatic hypotension observed with this drug.

12.2 Pharmacodynamics

Quetiapine is an antagonist at multiple neurotransmitter receptors in the brain: serotonin $5HT1_A$ and $5HT_2$ (IC_{50s}=717 & 148nM respectively), dopamine D_1 and D_2 (IC_{50s}=1268 & 329nM respectively), histamine H1 (IC_{50}=30nM), and adrenergic α_1 and α_2 receptors (IC_{50s}=94 & 271nM, respectively). Quetiapine has no appreciable affinity at cholinergic muscarinic and benzodiazepine receptors (IC_{50s}>5000 nM).

12.3 Pharmacokinetics

Following multiple dosing of quetiapine up to a total daily dose of 800 mg, administered in divided doses, the plasma concentration of quetiapine and N-desalkyl quetiapine, the major active metabolite of quetiapine, were proportional to the total daily dose. Accumulation is predictable upon multiple dosing. Steady-state mean C_{max} and AUC of N-desalkyl quetiapine are about 21-27% and 46-56%, respectively of that observed for quetiapine. Elimination of quetiapine is mainly via hepatic metabolism. The mean-terminal half-life is approximately 7 hours for quetiapine and 9 to 12 hours for N-desalkyl quetiapine within the clinical dose range. Steady-state concentrations are expected to be achieved within two days of dosing. SEROQUEL XR is unlikely to interfere with the metabolism of drugs metabolized by cytochrome P450 enzymes.

Absorption

Quetiapine fumarate reaches peak plasma concentrations approximately 6 hours following administration. SEROQUEL XR dosed once daily at steady-state has comparable bioavailability to an equivalent total daily dose of SEROQUEL administered in divided doses, twice daily. A high-fat meal (approximately 800 to 1000 calories) was found to produce statistically significant increases in the SEROQUEL XR C_{max} and AUC of 44% to 52% and 20% to 22%, respectively, for the 50-mg and 300-mg tablets. In comparison, a light meal (approximately 300 calories) had no significant effect on the C_{max} or AUC of quetiapine. It is recommended that SEROQUEL XR be taken without food or with a light meal [see *Dosage and Administration* (2)].

Distribution

Quetiapine is widely distributed throughout the body with an apparent volume of distribution of 10±4 L/kg. It is 83% bound to plasma proteins at therapeutic concentrations. *In vitro*, quetiapine did not affect the binding of warfarin or diazepam to human serum albumin. In turn, neither warfarin nor diazepam altered the binding of quetiapine.

Metabolism and Elimination

Following a single oral dose of ^{14}C-quetiapine, less than 1% of the administered dose was excreted as unchanged drug, indicating that quetiapine is highly metabolized. Approximately 73% and 20% of the dose was recovered in the urine and feces, respectively. The average dose fraction of free quetiapine and its major active metabolite is <5% excreted in the urine.

Quetiapine is extensively metabolized by the liver. The major metabolic pathways are sulfoxidation to the sulfoxide metabolite and oxidation to the parent acid metabolite; both metabolites are pharmacologically inactive. *In vitro* studies using human liver microsomes revealed that the cytochrome P450 3A4 isoenzyme is involved in the metabolism of quetiapine to its major, but inactive, sulfoxide metabolite and in the metabolism of its active metabolite N-desalkyl quetiapine.

Gender

There is no gender effect on the pharmacokinetics of quetiapine.

Race

There is no race effect on the pharmacokinetics of quetiapine.

Smoking

Smoking has no effect on the oral clearance of quetiapine.

Renal Insufficiency

Patients with severe renal impairment (CL_{cr}=10-30 mL/min/1.73m^2, n=8) had a 25% lower mean oral clearance than normal subjects (CL_{cr}>80 mL/min/1.73m^2, n=8), but plasma quetiapine concentrations in the subjects with renal insufficiency were within the range of concentrations seen in normal subjects receiving the same dose. Dosage adjustment is therefore not needed in these patients.

Hepatic Insufficiency

Hepatically impaired patients (n=8) had a 30% lower mean oral clearance of quetiapine than normal subjects. In 2 of the 8 hepatically impaired patients, AUC and C_{max} were 3 times higher than those observed typically in healthy subjects. Since quetiapine is extensively metabolized by the liver, higher plasma levels are expected in the hepatically impaired population, and dosage adjustment may be needed [see *Dosage and Administration* (2)].

Drug-Drug Interactions

In vitro enzyme inhibition data suggest that quetiapine and 9 of its metabolites would have little inhibitory effect on *in vivo* metabolism mediated by cytochromes P450 1A2, 2C9, 2C19, 2D6 and 3A4.

Quetiapine oral clearance is increased by the prototype cytochrome P450 3A4 inducer, phenytoin, and decreased by the prototype cytochrome P450 3A4 inhibitor, ketoconazole. Dose adjustment of quetiapine will be necessary if it is co-administered with phenytoin or ketoconazole [see *Drug Interactions* (7.1) and *Dosage and Administration* (2)].

Quetiapine oral clearance is not inhibited by the non-specific enzyme inhibitor, cimetidine.

Quetiapine at doses of 750 mg/day did not affect the single dose pharmacokinetics of antipyrine, lithium or lorazepam [see *Drug Interactions* (7.2)].

13 NONCLINICAL TOXICOLOGY

13.1 Carcinogenesis, Mutagenesis, Impairment of Fertility

Carcinogenesis

Carcinogenicity studies were conducted in C57BL mice and Wistar rats. Quetiapine was administered in the diet to mice at doses of 20, 75, 250, and 750 mg/kg and to rats by gavage at doses of 25, 75, and 250 mg/kg for two years. These doses are equivalent to 0.1, 0.5, 1.5, and 4.5 times the maximum human dose (800 mg/day) on a mg/m^2 basis (mice) or 0.3, 0.9, and 3.0 times the maximum human dose on a mg/m^2 basis (rats). There were statistically significant increases in thyroid gland follicular adenomas in male mice at doses of 250 and 750 mg/kg or 1.5 and 4.5 times the maximum human dose on a mg/m^2 basis and in male rats at a dose of 250 mg/kg or 3.0 times the maximum human dose on a mg/m^2 basis. Mammary gland adenocarcinomas were statistically significantly increased in female rats at all doses tested (25, 75, and 250 mg/kg or 0.3, 0.9, and 3.0 times the maximum recommended human dose on a mg/m^2 basis).

Thyroid follicular cell adenomas may have resulted from chronic stimulation of the thyroid gland by thyroid stimulating hormone (TSH) resulting from enhanced metabolism and clearance of thyroxine by rodent liver. Changes in TSH, thyroxine, and thyroxine clearance consistent with this mechanism were observed in subchronic toxicity studies in rat and mouse and in a 1-year toxicity study in rat; however, the results of these studies were not definitive. The relevance of the increases in thyroid follicular cell adenomas to human risk, through whatever mechanism, is unknown.

Continued on next page

Seroquel XR—Cont.

Antipsychotic drugs have been shown to chronically elevate prolactin levels in rodents. Serum measurements in a 1-yr toxicity study showed that quetiapine increased median serum prolactin levels a maximum of 32- and 13-fold in male and female rats, respectively. Increases in mammary neoplasms have been found in rodents after chronic administration of other antipsychotic drugs and are considered to be prolactin-mediated. The relevance of this increased incidence of prolactin-mediated mammary gland tumors in rats to human risk is unknown [see *Warnings and Precautions* (5.12)].

Mutagenesis

The mutagenic potential of quetiapine was tested in six *in vitro* bacterial gene mutation assays and in an *in vitro* mammalian gene mutation assay in Chinese Hamster Ovary cells. However, sufficiently high concentrations of quetiapine may not have been used for all tester strains. Quetiapine did produce a reproducible increase in mutations in one *Salmonella* typhimurium tester strain in the presence of metabolic activation. No evidence of clastogenic potential was obtained in an *in vitro* chromosomal aberration assay in cultured human lymphocytes or in the *in vivo* micronucleus assay in rats.

Impairment of Fertility

Quetiapine decreased mating and fertility in male Sprague-Dawley rats at oral doses of 50 and 150 mg/kg or 0.6 and 1.8 times the maximum human dose on a mg/m^2 basis. Drug related effects included increases in interval to mate and in the number of matings required for successful impregnation. These effects continued to be observed at 150 mg/kg even after a two-week period without treatment. The no-effect dose for impaired mating and fertility in male rats was 25 mg/kg, or 0.3 times the maximum human dose on a mg/m^2 basis. Quetiapine adversely affected mating and fertility in female Sprague-Dawley rats at an oral dose of 50 mg/kg, or 0.6 times the maximum human dose on a mg/m^2 basis. Drug-related effects included decreases in matings and in matings resulting in pregnancy, and an increase in the interval to mate. An increase in irregular estrus cycles was observed at doses of 10 and 50 mg/kg, or 0.1 and 0.6 times the maximum human dose on a mg/m^2 basis. The no effect dose in female rats was 1 mg/kg, or 0.01 times the maximum human dose on a mg/m^2 basis.

13.2 Animal Toxicology and/or Pharmacology

Quetiapine caused a dose-related increase in pigment deposition in thyroid gland in rat toxicity studies which were 4 weeks in duration or longer and in a mouse 2 year carcinogenicity study. Doses were 10-250 mg/kg in rats, 75-750 mg/kg in mice; these doses are 0.1-3.0, and 0.1-4.5 times the maximum recommended human dose (on a mg/m^2 basis), respectively. Pigment deposition was shown to be irreversible in rats. The identity of the pigment could not be determined, but was found to be co-localized with quetiapine in thyroid gland follicular epithelial cells. The functional effects and the relevance of this finding to human risk are unknown.

In dogs receiving quetiapine for 6 or 12 months, but not for 1 month, focal triangular cataracts occurred at the junction of posterior sutures in the outer cortex of the lens at a dose of 100 mg/kg, or 4 times the maximum recommended human dose on a mg/m^2 basis. This finding may be due to inhibition of cholesterol biosynthesis by quetiapine. Quetiapine caused a dose related reduction in plasma cholesterol levels in repeat-dose dog and monkey studies; however, there was no correlation between plasma cholesterol and the presence of cataracts in individual dogs. The appearance of delta 8 cholestanol in plasma is consistent with inhibition of a late stage in cholesterol biosynthesis in these species. There also was a 25% reduction in cholesterol content of the outer cortex of the lens observed in a special study in quetiapine treated female dogs. Drug-related cataracts have not been seen in any other species; however, in a 1-year study in monkeys, a striated appearance of the anterior lens surface was detected in 2/7 females at a dose of 225 mg/kg or 5.5 times the maximum recommended human dose on a mg/m^2 basis.

14 CLINICAL STUDIES

14.1 Schizophrenia

The efficacy of SEROQUEL XR in the treatment of schizophrenia was demonstrated in 1 short-term, 6-week, fixed-dose, placebo-controlled trial of inpatients and outpatients with schizophrenia (n=573) who met DSM IV criteria for schizophrenia. SEROQUEL XR (once daily) was administered as 300 mg on (Day 1), and the dose was increased to either 400 mg or 600 mg by Day 2, or 800 mg by Day 3. The primary endpoint was the change from baseline of the Positive and Negative Syndrome Scale (PANSS) total score at the end of treatment (Day 42). SEROQUEL XR doses of 400 mg, 600 mg and 800 mg once daily were superior to placebo in the PANSS total score at Day 42.

In a longer-term trial, clinically stable adult outpatients (n=171) meeting DSM-IV criteria for schizophrenia who remained stable following 16 weeks of open label treatment with flexible doses of SEROQUEL XR (400-800 mg/day) were randomized to placebo or to continue on their current SEROQUEL XR (400-800 mg/day) for observation for possible relapse during the double-blind continuation (maintenance) phase. Stabilization during the open label phase was defined as receiving a stable dose of SEROQUEL XR and having a CGI-S≤4 and a PANSS score ≤60 from beginning to end of this open-label phase (with no increase of ≥10 points in PANSS total score). Relapse during the double-blind phase was defined in terms of a ≥30% increase in the PANSS Total score, or CGI-Improvement score of ≥6, or hospitalization due to worsening of schizophrenia, or need for any other antipsychotic medication. Patients on SEROQUEL XR experienced a statistically significant longer time to relapse than did patients on placebo.

16 HOW SUPPLIED/STORAGE AND HANDLING

- 200 mg Tablets (NDC 0310-0282) yellow, film coated, capsule-shaped, biconvex, intagliated tablet with "SR 200" on one side and plain on the other are supplied in bottles of 60 tablets and 500 tablets and hospital unit dose packages of 100 tablets.
- 300 mg Tablets (NDC 0310-0283) pale yellow, film coated, capsule-shaped, biconvex, intagliated tablet with "SR 300" on one side and plain on the other are supplied in bottles of 60 tablets and 500 tablets and hospital unit dose packages of 100 tablets.
- 400 mg Tablets (NDC 0310-0284) white, film coated, capsule-shaped, biconvex, intagliated tablet with "SR 400" on one side and plain on the other are supplied in bottles of 60 tablets and 500 tablets and hospital unit dose packages of 100 tablets.

Store SEROQUEL XR at 25°C (77°F); excursions permitted to 15-30°C (59-86°F) [See USP].

17 PATIENT COUNSELING INFORMATION

Hyperglycemia and Diabetes Mellitus

Patients should be advised of the symptoms of hyperglycemia (high blood sugar, polydipsia, polyuria, polyphagia, and weakness) and be advised regarding the risk of diabetes mellitus. Patients who are diagnosed with diabetes, those with risk factors for diabetes, or those that develop these symptoms during treatment should be monitored [see *Warnings and Precautions* (5.3)].

Increased Mortality in Elderly Patients with Dementia-Related Psychosis

Patients and caregivers should be advised that elderly patients with dementia-related psychoses treated with atypical antipsychotic drugs are at increased risk of death compared with placebo. Quetiapine is not approved for elderly patients with dementia-related psychosis [see *Warnings and Precautions* (5.1)].

Clinical Worsening and Suicide Risk

Patients, their families, and their caregivers should be encouraged to be alert to the emergence of anxiety, agitation, panic attacks, insomnia, irritability, hostility, aggressiveness, impulsivity, akathisia (psychomotor restlessness), hypomania, mania, other unusual changes in behavior, worsening of depression, and suicidal ideation, especially early during antidepressant treatment and when the dose is adjusted up or down. Families and caregivers of patients should be advised to look for the emergence of such symptoms on a day-to-day basis, since changes may be abrupt. Such symptoms should be reported to the patient's prescriber or health professional, especially if they are severe, abrupt in onset, or were not part of the patient's presenting symptoms. Symptoms such as these may be associated with an increased risk for suicidal thinking and behavior and indicate a need for very close monitoring and possibly changes in the medication [see *Warnings and Precautions* (5.2)].

Prescribers or other health professionals should inform patients, their families, and their caregivers about the benefits and risks associated with treatment with SEROQUEL and should counsel them in its appropriate use. A patient Medication Guide about "Antidepressant Medicines, Depression and other Serious Mental Illness, and Suicidal Thoughts or Actions" is available for SEROQUEL. The prescriber or health professional should instruct patients, their families, and their caregivers to read the Medication Guide and should assist them in understanding its contents. Patients should be given the opportunity to discuss the contents of the Medication Guide and to obtain answers to any questions they may have. The complete text of the Medication Guide is reprinted at the end of this document. It should be noted that SEROQUEL XR is not approved for treatment of depression, however, an immediate release form of quetiapine (SEROQUEL) is approved for the treatment of bipolar depression.

Orthostatic Hypotension

Patients should be advised of the risk of orthostatic hypotension (symptoms include feeling dizzy or lightheaded upon standing) especially during the period of initial dose titration, and also at times of re-initiating treatment or increases in dose [see *Warnings and Precautions* (5.5)].

Leukopenia/Neutropenia

Patients with a pre-existing low WBC or a history of drug induced leukopenia/neutropenia should be advised that they should have their CBC monitored while taking SEROQUEL XR [see *Warnings and Precautions* (5.6)].

Interference with Cognitive and Motor Performance

Patients should be advised of the risk of somnolence or sedation, especially during the period of initial dose titration. Patients should be cautioned about performing any activity requiring mental alertness, such as operating a motor vehicle (including automobiles) or operating machinery, until they are reasonably certain quetiapine therapy does not affect them adversely. Patients should limit consumption of alcohol during treatment with quetiapine [see *Warnings and Precautions* (5.14)].

Pregnancy and Nursing

Patients should be advised to notify their physician if they become pregnant or intend to become pregnant during therapy. Patients should be advised not to breast feed if they are taking quetiapine [see *Use in Special Populations* (8.3)].

Concomitant Medication

As with other medications, patients should be advised to notify their physicians if they are taking, or plan to take, any prescription or over-the-counter drugs.

Heat Exposure and Dehydration

Patients should be advised regarding appropriate care in avoiding overheating and dehydration.

Neuroleptic Malignant Syndrome (NMS)

Patients should be advised to report to their physician any signs or symptoms that may be related to NMS. These may include muscle stiffness and high fever [see *Warnings and Precautions* (5.4)].

MEDICATION GUIDE

Antidepressant Medicines, Depression and other Serious Mental Illnesses, and Suicidal Thoughts or Actions

Read the Medication Guide that comes with your or your family member's antidepressant medicine. This Medication Guide is only about the risk of suicidal thoughts and actions with antidepressant medicines. **Talk to your, or your family member's, healthcare provider about:**

- all risks and benefits of treatment with antidepressant medicines
- all treatment choices for depression or other serious mental illness

What is the most important information I should know about antidepressant medicines, depression and other serious mental illnesses, and suicidal thoughts or actions?

1. **Antidepressant medicines may increase suicidal thoughts or actions in some children, teenagers, and young adults within the first few months of treatment.**
2. **Depression and other serious mental illnesses are the most important causes of suicidal thoughts and actions. Some people may have a particularly high risk of having suicidal thoughts or actions.** These include people who have (or have a family history of) bipolar illness (also called manic-depressive illness) or suicidal thoughts or actions.
3. **How can I watch for and try to prevent suicidal thoughts and actions in myself or a family member?**
   - Pay close attention to any changes, especially sudden changes, in mood, behaviors, thoughts, or feelings. This is very important when an antidepressant medicine is started or when the dose is changed.
   - Call the healthcare provider right away to report new or sudden changes in mood, behavior, thoughts, or feelings.
   - Keep all follow-up visits with the healthcare provider as scheduled. Call the healthcare provider between visits as needed, especially if you have concerns about symptoms.

Call a healthcare provider right away if you or your family member has any of the following symptoms, especially if they are new, worse, or worry you:

- thoughts about suicide or dying
- attempts to commit suicide
- new or worse depression
- new or worse anxiety
- feeling very agitated or restless
- panic attacks
- trouble sleeping (insomnia)
- new or worse irritability
- acting aggressive, being angry, or violent
- acting on dangerous impulses
- an extreme increase in activity and talking (mania)
- other unusual changes in behavior or mood

What else do I need to know about antidepressant medicines?

- **Never stop an antidepressant medicine without first talking to a healthcare provider.** Stopping an antidepressant medicine suddenly can cause other symptoms.
- **Antidepressants are medicines used to treat depression and other illnesses.** It is important to discuss all the risks of treating depression and also the risks of not treating it. Patients and their families or other caregivers should discuss all treatment choices with the healthcare provider, not just the use of antidepressants.
- **Antidepressant medicines have other side effects.** Talk to the healthcare provider about the side effects of the medicine prescribed for you or your family member.
- **Antidepressant medicines can interact with other medicines.** Know all of the medicines that you or your family member takes. Keep a list of all medicines to show the healthcare provider. Do not start new medicines without first checking with your healthcare provider.
- **Not all antidepressant medicines prescribed for children are FDA approved for use in children.** Talk to your child's healthcare provider for more information.

This Medication Guide has been approved by the U.S. Food and Drug Administration for all antidepressants.

It should be noted that SEROQUEL XR is not approved for treatment of depression, however, an immediate release form of quetiapine (SEROQUEL) is approved for the treatment of bipolar depression.

SEROQUEL XR is a trademark of the AstraZeneca group of companies

©AstraZeneca 2007

Distributed by:
AstraZeneca Pharmaceuticals LP
Wilmington, DE 19850
Made in United Kingdom
30420-05   11/07
257379

Boehringer Ingelheim
900 RIDGEBURY ROAD
P.O. BOX 368
RIDGEFIELD, CT 06877-0368

Direct inquiries to:
(800) 243-0127
TTY (800) 246-6196

For medical information or to report an adverse drug experience contact:
(800) 542-6257 (option 4)
TTY (800) 459-9906
us.boehringer-ingelheim.com

APTIVUS®   ℞
[ap-tĭ-vŭs]
(tipranavir)

Prescribing information for this product, which appears on pages 818–826 of the 2008 PDR, has been completely revised as follows. Please write "See Supplement A" next to the product heading.

HIGHLIGHTS OF PRESCRIBING INFORMATION
These highlights do not include all the information needed to use APTIVUS safely and effectively. See full prescribing information for APTIVUS.
APTIVUS® (tipranavir) capsules
Initial U.S. Approval: 2005

WARNING: HEPATOTOXICITY and INTRACRANIAL HEMORRHAGE
See full prescribing information for complete boxed warning.
- Clinical hepatitis and hepatic decompensation including some fatalities. Extra vigilance is warranted in patients with chronic hepatitis B or hepatitis C co-infection (5.1)
- Fatal and non-fatal intracranial hemorrhage (5.2)

RECENT MAJOR CHANGES
Indications and Usage (1)	10/2007
Warnings and Precautions	
Hepatic Impairment and Toxicity (5.1)	10/2007
Drug Interactions (5.3)	10/2007
Effects on Platelet Aggregation and Coagulation (5.4)	02/2007
Rash (5.5)	10/2007

INDICATIONS AND USAGE
APTIVUS, a protease inhibitor, co-administered with 200 mg of ritonavir, is indicated for combination antiretroviral treatment of HIV-1 infected adult patients who are treatment-experienced and infected with HIV-1 strains resistant to more than one protease inhibitor (1)
- Do not use APTIVUS/ritonavir in treatment-naïve patients (1)

DOSAGE AND ADMINISTRATION
- 500 mg APTIVUS, co-administered with 200 mg ritonavir, twice daily with food (2)
- Store unopened bottles in the refrigerator (16)

DOSAGE FORMS AND STRENGTHS
Capsules: 250 mg (3)

CONTRAINDICATIONS
- Patients with moderate or severe (Child-Pugh Class B or C) hepatic impairment (4.1, 5.1)
- Use with drugs highly dependent on CYP 3A for clearance or are potent CYP 3A inducers (4.2, 5.3, 7)

WARNINGS AND PRECAUTIONS
- Hepatic Impairment: Discontinue for signs and symptoms of clinical hepatitis or asymptomatic increases in ALT/AST > 10 times ULN or asymptomatic increases in ALT/AST 5–10 times ULN with concomitant increases in total bilirubin. Monitor liver function tests prior to therapy and frequently (5.1).
- Intracranial Hemorrhage/Platelet Aggregation and Coagulation: Use with caution in patients at risk for increased bleeding or who are receiving medications that increase the risk of bleeding (5.2, 5.4).
- Drug Interactions: Consider drug-drug interaction potential to reduce risk of serious or life-threatening adverse reactions (5.3).
- Rash: Discontinue and initiate appropriate treatment if severe skin reaction occurs or is suspected (5.5). Use with caution in patients with a known sulfonamide allergy (5.6).
- Patients may develop new onset or exacerbations of diabetes mellitus, hyperglycemia (5.7), immune reconstitution syndrome (5.8), redistribution/accumulation of body fat (5.9), and elevated lipids (5.10). Monitor cholesterol and triglycerides prior to therapy and periodically thereafter.
- Hemophilia: Spontaneous bleeding may occur, and additional factor VIII may be required (5.11)

Table 1   Drugs that are Contraindicated with APTIVUS Co-Administered with 200 mg of Ritonavir

Drug Class	Drugs within Class that are Contraindicated with APTIVUS Co-administered with 200 mg of Ritonavir	Clinical Comments:
Antiarrhythmics	Amiodarone, bepridil, flecainide, propafenone, quinidine	Potential for serious and/or life-threatening reactions such as cardiac arrhythmias secondary to increases in plasma concentrations of antiarrhythmics.
Antimycobacterials	Rifampin	May lead to loss of virologic response and possible resistance to APTIVUS or to the class of protease inhibitors or other co-administered antiretroviral agents.
Ergot derivatives	Dihydroergotamine, ergonovine, ergotamine, methylergonovine	Potential for acute ergot toxicity characterized by peripheral vasospasm and ischemia of the extremities and other tissues.
GI motility agent	Cisapride	Potential for cardiac arrhythmias.
Herbal Products	St. John's Wort (hypericum perforatum)	May lead to loss of virologic response and possible resistance to APTIVUS or to the class of protease inhibitors.
HMG CoA reductase inhibitors	Lovastatin, simvastatin	Potential for myopathy including rhabdomyolysis.
Neuroleptic	Pimozide	Potential for cardiac arrhythmias.
Sedatives/hypnotics	Midazolam, triazolam	Prolonged or increased sedation or respiratory depression.

ADVERSE REACTIONS
Most frequent adverse reactions (incidence > 4%) were diarrhea, nausea, pyrexia, vomiting, fatigue, headache, and abdominal pain (6)
To report SUSPECTED ADVERSE REACTIONS, contact Boehringer Ingelheim Pharmaceuticals, Inc. at (800) 542-6257 or (800) 459-9906 TTY or FDA at 1-800-FDA-1088 or www.fda.gov/medwatch.

DRUG INTERACTIONS
Coadministration of APTIVUS can alter the concentrations of other drugs and other drugs may alter the concentration of tipranavir. The potential for drug-drug interactions must be considered prior to and during therapy (4.2, 5.3, 7).

USE IN SPECIFIC POPULATIONS
The risk-benefit has not been established in pediatric patients (8.4)
See 17 for PATIENT COUNSELING INFORMATION and FDA-approved patient labeling.

Revised: 10/2007

FULL PRESCRIBING INFORMATION

WARNING: HEPATOTOXICITY and INTRACRANIAL HEMORRHAGE
Hepatotoxicity:
Clinical hepatitis and hepatic decompensation, including some fatalities, have been reported. Extra vigilance is warranted in patients with chronic hepatitis B or hepatitis C co-infection, as these patients have an increased risk of hepatotoxicity [see Warnings and Precautions (5.1)].
Intracranial Hemorrhage:
Both fatal and non-fatal intracranial hemorrhage have been reported [see Warnings and Precautions (5.2)].
---

1 INDICATIONS AND USAGE
APTIVUS (tipranavir), co-administered with 200 mg of ritonavir, is indicated for combination antiretroviral treatment of HIV-1 infected adult patients who are treatment-experienced and infected with HIV-1 strains resistant to more than one protease inhibitor (PI).
This indication is based on analyses of plasma HIV-1 RNA levels in two controlled studies of APTIVUS/ritonavir of 48 weeks duration. Both studies were conducted in clinically advanced, 3-class antiretroviral (NRTI, NNRTI, PI) treatment-experienced adults with evidence of HIV-1 replication despite ongoing antiretroviral therapy.
The following points should be considered when initiating therapy with APTIVUS/ritonavir:
- The use of APTIVUS/ritonavir in treatment-naïve patients is not recommended [see Warnings and Precautions (5.1)].
- The use of other active agents with APTIVUS/ritonavir is associated with a greater likelihood of treatment response [see Clinical Pharmacology (12.4) and Clinical Studies (14)].
- Genotypic or phenotypic testing and/or treatment history should guide the use of APTIVUS/ritonavir [see Clinical Pharmacology (12.4)]. The number of baseline primary protease inhibitor mutations affects the virologic response to APTIVUS/ritonavir [see Clinical Pharmacology (12.4)].
- Use caution when prescribing APTIVUS/ritonavir to patients with elevated transaminases, hepatitis B or C co-infection or patients with mild hepatic impairment [see Warnings and Precautions (5.1)].
- Liver function tests should be performed at initiation of therapy with APTIVUS/ritonavir and monitored frequently throughout the duration of treatment [see Warnings and Precautions (5.1)].
- The drug-drug interaction potential of APTIVUS/ritonavir when co-administered with other drugs must be considered prior to and during APTIVUS/ritonavir use [see Contraindications (4.2) and Drug Interactions (7)].
- Use caution when prescribing APTIVUS/ritonavir in patients who may be at risk for increased bleeding or who are receiving medications known to increase the risk of bleeding [see Warnings and Precautions (5.4)].

Continued on next page

Aptivus—Cont.

• The risk-benefit of APTIVUS/ritonavir has not been established in pediatric patients.

There are no study results demonstrating the effect of APTIVUS/ritonavir on clinical progression of HIV-1.

2 DOSAGE AND ADMINISTRATION

The recommended dose of APTIVUS (tipranavir) capsules is 500 mg (two 250 mg capsules), co-administered with 200 mg of ritonavir, twice daily.

APTIVUS capsules, co-administered with 200 mg of ritonavir should be taken with food. Bioavailability is increased with a high fat meal.

APTIVUS must be co-administered with 200 mg of ritonavir to exert its therapeutic effect. Failure to correctly co-administer APTIVUS with ritonavir will result in plasma levels of tipranavir that will be insufficient to achieve the desired antiviral effect and will alter some drug interactions.

3 DOSAGE FORMS AND STRENGTHS

250 mg, pink, oblong capsules imprinted with TPV 250

4 CONTRAINDICATIONS

4.1 Hepatic Impairment

APTIVUS is contraindicated in patients with moderate or severe (Child-Pugh Class B or C, respectively) hepatic impairment [*see Warnings and Precautions (5.1)*].

4.2 Drug Interactions

Co-administration of APTIVUS with 200 mg of ritonavir with drugs that are highly dependent on CYP 3A for clearance or are potent CYP 3A inducers are contraindicated (See Table 1). These recommendations are based on either drug interaction studies or they are predicted interactions due to the expected magnitude of interaction and potential for serious events or loss of efficacy. For information regarding clinical recommendations *see Drug Interactions (7.2)*.

[See table 1 at top of previous page]

Due to the need for co-administration of APTIVUS with 200 mg of ritonavir, please refer to the ritonavir prescribing information for a description of ritonavir contraindications.

5 WARNINGS AND PRECAUTIONS

Please refer to the ritonavir prescribing information for additional information on precautionary measures.

5.1 Hepatic Impairment and Toxicity

Clinical hepatitis and hepatic decompensation, including some fatalities, were reported with APTIVUS co-administered with 200 mg of ritonavir. These have generally occurred in patients with advanced HIV disease taking multiple concomitant medications. A causal relationship to APTIVUS/ritonavir could not be established. Physicians and patients should be vigilant for the appearance of signs or symptoms of hepatitis, such as fatigue, malaise, anorexia, nausea, jaundice, bilirubinuria, acholic stools, liver tenderness or hepatomegaly. Patients with signs or symptoms of clinical hepatitis should discontinue APTIVUS/ritonavir treatment and seek medical evaluation.

All patients should be followed closely with clinical and laboratory monitoring, especially those with chronic hepatitis B or C co-infection, as these patients have an increased risk of hepatotoxicity. Liver function tests should be performed prior to initiating therapy with APTIVUS/ritonavir, and frequently throughout the duration of treatment.

If asymptomatic elevations in AST or ALT greater than 10 times the upper limit of normal occur, APTIVUS/ritonavir therapy should be discontinued. If asymptomatic elevations in AST or ALT between 5–10 times the upper limit of normal and increases in total bilirubin greater than 2.5 times the upper limit of normal occur, APTIVUS/ritonavir therapy should be discontinued.

Treatment-experienced patients with chronic hepatitis B or hepatitis C co-infection or elevated transaminases are at approximately 2-fold risk for developing Grade 3 or 4 transaminase elevations or hepatic decompensation. In two large, randomized, open-label, controlled clinical trials with an active comparator (1182.12 and 1182.48) of treatment-experienced patients, Grade 3 and 4 increases in hepatic transaminases were observed in 10.3% (10.9/100 PEY) receiving APTIVUS/ritonavir through week 48. In a study of treatment-naïve patients, 20.3% (21/100 PEY) experienced Grade 3 or 4 hepatic transaminase elevations while receiving APTIVUS/ritonavir 500 mg/200 mg through week 48.

Tipranavir is principally metabolized by the liver. Caution should be exercised when administering APTIVUS/ritonavir to patients with mild hepatic impairment (Child-Pugh Class A) because tipranavir concentrations may be increased [*see Clinical Pharmacology (12.3)*].

5.2 Intracranial Hemorrhage

APTIVUS, co-administered with 200 mg of ritonavir, has been associated with reports of both fatal and non-fatal intracranial hemorrhage (ICH). Many of these patients had other medical conditions or were receiving concomitant medications that may have caused or contributed to these events. No pattern of abnormal coagulation parameters has been observed in patients in general, or preceding the development of ICH. Therefore, routine measurement of coagulation parameters is not currently indicated in the management of patients on APTIVUS.

5.3 Drug Interactions

See Table 1 for a listing of contraindicated drugs with APTIVUS due to potentially life-threatening adverse events, significant drug interactions, or due to loss of virologic activity [*see Contraindications (4.2)*].

Table 2 Adverse Reactions Reported in Randomized, Controlled Clinical Trials (1182.12 and 1182.48) Based on Treatment-Emergent Clinical Adverse Reactions of Moderate to Severe Intensity (Grades 2-4) in at least 2% of Treatment-Experienced Subjects in either Treatment Group[a] (48 week Analyses)

	Percentage of patients (rate per 100 patient-exposure years)	
	APTIVUS/ritonavir (500/200 mg BID) + OBR[c] (n=749; 757.4 patient-exposure years)	Comparator PI/ritonavir[b] + OBR (n=737; 503.9 patient-exposure years)
Blood and Lymphatic Disorders		
Anemia	3.3% (3.4)	2.3% (3.4)
Neutropenia	2.0% (2.0)	1.0% (1.4)
Gastrointestinal Disorders		
Diarrhea	15.0% (16.5)	13.4% (21.6)
Nausea	8.5% (9.0)	6.4% (9.7)
Vomiting	5.9% (6.0)	4.1% (6.1)
Abdominal pain	4.4% (4.5)	3.4% (5.1)
Abdominal pain upper	1.5% (1.5)	2.3% (3.4)
General Disorders		
Pyrexia	7.5% (7.7)	5.4% (8.2)
Fatigue	5.7% (5.9)	5.6% (8.4)
Investigations		
Weight decreased	3.1% (3.1)	2.2% (3.2)
ALT increased	2.0% (2.0)	0.5% (0.8)
GGT increased	2.0% (2.0)	0.4% (0.6)
Metabolism and Nutrition Disorders		
Hypertriglyceridemia	3.9% (4.0)	2.0% (3.0)
Hyperlipidemia	2.5% (2.6)	0.8% (1.2)
Dehydration	2.1% (2.1)	1.1% (1.6)
Musculoskeletal and Connective Tissue Disorders		
Myalgia	2.3% (2.3)	1.8% (2.6)
Nervous System Disorders		
Headache	5.2% (5.3)	4.2% (6.3)
Peripheral neuropathy	1.5% (1.5)	2.0% (3.0)
Psychiatric Disorders		
Insomnia	1.7% (1.7)	3.7% (5.5)
Respiratory, Thoracic and Mediastinal Disorders		
Dyspnea	2.1% (2.1)	1.0% (1.4)
Skin and Subcutaneous Tissue Disorders		
Rash	3.1% (3.1)	3.8% (5.7)

[a] Excludes laboratory abnormalities that were Adverse Events

[b] Comparator PI/ritonavir: lopinavir/ritonavir 400/100 mg BID, indinavir/ritonavir 800/100 mg BID, saquinavir/ritonavir 1000/100 mg BID, amprenavir/ritonavir 600/100 mg BID

[c] Optimized Background Regimen

5.4 Effects on Platelet Aggregation and Coagulation

APTIVUS/ritonavir should be used with caution in patients who may be at risk of increased bleeding from trauma, surgery or other medical conditions, or who are receiving medications known to increase the risk of bleeding such as antiplatelet agents and anticoagulants, or who are taking supplemental high doses of vitamin E.

In *in vitro* experiments, tipranavir was observed to inhibit human platelet aggregation at levels consistent with exposures observed in patients receiving APTIVUS/ritonavir.

In rats, co-administration with vitamin E increased the bleeding effects of tipranavir [*see Nonclinical Toxicology (13.2)*].

5.5 Rash

Rash, including urticarial rash, maculopapular rash, and possible photosensitivity, has been reported in subjects receiving APTIVUS/ritonavir. In some cases rash was accompanied by joint pain or stiffness, throat tightness, or generalized pruritus. In controlled clinical trials, rash (all grades, all causality) was observed in 10% of females and in 8% of males receiving APTIVUS/ritonavir through 48 weeks of treatment. The median time to onset of rash was 53 days and the median duration of rash was 22 days. The discontinuation rate for rash in clinical trials was 0.5%. In an uncontrolled compassionate use program (n=3920), cases of rash, some of which were severe, accompanied by myalgia, fever, erythema, desquamation, and mucosal erosions were reported. Discontinue and initiate appropriate treatment if severe skin rash develops.

5.6 Sulfa Allergy

APTIVUS (tipranavir) should be used with caution in patients with a known sulfonamide allergy. Tipranavir contains a sulfonamide moiety. The potential for cross-sensitivity between drugs in the sulfonamide class and APTIVUS is unknown.

5.7 Diabetes Mellitus/Hyperglycemia

New onset diabetes mellitus, exacerbation of pre-existing diabetes mellitus and hyperglycemia have been reported during post-marketing surveillance in HIV-1 infected patients receiving protease inhibitor therapy. Some patients required either initiation or dose adjustments of insulin or oral hypoglycemic agents for treatment of these events. In some cases, diabetic ketoacidosis has occurred. In those patients who discontinued protease inhibitor therapy, hyperglycemia persisted in some cases. Because these events have been reported voluntarily during clinical practice, estimates of frequency cannot be made and a causal relationship between protease inhibitor therapy and these events has not been established.

5.8 Immune Reconstitution Syndrome

Immune reconstitution syndrome has been reported in patients treated with combination antiretroviral therapy, including APTIVUS. During the initial phase of combination antiretroviral treatment, patients whose immune system responds may develop an inflammatory response to indolent or residual opportunistic infections (such as *Mycobacterium avium* infection, cytomegalovirus, *Pneumocystis jiroveci* pneumonia, tuberculosis, or reactivation of herpes simplex and herpes zoster), which may necessitate further evaluation and treatment.

5.9 Fat Redistribution

Redistribution/accumulation of body fat including central obesity, dorsocervical fat enlargement (buffalo hump), peripheral wasting, facial wasting, breast enlargement, and "cushingoid appearance" have been observed in patients receiving antiretroviral therapy. The mechanism and long-term consequences of these events are currently unknown. A causal relationship has not been established.

5.10 Elevated Lipids

Treatment with APTIVUS co-administered with 200 mg of ritonavir has resulted in large increases in the concentration of total cholesterol and triglycerides [*see Adverse Reactions (6)*]. Triglyceride and cholesterol testing should be performed prior to initiating APTIVUS/ritonavir therapy and at periodic intervals during therapy. Lipid disorders should be managed as clinically appropriate, taking into account any potential drug-drug interactions [*see Drug Interactions (7.2)*].

5.11 Patients with Hemophilia

There have been reports of increased bleeding, including spontaneous skin hematomas and hemarthrosis in patients with hemophilia type A and B treated with protease inhibitors. In some patients additional Factor VIII was given. In more than half of the reported cases, treatment with protease inhibitors was continued or reintroduced if treatment had been discontinued. A causal relationship between protease inhibitors and these events has not been established.

5.12 Resistance/Cross Resistance

Because the potential for HIV cross-resistance among protease inhibitors has not been fully explored in APTIVUS/ritonavir treated patients, it is unknown what effect therapy with APTIVUS will have on the activity of subsequently administered protease inhibitors.

6 ADVERSE REACTIONS

The following adverse reactions are discussed in greater detail in other sections of the labeling.

- Hepatic Impairment and Toxicity [*see Warnings and Precautions (5.1)*]
- Intracranial Hemorrhage [*see Warnings and Precautions (5.2)*]

6.1 Clinical Trials Experience

APTIVUS (tipranavir), co-administered with ritonavir, has been studied in a total of 6308 HIV-positive adults as combination therapy in clinical studies. Of these, 1299 treatment-experienced patients received the dose of 500/200 mg BID. Nine hundred nine (909) adults, including 541 in the 1182.12 and 1182.48 controlled clinical trials, have been treated for at least 48 weeks [*see Clinical Studies (14)*]. In 1182.12 and 1182.48 in the APTIVUS/ritonavir arm, the most frequent adverse reactions were diarrhea, nausea, pyrexia, vomiting, fatigue, headache, and abdominal pain. The 48 Week Kaplan-Meier rates of adverse reactions leading to discontinuation were 13.3% for APTIVUS/ritonavir-treated patients and 10.8% for the comparator arm patients.
Due to the need for co-administration of APTIVUS with 200 mg of ritonavir, please refer to ritonavir prescribing information for ritonavir-associated adverse reactions.
Adverse reactions reported in the controlled clinical trials 1182.12 and 1182.48, based on treatment-emergent clinical adverse reactions of moderate to severe intensity (Grades 2 - 4) in at least 2% of treatment-experienced subjects in either treatment group are summarized in Table 2 below.
Because clinical trials are conducted under widely varying conditions. adverse reaction rates observed in the clinical trials of a drug cannot be directly compared to rates in the clinical trials of another drug and may not reflect the rates observed in clinical practice.
[See table 2 at top of previous page]

Less Common Adverse Reactions

Other adverse reactions reported in < 2% of adult patients (n=1474) treated with APTIVUS/ritonavir 500/200 mg in Phase 2 and 3 clinical trials are listed below by body system:
Blood and Lymphatic System Disorders: thrombocytopenia
Gastrointestinal Disorders: abdominal distension, dyspepsia, flatulence, gastroesophageal reflux disease, pancreatitis
General Disorders: influenza like illness, malaise
Hepatobiliary Disorders: hepatitis, hepatic failure, hyperbilirubinemia, cytolytic hepatitis, toxic hepatitis, hepatic steatosis
Immune System Disorders: hypersensitivity
Investigations: hepatic enzymes increased, liver function test abnormal, lipase increased
Metabolism and Nutrition Disorders: anorexia, decreased appetite, diabetes mellitus, facial wasting, hyperamylasemia, hypercholesterolemia, hyperglycemia, mitochondrial toxicity
Musculoskeletal and Connective Tissue Disorders: muscle cramp
Nervous System Disorders: dizziness, intracranial hemorrhage, somnolence
Psychiatric Disorders: sleep disorder
Renal and Urinary Disorders: renal insufficiency
Skin and Subcutaneous System Disorders: exanthem, lipoatrophy, lipodystrophy acquired, lipohypertrophy, pruritus
Laboratory Abnormalities
Treatment emergent laboratory abnormalities reported at 48 weeks in the controlled clinical trials 1182.12 and 1182.48 in adults are summarized in Table 3 below.
[See table 3 above]
In controlled clinical trials 1182.12 and 1182.48 extending up to 96 weeks, the proportion of patients who developed Grade 2-4 ALT and/or AST elevations increased from 26% at week 48 to 32.1% at week 96 with APTIVUS/ritonavir. The risk of developing transaminase elevations is greater during the first year of therapy.

Table 3 Treatment Emergent Laboratory Abnormalities Reported in ≥ 2% of Adult Patients (48 week Analyses)

		Randomized, Controlled Clinical Trials 1182.12 and 1182.48	
		Percentage of patients (rate per 100 patient-exposure years)	
	Limit	APTIVUS/ritonavir (500/200 mg BID) + OBR (n=738)	Comparator PI/ritonavir + OBR* (n=724)
Hematology			
WBC count decrease			
Grade 3	< 2.0 × 10^3/μL	5.4% (5.6)	4.8% (7.7)
Grade 4	< 1.0 × 10^3/μL	0.3% (0.3)	1.1% (1.7)
Chemistry			
Amylase			
Grade 3	> 2.5 × ULN	5.7% (5.9)	6.4% (10.4)
Grade 4	> 5 × ULN	0.3% (0.3)	0.7% (1.1)
ALT			
Grade 2	> 2.5-5 × ULN	14.9% (16.5)	7.5% (12.4)
Grade 3	> 5-10 × ULN	5.6% (5.7)	1.7% (2.6)
Grade 4	> 10 × ULN	4.1% (4.1)	0.4% (0.7)
AST			
Grade 2	> 2.5-5 × ULN	9.9% (10.5)	8.0% (13.3)
Grade 3	> 5-10 × ULN	4.5% (4.6)	1.4% (2.2)
Grade 4	> 10 × ULN	1.6% (1.6)	0.4% (0.6)
ALT and/or AST			
Grade 2-4	> 2.5 × ULN	26.0% (31.5)	13.7% (23.8)
Cholesterol			
Grade 2	> 300-400 mg/dL	15.6% (17.7)	6.4% (10.5)
Grade 3	> 400-500 mg/dL	3.3% (3.3)	0.3% (0.4)
Grade 4	> 500 mg/dL	0.9% (1.0)	0.1% (0.2)
Triglycerides			
Grade 2	400-750 mg/dL	35.9% (49.9)	26.8% (51.0)
Grade 3	> 750-1200 mg/dL	16.9% (19.4)	8.7% (14.6)
Grade 4	> 1200 mg/dL	8.0% (8.4)	4.3% (7.0)

*Comparator PI/ritonavir: lopinavir/ritonavir 400/100 mg BID, indinavir/ritonavir 800/100 mg BID, saquinavir/ritonavir 1000/100 mg BID, amprenavir/ritonavir 600/100 mg BID

7 DRUG INTERACTIONS

See also *Contraindications (4.2), Warnings and Precautions (5.3), and Clinical Pharmacology (12.3).*

7.1 Potential for APTIVUS/ritonavir to Affect Other Drugs

APTIVUS co-administered with 200 mg of ritonavir at the recommended dose is a net inhibitor of CYP 3A and may increase plasma concentrations of agents that are primarily metabolized by CYP 3A. Thus, co-administration of APTIVUS/ritonavir with drugs highly dependent on CYP 3A for clearance and for which elevated plasma concentrations are associated with serious and/or life-threatening events is contraindicated [*see Contraindications (4.2)*]. Co-administration with other CYP 3A substrates may require a dose adjustment or additional monitoring [*see Drug Interactions (7)*].
Clinically significant drug-drug interactions of APTIVUS co-administered with 200 mg of ritonavir are summarized in Table 4 below.
A phenotypic cocktail study was conducted with 16 healthy volunteers to quantify the influence of 10 days of APTIVUS/ritonavir administration on the activity of hepatic CYP 1A2 (caffeine), 2C9 (warfarin), 2C19 (omeprazole), 2D6 (dextromethorphan) and the activity of intestinal and hepatic CYP3A4/5 (midazolam) and P-glycoprotein (P-gp) (digoxin). This study determined the first-dose and steady-state effects of 500 mg of APTIVUS co-administered with 200 mg of ritonavir twice-daily in capsule form.
There was no net effect on CYP2C9 or hepatic P-gp at first dose or steady state. There was no net effect after first dose on CYP1A2, but there was moderate induction at steady state. There was modest inhibition of CYP2C19 at the first dose, but there was marked induction at steady state. Potent inhibition of CYP2D6 and both hepatic and intestinal CYP3A4/5 activities were observed after first dose and steady state.
Intestinal and hepatic P-gp activity was assessed by administering oral and intravenous digoxin, respectively. The digoxin results indicate P-gp was inhibited after the first dose of APTIVUS/ritonavir followed by induction of P-gp over time. Thus, it is difficult to predict the net effect of APTIVUS administered with ritonavir on oral bioavailability and plasma concentrations of drugs that are dual substrates of CYP 3A and P-gp. The net effect will vary depending on the relative affinity of the co-administered drugs for CYP 3A and P-gp, and the extent of intestinal first-pass metabolism/efflux. An *in vitro* induction study in human hepatocytes showed an increase in UGT1A1 by tipranavir similar to that evoked by rifampin. The clinical consequences of this finding have not been established.

7.2 Potential for Other Drugs to Affect Tipranavir

Tipranavir is a CYP 3A substrate and a P-gp substrate. Co-administration of APTIVUS/ritonavir and drugs that induce CYP 3A and/or P-gp may decrease tipranavir plasma concentrations. Co-administration of APTIVUS/ritonavir and drugs that inhibit P-gp may increase tipranavir plasma concentrations. Co-administration of APTIVUS/ritonavir with drugs that inhibit CYP 3A may not further increase tipranavir plasma concentrations, because the level of metabolites is low following steady-state administration of APTIVUS/ritonavir 500/200 mg twice daily.
Clinically significant drug-drug interactions of APTIVUS co-administered with 200 mg of ritonavir are summarized in Table 4 below.
[See table 4 on pages 62 through 64]

8 USE IN SPECIFIC POPULATIONS

8.1 Pregnancy

Teratogenic Effects, Pregnancy Category C.
Investigation of fertility and early embryonic development with tipranavir disodium was performed in rats, teratogenicity studies were performed in rats and rabbits, and pre- and post-natal development were explored in rats.
No teratogenicity was detected in reproductive studies performed in pregnant rats and rabbits up to dose levels of 1000 mg/kg/day and 150 mg/kg/day tipranavir, respectively, at exposure levels approximately 1.1-fold and 0.1-fold human exposure. At 400 mg/kg/day and above in rats, fetal toxicity (decreased sternebrae ossification and body weights) was observed, corresponding to an AUC of 1310 μM·h or approximately 0.8-fold human exposure at the recommended dose. In rats and rabbits, fetal toxicity was not noted at 40 mg/kg/day and 150 mg/kg/day, respectively, corresponding accordingly to $C_{max}/AUC_{0\text{-}24h}$ levels of 30.4 μM/340 μM·h and 8.4 μM/120 μM·h. These exposure levels (AUC) are approximately 0.2-fold and 0.1-fold the exposure in humans at the recommended dose.
In pre- and post-development studies in rats, tipranavir showed no adverse effects at 40 mg/kg/day (~0.2-fold human exposure), but caused growth inhibition in pups and maternal toxicity at dose levels of 400 mg/kg/day (~0.8-fold human exposure). No post-weaning functions were affected at any dose level.
There are no adequate and well-controlled studies in pregnant women for the treatment of HIV-1 infection. APTIVUS should be used during pregnancy only if the potential benefit justifies the potential risk to the fetus.
Antiretroviral Pregnancy Registry
To monitor maternal-fetal outcomes of pregnant women exposed to APTIVUS, an Antiretroviral Pregnancy Registry has been established. Physicians are encouraged to register patients by calling (800) 258-4263.

8.3 Nursing Mothers

The Centers for Disease Control and Prevention recommend that HIV-infected mothers not breastfeed their infants to avoid risking postnatal transmission of HIV. Because of both the potential for HIV transmission and any possible adverse effects of APTIVUS, mothers should be instructed not to breastfeed if they are receiving APTIVUS.

8.4 Pediatric Use

Safety and effectiveness in pediatric patients have not been established.

8.5 Geriatric Use

Clinical studies of APTIVUS/ritonavir did not include sufficient numbers of subjects aged 65 and over to determine whether they respond differently than younger subjects. In general, caution should be exercised in the administration and monitoring of APTIVUS in elderly patients reflecting the greater frequency of decreased hepatic, renal, or cardiac function, and of concomitant disease or other drug therapy.

8.6 Hepatic Impairment

Tipranavir is principally metabolized by the liver. Caution should be exercised when administering APTIVUS/ritonavir to patients with mild (Child-Pugh Class A) hepatic impairment because tipranavir concentrations may be increased [*see Clinical Pharmacology (12.3)*]. APTIVUS/ritonavir is contraindicated in patients with moderate or severe (Child-Pugh Class B or Child-Pugh Class C) hepatic impairment [*see Contraindications (4.1)*].

10 OVERDOSAGE

There is no known antidote for APTIVUS overdose. Treatment of overdose should consist of general supportive measures, including monitoring of vital signs and observation of the patient's clinical status. If indicated, elimination of unabsorbed tipranavir should be achieved by emesis or gastric lavage. Administration of activated charcoal may also be used to aid in removal of unabsorbed drug. Since tipranavir is highly protein bound, dialysis is unlikely to provide significant removal of the drug.

11 DESCRIPTION

APTIVUS is a protease inhibitor of HIV belonging to the class of 4-hydroxy-5,6-dihydro-2-pyrone sulfonamides.
The chemical name of tipranavir is 2-Pyridinesulfonamide, N-[3-[(1R)-1-[(6R)-5,6-dihydro-4-hydroxy-2-oxo-6-(2-phenylethyl)-6-propyl-2H-pyran-3-yl]propyl]phenyl]-5-(trifluoromethyl). It has a molecular formula of $C_{31}H_{33}F_3N_2O_5S$ and a molecular weight of 602.7. Tipranavir has the following structural formula and is a single stereoisomer with the 1R, 6R configuration.
[See chemical structure at top of next column]
Tipranavir is a white to off-white to slightly yellow solid. It is freely soluble in dehydrated alcohol and propylene glycol, and insoluble in aqueous buffer at pH 7.5.

Continued on next page

Aptivus—Cont.

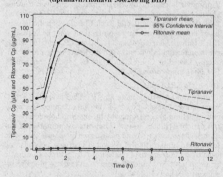

APTIVUS soft gelatin capsules are for oral administration. Each capsule contains 250 mg tipranavir. The major inactive ingredients in the capsule are dehydrated alcohol (7% w/w or 0.1 g per capsule), polyoxyl 35 castor oil, propylene glycol, mono/diglycerides of caprylic/capric acid and gelatin.

12 CLINICAL PHARMACOLOGY

12.1 Mechanism of Action
Tipranavir is an antiviral drug [see *Clinical Pharmacology (12.4)*].

12.2 Pharmacodynamics
Anitviral Activity
The median Inhibitory Quotient (IQ) determined from 264 treatment-experienced patients was about 80 (inter-quartile range: 31-226), from the controlled clinical trials 1182.12 and 1182.48. The IQ is defined as the tipranavir trough concentration divided by the viral EC_{50} value, corrected for protein binding. There was a relationship between the proportion of patients with a $\geq 1 \log_{10}$ reduction of viral load from baseline at week 48 and their IQ value. Among the 198 patients receiving APTIVUS/ritonavir with no new enfuvirtide use (e.g., new enfuvirtide, defined as initiation of enfuvirtide for the first time), the response rate was 23% in those with an IQ value < 80 and 59% in those with an IQ value $\geq$ 80. Among the 66 patients receiving APTIVUS/ritonavir with new enfuvirtide, the response rates in patients with an IQ value < 80 versus those with an IQ value $\geq$ 80 were 55% and 71%, respectively. These IQ groups are derived from a select population and are not meant to represent clinical breakpoints.

12.3 Pharmacokinetics
In order to achieve effective tipranavir plasma concentrations and a twice-daily dosing regimen, co-administration of APTIVUS with 200 mg of ritonavir is essential [see *Dosage and Administration (2)*]. Ritonavir inhibits hepatic cytochrome P450 3A (CYP 3A), the intestinal P-gp efflux pump and possibly intestinal CYP 3A. In a dose-ranging evaluation in 113 HIV-negative male and female volunteers, there was a 29-fold increase in the geometric mean morning steady-state trough plasma concentrations of tipranavir following APTIVUS co-administered with low-dose ritonavir (500/200 mg twice daily) compared to APTIVUS 500 mg twice daily without ritonavir. The mean systemic ritonavir concentration when 200 mg of ritonavir was given with APTIVUS was similar to the concentrations observed when 100 mg was given with the other protease inhibitors. Figure 1 displays mean plasma concentrations of tipranavir and ritonavir at steady state for 30 HIV-infected patients dosed with 500/200 mg tipranavir/ritonavir for 14 days.

Figure 1   **Mean Steady State Tipranavir Plasma Concentrations (95% CI) with Ritonavir Co-administration (tipranavir/ritonavir 500/200 mg BID)**

Absorption and Bioavailability
Absorption of tipranavir in humans is limited, although no absolute quantification of absorption is available. Tipranavir is a P-gp substrate, a weak P-gp inhibitor, and appears to be a potent P-gp inducer as well. *In vivo* data suggest that tipranavir/ritonavir, at the dose of 500/200 mg, is a P-gp inhibitor after the first dose and induction of P-gp occurs over time. Tipranavir trough concentrations at steady-state are about 70% lower than those on Day 1, presumably due to intestinal P-gp induction. Steady state is attained in most subjects after 7-10 days of dosing.
Dosing APTIVUS 500 mg with 200 mg ritonavir twice-daily for greater than 2 weeks and without meal restriction produced the pharmacokinetic parameters for male and female HIV-positive patients presented in Table 5.

Table 4   Established and Other Potentially Significant Drug Interactions: Alterations in Dose or Regimen May be Recommended Based on Drug Interaction Studies or Predicted Interaction

Concomitant Drug Class: Drug name	Effect on Concentration of Tipranavir or Concomitant Drug	Clinical Comment
HIV-Antiviral Agents		
Nucleoside reverse transcriptase inhibitors:		
Abacavir	↓ Abacavir AUC by approximately 40%	Clinical relevance of reduction in abacavir levels not established. Dose adjustment of abacavir cannot be recommended at this time.
Didanosine (EC)	↓ Didanosine	Clinical relevance of reduction in didanosine levels not established. For optimal absorption, didanosine should be separated from APTIVUS/ritonavir dosing by at least 2 hours.
Zidovudine	↓ Zidovudine AUC by approximately 35%. ZDV glucuronide concentrations were unaltered.	Clinical relevance of reduction in zidovudine levels not established. Dose adjustment of zidovudine cannot be recommended at this time.
Protease inhibitors (co-administered with 200 mg of ritonavir):		
Fosamprenavir	↓ Amprenavir,	Combining a protease inhibitor with APTIVUS/ritonavir is not recommended.
Lopinavir	↓ Lopinavir,	
Saquinavir	↓ Saquinavir	
Protease inhibitors (co-administered with 100 mg of ritonavir):		
Atazanavir	↓ Atazanavir, ↑ Tipranavir	
Agents for Opportunistic Infections		
Antifungals:		Fluconazole increases tipranavir concentrations but dose adjustments are not needed. Fluconazole doses > 200 mg/day are not recommended.
Fluconazole	↑ Tipranavir, ↔ Fluconazole	Based on theoretical considerations itraconazole and ketoconazole should be used with caution. High doses (> 200 mg/day) are not recommended.
Itraconazole	↑ Itraconazole (not studied)	
Ketoconazole	↑ Ketoconazole (not studied)	
Voriconazole	↕ Voriconazole (not studied)	Due to multiple enzymes involved with voriconazole metabolism, it is difficult to predict the interaction.
Antimycobacterials:		
Clarithromycin	↑ Tipranavir, ↑ Clarithromycin, ↓ 14-hydroxy-clarithromycin metabolite	No dose adjustment of APTIVUS or clarithromycin for patients with normal renal function is necessary. For patients with renal impairment the following dosage adjustments should be considered: • For patients with CL_{CR} 30 to 60 mL/min the dose of clarithromycin should be reduced by 50%. • For patients with CL_{CR} < 30 mL/min the dose of clarithromycin should be decreased by 75%.
Rifabutin	Tipranavir not changed, ↑ Rifabutin ↑ Desacetyl-rifabutin	Single dose study. Dosage reductions of rifabutin by 75% are recommended (e.g., 150 mg every other day). Increased monitoring for adverse events in patients receiving the combination is warranted. Further dosage reduction may be necessary.

(Table continued on next page)

Table 5   Pharmacokinetic Parameters[a] of tipranavir/ritonavir 500/200 mg for HIV+ Patients by Gender

	Females (n = 14)	Males (n = 106)
$C_{Ptrough}$ (µM)	41.6 ± 24.3	35.6 ± 16.7
C_{max} (µM)	94.8 ± 22.8	77.6 ± 16.6
T_{max} (h)	2.9	3.0
AUC_{0-12h} (µM·h)	851 ± 309	710 ± 207
CL (L/h)	1.15	1.27
V (L)	7.7	10.2
$t_{\frac{1}{2}}$ (h)	5.5	6.0

[a] Population pharmacokinetic parameters reported as mean ± standard deviation

Effects of Food on Oral Absorption
APTIVUS capsules co-administered with ritonavir should be taken with food. Bioavailability is increased with a high fat meal. APTIVUS capsules, administered under high fat meal conditions or with a light snack of toast and skimmed milk, were tested in a multiple dose study. High-fat meals (868 kcal, 53% derived from fat, 31% derived from carbohydrates) enhanced the extent of bioavailability (AUC point estimate 1.31, confidence interval 1.23-1.39), but had minimal effect on peak tipranavir concentrations (C_{max} point estimate 1.16, confidence interval 1.09-1.24).

Distribution
Tipranavir is extensively bound to plasma proteins (> 99.9%). It binds to both human serum albumin and α-1-acid glycoprotein. The mean fraction of tipranavir (dosed without ritonavir) unbound in plasma was similar in clinical samples from healthy volunteers and HIV-positive patients. Total plasma tipranavir concentrations for these samples ranged from 9 to 82 µM. The unbound fraction of tipranavir appeared to be independent of total drug concentration over this concentration range.
No studies have been conducted to determine the distribution of tipranavir into human cerebrospinal fluid or semen.

Metabolism
In vitro metabolism studies with human liver microsomes indicated that CYP 3A4 is the predominant CYP enzyme involved in tipranavir metabolism.
The oral clearance of tipranavir decreased after the addition of ritonavir, which may represent diminished first-pass clearance of the drug at the gastrointestinal tract as well as the liver.

there are no results from controlled studies evaluating the effect of APTIVUS/ritonavir on clinical progression of HIV. *APTIVUS/ritonavir 500/200 mg BID + optimized background regimen (OBR) vs. Comparator Protease Inhibitor/ritonavir BID + OBR*

The two clinical trials 1182.12 and 1182.48 (RESIST 1 and RESIST 2) are ongoing, randomized, controlled, open-label, multicenter studies in HIV-positive, triple antiretroviral class experienced patients. All patients were required to have previously received at least two protease inhibitor-based antiretroviral regimens and were failing a protease inhibitor-based regimen at the time of study entry with baseline HIV-1 RNA at least 1000 copies/mL and any CD4+ cell count. At least one primary protease gene mutation from among 30N, 46I, 46L, 48V, 50V, 82A, 82F, 82L, 82T, 84V or 90M had to be present at baseline, with not more than two mutations at codons 33, 82, 84 or 90.

These studies evaluated treatment response at 48 weeks in a total of 1483 patients receiving either APTIVUS co-administered with 200 mg of ritonavir plus OBR versus a control group receiving a ritonavir-boosted protease inhibitor (lopinavir, amprenavir, saquinavir or indinavir) plus OBR. Prior to randomization, OBR was individually defined for each patient based on genotypic resistance testing and patient history. The investigator had to declare OBR, comparator protease inhibitor, and use of new enfuvirtide prior to randomization. Randomization was stratified by choice of comparator protease inhibitor and use of new enfuvirtide.

After Week 8, patients in the control group who met the protocol defined criteria of initial lack of virologic response or confirmed virologic failure had the option of discontinuing treatment and switching to APTIVUS/ritonavir in a separate roll-over study.

Demographics and baseline characteristics were balanced between the APTIVUS/ritonavir arm and control arm. In both studies combined, the 1483 patients had a median age of 43 years (range 17-80), and were 86.3% male, 75.6% white, 12.9% black, and 0.9% Asian. The median baseline plasma HIV-1 RNA for both treatment groups was 4.8 (range 2.0 to 6.8) $\log_{10}$ copies/mL and median baseline CD4+ cell count was 162 (range 1 to 1894) cells/mm^3. Overall, 38.4% of patients had a baseline HIV-1 RNA of >100,000 copies/mL, 58.6% had a baseline CD4+ cell count $\leq$ 200 cells/mm^3, and 57.8% had experienced an AIDS defining Class C event at baseline.

Patients had prior exposure to a median of 6 NRTIs, 1 NNRTI, and 4 PIs. A total of 10.1% of patients had previously used enfuvirtide. In baseline patient samples (n=454), 97% of the HIV isolates were resistant to at least one protease inhibitor, 95% of the isolates were resistant to at least one NRTI, and > 75% of the isolates were resistant to at least one NNRTI.

The individually pre-selected protease inhibitor based on genotypic testing and the patient's medical history was lopinavir in 48.7%, amprenavir in 26.4%, saquinavir in 21.8% and indinavir in 3.1% of patients. A total of 85.1% were possibly resistant or resistant to the pre-selected comparator protease inhibitors. Approximately 21% of patients used enfuvirtide during the study of which 16.6% in the APTIVUS/ritonavir arm and 13.2% in the comparator/ritonavir arm represented first time use of enfuvirtide (new enfuvirtide). Treatment response and efficacy outcomes of randomized treatment through Week 48 of studies 1182.12 and 1182.48 are shown in Table 11.

[See table 11 at top of page 68]

Through 48 weeks of treatment, the proportion of patients in the APTIVUS/ritonavir arm compared to the comparator PI/ritonavir arm with HIV-1 RNA < 400 copies/mL was 30.3% and 13.6% respectively, and with HIV-1 RNA < 50 copies/mL was 22.7% and 10.2% respectively. Among all randomized and treated patients, the median change from baseline in HIV-1 RNA at the last measurement up to Week 48 was -0.64 $\log_{10}$ copies/mL in patients receiving APTIVUS/ritonavir versus -0.22 $\log_{10}$ copies/mL in the comparator PI/ritonavir arm.

Among all randomized and treated patients, the median change from baseline in CD4+ cell count at the last measurement up to Week 48 was +23 cells/mm^3 in patients receiving APTIVUS/ritonavir (N=740) versus +4 cells/mm^3 in the comparator PI/ritonavir (N=727) arm.

Patients in the APTIVUS/ritonavir arm achieved a significantly better virologic outcome when APTIVUS/ritonavir was combined with enfuvirtide. Among patients with new enfuvirtide use, the proportion of patients in the APTIVUS/ritonavir arm compared to the comparator PI/ritonavir arm with HIV-1 RNA < 400 copies/mL was 52.4 % and 19.6% respectively, and with HIV-1 RNA < 50 copies/mL was 37.3% and 14.4% respectively [*see Clinical Pharmacology (12.2, 12.4)*]. The median change from baseline in CD4+ cell count at the last measurement up to Week 48 was +89 cells/mm^3 in patients receiving APTIVUS/ritonavir in combination with newly introduced enfuvutide (N=124) and +18 cells/mm^3 in the comparator PI/ritonavir (N=96) arm.

16 HOW SUPPLIED/STORAGE AND HANDLING

APTIVUS (tipranavir) capsules 250 mg are pink, oblong soft gelatin capsules imprinted in black with "TPV 250". They are packaged in HDPE unit-of-use bottles with a child resistant closure and 120 capsules. (NDC 0597-0003-02)

Storage

APTIVUS capsules should be **stored in a refrigerator 2°-8°C (36°-46°F)** prior to opening the bottle. After opening the bot-

---

Table 6   Drug Interactions: Pharmacokinetic Parameters for Tipranavir in the Presence of Co-administered Drugs

Co-administered Drug	Co-administered Drug Dose (Schedule)	tipranavir/ ritonavir Drug Dose (Schedule)	n	PK	C_{max}	AUC	C_{min}
					Ratio (90% Confidence Interval) of Tipranavir Pharmacokinetic Parameters with/without Co-administered Drug; No Effect = 1.00		
Antacids (Maalox®)	20 mL (1 dose)	500/200 mg (1 dose)	23	↓	0.75 (0.63, 0.88)	0.73 (0.64, 0.84)	-
Atazanavir/ ritonavir	300/100 mg QD (9 doses)	500/100 mg BID (34 doses)	13	↑	1.08 (0.98, 1.20)	1.20 (1.09, 1.32)	1.75 (1.39, 2.20)
Atorvastatin	10 mg (1 dose)	500/200 mg BID (14 doses)	22	↔	0.96 (0.86, 1.07)	1.08 (1.00, 1.15)	1.04 (0.89, 1.22)
Clarithromycin	500 mg BID (25 doses)	500/200 mg BID*	24 (68)	↑	1.40 (1.24, 1.47)	1.66 (1.43, 1.73)	2.00 (1.58, 2.47)
Didanosine	400 mg (1 dose)	500/100 mg BID (27 doses)	5	↓	1.32 (1.09, 1.60)	1.08 (0.82, 1.42)	0.66 (0.31, 1.43)
Efavirenz	600 mg QD (8 doses)	500/100 mg BID*	21 (89)	↓	0.79 (0.69, 0.89)	0.69 (0.57, 0.83)	0.58 (0.36, 0.86)
		750/200 mg BID*	25 (100)	↔	0.97 (0.85, 1.09)	1.01 (0.85, 1.18)	0.97 (0.69, 1.28)
Ethinyl estradiol/ Norethindrone	0.035/1.0 mg (1 dose)	500/100 mg BID (21 doses)	21	↓	1.10 (0.98, 1.24)	0.98 (0.88, 1.11)	0.73 (0.59, 0.90)
		750/200 mg BID (21 doses)	13	↔	1.01 (0.96, 1.06)	0.98 (0.90, 1.07)	0.91 (0.69, 1.20)
Fluconazole	100 mg QD (12 doses)	500/200 mg BID*	20 (68)	↑	1.32 (1.18, 1.47)	1.50 (1.29, 1.73)	1.69 (1.33, 2.09)
Loperamide	16 mg (1 dose)	750/200 mg BID (21 doses)	24	↓	1.03 (0.92, 1.17)	0.98 (0.86, 1.12)	0.74 (0.62, 0.88)
Rifabutin	150 mg (1 dose)	500/200 mg BID (15 doses)	21	↔	0.99 (0.93, 1.07)	1.00 (0.96, 1.04)	1.16 (1.07, 1.27)
Tadalafil	10 mg (1 dose)	500/200 mg BID (17 doses)	17	↔	0.90 (0.80, 1.01)	0.85 (0.74, 0.97)	0.81 (0.70, 0.94)
Tenofovir	300 mg (1 dose)	500/100 mg BID	22	↓	0.83 (0.74, 0.94)	0.82 (0.75, 0.91)	0.79 (0.70, 0.90)
		750/200 mg BID (23 doses)	20	↔	0.89 (0.84, 0.96)	0.91 (0.85, 0.97)	0.88 (0.78, 1.00)
Zidovudine	300 mg (1 dose)	500/100 mg BID	29	↓	0.87 (0.80, 0.94)	0.82 (0.76, 0.89)	0.77 (0.68, 0.87)
		750/200 mg BID (23 doses)	25	↔	1.02 (0.94, 1.10)	1.02 (0.92, 1.13)	1.07 (0.86, 1.34)

* steady state comparison to historical data (n)
↑ increase, ↓ decrease, ↔ no change, ↕ unable to predict

---

tle, the capsules may be **stored at 25°C (77°F); excursions permitted to 15°-30°C (59°-86°F)** and must be used within 60 days.

Store in a safe place out of the reach of children.

17   PATIENT COUNSELING INFORMATION

See FDA-Approved Patient Labeling (17.9)

17.1   Hepatic Impairment and Toxicity

Patients should be informed that APTIVUS co-administered with 200 mg of ritonavir, has been associated with severe liver disease, including some deaths. Patients with signs or symptoms of clinical hepatitis should discontinue APTIVUS/ritonavir treatment and seek medical evaluation. Symptoms of hepatitis include fatigue, malaise, anorexia, nausea, jaundice, bilirubinuria, acholic stools, liver tenderness or hepatomegaly. Extra vigilance is needed for patients with chronic hepatitis B or C co-infection, as these patients have an increased risk of developing hepatotoxicity.

Liver function tests should be performed prior to initiating therapy with APTIVUS and 200 mg of ritonavir, and frequently throughout the duration of treatment. Patients with chronic hepatitis B or C co-infection or elevations in liver enzymes prior to treatment are at increased risk (approximately 2-fold) for developing further liver enzyme elevations or severe liver disease. Caution should be exercised when administering APTIVUS/ritonavir to patients with liver enzyme abnormalities or history of chronic liver disease. Increased liver function testing is warranted in these patients. APTIVUS should not be given to patients with moderate to severe hepatic impairment.

17.2   Intracranial Hemorrhage

Patients should be informed that APTIVUS co-administered with 200 mg of ritonavir has been associated with reports of both fatal and non-fatal intracranial hemorrhage. Patients should report any unusual or unexplained bleeding to their physician.

17.3   Drug Interactions

APTIVUS may interact with some drugs; therefore, patients should be advised to report to their health care provider the use of any other prescription or non-prescription medications or herbal products, particularly St. John's wort.

17.4   Rash

Rash, including flat or raised rashes or sensitivity to the sun, have been reported in approximately 10% of subjects receiving APTIVUS. Some patients who developed rash also had one or more of the following symptoms: joint pain or stiffness, throat tightness, generalized itching, muscle aches, fever, redness, blisters, or peeling of the skin. Women taking birth control pills may get a skin rash. Patients should be told to discontinue use of APTIVUS and call their physician right away if any of these symptoms develop.

17.5   Sulfa Allergy

Patients should be told to report any history of sulfonamide allergy to the physician.

17.6   Contraceptives

Women receiving estrogen-based hormonal contraceptives should be instructed that additional or alternative contraceptive measures should be used during therapy with APTIVUS/ritonavir. There may be an increased risk of rash when APTIVUS is given with hormonal contraceptives.

17.7   Fat Redistribution

Patients should be informed that redistribution or accumulation of body fat may occur in patients receiving antiretroviral therapy and that the cause and long-term health effects of these conditions are not known at this time.

17.8   Administration

Patients should be informed that APTIVUS must be co-administered with 200 mg ritonavir to ensure its therapeu-

Continued on next page

Table 7   Drug Interactions: Pharmacokinetic Parameters for Co-administered Drug in the Presence of APTIVUS/Ritonavir

Co-administered Drug	Co-administered Drug Dose (Schedule)	tipranavir/ritonavir Drug Dose (Schedule)	n	PK	C_{max}	AUC	C_{min}
Amprenavir/ritonavir[a]	600/100 mg BID (27 doses)	500/200 mg BID (28 doses)	16 74	↓ ↓	0.61 (0.51, 0.73)[d]	0.56 (0.49, 0.64)[d]	0.45 (0.38, 0.53)[d] 0.44 (0.39, 0.49)[e]
Abacavir[a]	300 mg BID (43 doses)	250/200 mg BID 750/100 mg BID 1250/100 mg BID (42 doses)	28 14 11	↓ ↓ ↓	0.56 (0.48, 0.66) 0.54 (0.47, 0.63) 0.48 (0.42, 0.53)	0.56 (0.49, 0.63) 0.64 (0.55, 0.74) 0.65 (0.55, 0.76)	- - -
Atazanavir/ritonavir	300/100 mg QD (9 doses)	500/100 mg BID (34 doses)	13	↓	0.43 (0.38, 0.50)	0.32 (0.29, 0.36)	0.19 (0.15, 0.24)
Atorvastatin	10 mg (1 dose)	500/200 mg BID (17 doses)	22	↑	8.61 (7.25, 10.21)	9.36 (8.02, 10.94)	5.19 (4.21, 6.40)
Orthohydroxy-atorvastatin			21, 12, 17	↓	0.02 (0.02, 0.03)	0.11 (0.08, 0.17)	0.07 (0.06, 0.08)
Parahydroxy-atorvastatin			13, 22, 1	↓	1.04 (0.87, 1.25)	0.18 (0.14, 0.24)	0.33 (NA)
Carbamazepine	100 mg BID (29 doses) (43 doses) 200 mg BID (29 doses) (43 doses)	500/200 mg (1 dose) (15 doses) 500/200 mg (1 dose) (15 doses)	7 7 17 17	↔ ↔ ↔ ↑	1.04 (1.00, 1.07) 1.10 (0.85, 1.42) 1.00 (0.96, 1.04) 1.22 (1.11, 1.34)	1.05 (1.02, 1.09) 1.08 (0.91, 1.27) 1.04 (1.00, 1.08) 1.26 (1.15, 1.38)	1.17 (1.11, 1.24) 1.07 (0.90–1.27) 1.16 (1.11, 1.22) 1.35 (1.22, 1.50)
Clarithromycin	500 mg BID (25 doses)	500/200 mg BID (15 doses)	21	↑	0.95 (0.83, 1.09)	1.19 (1.04, 1.37)	1.68 (1.42, 1.98)
14-OH-clarithromycin			21	↓	0.03 (0.02, 0.04)	0.03 (0.02, 0.04)	0.05 (0.04, 0.07)
Didanosine[b]	200 mg BID, ≥ 60 kg 125 mg BID, < 60 kg (43 doses)	250/200 mg BID 750/100 mg BID 1250/100 mg BID (42 doses)	10 8 9	↓ ↔ ↔	0.57 (0.42, 0.79) 0.76 (0.49, 1.17) 0.77 (0.47, 1.26)	0.67 (0.51, 0.88) 0.97 (0.64, 1.47) 0.87 (0.47, 1.65)	- - -
	400 mg (1 dose)	500/100 mg BID (27 doses)	5	↔	0.80 (0.63, 1.02)	0.90 (0.72, 1.11)	1.17 (0.62, 2.20)
Efavirenz[b]	600 mg QD (15 doses)	500/100 mg BID 750/200 mg BID (15 doses)	24 22	↔ ↔	1.09 (0.99, 1.19) 1.12 (0.98, 1.28)	1.04 (0.97, 1.12) 1.00 (0.93, 1.09)	1.02 (0.92, 1.12) 0.94 (0.84, 1.04)
Ethinyl estradiol	0.035 mg (1 dose)	500/100 mg BID 750/200 mg BID (21 doses)	21 13	↓ ↓	0.52 (0.47, 0.57) 0.48 (0.42, 0.57)	0.52 (0.48, 0.56) 0.57 (0.54, 0.60)	- -
Fluconazole	200 mg (Day 1) then 100 mg QD (6 or 12 doses)	500/200 mg BID (2 or 14 doses)	19 19	↔ ↔	0.97 (0.94, 1.01) 0.94 (0.91, 0.98)	0.99 (0.97, 1.02) 0.92 (0.88, 0.95)	0.98 (0.94, 1.02) 0.89 (0.85, 0.92)
Lopinavir/ritonavir[a]	400/100 mg BID (27 doses)	500/200 mg BID (28 doses)	21 69	↓ ↓	0.53 (0.40, 0.69)[d]	0.45 (0.32, 0.63)[d]	0.30 (0.17, 0.51)[d] 0.48 (0.40, 0.58)[e]
Loperamide	16 mg (1 dose)	750/200 mg BID (21 doses)	24	↓	0.39 (0.31, 0.48)	0.49 (0.40, 0.61)	
N-Demethyl-Loperamide			24	↓	0.21 (0.17, 0.25)	0.23 (0.19, 0.27)	
Lamivudine[a]	150 mg BID (43 doses)	250/200 mg BID 750/100 mg BID 1250/100 mg BID (42 doses)	64 46 35	↔ ↔ ↔	0.96 (0.89, 1.03) 0.86 (0.78, 0.94) 0.71 (0.62, 0.81)	0.95 (0.89, 1.02) 0.96 (0.90, 1.03) 0.82 (0.66, 1.00)	- - -
Methadone	5 mg (1 dose)	500/200 mg BID (16 doses)	14	↓	0.45 (0.41, 0.49)	0.47 (0.44, 0.51)	0.50 (0.46, 0.54)
R-methadone S-methadone					0.54 (0.50, 0.58) 0.38 (0.35, 0.43)	0.52 (0.49, 0.56) 0.37 (0.34, 0.41)	
Nevirapine[a]	200 mg BID (43 doses)	250/200 mg BID 750/100 mg BID 1250/100 mg BID (42 doses)	26 22 17	↔ ↔ ↔	0.97 (0.90, 1.04) 0.86 (0.76, 0.97) 0.71 (0.62, 0.82)	0.97 (0.91, 1.04) 0.89 (0.78, 1.01) 0.76 (0.63, 0.91)	0.96 (0.87, 1.05) 0.93 (0.80, 1.08) 0.77 (0.64, 0.92)
Norethindrone	1.0 mg (1 dose)	500/100 mg BID 750/200 mg BID (21 doses)	21 13	↔ ↔	1.03 (0.94, 1.13) 1.08 (0.97, 1.20)	1.14 (1.06, 1.22) 1.27 (1.13, 1.43)	- -

(Table continued on next page)

Aptivus—Cont.

tic effect. Failure to correctly co-administer APTIVUS with ritonavir will result in reduced plasma levels of tipranavir that may be insufficient to achieve the desired antiviral effect.

Patients should be told that sustained decreases in plasma HIV-1 RNA have been associated with a reduced risk of progression to AIDS and death. Patients should remain under the care of a physician while using APTIVUS. Patients should be advised to take APTIVUS and other concomitant antiretroviral therapy every day as prescribed. APTIVUS, co-administered with ritonavir, must be given in combination with other antiretroviral drugs. Patients should not alter the dose or discontinue therapy without consulting with their healthcare professional. If a dose of APTIVUS is

missed, patients should take the dose as soon as possible and then return to their normal schedule. However, if a dose is skipped the patient should not double the next dose.

Patients should be informed that APTIVUS is not a cure for HIV-1 infection and that they may continue to develop opportunistic infections and other complications associated with HIV disease. The long-term effects of APTIVUS are unknown at this time. Patients should be told that there are currently no data demonstrating that therapy with APTIVUS can reduce the risk of transmitting HIV to others through sexual contact.

APTIVUS should be taken with food to enhance absorption.

17.9   FDA-Approved Patient Labeling

Read the Patient Information that comes with APTIVUS before you start taking it and each time you get a refill. There may be new information. This leaflet does not take the place

of talking with your healthcare professional about your medical condition or treatment. You should stay under a healthcare professional's care while taking APTIVUS.

What is the most important information I should know about APTIVUS?

Patients taking APTIVUS, together with 200 mg NORVIR® (ritonavir), may develop severe liver disease that can cause death. If you develop any of the following symptoms of liver problems, you should stop taking APTIVUS and NORVIR® (ritonavir) and call your healthcare professional right away: tiredness, general ill feeling or "flu-like" symptoms, loss of appetite, nausea (feeling sick to your stomach), yellowing of your skin or whites of your eyes, dark (tea-colored) urine, pale stools (bowel movements), or pain, ache, or sensitivity on your right side below your ribs. If you have chronic hepatitis B or C infection, your health-

Table 7 *(cont.)* Drug Interactions: Pharmacokinetic Parameters for Co-administered Drug in the Presence of APTIVUS/Ritonavir

Co-administered Drug	Co-administered Drug Dose (Schedule)	tipranavir/ritonavir Drug Dose (Schedule)	n	PK	Ratio (90% Confidence Interval) of Co-administered Drug Pharmacokinetic Parameters with/without tipranavir/ritonavir; No Effect = 1.00		
					C_{max}	AUC	C_{min}
Rifabutin	150 mg (1 dose)	500/200 mg BID (15 doses)	20	↑	1.70 (1.49, 1.94)	2.90 (2.59, 3.26)	2.14 (1.90, 2.41)
25-O-desacetyl-rifabutin			20	↑	3.20 (2.78, 3.68)	20.71 (17.66, 24.28)	7.83 (6.70, 9.14)
Rifabutin + 25-O-desacetyl-rifabutin[c]			20	↑	1.86 (1.63, 2.12)	4.33 (3.86, 4.86)	2.76 (2.44, 3.12)
Saquinavir/ritonavir[a]	600/100 mg BID (27 doses)	500/200 mg BID (28 doses)	20	↓	0.30 (0.23, 0.40)[d]	0.24 (0.19, 0.32)[d]	0.18 (0.13, 0.26)[d]
			68	↓			0.20 (0.16, 0.25)[e]
Stavudine[a]	40 mg BID, ≥ 60 kg	250/200 mg BID	26	↔	0.90 (0.81, 1.02)	1.00 (0.91, 1.11)	
	30 mg BID, < 60 kg	750/100 mg BID	22	↔	0.76 (0.66, 0.89)	0.84 (0.74, 0.96)	
	(43 doses)	1250/100 mg BID (42 doses)	19	↔	0.74 (0.69, 0.80)	0.93 (0.83, 1.05)	
Tadalafil	10 mg (1 dose)	500/200 mg (1 dose)	17	↑	0.78 (0.72, 0.84)	2.33 (2.02, 2.69)	
	10 mg (1 dose)	500/200 mg BID (17 doses)	17	↔	0.70 (0.63, 0.78)	1.01 (0.83, 1.21)	
Tenofovir	300 mg (1 dose)	500/100 mg BID	22	↓	0.77 (0.68, 0.87)	0.98 (0.91, 1.05)	1.07 (0.98, 1.17)
		750/100 mg BID (23 doses)	20	↓	0.62 (0.54, 0.71)	1.02 (0.94, 1.10)	1.14 (1.01, 1.27)
Zidovudine[b]	300 mg BID	250/200 mg BID	48	↓	0.54 (0.47, 0.62)	0.58 (0.51, 0.66)	-
	300 mg BID	750/100 mg BID	31	↓	0.51 (0.44, 0.60)	0.64 (0.55, 0.75)	-
	300 mg BID (43 doses)	1250/100 mg BID (42 doses)	23	↓	0.49 (0.40, 0.59)	0.69 (0.49, 0.97)	-
	300 mg (1 dose)	500/100 mg BID	29	↓	0.39 (0.33, 0.45)	0.57 (0.52, 0.63)	0.89 (0.81, 0.99)
		750/100 mg BID (23 doses)	25	↔	0.44 (0.36, 0.54)	0.67 (0.62, 0.73)	1.25 (1.08, 1.44)
Zidovudine glucuronide		500/100 mg BID	29	↑	0.82 (0.74, 0.90)	1.02 (0.97, 1.06)	1.52 (1.34, 1.71)
		750/200 mg BID (23 doses)	25	↑	0.82 (0.73, 0.92)	1.09 (1.05, 1.14)	1.94 (1.62, 2.31)

[a] HIV+ patients
[b] HIV+ patients (tipranavir/ritonavir 250 mg/200 mg, 750 mg/200 mg and 1250 mg/100 mg) and healthy volunteers (tipranavir/ritonavir 500 mg/100 mg and 750 mg/200 mg)
[c] Normalized sum of parent drug (rifabutin) and active metabolite (25-O-desacetyl-rifabutin)
[d] Intensive PK analysis
[e] Drug levels obtained at 8-16 hrs post-dose
↑ increase, ↓ decrease, ↔ no change, ↕ unable to predict

care professional should check your blood tests more often because you have an increased chance of developing liver problems.

Patients taking APTIVUS together with 200 mg NORVIR® (ritonavir) may develop bleeding in the brain that can cause death.
You should report any unusual or unexplained bleeding to your healthcare professional if you are taking APTIVUS together with 200 mg of NORVIR® (ritonavir).

What is APTIVUS?
APTIVUS is a medicine called a "protease inhibitor" that is used to treat adults with Human Immunodeficiency Virus (HIV). APTIVUS blocks HIV protease, an enzyme which is needed for HIV to make more virus. When used with other anti-HIV medicines, APTIVUS may reduce the amount of HIV in your blood and increase the number of CD4+ cells. Reducing the amount of HIV in the blood may keep your immune system healthy, so it can help fight infections. APTIVUS is always taken with NORVIR® (ritonavir) and at the same time as NORVIR. When you take APTIVUS with NORVIR, you must always use at least 2 other anti-HIV medicines.

Does APTIVUS cure HIV or AIDS?
APTIVUS does not cure HIV infection or AIDS. The long-term effects of APTIVUS are not known at this time. People taking APTIVUS may still get infections or other conditions common in people with HIV (opportunistic infections). It is very important that you stay under the care of your doctor during treatment with APTIVUS.

Does APTIVUS lower the chance of passing HIV to other people?
APTIVUS does not reduce the chance of passing HIV to others through sexual contact, sharing needles, or being exposed to your blood. Continue to practice safer sex. Use a latex or polyurethane condom or other barrier method to lower the chance of sexual contact with any body fluids such as semen, vaginal secretions or blood. Never use or share dirty needles.
Ask your healthcare professional if you have any questions about safer sex or how to prevent passing HIV to other people.

Who should not take APTIVUS?
Do not take APTIVUS if you:
• are allergic to tipranavir or any of the other ingredients in APTIVUS. See the end of this leaflet for a list of major ingredients.
• are allergic to NORVIR® (ritonavir)
• have moderate to severe liver problems
• take any of the following types of medicines because **you could have serious side effects:**

◦ Migraine headache medicines called "ergot alkaloids". If you take migraine headache medicines, ask your healthcare professional or pharmacist if any of them are "ergot alkaloids".
◦ Halcion® (triazolam)
◦ Orap® (pimozide)
◦ Propulsid® (cisapride)
◦ Versed® (midazolam)
◦ Pacenone® (amiodarone)
◦ Vascor® (bepridil)
◦ Tambocor® (flecainide)
◦ Rythmol® (propafenone)
◦ Quinaglute dura® (quinidine)
◦ Zocor® (simvastatin)
◦ Mevacor® (lovastatin)
• take St. John's Wort or Rifampin. It may result in reduced virologic activity and possible resistance to tipranavir or to the class of protease inhibitors.

What should I tell my healthcare professional before I take APTIVUS?
Tell your healthcare professional about all of your medical conditions, including if you:
• **have hemophilia** or another medical condition that increases your chance of bleeding, or are taking medicines which increase your chance of bleeding. These patients may have an increased chance of bleeding.
• **have liver problems** or are infected with hepatitis B or hepatitis C. These patients may have worsening of their liver disease.
• **are allergic to sulfa medicines.**
• **have diabetes.** APTIVUS may worsen diabetes or high blood sugar levels.
• **are pregnant or planning to become pregnant.** It is not known if APTIVUS can harm your unborn baby. You and your healthcare professional will need to decide if APTIVUS is right for you. If you take APTIVUS while you are pregnant, talk to your healthcare professional about how you can be in the Antiretroviral Pregnancy Registry.
• **are breast-feeding.** Do not breast-feed if you are taking APTIVUS. You should not breast-feed if you have HIV because of the chance of passing the HIV virus to your baby. Talk with your healthcare professional about the best way to feed your baby.
• **are using estrogens for birth control or hormone replacement.** Women who use estrogens for birth control or hormone replacement have an increased chance of developing a skin rash while taking APTIVUS. If a rash occurs, it is usually mild to moderate, but you should talk to your healthcare professional as you may need to temporarily stop taking either APTIVUS or the other medicine that contains estrogen or female hormones.

Tell your healthcare professional about all the medicines you take including prescription and nonprescription medicines, vitamins and herbal supplements. APTIVUS and many other medicines can interact. Sometimes serious side effects will happen if APTIVUS is taken with certain other medicines (see "Who should not take APTIVUS?").
• Some medicines cannot be taken at all with APTIVUS.
• Some medicines will require a change in dosage if taken with APTIVUS.
• Some medicines will require close monitoring if taken with APTIVUS.
Do not take Flonase®, Viagra®, Cialis®, or Levitra® with Aptivus/ritonavir without first speaking with your healthcare professional.
Women taking birth control pills need to use another birth control method. APTIVUS makes birth control pills work less well.
Know all the medicines you take and keep a list of them with you. Show this list to all your healthcare professionals and pharmacists anytime you get a new medicine you take. They will tell you if you can take these other medicines with APTIVUS. **Do not start any new medicines while you are taking APTIVUS without first talking with your healthcare professional or pharmacist.** You can ask your healthcare professional or pharmacist for a list of medicines that can interact with APTIVUS.

How should I take APTIVUS?
• Take APTIVUS exactly as your healthcare professional has prescribed. You should check with your healthcare professional or pharmacist if you are not sure. **You must take APTIVUS at the same time as NORVIR® (ritonavir).** The usual dose is 500 mg (two 250 mg capsules) of APTIVUS, together with 200 mg (two 100 mg capsules or 2.5 mL of solution) of NORVIR, twice per day. APTIVUS with NORVIR must be used together with other anti-HIV medicines.
APTIVUS comes in a capsule form and you should **swallow APTIVUS capsules whole. Do not chew the capsules.**
• You should take APTIVUS with food.
• Do not change your dose or stop taking APTIVUS without first talking with your healthcare professional.
• If you take too much APTIVUS, call your healthcare professional or poison control center right away.
• If you forget to take APTIVUS, take the next dose of APTIVUS, together with NORVIR® (ritonavir), as soon as possible. Do not take a double dose to make up for a missed dose.
• It is very important to take all your anti-HIV medicines as prescribed and at the right times of day. This can help

Continued on next page

Aptivus—Cont.

your medicines work better. It also lowers the chance that your medicines will stop working to fight HIV (drug resistance).

- When your APTIVUS® supply starts to run low, get more from your healthcare professional or pharmacy. This is very important because the amount of virus in your blood may increase if the medicine is stopped for even a short period of time. The HIV virus may develop resistance to APTIVUS and become harder to treat. You should NEVER stop taking APTIVUS or your other HIV medicines without talking with your healthcare professional.

What are the possible side effects of APTIVUS?
APTIVUS may cause serious side effects, including:

- **liver problems, including liver failure and death.** Your healthcare professional should do blood tests to monitor your liver function during treatment with APTIVUS. Patients with liver diseases such as hepatitis B and hepatitis C may have worsening of their liver disease with APTIVUS and should have more frequent monitoring of blood tests.

- **bleeding in the brain.** This has occurred in patients treated with APTIVUS in clinical trials and can lead to permanent disability or death. Many of the patients experiencing bleeding in the brain had other medical conditions or were receiving other medications that may have caused or added to bleeding in the brain. Patients with hemophilia or another medical condition that increases the chance of bleeding, or patients taking medicines that may cause bleeding in the brain may have an increased chance of bleeding in the brain.

- **rash.** Rash, including flat or raised rashes or sensitivity to the sun, have been reported in approximately 10% of subjects receiving APTIVUS. Some patients who developed rash also had one or more of the following symptoms: joint pain or stiffness, throat tightness, generalized itching, muscle aches, fever, redness, blisters, or peeling of the skin. Women taking birth control pills may get a skin rash. If you develop any of these symptoms, stop using APTIVUS and call your healthcare professional right away.

- **increased bleeding in patients with hemophilia.** This can happen in patients taking APTIVUS or other protease inhibitor medicines.

- **diabetes and high blood sugar (hyperglycemia).** This can happen in patients taking APTIVUS or other protease inhibitor medicines. Some patients have diabetes before starting treatment with APTIVUS which gets worse. Some patients get diabetes during treatment with APTIVUS. Some patients will need changes in their diabetes medicine. Some patients will need new diabetes medicine.

- **increased blood fat (lipid) levels.** Your healthcare professional should do blood tests to monitor your blood fat (triglycerides and cholesterol) during treatment with APTIVUS. Some patients taking APTIVUS have large increases in triglycerides and cholesterol. The long-term chance of having a heart attack or stroke due to increases in blood fats caused by APTIVUS is not known at this time.

- **changes in body fat.** These changes have happened in patients taking APTIVUS and other anti-HIV medicines. The changes may include an increased amount of fat in the upper back and neck ("buffalo hump"), breast, and around the back, chest, and stomach area. Loss of fat from the legs, arms, and face may also happen. The cause and long-term health effects of these conditions are not known.

The most common side effects of APTIVUS include diarrhea, nausea, headache, fever, vomiting, tiredness, and stomach pain.

It may be hard to tell the difference between side effects caused by APTIVUS, by the other medicines you are also taking, or by the complications of HIV infection. For this reason it is very important that you tell your healthcare professional about any changes in your health. You should report any new or continuing symptoms to your healthcare professional right away. Your healthcare professional may be able to help you manage these side effects.

The list of side effects is **not** complete. Ask your healthcare professional or pharmacist for more information.

How should I store APTIVUS?

- Store APTIVUS capsules in a refrigerator at approximately **36°F to 46°F (2°C to 8°C).** Once the bottle is opened, the contents must be used within 60 days. Patients may take the bottle with them for use away from home so long as the bottle remains at a temperature of approximately **59°F to 86°F (15°C to 30°C).** You can write the date of opening the bottle on the label. Do not use after the expiration date written on the bottle.

- Keep APTIVUS and all medicines out of the reach of children.

General advice about APTIVUS
Medicines are sometimes prescribed for purposes other than those listed in a Patient Information leaflet. Do not use APTIVUS for a condition for which it was not prescribed. Do not give APTIVUS to other people, even if they have the same condition you have. It may harm them.

Table 8 Controlled Clinical Trials 1182.12 and 1182.48: Proportion of Responders (confirmed ≥ 1 log_{10} decrease at Week 48) by Number of Baseline Primary Protease Inhibitor (PI) Resistance Associated Substitutions

Number of Baseline Primary PI Mutations[a]	APTIVUS/ritonavir N = 578		Comparator PI/ritonavir N = 610	
	No New Enfuvirtide[b]	+ New Enfuvirtide[c]	No New Enfuvirtide[b]	+ New Enfuvirtide[c]
Overall	38% (180/470)	69% (75/108)	18% (92/524)	26% (22/86)
1-2	62% (24/39)	60% (3/5)	33% (14/43)	0% (0/1)
3-4	48% (96/202)	71% (27/38)	23% (45/193)	38% (13/34)
5+	26% (60/229)	69% (45/65)	11% (33/288)	18% (9/51)

[a] Primary PI mutations include any amino acid substitution at positions 30, 32, 36, 46, 47, 48, 50, 53, 54, 82, 84, 88 and 90
[b] No new enfuvirtide is defined as recycled or continued use of enfuvirtide or no use of enfuvirtide
[c] New enfuvirtide is defined as initiation of enfuvirtide for the first time

Table 9 Response by Baseline Tipranavir Phenotype at 48 weeks in the Controlled Clinical Trials 1182.12 and 1182.48

Baseline Tipranavir Phenotype (Fold Change)[a]	Proportion of Responders[b] with No New Enfuvirtide[c] Use N=211	Proportion of Responders[b] with New Enfuvirtide[d] Use N=68	Tipranavir Susceptibility
0-3	48% (73/153)	70% (33/47)	Susceptible
> 3-10	21% (10/48)	53% (8/15)	Decreased Susceptibility
> 10	10% (1/10)	50% (3/6)	Resistant

[a] Change in tipranavir EC_{50} value from wild-type reference
[b] Confirmed ≥ 1 log_{10} decrease at Week 48
[c] No new enfuvirtide is defined as recycled or continued use of enfuvirtide or no use of enfuvirtide
[d] New enfuvirtide is defined as initiation of enfuvirtide for the first time

Table 10 Correlation of Baseline Tipranavir Phenotype to Genotype using HIV isolates from Phase 2 and Phase 3 Clinical Trials

Baseline Tipranavir Phenotype (Fold Change)[a]	# of Baseline Protease Mutations at 33, 82, 84, 90	# of Baseline Tipranavir Resistance-Associated Mutations[b]	Tipranavir Susceptibility[c]
0-3	0-2	0-4	Susceptible
> 3-10	3	5-7	Decreased Susceptibility
> 10	4	8+	Resistant

[a] Change in tipranavir EC_{50} value from wild-type reference
[b] Number of amino acid substitutions in HIV protease among L10V, I13V, K20M/R/V, L33F, E35G, M36I, K43T, M46L, I47V, I54A/M/V, Q58E, H69K, T74P, V82L/T, N83D or I84V
[c] defined by week 48 response

Table 11 Outcomes of Randomized Treatment Through Week 48 (Pooled Studies 1182.12 and 1182.48)

Outcome	APTIVUS/ritonavir (500/200 mg BID) + OBR (N=746)	Comparator Protease Inhibitor*/ritonavir + OBR (N=737)
Virologic Responders[a] (confirmed at least 1 log_{10} HIV-1 RNA below baseline)	33.8%	14.9%
Virologic failures	55.1%	77.3%
Initial lack of virologic response by Week 8[b]	33.0%	57.9%
Rebound	18.9%	16.4%
Never suppressed	3.2%	3.0%
Death[c] or discontinued due to adverse events	5.9%	1.9%
Death	0.5%	0.3%
Discontinued due to adverse events	5.4%	1.6%
Discontinued due to other reasons[d]	5.2%	5.8%

*Comparator protease inhibitors were lopinavir, amprenavir, saquinavir or indinavir and 85.1% of patients were possibly resistant or resistant to the chosen protease inhibitors.
[a] Patients achieved and maintained a confirmed ≥ 1 log_{10} HIV-1 RNA drop from baseline through Week 48 without prior evidence of treatment failure.
[b] Patients did not achieve a 0.5 log_{10} HIV-1 RNA drop from baseline and did not have viral load < 100,000 copies/mL by Week 8.
[c] Death only counted if it was the reason for treatment failure.
[d] Includes patients who were lost to-follow-up, withdrawn consent, non-adherent, protocol violations, added/changed background antiretroviral drugs for reasons other than tolerability or toxicity, or discontinued while suppressed.

This leaflet summarizes the most important information about APTIVUS. If you would like more information, talk with your healthcare professional. You can ask your pharmacist or healthcare professional for information about APTIVUS that is written for health professionals.
For additional information, you may also call Boehringer Ingelheim Pharmaceuticals, Inc. at 1-800-542-6257, or (TTY) 1-800-459-9906.

What are the ingredients in APTIVUS?
Active Ingredient: tipranavir
Major Inactive Ingredients: dehydrated alcohol, polyoxyl 35 castor oil, propylene glycol, mono/diglycerides of caprylic/capric acid and gelatin.
Distributed by:
Boehringer Ingelheim Pharmaceuticals, Inc.
Ridgefield, CT 06877 USA

APTIVUS® is a registered trademark used under license from Boehringer Ingelheim International GmbH

APTIVUS capsules are covered by U.S. Patents 5,852,195; 6,147,095; 6,169,181 and 6,231,887
OT2000FJ0307 10003515/US/5 10003515/05

FLOMAX® ℞
[flō-măx]
(tamsulosin hydrochloride)
Capsules, 0.4 mg
Rx only

Prescribing information for this product, which appears on pages 840–844 of the 2008 PDR, has been completely revised as follows. Please write "See Supplement A" next to the product heading.

Prescribing Information

DESCRIPTION

Tamsulosin hydrochloride is an antagonist of alpha$_{1A}$ adrenoceptors in the prostate.

Tamsulosin hydrochloride is (-)-(*R*)-5-[2-[[2-(*o*-Ethoxyphenoxy) ethyl]amino]propyl]-2-methoxybenzenesulfonamide, monohydrochloride. Tamsulosin hydrochloride is a white crystalline powder that melts with decomposition at approximately 230°C. It is sparingly soluble in water and methanol, slightly soluble in glacial acetic acid and ethanol, and practically insoluble in ether.

The empirical formula of tamsulosin hydrochloride is $C_{20}H_{28}N_2O_5S$ • HCl. The molecular weight of tamsulosin hydrochloride is 444.98. Its structural formula is:

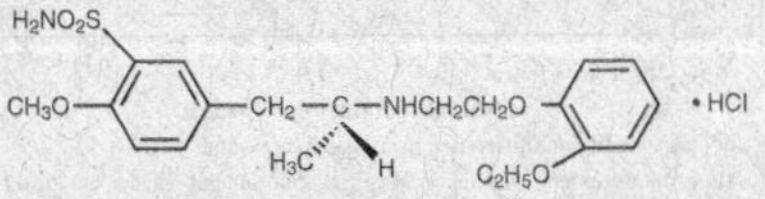

Each FLOMAX capsule for oral administration contains tamsulosin hydrochloride 0.4 mg, and the following inactive ingredients: methacrylic acid copolymer, microcrystalline cellulose, triacetin, calcium stearate, talc, FD&C blue No. 2, titanium dioxide, ferric oxide, gelatin, and trace amounts black edible ink.

CLINICAL PHARMACOLOGY

The symptoms associated with benign prostatic hyperplasia (BPH) are related to bladder outlet obstruction, which is comprised of two underlying components: static and dynamic. The static component is related to an increase in prostate size caused, in part, by a proliferation of smooth muscle cells in the prostatic stroma. However, the severity of BPH symptoms and the degree of urethral obstruction do not correlate well with the size of the prostate. The dynamic component is a function of an increase in smooth muscle tone in the prostate and bladder neck leading to constriction of the bladder outlet. Smooth muscle tone is mediated by the sympathetic nervous stimulation of alpha$_1$ adrenoceptors, which are abundant in the prostate, prostatic capsule, prostatic urethra, and bladder neck. Blockade of these adrenoceptors can cause smooth muscles in the bladder neck and prostate to relax, resulting in an improvement in urine flow rate and a reduction in symptoms of BPH.

Tamsulosin, an alpha$_1$ adrenoceptor blocking agent, exhibits selectivity for alpha$_1$ receptors in the human prostate. At least three discrete alpha$_1$-adrenoceptor subtypes have been identified: alpha$_{1A}$, alpha$_{1B}$ and alpha$_{1D}$; their distribution differs between human organs and tissue. Approximately 70% of the alpha$_1$-receptors in human prostate are of the alpha$_{1A}$ subtype.

Flomax® (tamsulosin hydrochloride) capsules are not intended for use as an antihypertensive drug.

Pharmacokinetics

The pharmacokinetics of tamsulosin hydrochloride have been evaluated in adult healthy volunteers and patients with BPH after single and/or multiple administration with doses ranging from 0.1 mg to 1 mg.

Absorption

Absorption of tamsulosin hydrochloride from FLOMAX capsules 0.4 mg is essentially complete (>90%) following oral administration under fasting conditions. Tamsulosin hydrochloride exhibits linear kinetics following single and multiple dosing, with achievement of steady-state concentrations by the fifth day of once-a-day dosing.

Effect of Food

The time to maximum concentration (T_{max}) is reached by four to five hours under fasting conditions and by six to seven hours when FLOMAX capsules are administered with food. Taking FLOMAX capsules under fasted conditions results in a 30% increase in bioavailability (AUC) and 40% to 70% increase in peak concentrations (C_{max}) compared to fed conditions (Figure 1).

[See figure 1 at top of next column]

The effects of food on the pharmacokinetics of tamsulosin hydrochloride are consistent regardless of whether a FLOMAX is taken with a light breakfast or a high-fat breakfast (Table 1).

[See table 1 above]

Distribution

The mean steady-state apparent volume of distribution of tamsulosin hydrochloride after intravenous administration to ten healthy male adults was 16L, which is suggestive of distribution into extracellular fluids in the body.

Table 1 Mean (± S.D.) Pharmacokinetic Parameters Following Flomax® (tamsulosin HCl) capsules 0.4 mg Once Daily or 0.8 mg Once Daily with a Light Breakfast, High-Fat Breakfast or Fasted

Pharmacokinetic Parameter	0.4 mg QD to healthy volunteers; n=23 (age range 18–32 years)		0.8 mg QD to healthy volunteers; n=22 (age range 55-75 years)		
	Light Breakfast	Fasted	Light Breakfast	High-Fat Breakfast	Fasted
Cmin (ng/mL)	4.0 ± 2.6	3.8 ± 2.5	12.3 ± 6.7	13.5 ± 7.6	13.3 ± 13.3
Cmax (ng/mL)	10.1 ± 4.8	17.1 ± 17.1	29.8 ± 10.3	29.1 ± 11.0	41.6 ± 15.6
Cmax/Cmin Ratio	3.1 ± 1.0	5.3 ± 2.2	2.7 ± 0.7	2.5 ± 0.8	3.6 ± 1.1
Tmax (hours)	6.0	4.0	7.0	6.6	5.0
T1/2 (hours)	-	-	-	-	14.9 ± 3.9
AUCτ (ng•hr/mL)	151 ± 81.5	199 ± 94.1	440 ± 195	449 ± 217	557 ± 257

Cmin = observed minimum concentration
Cmax = observed maximum tamsulosin hydrochloride plasma concentration
Tmax = median time-to-maximum concentration
T1/2 = observed half-life
AUCτ = Area under the tamsulosin hydrochloride plasma time curve over the dosing interval

Figure 1 Mean Plasma Tamsulosin Hydrochloride Concentrations Following Single-Dose Administration of FLOMAX capsules 0.4 mg Under Fasted and Fed Conditions (n=8)

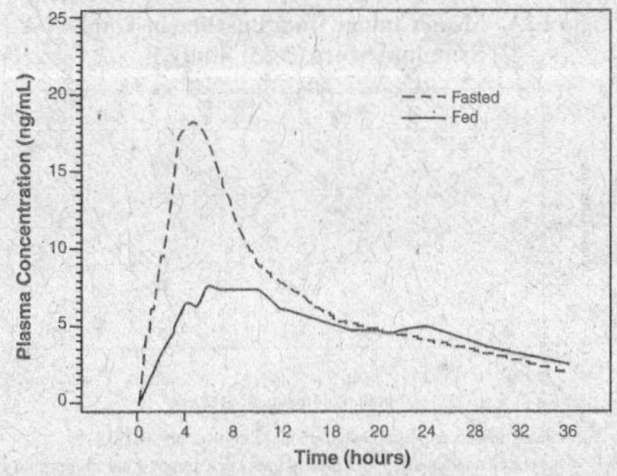

Tamsulosin hydrochloride is extensively bound to human plasma proteins (94% to 99%), primarily alpha-1 acid glycoprotein (AAG), with linear binding over a wide concentration range (20 to 600 ng/mL). The results of two-way *in vitro* studies indicate that the binding of tamsulosin hydrochloride to human plasma proteins is not affected by amitriptyline, diclofenac, glyburide, simvastatin plus simvastatin-hydroxy acid metabolite, warfarin, diazepam, propranolol, trichlormethiazide, or chlormadinone. Likewise, tamsulosin hydrochloride had no effect on the extent of binding of these drugs.

Metabolism

There is no enantiomeric bioconversion from tamsulosin hydrochloride [R(-) isomer] to the S(+) isomer in humans. Tamsulosin hydrochloride is extensively metabolized by cytochrome P450 enzymes in the liver and less than 10% of the dose is excreted in urine unchanged. However, the pharmacokinetic profile of the metabolites in humans has not been established. In vitro results indicate that CYP3A4 and CYP2D6 are involved in metabolism of tamsulosin as well as some minor participation of other CYP isoenzymes. Inhibition of hepatic drug metabolizing enzymes may lead to increased exposure to tamsulosin (see ***Drug-Drug Interactions**, Cytochrome P450 Inhibition*). The metabolites of tamsulosin hydrochloride undergo extensive conjugation to glucuronide or sulfate prior to renal excretion.

Incubations with human liver microsomes showed no evidence of clinically significant metabolic interactions between tamsulosin hydrochloride and amitriptyline, albuterol (beta agonist), glyburide (glibenclamide) and finasteride (5alpha-reductase inhibitor for treatment of BPH). However, results of the *in vitro* testing of the tamsulosin hydrochloride interaction with diclofenac and warfarin were equivocal.

Excretion

On administration of the radiolabeled dose of tamsulosin hydrochloride to four healthy volunteers, 97% of the administered radioactivity was recovered, with urine (76%) representing the primary route of excretion compared to feces (21%) over 168 hours.

Following intravenous or oral administration of an immediate-release formulation, the elimination half-life of tamsulosin hydrochloride in plasma range from five to seven hours. Because of absorption rate-controlled pharmacokinetics with Flomax® (tamsulosin hydrochloride) capsules, the apparent half-life of tamsulosin hydrochloride is approximately 9 to 13 hours in healthy volunteers and 14 to 15 hours in the target population.

Tamsulosin hydrochloride undergoes restrictive clearance in humans, with a relatively low systemic clearance (2.88 L/h).

Special Populations

Geriatrics (Age)

Cross-study comparison of FLOMAX capsules overall exposure (AUC) and half-life indicate that the pharmacokinetic disposition of tamsulosin hydrochloride may be slightly prolonged in geriatric males compared to young, healthy male volunteers. Intrinsic clearance is independent of tamsulosin hydrochloride binding to AAG, but diminishes with age, resulting in a 40% overall higher exposure (AUC) in subjects of age 55 to 75 years compared to subjects of age 20 to 32 years.

Renal Dysfunction

The pharmacokinetics of tamsulosin hydrochloride have been compared in 6 subjects with mild-moderate ($30 \le CL_{cr} < 70$ mL/min/1.73m^2) or moderate-severe ($10 \le CL_{cr} < 30$ mL/min/1.73m^2) renal impairment and 6 normal subjects (CL_{cr} <90 mL/min/1.73m^2). While a change in the overall plasma concentration of tamsulosin hydrochloride was observed as the result of altered binding to AAG, the unbound (active) concentration of tamsulosin hydrochloride, as well as the intrinsic clearance, remained relatively constant. Therefore, patients with renal impairment do not require an adjustment in FLOMAX dosing. However, patients with endstage renal disease (CL_{cr} <10 mL/min/1.73m^2) have not been studied.

Hepatic Dysfunction

The pharmacokinetics of tamsulosin hydrochloride have been compared in 8 subjects with moderate hepatic dysfunction (Child-Pugh's classification: Grades A and B) and 8 normal subjects. While a change in the overall plasma concentration of tamsulosin hydrochloride was observed as the result of altered binding to AAG, the unbound (active) concentration of tamsulosin hydrochloride does not change significantly with only a modest (32%) change in intrinsic clearance of unbound tamsulosin hydrochloride. Therefore, patients with moderate hepatic dysfunction do not require an adjustment in Flomax® (tamsulosin HCl) capsules dosage. FLOMAX has not been studied in patients with severe hepatic dysfunction.

Drug-Drug Interactions

Nifedipine, Atenolol, Enalapril

In three studies in hypertensive subjects (age range 47-79 years) whose blood pressure was controlled with stable doses of Procardia XL®, atenolol, or enalapril for at least three months, FLOMAX capsules 0.4 mg for seven days followed by FLOMAX capsules 0.8 mg for another seven days (n=8 per study) resulted in no clinically significant effects on blood pressure and pulse rate compared to placebo (n=4 per study). Therefore, dosage adjustments are not necessary when FLOMAX capsules are administered concomitantly with Procardia XL®, atenolol, or enalapril.

Warfarin

A definitive drug-drug interaction study between tamsulosin hydrochloride and warfarin was not conducted. Results from limited *in vitro* and *in vivo* studies are inconclusive. Therefore, caution should be exercised with concomitant administration of warfarin and FLOMAX capsules.

Digoxin and Theophylline

In two studies in healthy volunteers (n=10 per study; age range 19-39 years) receiving FLOMAX capsules 0.4 mg/day for two days, followed by FLOMAX capsules 0.8 mg/day for five to eight days, single intravenous doses of digoxin 0.5 mg or theophylline 5 mg/kg resulted in no change in the pharmacokinetics of digoxin or theophylline. Therefore, dosage adjustments are not necessary when a FLOMAX capsule is administered concomitantly with digoxin or theophylline.

Furosemide

The pharmacokinetic and pharmacodynamic interaction between FLOMAX 0.8 mg/day (steady-state) and furosemide 20 mg intravenously (single dose) was evaluated in ten healthy volunteers (age range 21-40 years). FLOMAX capsules had no effect on the pharmacodynamics (excretion of electrolytes) of furosemide. While furosemide produced an 11% to 12% reduction in tamsulosin hydrochloride C_{max} and AUC, these changes are expected to be clinically insignificant and do not require adjustment of the FLOMAX capsules dosage.

Cytochrome P450 Inhibition:

Cimetidine

The effects of cimetidine at the highest recommended dose (400 mg every six hours for six days) on the pharmacokinet-

Continued on next page

Table 2   Mean (±S.D.) Changes from Baseline to Week 13 in Total AUA Symptom Score** and Peak Urine Flow Rate (mL/sec)

	Total AUA Symptom Score		Peak Urine Flow Rate	
	Mean Baseline Value	Mean Change	Mean Baseline Value	Mean Change
Study 1†				
FLOMAX capsules 0.8 mg once daily	19.9 ± 4.9 n=247	-9.6*± 6.7 n=237	9.57 ± 2.51 n=247	1.78*± 3.35 n=247
FLOMAX capsules 0.4 mg once daily	19.8 ± 5.0 n=254	-8.3* ± 6.5 n=246	9.46 ± 2.49 n=254	1.75* ± 3.57 n=254
Placebo	19.6 ± 4.9 n=254	-5.5 ± 6.6 n=246	9.75 ± 2.54 n=254	0.52 ± 3.39 n=253
Study 2‡				
FLOMAX capsules 0.8 mg once daily	18.2 ± 5.6 n=244	-5.8*± 6.4 n=238	9.96 ± 3.16 n=244	1.79*± 3.36 n=237
FLOMAX capsules 0.4 mg once daily	17.9 ± 5.8 n=248	-5.1*± 6.4 n=244	9.94 ± 3.14 n=248	1.52 ± 3.64 n=244
Placebo	19.2 ± 6.0 n=239	-3.6 ± 5.7 n=235	9.95 ± 3.12 n=239	0.93 ± 3.28 n=235

* Statistically significant difference from placebo (p-value≤0.050; Bonferroni-Holm multiple test procedure);
** Total AUA Symptom Scores ranged from 0 to 35.
† Peak urine flow rate measured 4 to 8 hours post dose at Week 13.
‡ Peak urine flow rate measured 24 to 27 hours post dose at Week 13.
Week 13: For patients not completing the 13 week study the last observation was carried forward.

Flomax—Cont.

ics of a single FLOMAX capsule 0.4 mg dose was investigated in ten healthy volunteers (age range 21-38 years). Treatment with cimetidine resulted in a significant decrease (26%) in the clearance of tamsulosin hydrochloride which resulted in a moderate increase in tamsulosin hydrochloride AUC (44%). Therefore, FLOMAX capsules should be used with caution in combination with cimetidine, particularly at doses higher than 0.4 mg.

Strong and Moderate Inhibitors of CYP2D6 or CYP3A4
No studies have been conducted to examine the effect of concomitant administration of a strong or moderate inhibitor of CYP2D6 or CYP3A4 on the pharmacokinetics of tamsulosin.

CLINICAL STUDIES

Four placebo-controlled clinical studies and one active-controlled clinical study enrolled a total of 2296 patients (1003 received Flomax® (tamsulosin HCl) capsules 0.4 mg once daily, 491 received FLOMAX capsules 0.8 mg once daily, and 802 were control patients) in the U.S. and Europe.

In the two U.S. placebo-controlled, double-blind, 13-week, multicenter studies [Study 1 (US92-03A) and Study 2 (US93-01)], 1486 men with the signs and symptoms of BPH were enrolled. In both studies, patients were randomized to either placebo, FLOMAX capsules 0.4 mg once daily, or FLOMAX capsules 0.8 mg once daily. Patients in FLOMAX capsules 0.8 mg once daily treatment groups received a dose of 0.4 mg once daily for one week before increasing to the 0.8 mg once daily dose. The primary efficacy assessments included: 1) total American Urological Association (AUA) Symptom Score questionnaire, which evaluated irritative (frequency, urgency, and nocturia), and obstructive (hesitancy, incomplete emptying, intermittency, and weak stream) symptoms, where a decrease in score is consistent with improvement in symptoms; and 2) peak urine flow rate, where an increased peak urine flow rate value over baseline is consistent with decreased urinary obstruction.

Mean changes from baseline to week 13 in total AUA Symptom Score were significantly greater for groups treated with FLOMAX capsules 0.4 mg and 0.8 mg once daily compared to placebo in both U.S. studies (Table 2, Figures 2A and 2B). The changes from baseline in peak urine flow rate were also significantly greater for the FLOMAX capsules 0.4 mg and 0.8 mg once daily groups compared to placebo in Study 1, and for the FLOMAX capsules 0.8 mg once daily group in Study 2 (Table 2, Figures 3A and 3B). Overall there were no significant differences in improvement observed in total AUA Symptom Scores or peak urine flow rates between the 0.4 mg and the 0.8 mg dose groups with the exception that the 0.8 mg dose in Study 1 had a significantly greater improvement in total AUA Symptom Score compared to the 0.4 mg dose.

[See table 2 above]

Mean total AUA Symptom Scores for both Flomax® (tamsulosin hydrochloride) capsules 0.4 mg and 0.8 mg once daily groups showed a rapid decrease starting at one week after dosing and remained decreased through 13 weeks in both studies (Figures 2A and 2B).

In Study 1, 400 patients (53% of the originally randomized group) elected to continue in their originally assigned treatment groups in a double-blind, placebo controlled, 40 week extension trial (138 patients on 0.4 mg, 135 patients on 0.8 mg and 127 patients on placebo). Three hundred and twenty-three patients (43% of the originally randomized group) completed one year. Of these, 81% (97 patients) on 0.4 mg, 74% (75 patients) on 0.8 mg and 56% (57 patients) on placebo had a response ≥25% above baseline in total AUA Symptom Score at one year.

Figure 2A   Mean Change from Baseline in Total AUA Symptom Score (0-35) Study 1

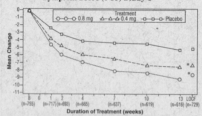

* indicates significant difference from placebo (p-value ≤0.050).
B = Baseline determined approximately one week prior to the initial dose of double-blind medication at Week 0. Subsequent values are observed cases.
LOCF= Last observation carried forward for patients not completing the 13-week study.
Note: Patients in the 0.8 mg treatment group received 0.4 mg for the first week.
Note: Total AUA Symptom Scores range from 0 to 35.

Figure 2B   Mean Change from Baseline in Total AUA Symptom Score (0-35) Study 2

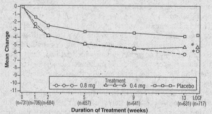

* indicates significant difference from placebo (p-value ≤0.050).
Baseline measurement was taken Week 0. Subsequent values are observed cases.
LOCF= Last observation carried forward for patients not completing the 13-week study.
Note: Patients in the 0.8 mg treatment group received 0.4 mg for the first week.
Note: Total AUA Symptom Scores range from 0 to 35.

[See figure 3A at top of next column]
[See figure 3B at top of next column]

INDICATIONS AND USAGE

Flomax® (tamsulosin hydrochloride) capsules are indicated for the treatment of the signs and symptoms of benign prostatic hyperplasia (BPH). FLOMAX capsules are not indicated for the treatment of hypertension.

CONTRAINDICATIONS

FLOMAX capsules are contraindicated in patients known to be hypersensitive to tamsulosin hydrochloride or any component of FLOMAX capsules.

WARNINGS

The signs and symptoms of orthostasis (postural hypotension, dizziness and vertigo) were detected more frequently in FLOMAX capsule treated patients than in placebo recipients. As with other alpha-adrenergic blocking agents there is a potential risk of syncope (see **ADVERSE REACTIONS**).
Patients beginning treatment with Flomax® (tamsulosin HCl) capsules should be cautioned to avoid situations where injury could result should syncope occur.

Figure 3A   Mean Increase in Peak Urine Flow Rate (mL/Sec) Study 1

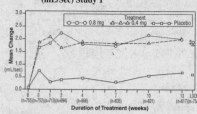

* indicates significant difference from placebo (p-value ≤0.050).
B = Baseline determined approximately one week prior to the initial dose of double-blind medication at Week 0. Subsequent values are observed cases.
LOCF= Last observation carried forward for patients not completing the 13-week study.
Note: The uroflowmetry assessments at week 0 were recorded 4-8 hours after patients received the first dose of double-blind medication.
Measurements at each visit were scheduled 4-8 hours after dosing (approximately peak plasma tamsulosin concentration).
Note: Patients in the 0.8 mg treatment groups received 0.4 for the first week.

Figure 3B   Mean Increase in Peak Urine Flow Rate (mL/Sec) Study 2

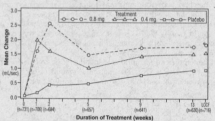

* indicates significant difference from placebo (p-value ≤0.050).
Baseline measurement was taken Week 0. Subsequent values are observed cases.
LOCF= Last observation carried forward for patients not completing the 13-week study.
Note: Patients in the 0.8 mg treatment group received 0.4 mg for the first week.
Note: Week 1 and Week 2 measurements were scheduled 4-8 hours after dosing (approximate peak plasma tamsulosin concentration).
All other visits were scheduled 24-27 hours after dosing (approximate trough tamsulosin concentration).

Rarely (probably less than one in fifty thousand patients), tamsulosin, like other alpha₁ antagonists, has been associated with priapism (persistent painful penile erection unrelated to sexual activity). Because this condition can lead to permanent impotence if not properly treated, patients must be advised about the seriousness of the condition (see **PRECAUTIONS, Information for Patients**).

PRECAUTIONS

General

1. *Carcinoma of the prostate:* Carcinoma of the prostate and BPH cause many of the same symptoms. These two diseases frequently co-exist. Patients should be evaluated prior to the start of FLOMAX capsules therapy to rule out the presence of carcinoma of the prostate.

2. *Intraoperative Floppy Iris Syndrome:* Intraoperative Floppy Iris Syndrome (IFIS) has been observed during cataract surgery in some patients treated with alpha-1 blockers, including FLOMAX capsules. Most reports were in patients taking the alpha-1 blocker when IFIS occurred, but in some cases, the alpha-1 blocker had been stopped prior to surgery. In most of these cases, the alpha-1-blocker had been stopped recently prior to surgery (2 to 14 days), but in a few cases, IFIS was reported after the patient had been off the alpha-1 blocker for a longer period (5 weeks to 9 months). IFIS is a variant of small pupil syndrome and is characterized by the combination of a flaccid iris that billows in response to intraoperative irrigation currents, progressive intraoperative miosis despite preoperative dilation with standard mydriatic drugs and potential prolapse of the iris toward the phacoemulsification incisions. The patient's ophthalmologist should be prepared for possible modifications to their surgical technique, such as the utilization of iris hooks, iris dilator rings, or viscoelastic substances. The benefit of stopping alpha-1 blocker therapy prior to cataract surgery has not been established.

3. *Sulfa Allergy:* In patients with sulfa allergy, allergic reaction to FLOMAX has been rarely reported. If a patient reports a serious or life threatening sulfa allergy, caution is warranted when administering FLOMAX capsules.

4. *Drug-Drug Interactions:* The pharmacokinetic and pharmacodynamic interactions between FLOMAX capsules and other alpha-adrenergic blocking agents have not been determined. However, interactions may be expected and FLOMAX capsules should NOT be used in combination with other alpha-adrenergic blocking agents.

The pharmacokinetic interaction between cimetidine, a mild inhibitor of several CYP enzymes, and FLOMAX capsules was investigated in 10 subjects (see **CLINICAL PHARMACOLOGY, *Drug-Drug Interactions***). The results indicate significant changes in both tamsulosin hydrochloride clearance (26% decrease) and exposure (44% increase in AUC). Therefore, FLOMAX capsules should be used with caution in combination with cimetidine, particularly at doses higher than 0.4 mg.

Additional pharmacokinetic interactions between strong or moderate CYP2D6 or CYP3A4 inhibitors with Flomax® (tamsulosin HCl) capsules have not been examined. As FLOMAX is extensively metabolized (mainly by CYP2D6 and CYP3A4) and as concomitant administration with cimetidine caused 44% increase in FLOMAX exposure, concomitant administration of FLOMAX and an inhibitor of CYP2D6 or CYP3A4 may lead to increased FLOMAX plasma exposure. FLOMAX capsules should be used with caution in combination with moderate or strong inhibitors of CYP2D6 (e.g., fluoxetine) or CYP3A4 (e.g., ketoconazole), particularly at doses higher than 0.4 mg.

Results from limited *in vitro* and *in vivo* drug-drug interaction studies between tamsulosin hydrochloride and warfarin are inconclusive. Therefore, caution should be exercised with concomitant administration of warfarin and FLOMAX capsules.

See also ***Drug-Drug Interactions*** studies in **CLINICAL PHARMACOLOGY, Pharmacokinetics** subsection.

Information for Patients (see **PATIENT INFORMATION ABOUT FLOMAX CAPSULES**)

Patients should be told about the possible occurrence of symptoms related to postural hypotension such as dizziness when taking FLOMAX capsules, and they should be cautioned about driving, operating machinery or performing hazardous tasks.

Patients should be advised not to crush, chew or open the FLOMAX capsules.

Patients should be advised about the possibility of priapism as a result of treatment with FLOMAX capsules and other similar medications. Patients should be informed that this reaction is extremely rare, but if not brought to immediate medical attention, can lead to permanent erectile dysfunction (impotence).

Patients should be advised that if they are considering cataract surgery, to tell their ophthalmologist that they have taken FLOMAX.

Laboratory Tests

No laboratory test interactions with FLOMAX capsules are known. Treatment with FLOMAX capsules for up to 12 months had no significant effect on prostate-specific antigen (PSA).

Pregnancy

Teratogenic Effects, *Pregnancy Category B.*

Administration of tamsulosin hydrochloride to pregnant female rats at dose levels up to 300 mg/kg/day (approximately 50 times the human therapeutic AUC exposure) revealed no evidence of harm to the fetus. Administration of tamsulosin hydrochloride to pregnant rabbits at dose levels up to 50 mg/kg/day produced no evidence of fetal harm. FLOMAX capsules are not indicated for use in women.

Geriatric Use

Of the total number of subjects (1,783) in clinical studies of tamsulosin, 36% were 65 years of age and over. No overall differences in safety or effectiveness were observed between these subjects and younger subjects, and the other reported clinical experience has not identified differences in responses between the elderly and younger patients, but greater sensitivity of some older individuals cannot be ruled out (see **CLINICAL PHARMACOLOGY, Pharmacokinetics, *Special Populations,*** *Geriatrics (Age)*).

Nursing Mothers

Flomax® (tamsulosin HCl) capsules are not indicated for use in women.

Pediatric Use

FLOMAX capsules are not indicated for use in pediatric populations.

Carcinogenesis, Mutagenesis, and Impairment of Fertility

Rats administered doses up to 43 mg/kg/day in males and 52 mg/kg/day in females had no increases in tumor incidence with the exception of a modest increase in the frequency of mammary gland fibroadenomas in female rats receiving doses ≥5.4 mg/kg (P <0.015). The highest doses of tamsulosin hydrochloride evaluated in the rat carcinogenicity study produced systemic exposures (AUC) in rats 3 times the exposures in men receiving the maximum therapeutic dose of 0.8 mg/day.

Mice were administered doses up to 127 mg/kg/day in males and 158 mg/kg/day in females. There were no significant tumor findings in male mice. Female mice treated for 2 years with the two highest doses of 45 and 158 mg/kg/day had statistically significant increases in the incidence of mammary gland fibroadenomas (P<0.0001) and adenocarcinomas (P<0.0075). The highest dose levels of tamsulosin hydrochloride evaluated in the mice carcinogenicity study produced systemic exposures (AUC) in mice 8 times the exposures in men receiving the maximum therapeutic dose of 0.8 mg/day.

The increased incidences of mammary gland neoplasms in female rats and mice were considered secondary to tamsulosin hydrochloride-induced hyperprolactinemia. It is not known if FLOMAX elevate prolactin in humans. The relevance for human risk of the findings of prolactin-mediated endocrine tumors in rodents is not known.

Tamsulosin hydrochloride produced no evidence of mutagenic potential *in vitro* in the Ames reverse mutation test, mouse lymphoma thymidine kinase assay, unscheduled DNA repair synthesis assay, and chromosomal aberration assays in Chinese hamster ovary cells or human lymphocytes. There were no mutagenic effects in the *in vivo* sister chromatid exchange and mouse micronucleus assay.

Studies in rats revealed significantly reduced fertility in males dosed with single or multiple daily doses of 300 mg/kg/day of tamsulosin hydrochloride (AUC exposure in rats about 50 times the human exposure with the maximum therapeutic dose). The mechanism of decreased fertility in male rats is considered to be an effect of the compound on the vaginal plug formation possibly due to changes of semen content or impairment of ejaculation. The effects on fertility were reversible showing improvement by 3 days after a single dose and 4 weeks after multiple dosing. Effects on fertility in males were completely reversed within nine weeks of discontinuation of multiple dosing. Multiple doses of 10 and 100 mg/kg/day tamsulosin hydrochloride (1/5 and 16 times the anticipated human AUC exposure) did not significantly alter fertility in male rats. Effects of tamsulosin hydrochloride on sperm counts or sperm function have not been evaluated.

Studies in female rats revealed significant reductions in fertility after single or multiple dosing with 300 mg/kg/day of the R-isomer or racemic mixture of tamsulosin hydrochloride, respectively. In female rats, the reductions in fertility after single doses were considered to be associated with impairments in fertilization. Multiple dosing with 10 or 100 mg/kg/day of the racemic mixture did not significantly alter fertility in female rats.

Table 3 Treatment Emergent[1] Adverse Events Occurring in ≥2% of Flomax® (tamsulosin hydrochloride) capsules or Placebo Patients in Two U.S. Short-Term Placebo-Controlled Clinical Studies

BODY SYSTEM/ ADVERSE EVENT	FLOMAX CAPSULES GROUPS 0.4 mg n=502	0.8 mg n=492	PLACEBO n=493
BODY AS WHOLE			
Headache	97 (19.3%)	104 (21.1%)	99 (20.1%)
Infection[2]	45 (9.0%)	53 (10.8%)	37 (7.5%)
Asthenia	39 (7.8%)	42 (8.5%)	27 (5.5%)
Back pain	35 (7.0%)	41 (8.3%)	27 (5.5%)
Chest Pain	20 (4.0%)	20 (4.1%)	18 (3.7%)
NERVOUS SYSTEM			
Dizziness	75 (14.9%)	84 (17.1%)	50 (10.1%)
Somnolence	15 (3.0%)	21 (4.3%)	8 (1.6%)
Insomnia	12 (2.4%)	7 (1.4%)	3 (0.6%)
Libido Decreased	5 (1.0%)	10 (2.0%)	6 (1.2%)
RESPIRATORY SYSTEM			
Rhinitis[3]	66 (13.1%)	88 (17.9%)	41 (8.3%)
Pharyngitis	29 (5.8%)	25 (5.1%)	23 (4.7%)
Cough Increased	17 (3.4%)	22 (4.5%)	12 (2.4%)
Sinusitis	11 (2.2%)	18 (3.7%)	8 (1.6%)
DIGESTIVE SYSTEM			
Diarrhea	31 (6.2%)	21 (4.3%)	22 (4.5%)
Nausea	13 (2.6%)	19 (3.9%)	16 (3.2%)
Tooth Disorder	6 (1.2%)	10 (2.0%)	7 (1.4%)
UROGENITAL SYSTEM			
Abnormal Ejaculation	42 (8.4%)	89 (18.1%)	1 (0.2%)
SPECIAL SENSES			
Blurred vision	1 (0.2%)	10 (2.0%)	2 (0.4%)

[1] A treatment-emergent adverse event was defined as any event satisfying one of the following criteria:
- The adverse event occurred for the first time after initial dosing with double-blind study medication.
- The adverse event was present prior to or at the time of initial dosing with double-blind study medication and subsequently increased in severity during double-blind treatment; or
- The adverse event was present prior to or at the time of initial dosing with double-blind study medication, disappeared completely, and then reappeared during double-blind treatment.

[2] Coding preferred terms also include cold, common cold, head cold, flu, and flu-like symptoms.
[3] Coding preferred terms also include nasal congestion, stuffy nose, runny nose, sinus congestion, and hay fever.

ADVERSE REACTIONS

The incidence of treatment-emergent adverse events has been ascertained from six short-term U.S. and European placebo-controlled clinical trials in which daily doses of 0.1 to 0.8 mg Flomax® (tamsulosin HCl) capsules were used. These studies evaluated safety in 1783 patients treated with FLOMAX capsules and 798 patients administered placebo. Table 3 summarizes the treatment-emergent adverse events that occurred in ≥2% of patients receiving either FLOMAX capsules 0.4 mg, or 0.8 mg and at an incidence numerically higher than that in the placebo group during two 13-week U.S. trials (US92-03A and US93-01) conducted in 1487 men.

[See table 3 above]

Signs and Symptoms of Orthostasis: In the two U.S. studies, symptomatic postural hypotension was reported by 0.2% of patients (1 of 502) in the 0.4 mg group, 0.4% of patients (2 of 492) in the 0.8 mg group, and by no patients in the placebo group. Syncope was reported by 0.2% of patients (1 of 502) in the 0.4 mg group, 0.4% of patients (2 of 492) in the 0.8 mg group and 0.6% of patients (3 of 493) in the placebo group. Dizziness was reported by 15% of patients (75 of 502) in the 0.4 mg group, 17% of patients (84 of 492) in the 0.8 mg group, and 10% of patients (50 of 493) in the placebo group. Vertigo was reported by 0.6% of patients (3 of 502) in the 0.4 mg group, 1% of patients (5 of 492) in the 0.8 mg group and by 0.6% of patients (3 of 493) in the placebo group.

Multiple testing for orthostatic hypotension was conducted in a number of studies. Such a test was considered positive if it met one or more of the following criteria: (1) a decrease in systolic blood pressure of ≥20 mmHg upon standing from the supine position during the orthostatic tests; (2) a decrease in diastolic blood pressure ≥10 mmHg upon standing, with the standing diastolic blood pressure <65 mmHg during the orthostatic test; (3) an increase in pulse rate of ≥20 bpm upon standing with a standing pulse rate ≥100 bpm during the orthostatic test; and (4) the presence of clinical symptoms (faintness, lightheadedness/lightheaded, dizziness, spinning sensation, vertigo, or postural hypotension) upon standing during the orthostatic test.

Following the first dose of double-blind medication in Study 1, a positive orthostatic test result at 4 hours post-dose was observed in 7% of patients (37 of 498) who received Flomax® (tamsulosin hydrochloride) capsules 0.4 mg once daily and in 3% of the patients (8 of 253) who received placebo. At 8 hours post-dose, a positive orthostatic test result was observed for 6% of the patients (31 of 498) who received FLOMAX capsules 0.4 mg once daily and 4% (9 of 250) who received placebo (Note: patients in the 0.8 mg group received 0.4 mg once daily for the first week of Study 1).

In Studies 1 and 2, at least one positive orthostatic test result was observed during the course of these studies for 81 of the 502 patients (16%) in the FLOMAX capsules 0.4 mg once daily group, 92 of the 491 patients (19%) in the FLOMAX capsules 0.8 mg once daily group and 54 of the 493 patients (11%) in the placebo group.

Because orthostasis was detected more frequently in FLOMAX capsule-treated patients than in placebo recipients, there is a potential risk of syncope (see **WARNINGS**).

Abnormal Ejaculation: Abnormal ejaculation includes ejaculation failure, ejaculation disorder, retrograde ejaculation and ejaculation decrease. As shown in Table 3, abnormal ejaculation was associated with FLOMAX capsules administration and was dose-related in the U.S. studies. Withdrawal from these clinical studies of FLOMAX capsules because of abnormal ejaculation was also dose-dependent with 8 of 492 patients (1.6%) in the 0.8 mg group,

Continued on next page

Flomax—Cont.

and no patients in the 0.4 mg or placebo groups discontinuing treatment due to abnormal ejaculation.

Post-Marketing Experience

The following adverse reactions have been identified during post-approval use of FLOMAX capsules. Because these reactions are reported voluntarily from a population of uncertain size, it is not always possible to reliably estimate their frequency or establish a causal relationship to drug exposure. Decisions to include these reactions in labeling are typically based on one or more of the following factors: (1) seriousness of the reaction, (2) frequency of reporting, or (3) strength of causal connection to Flomax® (tamsulosin HCl) capsules. Allergic-type reactions such as skin rash, urticaria, pruritus, angioedema and respiratory symptoms have been reported with positive rechallenge in some cases. Priapism has been reported rarely. Infrequent reports of palpitations, hypotension, skin desquamation, constipation and vomiting have been received during the post-marketing period.

During cataract surgery, a variant of small pupil syndrome known as Intraoperative Floppy Iris Syndrome (IFIS) has been reported in association with alpha-1 blocker therapy (see **PRECAUTIONS, General**).

OVERDOSAGE

Should overdosage of FLOMAX lead to hypotension (see **WARNINGS** and **ADVERSE REACTIONS**), support of the cardiovascular system is of first importance. Restoration of blood pressure and normalization of heart rate may be accomplished by keeping the patient in the supine position. If this measure is inadequate, then administration of intravenous fluids should be considered. If necessary, vasopressors should then be used and renal function should be monitored and supported as needed. Laboratory data indicate that tamsulosin hydrochloride is 94% to 99% protein bound; therefore, dialysis is unlikely to be of benefit.

One patient reported an overdose of thirty 0.4 mg FLOMAX capsules. Following the ingestion of the capsules, the patient reported a severe headache.

DOSAGE AND ADMINISTRATION

FLOMAX capsules 0.4 mg once daily is recommended as the dose for the treatment of the signs and symptoms of BPH. It should be administered approximately one-half hour following the same meal each day.

For those patients who fail to respond to the 0.4 mg dose after two to four weeks of dosing, the dose of FLOMAX capsules can be increased to 0.8 mg once daily. If FLOMAX capsules administration is discontinued or interrupted for several days at either the 0.4 mg or 0.8 mg dose, therapy should be started again with the 0.4 mg once daily dose.

HOW SUPPLIED

FLOMAX capsules 0.4 mg are supplied in high density polyethylene bottles containing 100 hard gelatin capsules with olive green opaque cap and orange opaque body. The capsules are imprinted on one side with "Flomax 0.4 mg" and on the other side with "BI 58."

FLOMAX capsules 0.4 mg, 100 capsules (NDC 0597-0058-01)

Store at 25°C (77°F); excursions permitted to 15°–30°C (59°–86°F) [see USP Controlled Room Temperature].

Keep FLOMAX capsules and all medicines out of reach of children.

Patients should be reminded to read and follow the accompanying "PATIENT INFORMATION ABOUT FLOMAX CAPSULES", which should be dispensed with the product.

Marketed by:
Boehringer Ingelheim Pharmaceuticals, Inc.
Ridgefield, CT 06877 USA
and
Astellas Pharma US, Inc.
Deerfield, IL 60015 USA
Manufactured by:
Astellas Pharma Inc.
Tokyo 103-8411, JAPAN
or
Astellas Pharma, Inc.
Norman, OK 73072
Licensed from:
Astellas Pharma Inc.
Tokyo 103-8411, JAPAN
Copyright©2007, ALL RIGHTS RESERVED
IT8004DJ1907
PRT42/US/1
Rev: October 2007   Printed in USA

Flomax®
(tamsulosin hydrochloride)
Capsules, 0.4 mg

PATIENT INFORMATION ABOUT FLOMAX CAPSULES

FLOMAX capsules are for use by men only. **FLOMAX capsules are not indicated for use in women.**

Please read this leaflet before you start taking FLOMAX capsules. Also, read it each time you renew your prescription, just in case new information has been added. Remember, this leaflet does not take the place of careful discussions with your doctor. You and your doctor should discuss FLOMAX capsules when you start taking your medication and at regular checkups.

Why has your doctor prescribed FLOMAX capsules?

Your doctor has prescribed FLOMAX capsules because you have a medical condition called benign prostatic hyperplasia (BPH) also commonly referred to as enlarged prostate. This occurs only in men.

What is BPH?

Benign prostatic hyperplasia is an enlargement of the prostate gland. After age 50, most men develop enlarged prostates. The prostate is located below the bladder. As the prostate enlarges, it may slowly restrict the flow of urine. This can lead to symptoms such as:
- a weak or interrupted urinary stream
- a feeling that you cannot empty your bladder completely
- a feeling of delay or hesitation when you start to urinate
- a need to urinate often, especially at night
- a feeling that you must urinate right away

Since cancer of the prostate may cause similar symptoms, you should be evaluated by your doctor to rule out prostate cancer. Your doctor will likely examine your prostate gland manually to detect abnormalities and may measure prostate-specific antigen (PSA) in your blood to help in evaluating for the presence of prostate cancer. FLOMAX capsules do not affect PSA levels.

Treatment Options for BPH

There are three main treatment options for BPH:
- Program of monitoring or "Watchful Waiting". Some men have an enlarged prostate gland, but no symptoms, or symptoms that are not bothersome. If this applies, you and your doctor may decide on a program of monitoring, including regular checkups, instead of medication or surgery.
- There are different kinds of medication used to treat BPH. Your doctor has prescribed Flomax® (tamsulosin hydrochloride) capsules for you (see **What a FLOMAX capsule does to treat BPH**) below.
- Surgery. Some patients may need surgery. Your doctor can describe several different surgical procedures to treat BPH. Which procedure is best depends on your symptoms and medical condition.

What a FLOMAX capsule does to treat BPH

FLOMAX capsules act by relaxing muscles in the prostate and bladder neck at the site of the obstruction, resulting in improved urine flow and reduced BPH symptoms.

What you need to know while taking FLOMAX capsules
- **You must see your doctor regularly.**
While taking FLOMAX capsules, you must have regular checkups. Follow your doctor's advice about when to have these checkups.
- **It is important for you to recognize that FLOMAX capsules can cause a sudden drop in blood pressure especially following the first dose or when changing doses of FLOMAX capsules.** Such a drop in blood pressure, although rare in occurrence, may be associated with fainting, dizziness, or lightheadedness. Therefore, get up slowly from a chair or bed at any time until you learn how you react to FLOMAX capsules. You should not drive or do any hazardous tasks until you are used to the side effects of FLOMAX capsules. If you begin to feel dizzy, sit down until you feel better. Although these symptoms are unlikely, you should avoid driving or hazardous tasks for 12 hours after the initial dose or after your doctor recommends an increase in dose. If you interrupt your treatment for several days or more, resume treatment at one capsule a day, after consulting with your physician. Other side effects may include sleeplessness, runny nose, or ejaculatory problems. In some cases, side effects may decrease or disappear when you continue to take FLOMAX capsules.
- Extremely rarely, FLOMAX capsules and similar medications have caused prolonged, painful erection of the penis, which is unrelieved by sexual intercourse or masturbation. This condition, if untreated, can lead to permanent inability to have an erection. If you have a prolonged erection, call your doctor or go to an Emergency Room as soon as possible.
- If you are contemplating cataract surgery, make certain to advise your eye surgeon that you have taken FLOMAX.

You should discuss side effects with your doctor before taking FLOMAX capsules and anytime you think you are having a side effect.

How to take FLOMAX capsules

Follow your doctor's advice about how to take FLOMAX capsules. You should take it approximately 30 minutes following the same meal every day.

Do not share Flomax® (tamsulosin HCl) capsules with anyone else; it was prescribed only for you.

Do not crush, chew, or open FLOMAX capsules.

Keep FLOMAX capsules and all medicines out of reach of children.

FOR MORE INFORMATION ABOUT FLOMAX CAPSULES AND BPH, TALK WITH YOUR DOCTOR. IN ADDITION, TALK TO YOUR PHARMACIST OR OTHER HEALTHCARE PROVIDER.

Marketed by:
Boehringer Ingelheim Pharmaceuticals, Inc.
Ridgefield, CT 06877 USA
and
Astellas Pharma US, Inc.
Deerfield, IL 60015 USA
Manufactured by:
Astellas Pharma Inc.
Tokyo 103-8411, JAPAN
or
Astellas Pharma, Inc.
Norman, OK 73072

Licensed from:
Astellas Pharma Inc.
Tokyo 103-8411, JAPAN
Copyright©2007, ALL RIGHTS RESERVED
IT8004DJ1907
PRT42/US/1
Rev: October 2007   Printed in USA

ATTENTION PHARMACIST: Detach "Patient's Instructions for Use" from package insert and dispense with the product.

SPIRIVA®   ℞
HANDIHALER®
(tiotropium bromide inhalation powder)
FOR ORAL INHALATION ONLY
DO NOT SWALLOW SPIRIVA CAPSULES
Rx only
Prescribing Information

Prescribing information for this product, which appears on pages 862–866 of the 2008 PDR, has been completely revised as follows. Please write "See Supplement A" next to the product heading.

DESCRIPTION

SPIRIVA® HandiHaler® (tiotropium bromide inhalation powder) consists of a capsule dosage form containing a dry powder formulation of SPIRIVA intended for oral inhalation only with the HandiHaler inhalation device.

Each light green, hard gelatin capsule contains 18 mcg tiotropium (equivalent to 22.5 mcg tiotropium bromide monohydrate) blended with lactose monohydrate as the carrier.

The dry powder formulation within the capsule is intended for oral inhalation only.

The active component of SPIRIVA is tiotropium. The drug substance, tiotropium bromide monohydrate, is an anticholinergic with specificity for muscarinic receptors. It is chemically described as (1α, 2ß, 4ß, 5α, 7ß)-7-[(Hydroxydi-2-thienylacetyl)oxy]-9,9-dimethyl-3-oxa-9-azoniatricyclo[3.3.1.0^{2,4}]nonane bromide monohydrate. It is a synthetic, nonchiral, quaternary ammonium compound. Tiotropium bromide is a white or yellowish white powder. It is sparingly soluble in water and soluble in methanol.

The structural formula is:

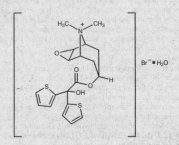

Tiotropium bromide (monohydrate) has a molecular mass of 490.4 and a molecular formula of $C_{19}H_{22}NO_4S_2Br \cdot H_2O$. The HandiHaler is an inhalation device used to inhale the dry powder contained in the SPIRIVA capsule. The dry powder is delivered from the HandiHaler device at flow rates as low as 20 L/min. Under standardized *in vitro* testing, the HandiHaler device delivers a mean of 10.4 mcg tiotropium when tested at a flow rate of 39 L/min for 3.1 seconds (2L total). In a study of 26 adult patients with chronic obstructive pulmonary disease (COPD) and severely compromised lung function [mean FEV_1 1.02 L (range 0.45 to 2.24 L); 37.6% of predicted (range 16%–65%)], the median peak inspiratory flow (PIF) through the HandiHaler device was 30.0 L/min (range 20.4 to 45.6 L/min). The amount of drug delivered to the lungs will vary depending on patient factors such as inspiratory flow and peak inspiratory flow through the HandiHaler device, which may vary from patient to patient, and may vary with the exposure time of the capsule outside the blister pack.

For administration of SPIRIVA, a capsule is placed into the center chamber of the HandiHaler device. The capsule is pierced by pressing and releasing the green piercing button on the side of the inhalation device. The tiotropium formulation is dispersed into the air stream when the patient inhales through the mouthpiece (see **Patient's Instructions for Use**).

CLINICAL PHARMACOLOGY
Mechanism of Action

Tiotropium is a long-acting, antimuscarinic agent, which is often referred to as an anticholinergic. It has similar affinity to the subtypes of muscarinic receptors, M_1 to M_5. In the airways, it exhibits pharmacological effects through inhibition of M_3-receptors at the smooth muscle leading to bronchodilation. The competitive and reversible nature of antagonism was shown with human and animal origin receptors and isolated organ preparations. In preclinical *in vitro* as well as *in vivo* studies prevention of methacholine-induced bronchoconstriction effects were dose-dependent and lasted longer than 24 hours. The bronchodilation following inhalation of tiotropium is predominantly a site-specific effect.

Pharmacokinetics

Tiotropium is administered by dry powder inhalation. In common with other inhaled drugs, the majority of the delivered dose is deposited in the gastrointestinal tract and, to a lesser extent, in the lung, the intended organ. Many of the pharmacokinetic data described below were obtained with higher doses than recommended for therapy.

Absorption

Following dry powder inhalation by young healthy volunteers, the absolute bioavailability of 19.5% suggests that the fraction reaching the lung is highly bioavailable. It is expected from the chemical structure of the compound (quaternary ammonium compound) that tiotropium is poorly absorbed from the gastrointestinal tract. Food is not expected to influence the absorption of tiotropium for the same reason. Oral solutions of tiotropium have an absolute bioavailability of 2–3%. Maximum tiotropium plasma concentrations were observed five minutes after inhalation.

Distribution

Tiotropium shows a volume of distribution of 32 L/kg indicating that the drug binds extensively to tissues. The drug is bound by 72% to plasma proteins. At steady state, peak tiotropium plasma levels in COPD patients were 17-19 pg/mL when measured 5 minutes after dry powder inhalation of an 18 mcg dose and decreased rapidly in a multicompartmental manner. Steady state trough plasma concentrations were 3–4 pg/mL. Local concentrations in the lung are not known, but the mode of administration suggests substantially higher concentrations in the lung. Studies in rats have shown that tiotropium does not readily penetrate the blood-brain barrier.

Biotransformation

The extent of biotransformation appears to be small. This is evident from a urinary excretion of 74% of unchanged substance after an intravenous dose to young healthy volunteers. Tiotropium, an ester, is nonenzymatically cleaved to the alcohol N-methylscopine and dithienylglycolic acid, neither of which bind to muscarinic receptors.

In $vitro$ experiments with human liver microsomes and human hepatocytes suggest that a fraction of the administered dose (74% of an intravenous dose is excreted unchanged in the urine, leaving 25% for metabolism) is metabolized by cytochrome P450-dependent oxidation and subsequent glutathione conjugation to a variety of Phase II metabolites. This enzymatic pathway can be inhibited by CYP450 2D6 and 3A4 inhibitors, such as quinidine, ketoconazole, and gestodene. Thus, CYP450 2D6 and 3A4 are involved in the metabolic pathway that is responsible for the elimination of a small part of the administered dose. In $vitro$ studies using human liver microsomes showed that tiotropium in supratherapeutic concentrations does not inhibit CYP450 1A1, 1A2, 2B6, 2C9, 2C19, 2D6, 2E1, or 3A4.

Elimination

The terminal elimination half-life of tiotropium is between 5 and 6 days following inhalation. Total clearance was 880 mL/min after an intravenous dose in young healthy volunteers with an inter-individual variability of 22%. Intravenously administered tiotropium is mainly excreted unchanged in urine (74%). After dry powder inhalation, urinary excretion is 14% of the dose, the remainder being mainly non-absorbed drug in the gut which is eliminated via the feces. The renal clearance of tiotropium exceeds the creatinine clearance, indicating active secretion into the urine. After chronic once-daily inhalation by COPD patients, pharmacokinetic steady state was reached after 2–3 weeks with no accumulation thereafter.

Drug Interactions

An interaction study with tiotropium (14.4 mcg intravenous infusion over 15 minutes) and cimetidine 400 mg three times daily or ranitidine 300 mg once daily was conducted. Concomitant administration of cimetidine with tiotropium resulted in a 20% increase in the AUC_{0-4h}, a 28% decrease in the renal clearance of tiotropium and no significant change in the C_{max} and amount excreted in urine over 96 hours. Co-administration of tiotropium with ranitidine did not affect the pharmacokinetics of tiotropium. Therefore, no clinically significant interaction occurred between tiotropium and cimetidine or ranitidine.

Electrophysiology

In a multicenter, randomized, double-blind trial that enrolled 198 patients with COPD, the number of subjects with changes from baseline-corrected QT interval of 30–60 msec was higher in the SPIRIVA group as compared with placebo. This difference was apparent using both the Bazett (QTcB) [20 (20%) patients vs. 12 (12%) patients] and Fredericia (QTcF) [16 (16%) patients vs. 1 (1%) patient] corrections of QT for heart rate. No patients in either group had either QTcB or QTcF of >500 msec. Other clinical studies with SPIRIVA did not detect an effect of the drug on QTc intervals.

Special Populations

Elderly Patients

As expected for drugs predominantly excreted renally, advanced age was associated with a decrease of tiotropium renal clearance (326 mL/min in COPD patients <58 years to 163 mL/min in COPD patients >70 years), which may be explained by decreased renal function. Tiotropium excretion in urine after inhalation decreased from 14% (young healthy volunteers) to about 7% (COPD patients). Plasma concentrations were numerically increased with advancing age within COPD patients (43% increase in AUC_{0-4} after dry powder inhalation), which was not significant when considered in relation to inter- and intra-individual variability (see DOSAGE AND ADMINISTRATION).

Figure 1: Mean FEV₁ Over Time (prior to and after administration of study drug) on Days 1 and 169 for Trial A (a Six-Month Placebo-Controlled Study)*

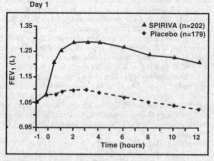
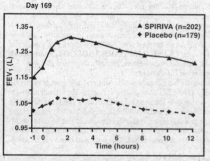

*Means adjusted for center, treatment, and baseline effect. On Day 169, a total of 183 and 149 patients in the SPIRIVA and placebo groups, respectively, completed the trial. The data for the remaining patients were imputed using last observation or least favorable observation carried forward.

Figure 2: Mean FEV₁ Over Time (0 to 6 hours post-dose) on Days 1 and 92, respectively, for one of the two Ipratropium-Controlled Studies*

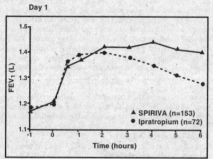
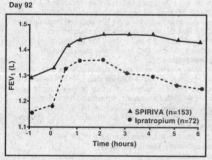

*Means adjusted for center, treatment, and baseline effect. On Day 92 (primary endpoint), a total of 151 and 69 patients in the SPIRIVA and ipratropium groups, respectively, completed through three months of observation. The data for the remaining patients were imputed using last observation or least favorable observation carried forward.

Hepatically-impaired Patients

The effects of hepatic impairment on the pharmacokinetics of tiotropium were not studied. However, hepatic insufficiency is not expected to have relevant influence on tiotropium pharmacokinetics. Tiotropium is predominantly cleared by renal elimination (74% in young healthy volunteers) and by simple non-enzymatic ester cleavage to products that do not bind to muscarinic receptors (see DOSAGE AND ADMINISTRATION).

Renally-impaired Patients

Since tiotropium is predominantly renally excreted, renal impairment was associated with increased plasma drug concentrations and reduced drug clearance after both intravenous infusion and dry powder inhalation. Mild renal impairment (CrCl 50–80 mL/min), which is often seen in elderly patients, increased tiotropium plasma concentrations (39% increase in AUC_{0-4} after intravenous infusion). In COPD patients with moderate to severe renal impairment (CrCl <50 mL/min), the intravenous administration of tiotropium resulted in doubling of the plasma concentrations (82% increase in AUC_{0-4}), which was confirmed by plasma concentrations after dry powder inhalation (see DOSAGE AND ADMINISTRATION and PRECAUTIONS).

CLINICAL STUDIES

The SPIRIVA HandiHaler (tiotropium bromide inhalation powder) clinical development program consisted of six Phase 3 studies in 2,663 patients with COPD (1,308 receiving SPIRIVA): two 1-year, placebo-controlled studies, two 6-month, placebo-controlled studies and two 1-year, ipratropium-controlled studies. These studies enrolled patients who had a clinical diagnosis of COPD, were 40 years of age or older, had a history of smoking greater than 10 pack-years, had an FEV₁ less than or equal to 60 or 65% of predicted, and a ratio of FEV₁/FVC of less than or equal to 0.7.

In these studies, SPIRIVA, administered once-daily in the morning, provided improvement in lung function (forced expiratory volume in one second, FEV₁), with peak effect occurring within 3 hours following the first dose.

In the 1-year, placebo-controlled trials, the mean improvement in FEV₁ at 30 minutes was 0.13 liters (13%) with a peak improvement of 0.24 liters (24%) relative to baseline after the first dose (Day 1). Further improvements in FEV₁ and FVC were observed with pharmacodynamic steady state reached by Day 8 with once-daily treatment. The mean peak improvement in FEV₁, relative to baseline, was 0.28 to 0.31 liters (28% to 31%), after 1 week (Day 8) of once-daily treatment. Improvement of lung function was maintained for 24 hours after a single dose and consistently maintained over the 1-year treatment period with no evidence of tolerance.

In the two 6-month, placebo-controlled trials, serial spirometric evaluations were performed throughout daytime hours in Trial A (12 hours) and limited to 3 hours in Trial B.

The serial FEV₁ values over 12 hours (Trial A) are displayed in Figure 1. These trials further support the improvement in pulmonary function (FEV₁) with SPIRIVA, which persisted over the spirometric observational period. Effectiveness was maintained for 24 hours after administration over the 6-month treatment period.

[See figure 1 above]

Results of each of the one-year ipratropium-controlled trials were similar to the results of the one-year placebo-controlled trials. The results of one of these trials are shown in Figure 2.

[See figure 2 above]

A randomized, placebo-controlled clinical study in 105 patients with COPD demonstrated that bronchodilation was maintained throughout the 24-hour dosing interval in comparison to placebo, regardless of whether SPIRIVA was administered in the morning or in the evening.

Throughout each week of the one-year treatment period in the two placebo-controlled trials, patients taking SPIRIVA had a reduced requirement for the use of rescue short-acting beta₂-agonists. Reduction in the use of rescue short-acting beta₂-agonists, as compared to placebo, was demonstrated in one of the two 6-month studies.

INDICATIONS AND USAGE

SPIRIVA HandiHaler (tiotropium bromide inhalation powder) is indicated for the long-term, once-daily, maintenance treatment of bronchospasm associated with chronic obstructive pulmonary disease (COPD), including chronic bronchitis and emphysema.

CONTRAINDICATIONS

SPIRIVA® HandiHaler® (tiotropium bromide inhalation powder) is contraindicated in patients with a history of hypersensitivity to atropine or its derivatives, including ipratropium, or to any component of this product.

WARNINGS

SPIRIVA HandiHaler (tiotropium bromide inhalation powder) is intended as a once-daily maintenance treatment for COPD and is not indicated for the initial treatment of acute episodes of bronchospasm, i.e., rescue therapy.

Immediate hypersensitivity reactions, including angioedema, may occur after administration of SPIRIVA. If such a reaction occurs, therapy with SPIRIVA should be stopped at once and alternative treatments should be considered. Inhaled medicines, including SPIRIVA, may cause paradoxical bronchospasm. If this occurs, treatment with SPIRIVA should be stopped and other treatments considered.

PRECAUTIONS

General

As an anticholinergic drug, SPIRIVA (tiotropium bromide inhalation powder) may potentially worsen symptoms and

Continued on next page

Spiriva—Cont.

signs associated with narrow-angle glaucoma, prostatic hyperplasia or bladder-neck obstruction and should be used with caution in patients with any of these conditions.

As a predominantly renally excreted drug, patients with moderate to severe renal impairment (creatinine clearance of ≤50 mL/min) treated with SPIRIVA should be monitored closely (see **CLINICAL PHARMACOLOGY, Pharmacokinetics, Special Populations,** *Renally-impaired Patients*).

Information for Patients

It is important for patients to understand how to correctly administer SPIRIVA capsules using the HandiHaler inhalation device (see **Patient's Instructions for Use**). SPIRIVA capsules should only be administered via the HandiHaler device and the HandiHaler device should not be used for administering other medications. **The contents of SPIRIVA capsules are for oral inhalation only and must not be swallowed.**

Capsules should always be stored in sealed blisters. Remove only one capsule immediately before use, or its effectiveness may be reduced. Additional capsules that are exposed to air (i.e., not intended for immediate use) should be discarded.

Eye pain or discomfort, blurred vision, visual halos or colored images in association with red eyes from conjunctival congestion and corneal edema may be signs of acute narrow-angle glaucoma. Should any of these signs and symptoms develop, consult a physician immediately. Miotic eye drops alone are not considered to be effective treatment.

Care must be taken not to allow the powder to enter into the eyes as this may cause blurring of vision and pupil dilation.

SPIRIVA HandiHaler is a once-daily maintenance bronchodilator and should not be used for immediate relief of breathing problems, i.e., as a rescue medication.

Drug Interactions

SPIRIVA has been used concomitantly with other drugs commonly used in COPD without increases in adverse drug reactions. These include short-acting and long-acting sympathomimetic (beta-agonists) bronchodilators, methylxanthines, and oral and inhaled steroids. However, the co-administration of SPIRIVA with other anticholinergic-containing drugs (e.g., ipratropium) has not been studied and is therefore not recommended.

Drug/Laboratory Test Interactions

None known.

Carcinogenesis, Mutagenesis, Impairment of Fertility

No evidence of tumorigenicity was observed in a 104-week inhalation study in rats at tiotropium doses up to 0.059 mg/kg/day, in an 83-week inhalation study in female mice at doses up to 0.145 mg/kg/day, and in a 101-week inhalation study in male mice at doses up to 0.002 mg/kg/day. These doses correspond to 25, 35, and 0.5 times the Recommended Human Daily Dose (RHDD) on a mg/m^2 basis, respectively. These dose multiples may be over-estimated due to difficulties in measuring deposited doses in animal inhalation studies.

Tiotropium bromide demonstrated no evidence of mutagenicity or clastogenicity in the following assays: the bacterial gene mutation assay, the V79 Chinese hamster cell mutagenesis assay, the chromosomal aberration assays in human lymphocytes *in vitro* and mouse micronucleus formation *in vivo*, and the unscheduled DNA synthesis in primary rat hepatocytes *in vitro* assay.

In rats, decreases in the number of corpora lutea and the percentage of implants were noted at inhalation tiotropium doses of 0.078 mg/kg/day or greater (approximately 35 times the RHDD on a mg/m^2 basis). No such effects were observed at 0.009 mg/kg/day (approximately 4 times than the RHDD on a mg/m^2 basis). The fertility index, however, was not affected at inhalation doses up to 1.689 mg/kg/day (approximately 760 times the RHDD on a mg/m^2 basis). These dose multiples may be over-estimated due to difficulties in measuring deposited doses in animal inhalation studies.

Pregnancy

Pregnancy Category C.

No evidence of structural alterations was observed in rats and rabbits at inhalation tiotropium doses of up to 1.471 and 0.007 mg/kg/day, respectively. These doses correspond to approximately 660 and 6 times the recommended human daily dose (RHDD) on a mg/m^2 basis. However, in rats, fetal resorption, litter loss, decreases in the number of live pups at birth and the mean pup weights, and a delay in pup sexual maturation were observed at inhalation tiotropium doses of ≥0.078 mg/kg (approximately 35 times the RHDD on a mg/m^2 basis). In rabbits, an increase in post-implantation loss was observed at an inhalation dose of 0.4 mg/kg/day (approximately 360 times the RHDD on a mg/m^2 basis). Such effects were not observed at inhalation doses of 0.009 and up to 0.088 mg/kg/day in rats and rabbits, respectively. These doses correspond to approximately 4 and 80 times the RHDD on a mg/m^2 basis, respectively. These dose multiples may be over-estimated due to difficulties in measuring deposited doses in animal inhalation studies.

There are no adequate and well-controlled studies in pregnant women. SPIRIVA should be used during pregnancy only if the potential benefit justifies the potential risk to the fetus.

Use in Labor and Delivery

The safety and effectiveness of SPIRIVA has not been studied during labor and delivery.

Nursing Mothers

Clinical data from nursing women exposed to tiotropium are not available. Based on lactating rodent studies, tiotropium is excreted into breast milk. It is not known whether tiotropium is excreted in human milk, but because many drugs are excreted in human milk and given these findings in rats, caution should be exercised if SPIRIVA is administered to a nursing woman.

Pediatric Use

SPIRIVA HandiHaler is approved for use in the maintenance treatment of bronchospasm associated with chronic obstructive pulmonary disease, including chronic bronchitis and emphysema. This disease does not normally occur in children. The safety and effectiveness of SPIRIVA in pediatric patients have not been established.

Geriatric Use

Of the total number of patients who received SPIRIVA in the 1-year clinical trials, 426 were <65 years, 375 were 65–74 years and 105 were ≥75 years of age. Within each age subgroup, there were no differences between the proportion of patients with adverse events in the SPIRIVA and the comparator groups for most events. Dry mouth increased with age in the SPIRIVA group (differences from placebo were 9.0%, 17.1%, and 16.2% in the aforementioned age subgroups). A higher frequency of constipation and urinary tract infections with increasing age was observed in the SPIRIVA group in the placebo-controlled studies. The differences from placebo for constipation were 0%, 1.8%, and 7.8% for each of the age groups. The differences from placebo for urinary tract infections were –0.6%, 4.6% and 4.5%. No overall differences in effectiveness were observed among these groups. Based on available data, no adjustment of SPIRIVA dosage in geriatric patients is warranted.

ADVERSE REACTIONS

Of the 2,663 patients in the four 1-year and two 6-month controlled clinical trials, 1,308 were treated with SPIRIVA (tiotropium bromide inhalation powder) at the recommended dose of 18 mcg once a day. Patients with narrow angle glaucoma, or symptomatic prostatic hypertrophy or bladder outlet obstruction were excluded from these trials. The most commonly reported adverse drug reaction was dry mouth. Dry mouth was usually mild and often resolved during continued treatment. Other reactions reported in individual patients and consistent with possible anticholinergic effects included constipation, increased heart rate, blurred vision, glaucoma, urinary difficulty, and urinary retention.

Four multicenter, 1-year, controlled studies evaluated SPIRIVA in patients with COPD. Table 1 shows all adverse events that occurred with a frequency of ≥3% in the SPIRIVA group in the 1-year placebo-controlled trials where the rates in the SPIRIVA group exceeded placebo by ≥1%. The frequency of corresponding events in the ipratropium-controlled trials is included for comparison.

[See table 1 below]

Table 1 Adverse Experience Incidence (% Patients) in One-Year-COPD Clinical Trials

Body System (Event)	Placebo-Controlled Trials SPIRIVA [n = 550]	Placebo [n = 371]	Ipratropium-Controlled Trials SPIRIVA [n = 356]	Ipratropium [n = 179]
Body as a Whole				
Accidents	13	11	5	8
Chest Pain (non-specific)	7	5	5	2
Edema, Dependent	5	4	3	5
Gastrointestinal System Disorders				
Abdominal Pain	5	3	6	6
Constipation	4	2	1	1
Dry Mouth	16	3	12	6
Dyspepsia	6	5	1	1
Vomiting	4	2	1	2
Musculoskeletal System				
Myalgia	4	3	4	3
Resistance Mechanism Disorders				
Infection	4	3	1	3
Moniliasis	4	2	3	2
Respiratory System (upper)				
Epistaxis	4	2	1	1
Pharyngitis	9	7	7	3
Rhinitis	6	5	3	2
Sinusitis	11	9	3	2
Upper Respiratory Tract Infection	41	37	43	35
Skin and Appendage Disorders				
Rash	4	2	2	2
Urinary System				
Urinary Tract Infection	7	5	4	2

Arthritis, coughing, and influenza-like symptoms occurred at a rate of ≥3% in the SPIRIVA treatment group, but were <1% in excess of the placebo group.

Other events that occurred in the SPIRIVA group at a frequency of 1–3% in the placebo-controlled trials where the rates exceeded that in the placebo group include: *Body as a Whole:* allergic reaction, leg pain; *Central and Peripheral Nervous System:* dysphonia, paresthesia; *Gastrointestinal System Disorders:* gastrointestinal disorder not otherwise specified (NOS), gastroesophageal reflux, stomatitis (including ulcerative stomatitis); *Metabolic and Nutritional Disorders:* hypercholesterolemia, hyperglycemia; *Musculoskeletal System Disorders:* skeletal pain; *Cardiac Events:* angina pectoris (including aggravated angina pectoris); *Psychiatric Disorder:* depression; *Infections:* herpes zoster; *Respiratory System Disorder (Upper):* laryngitis; *Vision Disorder:* cataract. In addition, among the adverse events observed in the clinical trials with an incidence of <1% were atrial fibrillation, supraventricular tachycardia, angioedema, and urinary retention.

In the 1-year trials, the incidence of dry mouth, constipation, and urinary tract infection increased with age (see **PRECAUTIONS, Geriatric Use**).

Two multicenter, 6-month, controlled studies evaluated SPIRIVA in patients with COPD. The adverse events and the incidence rates were similar to those seen in the 1-year controlled trials.

The following adverse reactions have been identified during worldwide post-approval use of SPIRIVA: application site irritation (glossitis, mouth ulceration, and pharyngolaryngeal pain), dizziness, dysphagia, epistaxis, hoarseness, intestinal obstruction including ileus paralytic, intraocular pressure increased, oral candidiasis, palpitations, pruritus, tachycardia, throat irritation, and urticaria.

OVERDOSAGE

High doses of tiotropium may lead to anticholinergic signs and symptoms. However, there were no systemic anticholinergic adverse effects following a single inhaled dose of up to 282 mcg tiotropium in 6 healthy volunteers. In a study of 12 healthy volunteers, bilateral conjunctivitis and dry mouth were seen following repeated once-daily inhalation of 141 mcg of tiotropium.

Accidental Ingestion

Acute intoxication by inadvertent oral ingestion of SPIRIVA (tiotropium bromide inhalation powder) capsules is unlikely since it is not well-absorbed systemically.

A case of overdose has been reported from post-marketing experience. A female patient was reported to have inhaled 30 capsules over a 2.5 day period, and developed altered mental status, tremors, abdominal pain, and severe constipation. The patient was hospitalized, SPIRIVA was discontinued, and the constipation was treated with an enema. The patient recovered and was discharged on the same day.

No mortality was observed at inhalation tiotropium doses up to 32.4 mg/kg in mice, 267.7 mg/kg in rats, and 0.6 mg/kg in dogs. These doses correspond to 7,300, 120,000, and 850 times the recommended human daily dose on a mg/m^2 basis, respectively. These dose multiples may be over-estimated due to difficulties in measuring deposited doses in animal inhalation studies.

DOSAGE AND ADMINISTRATION

SPIRIVA capsules must not be swallowed as the intended effects on the lungs will not be obtained. The contents of the capsules are for oral inhalation only (see OVERDOSAGE section).

The recommended dosage of SPIRIVA HandiHaler (tiotropium bromide inhalation powder) is the inhalation of the contents of one SPIRIVA capsule, once-daily, with the HandiHaler inhalation device (see **Patient's Instructions for Use**).

No dosage adjustment is required for geriatric, hepatically-impaired, or renally-impaired patients. However, patients with moderate to severe renal impairment given SPIRIVA should be monitored closely (see **CLINICAL PHARMACOLOGY, Pharmacokinetics, Special Populations** and **PRECAUTIONS**).

HOW SUPPLIED

SPIRIVA (tiotropium bromide inhalation powder) capsules, containing 18 mcg tiotropium, are light green, with TI 01 printed on one side of the capsule and the Boehringer Ingelheim company logo on the other side.

The HandiHaler inhalation device is gray colored with a green piercing button. It is imprinted with SPIRIVA HandiHaler (tiotropium bromide inhalation powder), the Boehringer Ingelheim company logo, and the Pfizer company logo. It is also imprinted to indicate that SPIRIVA capsules should not be stored in the HandiHaler device and that the HandiHaler device is only to be used with SPIRIVA capsules.

SPIRIVA capsules are packaged in an aluminum/aluminum blister card and joined along a perforated-cut line. Capsules should always be stored in the blister and only removed immediately before use. The drug should be used immediately after the packaging over an individual capsule is opened. The following packages are available:

carton containing 5 SPIRIVA capsules (1 unit-dose blister card) and 1 HandiHaler inhalation device (NDC 0597-0075-75)

carton containing 30 SPIRIVA capsules (3 unit-dose blister cards) and 1 HandiHaler inhalation device (NDC 0597-0075-41)

carton containing 90 SPIRIVA capsules (9 unit-dose blister cards) and 1 HandiHaler inhalation device (NDC 0597-0075-47)

Storage

Store at 25°C (77°F); excursions permitted to 15°–30°C (59°–86°F) [see USP Controlled Room Temperature].

The capsules should not be exposed to extreme temperature or moisture. Do not store capsules in the HandiHaler device.

Distributed by:
Boehringer Ingelheim Pharmaceuticals, Inc.
Ridgefield, CT 06877 USA
Marketed by:
Boehringer Ingelheim Pharmaceuticals, Inc.
Ridgefield, CT 06877 USA
and
Pfizer Inc
New York, NY 10017 USA
Licensed from:
Boehringer Ingelheim International GmbH
Address medical inquiries to: www.Spiriva.com, (800) 542-6257 or (800) 459-9906 TTY.
SPIRIVA® and HandiHaler® are registered trademarks and are used under license from Boehringer Ingelheim International GmbH

Patient's Instructions for Use

Spiriva®
HandiHaler®
(tiotropium bromide inhalation powder)
FOR ORAL INHALATION ONLY
DO NOT SWALLOW SPIRIVA CAPSULES
Read all instructions before use.

This leaflet provides summary information about SPIRIVA capsules and the HandiHaler inhalation device. Before you start to take SPIRIVA or use the HandiHaler, read this leaflet carefully and keep it for future use. You should read the leaflet that comes with your prescription every time you refill it because there may be new information.

For more information, ask your healthcare provider or pharmacist.

What should you know about SPIRIVA and the HandiHaler?
Each SPIRIVA capsule contains a dry powder blend of active drug (18 mcg tiotropium) and lactose monohydrate as the carrier. The dry powder in the capsule is inhaled from the HandiHaler inhalation device. **SPIRIVA capsules contain only a small amount of powder which makes the capsule appear almost empty.** When disposing of the capsule, you may notice that a dusting of this powder is left in the capsule. This is normal.

SPIRIVA is a once daily maintenance bronchodilator medicine that opens narrowed airways and helps keep them open for 24 hours. SPIRIVA HandiHaler should not be used for immediate relief of breathing problems, i.e., as a rescue medication.

Tell your doctor before you use SPIRIVA HandiHaler:
if you may be pregnant or wish to become pregnant;
if you are a breastfeeding mother;
if you are taking any medications including eye drops, this includes those you can buy without a prescription;
if you have any other medical problems such as difficulty urinating or an enlarged prostate;
if you are allergic to any medications.
USE THIS PRODUCT AS DIRECTED, UNLESS INSTRUCTED TO DO OTHERWISE BY YOUR PHYSICIAN.
SPIRIVA CAPSULES ARE INTENDED FOR ORAL INHALATION ONLY AND ARE TO BE USED ONLY WITH THE HANDIHALER INHALATION DEVICE.
SPIRIVA CAPSULES SHOULD NOT BE SWALLOWED.
The HandiHaler is an inhalation device that has been specially designed for use with SPIRIVA capsules. It must not be used to take any other medication.
Care must be taken not to allow the powder to enter into the eyes. If symptoms of eye pain, eye discomfort, blurred vision, visual halos, or colored images in association with red eyes occur, consult a physician immediately.

Becoming familiar with SPIRIVA HandiHaler:

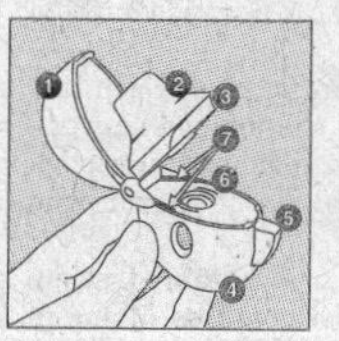

Remove the HandiHaler inhalation device from the pouch and become familiar with its components. (Figure A)
1. dust cap
2. mouthpiece
3. mouthpiece ridge
4. base
5. green piercing button
6. center chamber
7. air intake vents

Figure A

Each SPIRIVA capsule is packaged in a blister. Each blister can be separated from the blister card by tearing along the perforation. (Figure B)

Figure B

How do you take your dose of SPIRIVA using the HandiHaler?
Taking your dose of SPIRIVA, requires four main steps:
1. **OPEN** the HandiHaler device and the blister
2. **INSERT** the SPIRIVA capsule
3. **PRESS** the green piercing button
4. **INHALE** your medication
(See below for details)
Opening the HandiHaler device:

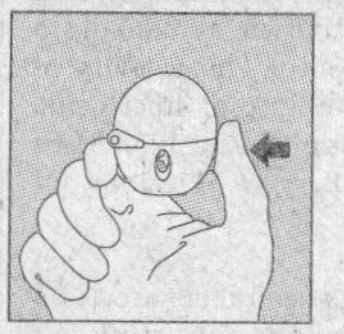

OPEN the dust cap by pressing the green piercing button. (Figure 1)

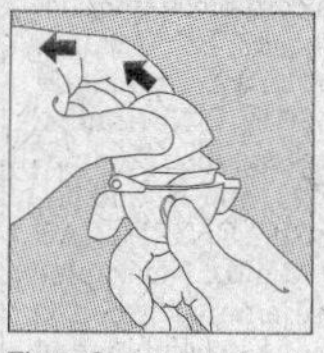

Figure 1

Pull the dust cap upwards to expose the mouthpiece. (Figure 2)

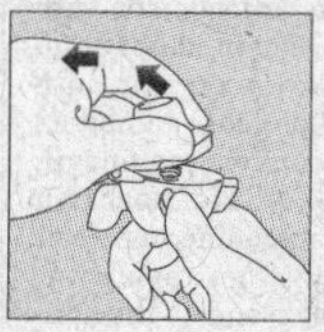

Figure 2

Open the mouthpiece by pulling the mouthpiece ridge upwards. (Figure 3)

Figure 3

Removing a SPIRIVA capsule:

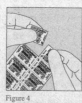

Prior to removing a SPIRIVA capsule from the blister, separate one of the blisters from the blister card by tearing along the perforation. (Figure 4)
Capsules should always be stored in the sealed blisters and only removed immediately before use. Do not store capsules in the HandiHaler device. The drug should be used immediately after the packaging of an individual capsule is opened, or else its effectiveness may be reduced.

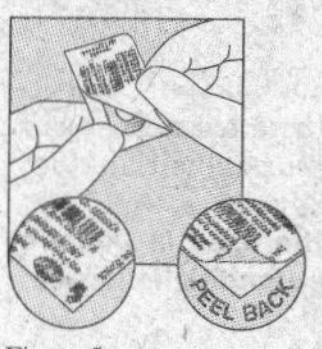

Figure 4

Immediately before you are ready to use your dose of SPIRIVA:
Bend back and forth one of the corners that has an arrow and with your finger separate the aluminum foil layers. Then carefully peel back the printed foil until the capsule is fully visible. (Figure 5)
Turn the blister upside down and tip the capsule out, tapping the back of the blister, if necessary.

Figure 5

DO NOT CUT THE FOIL OR USE SHARP INSTRUMENTS TO REMOVE THE CAPSULE FROM THE BLISTER.
If additional capsules are exposed to air, they should not be used and should be discarded.
Inserting the SPIRIVA capsule into the HandiHaler:

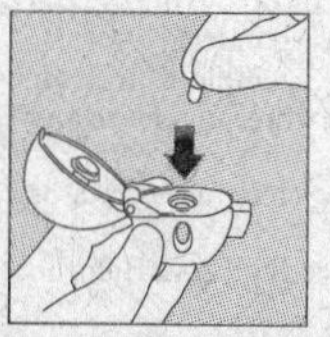

INSERT the capsule in the center chamber of the HandiHaler device. It does not matter which end of the capsule is placed in the chamber. (Figure 6)

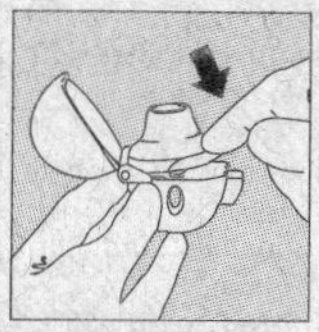

Figure 6

Close the mouthpiece **firmly until you hear a click**, leaving the dust cap open. (Figure 7)
Be sure that the mouthpiece sits firmly against the gray base.

Figure 7

Taking your dose of SPIRIVA:

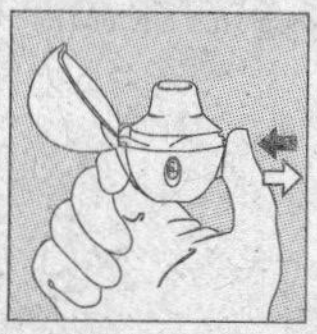

Hold the HandiHaler device with the mouthpiece upwards.
PRESS the green piercing button until it is flush against the base, and release. This makes holes in the capsule and allows the medication to be released when you breathe in. (Figure 8)
DO NOT PRESS THE GREEN PIERCING BUTTON MORE THAN ONE TIME.

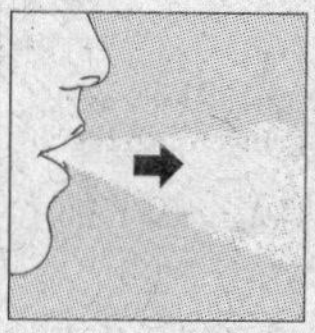

Figure 8

Breathe out completely. (Figure 9)
Important: Do not breathe (exhale) into the HandiHaler mouthpiece at any time.

Figure 9

INHALE
• Hold the HandiHaler by the gray base. Do not block the air intake vents.
• Raise the HandiHaler device to your mouth and close your lips tightly around the mouthpiece.
• **Keep your head in an upright position. The HandiHaler should be in a horizontal position.** (Figure 10)

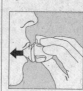

Figure 10

• Breathe in **slowly and deeply** but at a rate **sufficient to hear or feel the capsule vibrate.**
• Breathe in until your lungs are full.
• Hold your breath as long as is comfortable and at the same time take the HandiHaler device out of your mouth. Resume normal breathing.

To ensure you get the full dose of SPIRIVA, you must again breathe out completely and inhale once again as previously described (Figure 10).
DO NOT PRESS THE GREEN PIERCING BUTTON AGAIN.
If you do not hear or feel the capsule vibrate, **Do Not Press The Green Piercing Button Again** but instead tap the HandiHaler gently on a table, holding it in an upright position. Check to see that the mouthpiece is completely closed. Then breathe in again – slowly and deeply. If you still do not hear or feel the capsule vibrate after repeating the above steps, please consult your physician.

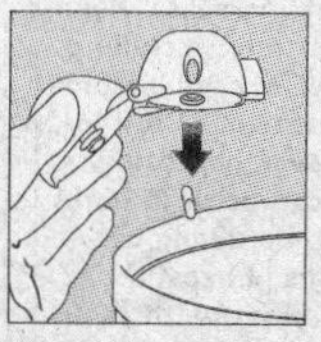

After you have finished taking your daily dose of SPIRIVA, open the mouthpiece again. Tip out the used capsule and discard. (Figure 11)

Figure 11

Continued on next page

Spiriva—Cont.

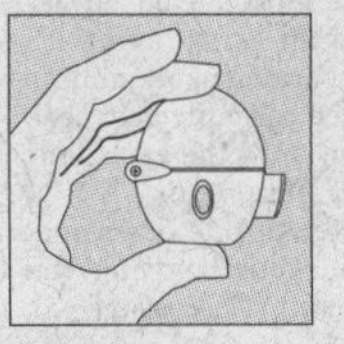

Close the mouthpiece and dust cap for storage of your HandiHaler device. (Figure 12)

Do not store the used or unused capsules in the HandiHaler device.

Figure 12

When and how should you clean your HandiHaler Device?

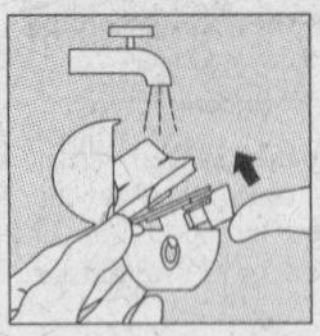

Clean the HandiHaler once a month. (Figure 13)

- Open the dust cap and mouthpiece.
- Open the base by lifting the green piercing button.
- Rinse the complete inhaler with warm water to remove any powder.
- Do not use cleaning agents or detergents.
- Do not place the HandiHaler in the dishwasher for cleaning.

Figure 13

- Dry the HandiHaler thoroughly by tipping the excess water out on a paper towel and air-dry afterwards, leaving the dust cap, mouthpiece, and base open.
- **It takes 24 hours to air dry, so clean it right after you use it and it will be ready for your next dose.**
- Do not use the HandiHaler device when it is wet. If needed, the outside of the mouthpiece may be cleaned with a moist but not wet tissue.

Where should you store SPIRIVA capsules and the HandiHaler Device?

Store at 25°C (77°F); excursions permitted to 15°–30°C (59°–86°F) [see USP Controlled Room Temperature].

The capsules should not be exposed to extreme temperature or moisture. Do not store capsules in the HandiHaler.

As with all prescription medications, keep this out of the reach of children.

Distributed by:
Boehringer Ingelheim Pharmaceuticals, Inc.
Ridgefield, CT 06877 USA
Marketed by:
Boehringer Ingelheim Pharmaceuticals, Inc.
Ridgefield, CT 06877 USA
and
Pfizer Inc
New York, NY 10017 USA
Licensed from:
Boehringer Ingelheim International GmbH

SPIRIVA® and HandiHaler® are registered trademarks and are used under license from Boehringer Ingelheim International GmbH
©Copyright Boehringer Ingelheim International GmbH 2007
ALL RIGHTS RESERVED

SPIRIVA® (tiotropium bromide inhalation powder) is covered by U.S. Patent Nos. RE38,912, RE39,820, 6,777,423, 6,908,928, and 7,070,800 with other patents pending. The HandiHaler® inhalation device is covered by U.S. Design Patent No. D355,029 with other patents pending.

IT1600MK2807
10004551/US/3 10004551/03
65626/US/3
Rev: December 2007

VIRAMUNE® ℞
[*vī-ră-mewn*]
(nevirapine) Tablets
VIRAMUNE® ℞
(nevirapine) Oral Suspension
Rx only

Prescribing information for this product, which appears on pages 866–872 of the 2008 PDR, has been revised as follows. Please write "See Supplement A" next to the product heading.

WARNING

Severe, life-threatening, and in some cases fatal hepatotoxicity, particularly in the first 18 weeks, has been reported in patients treated with VIRAMUNE®. In some cases, patients presented with non-specific prodromal signs or symptoms of hepatitis and progressed to hepatic failure. These events are often associated with rash. Female gender and higher CD4 counts at initiation of therapy place patients at increased risk; women with CD4 counts >250 cells/mm^3, including pregnant women receiving VIRAMUNE in combination with other antiretrovirals for the treatment of HIV infection, are at the greatest risk. However, hepatotoxicity associated with VIRAMUNE use can occur in both genders, all CD4 counts and at any time during treatment. Patients with signs or symptoms of hepatitis, or with increased transaminases combined with rash or other systemic symptoms, must discontinue VIRAMUNE and seek medical evaluation immediately (see WARNINGS).

Severe, life-threatening skin reactions, including fatal cases, have occurred in patients treated with VIRAMUNE. These have included cases of Stevens-Johnson syndrome, toxic epidermal necrolysis, and hypersensitivity reactions characterized by rash, constitutional findings, and organ dysfunction. Patients developing signs or symptoms of severe skin reactions or hypersensitivity reactions must discontinue VIRAMUNE and seek medical evaluation immediately (see WARNINGS).

It is essential that patients be monitored intensively during the first 18 weeks of therapy with VIRAMUNE to detect potentially life-threatening hepatotoxicity or skin reactions. Extra vigilance is warranted during the first 6 weeks of therapy, which is the period of greatest risk of these events. Do not restart VIRAMUNE following severe hepatic, skin or hypersensitivity reactions. In some cases, hepatic injury has progressed despite discontinuation of treatment. In addition, the 14-day lead-in period with VIRAMUNE 200 mg daily dosing must be strictly followed (see WARNINGS).

DESCRIPTION

VIRAMUNE is the brand name for nevirapine (NVP), a non-nucleoside reverse transcriptase inhibitor with activity against Human Immunodeficiency Virus Type 1 (HIV-1). Nevirapine is structurally a member of the dipyridodiazepin one chemical class of compounds.

VIRAMUNE Tablets are for oral administration. Each tablet contains 200 mg of nevirapine and the inactive ingredients microcrystalline cellulose, lactose monohydrate, povidone, sodium starch glycolate, colloidal silicon dioxide and magnesium stearate.

VIRAMUNE Oral Suspension is for oral administration. Each 5 mL of VIRAMUNE suspension contains 50 mg of nevirapine (as nevirapine hemihydrate). The suspension also contains the following excipients: carbomer 934P, methylparaben, propylparaben, sorbitol, sucrose, polysorbate 80, sodium hydroxide and purified water.

The chemical name of nevirapine is 11-cyclopropyl-5,11-dihydro-4-methyl-6H-dipyrido [3,2-b:2′,3′-e][1,4] diazepin-6-one. Nevirapine is a white to off-white crystalline powder with the molecular weight of 266.30 and the molecular formula $C_{15}H_{14}N_4O$. Nevirapine has the following structural formula:

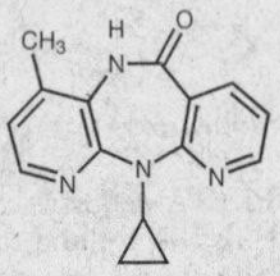

MICROBIOLOGY

Mechanism of Action

Nevirapine is a non-nucleoside reverse transcriptase inhibitor (NNRTI) of HIV-1. Nevirapine binds directly to reverse transcriptase (RT) and blocks the RNA-dependent and DNA-dependent DNA polymerase activities by causing a disruption of the enzyme's catalytic site. The activity of nevirapine does not compete with template or nucleoside triphosphates. HIV-2 RT and eukaryotic DNA polymerases (such as human DNA polymerases α, β, γ, or δ) are not inhibited by nevirapine.

Antiviral Activity

The antiviral activity of nevirapine has been measured in a variety of cell lines including peripheral blood mononuclear cells, monocyte derived macrophages, and lymphoblastoid cell lines. In recent studies using human cord blood lymphocytes and human embryonic kidney 293 cells, EC50 values (50% inhibitory concentration) ranged from 14-302 nM against laboratory and clinical isolates of HIV-1. Nevirapine exhibited antiviral activity in cell culture against group M HIV-1 isolates from clades A, B, C, D, F, G, and H, and circulating recombinant forms (CRF) CRF01_AE, CRF02_AG and CRF12_BF (median EC50 value of 63 nM). Nevirapine had no antiviral activity in cell culture against group O HIV-1 isolates or HIV-2 isolates. Nevirapine in combination with efavirenz exhibited strong antagonistic anti-HIV-1 activity in cell culture and was additive to antagonistic with the protease inhibitor ritonavir or the fusion inhibitor enfuvirtide. Nevirapine exhibited additive to synergistic anti-HIV-1 activity in combination with the protease inhibitors amprenavir, atazanavir, indinavir, lopinavir, nelfinavir, saquinavir and tipranavir, and the NRTIs abacavir, didanosine, emtricitabine, lamivudine, stavudine, tenofovir and zidovudine. The anti-HIV-1 activity of nevirapine was antagonized by the anti-HBV drug adefovir and by the anti-HCV drug ribavirin in cell culture.

Resistance

HIV-1 isolates with reduced susceptibility (100-250-fold) to nevirapine emerge in cell culture. Genotypic analysis showed mutations in the HIV-1 RT gene Y181C and/or V106A depending upon the virus strain and cell line employed. Time to emergence of nevirapine resistance in cell culture was not altered when selection included nevirapine in combination with several other NNRTIs.

Phenotypic and genotypic changes in HIV-1 isolates from treatment-naïve patients receiving either nevirapine (n=24) or nevirapine and ZDV (n=14) were monitored in Phase I/II trials over 1 to ≥12 weeks. After 1 week of nevirapine monotherapy, isolates from 3/3 patients had decreased susceptibility to nevirapine in cell culture. One or more of the RT mutations resulting in amino acid substitutions K103N, V106A, V108I, Y181C, Y188C and G190A were detected in HIV-1 isolates from some patients as early as 2 weeks after therapy initiation. By week eight of nevirapine monotherapy, 100% of the patients tested (n=24) had HIV-1 isolates with a >100-fold decrease in susceptibility to nevirapine in cell culture compared to baseline, and had one or more of the nevirapine-associated RT resistance mutations. Nineteen of these patients (80%) had isolates with Y181C mutations regardless of dose.

Genotypic analysis of isolates from antiretroviral naïve patients experiencing virologic failure (n=71) receiving nevirapine once daily (n=25) or twice daily (n=46) in combination with lamivudine and stavudine (study 2NN) for 48 weeks showed that isolates from 8/25 and 23/46 patients, respectively, contained one or more of the following NNRTI resistance-associated mutations: Y181C, K101E, G190A/S, K103N, V106A/M, V108I, Y188C/L, A98G, F227L and M230L.

Cross-resistance

Rapid emergence of HIV-1 strains which are cross-resistant to NNRTIs has been observed in cell culture. Nevirapine-resistant HIV-1 isolates were cross-resistant to the NNRTIs delavirdine and efavirenz. However, nevirapine-resistant isolates were susceptible to the NRTI's ddI and ZDV. Similarly, ZDV-resistant isolates were susceptible to nevirapine in cell culture.

ANIMAL PHARMACOLOGY

Animal studies have shown that nevirapine is widely distributed to nearly all tissues and readily crosses the blood-brain barrier.

CLINICAL PHARMACOLOGY

Pharmacokinetics in Adults

Absorption and Bioavailability: Nevirapine is readily absorbed (>90%) after oral administration in healthy volunteers and in adults with HIV-1 infection. Absolute bioavailability in 12 healthy adults following single-dose administration was 93 ± 9% (mean ± SD) for a 50 mg tablet and 91 ± 8% for an oral solution. Peak plasma nevirapine concentrations of 2 ± 0.4 µg/mL (7.5 µM) were attained by 4 hours following a single 200 mg dose. Following multiple doses, nevirapine peak concentrations appear to increase linearly in the dose range of 200 to 400 mg/day. Steady state trough nevirapine concentrations of 4.5 ± 1.9 µg/mL (17 ± 7 µM), (n = 242) were attained at 400 mg/day. Nevirapine tablets and suspension have been shown to be comparably bioavailable and interchangeable at doses up to 200 mg. When VIRAMUNE (200 mg) was administered to 24 healthy adults (12 female, 12 male), with either a high fat breakfast (857 kcal, 50 g fat, 53% of calories from fat) or antacid (Maalox® 30 mL), the extent of nevirapine absorption (AUC) was comparable to that observed under fasting conditions. In a separate study in HIV-1 infected patients (n=6), nevirapine steady-state systemic exposure (AUC_T) was not significantly altered by didanosine, which is formulated with an alkaline buffering agent. VIRAMUNE may be administered with or without food, antacid or didanosine.

Distribution: Nevirapine is highly lipophilic and is essentially nonionized at physiologic pH. Following intravenous administration to healthy adults, the apparent volume of distribution (Vdss) of nevirapine was 1.21 ± 0.09 L/kg, suggesting that nevirapine is widely distributed in humans. Nevirapine readily crosses the placenta and is also found in breast milk (see **PRECAUTIONS, *Nursing Mothers***). Nevirapine is about 60% bound to plasma proteins in the plasma concentration range of 1-10 µg/mL. Nevirapine concentrations in human cerebrospinal fluid (n=6) were 45% (± 5%) of the concentrations in plasma; this ratio is approximately equal to the fraction not bound to plasma protein.

Metabolism/Elimination: *In vivo* studies in humans and *in vitro* studies with human liver microsomes have shown that nevirapine is extensively biotransformed via cytochrome P450 (oxidative) metabolism to several hydroxylated metabolites. *In vitro* studies with human liver microsomes suggest that oxidative metabolism of nevirapine is mediated primarily by cytochrome P450 (CYP) isozymes from the CYP3A4 and CYP2B6 families, although other isozymes may have a secondary role. In a mass balance/excretion study in eight healthy male volunteers dosed to steady state with nevirapine 200 mg given twice daily followed by a single 50 mg dose of ^{14}C-nevirapine, approximately 91.4 ±10.5% of the radiolabeled dose was recovered, with urine (81.3 ± 11.1%) representing the primary route of excretion compared to feces (10.1 ± 1.5%). Greater than 80% of the radioactivity in urine was made up of glucuronide conjugates of hydroxylated metabolites. Thus cytochrome P450 metabolism, glucuronide conjugation, and urinary excretion of glucuronidated metabolites represent the primary route of nevirapine biotransformation and elimination in humans. Only a small fraction (<5%) of the radioactivity in urine (representing <3% of the total dose) was made up of parent compound; therefore, renal excretion plays a minor role in elimination of the parent compound.

Nevirapine is an inducer of hepatic cytochrome P450 (CYP) metabolic enzymes 3A4 and 2B6. Nevirapine induces CYP3A4 and CYP2B6 by approximately 20-25%, as indicated by erythromycin breath test results and urine metabolites. Autoinduction of CYP3A4 and CYP2B6 mediated metabolism leads to an approximately 1.5 to 2 fold increase in the apparent oral clearance of nevirapine as treatment con-

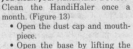

tinues from a single dose to two-to-four weeks of dosing with 200-400 mg/day. Autoinduction also results in a corresponding decrease in the terminal phase half-life of nevirapine in plasma, from approximately 45 hours (single dose) to approximately 25-30 hours following multiple dosing with 200-400 mg/day.

Pharmacokinetics in Special Populations

Renal Impairment: HIV seronegative adults with mild (CrCL 50-79 mL/min; n=7), moderate (CrCL 30-49 mL/min; n=6), or severe (CrCL <30 mL/min; n=4) renal impairment received a single 200 mg dose of nevirapine in a pharmacokinetic study. These subjects did not require dialysis. The study included six additional subjects with renal failure requiring dialysis.

In subjects with renal impairment (mild, moderate or severe), there were no significant changes in the pharmacokinetics of nevirapine. However, subjects requiring dialysis exhibited a 44% reduction in nevirapine AUC over a one-week exposure period. There was also evidence of accumulation of nevirapine hydroxy-metabolites in plasma in subjects requiring dialysis. An additional 200 mg dose following each dialysis treatment is indicated (see **DOSAGE AND ADMINISTRATION** and **PRECAUTIONS**).

Hepatic Impairment: HIV seronegative adults with mild (Child-Pugh Class A; n=6) or moderate (Child-Pugh Class B; n=4) hepatic impairment received a single 200 mg dose of nevirapine in a pharmacokinetic study.

In the majority of patients with mild or moderate hepatic impairment, no significant changes were seen in the pharmacokinetics of nevirapine. However, a significant increase in the AUC of nevirapine observed in one patient with Child-Pugh Class B and ascites suggests that patients with worsening hepatic function and ascites may be at risk of accumulating nevirapine in the systemic circulation. Because nevirapine induces its own metabolism with multiple dosing, a single dose study may not reflect the impact of hepatic impairment on multiple dose pharmacokinetics (see **PRECAUTIONS**). Nevirapine should not be administered to patients with severe hepatic impairment (see **WARNINGS**).

Gender: In the multinational 2NN study, a population pharmacokinetic substudy of 1077 patients was performed that included 391 females. Female patients showed a 13.8% lower clearance of nevirapine than did men. Since neither body weight nor Body Mass Index (BMI) had an influence on the clearance of nevirapine, the effect of gender cannot solely be explained by body size.

Race: An evaluation of nevirapine plasma concentrations (pooled data from several clinical trials) from HIV-1-infected patients (27 Black, 24 Hispanic, 189 Caucasian) revealed no marked difference in nevirapine steady-state trough concentrations (median C_{minss} = 4.7 µg/mL Black, 3.8 µg/mL Hispanic, 4.3 µg/mL Caucasian) with long-term nevirapine treatment at 400 mg/day. However, the pharmacokinetics of nevirapine have not been evaluated specifically for the effects of ethnicity.

Geriatric Patients: Nevirapine pharmacokinetics in HIV-1-infected adults do not appear to change with age (range 18–68 years); however, nevirapine has not been extensively evaluated in patients beyond the age of 55 years.

Pediatric Patients: The pharmacokinetics of nevirapine have been studied in two open-label studies in children with HIV-1 infection. In one study (BI 853; ACTG 165), nine HIV-1-infected children ranging in age from 9 months to 14 years were administered a single dose (7.5 mg, 30 mg, or 120 mg per m²; n=3 per dose) of nevirapine suspension after an overnight fast. The mean nevirapine apparent clearance adjusted for body weight was greater in children compared to adults.

In a multiple dose study (BI 882; ACTG 180), nevirapine suspension or tablets (240 or 400 mg/m²/day) were administered as monotherapy or in combination with ZDV or ZDV+ddI to 37 HIV-1-infected pediatric patients with the following demographics: male (54%), racial minority groups (73%), median age of 11 months (range: 2 months-15 years). The majority of these patients received 120 mg/m²/day of nevirapine for approximately 4 weeks followed by 120 mg/m²/BID (patients > 9 years of age) or 200 mg/m²/BID (patients ≤ 9 years of age). Nevirapine apparent clearance adjusted for body weight reached maximum values by age 1 to 2 years and then decreased with increasing age. Nevirapine apparent clearance adjusted for body weight was at least two-fold greater in children younger than 8 years compared to adults. The relationship between nevirapine clearance with long term drug administration and age is shown in Figure 1. The pediatric dosing regimens were selected in order to achieve steady-state plasma concentrations in pediatric patients that approximate those in adults (see **DOSAGE AND ADMINISTRATION**, *Pediatric Patients*).

[See figure 1 at top of next column]

Drug Interactions: (see **PRECAUTIONS**, *Drug Interactions*) Nevirapine induces hepatic cytochrome P450 metabolic isoenzymes 3A4 and 2B6. Co-administration of VIRAMUNE and drugs primarily metabolized by CYP3A4 or CYP2B6 may result in decreased plasma concentrations of these drugs and could attenuate their therapeutic effects.

While primarily an inducer of cytochrome P450 3A4 and 2B6 enzymes, nevirapine may also inhibit this system. Among human hepatic cytochrome P450s, nevirapine is capable *in vitro* of inhibiting the 10-hydroxylation of (R)-warfarin (CYP3A4). The estimated K_i for the inhibition of CYP3A4 was 270 µM, a concentration that is unlikely to be achieved in patients as the therapeutic range is <25 µM. Therefore, nevirapine may have minimal inhibitory effect on other substrates of CYP3A4.

Table 1 Drug Interactions: Changes in Pharmacokinetic Parameters for Co-administered Drug in the Presence of VIRAMUNE (All interaction studies were conducted in HIV-1 positive patients)

Co-administered Drug	Dose of Co-administered Drug	Dose Regimen of VIRAMUNE	n	% Change of Co-administered Drug Pharmacokinetic Parameters (90% CI)		
Antiretrovirals				AUC	C_{max}	C_{min}
Didanosine	100-150 mg BID	200 mg QD × 14 days; 200 mg BID × 14 days	18	⇔	⇔	§
Efavirenz[a]	600 mg QD	200 mg QD × 14 days; 400 mg QD × 14 days	17	↓28 (↓34 to ↓14)	↓12 (↓23 to ↑1)	↓32 (↓35 to ↓19)
Indinavir[a]	800 mg q8H	200 mg QD × 14 days; 200 mg BID × 14 days	19	↓31 (↓39 to ↓22)	↓15 (↓24 to ↓4)	↓44 (↓53 to ↓33)
Lopinavir[a, b]	300/75 mg/m² (lopinavir/ritonavir)[b]	7 mg/kg or 4 mg/kg QD × 2 weeks; BID × 1 week	12, 15[c]	↓22 (↓44 to ↑9)	↓14 (↓36 to ↑16)	↓55 (↓75 to ↓19)
Lopinavir[a]	400/100 mg BID (lopinavir/ritonavir)	200 mg QD × 14 days; 200 mg BID > 1 year	22, 19[c]	↓27 (↓47 to ↓2)	↓19 (↓38 to ↑5)	↓51 (↓72 to ↓26)
Nelfinavir[a]	750 mg TID	200 mg QD × 14 days; 200 mg BID × 14 days	23	⇔	⇔	↓32 (↓50 to ↑5)
Nelfinavir-M8 metabolite				↓62 (↓70 to ↓53)	↓59 (↓68 to ↓48)	↓66 (↓74 to ↓55)
Ritonavir	600 mg BID	200 mg QD × 14 days; 200 mg BID × 14 days	18	⇔	⇔	⇔
Saquinavir[a]	600 mg TID	200 mg QD × 14 days; 200 mg BID × 21 days	23	↓38 (↓47 to ↓11)	↓32 (↓44 to ↓6)	§
Stavudine	30-40 mg BID	200 mg QD × 14 days; 200 mg BID × 14 days	22	⇔	⇔	§
Zalcitabine	0.125-0.25 mg TID	200 mg QD × 14 days; 200 mg BID × 14 days	6	⇔	⇔	§
Zidovudine	100-200 mg TID	200 mg QD × 14 days; 200 mg BID × 14 days	11	↓28 (↓40 to ↓4)	↓30 (↓51 to ↑14)	§
Other Medications				AUC	C_{max}	C_{min}
Clarithromycin[a]	500 mg BID	200 mg QD × 14 days; 200 mg BID × 14 days	15	↓31 (↓38 to ↓24)	↓23 (↓31 to ↓14)	↓56 (↓70 to ↓36)
Metabolite 14-OH-clarithromycin				↑42 (↑16 to ↑73)	↑47 (↑21 to ↑80)	⇔
Ethinyl estradiol[a] and	0.035 mg (as Ortho-Novum® 1/35)	200 mg QD × 14 days; 200 mg BID × 14 days	10	↓20 (↓33 to ↓3)	⇔	§
Norethindrone[a]	1 mg (as Ortho-Novum® 1/35)			↓19 (↓30 to ↓7)	↓16 (↓27 to ↓3)	§
Fluconazole	200 mg QD	200 mg QD × 14 days; 200 mg BID × 14 days	19	⇔	⇔	⇔
Ketoconazole[a]	400 mg QD	200 mg QD × 14 days; 200 mg BID × 14 days	21	↓72 (↓80 to ↓60)	↓44 (↓58 to ↓27)	§

(Table continued on next page)

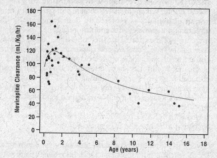

Figure 1: Nevirapine Apparent Clearance (mL/kg/hr) in Pediatric Patients

Nevirapine does not appear to affect the plasma concentrations of drugs that are substrates of other CYP450 enzyme systems, such as 1A2, 2D6, 2A6, 2E1, 2C9 or 2C19.

Table 1 (see below) contains the results of drug interaction studies performed with VIRAMUNE and other drugs likely to be co-administered. The effects of VIRAMUNE on the AUC, C_{max}, and C_{min} of co-administered drugs are summarized. To measure the full potential pharmacokinetic interaction effect following induction, patients on the concomitant drug at steady state were reassessed 28 days of VIRAMUNE (200 mg QD for 14 days followed by 200 mg BID for 14 days) followed by a steady state reassessment of the concomitant drug.

[See table 1 above and on next page]

Because of the design of the drug interaction trials (addition of 28 days of VIRAMUNE therapy to existing HIV therapy) the effect of the concomitant drug on plasma nevirapine steady state concentrations was estimated by comparison to historical controls.

Administration of rifampin had a clinically significant effect on nevirapine pharmacokinetics, decreasing AUC and C_{max} by greater than 50%. Administration of fluconazole resulted in an approximate 100% increase in nevirapine exposure, based on a comparison to historic data (see **PRECAUTIONS**, *Drug Interactions*, Table 3). The effect of other drugs listed in Table 1 on nevirapine pharmacokinetics was not significant.

INDICATIONS AND USAGE

VIRAMUNE (nevirapine) is indicated for use in combination with other antiretroviral agents for the treatment of HIV-1-infection. This indication is based on one principal clinical trial (BI 1090) that demonstrated prolonged suppression of HIV-RNA and two smaller supportive studies, one of which (BI 1046) is described below.

Additional important information regarding the use of VIRAMUNE for the treatment of HIV-1 infection:

• Based on serious and life-threatening hepatotoxicity observed in controlled and uncontrolled studies, VIRAMUNE should not be initiated in adult females with CD4+ cell counts greater than 250 cells/mm³ or in adult males with CD4+ cell counts greater than 400 cells/mm³ unless the benefit outweighs the risk (see **WARNINGS**).

• The 14-day lead-in period with VIRAMUNE 200 mg daily dosing has been demonstrated to reduce the frequency of rash (see **WARNINGS** and **DOSAGE AND ADMINISTRATION**).

Description of Clinical Studies

Trial BI 1090, was a placebo-controlled, double-blind, randomized trial in 2249 HIV-1-infected patients with <200

Viramune—Cont.

CD4+ cells/mm[3] at screening. Initiated in 1995, BI 1090 compared treatment with VIRAMUNE + lamivudine + background therapy versus lamivudine + background therapy in NNRTI naïve patients. Treatment doses were VIRAMUNE, 200 mg daily for two weeks followed by 200 mg twice daily or placebo, and lamivudine 150 mg twice daily. Other antiretroviral agents were given at approved doses. Initial background therapy (in addition to lamivudine) was one NRTI in 1309 patients (58%), two or more NRTIs in 771 (34%), and PIs and NRTIs in 169 (8%). The patients (median age 36.5 years, 70% Caucasian, 79% male) had advanced HIV infection, with a median baseline CD4+ cell count of 96 cells/mm[3] and a baseline HIV RNA of 4.58 $\log_{10}$ copies/mL (38,291 copies/mL). Prior to entering the trial, 45% had previously experienced an AIDS-defining clinical event. Eighty-nine percent had antiretroviral treatment prior to entering the trial. BI 1090 was originally designed as a clinical endpoint study. Prior to unblinding the trial, the primary endpoint was changed to proportion of patients with HIV RNA <50 copies/mL and not previously failed at 48 weeks. Treatment response and outcomes are shown in Table 2.

Table 2 BI 1090 Outcomes through 48 weeks

Outcome	VIRAMUNE (N=1121) %	Placebo (N=1128) %
Responders at 48 weeks: HIV RNA <50 copies/mL	18.0	1.6
Treatment Failure	82.0	98.4
Never suppressed viral load	44.6	66.4
Virologic failure after response	7.2	4.3
CDC category C event or death	9.6	11.2
Added antiretroviral therapy[1] while <50 copies/mL	5.0	0.9
Discontinued trial therapy due to AE	7.0	5.9
Discontinued trial <48 weeks[2]	8.5	9.8

[1] including change to open-label NVP
[2] includes withdrawal of consent, lost to follow-up, non-compliance with protocol, other administrative reasons

The change from baseline in CD4+ cell count through one year of therapy was significantly greater for the VIRAMUNE group compared to the placebo group for the overall study population (64 cells/mm[3] vs 22 cells/mm[3], respectively), as well as for patients who entered the trial as treatment naïve or having received only ZDV (85 cells/mm[3] vs 25 cells/mm[3], respectively).

At two years into the study, 16% of subjects on VIRAMUNE had experienced class C CDC events as compared to 21% of subjects on the control arm.

Trial BI 1046 (INCAS) was a double-blind, placebo-controlled, randomized, three arm trial with 151 HIV-1 infected patients with CD4+ cell counts of 200-600 cells/mm[3] at baseline. BI 1046 compared treatment with VIRAMUNE+zidovudine+didanosine to VIRAMUNE+zidovudine and zidovudine+didanosine. Treatment doses were VIRAMUNE at 200 mg daily for two weeks followed by 200 mg twice daily or placebo, zidovudine at 200 mg three times daily, and didanosine at 125 or 200 mg twice daily (depending on body weight). The patients had mean baseline HIV RNA of 4.41 $\log_{10}$ copies/mL (25,704 copies/mL) and mean baseline CD4+ cell count of 376 cells/mm[3]. The primary endpoint was the proportion of patients with HIV-RNA <400 copies/mL and not previously failed at 48 weeks. The virologic responder rates at 48 weeks were 45% for patients treated with VIRAMUNE+zidovudine+didanosine, 19% for patients treated with zidovudine+didanosine, and 0% for patients treated with VIRAMUNE+zidovudine. CD4+ cell counts in the VIRAMUNE+ZDV+ddI group increased above baseline by a mean of 139 cells/mm[3] at one year, significantly greater than the increase of 87 cells/mm[3] in the ZDV+ddI patients. The VIRAMUNE+ZDV group mean decreased by 6 cells/mm[3] below baseline.

CONTRAINDICATIONS

VIRAMUNE (nevirapine) is contraindicated in patients with clinically significant hypersensitivity to any of the components contained in the tablet or the oral suspension.

WARNINGS

General

The most serious adverse reactions associated with VIRAMUNE (nevirapine) are hepatitis/hepatic failure, Stevens-Johnson syndrome, toxic epidermal necrolysis, and hypersensitivity reactions. Hepatitis/hepatic failure may be associated with signs of hypersensitivity which can include severe rash or rash accompanied by fever, general malaise, fatigue, muscle or joint aches, blisters, oral lesions, conjunctivitis, facial edema, eosinophilia, granulocytopenia, lymphadenopathy, or renal dysfunction.

Table 1 (cont.) Drug Interactions: Changes in Pharmacokinetic Parameters for Co-administered Drug in the Presence of VIRAMUNE (All interaction studies were conducted in HIV-1 positive patients)

Co-administered Drug	Dose of Co-administered Drug	Dose Regimen of VIRAMUNE	n	% Change of Co-administered Drug Pharmacokinetic Parameters (90% CI)		
Antiretrovirals				AUC	C_{max}	C_{min}
Methadone[a]	Individual Patient Dosing	200 mg QD × 14 days; 200 mg BID ≥ 7 days	9	In a controlled pharmacokinetic study with 9 patients receiving chronic methadone to whom steady state nevirapine therapy was added, the clearance of methadone was increased by 3-fold resulting in symptoms of withdrawal, requiring dose adjustments in 10 mg segments, in 7 of the 9 patients. Methadone did not have any effect on nevirapine clearance.		
Rifabutin[a]	150 or 300 mg QD	200 mg QD × 14 days; 200 mg BID × 14 days	19	↑17 (↓2 to ↑40)	↑28 (↑9 to ↑51)	⇔
Metabolite 25-O-desacetyl-rifabutin				↑24 (↓16 to ↑84)	↑29 (↓2 to ↑68)	↑22 (↓14 to ↑74)
Rifampin[a]	600 mg QD	200 mg QD × 14 days; 200 mg BID × 14 days	14	↑11 (↓4 to ↑28)	⇔	§

§ = C_{min} below detectable level of the assay
↑ = Increase, ↓ = Decrease, ⇔ = No Effect
[a] For information regarding clinical recommendations see **PRECAUTIONS, Drug Interactions, Table 3.**
[b] Pediatric subjects ranging in age from 6 months to 12 years
[c] Parallel group design; n for VIRAMUNE +lopinavir/ritonavir, n for lopinavir/ritonavir alone

Table 3 Established Drug Interactions: Alteration in Dose or Regimen May Be Recommended Based on Drug Interaction Studies (See CLINICAL PHARMACOLOGY, Table 1 for Magnitude of Interaction)

Drug Name	Effect on Concentration of Nevirapine or Concomitant Drug	Clinical Comment
Clarithromycin	↓ Clarithromycin ↑ 14-OH clarithromycin	Clarithromycin exposure was significantly decreased by nevirapine; however, 14-OH metabolite concentrations were increased. Because clarithromycin active metabolite has reduced activity against Mycobacterium avium-intracellulare complex, overall activity against this pathogen may be altered. Alternatives to clarithromycin, such as azithromycin, should be considered.
Efavirenz	↓ Efavirenz	Appropriate doses for this combination are not established.
Ethinyl estradiol and Norethindrone	↓ Ethinyl estradiol ↓ Norethindrone	Oral contraceptives and other hormonal methods of birth control should not be used as the sole method of contraception in women taking nevirapine, since nevirapine may lower the plasma levels of these medications. An alternative or additional method of contraception is recommended.
Fluconazole	↑ Nevirapine	Because of the risk of increased exposure to nevirapine, caution should be used in concomitant administration, and patients should be monitored closely for nevirapine-associated adverse events.

(Table continued on next page)

The first 18 weeks of therapy with VIRAMUNE are a critical period during which intensive clinical and laboratory monitoring of patients is required to detect potentially life-threatening hepatic events and skin reactions. The optimal frequency of monitoring during this time period has not been established. Some experts recommend clinical and laboratory monitoring more often than once per month and in particular, would include monitoring of liver function tests at baseline, prior to dose escalation and at two weeks post-dose escalation. After the initial 18 week period, frequent clinical and laboratory monitoring should continue throughout VIRAMUNE treatment. In addition, the 14-day lead-in period with VIRAMUNE 200 mg daily dosing has been demonstrated to reduce the frequency of rash.

Hepatic Events

Severe, life-threatening, and in some cases fatal hepatotoxicity, including fulminant and cholestatic hepatitis, hepatic necrosis and hepatic failure, have been reported in patients treated with VIRAMUNE. In controlled clinical trials, symptomatic hepatic events regardless of severity occurred in 4% (range 0% to 11.0%) of patients who received VIRAMUNE and 1.2% of patients in control groups.

The risk of symptomatic hepatic events regardless of severity was greatest in the first 6 weeks of therapy. The risk continued to be greater in the VIRAMUNE groups compared to controls through 18 weeks of treatment. However, hepatic events may occur at any time during treatment. In some cases, patients presented with non-specific, prodromal signs or symptoms of fatigue, malaise, anorexia, nausea, jaundice, liver tenderness or hepatomegaly, with or without initially abnormal serum transaminase levels. Rash was observed in approximately half of the patients with symptomatic hepatic adverse events. Fever and flu-like symptoms accompanied some of these hepatic events. Some events, particularly those with rash and other symptoms, have progressed to hepatic failure with transaminase elevation, with or without hyperbilirubinemia, hepatic encephalopathy, prolonged partial thromboplastin time, or eosinophilia. Rhabdomyolysis has been observed in some patients experiencing skin and/or liver reactions associated with VIRAMUNE use. Patients with signs or symptoms of hepatitis must be advised to discontinue VIRAMUNE and immediately seek medical evaluation, which should include liver function tests.

Liver function tests should be performed immediately if a patient experiences signs or symptoms suggestive of hepatitis and/or hypersensitivity reaction. Liver function tests should also be obtained immediately for all patients who develop a rash in the first 18 weeks of treatment. Physicians and patients should be vigilant for the appearance of signs or symptoms of hepatitis, such as fatigue, malaise, anorexia, nausea, jaundice, bilirubinuria, acholic stools, liver tenderness or hepatomegaly. The diagnosis of hepatotoxicity should be considered in this setting, even if liver function tests are initially normal or alternative diagnoses are possible (see PRECAUTIONS, Information for Patients and DOSAGE AND ADMINISTRATION).

If clinical hepatitis or transaminase elevations combined with rash or other systemic symptoms occur, VIRAMUNE should be permanently discontinued. Do not restart VIRAMUNE after recovery. In some cases, hepatic injury progresses despite discontinuation of treatment. The patients at greatest risk of hepatic events, including potentially fatal events, are women with high CD4 counts. In general, during the first 6 weeks of treatment, women have a three fold higher risk than men for symptomatic, often rash-associated, hepatic events (5.8% versus 2.2%), and patients with higher CD4 counts at initiation of VIRAMUNE therapy are at higher risk for symptomatic hepatic events with VIRAMUNE. In a retrospective review, women with CD4 counts >250 cells/mm^3 had a 12 fold higher risk of symptomatic hepatic adverse events compared to women with CD4 counts <250 cells/mm^3 (11.0% versus 0.9%). An increased risk was observed in men with CD4 counts >400 cells/mm^3 (6.3% versus 1.2% for men with CD4 counts <400 cells/mm^3). However, all patients, regardless of gender, CD4 count, or antiretroviral treatment history, should be monitored for hepatotoxicity since symptomatic hepatic adverse events have been reported at all CD4 counts. Co-infection with hepatitis B or C and/or increased liver function tests at the start of therapy with VIRAMUNE® are associated with a greater risk of later symptomatic events (6 weeks or more after starting VIRAMUNE) and asymptomatic increases in AST or ALT.

In addition, serious hepatotoxicity (including liver failure requiring transplantation in one instance) has been reported in HIV-uninfected individuals receiving multiple doses of VIRAMUNE in the setting of post-exposure prophylaxis, an unapproved use.

Because increased nevirapine levels and nevirapine accumulation may be observed in patients with serious liver disease, VIRAMUNE should not be administered to patients with severe hepatic impairment (see **CLINICAL PHARMACOLOGY**, *Pharmacokinetics in Special Populations*: **Hepatic Impairment**; **PRECAUTIONS**, *General*).

Skin Reactions

Severe and life-threatening skin reactions, including fatal cases, have been reported, occurring most frequently during the first 6 weeks of therapy. These have included cases of Stevens-Johnson syndrome, toxic epidermal necrolysis, and hypersensitivity reactions characterized by rash, constitutional findings, and organ dysfunction including hepatic failure. Rhabdomyolysis has been observed in some patients experiencing skin and/or liver reactions associated with VIRAMUNE use. In controlled clinical trials, Grade 3 and 4 rashes were reported during the first 6 weeks in 1.5% of VIRAMUNE recipients compared to 0.1% of placebo subjects.

Patients developing signs or symptoms of severe skin reactions or hypersensitivity reactions (including, but not limited to, severe rash or rash accompanied by fever, general malaise, fatigue, muscle or joint aches, blisters, oral lesions, conjunctivitis, facial edema, and/or hepatitis, eosinophilia, granulocytopenia, lymphadenopathy, and renal dysfunction) must permanently discontinue VIRAMUNE and seek medical evaluation immediately (see **PRECAUTIONS**, *Information for Patients*). Do not restart VIRAMUNE following severe skin rash, skin rash combined with increased transaminases or other symptoms, or hypersensitivity reaction.

If patients present with a suspected VIRAMUNE-associated rash, liver function tests should be performed. Patients with rash-associated AST or ALT elevations should be permanently discontinued from VIRAMUNE.

Therapy with VIRAMUNE must be initiated with a 14-day lead-in period of 200 mg/day (4 mg/kg/day in pediatric patients), which has been shown to reduce the frequency of rash. If rash is observed during this lead-in period, dose escalation should not occur until the rash has resolved (see **DOSAGE AND ADMINISTRATION**). Patients should be monitored closely if isolated rash of any severity occurs. Delay in stopping VIRAMUNE treatment after the onset of rash may result in a more serious reaction.

Women appear to be at higher risk than men of developing rash with VIRAMUNE.

In a clinical trial, concomitant prednisone use (40 mg/day for the first 14 days of VIRAMUNE administration) was associated with an increase in incidence and severity of rash during the first 6 weeks of VIRAMUNE therapy. Therefore, use of prednisone to prevent VIRAMUNE-associated rash is not recommended.

Resistance

VIRAMUNE must not be used as a single agent to treat HIV or added on as a sole agent to a failing regimen. As with all other non-nucleoside reverse transcriptase inhibitors, resistant virus emerges rapidly when nevirapine is administered as monotherapy. The choice of new antiretroviral agents to be used in combination with nevirapine should take into consideration the potential for cross resistance. When discontinuing an antiretroviral regimen containing VIRAMUNE, the long half-life of nevirapine should be taken into account; if antiretrovirals with shorter half-lives than VIRAMUNE are stopped concurrently, low plasma concentrations of nevirapine alone may persist for a week or longer and virus resistance may subsequently develop.

St. John's wort

Concomitant use of St. John's wort (*Hypericum perforatum*) or St. John's wort containing products and VIRAMUNE is not recommended. Co-administration of non-nucleoside reverse transcriptase inhibitors (NNRTIs), including VIRAMUNE, with St. John's wort is expected to substantially decrease NNRTI concentrations and may result in sub-optimal levels of VIRAMUNE and lead to loss of virologic response and possible resistance to VIRAMUNE or to the class of NNRTIs.

PRECAUTIONS

General

The most serious adverse reactions associated with VIRAMUNE (nevirapine) are hepatitis/hepatic failure, Stevens-Johnson syndrome, toxic epidermal necrolysis, and

Table 3 *(cont.)* *Established* Drug Interactions: Alteration in Dose or Regimen May Be Recommended Based on Drug Interaction Studies (See CLINICAL PHARMACOLOGY, Table 1 for Magnitude of Interaction)

Drug Name	Effect on Concentration of Nevirapine or Concomitant Drug	Clinical Comment
Indinavir	↓ Indinavir	Appropriate doses for this combination are not established, but an increase in the dosage of indinavir may be required.
Ketoconazole	↓ Ketoconazole	Nevirapine and ketoconazole should not be administered concomitantly because decreases in ketoconazole plasma concentrations may reduce the efficacy of the drug.
Lopinavir/Ritonavir	↓ Lopinavir	KALETRA 400/100 mg tablets can be used twice-daily in combination with nevirapine with no dose adjustment in antiretroviral-naïve patients. A dose increase of KALETRA tablets to 600/150 mg (3 tablets) twice daily may be considered when used in combination with nevirapine in treatment experienced patients where decreased susceptibility to lopinavir is clinically suspected (by treatment history or laboratory evidence). A dose increase of lopinavir/ritonavir oral solution to 533/133 mg twice daily with food is recommended in combination with nevirapine. In children 6 months to 12 years of age, consideration should be given to increasing the dose of lopinavir/ritonavir to 13/3.25 mg/kg for those 7 to < 15 kg; 11/2.75 mg/kg for those 15 to 45 kg; and up to a maximum dose of 533/133 mg for those > 45 kg twice daily when used in combination with nevirapine, particularly for patients in whom reduced susceptibility to lopinavir/ritonavir is suspected.
Methadone	↓ Methadone	Methadone levels may be decreased; increased dosages may be required to prevent symptoms of opiate withdrawal. Methadone maintained patients beginning nevirapine therapy should be monitored for evidence of withdrawal and methadone dose should be adjusted accordingly.
Nelfinavir	↓ Nelfinavir M8 Metabolite ↓ Nelfinavir C_{min}	The appropriate dose for nelfinavir in combination with nevirapine, with respect to safety and efficacy, has not been established.
Rifabutin	↑ Rifabutin	Rifabutin and its metabolite concentrations were moderately increased. Due to high intersubject variability, however, some patients may experience large increases in rifabutin exposure and may be at higher risk for rifabutin toxicity. Therefore, caution should be used in concomitant administration.
Rifampin	↓ Nevirapine	Nevirapine and rifampin should not be administered concomitantly because decreases in nevirapine plasma concentrations may reduce the efficacy of the drug. Physicians needing to treat patients co-infected with tuberculosis and using a nevirapine containing regimen may use rifabutin instead.
Saquinavir	↓ Saquinavir	Appropriate doses for this combination are not established, but an increase in the dosage of saquinavir may be required.

hypersensitivity reactions. Hepatitis/hepatic failure may be isolated or associated with signs of hypersensitivity which may include severe rash or rash accompanied by fever, general malaise, fatigue, muscle or joint aches, blisters, oral lesions, conjunctivitis, facial edema, eosinophilia, granulocytopenia, lymphadenopathy, or renal dysfunction (see **WARNINGS**).

Nevirapine is extensively metabolized by the liver and nevirapine metabolites are extensively eliminated by the kidney. No adjustment in nevirapine dosing is required in patients with CrCL ≥20 mL/min. In patients undergoing chronic hemodialysis, an additional 200 mg dose following each dialysis treatment is indicated. Nevirapine metabolites may accumulate in patients receiving dialysis; however, the clinical significance of this accumulation is not known (see **CLINICAL PHARMACOLOGY**, *Pharmacokinetics in Special Populations*: **Renal Impairment**; **DOSAGE AND ADMINISTRATION**, *Dosage Adjustment*).

It is not clear whether a dosing adjustment is needed for patients with mild to moderate hepatic impairment, because multiple dose pharmacokinetic data are not available for this population. However, patients with moderate hepatic impairment and ascites may be at risk of accumulating nevirapine in the systemic circulation. Caution should be exercised when nevirapine is administered to patients with moderate hepatic impairment. Nevirapine should not be administered to patients with severe hepatic impairment (see **WARNINGS**; **CLINICAL PHARMACOLOGY**, *Pharmacokinetics in Special Populations*: **Hepatic Impairment**). The duration of clinical benefit from antiretroviral therapy may be limited. Patients receiving VIRAMUNE or any other antiretroviral therapy may continue to develop opportunistic infections and other complications of HIV infection, and

therefore should remain under close clinical observation by physicians experienced in the treatment of patients with associated HIV diseases.

When administering VIRAMUNE as part of an antiretroviral regimen, the complete product information for each therapeutic component should be consulted before initiation of treatment.

Drug Interactions

Nevirapine is principally metabolized by the liver via the cytochrome P450 isoenzymes, 3A4 and 2B6. Nevirapine is known to be an inducer of these enzymes. As a result, drugs that are metabolized by these enzyme systems may have lower than expected plasma levels when co-administered with nevirapine.

The specific pharmacokinetic changes that occur with co-administration of nevirapine and other drugs are listed in **CLINICAL PHARMACOLOGY**, Table 1. Clinical comments about possible dosage modifications based on these pharmacokinetic changes are listed in Table 3. The data in Tables 1 and 3 are based on the results of drug interaction studies conducted in HIV-1 seropositive subjects unless otherwise indicated.

In addition to established drug interactions, there may be potential pharmacokinetic interactions between nevirapine and other drug classes that are metabolized by the cytochrome P450 system. These potential drug interactions are listed in Table 4. Although specific drug interaction studies in HIV-1 seropositive subjects have not been conducted for the classes of drugs listed in Table 4, additional clinical monitoring may be warranted when co-administering these drugs.

Continued on next page

Viramune—Cont.

The *in vitro* interaction between nevirapine and the antithrombotic agent warfarin is complex. As a result, when giving these drugs concomitantly, plasma warfarin levels may change with the potential for increases in coagulation time. When warfarin is co-administered with nevirapine, anticoagulation levels should be monitored frequently.
[See table 3 on pages 78 and 79]

Table 4 *Potential* Drug Interactions: Use With Caution, Dose Adjustment of Co-administered Drug May Be Needed due to Possible Decrease in Clinical Effect

Examples of Drugs in Which Plasma Concentrations May Be Decreased By Co-administration With Nevirapine

Drug Class	Examples of Drugs
Antiarrhythmics	Amiodarone, disopyramide, lidocaine
Anticonvulsants	Carbamazepine, clonazepam, ethosuximide
Antifungals	Itraconazole
Calcium channel blockers	Diltiazem, nifedipine, verapamil
Cancer chemotherapy	Cyclophosphamide
Ergot alkaloids	Ergotamine
Immunosuppressants	Cyclosporin, tacrolimus, sirolimus
Motility agents	Cisapride
Opiate agonists	Fentanyl

Examples of Drugs in Which Plasma Concentrations May Be Increased By Co-administration With Nevirapine

Antithrombotics	Warfarin Potential effect on anticoagulation. Monitoring of anticoagulation levels is recommended.

Fat Redistribution
Redistribution/accumulation of body fat including central obesity, dorsocervical fat enlargement (buffalo hump), peripheral wasting, facial wasting, breast enlargement, and "cushingoid appearance" have been observed in patients receiving antiretroviral therapy. The mechanism and long-term consequences of these events are currently unknown. A causal relationship has not been established.

Immune Reconstitution Syndrome
Immune reconstitution syndrome has been reported in patients treated with combination antiretroviral therapy, including VIRAMUNE. During the initial phase of combination antiretroviral treatment, patients whose immune system responds may develop an inflammatory response to indolent or residual opportunistic infections (such as *Mycobacterium avium* infection, cytomegalovirus, *Pneumocystis jirovecii* pneumonia (PCP), or tuberculosis), which may necessitate further evaluation and treatment.

Information for Patients
Patients should be informed of the possibility of severe liver disease or skin reactions associated with VIRAMUNE that may result in death. Patients developing signs or symptoms of liver disease or severe skin reactions should be instructed to discontinue VIRAMUNE and seek medical attention immediately, including performance of laboratory monitoring. Symptoms of liver disease include fatigue, malaise, anorexia, nausea, jaundice, acholic stools, liver tenderness or hepatomegaly. Symptoms of severe skin or hypersensitivity reactions include rash accompanied by fever, general malaise, fatigue, muscle or joint aches, blisters, oral lesions, conjunctivitis, facial edema and/or hepatitis.

Intensive clinical and laboratory monitoring, including liver function tests, is essential during the first 18 weeks of therapy with VIRAMUNE to detect potentially life-threatening hepatotoxicity and skin reactions. However, liver disease can occur after this period, therefore monitoring should continue at frequent intervals throughout VIRAMUNE treatment. Extra vigilance is warranted during the first 6 weeks of therapy, which is the period of greatest risk of hepatic events and skin reactions. Patients with signs and symptoms of hepatitis should discontinue VIRAMUNE and seek medical evaluation immediately. If VIRAMUNE is discontinued due to hepatotoxicity, do not restart it. Patients, particularly women, with increased CD4+ cell count at initiation of VIRAMUNE therapy (>250 cells/mm^3 in women and >400 cells/mm^3 in men) are at substantially higher risk for development of symptomatic hepatic events, often associated with rash. Patients should be advised that co-infection with hepatitis B or C and/or increased liver function tests at the start of therapy with VIRAMUNE are associated with a greater risk of later symptomatic events (6 weeks or more after starting VIRAMUNE) and asymptomatic increases in AST or ALT (see **WARNINGS, Hepatic Events**).

The majority of rashes associated with VIRAMUNE occur within the first 6 weeks of initiation of therapy. Patients should be instructed that if any rash occurs during the two-week lead-in period, the VIRAMUNE dose should not be escalated until the rash resolves. Any patient experiencing a rash should have their liver function evaluated immediately. Patients with severe rash or hypersensitivity reactions should discontinue VIRAMUNE immediately and consult a physician. VIRAMUNE should not be restarted following severe skin rash or hypersensitivity reaction. Women tend to be at higher risk for development of VIRAMUNE associated rash.

Oral contraceptives and other hormonal methods of birth control should not be used as the sole method of contraception in women taking VIRAMUNE, since VIRAMUNE may lower the plasma levels of these medications. Additionally, when oral contraceptives are used for hormonal regulation during VIRAMUNE therapy, the therapeutic effect of the hormonal therapy should be monitored (see **PRECAUTIONS, Drug Interactions**).

VIRAMUNE may decrease plasma concentrations of methadone by increasing its hepatic metabolism. Narcotic withdrawal syndrome has been reported in patients treated with VIRAMUNE and methadone concomitantly. Methadone-maintained patients beginning nevirapine therapy should be monitored for evidence of withdrawal and methadone dose should be adjusted accordingly.

VIRAMUNE may interact with some drugs, therefore, patients should be advised to report to their doctor the use of any other prescription, non-prescription medication or herbal products, particularly St. John's wort.

Patients should be informed that VIRAMUNE therapy has not been shown to reduce the risk of transmission of HIV-1 to others through sexual contact or blood contamination. The long-term effects of VIRAMUNE are unknown at this time.

VIRAMUNE is not a cure for HIV-1 infection; patients may continue to experience illnesses associated with advanced HIV-1 infection, including opportunistic infections. Patients should be advised to remain under the care of a physician when using VIRAMUNE.

Patients should be informed to take VIRAMUNE every day as prescribed. Patients should not alter the dose without consulting their doctor. If a dose is missed, patients should take the next dose as soon as possible. However, if a dose is skipped, the patient should not double the next dose. Patients should be advised to report to their doctor the use of any other medications.

Patients should be informed that redistribution or accumulation of body fat may occur in patients receiving antiretroviral therapy and that the cause and long term health effects of these conditions are not known at this time.

The Medication Guide provides written information for the patient, and should be dispensed with each new prescription and refill.

Carcinogenesis, Mutagenesis, Impairment of Fertility
Long-term carcinogenicity studies in mice and rats were carried out with nevirapine. Mice were dosed with 0, 50, 375 or 750 mg/kg/day for two years. Hepatocellular adenomas and carcinomas were increased at all doses in males and at the two high doses in females. In studies in which rats were administered nevirapine at doses of 0, 3.5, 17.5 or 35 mg/kg/day for two years, an increase in hepatocellular adenomas was seen in males at all doses and in females at the high dose. The systemic exposure (based on AUCs) at all doses in the two animal studies were lower than that measured in humans at the 200 mg BID dose. The mechanism of the carcinogenic potential is unknown. However, in genetic toxicology assays, nevirapine showed no evidence of mutagenic or clastogenic activity in a battery of *in vitro* and *in vivo* studies. These included microbial assays for gene mutation (Ames: Salmonella strains and *E. coli*), mammalian cell gene mutation assay (CHO/HGPRT), cytogenetic assays using a Chinese hamster ovary cell line and a mouse bone marrow micronucleus assay following oral administration. Given the lack of genotoxic activity of nevirapine, the relevance to humans of hepatocellular neoplasms in nevirapine treated mice and rats is not known. In reproductive toxicology studies, evidence of impaired fertility was seen in female rats at doses providing systemic exposure, based on AUC, approximately equivalent to that provided with the recommended clinical dose of VIRAMUNE.

Pregnancy: Pregnancy Category B
No observable teratogenicity was detected in reproductive studies performed in pregnant rats and rabbits. The maternal and developmental no-observable-effect level dosages produced systemic exposures approximately equivalent to or approximately 50% higher in rats and rabbits, respectively, than those seen at the recommended daily human dose (based on AUC). In rats, decreased fetal body weights were observed due to administration of a maternally toxic dose (exposures approximately 50% higher than that seen at the recommended human clinical dose).

There are no adequate and well-controlled studies of VIRAMUNE in pregnant women. The Antiretroviral Pregnancy Registry, which has been surveying pregnancy outcomes since January 1989, has not found an increased risk of birth defects following first trimester exposures to nevirapine. The prevalence of birth defects after any trimester exposure to nevirapine is comparable to the prevalence observed in the general population.

Severe hepatic events, including fatalities, have been reported in pregnant women receiving chronic VIRAMUNE therapy as part of combination treatment of HIV infection. Regardless of pregnancy status women with CD4 counts >250 cells/mm^3 should not initiate VIRAMUNE unless the benefit outweighs the risk. It is unclear if pregnancy augments the risk observed in non-pregnant women (see **Boxed WARNING**).

VIRAMUNE should be used during pregnancy only if the potential benefit justifies the potential risk to the fetus.

Antiretroviral Pregnancy Registry
To monitor maternal-fetal outcomes of pregnant women exposed to VIRAMUNE, an Antiretroviral Pregnancy Registry has been established. Physicians are encouraged to register patients by calling (800) 258-4263.

Nursing Mothers
The Centers for Disease Control and Prevention recommend that HIV-infected mothers not breast-feed their infants to avoid risking postnatal transmission of HIV. Nevirapine is excreted in breast milk. Because of both the potential for HIV transmission and the potential for serious adverse reactions in nursing infants, mothers should be instructed not to breast-feed if they are receiving VIRAMUNE.

Pediatric Use
The pharmacokinetics of nevirapine have been studied in two open-label studies in children with HIV-1 infection (see **CLINICAL PHARMACOLOGY, Pharmacokinetics in Special Populations**). For dose recommendations for pediatric patients see **DOSAGE AND ADMINISTRATION**. The most frequently reported adverse events related to VIRAMUNE in pediatric patients were similar to those observed in adults, with the exception of granulocytopenia, which was more commonly observed in children receiving both zidovudine and VIRAMUNE (see **ADVERSE REACTIONS, Pediatric Patients**). The evaluation of the antiviral activity of VIRAMUNE in pediatric patients is ongoing.

Geriatric Use
Clinical studies of VIRAMUNE did not include sufficient numbers of subjects aged 65 and older to determine whether elderly subjects respond differently from younger subjects. In general, dose selection for an elderly patient should be cautious, reflecting the greater frequency of decreased hepatic, renal or cardiac function, and of concomitant disease or other drug therapy.

ADVERSE REACTIONS
The most serious adverse reactions associated with VIRAMUNE (nevirapine) are hepatitis/hepatic failure, Stevens-Johnson syndrome, toxic epidermal necrolysis, and hypersensitivity reactions. Hepatitis/hepatic failure may be isolated or associated with signs of hypersensitivity which may include severe rash or rash accompanied by fever, general malaise, fatigue, muscle or joint aches, blisters, oral lesions, conjunctivitis, facial edema, eosinophilia, granulocytopenia, lymphadenopathy, or renal dysfunction (see **WARNINGS**).

Adults
The most common clinical toxicity of VIRAMUNE is rash, which can be severe or life-threatening (see **WARNINGS**). Rash occurs most frequently within the first 6 weeks of therapy. Rashes are usually mild to moderate, maculopapular erythematous cutaneous eruptions, with or without pruritus, located on the trunk, face and extremities. In controlled clinical trials, Grade 1 and 2 rashes were reported in 13.3% of patients receiving VIRAMUNE compared to 5.8% receiving placebo during the first 6 weeks of therapy. Grade 3 and 4 rashes were reported in 1.5% of VIRAMUNE recipients compared to 0.1% of subjects receiving placebo. Women tend to be at higher risk for development of VIRAMUNE associated rash.

In controlled clinical trials, symptomatic hepatic events regardless of severity occurred in 4.0% (range 0% to 11.0%) of patients who received VIRAMUNE and 1.2% of patients in control groups. Female gender and higher CD4 counts (>250 cells/mm^3 in women and >400 cells/mm^3 in men) place patients at increased risk of these events (see **WARNINGS**).

Asymptomatic transaminase elevations (AST or ALT > 5X ULN) were observed in 5.8% (range 0% to 9.2%) of patients who received VIRAMUNE and 5.5% of patients in control groups. Co-infection with hepatitis B or C and/or increased liver function tests at the start of therapy with VIRAMUNE are associated with a greater risk of later symptomatic events (6 weeks or more after starting VIRAMUNE) and asymptomatic increases in AST or ALT.

Treatment related, adverse experiences of moderate or severe intensity observed in >2% of patients receiving VIRAMUNE in placebo-controlled trials are shown in Table 5.
[See table 5 at bottom of next page]

Laboratory Abnormalities: Liver function test abnormalities (AST, ALT) were observed more frequently in patients receiving VIRAMUNE than in controls (Table 6). Asymptomatic elevations in GGT occur frequently but are not a contraindication to continue VIRAMUNE therapy in the absence of elevations in other liver function tests. Other laboratory abnormalities (bilirubin, anemia, neutropenia, thrombocytopenia) were observed with similar frequencies in clinical trials comparing VIRAMUNE and control regimens (see Table 6).
[See table 6 at bottom of next page]

Post Marketing Surveillance: In addition to the adverse events identified during clinical trials, the following events have been reported with the use of VIRAMUNE in clinical practice:

   Body as a Whole: fever, somnolence, drug withdrawal (see **PRECAUTIONS: Drug Interactions**), redistribution/accumulation of body fat (see **PRECAUTIONS, Fat Redistribution**)

Gastrointestinal: vomiting
Liver and Biliary: jaundice, fulminant and cholestatic hepatitis, hepatic necrosis, hepatic failure
Hematology: anemia, eosinophilia, neutropenia
Musculoskeletal: arthralgia, rhabdomyolysis associated with skin and/or liver reactions
Neurologic: paraesthesia
Skin and Appendages: allergic reactions including anaphylaxis, angioedema, bullous eruptions, ulcerative stomatitis and urticaria have all been reported. In addition, hypersensitivity syndrome and hypersensitivity reactions with rash associated with constitutional findings such as fever, blistering, oral lesions, conjunctivitis, facial edema, muscle or joint aches, general malaise, fatigue or significant hepatic abnormalities (see **WARNINGS**). plus one or more of the following: hepatitis, eosinophilia, granulocytopenia, lymphadenopathy and/or renal dysfunction have been reported with the use of VIRAMUNE.

Pediatric Patients
Safety was assessed in trial BI 882 in which patients were followed for a mean duration of 33.9 months (range: 6.8 months to 5.3 years, including long-term follow-up in 29 of these patients in trial BI 892). The most frequently reported adverse events related to VIRAMUNE in pediatric patients were similar to those observed in adults, with the exception of granulocytopenia, which was more commonly observed in children receiving both zidovudine and VIRAMUNE. Serious adverse events were assessed in ACTG 245, a double-blind, placebo-controlled trial of VIRAMUNE (n = 305) in which pediatric patients received combination treatment with VIRAMUNE. In this trial two patients were reported to experience Stevens-Johnson syndrome or Stevens-Johnson/toxic epidermal necrolysis transition syndrome. Cases of allergic reaction, including one case of anaphylaxis, were also reported. In post-marketing surveillance anemia has been more commonly observed in children although development of anemia due to concomitant medication use cannot be ruled out.

OVERDOSAGE

There is no known antidote for VIRAMUNE (nevirapine) overdosage. Cases of VIRAMUNE overdose at doses ranging from 800 to 1800 mg per day for up to 15 days have been reported. Patients have experienced events including edema, erythema nodosum, fatigue, fever, headache, insomnia, nausea, pulmonary infiltrates, rash, vertigo, vomiting and weight decrease. All events subsided following discontinuation of VIRAMUNE.

DOSAGE AND ADMINISTRATION
Adults
The recommended dose for VIRAMUNE (nevirapine) is one 200 mg tablet daily for the first 14 days **(this lead-in period should be used because it has been found to lessen the frequency of rash)**, followed by one 200 mg tablet twice daily, in combination with other antiretroviral agents. For concomitantly administered antiretroviral therapy, the manufacturer's recommended dosage and monitoring should be followed.

Pediatric Patients
The recommended oral dose of VIRAMUNE for pediatric patients 2 months up to 8 years of age is 4 mg/kg once daily for the first 14 days followed by 7 mg/kg twice daily thereafter. For patients 8 years and older the recommended dose is 4 mg/kg once daily for two weeks followed by 4 mg/kg twice daily thereafter. The total daily dose should not exceed 400 mg for any patient.
VIRAMUNE suspension should be shaken gently prior to administration. It is important to administer the entire measured dose of suspension by using an oral dosing syringe or dosing cup. An oral dosing syringe is recommended, particularly for volumes of 5 mL or less. If a dosing cup is used, it should be thoroughly rinsed with water and the rinse should also be administered to the patient.

Monitoring of Patients
Intensive clinical and laboratory monitoring, including liver function tests, is essential at baseline and during the first 18 weeks of treatment with VIRAMUNE. The optimal frequency of monitoring during this period has not been established. Some experts recommend clinical and laboratory monitoring more often than once per month, and in particular, would include monitoring of liver function tests at baseline, prior to dose escalation, and at two weeks post dose escalation. After the initial 18 week period, frequent clinical and laboratory monitoring should continue throughout VIRAMUNE treatment (see **WARNINGS**). In some cases, hepatic injury has progressed despite discontinuation of treatment.

Dosage Adjustment
VIRAMUNE should be discontinued if patients experience severe rash or a rash accompanied by constitutional findings (see WARNINGS). Patients experiencing rash during the 14-day lead-in period of 200 mg/day (4 mg/kg/day in pediatric patients) should not have their VIRAMUNE dose increased until the rash has resolved (see PRECAUTIONS, *Information for Patients*).
If a clinical (symptomatic) hepatic event occurs, VIRAMUNE should be permanently discontinued. Do not restart VIRAMUNE after recovery (see WARNINGS).
Patients who interrupt VIRAMUNE dosing for more than 7 days should restart the recommended dosing, using one 200 mg tablet daily (4 mg/kg/day in pediatric patients) for the first 14 days (lead-in) followed by one 200 mg tablet twice daily (4 or 7 mg/kg twice daily, according to age, for pediatric patients).
An additional 200 mg dose of VIRAMUNE following each dialysis treatment is indicated in patients requiring dialysis. Nevirapine metabolites may accumulate in patients receiving dialysis; however, the clinical significance of this accumulation is not known (see **CLINICAL PHARMACOLOGY**, *Pharmacokinetics in Special Populations:Renal Impairment*). Patients with CrCL ≥20 mL/min do not require an adjustment in VIRAMUNE dosing.

HOW SUPPLIED

VIRAMUNE (nevirapine) Tablets, 200 mg, are white, oval, biconvex tablets, 9.3 mm × 19.1 mm. One side is embossed with "54 193", with a single bisect separating the "54" and "193". The opposite side has a single bisect. VIRAMUNE Tablets are supplied in bottles of 60 (NDC 0597-0046-60).
VIRAMUNE (nevirapine) Oral Suspension is a white to off-white preserved suspension containing 50 mg nevirapine (as nevirapine hemihydrate) in each 5 mL. VIRAMUNE suspension is supplied in plastic bottles with child-resistant closures containing 240 mL of suspension (NDC 0597-0047-24).
Store at 25°C (77°F); excursions permitted to 15°–30°C (59°–86°F) [see USP Controlled Room Temperature]. Store in a safe place out of the reach of children.
Distributed by:
Boehringer Ingelheim Pharmaceuticals, Inc.
Ridgefield, CT 06877 USA
©Copyright Boehringer Ingelheim Pharmaceuticals, Inc. 2007, ALL RIGHTS RESERVED
Rev: June 2007
10003354/02
10003354/US/2
OT1801DF2507

MEDICATION GUIDE

VIRAMUNE® (VIH-rah-mune) Tablets
VIRAMUNE® Oral Suspension
Generic name: nevirapine tablets and oral suspension
Read this Medication Guide before you start taking VIRAMUNE® and each time you get a refill because there may be new information. This information does not take the place of talking with your doctor. You and your doctor should discuss VIRAMUNE when you start taking your medicine and at regular checkups. You should stay under a doctor's care while using VIRAMUNE. You should consult with your doctor before making any changes to your medications, except in any of the special circumstances described below regarding rash or liver problems.
What is the most important information I should know about VIRAMUNE?
Patients taking VIRAMUNE may develop severe liver disease or skin reactions that can cause death. The risk of these reactions is greatest during the first 18 weeks of treatment, but these reactions also can occur later.
Liver Reactions
Any patient can experience liver problems while taking VIRAMUNE. However, women and patients who have higher CD4 counts when they begin VIRAMUNE treatment have a greater chance of developing liver damage. Women with CD4 counts higher than 250 cells/mm³ are at the greatest risk of these events. If you are a woman with CD4>250 cells/mm³ or a man with CD4>400 cells/mm³ you should not begin taking VIRAMUNE unless you and your doctor have decided that the benefit of doing so outweighs the risk. Liver problems are often accompanied by a rash. Patients starting VIRAMUNE with abnormal liver function tests and patients with hepatitis B or C have a greater chance of developing further increases in liver function tests after starting VIRAMUNE and throughout therapy.
In rare cases liver problems have led to liver failure and can lead to a liver transplant or death. Therefore, if you develop any of the following symptoms of liver problems stop taking VIRAMUNE and call your doctor right away:
- general ill feeling or "flu-like" symptoms
- tiredness
- nausea (feeling sick to your stomach)
- lack of appetite
- yellowing of your skin or whites of your eyes
- dark urine (tea colored)
- pale stools (bowel movements)
- pain, ache, or sensitivity to touch on your right side below your ribs

Table 5   Percentage of Patients with Moderate or Severe Drug Related Events in Adult Placebo Controlled Trials

	Trial 1090[1]		Trials 1037, 1038, 1046[2]	
	VIRAMUNE	Placebo	VIRAMUNE	Placebo
	(n=1121)	(n=1128)	(n=253)	(n=203)
Median exposure (weeks)	58	52	28	28
Any adverse event	14.5%	11.1%	31.6%	13.3%
Rash	5.1	1.8	6.7	1.5
Nausea	0.5	1.1	8.7	3.9
Granulocytopenia	1.8	2.8	0.4	0
Headache	0.7	0.4	3.6	0.5
Fatigue	0.2	0.3	4.7	3.9
Diarrhea	0.2	0.8	2.0	0.5
Abdominal pain	0.1	0.4	2.0	0
Myalgia	0.2	0	1.2	2.0

[1] Background therapy included 3TC for all patients and combinations of NRTIs and PIs. Patients had CD4+ cell counts <200 cells/mm³.
[2] Background therapy included ZDV and ZDV+ddI; VIRAMUNE monotherapy was administered in some patients. Patients had CD4+ cell count ≥200 cells/mm³.

Table 6   Percentage of Adult Patients with Laboratory Abnormalities

	Trial 1090[1]		Trials 1037, 1038, 1046[2]	
	VIRAMUNE	Placebo	VIRAMUNE	Placebo
Laboratory Abnormality	n=1121	n=1128	n=253	n=203
Blood Chemistry				
SGPT (ALT) >250 U/L	5.3%	4.4%	14.0%	4.0%
SGOT (AST) >250 U/L	3.7	2.5	7.6	1.5
Bilirubin >2.5 mg/dL	1.7	2.2	1.7	1.5
Hematology				
Hemoglobin <8.0 g/dL	3.2	4.1	0	0
Platelets <50,000/mm³	1.3	1.0	0.4	1.5
Neutrophils <750/mm³	13.3	13.5	3.6	1.0

[1] Background therapy included 3TC for all patients and combinations of NRTIs and PIs. Patients had CD4+ cell counts <200 cells/mm³.
[2] Background therapy included ZDV and ZDV+ddI; VIRAMUNE monotherapy was administered in some patients. Patients had CD4+ cell count ≥200 cells/mm³.

Continued on next page

Viramune—Cont.

Your doctor should check you and do blood tests often to check your liver function during the first 18 weeks of therapy. Checks for liver problems should continue regularly during treatment with VIRAMUNE.

Skin Reactions

Skin rash is the most common side effect of VIRAMUNE. Most rashes occur in the first 6 weeks of treatment. In a small number of patients, **rash can be serious and result in death**. Therefore, **if you develop a rash with any of the following symptoms stop using VIRAMUNE and call your doctor right away:**

- general ill feeling or "flu-like" symptoms
- fever
- muscle or joint aches
- conjunctivitis (red or inflamed eyes, like "pink eye")
- any of the symptoms of liver problems discussed above
- blisters
- mouth sores
- swelling of your face
- tiredness

If your doctor tells you to stop treatment with VIRAMUNE because you have experienced the serious liver or skin reactions described above, never take VIRAMUNE again.

These are not all the side effects of VIRAMUNE. See the section "**What are the possible side effects of VIRAMUNE?**" for more information. Tell your doctor if you have any side effects from VIRAMUNE.

What is VIRAMUNE?

VIRAMUNE is a medicine used to treat Human Immunodeficiency Virus (HIV), the virus that causes AIDS (Acquired Immune Deficiency Syndrome).

VIRAMUNE is a type of anti-HIV medicine called a "non-nucleoside reverse transcriptase inhibitor" (NNRTI). It works by lowering the amount of HIV in the blood ("viral load"). You must take VIRAMUNE with other anti-HIV medicines. When taken with other anti-HIV medicines, VIRAMUNE can reduce viral load and increase the number of CD4 cells ("T cells"). CD4 cells are a type of immune helper cell in the blood. VIRAMUNE may not have these effects in every patient.

VIRAMUNE does not cure HIV or AIDS, and it is not known if it will help you live longer with HIV. People taking VIRAMUNE may still get infections common in people with HIV (opportunistic infections). Therefore, it is very important that you stay under the care of your doctor.

Who should not take VIRAMUNE?

- Do not take VIRAMUNE if you are allergic to VIRAMUNE or any of its ingredients. The active ingredient is nevirapine. Your doctor or pharmacist can tell you about the inactive ingredients.
- Do not restart VIRAMUNE after you recover from serious liver or skin reactions that happened when you took VIRAMUNE.
- Do not take VIRAMUNE if you take certain medicines. (See "**Can I take other medicines with VIRAMUNE?**" for a list of medicines.)
- Do not take VIRAMUNE if you are not infected with HIV.

What should I tell my doctor before taking VIRAMUNE?

Before starting VIRAMUNE, tell your doctor about all of your medical conditions, including if you:

- have problems with your liver or have had hepatitis
- are undergoing dialysis
- have skin conditions, such as a rash
- are pregnant, planning to become pregnant, or are breast feeding

How should I take VIRAMUNE?

- Take the exact amount of VIRAMUNE your doctor prescribes. The usual dose for adults is one tablet daily for the first 14 days followed by one tablet twice daily. Starting with one dose a day lowers the chance of rash, which could be serious. Therefore, it is important to strictly follow the once daily dose for the first 14 days. Do not start taking VIRAMUNE twice a day if you have any symptoms of liver problems or skin rash. See the first section "**What is the most important information I should know about VIRAMUNE?**"
- The dose of VIRAMUNE for children is based on their age and weight. Children's dosing also starts with once a day for 14 days and then twice a day after that.
- You may take VIRAMUNE with water, milk, or soda, with or without food.
- If you or your child uses VIRAMUNE suspension (liquid), shake it gently before use. Use an oral dosing syringe or dosing cup to measure the right dose. After drinking the medicine, fill the dosing cup with water and drink it to make sure you get all the medicine. If the dose is less than 5 mL (one teaspoon), use the syringe.
- Do not miss a dose of VIRAMUNE, because this could make the virus harder to treat. If you forget to take VIRAMUNE, take the missed dose right away. If it is almost time for your next dose, do not take the missed dose. Instead, follow your regular dosing schedule by taking the next dose at its regular time.
- If you stop taking VIRAMUNE for more than 7 days, ask your doctor how much to take before you start taking it again. You may need to start with once-a-day dosing.
- If you suspect that you have taken too much VIRAMUNE, contact your local poison control center or emergency room right away.

Can I take other medicines with VIRAMUNE?

- VIRAMUNE may change the effect of other medicines, and other medicines can change the effect of VIRAMUNE.

Tell your doctors and pharmacists about **all** medicines you take, including non-prescription medicines, vitamins and herbal supplements.

- Do **not** take Nizoral® (ketoconazole) or Rifadin®/Rifamate®/Rifater® (rifampin) with VIRAMUNE.
- Tell your doctor if you take Biaxin® (clarithromycin), Diflucan® (fluconazole), methadone, or Mycobutin® (rifabutin). VIRAMUNE may not be right for you, or you may need careful monitoring.
- It is recommended that you not take products containing St. John's wort, which can reduce the amount of VIRAMUNE in your body.
- If you take birth control pills, you should not rely on them to prevent pregnancy. They may not work if you take VIRAMUNE. Talk with your doctor about other types of birth control that you can use.

What should I avoid while taking VIRAMUNE?

Avoid doing things that can spread HIV infection, as VIRAMUNE does not stop you from passing HIV infection to others. Do not share needles, other injection equipment or personal items that can have blood or body fluids on them, like toothbrushes and razor blades. Always practice safe sex by using a latex or polyurethane condom to lower the chance of sexual contact with semen, vaginal secretions, or blood.

The Centers for Disease Control and Prevention advises mothers with HIV not to breast feed so they will not pass HIV to the infant through their milk. Ask your doctor about the best way to feed your infant.

What are the possible side effects of VIRAMUNE?

VIRAMUNE can cause serious liver damage and skin reactions that can cause death. Any patient can experience such side effects, but some patients are more at risk than others. See "**What is the most important information I should know about VIRAMUNE?**" at the beginning of this Medication Guide.

Other common side effects of VIRAMUNE include nausea, fatigue, fever, headache, vomiting, diarrhea, abdominal pain, and myalgia. This list of side effects is not complete. Ask your doctor or pharmacist for more information.

Changes in body fat have also been seen in some patients taking antiretroviral therapy. The changes may include increased amount of fat in the upper back and neck ("buffalo hump"), breast, and around the trunk. Loss of fat from the legs, arms, and face may also happen. The cause and long-term health effects of these conditions are not known at this time.

How do I store VIRAMUNE?

Store VIRAMUNE at room temperature, between 59° to 86°F (15° to 30°C).

Throw away VIRAMUNE that is no longer needed or out-of-date.

Keep VIRAMUNE and all medicines out of the reach of children.

General information about VIRAMUNE

Medicines are sometimes prescribed for purposes other than those listed in a Medication Guide. Do not use VIRAMUNE for a condition for which it was not prescribed. Do not give VIRAMUNE to other people, even if they have the same condition you have. It may harm them.

This Medication Guide summarizes the most important information about VIRAMUNE. If you would like more information, talk with your doctor. You can ask your pharmacist or doctor for information about VIRAMUNE that is written for health professionals, or you can visit www.viramune.com or call 1-800-542-6257 for additional information.

Distributed by:

Boehringer Ingelheim Pharmaceuticals, Inc.
Ridgefield, CT 06877 USA

©Copyright Boehringer Ingelheim Pharmaceuticals, Inc. 2007, ALL RIGHTS RESERVED

Biaxin is a trademark of Abbott Laboratories. Diflucan is a trademark of Pfizer, Inc. Mycobutin is a trademark of Pharmacia & Upjohn Company. Nizoral is a trademark of Janssen Pharmaceutica. Rifadin, Rifamate and Rifater are trademarks of Aventis Pharmaceuticals Inc.

Rev: June 2007
10003354/02   10003354/US/2
OT1801DF2507

This Medication Guide has been approved by the US Food and Drug Administration.

To keep your **PDR** up to date throughout the year, note these revisions on the corresponding pages of the annual volume. Simply write "**See Supplement A**" next to the product heading.

Bristol-Myers Squibb Company

P.O. BOX 4500
PRINCETON, NJ 08543-4500
NOUS08AB00401

For Medical Information Contact:

Generally:

Bristol-Myers Squibb Medical Information Department
P.O. Box 4500
Princeton, NJ 08543-4500
(800) 321-1335

To report SUSPECTED ADVERSE REACTIONS, contact Bristol-Myers Squibb at 1-800-721-5072 between 8:00 AM–5:00 PM EST

Sales and Ordering:

Orders may be placed by:

1. Calling your purchase orders in toll-free between 8:30 AM–6:00 PM EST:
(800) 631-5244
2. Mailing your purchase orders to:
Bristol-Myers Squibb U.S. Pharmaceuticals
Attn: Customer Service
P.O. Box 4500
Princeton, NJ 08543-4500
3. Faxing your purchase orders to:
(800) 523-2965
4. Transmitting computer-to-computer on the NWDA and UCS formats through Ordernet Services use:
DEA#PE0048579
NOUS08AB00402

ABILIFY®   ℞

[ă-bĭl-ĭfĭ]

(aripiprazole)

Prescribing information for this product, which appears on page(s) 872-879 of the 2008 PDR, has been completely revised as follows. Please write "See Supplement A" next to the product heading.

HIGHLIGHTS OF PRESCRIBING INFORMATION

These highlights do not include all the information needed to use ABILIFY safely and effectively. See full prescribing information for ABILIFY.

ABILIFY® (aripiprazole) Tablets
ABILIFY® DISCMELT™ (aripiprazole) Orally Disintegrating Tablets
ABILIFY® (aripiprazole) Oral Solution
ABILIFY® (aripiprazole) Injection FOR INTRAMUSCULAR USE ONLY
Initial U.S. Approval: 2002

> **WARNINGS: INCREASED MORTALITY IN ELDERLY PATIENTS WITH DEMENTIA-RELATED PSYCHOSIS and SUICIDALITY AND ANTIDEPRESSANT DRUGS**
> *See full prescribing information for complete boxed warning.*
>
> - Elderly patients with dementia-related psychosis treated with atypical antipsychotic drugs are at an increased risk of death compared to placebo. ABILIFY is not approved for the treatment of patients with dementia-related psychosis. (5.1)
> - Children, adolescents, and young adults taking antidepressants for Major Depressive Disorder (MDD) and other psychiatric disorders are at increased risk of suicidal thinking and behavior. (5.2)

-------------- **RECENT MAJOR CHANGES** --------------

Boxed Warning, Suicidality and Antidepressant Drugs	11/2007
Indications and Usage,	
Pediatric (13 to 17 years) Schizophrenia (1.1)	10/2007
Pediatric (10 to 17 years) Bipolar Mania (1.2)	02/2008
Adjunctive Treatment in Adults with MDD (1.3)	11/2007
Dosage and Administration,	
Pediatric Schizophrenia (2.1)	10/2007
Pediatric Bipolar Mania (2.2)	02/2008
Adjunctive Treatment in Adults with MDD (2.3)	11/2007
Warnings and Precautions, Clinical Worsening of Depression and Suicide Risk (5.2)	11/2007

-------------- **INDICATIONS AND USAGE** --------------

ABILIFY is an atypical antipsychotic indicated as oral formulations for:

- Treatment of Schizophrenia in adults and adolescents aged 13 to 17 years (1.1)
- Treatment of acute manic or mixed episodes associated with Bipolar I Disorder in adults and pediatric patients aged 10 to 17 years (1.2)
- Adjunctive treatment of Major Depressive Disorder in adults (1.3)

as an injection for:

- Treatment of adults with agitation associated with Schizophrenia or Bipolar I Disorder, manic or mixed (1.4)

DOSAGE AND ADMINISTRATION

	Initial Dose	Recommended Dose	Maximum Dose
Schizophrenia – adults (2.1)	10-15 mg/day	10-15 mg/day	30 mg/day
Schizophrenia – adolescents (2.1)	2 mg/day	10 mg/day	30 mg/day
Bipolar Mania – adults (2.2)	15-30 mg/day	15-30 mg/day	30 mg/day
Bipolar Mania – pediatric patients (2.2)	2 mg/day	10 mg/day	30 mg/day
As an adjunct to antidepressants for the treatment of Major Depressive Disorder (2.3)	2-5 mg/day	5-10 mg/day	15 mg/day
Agitation associated with Schizophrenia or Bipolar Mania – adults (2.4)	9.75 mg/1.3 mL injected IM		30 mg/day injected IM

- Oral formulations: Administer once daily without regard to meals (2)
- IM injection: Wait at least 2 hours between doses. Maximum daily dose 30 mg (2.4)

DOSAGE FORMS AND STRENGTHS

- Tablets: 2 mg, 5 mg, 10 mg, 15 mg, 20 mg, and 30 mg (3)
- Orally Disintegrating Tablets: 10 mg and 15 mg (3)
- Oral Solution: 1 mg/mL (3)
- Injection: 9.75 mg/1.3 mL single-dose vial (3)

CONTRAINDICATIONS

Known hypersensitivity to ABILIFY (4)

WARNINGS AND PRECAUTIONS

- *Elderly Patients with Dementia-Related Psychosis:* Increased incidence of cerebrovascular adverse events (eg, stroke, transient ischemic attack, including fatalities) (5.1)
- *Suicidality and Antidepressants:* Increased risk of suicidality in children, adolescents, and young adults with Major Depressive Disorder (5.2)
- *Neuroleptic Malignant Syndrome:* Manage with immediate discontinuation and close monitoring (5.3)
- *Tardive Dyskinesia:* Discontinue if clinically appropriate (5.4)
- *Hyperglycemia and Diabetes Mellitus:* Monitor glucose regularly in patients with and at risk for diabetes (5.5)
- *Orthostatic Hypotension:* Use with caution in patients with known cardiovascular or cerebrovascular disease (5.6)
- *Seizures/Convulsions:* Use cautiously in patients with a history of seizures or with conditions that lower the seizure threshold (5.7)
- *Potential for Cognitive and Motor Impairment:* Use caution when operating machinery (5.8)
- *Suicide:* Closely supervise high-risk patients (5.10)

ADVERSE REACTIONS

Commonly observed adverse reactions (incidence ≥5% and at least twice that for placebo) were (6.2):
- Adult patients with Schizophrenia: akathisia
- Pediatric patients (13 to 17 years) with Schizophrenia: extrapyramidal disorder, somnolence, and tremor
- Adult patients with Bipolar Mania: constipation, akathisia, sedation, tremor, restlessness, and extrapyramidal disorder
- Pediatric patients (10 to 17 years) with Bipolar Mania: somnolence, extrapyramidal disorder, fatigue, nausea, akathisia, blurred vision, salivary hypersecretion, and dizziness
- Adult patients with Major Depressive Disorder (adjunctive treatment to antidepressant therapy): akathisia, restlessness, insomnia, constipation, fatigue, and blurred vision
- Adult patients with agitation associated with Schizophrenia or Bipolar Mania: nausea.

To report SUSPECTED ADVERSE REACTIONS, contact Bristol-Myers Squibb at 1-800-721-5072 or FDA at 1-800-FDA-1088 or www.fda.gov/medwatch

DRUG INTERACTIONS

- *Strong CYP3A4 (eg, ketoconazole) or CYP2D6 (eg, fluoxetine) inhibitors* will increase ABILIFY drug concentrations; reduce ABILIFY dose by one-half when used concomitantly (2.5, 7.1), except when used as adjunctive treatment with antidepressants (2.5)
- *CYP3A4 inducers (eg, carbamazepine)* will decrease ABILIFY drug concentrations; double ABILIFY dose when used concomitantly (2.5, 7.1)

See 17 for PATIENT COUNSELING INFORMATION and Medication Guide

Revised: 02/2008

FULL PRESCRIBING INFORMATION: CONTENTS*
WARNINGS: INCREASED MORTALITY IN ELDERLY PATIENTS WITH DEMENTIA-RELATED PSYCHOSIS and SUICIDALITY AND ANTIDEPRESSANT DRUGS

FULL PRESCRIBING INFORMATION

WARNINGS: INCREASED MORTALITY IN ELDERLY PATIENTS WITH DEMENTIA-RELATED PSYCHOSIS and SUICIDALITY AND ANTIDEPRESSANT DRUGS
Elderly patients with dementia-related psychosis treated with atypical antipsychotic drugs are at an increased risk of death compared to placebo. Analyses of seventeen placebo-controlled trials (modal duration of 10 weeks) in these patients revealed a risk of death in the drug-treated patients of between 1.6 to 1.7 times that seen in placebo-treated patients. Over the course of a typical 10-week controlled trial, the rate of death in drug-treated patients was about 4.5%, compared to a rate of about 2.6% in the placebo group. Although the causes of death were varied, most of the deaths appeared to be either cardiovascular (eg, heart failure, sudden death) or infectious (eg, pneumonia) in nature. ABILIFY (aripiprazole) is not approved for the treatment of patients with dementia-related psychosis *[see WARNINGS AND PRECAUTIONS (5.1)].*
Antidepressants increased the risk compared to placebo of suicidal thinking and behavior (suicidality) in children, adolescents, and young adults in short-term studies of Major Depressive Disorder (MDD) and other psychiatric disorders. Anyone considering the use of adjunctive ABILIFY or any other antidepressant in a child, adolescent, or young adult must balance this risk with the clinical need. Short-term studies did not show an increase in the risk of suicidality with antidepressants compared to placebo in adults beyond age 24; there was a reduction in risk with antidepressants compared to placebo in adults aged 65 and older. Depression and certain other psychiatric disorders are themselves associated with increases in the risk of suicide. Patients of all ages who are started on antidepressant therapy should be monitored appropriately and observed closely for clinical worsening, suicidality, or unusual changes in behavior. Families and caregivers should be advised of the need for close observation and communication with the prescriber. ABILIFY is not approved for use in pediatric patients with depression *[see WARNINGS AND PRECAUTIONS (5.2)].*

1 INDICATIONS AND USAGE

1.1 Schizophrenia
Adults
ABILIFY (aripiprazole) is indicated for acute and maintenance treatment of Schizophrenia *[see CLINICAL STUDIES (14.1)].*
Adolescents
ABILIFY is indicated for the treatment of Schizophrenia in adolescents 13 to 17 years of age *[see CLINICAL STUDIES (14.1)].*

1.2 Bipolar Disorder
Adults
ABILIFY is indicated for acute and maintenance treatment of manic and mixed episodes associated with Bipolar I Disorder with or without psychotic features *[see CLINICAL STUDIES (14.2)].*
Pediatric Patients
ABILIFY is indicated for the acute treatment of manic and mixed episodes associated with Bipolar Disorder with or without psychotic features in pediatric patients 10 to 17 years of age *[see CLINICAL STUDIES (14.2)].*

1.3 Adjunctive Treatment of Major Depressive Disorder
Adults
ABILIFY is indicated for use as an adjunctive treatment to antidepressants for Major Depressive Disorder *[see CLINICAL STUDIES (14.3)].*

1.4 Agitation Associated with Schizophrenia or Bipolar Mania
Adults
ABILIFY Injection is indicated for the treatment of agitation associated with Schizophrenia or Bipolar Disorder, manic or mixed. "Psychomotor agitation" is defined in DSM-IV as "excessive motor activity associated with a feeling of inner tension." Patients experiencing agitation often manifest behaviors that interfere with their diagnosis and care (eg, threatening behaviors, escalating or urgently distressing behavior, or self-exhausting behavior), leading clinicians to the use of intramuscular antipsychotic medications to achieve immediate control of the agitation *[see CLINICAL STUDIES (14.4)].*

2 DOSAGE AND ADMINISTRATION

2.1 Schizophrenia
Usual Dose
Adults
The recommended starting and target dose for ABILIFY is 10 mg/day or 15 mg/day administered on a once-a-day schedule without regard to meals. ABILIFY has been systematically evaluated and shown to be effective in a dose range of 10 mg/day to 30 mg/day, when administered as the tablet formulation; however, doses higher than 10 mg/day or 15 mg/day were not more effective than 10 mg/day or 15 mg/day. Dosage increases should not be made before 2 weeks, the time needed to achieve steady-state *[see CLINICAL STUDIES (14.1)].*
Adolescents
The recommended target dose of ABILIFY is 10 mg/day. Aripiprazole was studied in pediatric patients 13 to 17 years of age with Schizophrenia at daily doses of 10 mg and 30 mg. The starting daily dose of the tablet formulation in these patients was 2 mg, which was titrated to 5 mg after 2 days and to the target dose of 10 mg after 2 additional days. Subsequent dose increases should be administered in 5 mg increments. The 30 mg/day dose was not shown to be more efficacious than the 10 mg/day dose. ABILIFY can be administered without regard to meals *[see CLINICAL STUDIES (14.1)].*
Maintenance Therapy
Adults
While there is no body of evidence available to answer the question of how long a patient treated with aripiprazole

Continued on next page

Product information on these pages reflects product labeling on June 1, 2007. Current information on products of Bristol-Myers Squibb may be obtained at 1-800-321-1335 or www.bms.com.
NOUS08AB00403

Abilify—Cont.

should remain on it, systematic evaluation of patients with Schizophrenia who had been symptomatically stable on other antipsychotic medications for periods of 3 months or longer, were discontinued from those medications, and were then administered ABILIFY (aripiprazole) 15 mg/day and observed for relapse during a period of up to 26 weeks, has demonstrated a benefit of such maintenance treatment [see CLINICAL STUDIES (14.1)]. Patients should be periodically reassessed to determine the need for maintenance treatment.

Pediatric Patients
The efficacy of ABILIFY for the maintenance treatment of Schizophrenia in the pediatric population has not been evaluated.

Switching from Other Antipsychotics
There are no systematically collected data to specifically address switching patients with Schizophrenia from other antipsychotics to ABILIFY or concerning concomitant administration with other antipsychotics. While immediate discontinuation of the previous antipsychotic treatment may be acceptable for some patients with Schizophrenia, more gradual discontinuation may be most appropriate for others. In all cases, the period of overlapping antipsychotic administration should be minimized.

2.2 Bipolar Disorder
Usual Dose
Adults
In clinical trials, the starting dose was 30 mg given once a day, without regard to meals. A dose of 30 mg/day was found to be effective when administered as the tablet formulation. Approximately 15% of patients had their dose decreased to 15 mg based on assessment of tolerability. The safety of doses above 30 mg/day has not been evaluated in clinical trials [see CLINICAL STUDIES (14.2)].

Pediatric Patients
The efficacy of aripiprazole has been established in the treatment of pediatric patients 10 to 17 years of age with Bipolar I Disorder at doses of 10 mg/day or 30 mg/day. The recommended target dose of ABILIFY is 10 mg/day. The starting daily dose of the tablet formulation in these patients was 2 mg/day, which was titrated to 5 mg/day after 2 days and to the target dose of 10 mg/day after 2 additional days. Subsequent dose increases should be administered in 5 mg/day increments. ABILIFY can be administered without regard to meals. [See CLINICAL STUDIES (14.2).]

Maintenance Therapy
Adults
While there is no body of evidence available to answer the question of how long a patient treated with aripiprazole should remain on it, adult patients with Bipolar I Disorder who had been symptomatically stable on ABILIFY Tablets (15 mg/day or 30 mg/day with a starting dose of 30 mg/day) for at least 6 consecutive weeks and then randomized to ABILIFY Tablets (15 mg/day or 30 mg/day) or placebo and monitored for relapse, demonstrated a benefit of such maintenance treatment [see CLINICAL STUDIES (14.2)]. While it is generally agreed that pharmacological treatment beyond an acute response in Mania is desirable, both for maintenance of the initial response and for prevention of new manic episodes, there are no systematically obtained data to support the use of aripiprazole in such longer-term treatment (beyond 6 weeks). Physicians who elect to use ABILIFY for extended periods, that is, longer than 6 weeks, should periodically re-evaluate the long-term usefulness of the drug for the individual.

Pediatric Patients
The efficacy of ABILIFY for the maintenance treatment of Bipolar I Disorder in the pediatric population has not been evaluated.

2.3 Adjunctive Treatment of Major Depressive Disorder
Usual Dose
Adults
The recommended starting dose for ABILIFY as adjunctive treatment for patients already taking an antidepressant is 2 mg/day to 5 mg/day. The efficacy of ABILIFY as an adjunctive therapy for Major Depressive Disorder was established within a dose range of 2 mg/day to 15 mg/day. Dose adjustments of up to 5 mg/day should occur gradually, at intervals of no less than 1 week. The long-term efficacy of ABILIFY for the adjunctive treatment of Major Depressive Disorder has not been established [see CLINICAL STUDIES (14.3)].

Pediatric Patients
The efficacy of ABILIFY for the adjunctive treatment of Major Depressive Disorder in the pediatric population has not been evaluated.

2.4 Agitation Associated with Schizophrenia or Bipolar Mania (Intramuscular Injection)
Usual Dose
Adults
The recommended dose in these patients is 9.75 mg. The effectiveness of aripiprazole injection in controlling agitation in Schizophrenia and Bipolar Mania was demonstrated over a dose range of 5.25 mg to 15 mg. No additional benefit was demonstrated for 15 mg compared to 9.75 mg. A lower dose of 5.25 mg may be considered when clinical factors warrant. If agitation warranting a second dose persists following the initial dose, cumulative doses up to a total of 30 mg/day may be given. However, the efficacy of repeated doses of aripiprazole injection in agitated patients has not been systematically evaluated in controlled clinical trials. The safety of total daily doses greater than 30 mg or injec-

tions given more frequently than every 2 hours have not been adequately evaluated in clinical trials [see CLINICAL STUDIES (14.4)].
If ongoing aripiprazole therapy is clinically indicated, oral aripiprazole in a range of 10 mg/day to 30 mg/day should replace aripiprazole injection as soon as possible [see DOSAGE AND ADMINISTRATION (2.1 and 2.2)].

Administration of ABILIFY Injection
To administer ABILIFY (aripiprazole) Injection, draw up the required volume of solution into the syringe as shown in Table 1. Discard any unused portion.

Table 1:   ABILIFY Injection Dosing Recommendations

Single-Dose	Required Volume of Solution
5.25 mg	0.7 mL
9.75 mg	1.3 mL
15 mg	2 mL

ABILIFY Injection is intended for intramuscular use only. Do not administer intravenously or subcutaneously. Inject slowly, deep into the muscle mass.
Parenteral drug products should be inspected visually for particulate matter and discoloration prior to administration, whenever solution and container permit.

Pediatric Patients
ABILIFY Intramuscular Injection has not been evaluated in pediatric patients.

2.5 Dosage Adjustment
Dosage adjustments in adults are not routinely indicated on the basis of age, gender, race, or renal or hepatic impairment status [see USE IN SPECIFIC POPULATIONS (8.4-8.10)].

Dosage adjustment for patients taking aripiprazole concomitantly with strong CYP3A4 inhibitors: When concomitant administration of aripiprazole with strong CYP3A4 inhibitors such as ketoconazole or clarithromycin is indicated, the aripiprazole dose should be reduced to one-half the usual dose. When the CYP3A4 inhibitor is withdrawn from the combination therapy, the aripiprazole dose should then be increased [see DRUG INTERACTIONS (7.1)].

Dosage adjustment for patients taking aripiprazole concomitantly with potential CYP2D6 inhibitors: When concomitant administration of potential CYP2D6 inhibitors such as quinidine, fluoxetine, or paroxetine with aripiprazole occurs, aripiprazole dose should be reduced at least to one-half of its normal dose. When the CYP2D6 inhibitor is withdrawn from the combination therapy, the aripiprazole dose should then be increased [see DRUG INTERACTIONS (7.1)]. When adjunctive ABILIFY is administered to patients with Major Depressive Disorder, ABILIFY should be administered without dosage adjustment as specified in DOSAGE AND ADMINISTRATION (2.3).

Dosage adjustment for patients taking potential CYP3A4 inducers: When a potential CYP3A4 inducer such as carbamazepine is added to aripiprazole therapy, the aripiprazole dose should be doubled. Additional dose increases should be based on clinical evaluation. When the CYP3A4 inducer is withdrawn from the combination therapy, the aripiprazole dose should be reduced to 10 mg to 15 mg [see DRUG INTERACTIONS (7.1)].

2.6 Dosing of Oral Solution
The oral solution can be substituted for tablets on a mg-per-mg basis up to the 25 mg dose level. Patients receiving 30 mg tablets should receive 25 mg of the solution [see CLINICAL PHARMACOLOGY (12.3)].

2.7 Dosing of Orally Disintegrating Tablets
The dosing for ABILIFY Orally Disintegrating Tablets is the same as for the oral tablets [see DOSAGE AND ADMINISTRATION (2.1, 2.2 and 2.3)].

3 DOSAGE FORMS AND STRENGTHS
ABILIFY® (aripiprazole) Tablets are available as described in Table 2.

Table 2:   ABILIFY Tablet Presentations

Tablet Strength	Tablet Color/Shape	Tablet Markings
2 mg	green modified rectangle	"A-006" and "2"
5 mg	blue modified rectangle	"A-007" and "5"
10 mg	pink modified rectangle	"A-008" and "10"
15 mg	yellow round	"A-009" and "15"
20 mg	white round	"A-010" and "20"
30 mg	pink round	"A-011" and "30"

ABILIFY® DISCMELT™ (aripiprazole) Orally Disintegrating Tablets are available as described in Table 3.

Table 3:   ABILIFY DISCMELT Orally Disintegrating Tablet Presentations

Tablet Strength	Tablet Color/Shape	Tablet Markings
10 mg	pink (with scattered specks) round	"A" and "640" "10"
15 mg	yellow (with scattered specks) round	"A" and "641" "15"

ABILIFY® (aripiprazole) Oral Solution (1 mg/mL) is a clear, colorless to light yellow solution, supplied in child-resistant bottles along with a calibrated oral dosing cup.
ABILIFY® (aripiprazole) Injection for Intramuscular Use is a clear, colorless solution available as a ready-to-use, 9.75 mg/1.3 mL (7.5 mg/mL) solution in clear, Type 1 glass vials.

4 CONTRAINDICATIONS
Known hypersensitivity reaction to ABILIFY. Reactions have ranged from pruritus/urticaria to anaphylaxis [see ADVERSE REACTIONS (6.3)].

5 WARNINGS AND PRECAUTIONS
5.1 Use in Elderly Patients with Dementia-Related Psychosis
Increased Mortality
Elderly patients with dementia-related psychosis treated with atypical antipsychotic drugs are at an increased risk of death compared to placebo. ABILIFY (aripiprazole) is not approved for the treatment of patients with dementia-related psychosis [see BOXED WARNING].
Cerebrovascular Adverse Events, Including Stroke
In placebo-controlled clinical studies (two flexible dose and one fixed dose study) of dementia-related psychosis, there was an increased incidence of cerebrovascular adverse events (eg, stroke, transient ischemic attack), including fatalities, in aripiprazole-treated patients (mean age: 84 years; range: 78-88 years). In the fixed-dose study, there was a statistically significant dose response relationship for cerebrovascular adverse events in patients treated with aripiprazole. Aripiprazole is not approved for the treatment of patients with dementia-related psychosis [see also BOXED WARNING].
Safety Experience in Elderly Patients with Psychosis Associated with Alzheimer's Disease
In three, 10-week, placebo-controlled studies of aripiprazole in elderly patients with psychosis associated with Alzheimer's disease (n=938; mean age: 82.4 years; range: 56-99 years), the treatment-emergent adverse events that were reported at an incidence of ≥3% and aripiprazole incidence at least twice that for placebo were lethargy [placebo 2%, aripiprazole 5%], somnolence (including sedation) [placebo 3%, aripiprazole 8%], and incontinence (primarily, urinary incontinence) [placebo 1%, aripiprazole 5%], excessive salivation (placebo 0%, aripiprazole 4%), and lightheadedness (placebo 1%, aripiprazole 4%).
The safety and efficacy of ABILIFY in the treatment of patients with psychosis associated with dementia have not been established. If the prescriber elects to treat such patients with ABILIFY, vigilance should be exercised, particularly for the emergence of difficulty swallowing or excessive somnolence, which could predispose to accidental injury or aspiration [see also BOXED WARNING].

5.2 Clinical Worsening of Depression and Suicide Risk
Patients with Major Depressive Disorder (MDD), both adult and pediatric, may experience worsening of their depression and/or the emergence of suicidal ideation and behavior (suicidality) or unusual changes in behavior, whether or not they are taking antidepressant medications, and this risk may persist until significant remission occurs. Suicide is a known risk of depression and certain other psychiatric disorders, and these disorders themselves are the strongest predictors of suicide. There has been a long-standing concern, however, that antidepressants may have a role in inducing worsening of depression and the emergence of suicidality in certain patients during the early phases of treatment. Pooled analyses of short-term placebo-controlled trials of antidepressant drugs (SSRIs and others) showed that these drugs increase the risk of suicidal thinking and behavior (suicidality) in children, adolescents, and young adults (ages 18-24) with Major Depressive Disorder (MDD) and other psychiatric disorders. Short-term studies did not show an increase in the risk of suicidality with antidepressants compared to placebo in adults beyond age 24; there was a reduction with antidepressants compared to placebo in adults aged 65 and older.
The pooled analyses of placebo-controlled trials in children and adolescents with MDD, Obsessive Compulsive Disorder (OCD), or other psychiatric disorders included a total of 24 short-term trials of 9 antidepressant drugs in over 4400 patients. The pooled analyses of placebo-controlled trials in adults with MDD or other psychiatric disorders included a total of 295 short-term trials (median duration of 2 months) of 11 antidepressant drugs in over 77,000 patients. There was considerable variation in risk of suicidality among drugs, but a tendency toward an increase in the younger patients for almost all drugs studied. There were differences in absolute risk of suicidality across the different indications, with the highest incidence in MDD. The risk differences (drug vs. placebo), however, were relatively stable within age strata and across indications. These risk differ-

ences (drug-placebo difference in the number of cases of suicidality per 1000 patients treated) are provided in Table 4.

Table 4:

Age Range	Drug-Placebo Difference in Number of Cases of Suicidality per 1000 Patients Treated
	Increases Compared to Placebo
<18	14 additional cases
18-24	5 additional cases
	Decreases Compared to Placebo
25-64	1 fewer case
≥65	6 fewer cases

No suicides occurred in any of the pediatric trials. There were suicides in the adult trials, but the number was not sufficient to reach any conclusion about drug effect on suicide.

It is unknown whether the suicidality risk extends to longer-term use, ie, beyond several months. However, there is substantial evidence from placebo-controlled maintenance trials in adults with depression that the use of antidepressants can delay the recurrence of depression.

All patients being treated with antidepressants for any indication should be monitored appropriately and observed closely for clinical worsening, suicidality, and unusual changes in behavior, especially during the initial few months of a course of drug therapy, or at times of dose changes, either increases or decreases.

The following symptoms, anxiety, agitation, panic attacks, insomnia, irritability, hostility, aggressiveness, impulsivity, akathisia (psychomotor restlessness), hypomania, and mania, have been reported in adult and pediatric patients being treated with antidepressants for Major Depressive Disorder as well as for other indications, both psychiatric and nonpsychiatric. Although a causal link between the emergence of such symptoms and either the worsening of depression and/or the emergence of suicidal impulses has not been established, there is concern that such symptoms may represent precursors to emerging suicidality.

Consideration should be given to changing the therapeutic regimen, including possibly discontinuing the medication, in patients whose depression is persistently worse, or who are experiencing emergent suicidality or symptoms that might be precursors to worsening depression or suicidality, especially if these symptoms are severe, abrupt in onset, or were not part of the patient's presenting symptoms.

Families and caregivers of patients being treated with antidepressants for Major Depressive Disorder or other indications, both psychiatric and nonpsychiatric, should be alerted about the need to monitor patients for the emergence of agitation, irritability, unusual changes in behavior, and the other symptoms described above, as well as the emergence of suicidality, and to report such symptoms immediately to healthcare providers. Such monitoring should include daily observation by families and caregivers. Prescriptions for ABILIFY (aripiprazole) should be written for the smallest quantity of tablets consistent with good patient management, in order to reduce the risk of overdose.

Screening Patients for Bipolar Disorder: A major depressive episode may be the initial presentation of Bipolar Disorder. It is generally believed (though not established in controlled trials) that treating such an episode with an antidepressant alone may increase the likelihood of precipitation of a mixed/manic episode in patients at risk for Bipolar Disorder. Whether any of the symptoms described above represent such a conversion is unknown. However, prior to initiating treatment with an antidepressant, patients with depressive symptoms should be adequately screened to determine if they are at risk for Bipolar Disorder; such screening should include a detailed psychiatric history, including a family history of suicide, Bipolar Disorder, and depression. It should be noted that ABILIFY is not approved for use in treating depression in the pediatric population.

5.3   Neuroleptic Malignant Syndrome (NMS)
A potentially fatal symptom complex sometimes referred to as Neuroleptic Malignant Syndrome (NMS) may occur with administration of antipsychotic drugs, including aripiprazole. Rare cases of NMS occurred during aripiprazole treatment in the worldwide clinical database. Clinical manifestations of NMS are hyperpyrexia, muscle rigidity, altered mental status, and evidence of autonomic instability (irregular pulse or blood pressure, tachycardia, diaphoresis, and cardiac dysrhythmia). Additional signs may include elevated creatine phosphokinase, myoglobinuria (rhabdomyolysis), and acute renal failure.

The diagnostic evaluation of patients with this syndrome is complicated. In arriving at a diagnosis, it is important to exclude cases where the clinical presentation includes both serious medical illness (eg, pneumonia, systemic infection) and untreated or inadequately treated extrapyramidal signs and symptoms (EPS). Other important considerations in the differential diagnosis include central anticholinergic toxicity, heat stroke, drug fever, and primary central nervous system pathology.

The management of NMS should include: 1) immediate discontinuation of antipsychotic drugs and other drugs not essential to concurrent therapy; 2) intensive symptomatic treatment and medical monitoring; and 3) treatment of any concomitant serious medical problems for which specific treatments are available. There is no general agreement about specific pharmacological treatment regimens for uncomplicated NMS.

If a patient requires antipsychotic drug treatment after recovery from NMS, the potential reintroduction of drug therapy should be carefully considered. The patient should be carefully monitored, since recurrences of NMS have been reported.

5.4   Tardive Dyskinesia
A syndrome of potentially irreversible, involuntary, dyskinetic movements may develop in patients treated with antipsychotic drugs. Although the prevalence of the syndrome appears to be highest among the elderly, especially elderly women, it is impossible to rely upon prevalence estimates to predict, at the inception of antipsychotic treatment, which patients are likely to develop the syndrome. Whether antipsychotic drug products differ in their potential to cause tardive dyskinesia is unknown.

The risk of developing tardive dyskinesia and the likelihood that it will become irreversible are believed to increase as the duration of treatment and the total cumulative dose of antipsychotic drugs administered to the patient increase. However, the syndrome can develop, although much less commonly, after relatively brief treatment periods at low doses.

There is no known treatment for established cases of tardive dyskinesia, although the syndrome may remit, partially or completely, if antipsychotic treatment is withdrawn. Antipsychotic treatment, itself, however, may suppress (or partially suppress) the signs and symptoms of the syndrome and, thereby, may possibly mask the underlying process. The effect that symptomatic suppression has upon the long-term course of the syndrome is unknown.

Given these considerations, ABILIFY (aripiprazole) should be prescribed in a manner that is most likely to minimize the occurrence of tardive dyskinesia. Chronic antipsychotic treatment should generally be reserved for patients who suffer from a chronic illness that (1) is known to respond to antipsychotic drugs and (2) for whom alternative, equally effective, but potentially less harmful treatments are not available or appropriate. In patients who do require chronic treatment, the smallest dose and the shortest duration of treatment producing a satisfactory clinical response should be sought. The need for continued treatment should be reassessed periodically.

If signs and symptoms of tardive dyskinesia appear in a patient on ABILIFY, drug discontinuation should be considered. However, some patients may require treatment with ABILIFY despite the presence of the syndrome.

5.5   Hyperglycemia and Diabetes Mellitus
Hyperglycemia, in some cases extreme and associated with ketoacidosis or hyperosmolar coma or death, has been reported in patients treated with atypical antipsychotics. There have been few reports of hyperglycemia in patients treated with ABILIFY *[see ADVERSE REACTIONS (6.2, 6.3)]*. Although fewer patients have been treated with ABILIFY, it is not known if this more limited experience is the sole reason for the paucity of such reports. Assessment of the relationship between atypical antipsychotic use and glucose abnormalities is complicated by the possibility of an increased background risk of diabetes mellitus in patients with Schizophrenia and the increasing incidence of diabetes mellitus in the general population. Given these confounders, the relationship between atypical antipsychotic use and hyperglycemia-related adverse events is not completely understood. However, epidemiological studies which did not include ABILIFY suggest an increased risk of treatment-emergent hyperglycemia-related adverse events in patients treated with the atypical antipsychotics included in these studies. Because ABILIFY was not marketed at the time these studies were performed, it is not known if ABILIFY is associated with this increased risk. Precise risk estimates for hyperglycemia-related adverse events in patients treated with atypical antipsychotics are not available.

Patients with an established diagnosis of diabetes mellitus who are started on atypical antipsychotics should be monitored regularly for worsening of glucose control. Patients with risk factors for diabetes mellitus (eg, obesity, family history of diabetes) who are starting treatment with atypical antipsychotics should undergo fasting blood glucose testing at the beginning of treatment and periodically during treatment. Any patient treated with atypical antipsychotics should be monitored for symptoms of hyperglycemia including polydipsia, polyuria, polyphagia, and weakness. Patients who develop symptoms of hyperglycemia during treatment with atypical antipsychotics should undergo fasting blood glucose testing. In some cases, hyperglycemia has resolved when the atypical antipsychotic was discontinued; however, some patients required continuation of antidiabetic treatment despite discontinuation of the suspect drug.

5.6   Orthostatic Hypotension
Aripiprazole may cause orthostatic hypotension, perhaps due to its α_1-adrenergic receptor antagonism. The incidence of orthostatic hypotension-associated events from short-term, placebo-controlled trials of adult patients on oral ABILIFY (n=1894) included (aripiprazole incidence, placebo incidence) orthostatic hypotension (1.2%, 0.3%), postural dizziness (0.6%, 0.4%), and syncope (0.6%, 0.5%); of pediatric patients 10 to 17 years of age (n=399) on oral ABILIFY included orthostatic hypotension (1.0%, 0%), postural dizziness (0.5%, 0%), and syncope (0.3%, 0%); and of patients on ABILIFY Injection (n=501) included orthostatic hypotension (0.6%, 0%), postural dizziness (0.2%, 0.5%), and syncope (0.4%, 0%).

The incidence of a significant orthostatic change in blood pressure (defined as a decrease in systolic blood pressure ≥20 mmHg accompanied by an increase in heart rate ≥25

when comparing standing to supine values) for aripiprazole was not meaningfully different from placebo (aripiprazole incidence, placebo incidence): in adult oral aripiprazole-treated patients (5%, 3%), in pediatric oral aripiprazole-treated patients aged 10 to 17 years (0%, 0.5%), or in aripiprazole injection-treated patients (3%, 2%).

Aripiprazole should be used with caution in patients with known cardiovascular disease (history of myocardial infarction or ischemic heart disease, heart failure or conduction abnormalities), cerebrovascular disease, or conditions which would predispose patients to hypotension (dehydration, hypovolemia, and treatment with antihypertensive medications).

If parenteral benzodiazepine therapy is deemed necessary in addition to aripiprazole injection treatment, patients should be monitored for excessive sedation and for orthostatic hypotension *[see DRUG INTERACTIONS (7.3)]*.

5.7   Seizures/Convulsions
In short-term, placebo-controlled trials, seizures/convulsions occurred in 0.2% (3/1894) of adult patients treated with oral aripiprazole, in 0.3% (1/399) of pediatric patients (10 to 17 years), and in 0.2% (1/501) of adult aripiprazole injection-treated patients.

As with other antipsychotic drugs, aripiprazole should be used cautiously in patients with a history of seizures or with conditions that lower the seizure threshold, eg, Alzheimer's dementia. Conditions that lower the seizure threshold may be more prevalent in a population of 65 years or older.

5.8   Potential for Cognitive and Motor Impairment
ABILIFY (aripiprazole), like other antipsychotics, may have the potential to impair judgment, thinking, or motor skills. For example, in short-term, placebo-controlled trials, somnolence (including sedation) was reported as follows (aripiprazole incidence, placebo incidence): in adult patients (n=1894) treated with oral ABILIFY (11%, 7%), in pediatric patients ages 10 to 17 (21%, 5%), and in adult patients on ABILIFY Injection (9%, 6%). Somnolence (including sedation) led to discontinuation in 0.2% (4/1894) of adult patients, and 1% (4/399) of pediatric patients (10 to 17 years) on oral ABILIFY in short-term, placebo-controlled trials, but did not lead to discontinuation of any adult patients on ABILIFY Injection.

Despite the relatively modest increased incidence of these events compared to placebo, patients should be cautioned about operating hazardous machinery, including automobiles, until they are reasonably certain that therapy with ABILIFY does not affect them adversely.

5.9   Body Temperature Regulation
Disruption of the body's ability to reduce core body temperature has been attributed to antipsychotic agents. Appropriate care is advised when prescribing aripiprazole for patients who will be experiencing conditions which may contribute to an elevation in core body temperature, (eg, exercising strenuously, exposure to extreme heat, receiving concomitant medication with anticholinergic activity, or being subject to dehydration) *[see ADVERSE REACTIONS (6.3)]*.

5.10   Suicide
The possibility of a suicide attempt is inherent in psychotic illnesses, Bipolar Disorder, and Major Depressive Disorder, and close supervision of high-risk patients should accompany drug therapy. Prescriptions for ABILIFY should be written for the smallest quantity consistent with good patient management in order to reduce the risk of overdose *[see ADVERSE REACTIONS (6.2, 6.3)]*.

In two 6-week placebo-controlled studies of aripiprazole as adjunctive treatment of Major Depressive Disorder, the incidences of suicidal ideation and suicide attempts were 0% (0/371) for aripiprazole and 0.5% (2/366) for placebo.

5.11   Dysphagia
Esophageal dysmotility and aspiration have been associated with antipsychotic drug use, including ABILIFY. Aspiration pneumonia is a common cause of morbidity and mortality in elderly patients, in particular those with advanced Alzheimer's dementia. Aripiprazole and other antipsychotic drugs should be used cautiously in patients at risk for aspiration pneumonia *[see WARNINGS AND PRECAUTIONS (5.1) and ADVERSE REACTIONS (6.3)]*.

5.12   Use in Patients with Concomitant Illness
Clinical experience with ABILIFY in patients with certain concomitant systemic illnesses is limited *[see USE IN SPECIFIC POPULATIONS (8.6, 8.7)]*.

ABILIFY has not been evaluated or used to any appreciable extent in patients with a recent history of myocardial infarction or unstable heart disease. Patients with these diagnoses were excluded from premarketing clinical studies *[see WARNINGS AND PRECAUTIONS (5.1, 5.6)]*.

6   ADVERSE REACTIONS
6.1   Overall Adverse Reactions Profile
The following are discussed in more detail in other sections of the labeling:
• Use in Elderly Patients with Dementia-Related Psychosis *[see BOXED WARNING and WARNINGS AND PRECAUTIONS (5.1)]*

Continued on next page

Product information on these pages reflects product labeling on June 1, 2007. Current information on products of Bristol-Myers Squibb may be obtained at 1-800-321-1335 or www.bms.com.
NOUS08AB00403

Abilify—Cont.

- Clinical Worsening of Depression and Suicide Risk *[see BOXED WARNING and WARNINGS AND PRECAUTIONS (5.2)]*
- Neuroleptic Malignant Syndrome (NMS) *[see WARNINGS AND PRECAUTIONS (5.3)]*
- Tardive Dyskinesia *[see WARNINGS AND PRECAUTIONS (5.4)]*
- Hyperglycemia and Diabetes Mellitus *[see WARNINGS AND PRECAUTIONS (5.5)]*
- Orthostatic Hypotension *[see WARNINGS AND PRECAUTIONS (5.6)]*
- Seizures/Convulsions *[see WARNINGS AND PRECAUTIONS (5.7)]*
- Potential for Cognitive and Motor Impairment *[see WARNINGS AND PRECAUTIONS (5.8)]*
- Body Temperature Regulation *[see WARNINGS AND PRECAUTIONS (5.9)]*
- Suicide *[see WARNINGS AND PRECAUTIONS (5.10)]*
- Dysphagia *[see WARNINGS AND PRECAUTIONS (5.11)]*
- Use in Patients with Concomitant Illness *[see WARNINGS AND PRECAUTIONS (5.12)]*

The most common adverse reactions in adult patients in clinical trials (≥10%) were nausea, vomiting, constipation, headache, dizziness, akathisia, anxiety, insomnia, and restlessness.

The most common adverse reactions in the pediatric clinical trials (≥10%) were somnolence, extrapyramidal disorder, headache, and nausea.

Aripiprazole has been evaluated for safety in 12,925 adult patients who participated in multiple-dose, clinical trials in Schizophrenia, Bipolar Disorder, Major Depressive Disorder, and Dementia of the Alzheimer's type, and who had approximately 7482 patient-years of exposure to oral aripiprazole and 749 patients with exposure to aripiprazole injection. A total of 3338 patients were treated with oral aripiprazole for at least 180 days and 1898 patients treated with oral aripiprazole had at least 1 year of exposure.

Aripiprazole has been evaluated for safety in 514 patients (10 to 17 years) who participated in multiple-dose, clinical trials in Schizophrenia or Bipolar Mania and who had approximately 205 patient-years of exposure to oral aripiprazole. A total of 278 pediatric patients were treated with oral aripiprazole for at least 180 days.

The conditions and duration of treatment with aripiprazole included (in overlapping categories) double-blind, comparative and noncomparative open-label studies, inpatient and outpatient studies, fixed- and flexible-dose studies, and short- and longer-term exposure.

Adverse events during exposure were obtained by collecting volunteered adverse events, as well as results of physical examinations, vital signs, weights, laboratory analyses, and ECG. Adverse experiences were recorded by clinical investigators using terminology of their own choosing. In the tables and tabulations that follow, MedDRA dictionary terminology has been used to classify reported adverse events into a smaller number of standardized event categories, in order to provide a meaningful estimate of the proportion of individuals experiencing adverse events.

The stated frequencies of adverse reactions represent the proportion of individuals who experienced at least once, a treatment-emergent adverse event of the type listed. An event was considered treatment emergent if it occurred for the first time or worsened while receiving therapy following baseline evaluation. There was no attempt to use investigator causality assessments; ie, all events meeting the defined criteria, regardless of investigator causality are included.

Throughout this section, adverse reactions are reported. These are adverse events that were considered to be reasonably associated with the use of ABILIFY (aripiprazole) (adverse drug reactions) based on the comprehensive assessment of the available adverse event information. A causal association for ABILIFY often cannot be reliably established in individual cases.

The figures in the tables and tabulations cannot be used to predict the incidence of side effects in the course of usual medical practice where patient characteristics and other factors differ from those that prevailed in the clinical trials. Similarly, the cited frequencies cannot be compared with figures obtained from other clinical investigations involving different treatment, uses, and investigators. The cited figures, however, do provide the prescriber with some basis for estimating the relative contribution of drug and nondrug factors to the adverse reaction incidence in the population studied.

6.2 Clinical Studies Experience

Adult Patients with Schizophrenia

The following findings are based on a pool of five placebo-controlled trials (four 4-week and one 6-week) in which oral aripiprazole was administered in doses ranging from 2 mg/day to 30 mg/day.

Adverse Reactions Associated with Discontinuation of Treatment

Overall, there was little difference in the incidence of discontinuation due to adverse reactions between aripiprazole-treated (7%) and placebo-treated (9%) patients. The types of adverse reactions that led to discontinuation were similar for the aripiprazole- and placebo-treated patients.

Commonly Observed Adverse Reactions

The only commonly observed adverse reaction associated with the use of aripiprazole in patients with Schizophrenia (incidence of 5% or greater and aripiprazole incidence at least twice that for placebo) was akathisia (aripiprazole 8%; placebo 4%).

Adult Patients with Bipolar Mania

The following findings are based on a pool of 3-week, placebo-controlled, Bipolar Mania trials in which oral aripiprazole was administered at doses of 15 mg/day or 30 mg/day.

Adverse Reactions Associated with Discontinuation of Treatment

Overall, in patients with Bipolar Mania, there was little difference in the incidence of discontinuation due to adverse reactions between aripiprazole-treated (11%) and placebo-treated (9%) patients. The types of adverse reactions that led to discontinuation were similar between the aripiprazole- and placebo-treated patients.

Commonly Observed Adverse Reactions

Commonly observed adverse reactions associated with the use of aripiprazole in patients with Bipolar Mania (incidence of 5% or greater and aripiprazole incidence at least twice that for placebo) are shown in Table 5.

Table 5: Commonly Observed Adverse Reactions in Short-Term, Placebo-Controlled Trials of Adult Patients with Bipolar Mania Treated with Oral ABILIFY

Preferred Term	Percentage of Patients Reporting Reaction Aripiprazole (n=597)	Placebo (n=436)
Constipation	13	6
Akathisia	15	3
Sedation	8	3
Tremor	7	3
Restlessness	6	3
Extrapyramidal Disorder	5	2

Less Common Adverse Reactions in Adults

Table 6 enumerates the pooled incidence, rounded to the nearest percent, of adverse reactions that occurred during acute therapy (up to 6 weeks in Schizophrenia and up to 3 weeks in Bipolar Mania), including only those reactions that occurred in 2% or more of patients treated with aripiprazole (doses ≥2 mg/day) and for which the incidence in patients treated with aripiprazole was greater than the incidence in patients treated with placebo in the combined dataset.

Table 6: Adverse Reactions in Short-Term, Placebo-Controlled Trials in Adult Patients Treated with Oral ABILIFY

System Organ Class Preferred Term	Percentage of Patients Reporting Reaction[a] Aripiprazole (n=1523)	Placebo (n=849)
Eye Disorders		
Blurred Vision	3	1
Gastrointestinal Disorders		
Nausea	16	12
Vomiting	12	6
Constipation	11	7
Dyspepsia	10	8
Dry Mouth	5	4
Abdominal Discomfort	3	2
Stomach Discomfort	3	2
Salivary Hypersecretion	2	1
General Disorders and Administration Site Conditions		
Fatigue	6	5
Pain	3	2
Peripheral Edema	2	1
Musculoskeletal and Connective Tissue Disorders		
Arthralgia	5	4
Pain in Extremity	4	2
Nervous System Disorders		
Headache	30	25
Dizziness	11	8
Akathisia	10	4
Sedation	7	4
Extrapyramidal Disorder	6	4
Tremor	5	3
Somnolence	5	4
Psychiatric Disorders		
Anxiety	20	17
Insomnia	19	14
Restlessness	5	3
Respiratory, Thoracic, and Mediastinal Disorders		
Pharyngolaryngeal Pain	4	3
Cough	3	2
Nasal Congestion	3	2
Vascular Disorders		
Hypertension[b]	2	1

[a] Adverse reactions reported by at least 2% of patients treated with oral aripiprazole, except adverse reactions which had an incidence equal to or less than placebo.
[b] Including blood pressure increased.

An examination of population subgroups did not reveal any clear evidence of differential adverse reaction incidence on the basis of age, gender, or race.

Pediatric Patients (13 to 17 years) with Schizophrenia

The following findings are based on one 6-week placebo-controlled trial in which oral aripiprazole was administered in doses ranging from 2 mg/day to 30 mg/day.

Adverse Reactions Associated with Discontinuation of Treatment

The incidence of discontinuation due to adverse reactions between aripiprazole-treated and placebo-treated pediatric patients (13 to 17 years) was 5% and 2%, respectively.

Commonly Observed Adverse Reactions

Commonly observed adverse reactions associated with the use of aripiprazole in adolescent patients with Schizophrenia (incidence of 5% or greater and aripiprazole incidence at least twice that for placebo) were extrapyramidal disorder, somnolence, and tremor.

Pediatric Patients (10 to 17 years) with Bipolar Mania

The following findings are based on one 4-week placebo-controlled trial in which oral aripiprazole was administered in doses of 10 mg/day or 30 mg/day.

Adverse Reactions Associated with Discontinuation of Treatment

The incidence of discontinuation due to adverse reactions between aripiprazole- and placebo-treated pediatric patients (10 to 17 years) was 7% and 2%, respectively.

Commonly Observed Adverse Reactions

Commonly observed adverse reactions associated with the use of aripiprazole in pediatric patients with Bipolar Mania (incidence of 5% or greater and aripiprazole incidence at least twice that for placebo) are shown in Table 7.

Table 7: Commonly Observed Adverse Reactions in Short-Term, Placebo-Controlled Trials of Pediatric Patients (10 to 17 years) with Bipolar Mania Treated with Oral ABILIFY

Preferred Term	Percentage of Patients Reporting Reaction Aripiprazole (n=197)	Placebo (n=97)
Somnolence	23	3
Extrapyramidal Disorder	20	3
Fatigue	11	4
Nausea	11	4
Akathisia	10	2
Blurred Vision	8	0
Salivary Hypersecretion	6	0
Dizziness	5	1

Less Common Adverse Reactions in Pediatric Patients (10 to 17 years) with Schizophrenia or Bipolar Mania

Table 8 enumerates the pooled incidence, rounded to the nearest percent, of adverse reactions that occurred during acute therapy (up to 6 weeks in Schizophrenia and up to 4 weeks in Bipolar Mania), including only those reactions that occurred in 1% or more of pediatric patients treated with aripiprazole (doses ≥2 mg/day) and for which the incidence in patients treated with aripiprazole was greater than the incidence in patients treated with placebo.

Table 8: Adverse Reactions in Short-Term, Placebo-Controlled Trials of Pediatric Patients (10 to 17 years) Treated with Oral ABILIFY

System Organ Class Preferred Term	Percentage of Patients Reporting Reaction[a] Aripiprazole (n=399)	Placebo (n=197)
Eye Disorders		
Blurred Vision	5	0
Gastrointestinal Disorders		
Nausea	10	5
Salivary Hypersecretion	4	1
Diarrhea	3	0
Stomach Discomfort	2	1
Dry Mouth	2	1
General Disorders and Administration Site Conditions		
Fatigue	7	3
Pyrexia	3	1
Infections and Infestations		
Nasopharyngitis	4	3
Investigations		
Weight Increased	3	1
Metabolism and Nutrition Disorders		
Increased Appetite	4	2
Musculoskeletal and Connective Tissue Disorders		
Arthralgia	2	0
Nervous System Disorders		
Somnolence	20	5
Extrapyramidal Disorder	19	4
Headache	16	13
Akathisia	9	4
Dizziness	5	2
Tremor	5	2
Dystonia	2	0
Dyskinesia	1	0
Sedation	1	0
Skin and Subcutaneous Disorders		
Rash	2	1

Vascular Disorders

Orthostatic Hypotension	1	0

[a] Adverse reactions reported by at least 1% of pediatric patients treated with oral aripiprazole, except adverse reactions which had an incidence equal to or less than placebo.

Adult Patients Receiving ABILIFY as Adjunctive Treatment of Major Depressive Disorder

The following findings are based on a pool of two placebo-controlled trials of patients with Major Depressive Disorder in which aripiprazole was administered at doses of 2 mg to 20 mg as adjunctive treatment to continued antidepressant therapy.

Adverse Reactions Associated with Discontinuation of Treatment

The incidence of discontinuation due to adverse reactions was 6% for adjunctive aripiprazole-treated patients and 2% for adjunctive placebo-treated patients.

Commonly Observed Adverse Reactions

The commonly observed adverse reactions associated with the use of adjunctive aripiprazole in patients with Major Depressive Disorder (incidence of 5% or greater and aripiprazole incidence at least twice that for placebo) were: akathisia, restlessness, insomnia, constipation, fatigue, and blurred vision.

Less Common Adverse Reactions in Adult Patients with Major Depressive Disorder

Table 9 enumerates the pooled incidence, rounded to the nearest percent, of adverse reactions that occurred during acute therapy (up to 6 weeks), including only those adverse reactions that occurred in 2% or more of patients treated with adjunctive aripiprazole (doses ≥2 mg/day) and for which the incidence in patients treated with adjunctive aripiprazole was greater than the incidence in patients treated with adjunctive placebo in the combined dataset.

Table 9: Adverse Reactions in Short-Term, Placebo-Controlled Adjunctive Trials in Patients with Major Depressive Disorder

System Organ Class Preferred Term	Percentage of Patients Reporting Reaction[a]	
	Aripiprazole +ADT* (n=371)	Placebo +ADT* (n=366)
Eye Disorders		
Blurred Vision	6	1
Gastrointestinal Disorders		
Constipation	5	2
General Disorders and Administration Site Conditions		
Fatigue	8	4
Feeling Jittery	3	1
Infections and Infestations		
Upper Respiratory Tract Infection	6	4
Investigations		
Weight Increased	3	2
Metabolism and Nutrition Disorders		
Increased Appetite	3	2
Musculoskeletal and Connective Tissue Disorders		
Arthralgia	4	3
Myalgia	3	1
Nervous System Disorders		
Akathisia	25	4
Somnolence	6	4
Tremor	5	4
Sedation	4	2
Dizziness	4	2
Disturbance in Attention	3	1
Extrapyramidal Disorder	2	0
Psychiatric Disorders		
Restlessness	12	2
Insomnia	8	2

[a] Adverse reactions reported by at least 2% of patients treated with adjunctive aripiprazole, except adverse reactions which had an incidence equal to or less than placebo.
* Antidepressant Therapy

Patients with Agitation Associated with Schizophrenia or Bipolar Mania (Intramuscular Injection)

The following findings are based on a pool of three placebo-controlled trials of patients with agitation associated with Schizophrenia or Bipolar Mania in which aripiprazole injection was administered at doses of 5.25 mg to 15 mg.

Adverse Reactions Associated with Discontinuation of Treatment

Overall, in patients with agitation associated with Schizophrenia or Bipolar Mania, there was little difference in the incidence of discontinuation due to adverse reactions between aripiprazole-treated (0.8%) and placebo-treated (0.5%) patients.

Commonly Observed Adverse Reactions

There was one commonly observed adverse reaction (nausea) associated with the use of aripiprazole injection in patients with agitation associated with Schizophrenia and Bipolar Mania (incidence of 5% or greater and aripiprazole incidence at least twice that for placebo).

Less Common Adverse Reactions in Patients with Agitation Associated with Schizophrenia or Bipolar Mania

Table 10 enumerates the pooled incidence, rounded to the nearest percent, of adverse reactions that occurred during

acute therapy (24-hour), including only those adverse reactions that occurred in 2% or more of patients treated with aripiprazole injection (doses ≥5.25 mg/day) and for which the incidence in patients treated with aripiprazole injection was greater than the incidence in patients treated with placebo in the combined dataset.

Table 10: Adverse Reactions in Short-Term, Placebo-Controlled Trials in Patients Treated with ABILIFY Injection

System Organ Class Preferred Term	Percentage of Patients Reporting Reaction[a]	
	Aripiprazole (n=501)	Placebo (n=220)
Cardiac Disorders		
Tachycardia	2	<1
Gastrointestinal Disorders		
Nausea	9	3
Vomiting	3	1
General Disorders and Administration Site Conditions		
Fatigue	2	1
Nervous System Disorders		
Headache	12	7
Dizziness	8	5
Somnolence	7	4
Sedation	3	2
Akathisia	2	0

[a] Adverse reactions reported by at least 2% of patients treated with aripiprazole injection, except adverse reactions which had an incidence equal to or less than placebo.

Dose-Related Adverse Reactions
Schizophrenia

Dose response relationships for the incidence of treatment-emergent adverse events were evaluated from four trials in adult patients with Schizophrenia comparing various fixed doses (2 mg/day, 5 mg/day, 10 mg/day, 15 mg/day, 20 mg/day, and 30 mg/day) of oral aripiprazole to placebo. This analysis, stratified by study, indicated that the only adverse reaction to have a possible dose response relationship, and then most prominent only with 30 mg, was somnolence [including sedation]; (incidences were placebo, 7.1%; 10 mg, 8.5%; 15 mg, 8.7%; 20 mg, 7.5%; 30 mg, 12.6%).

In the study of pediatric patients (13 to 17 years of age) with Schizophrenia, three common adverse reactions appeared to have a possible dose response relationship: extrapyramidal disorder (incidences were placebo, 5.0%; 10 mg, 13.0%; 30 mg, 21.6%); somnolence (incidences were placebo, 6.0%; 10 mg, 11.0%; 30 mg, 21.6%); and tremor (incidences were placebo, 2.0%; 10 mg, 2.0%; 30 mg, 11.8%).

Bipolar Mania

In the study of pediatric patients (10 to 17 years of age) with Bipolar Mania, four common adverse reactions had a possible dose response relationship at 4 weeks: extrapyramidal disorder (incidences were placebo, 3.1%; 10 mg, 12.2%; 30 mg, 27.3%); somnolence (incidences were placebo, 3.1%; 10 mg, 19.4%; 30 mg, 26.3%); akathisia (incidences were placebo, 2.1%; 10 mg, 8.2%; 30 mg, 11.1%); and salivary hypersecretion (incidences were placebo, 0%; 10 mg, 3.1%; 30 mg, 8.1%).

Extrapyramidal Symptoms

In short-term, placebo-controlled trials in Schizophrenia in adults, the incidence of reported EPS-related events, excluding events related to akathisia, for aripiprazole-treated patients was 13% vs. 12% for placebo; and the incidence of akathisia-related events for aripiprazole-treated patients was 8% vs. 4% for placebo. In the short-term, placebo-controlled trial of Schizophrenia in pediatric (13 to 17 years) patients, the incidence of reported EPS-related events, excluding events related to akathisia, for aripiprazole-treated patients was 25% vs. 7% for placebo; and the incidence of akathisia-related events for aripiprazole-treated patients was 9% vs. 6% for placebo. In the short-term, placebo-controlled trials in Bipolar Mania in adults, the incidence of reported EPS-related events, excluding events related to akathisia, for aripiprazole-treated patients was 15% vs. 8% for placebo and the incidence of akathisia-related events for aripiprazole-treated patients was 15% vs. 4% for placebo. In the short-term, placebo-controlled trial in Bipolar Mania in pediatric (10 to 17 years) patients, the incidence of reported EPS-related events, excluding events related to akathisia, for aripiprazole-treated patients was 26% vs. 5% for placebo and the incidence of akathisia-related events for aripiprazole-treated patients was 10% vs. 2% for placebo. In the short-term, placebo-controlled trials in Major Depressive Disorder, the incidence of reported EPS-related events, excluding events related to akathisia, for adjunctive aripiprazole-treated patients was 8% vs. 5% for adjunctive placebo-treated patients; and the incidence of akathisia-related events for adjunctive aripiprazole-treated patients was 25% vs. 4% for adjunctive placebo-treated patients.

Objectively collected data from those trials was collected on the Simpson Angus Rating Scale (for EPS), the Barnes Akathisia Scale (for akathisia), and the Assessments of Involuntary Movement Scales (for dyskinesias). In the adult Schizophrenia trials, the objectively collected data did not show a difference between aripiprazole and placebo, with the exception of the Barnes Akathisia Scale (aripiprazole, 0.08; placebo, -0.05). In the pediatric (13 to 17 years) Schizophrenia trial, the objectively collected data did not show a difference between aripiprazole and placebo,

with the exception of the Simpson Angus Rating Scale (aripiprazole, 0.24; placebo, -0.29). In the adult Bipolar Mania trials, the Simpson Angus Rating Scale and the Barnes Akathisia Scale showed a significant difference between aripiprazole and placebo (aripiprazole, 0.61; placebo, 0.03 and aripiprazole, 0.25; placebo, -0.06). Changes in the Assessments of Involuntary Movement Scales were similar for the aripiprazole and placebo groups. In the pediatric (10 to 17 years) short-term Bipolar Mania trial, the Simpson Angus Rating Scale showed a significant difference between aripiprazole and placebo (aripiprazole, 0.90; placebo, -0.05). Changes in the Barnes Akathisia Scale and the Assessments of Involuntary Movement Scales were similar for the aripiprazole and placebo groups. In the Major Depressive Disorder trials, the Simpson Angus Rating Scale and the Barnes Akathisia Scale showed a significant difference between adjunctive aripiprazole and adjunctive placebo (aripiprazole, 0.31; placebo, 0.03 and aripiprazole, 0.22; placebo, 0.02). Changes in the Assessments of Involuntary Movement Scales were similar for the adjunctive aripiprazole and adjunctive placebo groups.

Similarly, in a long-term (26-week), placebo-controlled trial of Schizophrenia in adults, objectively collected data on the Simpson Angus Rating Scale (for EPS), the Barnes Akathisia Scale (for akathisia), and the Assessments of Involuntary Movement Scales (for dyskinesias) did not show a difference between aripiprazole and placebo.

In the placebo-controlled trials in patients with agitation associated with Schizophrenia or Bipolar Mania, the incidence of reported EPS-related events excluding events related to akathisia for aripiprazole-treated patients was 2% vs. 2% for placebo and the incidence of akathisia-related events for aripiprazole-treated patients was 2% vs. 0% for placebo. Objectively collected data on the Simpson Angus Rating Scale (for EPS) and the Barnes Akathisia Scale (for akathisia) for all treatment groups did not show a difference between aripiprazole and placebo.

Dystonia

Class Effect: Symptoms of dystonia, prolonged abnormal contractions of muscle groups, may occur in susceptible individuals during the first few days of treatment. Dystonic symptoms include: spasm of the neck muscles, sometimes progressing to tightness of the throat, swallowing difficulty, difficulty breathing, and/or protrusion of the tongue. While these symptoms can occur at low doses, they occur more frequently and with greater severity with high potency and at higher doses of first generation antipsychotic drugs. An elevated risk of acute dystonia is observed in males and younger age groups.

Laboratory Test Abnormalities

A between group comparison for 3-week to 6-week, placebo-controlled trials in adults or 4-week to 6-week, placebo-controlled trials in pediatric patients (10 to 17 years) revealed no medically important differences between the aripiprazole and placebo groups in the proportions of patients experiencing potentially clinically significant changes in routine serum chemistry, hematology, or urinalysis parameters. Similarly, there were no aripiprazole/placebo differences in the incidence of discontinuations for changes in serum chemistry, hematology, or urinalysis in adult or pediatric patients.

In the 6-week trials of aripiprazole as adjunctive therapy for Major Depressive Disorder, there were no clinically important differences between the adjunctive aripiprazole-treated and adjunctive placebo-treated patients in the median change from baseline in prolactin, fasting glucose, HDL, LDL, or total cholesterol measurements. The median % change from baseline in triglycerides was 5% for adjunctive aripiprazole-treated patients vs. 0% for adjunctive placebo-treated patients.

In a long-term (26-week), placebo-controlled trial there were no medically important differences between the aripiprazole and placebo patients in the mean change from baseline in prolactin, fasting glucose, triglyceride, HDL, LDL, or total cholesterol measurements.

Weight Gain

In 4-week to 6-week trials in adults with Schizophrenia, there was a slight difference in mean weight gain between aripiprazole and placebo patients (+0.7 kg vs. -0.05 kg, respectively) and also a difference in the proportion of patients meeting a weight gain criterion of ≥7% of body weight [aripiprazole (8%) compared to placebo (3%)]. In a 6-week trial in pediatric patients (13 to 17 years) with Schizophrenia, there was a slight difference in mean weight gain between aripiprazole and placebo patients (+0.13 kg vs. -0.83 kg, respectively) and also a difference in the proportion of patients meeting a weight gain criterion of ≥7% of body weight [aripiprazole (5%) compared to placebo (1%)]. In 3-week trials in adults with Mania, the mean weight gain for aripiprazole and placebo patients was 0.0 kg vs. -0.2 kg, respectively. The proportion of patients meeting a weight gain criterion of ≥7% of body weight was aripiprazole (3%) compared to placebo (2%).

In the trials adding aripiprazole to antidepressants, patients first received 8 weeks of antidepressant treatment followed by 6 weeks of adjunctive aripiprazole or placebo in addition to their ongoing antidepressant treatment. The

Continued on next page

Product information on these pages reflects product labeling on June 1, 2007. Current information on products of Bristol-Myers Squibb may be obtained at 1-800-321-1335 or www.bms.com.
NOUS08AB00403

Table 11: Weight Change Results Categorized by BMI at Baseline: Placebo-Controlled Study in Schizophrenia, Safety Sample

	BMI <23		BMI 23-27		BMI >27	
	Placebo (n=54)	Aripiprazole (n=59)	Placebo (n=48)	Aripiprazole (n=39)	Placebo (n=49)	Aripiprazole (n=53)
Mean change from baseline (kg)	-0.5	-0.5	-0.6	-1.3	-1.5	-2.1
% with ≥7% increase BW	3.7%	6.8%	4.2%	5.1%	4.1%	5.7%

Abilify—Cont.

mean weight gain with adjunctive aripiprazole was 1.7 kg vs. 0.4 kg with adjunctive placebo. The proportion of patients meeting a weight gain criterion of ≥7% of body weight was 5% with adjunctive aripiprazole compared to 1% with adjunctive placebo.

Table 11 provides the weight change results from a long-term (26-week), placebo-controlled study of aripiprazole, both mean change from baseline and proportions of patients meeting a weight gain criterion of ≥7% of body weight relative to baseline, categorized by BMI at baseline. Although there was no mean weight increase, the aripiprazole group tended to show more patients with a ≥7% weight gain.

[See table 11 above]

Table 12 provides the weight change results from a long-term (52-week) study of aripiprazole, both mean change from baseline and proportions of patients meeting a weight gain criterion of ≥7% of body weight relative to baseline, categorized by BMI at baseline:

Table 12: Weight Change Results Categorized by BMI at Baseline: Active-Controlled Study in Schizophrenia, Safety Sample

	BMI <23 (n=314)	BMI 23-27 (n=265)	BMI >27 (n=260)
Mean change from baseline (kg)	2.6	1.4	-1.2
% with ≥7% increase BW	30%	19%	8%

ECG Changes

Between group comparisons for a pooled analysis of placebo-controlled trials in patients with Schizophrenia, Bipolar Mania, or Major Depressive Disorder revealed no significant differences between oral aripiprazole and placebo in the proportion of patients experiencing potentially important changes in ECG parameters. Aripiprazole was associated with a median increase in heart rate of 3 beats per minute compared to no increase among placebo patients.

In the pooled, placebo-controlled trials in patients with agitation associated with Schizophrenia or Bipolar Mania, there were no significant differences between aripiprazole injection and placebo in the proportion of patients experiencing potentially important changes in ECG parameters, as measured by standard 12-lead ECGs.

Additional Findings Observed in Clinical Trials

Adverse Reactions in Long-Term, Double-Blind, Placebo-Controlled Trials

The adverse reactions reported in a 26-week, double-blind trial comparing oral ABILIFY (aripiprazole) and placebo in patients with Schizophrenia were generally consistent with those reported in the short-term, placebo-controlled trials, except for a higher incidence of tremor [8% (12/153) for ABILIFY vs. 2% (3/153) for placebo]. In this study, the majority of the cases of tremor were of mild intensity (8/12 mild and 4/12 moderate), occurred early in therapy (9/12 ≤49 days), and were of limited duration (7/12 ≤10 days). Tremor infrequently led to discontinuation (<1%) of ABILIFY. In addition, in a long-term (52-week), active-controlled study, the incidence of tremor was 5% (40/859) for ABILIFY. A similar profile was observed in a long-term study in Bipolar Disorder.

Other Adverse Reactions Observed During the Premarketing Evaluation of Aripiprazole

Following is a list of MedDRA terms that reflect adverse reactions as defined in *ADVERSE REACTIONS (6.1)* reported by patients treated with oral aripiprazole at multiple doses ≥2 mg/day during any phase of a trial within the database of 12,925 adult patients. All events assessed as possible adverse drug reactions have been included with the exception of more commonly occurring events. In addition, medically/clinically meaningful adverse reactions, particularly those that are likely to be useful to the prescriber or that have pharmacologic plausibility, have been included. Events already listed in other parts of *ADVERSE REACTIONS (6)*, or those considered in *WARNINGS AND PRECAUTIONS (5)* or *OVERDOSAGE (10)* have been excluded. Although the reactions reported occurred during treatment with aripiprazole, they were not necessarily caused by it.

Events are further categorized by MedDRA system organ class and listed in order of decreasing frequency according to the following definitions: those occurring in at least 1/100 patients (only those not already listed in the tabulated results from placebo-controlled trials appear in this listing); those occurring in 1/100 to 1/1000 patients; and those occurring in fewer than 1/1000 patients.

Adults - Oral Administration

Blood and Lymphatic System Disorders:
≥1/1000 patients and <1/100 patients - leukopenia, neutropenia; *<1/1000 patients* - thrombocytopenia, agranulocytosis, idiopathic thrombocytopenic purpura

Cardiac Disorders:
≥1/1000 patients and <1/100 patients - cardiopulmonary failure, bradycardia, cardio-respiratory arrest, atrioventricular block, atrial fibrillation, angina pectoris, bundle branch block; *<1/1000 patients* - atrial flutter, ventricular tachycardia, complete atrioventricular block, supraventricular tachycardia

Eye Disorders:
≥1/1000 patients and <1/100 patients - eyelid edema, photophobia, diplopia, photopsia; *<1/1000 patients* - excessive blinking

Gastrointestinal Disorders:
≥1/1000 patients and <1/100 patients - dysphagia, gastroesophageal reflux disease, gastrointestinal hemorrhage, swollen tongue, ulcer, esophagitis, angioedema; *<1/1000 patients* - pancreatitis

General Disorders and Administration Site Conditions:
≥1/100 patients - asthenia; *≥1/1000 patients and <1/100 patients* - mobility decreased, face edema; *<1/1000 patients* - hypothermia

Hepatobiliary Disorders:
≥1/1000 patients and <1/100 patients - cholecystitis, cholelithiasis; *<1/1000 patients* - hepatitis, jaundice

Injury, Poisoning, and Procedural Complications:
≥1/100 patients - fall; *≥1/1000 patients and <1/100 patients* - self mutilation; *<1/1000 patients* - heat stroke

Investigations:
≥1/100 patients - creatine phosphokinase increased; *≥1/1000 patients and <1/100 patients* - hepatic enzyme increased, blood urea increased, blood bilirubin increased, blood creatinine increased, electrocardiogram QT corrected interval prolonged, blood prolactin increased; *<1/1000 patients* - blood lactate dehydrogenase increased, glycosylated hemoglobin increased, GGT increased

Metabolism and Nutrition Disorders:
≥1/1000 patients and <1/100 patients - anorexia, hyperlipidemia

Musculoskeletal and Connective Tissue Disorders:
≥1/100 patients - muscle spasms; *≥1/1000 patients and <1/100 patients* - muscle rigidity; *<1/1000 patients* - rhabdomyolysis

Nervous System Disorders:
≥1/100 patients - coordination abnormal; *≥1/1000 patients and <1/100 patients* - speech disorder, parkinsonism, cogwheel rigidity, memory impairment, cerebrovascular accident, hypokinesia, tardive dyskinesia, hypotonia, hypertonia, akinesia, myoclonus, bradykinesia; *<1/1000 patients* - Grand Mal convulsion, choreoathetosis

Psychiatric Disorders:
≥1/100 patients - agitation, irritability, suicidal ideation; *≥1/1000 patients and <1/100 patients* - aggression, loss of libido, libido decreased, hostility, suicide attempt, libido increased, anger, anorgasmia, delirium, intentional self injury, completed suicide, tic, homicidal ideation; *<1/1000 patients* - psychomotor agitation, premature ejaculation, catatonia, sleep walking

Renal and Urinary Disorders:
≥1/1000 patients and <1/100 patients - urinary retention, polyuria, nocturia

Reproductive System and Breast Disorders:
≥1/1000 patients and <1/100 patients - erectile dysfunction, amenorrhea, menstruation irregular, breast pain; *<1/1000 patients* - gynaecomastia, priapism, galactorrhea

Respiratory, Thoracic, and Mediastinal Disorders:
≥1/100 patients - dyspnea; *≥1/1000 patients and <1/100 patients* - pneumonia aspiration, respiratory distress; *<1/1000 patients* - pulmonary embolism, asphyxia

Skin and Subcutaneous Tissue Disorders:
≥1/100 patients - hyperhydrosis; *≥1/1000 patients and <1/100 patients* - erythema, pruritus, ecchymosis, face edema, photosensitivity reaction, alopecia, urticaria

Vascular Disorders:
≥1/1000 patients and <1/100 patients - hypotension, deep vein thrombosis, phlebitis; *<1/1000 patients* - shock, thrombophlebitis

Pediatric Patients - Oral Administration

Most adverse events observed in the pooled database of 514 pediatric patients aged 10 to 17 years were also observed in the adult population. Additional adverse reactions observed in the pediatric population are listed below.

Gastrointestinal Disorders:
≥1/1000 patients and <1/100 patients - tongue dry, tongue spasm

Investigations:
≥1/100 patients - blood insulin increased

Nervous System Disorders:
≥1/1000 patients and <1/100 patients - sleep talking

Skin and Subcutaneous Tissue Disorders:
≥1/1000 patients and <1/100 patients - hirsutism

Adults - Intramuscular Injection

All adverse reactions observed in the pooled database of 749 adult patients treated with aripiprazole injection, were also observed in the adult population treated with oral aripiprazole. Additional adverse reactions observed in the aripiprazole injection population are listed below.

General Disorders and Administration Site Conditions:
≥1/100 patients - injection site reaction; *≥1/1000 patients and <1/100 patients* - venipuncture site bruise

6.3 Postmarketing Experience

The following adverse reactions have been identified during postapproval use of ABILIFY (aripiprazole). Because these reactions are reported voluntarily from a population of uncertain size, it is not always possible to establish a causal relationship to drug exposure: rare occurrences of allergic reaction (anaphylactic reaction, angioedema, laryngospasm, pruritus/urticaria, or oropharyngeal spasm), and blood glucose fluctuation.

7 DRUG INTERACTIONS

Given the primary CNS effects of aripiprazole, caution should be used when ABILIFY is taken in combination with other centrally-acting drugs or alcohol.

Due to its alpha adrenergic antagonism, aripiprazole has the potential to enhance the effect of certain antihypertensive agents.

7.1 Potential for Other Drugs to Affect ABILIFY

Aripiprazole is not a substrate of CYP1A1, CYP1A2, CYP2A6, CYP2B6, CYP2C8, CYP2C9, CYP2C19, or CYP2E1 enzymes. Aripiprazole also does not undergo direct glucuronidation. This suggests that an interaction of aripiprazole with inhibitors or inducers of these enzymes, or other factors, like smoking, is unlikely.

Both CYP3A4 and CYP2D6 are responsible for aripiprazole metabolism. Agents that induce CYP3A4 (eg, carbamazepine) could cause an increase in aripiprazole clearance and lower blood levels. Inhibitors of CYP3A4 (eg, ketoconazole) or CYP2D6 (eg, quinidine, fluoxetine, or paroxetine) can inhibit aripiprazole elimination and cause increased blood levels.

Ketoconazole and Other CYP3A4 Inhibitors

Coadministration of ketoconazole (200 mg/day for 14 days) with a 15 mg single dose of aripiprazole increased the AUC of aripiprazole and its active metabolite by 63% and 77%, respectively. The effect of a higher ketoconazole dose (400 mg/day) has not been studied. When ketoconazole is given concomitantly with aripiprazole, the aripiprazole dose should be reduced to one-half of its normal dose. Other strong inhibitors of CYP3A4 (itraconazole) would be expected to have similar effects and need similar dose reductions; moderate inhibitors (erythromycin, grapefruit juice) have not been studied. When the CYP3A4 inhibitor is withdrawn from the combination therapy, the aripiprazole dose should be increased.

Quinidine and Other CYP2D6 Inhibitors

Coadministration of a 10 mg single dose of aripiprazole with quinidine (166 mg/day for 13 days), a potent inhibitor of CYP2D6, increased the AUC of aripiprazole by 112% but decreased the AUC of its active metabolite, dehydro-aripiprazole, by 35%. Aripiprazole dose should be reduced to one-half of its normal dose when quinidine is given concomitantly with aripiprazole. Other significant inhibitors of CYP2D6, such as fluoxetine or paroxetine, would be expected to have similar effects and should lead to similar dose reductions. When the CYP2D6 inhibitor is withdrawn from the combination therapy, the aripiprazole dose should be increased. When adjunctive ABILIFY is administered to patients with Major Depressive Disorder, ABILIFY should be administered without dosage adjustment as specified in *DOSAGE AND ADMINISTRATION (2.3)*.

Carbamazepine and Other CYP3A4 Inducers

Coadministration of carbamazepine (200 mg twice daily), a potent CYP3A4 inducer, with aripiprazole (30 mg/day) resulted in an approximate 70% decrease in C_{max} and AUC values of both aripiprazole and its active metabolite, dehydro-aripiprazole. When carbamazepine is added to aripiprazole therapy, aripiprazole dose should be doubled. Additional dose increases should be based on clinical evaluation. When carbamazepine is withdrawn from the combination therapy, the aripiprazole dose should be reduced.

7.2 Potential for ABILIFY to Affect Other Drugs

Aripiprazole is unlikely to cause clinically important pharmacokinetic interactions with drugs metabolized by cytochrome P450 enzymes. In *in vivo* studies, 10 mg/day to 30 mg/day doses of aripiprazole had no significant effect on metabolism by CYP2D6 (dextromethorphan), CYP2C9 (warfarin), CYP2C19 (omeprazole, warfarin), and CYP3A4 (dextromethorphan) substrates. Additionally, aripiprazole and dehydro-aripiprazole did not show potential for altering CYP1A2-mediated metabolism *in vitro*.

Alcohol

There was no significant difference between aripiprazole coadministered with ethanol and placebo coadministered with ethanol on performance of gross motor skills or stimulus response in healthy subjects. As with most psychoactive medications, patients should be advised to avoid alcohol while taking ABILIFY.

7.3 Drugs Having No Clinically Important Interactions with ABILIFY

Famotidine

Coadministration of aripiprazole (given in a single dose of 15 mg) with a 40 mg single dose of the H_2 antagonist famotidine, a potent gastric acid blocker, decreased the solubility of aripiprazole and, hence, its rate of absorption, reducing by 37% and 21% the C_{max} of aripiprazole and dehydro-aripiprazole, respectively, and by 13% and 15%, respectively, the extent of absorption (AUC). No dosage adjustment of aripiprazole is required when administered concomitantly with famotidine.

Valproate

When valproate (500 mg/day-1500 mg/day) and aripiprazole (30 mg/day) were coadministered, at steady-state the C_{max} and AUC of aripiprazole were decreased by 25%. No dosage adjustment of aripiprazole is required when administered concomitantly with valproate.

When aripiprazole (30 mg/day) and valproate (1000 mg/day) were coadministered, at steady-state there were no clinically significant changes in the C_{max} or AUC of valproate. No dosage adjustment of valproate is required when administered concomitantly with aripiprazole.

Lithium

A pharmacokinetic interaction of aripiprazole with lithium is unlikely because lithium is not bound to plasma proteins, is not metabolized, and is almost entirely excreted unchanged in urine. Coadministration of therapeutic doses of lithium (1200 mg/day-1800 mg/day) for 21 days with aripiprazole (30 mg/day) did not result in clinically significant changes in the pharmacokinetics of aripiprazole or its active metabolite, dehydro-aripiprazole (C_{max} and AUC increased by less than 20%). No dosage adjustment of aripiprazole is required when administered concomitantly with lithium.

Coadministration of aripiprazole (30 mg/day) with lithium (900 mg/day) did not result in clinically significant changes in the pharmacokinetics of lithium. No dosage adjustment of lithium is required when administered concomitantly with aripiprazole.

Dextromethorphan

Aripiprazole at doses of 10 mg/day to 30 mg/day for 14 days had no effect on dextromethorphan's O-dealkylation to its major metabolite, dextrorphan, a pathway dependent on CYP2D6 activity. Aripiprazole also had no effect on dextromethorphan's N-demethylation to its metabolite 3-methoxymorphinan, a pathway dependent on CYP3A4 activity. No dosage adjustment of dextromethorphan is required when administered concomitantly with aripiprazole.

Warfarin

Aripiprazole 10 mg/day for 14 days had no effect on the pharmacokinetics of R-warfarin and S-warfarin or on the pharmacodynamic end point of International Normalized Ratio, indicating the lack of a clinically relevant effect of aripiprazole on CYP2C9 and CYP2C19 metabolism or the binding of highly protein-bound warfarin. No dosage adjustment of warfarin is required when administered concomitantly with aripiprazole.

Omeprazole

Aripiprazole 10 mg/day for 15 days had no effect on the pharmacokinetics of a single 20 mg dose of omeprazole, a CYP2C19 substrate, in healthy subjects. No dosage adjustment of omeprazole is required when administered concomitantly with aripiprazole.

Lorazepam

Coadministration of lorazepam injection (2 mg) and aripiprazole injection (15 mg) to healthy subjects (n=40: 35 males and 5 females; ages 19-45 years old) did not result in clinically important changes in the pharmacokinetics of either drug. No dosage adjustment of aripiprazole is required when administered concomitantly with lorazepam. However, the intensity of sedation was greater with the combination as compared to that observed with aripiprazole alone and the orthostatic hypotension observed was greater with the combination as compared to that observed with lorazepam alone [see WARNINGS AND PRECAUTIONS (5.6)].

Escitalopram

Coadministration of 10 mg/day oral doses of aripiprazole for 14 days to healthy subjects had no effect on the steady-state pharmacokinetics of 10 mg/day escitalopram, a substrate of CYP2C19 and CYP3A4. No dosage adjustment of escitalopram is required when aripiprazole is added to escitalopram.

Venlafaxine

Coadministration of 10 mg/day to 20 mg/day oral doses of aripiprazole for 14 days to healthy subjects had no effect on the steady-state pharmacokinetics of venlafaxine and O-desmethylvenlafaxine following 75 mg/day venlafaxine XR, a CYP2D6 substrate. No dosage adjustment of venlafaxine is required when aripiprazole is added to venlafaxine.

Fluoxetine, Paroxetine, and Sertraline

A population pharmacokinetic analysis in patients with Major Depressive Disorder showed no substantial change in plasma concentrations of fluoxetine (20 mg/day or 40 mg/day), paroxetine CR (37.5 mg/day or 50 mg/day), or sertraline (100 mg/day or 150 mg/day) dosed to steady-state. The steady-state plasma concentrations of fluoxetine and norfluoxetine increased by about 18% and 36%, respectively, and concentrations of paroxetine decreased by about 27%. The steady-state plasma concentrations of sertraline and desmethylsertraline were not substantially changed when these antidepressant therapies were coadministered with

aripiprazole. Aripiprazole dosing was 2 mg/day to 15 mg/day (when given with fluoxetine or paroxetine) or 2 mg/day to 20 mg/day (when given with sertraline).

8 USE IN SPECIFIC POPULATIONS

In general, no dosage adjustment for ABILIFY is required on the basis of a patient's age, gender, race, smoking status, hepatic function, or renal function [see DOSAGE AND ADMINISTRATION (2.5)].

8.1 Pregnancy

Pregnancy Category C: In animal studies, aripiprazole demonstrated developmental toxicity, including possible teratogenic effects in rats and rabbits.

Pregnant rats were treated with oral doses of 3 mg/kg/day, 10 mg/kg/day, and 30 mg/kg/day (1 times, 3 times, and 10 times the maximum recommended human dose [MRHD] on a mg/m^2 basis) of aripiprazole during the period of organogenesis. Gestation was slightly prolonged at 30 mg/kg. Treatment caused a slight delay in fetal development, as evidenced by decreased fetal weight (30 mg/kg), undescended testes (30 mg/kg), and delayed skeletal ossification (10 mg/kg and 30 mg/kg). There were no adverse effects on embryofetal or pup survival. Delivered offspring had decreased bodyweights (10 mg/kg and 30 mg/kg), and increased incidences of hepatodiaphragmatic nodules and diaphragmatic hernia at 30 mg/kg (the other dose groups were not examined for these findings). A low incidence of diaphragmatic hernia was also seen in the fetuses exposed to 30 mg/kg. Postnatally, delayed vaginal opening was seen at 10 mg/kg and 30 mg/kg and impaired reproductive performance (decreased fertility rate, corpora lutea, implants, live fetuses, and increased post-implantation loss, likely mediated through effects on female offspring) was seen at 30 mg/kg. Some maternal toxicity was seen at 30 mg/kg; however, there was no evidence to suggest that these developmental effects were secondary to maternal toxicity.

In pregnant rats receiving aripiprazole injection intravenously (3 mg/kg/day, 9 mg/kg/day, and 27 mg/kg/day) during the period of organogenesis, decreased fetal weight and delayed skeletal ossification were seen at the highest dose, which also caused some maternal toxicity.

Pregnant rabbits were treated with oral doses of 10 mg/kg/day, 30 mg/kg/day, and 100 mg/kg/day (2 times, 3 times, and 11 times human exposure at MRHD based on AUC and 6 times, 19 times, and 65 times the MRHD based on mg/m^2) of aripiprazole during the period of organogenesis. Decreased maternal food consumption and increased abortions were seen at 100 mg/kg. Treatment caused increased fetal mortality (100 mg/kg), decreased fetal weight (30 mg/kg and 100 mg/kg), increased incidence of a skeletal abnormality (fused sternebrae at 30 mg/kg and 100 mg/kg), and minor skeletal variations (100 mg/kg).

In pregnant rabbits receiving aripiprazole injection intravenously (3 mg/kg/day, 10 mg/kg/day, and 30 mg/kg/day) during the period of organogenesis, the highest dose, which caused pronounced maternal toxicity, resulted in decreased fetal weight, increased fetal abnormalities (primarily skeletal), and decreased fetal skeletal ossification. The fetal no-effect dose was 10 mg/kg, which produced 5 times the human exposure at the MRHD based on AUC and is 6 times the MRHD based on mg/m^2.

In a study in which rats were treated with oral doses of 3 mg/kg/day, 10 mg/kg/day, and 30 mg/kg/day (1 times, 3 times, and 10 times the MRHD on a mg/m^2 basis) of aripiprazole perinatally and postnatally (from day 17 of gestation through day 21 postpartum), slight maternal toxicity and slightly prolonged gestation were seen at 30 mg/kg. An increase in stillbirths and decreases in pup weight (persisting into adulthood) and survival were seen at this dose.

In rats receiving aripiprazole injection intravenously (3 mg/kg/day, 8 mg/kg/day, and 20 mg/kg/day) from day 6 of gestation through day 20 postpartum, an increase in stillbirths was seen at 8 mg/kg and 20 mg/kg, and decreases in early postnatal pup weights and survival were seen at 20 mg/kg. These doses produced some maternal toxicity. There were no effects on postnatal behavioral and reproductive development.

There are no adequate and well-controlled studies in pregnant women. It is not known whether aripiprazole can cause fetal harm when administered to a pregnant woman or can affect reproductive capacity. Aripiprazole should be used during pregnancy only if the potential benefit outweighs the potential risk to the fetus.

8.2 Labor and Delivery

The effect of aripiprazole on labor and delivery in humans is unknown.

8.3 Nursing Mothers

Aripiprazole was excreted in milk of rats during lactation. It is not known whether aripiprazole or its metabolites are excreted in human milk. It is recommended that women receiving aripiprazole should not breast-feed.

8.4 Pediatric Use

Safety and effectiveness in pediatric patients with Major Depressive Disorder or agitation associated with Schizophrenia or Bipolar Mania have not been established.

Safety and effectiveness in pediatric patients with Schizophrenia were established in a 6-week, placebo-controlled clinical trial in 202 pediatric patients aged 13 to 17 years [see INDICATIONS AND USAGE (1.1), DOSAGE AND ADMINISTRATION (2.1), ADVERSE REACTIONS (6.2), and CLINICAL STUDIES (14.1)].

Safety and effectiveness in pediatric patients with Bipolar Mania were established in a 4-week, placebo-controlled clinical trial in 197 pediatric patients aged 10 to 17 years. [See

INDICATIONS AND USAGE (1.2), DOSAGE AND ADMINISTRATION (2.2), ADVERSE REACTIONS (6.2), and CLINICAL STUDIES (14.2)].

The pharmacokinetics of aripiprazole and dehydro-aripiprazole in pediatric patients 10 to 17 years of age were similar to those in adults after correcting for the differences in body weights.

8.5 Geriatric Use

In formal single-dose pharmacokinetic studies (with aripiprazole given in a single dose of 15 mg), aripiprazole clearance was 20% lower in elderly (≥65 years) subjects compared to younger adult subjects (18 to 64 years). There was no detectable age effect, however, in the population pharmacokinetic analysis in Schizophrenia patients. Also, the pharmacokinetics of aripiprazole after multiple doses in elderly patients appeared similar to that observed in young, healthy subjects. No dosage adjustment is recommended for elderly patients [see also BOXED WARNING and WARNINGS AND PRECAUTIONS (5.1)].

Of the 12,925 patients treated with oral aripiprazole in clinical trials, 1061 (8%) were ≥65 years old and 799 (6%) were ≥75 years old. The majority (97%) of the 799 patients were diagnosed with Dementia of the Alzheimer's type.

Placebo-controlled studies of oral aripiprazole in Schizophrenia, Bipolar Mania, or Major Depressive Disorder did not include sufficient numbers of subjects aged 65 and over to determine whether they respond differently from younger subjects.

Of the 749 patients treated with aripiprazole injection in clinical trials, 99 (13%) were ≥65 years old and 78 (10%) were ≥75 years old. Placebo-controlled studies of aripiprazole injection in patients with agitation associated with Schizophrenia or Bipolar Mania did not include sufficient numbers of subjects aged 65 and over to determine whether they respond differently from younger subjects.

Studies of elderly patients with psychosis associated with Alzheimer's disease have suggested that there may be a different tolerability profile in this population compared to younger patients with Schizophrenia [see also BOXED WARNING and WARNINGS AND PRECAUTIONS (5.1)]. The safety and efficacy of ABILIFY in the treatment of patients with psychosis associated with Alzheimer's disease has not been established. If the prescriber elects to treat such patients with ABILIFY (aripiprazole), vigilance should be exercised.

8.6 Renal Impairment

In patients with severe renal impairment (creatinine clearance <30 mL/min), C_{max} of aripiprazole (given in a single dose of 15 mg) and dehydro-aripiprazole increased by 36% and 53%, respectively, but AUC was 15% lower for aripiprazole and 7% higher for dehydro-aripiprazole. Renal excretion of both unchanged aripiprazole and dehydro-aripiprazole is less than 1% of the dose. No dosage adjustment is required in subjects with renal impairment.

8.7 Hepatic Impairment

In a single-dose study (15 mg of aripiprazole) in subjects with varying degrees of liver cirrhosis (Child-Pugh Classes A, B, and C), the AUC of aripiprazole, compared to healthy subjects, increased 31% in mild HI, increased 8% in moderate HI, and decreased 20% in severe HI. None of these differences would require dose adjustment.

8.8 Gender

C_{max} and AUC of aripiprazole and its active metabolite, dehydro-aripiprazole, are 30% to 40% higher in women than in men, and correspondingly, the apparent oral clearance of aripiprazole is lower in women. These differences, however, are largely explained by differences in body weight (25%) between men and women. No dosage adjustment is recommended based on gender.

8.9 Race

Although no specific pharmacokinetic study was conducted to investigate the effects of race on the disposition of aripiprazole, population pharmacokinetic evaluation revealed no evidence of clinically significant race-related differences in the pharmacokinetics of aripiprazole. No dosage adjustment is recommended based on race.

8.10 Smoking

Based on studies utilizing human liver enzymes *in vitro*, aripiprazole is not a substrate for CYP1A2 and also does not undergo direct glucuronidation. Smoking should, therefore, not have an effect on the pharmacokinetics of aripiprazole. Consistent with these *in vitro* results, population pharmacokinetic evaluation did not reveal any significant pharmacokinetic differences between smokers and nonsmokers. No dosage adjustment is recommended based on smoking status.

9 DRUG ABUSE AND DEPENDENCE

9.1 Controlled Substance

ABILIFY is not a controlled substance.

9.2 Abuse and Dependence

Aripiprazole has not been systematically studied in humans for its potential for abuse, tolerance, or physical dependence. In physical dependence studies in monkeys, withdrawal symptoms were observed upon abrupt cessation of dosing. While the clinical trials did not reveal any tendency for any drug-seeking behavior, these observations were not

Continued on next page

Product information on these pages reflects product labeling on June 1, 2007. Current information on products of Bristol-Myers Squibb may be obtained at 1-800-321-1335 or www.bms.com.

NOUS08AB00403

Abilify—Cont.

systematic and it is not possible to predict on the basis of this limited experience the extent to which a CNS-active drug will be misused, diverted, and/or abused once marketed. Consequently, patients should be evaluated carefully for a history of drug abuse, and such patients should be observed closely for signs of ABILIFY misuse or abuse (eg, development of tolerance, increases in dose, drug-seeking behavior).

10 OVERDOSAGE

MedDRA terminology has been used to classify the adverse reactions.

10.1 Human Experience

A total of 76 cases of deliberate or accidental overdosage with oral aripiprazole have been reported worldwide. These include overdoses with oral aripiprazole alone and in combination with other substances. No fatality was reported from these cases. Of the 44 cases with known outcome, 33 cases recovered without sequelae and one case recovered with sequelae (mydriasis and feeling abnormal). The largest known case of acute ingestion with a known outcome involved 1080 mg of oral aripiprazole (36 times the maximum recommended daily dose) in a patient who fully recovered. Included in the 76 cases are 10 cases of deliberate or accidental overdosage in children (age 12 and younger) involving oral aripiprazole ingestions up to 195 mg with no fatalities.

Common adverse reactions (reported in at least 5% of all overdose cases) reported with oral aripiprazole overdosage (alone or in combination with other substances) include vomiting, somnolence, and tremor. Other clinically important signs and symptoms observed in one or more patients with aripiprazole overdoses (alone or with other substances) include acidosis, aggression, aspartate aminotransferase increased, atrial fibrillation, bradycardia, coma, confusional state, convulsion, blood creatine phosphokinase increased, depressed level of consciousness, hypertension, hypokalemia, hypotension, lethargy, loss of consciousness, QRS complex prolonged, QT prolonged, pneumonia aspiration, respiratory arrest, status epilepticus, and tachycardia.

10.2 Management of Overdosage

No specific information is available on the treatment of overdose with aripiprazole. An electrocardiogram should be obtained in case of overdosage and if QT interval prolongation is present, cardiac monitoring should be instituted. Otherwise, management of overdose should concentrate on supportive therapy, maintaining an adequate airway, oxygenation and ventilation, and management of symptoms. Close medical supervision and monitoring should continue until the patient recovers.

Charcoal: In the event of an overdose of ABILIFY (aripiprazole), an early charcoal administration may be useful in partially preventing the absorption of aripiprazole. Administration of 50 g of activated charcoal, one hour after a single 15 mg oral dose of aripiprazole, decreased the mean AUC and C_{max} of aripiprazole by 50%.

Hemodialysis: Although there is no information on the effect of hemodialysis in treating an overdose with aripiprazole, hemodialysis is unlikely to be useful in overdose management since aripiprazole is highly bound to plasma proteins.

11 DESCRIPTION

Aripiprazole is a psychotropic drug that is available as ABILIFY® (aripiprazole) tablets, ABILIFY® DISCMELT™ (aripiprazole) orally disintegrating tablets, ABILIFY® (aripiprazole) oral solution, and ABILIFY® (aripiprazole) injection, a solution for intramuscular injection. Aripiprazole is 7-[4-[4-(2,3-dichlorophenyl)-1-piperazinyl] butoxy]-3,4-dihydrocarbostyril. The empirical formula is $C_{23}H_{27}Cl_2N_3O_2$ and its molecular weight is 448.38. The chemical structure is:

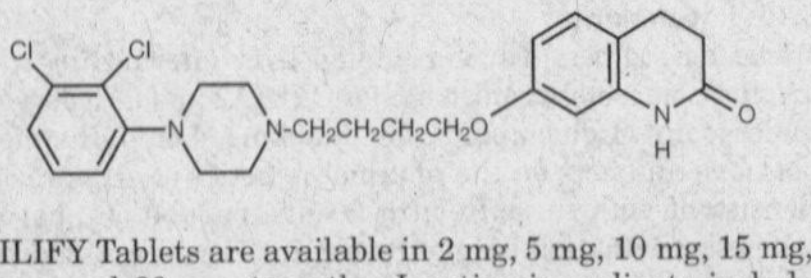

ABILIFY Tablets are available in 2 mg, 5 mg, 10 mg, 15 mg, 20 mg, and 30 mg strengths. Inactive ingredients include cornstarch, hydroxypropyl cellulose, lactose monohydrate, magnesium stearate, and microcrystalline cellulose. Colorants include ferric oxide (yellow or red) and FD&C Blue No. 2 Aluminum Lake.

ABILIFY DISCMELT Orally Disintegrating Tablets are available in 10 mg and 15 mg strengths. Inactive ingredients include acesulfame potassium, aspartame, calcium silicate, croscarmellose sodium, crospovidone, crème de vanilla (natural and artificial flavors), magnesium stearate, microcrystalline cellulose, silicon dioxide, tartaric acid, and xylitol. Colorants include ferric oxide (yellow or red) and FD&C Blue No. 2 Aluminum Lake.

ABILIFY Oral Solution is a clear, colorless to light yellow solution available in a concentration of 1 mg/mL. The inactive ingredients for this solution include disodium edetate, fructose, glycerin, dl-lactic acid, methylparaben, propylene glycol, propylparaben, sodium hydroxide, sucrose, and purified water. The oral solution is flavored with natural orange cream and other natural flavors.

ABILIFY Injection is available in single-dose vials as a ready-to-use, 9.75 mg/1.3 mL (7.5 mg/mL) clear, colorless, sterile, aqueous solution for intramuscular use only. Inactive ingredients for this solution include 150 mg/mL of sulfobutylether β-cyclodextrin (SBECD), tartaric acid, sodium hydroxide, and water for injection.

12 CLINICAL PHARMACOLOGY

12.1 Mechanism of Action

The mechanism of action of aripiprazole, as with other drugs having efficacy in Schizophrenia, Bipolar Disorder, Major Depressive Disorder, and agitation associated with Schizophrenia or Bipolar Disorder, is unknown. However, it has been proposed that the efficacy of aripiprazole is mediated through a combination of partial agonist activity at D_2 and 5-HT_{1A} receptors and antagonist activity at 5-HT_{2A} receptors. Actions at receptors other than D_2, 5-HT_{1A}, and 5-HT_{2A} may explain some of the other clinical effects of aripiprazole (eg, the orthostatic hypotension observed with aripiprazole may be explained by its antagonist activity at adrenergic $alpha_1$ receptors).

12.2 Pharmacodynamics

Aripiprazole exhibits high affinity for dopamine D_2 and D_3, serotonin 5-HT_{1A} and 5-HT_{2A} receptors (K_i values of 0.34 nM, 0.8 nM, 1.7 nM, and 3.4 nM, respectively), moderate affinity for dopamine D_4, serotonin 5-HT_{2C} and 5-HT_7, $alpha_1$-adrenergic and histamine H_1 receptors (K_i values of 44 nM, 15 nM, 39 nM, 57 nM, and 61 nM, respectively), and moderate affinity for the serotonin reuptake site (K_i=98 nM). Aripiprazole has no appreciable affinity for cholinergic muscarinic receptors (IC_{50}>1000 nM). Aripiprazole functions as a partial agonist at the dopamine D_2 and the serotonin 5-HT_{1A} receptors, and as an antagonist at serotonin 5-HT_{2A} receptor.

12.3 Pharmacokinetics

ABILIFY activity is presumably primarily due to the parent drug, aripiprazole, and to a lesser extent, to its major metabolite, dehydro-aripiprazole, which has been shown to have affinities for D_2 receptors similar to the parent drug and represents 40% of the parent drug exposure in plasma. The mean elimination half-lives are about 75 hours and 94 hours for aripiprazole and dehydro-aripiprazole, respectively. Steady-state concentrations are attained within 14 days of dosing for both active moieties. Aripiprazole accumulation is predictable from single-dose pharmacokinetics. At steady-state, the pharmacokinetics of aripiprazole are dose-proportional. Elimination of aripiprazole is mainly through hepatic metabolism involving two P450 isozymes, CYP2D6 and CYP3A4.

Pharmacokinetic studies showed that ABILIFY DISCMELT Orally Disintegrating Tablets are bioequivalent to ABILIFY Tablets.

ORAL ADMINISTRATION

Absorption

Tablet: Aripiprazole is well absorbed after administration of the tablet, with peak plasma concentrations occurring within 3 hours to 5 hours; the absolute oral bioavailability of the tablet formulation is 87%. ABILIFY (aripiprazole) can be administered with or without food. Administration of a 15 mg ABILIFY Tablet with a standard high-fat meal did not significantly affect the C_{max} or AUC of aripiprazole or its active metabolite, dehydro-aripiprazole, but delayed T_{max} by 3 hours for aripiprazole and 12 hours for dehydro-aripiprazole.

Oral Solution: Aripiprazole is well absorbed when administered orally as the solution. At equivalent doses, the plasma concentrations of aripiprazole from the solution were higher than that from the tablet formulation. In a relative bioavailability study comparing the pharmacokinetics of 30 mg aripiprazole as the oral solution to 30 mg aripiprazole tablets in healthy subjects, the solution to tablet ratios of geometric mean C_{max} and AUC values were 122% and 114%, respectively *[see DOSAGE AND ADMINISTRATION (2.6)]*. The single-dose pharmacokinetics of aripiprazole were linear and dose-proportional between the doses of 5 mg to 30 mg.

Distribution

The steady-state volume of distribution of aripiprazole following intravenous administration is high (404 L or 4.9 L/kg), indicating extensive extravascular distribution. At therapeutic concentrations, aripiprazole and its major metabolite are greater than 99% bound to serum proteins, primarily to albumin. In healthy human volunteers administered 0.5 mg/day to 30 mg/day aripiprazole for 14 days, there was dose-dependent D_2 receptor occupancy indicating brain penetration of aripiprazole in humans.

Metabolism and Elimination

Aripiprazole is metabolized primarily by three biotransformation pathways: dehydrogenation, hydroxylation, and N-dealkylation. Based on *in vitro* studies, CYP3A4 and CYP2D6 enzymes are responsible for dehydrogenation and hydroxylation of aripiprazole, and N-dealkylation is catalyzed by CYP3A4. Aripiprazole is the predominant drug moiety in the systemic circulation. At steady-state, dehydro-aripiprazole, the active metabolite, represents about 40% of aripiprazole AUC in plasma.

Approximately 8% of Caucasians lack the capacity to metabolize CYP2D6 substrates and are classified as poor metabolizers (PM), whereas the rest are extensive metabolizers (EM). PMs have about an 80% increase in aripiprazole exposure and about a 30% decrease in exposure to the active metabolite compared to EMs, resulting in about a 60% higher exposure to the total active moieties from a given dose of aripiprazole compared to EMs. Coadministration of ABILIFY with known inhibitors of CYP2D6, such as quinidine or fluoxetine in EMs, approximately doubles aripiprazole plasma exposure, and dose adjustment is needed *[see DRUG INTERACTIONS (7.1)]*. The mean elimination half-lives are about 75 hours and 146 hours for aripiprazole in EMs and PMs, respectively. Aripiprazole does not inhibit or induce the CYP2D6 pathway.

Following a single oral dose of [^{14}C]-labeled aripiprazole, approximately 25% and 55% of the administered radioactivity was recovered in the urine and feces, respectively. Less than 1% of unchanged aripiprazole was excreted in the urine and approximately 18% of the oral dose was recovered unchanged in the feces.

INTRAMUSCULAR ADMINISTRATION

In two pharmacokinetic studies of aripiprazole injection administered intramuscularly to healthy subjects, the median times to the peak plasma concentrations were at 1 hour and 3 hours. A 5 mg intramuscular injection of aripiprazole had an absolute bioavailability of 100%. The geometric mean maximum concentration achieved after an intramuscular dose was on average 19% higher than the C_{max} of the oral tablet. While the systemic exposure over 24 hours was generally similar between aripiprazole injection given intramuscularly and after oral tablet administration, the aripiprazole AUC in the first 2 hours after an intramuscular injection was 90% greater than the AUC after the same dose as a tablet. In stable patients with Schizophrenia or Schizoaffective Disorder, the pharmacokinetics of aripiprazole after intramuscular administration were linear over a dose range of 1 mg to 45 mg. Although the metabolism of aripiprazole injection was not systematically evaluated, the intramuscular route of administration would not be expected to alter the metabolic pathways.

13 NONCLINICAL TOXICOLOGY

13.1 Carcinogenesis, Mutagenesis, Impairment of Fertility

Carcinogenesis

Lifetime carcinogenicity studies were conducted in ICR mice and in Sprague-Dawley (SD) and F344 rats. Aripiprazole was administered for 2 years in the diet at doses of 1 mg/kg/day, 3 mg/kg/day, 10 mg/kg/day, and 30 mg/kg/day to ICR mice and 1 mg/kg/day, 3 mg/kg/day, and 10 mg/kg/day to F344 rats (0.2 times to 5 times and 0.3 times to 3 times the maximum recommended human dose [MRHD] based on mg/m^2, respectively). In addition, SD rats were dosed orally for 2 years at 10 mg/kg/day, 20 mg/kg/day, 40 mg/kg/day, and 60 mg/kg/day (3 times to 19 times the MRHD based on mg/m^2). Aripiprazole did not induce tumors in male mice or rats. In female mice, the incidences of pituitary gland adenomas and mammary gland adenocarcinomas and adenoacanthomas were increased at dietary doses of 3 mg/kg/day to 30 mg/kg/day (0.1 times to 0.9 times human exposure at MRHD based on AUC and 0.5 times to 5 times the MRHD based on mg/m^2). In female rats, the incidence of mammary gland fibroadenomas was increased at a dietary dose of 10 mg/kg/day (0.1 times human exposure at MRHD based on AUC and 3 times the MRHD based on mg/m^2); and the incidences of adrenocortical carcinomas and combined adrenocortical adenomas/carcinomas were increased at an oral dose of 60 mg/kg/day (14 times human exposure at MRHD based on AUC and 19 times the MRHD based on mg/m^2).

Proliferative changes in the pituitary and mammary gland of rodents have been observed following chronic administration of other antipsychotic agents and are considered prolactin-mediated. Serum prolactin was not measured in the aripiprazole carcinogenicity studies. However, increases in serum prolactin levels were observed in female mice in a 13-week dietary study at the doses associated with mammary gland and pituitary tumors. Serum prolactin was not increased in female rats in 4-week and 13-week dietary studies at the dose associated with mammary gland tumors. The relevance for human risk of the findings of prolactin-mediated endocrine tumors in rodents is unknown.

Mutagenesis

The mutagenic potential of aripiprazole was tested in the *in vitro* bacterial reverse-mutation assay, the *in vitro* bacterial DNA repair assay, the *in vitro* forward gene mutation assay in mouse lymphoma cells, the *in vitro* chromosomal aberration assay in Chinese hamster lung (CHL) cells, the *in vivo* micronucleus assay in mice, and the unscheduled DNA synthesis assay in rats. Aripiprazole and a metabolite (2,3-DCPP) were clastogenic in the *in vitro* chromosomal aberration assay in CHL cells with and without metabolic activation. The metabolite, 2,3-DCPP, produced increases in numerical aberrations in the *in vitro* assay in CHL cells in the absence of metabolic activation. A positive response was obtained in the *in vivo* micronucleus assay in mice; however, the response was due to a mechanism not considered relevant to humans.

Impairment of Fertility

Female rats were treated with oral doses of 2 mg/kg/day, 6 mg/kg/day, and 20 mg/kg/day (0.6 times, 2 times, and 6 times the maximum recommended human dose [MRHD] on a mg/m^2 basis) of aripiprazole from 2 weeks prior to mating through day 7 of gestation. Estrus cycle irregularities and increased corpora lutea were seen at all doses, but no impairment of fertility was seen. Increased pre-implantation loss was seen at 6 mg/kg and 20 mg/kg and decreased fetal weight was seen at 20 mg/kg.

Male rats were treated with oral doses of 20 mg/kg/day, 40 mg/kg/day, and 60 mg/kg/day (6 times, 13 times, and 19 times the MRHD on a mg/m^2 basis) of aripiprazole from 9 weeks prior to mating through mating. Disturbances in spermatogenesis were seen at 60 mg/kg and prostate atrophy was seen at 40 mg/kg and 60 mg/kg, but no impairment of fertility was seen.

13.2 Animal Toxicology and/or Pharmacology

Aripiprazole produced retinal degeneration in albino rats in a 26-week chronic toxicity study at a dose of 60 mg/kg and in a 2-year carcinogenicity study at doses of 40 mg/kg and 60 mg/kg. The 40 mg/kg and 60 mg/kg doses are 13 times and 19 times the maximum recommended human dose (MRHD) based on mg/m^2 and 7 times to 14 times human exposure at MRHD based on AUC. Evaluation of the retinas of albino mice and of monkeys did not reveal evidence of retinal degeneration. Additional studies to further evaluate the mechanism have not been performed. The relevance of this finding to human risk is unknown.

14 CLINICAL STUDIES

14.1 Schizophrenia

Adult

The efficacy of ABILIFY (aripiprazole) in the treatment of Schizophrenia was evaluated in five short-term (4-week and 6-week), placebo-controlled trials of acutely relapsed inpatients who predominantly met DSM-III/IV criteria for Schizophrenia. Four of the five trials were able to distinguish aripiprazole from placebo, but one study, the smallest, did not. Three of these studies also included an active control group consisting of either risperidone (one trial) or haloperidol (two trials), but they were not designed to allow for a comparison of ABILIFY and the active comparators.

In the four positive trials for ABILIFY, four primary measures were used for assessing psychiatric signs and symptoms. The Positive and Negative Syndrome Scale (PANSS) is a multi-item inventory of general psychopathology used to evaluate the effects of drug treatment in Schizophrenia. The PANSS positive subscale is a subset of items in the PANSS that rates seven positive symptoms of Schizophrenia (delusions, conceptual disorganization, hallucinatory behavior, excitement, grandiosity, suspiciousness/persecution, and hostility). The PANSS negative subscale is a subset of items in the PANSS that rates seven negative symptoms of Schizophrenia (blunted affect, emotional withdrawal, poor rapport, passive apathetic withdrawal, difficulty in abstract thinking, lack of spontaneity/flow of conversation, stereotyped thinking). The Clinical Global Impression (CGI) assessment reflects the impression of a skilled observer, fully familiar with the manifestations of Schizophrenia, about the overall clinical state of the patient.

In a 4-week trial (n=414) comparing two fixed doses of ABILIFY (15 mg/day or 30 mg/day) and haloperidol (10 mg/day) to placebo, both doses of ABILIFY were superior to placebo in the PANSS total score, PANSS positive subscale, and CGI-severity score. In addition, the 15 mg dose was superior to placebo in the PANSS negative subscale.

In a 4-week trial (n=404) comparing two fixed doses of ABILIFY (20 mg/day or 30 mg/day) and risperidone (6 mg/day) to placebo, both doses of ABILIFY were superior to placebo in the PANSS total score, PANSS positive subscale, PANSS negative subscale, and CGI-severity score.

In a 6-week trial (n=420) comparing three fixed doses of ABILIFY (10 mg/day, 15 mg/day, or 20 mg/day) to placebo, all three doses of ABILIFY were superior to placebo in the PANSS total score, PANSS positive subscale, and the PANSS negative subscale.

In a 6-week trial (n=367) comparing three fixed doses of ABILIFY (2 mg/day, 5 mg/day, or 10 mg/day) to placebo, the 10 mg dose of ABILIFY was superior to placebo in the PANSS total score, the primary outcome measure of the study. The 2 mg and 5 mg doses did not demonstrate superiority to placebo on the primary outcome measure.

In a fifth study, a 4-week trial (n=103) comparing ABILIFY in a range of 5 mg/day to 30 mg/day or haloperidol 5 mg/day to 20 mg/day to placebo, haloperidol was superior to placebo, in the Brief Psychiatric Rating Scale (BPRS), a multi-item inventory of general psychopathology traditionally used to evaluate the effects of drug treatment in psychosis, and in a responder analysis based on the CGI-severity score, the primary outcomes for that trial. ABILIFY was only significantly different compared to placebo in a responder analysis based on the CGI-severity score.

Thus, the efficacy of 10 mg, 15 mg, 20 mg, and 30 mg daily doses was established in two studies for each dose. Among these doses, there was no evidence that the higher dose groups offered any advantage over the lowest dose group of these studies.

An examination of population subgroups did not reveal any clear evidence of differential responsiveness on the basis of age, gender, or race.

A longer-term trial enrolled 310 inpatients or outpatients meeting DSM-IV criteria for Schizophrenia who were, by history, symptomatically stable on other antipsychotic medications for periods of 3 months or longer. These patients were discontinued from their antipsychotic medications and randomized to ABILIFY 15 mg/day or placebo for up to 26 weeks of observation for relapse. Relapse during the double-blind phase was defined as CGI-Improvement score of ≥5 (minimally worse), scores ≥5 (moderately severe) on the hostility or uncooperativeness items of the PANSS, or ≥20% increase in the PANSS total score. Patients receiving ABILIFY 15 mg/day experienced a significantly longer time to relapse over the subsequent 26 weeks compared to those receiving placebo.

Pediatric

The efficacy of ABILIFY (aripiprazole) in the treatment of Schizophrenia in pediatric patients (13 to 17 years of age) was evaluated in one 6-week, placebo-controlled trial of outpatients who met DSM-IV criteria for Schizophrenia and had a PANSS score ≥70 at baseline. In this trial (n=302) comparing two fixed doses of ABILIFY (aripiprazole) (10 mg/day or 30 mg/day) to placebo, ABILIFY was titrated starting from 2 mg/day to the target dose in 5 days in the 10 mg/day treatment arm and in 11 days in the 30 mg/day treatment arm. Both doses of ABILIFY were superior to placebo in the PANSS total score, the primary outcome measure of the study. The 30 mg/day dosage was not shown to be more efficacious than the 10 mg/day dose.

14.2 Bipolar Disorder

Adults

The efficacy of ABILIFY in the treatment of acute manic episodes was established in two 3-week, placebo-controlled trials in hospitalized patients who met the DSM-IV criteria for Bipolar I Disorder with manic or mixed episodes (in one trial, 21% of placebo and 42% of ABILIFY-treated patients had data beyond two weeks). These trials included patients with or without psychotic features and with or without a rapid-cycling course.

The primary instrument used for assessing manic symptoms was the Young Mania Rating Scale (Y-MRS), an 11-item clinician-rated scale traditionally used to assess the degree of manic symptomatology (irritability, disruptive/aggressive behavior, sleep, elevated mood, speech, increased activity, sexual interest, language/thought disorder, thought content, appearance, and insight) in a range from 0 (no manic features) to 60 (maximum score). A key secondary instrument included the Clinical Global Impression - Bipolar (CGI-BP) Scale.

In the two positive, 3-week, placebo-controlled trials (n=268; n=248) which evaluated ABILIFY 30 mg, once daily (with a starting dose of 30 mg/day and an allowed reduction to 15 mg/day), ABILIFY was superior to placebo in the reduction of Y-MRS total score and CGI-BP Severity of Illness score (mania).

A trial was conducted in patients meeting DSM-IV criteria for Bipolar I Disorder with a recent manic or mixed episode who had been stabilized on open-label ABILIFY and who had maintained a clinical response for at least 6 weeks. The first phase of this trial was an open-label stabilization period in which inpatients and outpatients were clinically stabilized and then maintained on open-label ABILIFY (15 mg/day or 30 mg/day, with a starting dose of 30 mg/day) for at least 6 consecutive weeks. One hundred sixty-one outpatients were then randomized in a double-blind fashion, to either the same dose of ABILIFY they were on at the end of the stabilization and maintenance period or placebo and were then monitored for manic or depressive relapse. During the randomization phase, ABILIFY was superior to placebo on time to the number of combined affective relapses (manic plus depressive), the primary outcome measure for this study. The majority of these relapses were due to manic rather than depressive symptoms. There is insufficient data to know whether ABILIFY is effective in delaying the time to occurrence of depression in patients with Bipolar I Disorder.

An examination of population subgroups did not reveal any clear evidence of differential responsiveness on the basis of age and gender; however, there were insufficient numbers of patients in each of the ethnic groups to adequately assess inter-group differences.

Pediatric Patients

The efficacy of ABILIFY in the treatment of Bipolar I Disorder in pediatric patients (10 to 17 years of age) was evaluated in one four-week placebo-controlled trial (n=296) of outpatients who met DSM-IV criteria for Bipolar I Disorder manic or mixed episodes with or without psychotic features and had a Y-MRS score ≥20 at baseline. This double-blind, placebo-controlled trial compared two fixed doses of ABILIFY (10 mg/day or 30 mg/day) to placebo. The ABILIFY dose was started at 2 mg/day, which was titrated to 5 mg/day after 2 days, and to the target dose in 5 days in the 10 mg/day treatment arm and in 13 days in the 30 mg/day treatment arm. Both doses of ABILIFY were superior to placebo in change from baseline to week 4 on the Y-MRS total score.

14.3 Adjunctive Treatment of Major Depressive Disorder

The efficacy of ABILIFY in the adjunctive treatment of Major Depressive Disorder was demonstrated in two short-term (6-week), placebo-controlled trials of adult patients meeting DSM-IV criteria for Major Depressive Disorder who had had an inadequate response to prior antidepressant therapy (1 to 3 courses) in the current episode and who had also demonstrated an inadequate response to 8 weeks of prospective antidepressant therapy (paroxetine controlled-release, venlafaxine extended-release, fluoxetine, escitalopram, or sertraline). Inadequate response for prospective treatment was defined as less than 50% improvement on the 17-item version of the Hamilton Depression Rating Scale (HAMD17), minimal HAMD17 score of 14, and a Clinical Global Impressions Improvement rating of no better than minimal improvement. Inadequate response to prior treatment was defined as less than 50% improvement as perceived by the patient after a minimum of 6 weeks of antidepressant therapy at or above the minimal effective dose.

The primary instrument used for assessing depressive symptoms was the Montgomery-Asberg Depression Rating Scale (MADRS), a 10-item clinician-rated scale used to assess the degree of depressive symptomatology (apparent sadness, reported sadness, inner tension, reduced sleep, reduced appetite, concentration difficulties, lassitude, inability to feel, pessimistic thoughts, and suicidal thoughts). The key secondary instrument was the Sheehan Disability Scale (SDS), a 3-item self-rated instrument used to assess the impact of depression on three domains of functioning (work/school, social life, and family life) with each item scored from 0 (not at all) to 10 (extreme).

In the two trials (n=381, n=362), ABILIFY (aripiprazole) was superior to placebo in reducing mean MADRS total scores. In one study, ABILIFY was also superior to placebo in reducing the mean SDS score.

In both trials, patients received ABILIFY adjunctive to antidepressants at a dose of 5 mg/day. Based on tolerability and efficacy, doses could be adjusted by 5 mg increments, one week apart. Allowable doses were: 2 mg/day, 5 mg/day, 10 mg/day, 15 mg/day, and for patients who were not on potent CYP2D6 inhibitors fluoxetine and paroxetine, 20 mg/day. The mean final dose at the end point for the two trials was 10.7 mg/day and 11.4 mg/day.

An examination of population subgroups did not reveal evidence of differential response based on age, choice of prospective antidepressant, or race. With regard to gender, a smaller mean reduction on the MADRS total score was seen in males than in females.

14.4 Agitation Associated with Schizophrenia or Bipolar Mania

The efficacy of intramuscular aripiprazole for injection for the treatment of agitation was established in three short-term (24-hour), placebo-controlled trials in agitated inpatients from two diagnostic groups: Schizophrenia and Bipolar I Disorder (manic or mixed episodes, with or without psychotic features). Each of the trials included a single active comparator treatment arm of either haloperidol injection (Schizophrenia studies) or lorazepam injection (Bipolar Mania study). Patients could receive up to three injections during the 24-hour treatment periods; however, patients could not receive the second injection until after the initial 2-hour period when the primary efficacy measure was assessed. Patients enrolled in the trials needed to be: (1) judged by the clinical investigators as clinically agitated and clinically appropriate candidates for treatment with intramuscular medication, and (2) exhibiting a level of agitation that met or exceeded a threshold score of ≥15 on the five items comprising the Positive and Negative Syndrome Scale (PANSS) Excited Component (ie, poor impulse control, tension, hostility, uncooperativeness, and excitement items) with at least two individual item scores ≥4 using a 1-7 scoring system (1 = absent, 4 = moderate, 7 = extreme). In the studies, the mean baseline PANSS Excited Component score was 19, with scores ranging from 15 to 34 (out of a maximum score of 35), thus suggesting predominantly moderate levels of agitation with some patients experiencing mild or severe levels of agitation. The primary efficacy measure used for assessing agitation signs and symptoms in these trials was the change from baseline in the PANSS Excited Component at 2 hours post-injection. A key secondary measure was the Clinical Global Impression of Improvement (CGI-I) Scale. The results of the trials follow:

In a placebo-controlled trial in agitated inpatients predominantly meeting DSM-IV criteria for Schizophrenia (n=350), four fixed aripiprazole injection doses of 1 mg, 5.25 mg, 9.75 mg, and 15 mg were evaluated. At 2 hours post-injection, the 5.25 mg, 9.75 mg, and 15 mg doses were statistically superior to placebo in the PANSS Excited Component and on the CGI-I Scale.

In a second placebo-controlled trial in agitated inpatients predominantly meeting DSM-IV criteria for Schizophrenia (n=445), one fixed aripiprazole injection dose of 9.75 mg was evaluated. At 2 hours post-injection, aripiprazole for injection was statistically superior to placebo in the PANSS Excited Component and on the CGI-I Scale.

In a placebo-controlled trial in agitated inpatients meeting DSM-IV criteria for Bipolar I Disorder (manic or mixed) (n=291), two fixed aripiprazole injection doses of 9.75 mg and 15 mg were evaluated. At 2 hours post-injection, both doses were statistically superior to placebo in the PANSS Excited Component.

Examination of population subsets (age, race, and gender) did not reveal any differential responsiveness on the basis of these subgroupings.

16 HOW SUPPLIED/STORAGE AND HANDLING

16.1 How Supplied

ABILIFY® (aripiprazole) Tablets have markings on one side and are available in the strengths and packages listed in Table 13.

[See table 13 at top of next page]

ABILIFY® DISCMELT™ (aripiprazole) Orally Disintegrating Tablets are round tablets with markings on either side. ABILIFY DISCMELT is available in the strengths and packages listed in Table 14.

[See table 14 at top of next page]

ABILIFY® (aripiprazole) Oral Solution (1 mg/mL) is supplied in child-resistant bottles along with a calibrated oral dosing cup. ABILIFY Oral Solution is available as follows:

150 mL bottle NDC 59148-013-15

Continued on next page

Product information on these pages reflects product labeling on June 1, 2007. Current information on products of Bristol-Myers Squibb may be obtained at 1-800-321-1335 or www.bms.com.

NOUS08AB00403

Abilify—Cont.

ABILIFY® (aripiprazole) Injection for intramuscular use is available as a ready-to-use, 9.75 mg/1.3 mL (7.5 mg/mL) solution in clear, Type 1 glass vials as follows:

9.75 mg/1.3 mL single-dose vial   NDC 59148-016-65

16.2   Storage

Tablets
Store at 25° C (77° F); excursions permitted between 15° C to 30° C (59° F to 86° F) [see USP Controlled Room Temperature].

Oral Solution
Store at 25° C (77° F); excursions permitted between 15° C to 30° C (59° F to 86° F) [see USP Controlled Room Temperature]. Opened bottles of ABILIFY Oral Solution can be used for up to 6 months after opening, but not beyond the expiration date on the bottle. The bottle and its contents should be discarded after the expiration date.

Injection
Store at 25° C (77° F); excursions permitted between 15° C to 30° C (59° F to 86° F) [see USP Controlled Room Temperature]. Protect from light by storing in the original container. Retain in carton until time of use.

17   PATIENT COUNSELING INFORMATION

See Medication Guide (17.2)

17.1   Information for Patients
Physicians are advised to discuss the following issues with patients for whom they prescribe ABILIFY:

Increased Mortality in Elderly Patients with Dementia-Related Psychosis
Patients and caregivers should be advised that elderly patients with dementia-related psychoses treated with atypical antipsychotic drugs are at increased risk of death compared with placebo. ABILIFY is not approved for elderly patients with dementia-related psychosis [see *WARNINGS AND PRECAUTIONS (5.1)*].

Clinical Worsening of Depression and Suicide Risk
Patients, their families, and their caregivers should be encouraged to be alert to the emergence of anxiety, agitation, panic attacks, insomnia, irritability, hostility, aggressiveness, impulsivity, akathisia (psychomotor restlessness), hypomania, mania, other unusual changes in behavior, worsening of depression, and suicidal ideation, especially early during antidepressant treatment and when the dose is adjusted up or down. Families and caregivers of patients should be advised to look for the emergence of such symptoms on a day-to-day basis, since changes may be abrupt. Such symptoms should be reported to the patient's prescriber or health professional, especially if they are severe, abrupt in onset, or were not part of the patient's presenting symptoms. Symptoms such as these may be associated with an increased risk for suicidal thinking and behavior and indicate a need for very close monitoring and possibly changes in the medication [see *WARNINGS AND PRECAUTIONS (5.2)*].

Prescribers or other health professionals should inform patients, their families, and their caregivers about the benefits and risks associated with treatment with ABILIFY and should counsel them in its appropriate use. A patient Medication Guide about "Antidepressant Medicines, Depression and other Serious Mental Illness, and Suicidal Thoughts or Actions" is available for ABILIFY. The prescriber or health professional should instruct patients, their families, and their caregivers to read the Medication Guide and should assist them in understanding its contents. Patients should be given the opportunity to discuss the contents of the Medication Guide and to obtain answers to any questions they may have. It should be noted that ABILIFY is not approved as a single agent for treatment of depression and has not been evaluated in pediatric Major Depressive Disorder.

Use of Orally Disintegrating Tablet
Do not open the blister until ready to administer. For single tablet removal, open the package and peel back the foil on the blister to expose the tablet. Do not push the tablet through the foil because this could damage the tablet. Immediately upon opening the blister, using dry hands, remove the tablet and place the entire ABILIFY DISCMELT Orally Disintegrating Tablet on the tongue. Tablet disintegration occurs rapidly in saliva. It is recommended that ABILIFY DISCMELT be taken without liquid. However, if needed, it can be taken with liquid. Do not attempt to split the tablet.

Interference with Cognitive and Motor Performance
Because aripiprazole may have the potential to impair judgment, thinking, or motor skills, patients should be cautioned about operating hazardous machinery, including automobiles, until they are reasonably certain that aripiprazole therapy does not affect them adversely [see *WARNINGS AND PRECAUTIONS (5.8)*].

Pregnancy
Patients should be advised to notify their physician if they become pregnant or intend to become pregnant during therapy with ABILIFY [see *USE IN SPECIFIC POPULATIONS (8.1)*].

Nursing
Patients should be advised not to breast-feed an infant if they are taking ABILIFY [see *USE IN SPECIFIC POPULATIONS (8.3)*].

Concomitant Medication
Patients should be advised to inform their physicians if they are taking, or plan to take, any prescription or over-the-counter drugs, since there is a potential for interactions [see *DRUG INTERACTIONS (7)*].

Table 13:   ABILIFY Tablet Presentations

Tablet Strength	Tablet Color/Shape	Tablet Markings	Pack Size	NDC Code
2 mg	green modified rectangle	"A-006" and "2"	Bottle of 30	59148-006-13
5 mg	blue modified rectangle	"A-007" and "5"	Bottle of 30 Blister of 100	59148-007-13 59148-007-35
10 mg	pink modified rectangle	"A-008" and "10"	Bottle of 30 Blister of 100	59148-008-13 59148-008-35
15 mg	yellow round	"A-009" and "15"	Bottle of 30 Blister of 100	59148-009-13 59148-009-35
20 mg	white round	"A-010" and "20"	Bottle of 30 Blister of 100	59148-010-13 59148-010-35
30 mg	pink round	"A-011" and "30"	Bottle of 30 Blister of 100	59148-011-13 59148-011-35

Table 14:   ABILIFY DISCMELT Orally Disintegrating Tablet Presentations

Tablet Strength	Tablet Color	Tablet Markings	Pack Size	NDC Code
10 mg	pink (with scattered specks)	"A" and "640" "10"	Blister of 30	59148-640-23
15 mg	yellow (with scattered specks)	"A" and "641" "15"	Blister of 30	59148-641-23

Alcohol
Patients should be advised to avoid alcohol while taking ABILIFY (aripiprazole) [see *DRUG INTERACTIONS (7.2)*].

Heat Exposure and Dehydration
Patients should be advised regarding appropriate care in avoiding overheating and dehydration [see *WARNINGS AND PRECAUTIONS (5.9)*].

Sugar Content
Patients should be advised that each mL of ABILIFY Oral Solution contains 400 mg of sucrose and 200 mg of fructose.

Phenylketonurics
Phenylalanine is a component of aspartame. Each ABILIFY DISCMELT Orally Disintegrating Tablet contains the following amounts: 10 mg - 1.12 mg phenylalanine and 15 mg - 1.68 mg phenylalanine.

Tablets manufactured by Otsuka Pharmaceutical Co, Ltd, Tokyo, 101-8535 Japan or Bristol-Myers Squibb Company, Princeton, NJ 08543 USA

Orally Disintegrating Tablets, Oral Solution, and Injection manufactured by Bristol-Myers Squibb Company, Princeton, NJ 08543 USA

Distributed and marketed by Otsuka America Pharmaceutical, Inc, Rockville, MD 20850 USA

Marketed by Bristol-Myers Squibb Company, Princeton, NJ 08543 USA

Bristol-Myers Squibb Company
Otsuka
Otsuka America Pharmaceutical, Inc.
US Patent Nos: 5,006,528; 6,977,257; and 7,115,587

Rev February 2008
© 2008, Otsuka Pharmaceutical Co, Ltd, Tokyo, 101-8535 Japan
1239550A1   0308L-0818
D6-B0001-02-08

17.2   Medication Guide

MEDICATION GUIDE
ABILIFY® (a-BIL-ĭ-fĭ)
Generic name: aripiprazole
Antidepressant Medicines, Depression and other Serious Mental Illnesses, and Suicidal Thoughts or Actions
Read the Medication Guide that comes with your or your family member's antidepressant medicine. This Medication Guide is only about the risk of suicidal thoughts and actions with antidepressant medicines. **Talk to your, or your family member's, healthcare provider about:**
• all risks and benefits of treatment with antidepressant medicines
• all treatment choices for depression or other serious mental illness

What is the most important information I should know about antidepressant medicines, depression and other serious mental illnesses, and suicidal thoughts or actions?
1. Antidepressant medicines may increase suicidal thoughts or actions in some children, teenagers, and young adults within the first few months of treatment.
2. Depression and other serious mental illnesses are the most important causes of suicidal thoughts and actions. Some people may have a particularly high risk of having suicidal thoughts or actions. These include people who have (or have a family history of) bipolar illness (also called manic-depressive illness) or suicidal thoughts or actions.
3. How can I watch for and try to prevent suicidal thoughts and actions in myself or a family member?
• Pay close attention to any changes, especially sudden changes, in mood, behaviors, thoughts, or feelings. This is very important when an antidepressant medicine is started or when the dose is changed.
• Call the healthcare provider right away to report new or sudden changes in mood, behavior, thoughts, or feelings.

• Keep all follow-up visits with the healthcare provider as scheduled. Call the healthcare provider between visits as needed, especially if you have concerns about symptoms.
Call a healthcare provider right away if you or your family member has any of the following symptoms, especially if they are new, worse, or worry you:
• thoughts about suicide or dying
• attempts to commit suicide
• new or worse depression
• new or worse anxiety
• feeling very agitated or restless
• panic attacks
• trouble sleeping (insomnia)
• new or worse irritability
• acting aggressive, being angry, or violent
• acting on dangerous impulses
• an extreme increase in activity and talking (mania)
• other unusual changes in behavior or mood
What else do I need to know about antidepressant medicines?
• **Never stop an antidepressant medicine without first talking to a healthcare provider.** Stopping an antidepressant medicine suddenly can cause other symptoms.
• **Antidepressants are medicines used to treat depression and other illnesses.** It is important to discuss all the risks of treating depression and also the risks of not treating it. Patients and their families or other caregivers should discuss all treatment choices with the healthcare provider, not just the use of antidepressants.
• **Antidepressant medicines have other side effects.** Talk to the healthcare provider about the side effects of the medicine prescribed for you or your family member.
• **Antidepressant medicines can interact with other medicines.** Know all of the medicines that you or your family member takes. Keep a list of all medicines to show the healthcare provider. Do not start new medicines without first checking with your healthcare provider.
• **Not all antidepressant medicines prescribed for children are FDA approved for use in children.** Talk to your child's healthcare provider for more information.
This Medication Guide has been approved by the U.S. Food and Drug Administration for all antidepressants.
It should be noted that ABILIFY (aripiprazole) is approved to be added to an antidepressant when the response from the antidepressant alone is not adequate. ABILIFY is not approved for pediatric patients with depression.
Call your doctor for medical advice about side effects. You may report side effects to FDA at 1-800-FDA-1088.
ABILIFY is a trademark of Otsuka Pharmaceutical Company.
1239550A1   0308L-0818   Rev February 2008
© 2008, Otsuka Pharmaceutical Co, Ltd, Tokyo, 101-8535 Japan
570US08LC10701
D6-B0001-02-08

PLAVIX®
clopidogrel bisulfate tablets
Rx only

Rx

DESCRIPTION

PLAVIX (clopidogrel bisulfate) is an inhibitor of ADP-induced platelet aggregation acting by direct inhibition of adenosine diphosphate (ADP) binding to its receptor and of the subsequent ADP-mediated activation of the glycoprotein GPIIb/IIIa complex. Chemically it is methyl (+)-(S)-α-(2-chlorophenyl)-6,7-dihydrothieno[3,2-c]pyridine-5(4H)-

acetate sulfate (1:1). The empirical formula of clopidogrel bisulfate is $C_{16}H_{16}ClNO_2S \cdot H_2SO_4$ and its molecular weight is 419.9.

The structural formula is as follows:

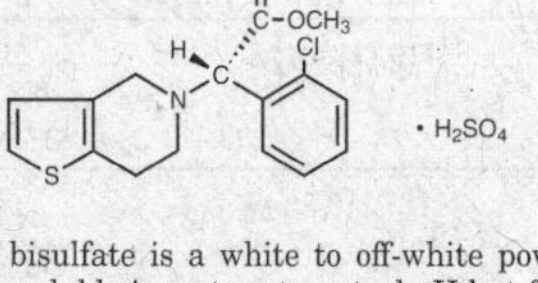

Clopidogrel bisulfate is a white to off-white powder. It is practically insoluble in water at neutral pH but freely soluble at pH 1. It also dissolves freely in methanol, dissolves sparingly in methylene chloride, and is practically insoluble in ethyl ether. It has a specific optical rotation of about +56°.

PLAVIX for oral administration is provided as either pink, round, biconvex, debossed film-coated tablets containing 97.875 mg of clopidogrel bisulfate which is the molar equivalent of 75 mg of clopidogrel base or pink, oblong, debossed film-coated tablets containing 391.5 mg of clopidogrel bisulfate which is the molar equivalent of 300 mg of clopidogrel base.

Each tablet contains hydrogenated castor oil, hydroxypropylcellulose, mannitol, microcrystalline cellulose and polyethylene glycol 6000 as inactive ingredients. The pink film coating contains ferric oxide, hypromellose 2910, lactose monohydrate, titanium dioxide and triacetin. The tablets are polished with Carnauba wax.

CLINICAL PHARMACOLOGY

Mechanism of Action

Clopidogrel is an inhibitor of platelet aggregation. A variety of drugs that inhibit platelet function have been shown to decrease morbid events in people with established cardiovascular atherosclerotic disease as evidenced by stroke or transient ischemic attacks, myocardial infarction, unstable angina or the need for vascular bypass or angioplasty. This indicates that platelets participate in the initiation and/or evolution of these events and that inhibiting them can reduce the event rate.

Pharmacodynamic Properties

Clopidogrel selectively inhibits the binding of adenosine diphosphate (ADP) to its platelet receptor and the subsequent ADP-mediated activation of the glycoprotein GPIIb/IIIa complex, thereby inhibiting platelet aggregation. Biotransformation of clopidogrel is necessary to produce inhibition of platelet aggregation, but an active metabolite responsible for the activity of the drug has not been isolated. Clopidogrel also inhibits platelet aggregation induced by agonists other than ADP by blocking the amplification of platelet activation by released ADP. Clopidogrel does not inhibit phosphodiesterase activity.

Clopidogrel acts by irreversibly modifying the platelet ADP receptor. Consequently, platelets exposed to clopidogrel are affected for the remainder of their lifespan.

Dose dependent inhibition of platelet aggregation can be seen 2 hours after single oral doses of PLAVIX (clopidogrel bisulfate). Repeated doses of 75 mg PLAVIX per day inhibit ADP-induced platelet aggregation on the first day, and inhibition reaches steady state between Day 3 and Day 7. At steady state, the average inhibition level observed with a dose of 75 mg PLAVIX per day was between 40% and 60%. Platelet aggregation and bleeding time gradually return to baseline values after treatment is discontinued, generally in about 5 days.

Pharmacokinetics and Metabolism

After repeated 75-mg oral doses of clopidogrel (base), plasma concentrations of the parent compound, which has no platelet inhibiting effect, are very low and are generally below the quantification limit (0.00025 mg/L) beyond 2 hours after dosing. Clopidogrel is extensively metabolized by the liver. The main circulating metabolite is the carboxylic acid derivative, and it too has no effect on platelet aggregation. It represents about 85% of the circulating drug-related compounds in plasma.

Following an oral dose of ^{14}C-labeled clopidogrel in humans, approximately 50% was excreted in the urine and approximately 46% in the feces in the 5 days after dosing. The elimination half-life of the main circulating metabolite was 8 hours after single and repeated administration. Covalent binding to platelets accounted for 2% of radiolabel with a half-life of 11 days.

Effect of Food: Administration of PLAVIX (clopidogrel bisulfate) with meals did not significantly modify the bioavailability of clopidogrel as assessed by the pharmacokinetics of the main circulating metabolite.

Absorption and Distribution: Clopidogrel is rapidly absorbed after oral administration of repeated doses of 75 mg clopidogrel (base), with peak plasma levels (≅ 3 mg/L) of the main circulating metabolite occurring approximately 1 hour after dosing. The pharmacokinetics of the main circulating metabolite are linear (plasma concentrations increased in proportion to dose) in the dose range of 50 to 150 mg of clopidogrel. Absorption is at least 50% based on urinary excretion of clopidogrel-related metabolites.

Clopidogrel and the main circulating metabolite bind reversibly *in vitro* to human plasma proteins (98% and 94%, respectively). The binding is nonsaturable *in vitro* up to a concentration of 100 μg/mL.

Metabolism and Elimination: *In vitro* and *in vivo*, clopidogrel undergoes rapid hydrolysis into its carboxylic acid derivative. In plasma and urine, the glucuronide of the carboxylic acid derivative is also observed.

Special Populations

Geriatric Patients: Plasma concentrations of the main circulating metabolite are significantly higher in elderly (≥75 years) compared to young healthy volunteers but these higher plasma levels were not associated with differences in platelet aggregation and bleeding time. No dosage adjustment is needed for the elderly.

Renally Impaired Patients: After repeated doses of 75 mg PLAVIX (clopidogrel bisulfate) per day, plasma levels of the main circulating metabolite were lower in patients with severe renal impairment (creatinine clearance from 5 to 15 mL/min) compared to subjects with moderate renal impairment (creatinine clearance 30 to 60 mL/min) or healthy subjects. Although inhibition of ADP-induced platelet aggregation was lower (25%) than that observed in healthy volunteers, the prolongation of bleeding time was similar to healthy volunteers receiving 75 mg of PLAVIX per day.

Gender: No significant difference was observed in the plasma levels of the main circulating metabolite between males and females. In a small study comparing men and women, less inhibition of ADP-induced platelet aggregation was observed in women, but there was no difference in prolongation of bleeding time. In the large, controlled clinical study (Clopidogrel vs. Aspirin in Patients at Risk of Ischemic Events; CAPRIE), the incidence of clinical outcome events, other adverse clinical events, and abnormal clinical laboratory parameters was similar in men and women.

Race: Pharmacokinetic differences due to race have not been studied.

CLINICAL STUDIES

The clinical evidence for the efficacy of PLAVIX is derived from four double-blind trials involving 81,090 patients: the CAPRIE study (Clopidogrel vs. Aspirin in Patients at Risk of Ischemic Events), a comparison of PLAVIX to aspirin, and the CURE (Clopidogrel in Unstable Angina to Prevent Recurrent Ischemic Events), the COMMIT/CCS-2 (Clopidogrel and Metoprolol in Myocardial Infarction Trial / Second Chinese Cardiac Study) studies comparing PLAVIX to placebo, both given in combination with aspirin and other standard therapy and CLARITY-TIMI 28 (Clopidogrel as Adjunctive Reperfusion Therapy – Thrombolysis in Myocardial Infarction).

Recent Myocardial Infarction (MI), Recent Stroke or Established Peripheral Arterial Disease

The CAPRIE trial was a 19,185-patient, 304-center, international, randomized, double-blind, parallel-group study comparing PLAVIX (75 mg daily) to aspirin (325 mg daily). The patients randomized had: 1) recent histories of myocardial infarction (within 35 days); 2) recent histories of ischemic stroke (within 6 months) with at least a week of residual neurological signs; or 3) objectively established peripheral arterial disease. Patients received randomized treatment for an average of 1.6 years (maximum of 3 years). The trial's primary outcome was the time to first occurrence of new ischemic stroke (fatal or not), new myocardial infarction (fatal or not), or other vascular death. Deaths not easily attributable to nonvascular causes were all classified as vascular.

Table 1: Outcome Events in the CAPRIE Primary Analysis

Patients	PLAVIX 9599	aspirin 9586
IS (fatal or not)	438 (4.6%)	461 (4.8%)
MI (fatal or not)	275 (2.9%)	333 (3.5%)
Other vascular death	226 (2.4%)	226 (2.4%)
Total	939 (9.8%)	1020 (10.6%)

As shown in the table, PLAVIX (clopidogrel bisulfate) was associated with a lower incidence of outcome events of every kind. The overall risk reduction (9.8% vs. 10.6%) was 8.7%, P=0.045. Similar results were obtained when all-cause mortality and all-cause strokes were counted instead of vascular mortality and ischemic strokes (risk reduction 6.9%). In patients who survived an on-study stroke or myocardial infarction, the incidence of subsequent events was again lower in the PLAVIX group.

The curves showing the overall event rate are shown in Figure 1. The event curves separated early and continued to diverge over the 3-year follow-up period.

Figure 1: Fatal or Non-Fatal Vascular Events in the CAPRIE Study

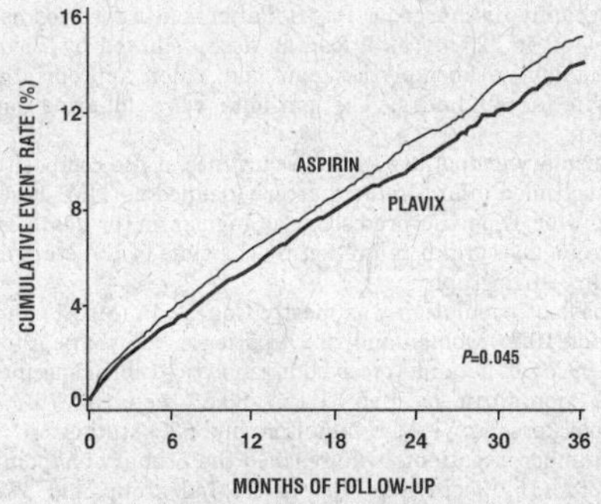

Although the statistical significance favoring PLAVIX over aspirin was marginal (P=0.045), and represents the result of a single trial that has not been replicated, the comparator drug, aspirin, is itself effective (vs. placebo) in reducing cardiovascular events in patients with recent myocardial infarction or stroke. Thus, the difference between PLAVIX (clopidogrel bisulfate) and placebo, although not measured directly, is substantial.

The CAPRIE trial included a population that was randomized on the basis of 3 entry criteria. The efficacy of PLAVIX relative to aspirin was heterogeneous across these randomized subgroups (P=0.043). It is not clear whether this difference is real or a chance occurrence. Although the CAPRIE trial was not designed to evaluate the relative benefit of PLAVIX over aspirin in the individual patient subgroups, the benefit appeared to be strongest in patients who were enrolled because of peripheral vascular disease (especially those who also had a history of myocardial infarction) and weaker in stroke patients. In patients who were enrolled in the trial on the sole basis of a recent myocardial infarction, PLAVIX was not numerically superior to aspirin.

In the meta-analyses of studies of aspirin vs. placebo in patients similar to those in CAPRIE, aspirin was associated with a reduced incidence of thrombotic events. There was a suggestion of heterogeneity in these studies too, with the effect strongest in patients with a history of myocardial infarction, weaker in patients with a history of stroke, and not discernible in patients with a history of peripheral vascular disease. With respect to the inferred comparison of PLAVIX to placebo, there is no indication of heterogeneity.

Acute Coronary Syndrome

The CURE study included 12,562 patients with acute coronary syndrome without ST segment elevation (unstable angina or non-Q-wave myocardial infarction) and presenting within 24 hours of onset of the most recent episode of chest pain or symptoms consistent with ischemia. Patients were required to have either ECG changes consistent with new ischemia (without ST segment elevation) or elevated cardiac enzymes or troponin I or T to at least twice the upper limit of normal. The patient population was largely Caucasian (82%) and included 38% women, and 52% patients ≥65 years of age.

Patients were randomized to receive PLAVIX (300 mg loading dose followed by 75 mg/day) or placebo, and were treated for up to one year. Patients also received aspirin (75-325 mg once daily) and other standard therapies such as heparin. The use of GPIIb/IIIa inhibitors was not permitted for three days prior to randomization.

The number of patients experiencing the primary outcome (CV death, MI, or stroke) was 582 (9.30%) in the PLAVIX-treated group and 719 (11.41%) in the placebo-treated group, a 20% relative risk reduction (95% CI of 10%-28%; p=0.00009) for the PLAVIX-treated group (see Table 2).

At the end of 12 months, the number of patients experiencing the co-primary outcome (CV death, MI, stroke or refractory ischemia) was 1035 (16.54%) in the PLAVIX-treated group and 1187 (18.83%) in the placebo-treated group, a 14% relative risk reduction (95% CI of 6%-21%, p=0.0005) for the PLAVIX-treated group (see Table 2).

In the PLAVIX-treated group, each component of the two primary endpoints (CV death, MI, stroke, refractory ischemia) occurred less frequently than in the placebo-treated group.

[See table 2 at top of next page]

The benefits of PLAVIX (clopidogrel bisulfate) were maintained throughout the course of the trial (up to 12 months).

Figure 2: Cardiovascular Death, Myocardial Infarction, and Stroke in the CURE Study

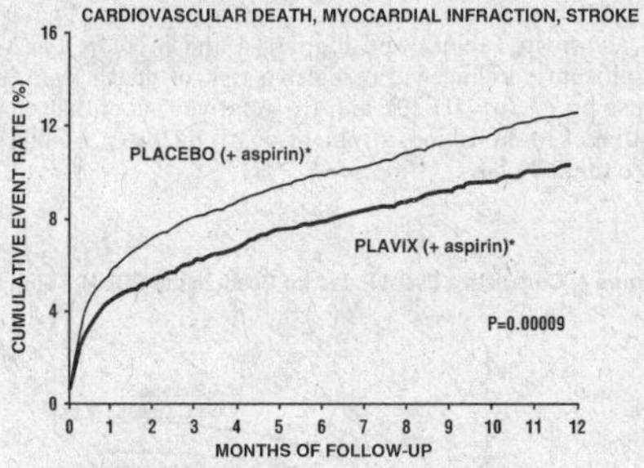

*Other standard therapies were used as appropriate

In CURE, the use of PLAVIX was associated with a lower incidence of CV death, MI or stroke in patient populations with different characteristics, as shown in Figure 3. The benefits associated with PLAVIX were independent of the use of other acute and long-term cardiovascular therapies, including heparin/LMWH (low molecular weight heparin), IV glycoprotein IIb/IIIa (GPIIb/IIIa) inhibitors, lipid-lowering drugs, beta-blockers, and ACE-inhibitors. The efficacy of PLAVIX was observed independently of the dose of aspirin (75-325 mg once daily). The use of oral anticoagu-

Continued on next page

Product information on these pages reflects product labeling on June 1, 2007. Current information on products of Bristol-Myers Squibb may be obtained at 1-800-321-1335 or www.bms.com.
NOUS08AB00403

Plavix—Cont.

lants, non-study anti-platelet drugs and chronic NSAIDs was not allowed in CURE.

Figure 3: Hazard Ratio for Patient Baseline Characteristics and On-Study Concomitant Medications/Interventions for the CURE Study

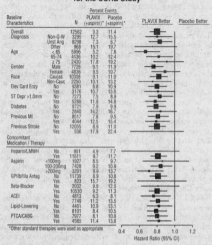

*Other standard therapies were used as appropriate

The use of PLAVIX (clopidogrel bisulfate) in CURE was associated with a decrease in the use of thrombolytic therapy (71 patients [1.1%] in the PLAVIX group, 126 patients [2.0%] in the placebo group; relative risk reduction of 43%, P=0.0001), and GPIIb/IIIa inhibitors (369 patients [5.9%] in the PLAVIX group, 454 patients [7.2%] in the placebo group, relative risk reduction of 18%, P=0.003). The use of PLAVIX in CURE did not impact the number of patients treated with CABG or PCI (with or without stenting), (2253 patients [36.0%] in the PLAVIX group, 2324 patients [36.9%] in the placebo group; relative risk reduction of 4.0%, P=0.1658).

In patients with ST-segment elevation acute myocardial infarction, safety and efficacy of clopidogrel have been evaluated in two randomized, placebo-controlled, double-blind studies, COMMIT- a large outcome study conducted in China - and CLARITY- a supportive study of a surrogate endpoint conducted internationally.

The randomized, double-blind, placebo-controlled, 2x2 factorial design COMMIT trial included 45,852 patients presenting within 24 hours of the onset of the symptoms of suspected myocardial infarction with supporting ECG abnormalities (i.e., ST elevation, ST depression or left bundle-branch block). Patients were randomized to receive PLAVIX (75 mg/day) or placebo, in combination with aspirin (162 mg/day), for 28 days or until hospital discharge whichever came first.

The co-primary endpoints were death from any cause and the first occurrence of re-infarction, stroke or death.

The patient population included 28% women, 58% patients ≥60 years (26% patients ≥70 years) and 55% patients who received thrombolytics, 68% received ace-inhibitors, and only 3% had percutaneous coronary intervention (PCI).

As shown in Table 3 and Figures 4 and 5 below, PLAVIX significantly reduced the relative risk of death from any cause by 7% (p = 0.029), and the relative risk of the combination of re-infarction, stroke or death by 9% (p = 0.002). [See table 3 above]

Figure 4: Cumulative Event Rates for Death in the COMMIT Study*

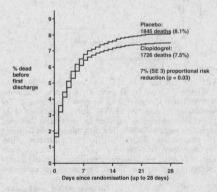

* All treated patients received aspirin.

[See figure 5 at top of next column]

The effect of PLAVIX did not differ significantly in various pre-specified subgroups as shown in Figure 6. Additionally, the effect was similar in non-prespecified subgroups including those based on infarct location, Killip class or prior MI

Table 2: Outcome Events in the CURE Primary Analysis

Outcome	PLAVIX (+ aspirin)* (n=6259)	Placebo (+ aspirin)* (n=6303)	Relative Risk Reduction (%) (95% CI)
Primary outcome (Cardiovascular death, MI, Stroke)	582 (9.3%)	719 (11.4%)	20% (10.3, 27.9) P=0.00009
Co-primary outcome (Cardiovascular death, MI, Stroke, Refractory Ischemia)	1035 (16.5%)	1187 (18.8%)	14% (6.2, 20.6) P=0.00052
All Individual Outcome Events:†			
CV death	318 (5.1%)	345 (5.5%)	7% (−7.7, 20.6)
MI	324 (5.2%)	419 (6.6%)	23% (11.0, 33.4)
Stroke	75 (1.2%)	87 (1.4%)	14% (−17.7, 36.6)
Refractory ischemia	544 (8.7%)	587 (9.3%)	7% (−4.0, 18.0)

* Other standard therapies were used as appropriate.

† The individual components do not represent a breakdown of the primary and co-primary outcomes, but rather the total number of subjects experiencing an event during the course of the study.

Table 3: Outcome Events in the COMMIT Analysis

Event	PLAVIX (+ aspirin) (N=22961)	Placebo (+ aspirin) (N=22891)	Odds ratio (95% CI)	p-value
Composite endpoint: Death, MI, or Stroke*	2121 (9.2%)	2310 (10.1%)	0.91 (0.86, 0.97)	0.002
Death	1726 (7.5%)	1845 (8.1%)	0.93 (0.87, 0.99)	0.029
Non-fatal MI**	270 (1.2%)	330 (1.4%)	0.81 (0.69, 0.95)	0.011
Non-fatal Stroke**	127 (0.6%)	142 (0.6%)	0.89 (0.70, 1.13)	0.33

* The difference between the composite endpoint and the sum of death+non-fatal MI+non-fatal stroke indicates that 9 patients (2 clopidogrel and 7 placebo) suffered both a non-fatal stroke and a non-fatal MI.

** Non-fatal MI and non-fatal stroke exclude patients who died (of any cause).

Figure 5: Cumulative Event Rates for the Combined Endpoint Re-Infarction, Stroke or Death in the COMMIT Study*

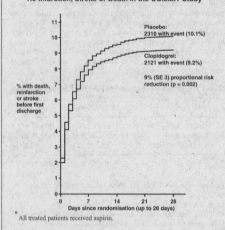

* All treated patients received aspirin.

history (see Figure 7). Such subgroup analyses should be interpreted very cautiously.
[See figure 6 at top of next column]
[See figure 7 at top of next column]

The randomized, double-blind, placebo-controlled CLARITY trial included 3,491 patients, 5% U.S., presenting within 12 hours of the onset of a ST elevation myocardial infarction and planned for thrombolytic therapy. Patients were randomized to receive PLAVIX (clopidogrel bisulfate) (300-mg loading dose, followed by 75 mg/day) or placebo until angiography, discharge, or Day 8. Patients also received aspirin (150 to 325 mg as a loading dose, followed by 75 to 162 mg/day), a fibrinolytic agent and, when appropriate, heparin for 48 hours. The patients were followed for 30 days.

The primary endpoint was the occurrence of the composite of an occluded infarct-related artery (defined as TIMI Flow Grade 0 or 1) on the predischarge angiogram, or death or recurrent myocardial infarction by the time of the start of coronary angiography. The patient population was mostly Caucasian (89.5%) and included 19.7% women and 29.2% patients ≥65 years. A total of 99.7% of patients received fibrinolytics (fibrin specific: 68.7%, non-fibrin specific: 31.1%), 89.5% heparin, 78.7% beta-blockers, 54.7% ACE inhibitors and 63% statins.

The number of patients who reached the primary endpoint was 262 (15.0%) in the PLAVIX-treated group and 377 (21.7%) in the placebo group, but most of the events related to the surrogate endpoint of vessel patency.
[See table 4 at top of next page]

Figure 6: Effects of Adding PLAVIX to Aspirin on the Combined Primary Endpoint across Baseline and Concomitant Medication Subgroups for the COMMIT Study

(See figure for detailed subgroup data.)

Figure 7: Effects of Adding PLAVIX to Aspirin in the Non-Prespecified Subgroups in the Commit Study

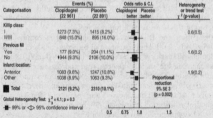

INDICATIONS AND USAGE

PLAVIX (clopidogrel bisulfate) is indicated for the reduction of atherothrombotic events as follows:

• **Recent MI, Recent Stroke or Established Peripheral Arterial Disease**

For patients with a history of recent myocardial infarction (MI), recent stroke, or established peripheral arterial disease, PLAVIX has been shown to reduce the rate of a combined endpoint of new ischemic stroke (fatal or not), new MI (fatal or not), and other vascular death.

- **Acute Coronary Syndrome**

  -For patients with non-ST-segment elevation acute coronary syndrome (unstable angina/non-Q-wave MI) including patients who are to be managed medically and those who are to be managed with percutaneous coronary intervention (with or without stent) or CABG, PLAVIX (clopidogrel bisulfate) has been shown to decrease the rate of a combined endpoint of cardiovascular death, MI, or stroke as well as the rate of a combined endpoint of cardiovascular death, MI, stroke, or refractory ischemia.

  -For patients with ST-segment elevation acute myocardial infarction, PLAVIX has been shown to reduce the rate of death from any cause and the rate of a combined endpoint of death, re-infarction or stroke. This benefit is not known to pertain to patients who receive primary angioplasty.

CONTRAINDICATIONS

The use of PLAVIX is contraindicated in the following conditions:

Hypersensitivity to the drug substance or any component of the product.

Active pathological bleeding such as peptic ulcer or intracranial hemorrhage.

WARNINGS

Thrombotic thrombocytopenic purpura (TTP):

TTP has been reported rarely following use of PLAVIX, sometimes after a short exposure (<2 weeks). TTP is a serious condition that can be fatal and requires urgent treatment including plasmapheresis (plasma exchange). It is characterized by thrombocytopenia, microangiopathic hemolytic anemia (schistocytes [fragmented RBCs] seen on peripheral smear), neurological findings, renal dysfunction, and fever. (See **ADVERSE REACTIONS**.)

PRECAUTIONS

General

PLAVIX prolongs the bleeding time and therefore should be used with caution in patients who may be at risk of increased bleeding from trauma, surgery, or other pathological conditions (particularly gastrointestinal and intraocular). If a patient is to undergo elective surgery and an antiplatelet effect is not desired, PLAVIX should be discontinued 5 days prior to surgery.

Due to the risk of bleeding and undesirable hematological effects, blood cell count determination and/or other appropriate testing should be promptly considered, whenever such suspected clinical symptoms arise during the course of treatment (see **ADVERSE REACTIONS**).

In patients with recent TIA or stroke who are at high risk for recurrent ischemic events, the combination of aspirin and PLAVIX has not been shown to be more effective than PLAVIX alone, but the combination has been shown to increase major bleeding.

GI Bleeding: In CAPRIE, PLAVIX was associated with a rate of gastrointestinal bleeding of 2.0%, vs. 2.7% on aspirin. In CURE, the incidence of major gastrointestinal bleeding was 1.3% vs. 0.7% (PLAVIX + aspirin vs. placebo + aspirin, respectively). PLAVIX should be used with caution in patients who have lesions with a propensity to bleed (such as ulcers). Drugs that might induce such lesions should be used with caution in patients taking PLAVIX.

Use in Hepatically Impaired Patients: Experience is limited in patients with severe hepatic disease, who may have bleeding diatheses. PLAVIX should be used with caution in this population.

Use in Renally-impaired Patients: Experience is limited in patients with severe renal impairment. PLAVIX should be used with caution in this population.

Information for Patients

Patients should be told that it may take them longer than usual to stop bleeding, that they may bruise and/or bleed more easily when they take PLAVIX or PLAVIX combined with aspirin, and that they should report any unusual bleeding to their physician. Patients should inform physicians and dentists that they are taking PLAVIX and/or any other product known to affect bleeding before any surgery is scheduled and before any new drug is taken.

Drug Interactions

Study of specific drug interactions yielded the following results:

Aspirin: Aspirin did not modify the clopidogrel-mediated inhibition of ADP-induced platelet aggregation. Concomitant administration of 500 mg of aspirin twice a day for 1 day did not significantly increase the prolongation of bleeding time induced by PLAVIX. PLAVIX potentiated the effect of aspirin on collagen-induced platelet aggregation. PLAVIX and aspirin have been administered together for up to one year.

Heparin: In a study in healthy volunteers, PLAVIX did not necessitate modification of the heparin dose or alter the effect of heparin on coagulation. Coadministration of heparin had no effect on inhibition of platelet aggregation induced by PLAVIX.

Nonsteroidal Anti-Inflammatory Drugs (NSAIDs): In healthy volunteers receiving naproxen, concomitant administration of PLAVIX was associated with increased occult gastrointestinal blood loss. NSAIDs and PLAVIX should be coadministered with caution.

Warfarin: Because of the increased risk of bleeding, the concomitant administration of warfarin with PLAVIX should be undertaken with caution. (See **PRECAUTIONS–General.**)

Table 4: Event Rates for the Primary Composite Endpoint in the CLARITY Study

	Clopidogrel 1752	Placebo 1739	OR	95% CI
Number (%) of patients reporting the composite endpoint	262 (15.0%)	377 (21.7%)	0.64	0.53, 0.76
Occluded IRA				
N (subjects undergoing angiography)	1640	1634		
n (%) patients reporting endpoint	192 (11.7%)	301 (18.4%)	0.59	0.48, 0.72
Death				
n (%) patients reporting endpoint	45 (2.6%)	38 (2.2%)	1.18	0.76, 1.83
Recurrent MI				
n (%) patients reporting endpoint	44 (2.5%)	62 (3.6%)	0.69	0.47, 1.02

*The total number of patients with a component event (occluded IRA, death, or recurrent MI) is greater than the number of patients with a composite event because some patients had more than a single type of component event.

Table 5: CURE Incidence of bleeding complications (% patients)

Event	PLAVIX (+ aspirin)* (n=6259)	Placebo (+ aspirin)* (n=6303)	P-value
Major bleeding †	3.7 ‡	2.7 §	0.001
Life-threatening bleeding	2.2	1.8	0.13
Fatal	0.2	0.2	
5 g/dL hemoglobin drop	0.9	0.9	
Requiring surgical intervention	0.7	0.7	
Hemorrhagic strokes	0.1	0.1	
Requiring inotropes	0.5	0.5	
Requiring transfusion (≥4 units)	1.2	1.0	
Other major bleeding	1.6	1.0	0.005
Significantly disabling	0.4	0.3	
Intraocular bleeding with significant loss of vision	0.05	0.03	
Requiring 2–3 units of blood	1.3	0.9	
Minor bleeding ¶	5.1	2.4	<0.001

* Other standard therapies were used as appropriate.

† Life threatening and other major bleeding.

‡ Major bleeding event rate for PLAVIX + aspirin was dose-dependent on aspirin: <100 mg=2.6%; 100-200 mg= 3.5%; >200 mg=4.9%

Major bleeding event rates for PLAVIX + aspirin by age were: <65 years = 2.5%, ≥65 to <75 years = 4.1%, ≥75 years 5.9%

§ Major bleeding event rate for placebo + aspirin was dose-dependent on aspirin: <100 mg=2.0%; 100-200 mg= 2.3%; >200 mg=4.0%

Major bleeding event rates for placebo + aspirin by age were: <65 years = 2.1%, ≥65 to <75 years = 3.1%, ≥75 years 3.6%

¶ Led to interruption of study medication.

Other Concomitant Therapy: No clinically significant pharmacodynamic interactions were observed when PLAVIX (clopidogrel bisulfate) was coadministered with **atenolol, nifedipine,** or both atenolol and nifedipine. The pharmacodynamic activity of PLAVIX was also not significantly influenced by the coadministration of **phenobarbital, cimetidine** or **estrogen**.

The pharmacokinetics of **digoxin** or **theophylline** were not modified by the coadministration of PLAVIX (clopidogrel bisulfate).

At high concentrations *in vitro*, clopidogrel inhibits P_{450} (2C9). Accordingly, PLAVIX may interfere with the metabolism of **phenytoin, tamoxifen, tolbutamide, warfarin, torsemide, fluvastatin,** and many **non-steroidal anti-inflammatory agents,** but there are no data with which to predict the magnitude of these interactions. Caution should be used when any of these drugs is coadministered with PLAVIX.

In addition to the above specific interaction studies, patients entered into clinical trials with PLAVIX received a variety of concomitant medications including **diuretics, beta-blocking agents, angiotensin converting enzyme inhibitors, calcium antagonists, cholesterol lowering agents, coronary vasodilators, antidiabetic agents** (including **insulin**), **thrombolytics, heparins** (unfractionated and LMWH) **GPIIb/IIIa antagonists, antiepileptic agents** and **hormone replacement therapy** without evidence of clinically significant adverse interactions.

There are no data on the concomitant use of oral anticoagulants, non-study oral anti-platelet drugs and chronic NSAIDs with clopidogrel.

Drug/Laboratory Test Interactions

None known.

Carcinogenesis, Mutagenesis, Impairment of Fertility

There was no evidence of tumorigenicity when clopidogrel was administered for 78 weeks to mice and 104 weeks to rats at dosages up to 77 mg/kg per day, which afforded plasma exposures >25 times that in humans at the recommended daily dose of 75 mg.

Clopidogrel was not genotoxic in four *in vitro* tests (Ames test, DNA-repair test in rat hepatocytes, gene mutation assay in Chinese hamster fibroblasts, and metaphase chromosome analysis of human lymphocytes) and in one *in vivo* test (micronucleus test by oral route in mice).

Clopidogrel was found to have no effect on fertility of male and female rats at oral doses up to 400 mg/kg per day (52 times the recommended human dose on a mg/m^2 basis).

Pregnancy

Pregnancy Category B. Reproduction studies performed in rats and rabbits at doses up to 500 and 300 mg/kg/day (respectively, 65 and 78 times the recommended daily human dose on a mg/m^2 basis), revealed no evidence of impaired fertility or fetotoxicity due to clopidogrel. There are, however, no adequate and well-controlled studies in pregnant women. Because animal reproduction studies are not always predictive of a human response, PLAVIX should be used during pregnancy only if clearly needed.

Nursing Mothers

Studies in rats have shown that clopidogrel and/or its metabolites are excreted in the milk. It is not known whether this drug is excreted in human milk. Because many drugs are excreted in human milk and because of the potential for serious adverse reactions in nursing infants, a decision should be made whether to discontinue nursing or to discontinue the drug, taking into account the importance of the drug to the nursing woman.

Pediatric Use

Safety and effectiveness in the pediatric population have not been established.

Geriatric Use

Of the total number of subjects in the CAPRIE, CURE and CLARITY controlled clinical studies, approximately 50% of patients treated with PLAVIX were 65 years of age and older, and 15% were 75 years of age and older. In COMMIT, approximately 58% of the patients treated with PLAVIX (clopidogrel bisulfate) were 60 years and older, 26% of whom were 70 years and older.

The observed risk of thrombotic events with clopidogrel plus aspirin versus placebo plus aspirin by age category is provided in Figures 3 and 6 for the CURE and COMMIT trials, respectively (see **CLINICAL STUDIES**). The observed risk of bleeding events with clopidogrel plus aspirin versus placebo plus aspirin by age category is provided in Tables 5 and 6 for the CURE and COMMIT trials, respectively (see **ADVERSE REACTIONS**).

ADVERSE REACTIONS

PLAVIX has been evaluated for safety in more than 42,000 patients, including over 9,000 patients treated for 1 year or more. The clinically important adverse events observed in CAPRIE, CURE, CLARITY and COMMIT are discussed below.

The overall tolerability of PLAVIX in CAPRIE was similar to that of aspirin regardless of age, gender and race, with an approximately equal incidence (13%) of patients withdrawing from treatment because of adverse reactions.

Continued on next page

Product information on these pages reflects product labeling on June 1, 2007. Current information on products of Bristol-Myers Squibb may be obtained at 1-800-321-1335 or www.bms.com.
NOUS08AB00403

Table 6: Number (%) of Patients with Bleeding Events in COMMIT

Type of bleeding	PLAVIX (+ aspirin) (N=22961)	Placebo (+ aspirin) (N=22891)	P-value
Major* noncerebral or cerebral bleeding**	134 (0.6%)	125 (0.5%)	0.59
Major noncerebral	82 (0.4%)	73 (0.3%)	0.48
Fatal	36 (0.2%)	37 (0.2%)	0.90
Hemorrhagic stroke	55 (0.2%)	56 (0.2%)	0.91
Fatal	39 (0.2%)	41 (0.2%)	0.81
Other noncerebral bleeding (non-major)	831 (3.6%)	721 (3.1%)	0.005
Any noncerebral bleeding	896 (3.9%)	777 (3.4%)	0.004

* Major bleeds are cerebral bleeds or non-cerebral bleeds thought to have caused death or that required transfusion.
** The relative rate of major noncerebral or cerebral bleeding was independent of age. Event rates for PLAVIX + aspirin by age were: <60 years = 0.3%, ≥60 to <70 years = 0.7%, ≥70 years 0.8%. Event rates for placebo + aspirin by age were: <60 years = 0.4%, ≥60 to <70 years = 0.6%, ≥70 years 0.7%.

Plavix—Cont.

Hemorrhagic: In CAPRIE patients receiving PLAVIX (clopidogrel bisulfate), gastrointestinal hemorrhage occurred at a rate of 2.0%, and required hospitalization in 0.7%. In patients receiving aspirin, the corresponding rates were 2.7% and 1.1%, respectively. The incidence of intracranial hemorrhage was 0.4% for PLAVIX compared to 0.5% for aspirin.

In CURE, PLAVIX use with aspirin was associated with an increase in bleeding compared to placebo with aspirin (see Table 5). There was an excess in major bleeding in patients receiving PLAVIX plus aspirin compared with placebo plus aspirin, primarily gastrointestinal and at puncture sites. The incidence of intracranial hemorrhage (0.1%), and fatal bleeding (0.2%), were the same in both groups.

The overall incidence of bleeding is described in Table 5 for patients receiving both PLAVIX and aspirin in CURE.

[See table 5 at top of previous page]

Ninety-two percent (92%) of the patients in the CURE study received heparin/LMWH, and the rate of bleeding in these patients was similar to the overall results.

There was no excess in major bleeds within seven days after coronary bypass graft surgery in patients who stopped therapy more than five days prior to surgery (event rate 4.4% PLAVIX + aspirin; 5.3% placebo + aspirin). In patients who remained on therapy within five days of bypass graft surgery, the event rate was 9.6% for PLAVIX + aspirin, and 6.3% for placebo + aspirin.

In CLARITY, the incidence of major bleeding (defined as intracranial bleeding or bleeding associated with a fall in hemoglobin > 5 g/dL) was similar between groups (1.3% versus 1.1% in the PLAVIX + aspirin and in the placebo + aspirin groups, respectively). This was consistent across subgroups of patients defined by baseline characteristics, and type of fibrinolytics or heparin therapy. The incidence of fatal bleeding (0.8% versus 0.6% in the PLAVIX + aspirin and in the placebo + aspirin groups, respectively) and intracranial hemorrhage (0.5% versus 0.7%, respectively) was low and similar in both groups.

The overall rate of noncerebral major bleeding or cerebral bleeding in COMMIT was low and similar in both groups as shown in Table 6 below.

[See table 6 above]

Adverse events occurring in ≥2.5% of patients on PLAVIX in the CAPRIE controlled clinical trial are shown below regardless of relationship to PLAVIX. The median duration of therapy was 20 months, with a maximum of 3 years.

Table 7: Adverse Events Occurring in ≥2.5% of PLAVIX Patients in CAPRIE

Body System Event	% Incidence (% Discontinuation) PLAVIX [n=9599]	Aspirin [n=9586]
Body as a Whole – general disorders		
Chest Pain	8.3 (0.2)	8.3 (0.3)
Accidental/Inflicted Injury	7.9 (0.1)	7.3 (0.1)
Influenza-like symptoms	7.5 (<0.1)	7.0 (<0.1)
Pain	6.4 (0.1)	6.3 (0.1)
Fatigue	3.3 (0.1)	3.4 (0.1)
Cardiovascular disorders, general		
Edema	4.1 (<0.1)	4.5 (<0.1)
Hypertension	4.3 (<0.1)	5.1 (<0.1)
Central & peripheral nervous system disorders		
Headache	7.6 (0.3)	7.2 (0.2)
Dizziness	6.2 (0.2)	6.7 (0.3)
Gastrointestinal system disorders		
Any event	27.1 (3.2)	29.8 (4.0)
Abdominal pain	5.6 (0.7)	7.1 (1.0)
Dyspepsia	5.2 (0.6)	6.1 (0.7)
Diarrhea	4.5 (0.4)	3.4 (0.3)
Nausea	3.4 (0.5)	3.8 (0.4)
Metabolic & nutritional disorders		
Hypercholesterolemia	4.0 (0)	4.4 (<0.1)
Musculo-skeletal system disorders		
Arthralgia	6.3 (0.1)	6.2 (0.1)
Back Pain	5.8 (0.1)	5.3 (<0.1)
Platelet, bleeding, & clotting disorders		
Purpura/Bruise	5.3 (0.3)	3.7 (0.1)
Epistaxis	2.9 (0.2)	2.5 (0.1)
Psychiatric disorders		
Depression	3.6 (0.1)	3.9 (0.2)
Respiratory system disorders		
Upper resp tract infection	8.7 (<0.1)	8.3 (<0.1)
Dyspnea	4.5 (0.1)	4.7 (0.1)
Rhinitis	4.2 (0.1)	4.2 (<0.1)
Bronchitis	3.7 (0.1)	3.7 (0)
Coughing	3.1 (<0.1)	2.7 (<0.1)
Skin & appendage disorders		
Any event	15.8 (1.5)	13.1 (0.8)
Rash	4.2 (0.5)	3.5 (0.2)
Pruritus	3.3 (0.3)	1.6 (0.1)
Urinary system disorders		
Urinary tract infection	3.1 (0)	3.5 (0.1)

No additional clinically relevant events to those observed in CAPRIE with a frequency ≥2.5%, have been reported during the CURE and CLARITY controlled studies. COMMIT collected only limited safety data.

Other adverse experiences of potential importance occurring in 1% to 2.5% of patients receiving PLAVIX (clopidogrel bisulfate) in the controlled clinical trials are listed below regardless of relationship to PLAVIX. In general, the incidence of these events was similar to that in patients receiving aspirin (in CAPRIE) or placebo + aspirin (in the other clinical trials).

Autonomic Nervous System Disorders: Syncope, Palpitation. *Body as a Whole-general disorders:* Asthenia, Fever, Hernia. *Cardiovascular disorders:* Cardiac failure. *Central and peripheral nervous system disorders:* Cramps legs, Hypoaesthesia, Neuralgia, Paraesthesia, Vertigo. *Gastrointestinal system disorders:* Constipation, Vomiting. *Heart rate and rhythm disorders:* Fibrillation atrial. *Liver and biliary system disorders:* Hepatic enzymes increased. *Metabolic and nutritional disorders:* Gout, hyperuricemia, non-protein nitrogen (NPN) increased. *Musculo-skeletal system disorders:* Arthritis, Arthrosis. *Platelet, bleeding & clotting disorders:* GI hemorrhage, hematoma, platelets decreased. *Psychiatric disorders:* Anxiety, Insomnia. *Red blood cell disorders:* Anemia. *Respiratory system disorders:* Pneumonia, Sinusitis. *Skin and appendage disorders:* Eczema, Skin ulceration. *Urinary system disorders:* Cystitis. *Vision disorders:* Cataract, Conjunctivitis.

Other potentially serious adverse events which may be of clinical interest but were rarely reported (<1%) in patients who received PLAVIX in the controlled clinical trials are listed below regardless of relationship to PLAVIX. In general, the incidence of these events was similar to that in patients receiving aspirin (in CAPRIE) or placebo + aspirin (in the other clinical trials).

Body as a whole: Allergic reaction, necrosis ischemic. *Cardiovascular disorders:* Edema generalized. *Gastrointestinal system disorders:* Peptic, gastric or duodenal ulcer, gastritis, gastric ulcer perforated, gastritis hemorrhagic, upper GI ulcer hemorrhagic. *Liver and Biliary system disorders:* Bilirubinemia, hepatitis infectious, liver fatty. *Platelet, bleeding and clotting disorders:* hemarthrosis, hematuria, hemoptysis, hemorrhage intracranial, hemorrhage retroperitoneal, hemorrhage of operative wound, ocular hemorrhage, pulmonary hemorrhage, purpura allergic, thrombocytopenia. *Red blood cell disorders:* Anemia aplastic, anemia hypochromic. *Reproductive disorders, female:* Menorrhagia. *Respiratory system disorders:* Hemothorax. *Skin and appendage disorders:* Bullous eruption, rash erythematous, rash maculopapular, urticaria. *Urinary system disorders:* Abnormal renal function, acute renal failure. *White cell and reticuloendothelial system disorders:* Agranulocytosis, granulocytopenia, leukemia, leukopenia, neutropenia.

Postmarketing Experience

The following events have been reported spontaneously from worldwide postmarketing experience:

- *Body as a whole:*
  - hypersensitivity reactions, anaphylactoid reactions, serum sickness
- *Central and Peripheral Nervous System disorders:*
  - confusion, hallucinations, taste disorders
- *Hepato-biliary disorders:*
  - abnormal liver function test, hepatitis (non-infectious), acute liver failure
- *Platelet, Bleeding and Clotting disorders:*
  - cases of bleeding with fatal outcome (especially intracranial, gastrointestinal and retroperitoneal hemorrhage)
  - thrombotic thrombocytopenic purpura (TTP) – some cases with fatal outcome – (see **WARNINGS**)
  - agranulocytosis, aplastic anemia/pancytopenia
  - conjunctival, ocular and retinal bleeding
- *Respiratory, thoracic and mediastinal disorders:*
  - bronchospasm, interstitial pneumonitis
- *Skin and subcutaneous tissue disorders:*
  - angioedema, erythema multiforme, Stevens-Johnson syndrome, toxic epidermal necrolysis, lichen planus
- *Renal and urinary disorders:*
  - glomerulopathy, increased creatinine levels
- *Vascular disorders:*
  - vasculitis, hypotension
- *Gastrointestinal disorders:*
  - colitis (including ulcerative or lymphocytic colitis), pancreatitis, stomatitis
- *Musculoskeletal, connective tissue and bone disorders:*
  - myalgia

OVERDOSAGE

Overdose following clopidogrel administration may lead to prolonged bleeding time and subsequent bleeding complications. A single oral dose of clopidogrel at 1500 or 2000 mg/kg was lethal to mice and to rats and at 3000 mg/kg to baboons. Symptoms of acute toxicity were vomiting (in baboons), prostration, difficult breathing, and gastrointestinal hemorrhage in all species.

Recommendations About Specific Treatment:

Based on biological plausibility, platelet transfusion may be appropriate to reverse the pharmacological effects of PLAVIX (clopidogrel bisulfate) if quick reversal is required.

DOSAGE AND ADMINISTRATION

Recent MI, Recent Stroke, or Established Peripheral Arterial Disease

The recommended daily dose of PLAVIX is 75 mg once daily.

Acute Coronary Syndrome

For patients with non-ST-segment elevation acute coronary syndrome (unstable angina/non-Q-wave MI), PLAVIX should be initiated with a single 300-mg loading dose and then continued at 75 mg once daily. Aspirin (75 mg-325 mg once daily) should be initiated and continued in combination with PLAVIX. In CURE, most patients with Acute Coronary Syndrome also received heparin acutely (see **CLINICAL STUDIES**).

For patients with ST-segment elevation acute myocardial infarction, the recommended dose of PLAVIX is 75 mg once daily, administered in combination with aspirin, with or without thrombolytics. PLAVIX may be initiated with or without a loading dose (300 mg was used in CLARITY; see **CLINICAL STUDIES**).

PLAVIX can be administered with or without food.

No dosage adjustment is necessary for elderly patients or patients with renal disease. (See **Clinical Pharmacology: Special Populations.**)

HOW SUPPLIED

PLAVIX (clopidogrel bisulfate) 75-mg tablets are available as pink, round, biconvex, film-coated tablets debossed with "75" on one side and "1171" on the other. Tablets are provided as follows:

NDC 63653-1171-6 bottles of 30
NDC 63653-1171-1 bottles of 90
NDC 63653-1171-5 bottles of 500
NDC 63653-1171-3 blisters of 100

PLAVIX (clopidogrel bisulfate) 300-mg tablets are available as pink, oblong, film-coated tablets debossed with "300" on one side and "1332" on the other. Tablets are provided as follows:

NDC 63653-1332-3 unit-dose packages of 100

Storage

Store at 25° C (77° F); excursions permitted to 15°–30° C (59°–86° F) [See USP Controlled Room Temperature].

Distributed by:
Bristol-Myers Squibb/Sanofi Pharmaceuticals Partnership
Bridgewater, NJ 08807
PLAVIX® is a registered trademark.
Revised October 2007
264US08LC12801
PLA-OCT07-F-Aa

To keep your **PDR** up to date throughout the year, note these revisions on the corresponding pages of the annual volume. Simply write **"See Supplement A"** next to the product heading.

Cephalon, Inc.
41 MOORES ROAD
PO BOX 4011
FRAZER, PA 19355

For Medical Information and Adverse Drug Experience/ Product Complaint Reporting Contact:
(800) 896-5855
Fax 610-738-6669

FENTORA® ℂ ℞

[fen-tor'-ah]
(fentanyl buccal tablet)
Each tablet contains fentanyl citrate equivalent to fentanyl base: 100, 200, 300, 400, 600 and 800 mcg

Prescribing information for this product, which appears on page(s) 960-964 of the 2008 PDR, has been completely revised as follows. Please write "See Supplement A" next to the product heading.

PHYSICIANS AND OTHER HEALTHCARE PROVIDERS MUST BECOME FAMILIAR WITH THE IMPORTANT WARNINGS IN THIS LABEL.

Reports of serious adverse events, including deaths in patients treated with *FENTORA* have been reported. Deaths occurred as a result of improper patient selection (e.g., use in opioid non-tolerant patients) and/or improper dosing. The substitution of *FENTORA* for any other fentanyl product may result in fatal overdose.

***FENTORA* is indicated only for the management of breakthrough pain in patients with cancer who are already receiving and who are tolerant to around-the-clock opioid therapy for their underlying persistent cancer pain.** Patients considered opioid tolerant are those who are taking around-the-clock medicine consisting of at least 60 mg of oral morphine daily, at least 25 mcg of transdermal fentanyl/hour, at least 30 mg of oxycodone daily, at least 8 mg of oral hydromorphone daily or an equianalgesic dose of another opioid daily for a week or longer.

***FENTORA* is not indicated for use in opioid non-tolerant patients including those with only as needed (PRN) prior exposure.**

***FENTORA* is contraindicated in the management of acute or postoperative pain including headache/migraine. Life-threatening respiratory depression could occur at any dose in opioid non-tolerant patients. Deaths have occurred in opioid non-tolerant patients.**

When prescribing, do not convert patients on a mcg per mcg basis from Actiq® to *FENTORA*. Carefully consult the Initial Dosing Recommendations table. (See DOSAGE AND ADMINISTRATION, Table 7.)

When dispensing, do not substitute a *FENTORA* prescription for other fentanyl products. Substantial differences exist in the pharmacokinetic profile of *FENTORA* compared to other fentanyl products that result in clinically important differences in the extent of absorption of fentanyl. As a result of these differences, the substitution of *FENTORA* for any other fentanyl product may result in fatal overdose.

Special care must be used when dosing *FENTORA*. If the breakthrough pain episode is not relieved after 30 minutes, patients may take ONLY one additional dose using the same strength and must wait at least 4 hours before taking another dose. (See **DOSAGE AND ADMINISTRATION.**)

***FENTORA* contains fentanyl, an opioid agonist and a Schedule II controlled substance, with an abuse liability similar to other opioid analgesics. *FENTORA* can be abused in a manner similar to other opioid agonists, legal or illicit. This should be considered when prescribing or dispensing *FENTORA* in situations where the physician or pharmacist is concerned about an increased risk of misuse, abuse or diversion. Schedule II opioid substances which include morphine, oxycodone, hydromorphone, oxymorphone, and methadone have the highest potential for abuse and risk of fatal overdose due to respiratory depression.**

Patients and their caregivers must be instructed that *FENTORA* contains a medicine in an amount which can be fatal to a child. Patients and their caregivers must be instructed to keep all tablets out of the reach of children. (See Information for Patients and Caregivers for disposal instructions.)

***FENTORA* is intended to be used only in the care of opioid tolerant cancer patients and only by healthcare professionals who are knowledgeable of and skilled in the use of Schedule II opioids to treat cancer pain.**

The concomitant use of *FENTORA* with strong and moderate cytochrome P450 3A4 inhibitors may result in an increase in fentanyl plasma concentrations, and may cause potentially fatal respiratory depression.

DESCRIPTION

FENTORA (fentanyl buccal tablet) is a potent opioid analgesic, intended for buccal mucosal administration. *FENTORA* is formulated as a flat-faced, round, beveled-edge white tablet.

FENTORA is designed to be placed and retained within the buccal cavity for a period sufficient to allow disintegration of the tablet and absorption of fentanyl across the oral mucosa.

FENTORA employs the OraVescent® drug delivery technology, which generates a reaction that releases carbon dioxide when the tablet comes in contact with saliva. It is believed that transient pH changes accompanying the reaction may optimize dissolution (at a lower pH) and membrane permeation (at a higher pH) of fentanyl through the buccal mucosa.

Active Ingredient: Fentanyl citrate, USP is N-(1-Phenethyl-4-piperidyl) propionanilide citrate (1:1). Fentanyl is a highly lipophilic compound (octanol-water partition coefficient at pH 7.4 is 816:1) that is freely soluble in organic solvents and sparingly soluble in water (1:40). The molecular weight of the free base is 336.5 (the citrate salt is 528.6). The pKa of the tertiary nitrogens are 7.3 and 8.4. The compound has the following structural formula:

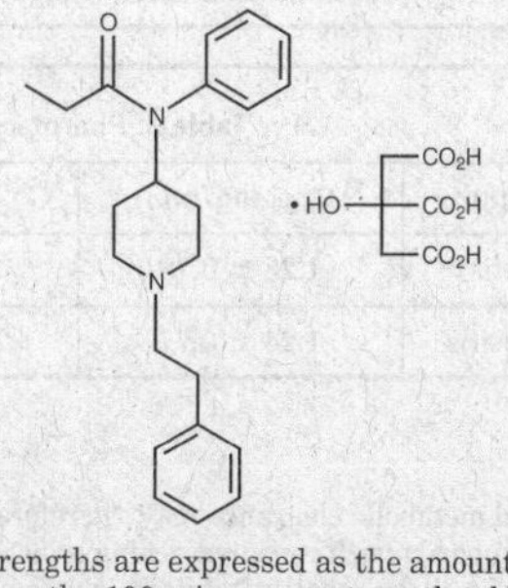

All tablet strengths are expressed as the amount of fentanyl free base, e.g., the 100 microgram strength tablet contains 100 micrograms of fentanyl free base.

Inactive Ingredients: Mannitol, sodium starch glycolate, sodium bicarbonate, sodium carbonate, citric acid, and magnesium stearate.

CLINICAL PHARMACOLOGY

Pharmacology:

Fentanyl is a pure opioid agonist whose principal therapeutic action is analgesia. Other members of the class known as opioid agonists include substances such as morphine, oxycodone, hydromorphone, codeine, and hydrocodone. Pharmacological effects of opioid agonists include anxiolysis, euphoria, feelings of relaxation, respiratory depression, constipation, miosis, cough suppression, and analgesia. Like all pure opioid agonist analgesics, with increasing doses there is increasing analgesia, unlike with mixed agonist/antagonists or non-opioid analgesics, where there is a limit to the analgesic effect with increasing doses. With pure opioid agonist analgesics, there is no defined maximum dose; the ceiling to analgesic effectiveness is imposed only by side effects, the more serious of which may include somnolence and respiratory depression.

Analgesia

The analgesic effects of fentanyl are related to the blood level of the drug, if proper allowance is made for the delay into and out of the CNS (a process with a 3-to-5-minute half-life).

In general, the effective concentration and the concentration at which toxicity occurs increase with increasing tolerance with any and all opioids. The rate of development of tolerance varies widely among individuals. As a result, the dose of *FENTORA* should be individually titrated to achieve the desired effect. (See **DOSAGE AND ADMINISTRATION.**)

Central Nervous System

The precise mechanism of the analgesic action is unknown although fentanyl is known to be a mu opioid receptor agonist. Specific CNS opioid receptors for endogenous compounds with opioid-like activity have been identified throughout the brain and spinal cord and play a role in the analgesic effects of this drug.

Fentanyl produces respiratory depression by direct action on brain stem respiratory centers. The respiratory depression involves both a reduction in the responsiveness of the brain stem to increases in carbon dioxide and to electrical stimulation.

Fentanyl depresses the cough reflex by direct effect on the cough center in the medulla. Antitussive effects may occur with doses lower than those usually required for analgesia. Fentanyl causes miosis even in total darkness. Pinpoint pupils are a sign of opioid overdose but are not pathognomonic (e.g., pontine lesions of hemorrhagic or ischemic origin may produce similar findings).

Gastrointestinal System

Fentanyl causes a reduction in motility associated with an increase in smooth muscle tone in the antrum of the stomach and in the duodenum. Digestion of food is delayed in the small intestine and propulsive contractions are decreased. Propulsive peristaltic waves in the colon are decreased, while tone may be increased to the point of spasm resulting in constipation. Other opioid-induced effects may include a reduction in gastric, biliary and pancreatic secretions, spasm of the sphincter of Oddi, and transient elevations in serum amylase.

Cardiovascular System

Fentanyl may produce release of histamine with or without associated peripheral vasodilation. Manifestations of histamine release and/or peripheral vasodilation may include pruritus, flushing, red eyes, sweating, and/or orthostatic hypotension.

Endocrine System

Opioid agonists have been shown to have a variety of effects on the secretion of hormones. Opioids inhibit the secretion of ACTH, cortisol, and luteinizing hormone (LH) in humans. They also stimulate prolactin, growth hormone (GH) secretion, and pancreatic secretion of insulin and glucagon in humans and other species, rats and dogs. Thyroid stimulating hormone (TSH) has been shown to be both inhibited and stimulated by opioids.

Respiratory System

All opioid mu-receptor agonists, including fentanyl, produce dose dependent respiratory depression. The risk of respiratory depression is less in patients receiving chronic opioid therapy who develop tolerance to respiratory depression and other opioid effects. During the titration phase of the clinical trials, somnolence, which may be a precursor to respiratory depression, did increase in patients who were treated with higher doses of another oral transmucosal fentanyl citrate (Actiq®). Peak respiratory depressive effects may be seen as early as 15 to 30 minutes from the start of oral transmucosal fentanyl citrate product administration and may persist for several hours.

Serious or fatal respiratory depression can occur even at recommended doses. Fentanyl depresses the cough reflex as a result of its CNS activity. Although not observed with oral transmucosal fentanyl products in clinical trials, fentanyl given rapidly by intravenous injection in large doses may interfere with respiration by causing rigidity in the muscles of respiration. Therefore, physicians and other healthcare providers should be aware of this potential complication. (See **BOXED WARNING, CONTRAINDICATIONS, WARNINGS, PRECAUTIONS, ADVERSE REACTIONS,** and **OVERDOSAGE** for additional information on hypoventilation.)

PHARMACOKINETICS

Fentanyl exhibits linear pharmacokinetics. Systemic exposure to fentanyl following administration of *FENTORA* increases linearly in an approximate dose-proportional manner over the 100- to 800-mcg dose range.

Absorption:

Following buccal administration of *FENTORA*, fentanyl is readily absorbed with an absolute bioavailability of 65%. The absorption profile of *FENTORA* is largely the result of an initial absorption from the buccal mucosa, with peak plasma concentrations following venous sampling generally attained within an hour after buccal administration. Approximately 50% of the total dose administered is absorbed transmucosally and becomes systemically available. The remaining half of the total dose is swallowed and undergoes more prolonged absorption from the gastrointestinal tract. In a study that compared the absolute and relative bioavailability of *FENTORA* and Actiq (oral transmucosal fentanyl citrate), the rate and extent of fentanyl absorption were considerably different (approximately 30% greater exposure with *FENTORA*) (Table 1).

Table 1. Pharmacokinetic Parameters* in Adult Subjects Receiving *FENTORA* or Actiq

Pharmacokinetic Parameter (mean)	*FENTORA* 400 mcg	Actiq 400 mcg (adjusted dose)***
Absolute Bioavailability	65% ± 20%	47% ± 10.5%
Fraction Absorbed Transmucosally	48% ± 31.8%	22% ± 17.3%
T_{max} (minute)**	46.8 (20-240)	90.8 (35-240)
C_{max} (ng/mL)	1.02 ± 0.42	0.63 ± 0.21
$AUC_{0\text{-}tmax}$ (ng•hr/mL)	0.40 ± 0.18	0.14 ± 0.05
$AUC_{0\text{-}inf}$ (ng•hr/mL)	6.48 ± 2.98	4.79 ± 1.96

* Based on venous blood samples.
** Data for T_{max} presented as median (range).
***Actiq data was dose adjusted (800 mcg to 400 mcg).

Similarly, in another bioavailability study exposure following administration of *FENTORA* was also greater (approximately 50%) compared to Actiq.

Due to differences in drug delivery, measures of exposure (C_{max}, $AUC_{0\text{-}tmax}$, $AUC_{0\text{-}inf}$) associated with a given dose of fentanyl were substantially greater with *FENTORA* compared to Actiq (see Figure 1). Therefore, caution must be exercised when switching patients from one product to another. (See **DOSAGE AND ADMINISTRATION.**) Figure 1 includes an inset which shows the mean plasma concentration versus time profile to 6 hours. The vertical line denotes the median T_{max} for *FENTORA*.

[See figure 1 at top of next column]

Systemic exposure to fentanyl following administration of *FENTORA* increases linearly in an approximate dose-proportional manner over the 100- to 800-mcg dose range. Mean pharmacokinetic parameters are presented in Table 2. Mean plasma concentration versus time profiles are presented in Figure 2.

[See table 2 at top of next page]
[See figure 2 at top of next column]

Dwell time (defined as the length of time that the tablet takes to fully disintegrate following buccal administration), does not appear to affect early systemic exposure to fentanyl.

Continued on next page

Fentora—Cont.

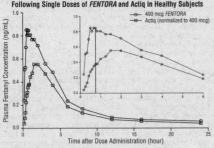

Figure 1. Mean Plasma Concentration Versus Time Profiles Following Single Doses of *FENTORA* and Actiq in Healthy Subjects

Actiq data was dose adjusted (800 mcg to 400 mcg).

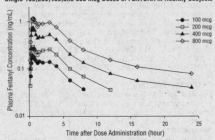

Figure 2. Mean Plasma Concentration Versus Time Profiles Following Single 100,200,400,and 800 mcg Doses of *FENTORA* in Healthy Subjects

The effect of mucositis (Grade 1) on the pharmacokinetic profile of *FENTORA* was studied in a group of patients with (N = 8) and without mucositis (N = 8) who were otherwise matched. A single 200 mcg tablet was administered, followed by sampling at appropriate intervals. Mean summary statistics (standard deviation in parentheses, expected t_{max} where range was used) are presented in Table 3.

[See table 3 above]

Distribution:

Fentanyl is highly lipophilic. The plasma protein binding of fentanyl is 80-85%. The main binding protein is alpha-1-acid glycoprotein, but both albumin and lipoproteins contribute to some extent. The mean oral volume of distribution at steady state (Vss/F) was 25.4 L/kg.

Metabolism:

The metabolic pathways following buccal administration of *FENTORA* have not been characterized in clinical studies. The progressive decline of fentanyl plasma concentrations results from the uptake of fentanyl in the tissues and biotransformation in the liver. Fentanyl is metabolized in the liver and in the intestinal mucosa to norfentanyl by cytochrome P450 3A4 isoform. In animal studies, norfentanyl was not found to be pharmacologically active. (See **PRECAUTIONS: Drug Interactions** for additional information.)

Elimination:

Disposition of fentanyl following buccal administration of *FENTORA* has not been characterized in a mass balance study. Fentanyl is primarily (more than 90%) eliminated by biotransformation to N-dealkylated and hydroxylated inactive metabolites. Less than 7% of the administered dose is excreted unchanged in the urine, and only about 1% is excreted unchanged in the feces. The metabolites are mainly excreted in the urine, while fecal excretion is less important.

The total plasma clearance of fentanyl following intravenous administration is approximately 42 L/h.

Special Populations:

The pharmacokinetics of *FENTORA* has not been studied in Special Populations.

Race

The pharmacokinetic effects of race with the use of *FENTORA* have not been systematically evaluated. In studies conducted in healthy Japanese subjects, systemic exposure was generally higher than that observed in US subjects (mean C_{max} and AUC values were approximately 50% and 20% higher, respectively). The observed differences were largely attributed to the lower mean weight of the Japanese subjects compared to US subjects (57.4 kg versus 73 kg).

Age

The effect of age on the pharmacokinetics of *FENTORA* has not been studied.

Gender

Systemic exposure was higher for women than men (mean C_{max} and AUC values were approximately 28% and 22% higher, respectively). The observed differences between men and women were largely attributable to differences in weight.

Renal or Hepatic Impairment:

The effect of renal or hepatic impairment on the pharmacokinetics of *FENTORA* has not been studied. Although fentanyl kinetics are known to be altered as a result of hepatic and renal disease due to alterations in metabolic clearance and plasma protein binding, the duration of effect for the initial dose of fentanyl is largely determined by the rate of distribution of the drug.

Table 2. Pharmacokinetic Parameters* Following Single 100, 200, 400, and 800 mcg Doses of *FENTORA* in Healthy Subjects

Pharmacokinetic Parameter (mean ± SD)	100 mcg	200 mcg	400 mcg	800 mcg
C_{max} (ng/mL)	0.25 ± 0.14	0.40 ± 0.18	0.97 ± 0.53	1.59 ± 0.90
T_{max}, minute** (range)	45.0 (25.0-181.0)	40.0 (20.0-180.0)	35.0 (20.0-180.0)	40.0 (25.0-180.0)
AUC_{0-inf} (ng•hr/mL)	0.98 ± 0.37	2.11 ± 1.13	4.72 ± 1.95	9.05 ± 3.72
AUC_{0-tmax} (ng•hr/mL)	0.09 ± 0.06	0.13 ± 0.09	0.34 ± 0.23	0.52 ± 0.38
T1/2, hr**	2.63 (1.47-13.57)	4.43 (1.85-20.76)	11.09 (4.63-20.59)	11.70 (4.63-28.63)

* Based on venous sampling.
** Data for T_{max} presented as median (range).

Table 3. Pharmacokinetic Parameters in Patients with Mucositis

Patient status	C_{max} (ng/mL)	t_{max} (min)	AUC_{0-tmax} (ng·hr/mL)	AUC_{0-8} (ng·hr/mL)
Mucositis	1.25 ± 0.78	25.0 (15-45)	0.21 ± 0.16	2.33 ± 0.93
No mucositis	1.24 ± 0.77	22.5 (10-121)	0.25 ± 0.24	1.86 ± 0.86

Diminished metabolic clearance may, therefore, become significant, primarily with repeated dosing or at very high single doses. For these reasons, while it is recommended that *FENTORA* is titrated to clinical effect for all patients, special care should be taken in patients with severe hepatic or renal disease. (See **PRECAUTIONS**.)

Drug Interactions

The interaction between ritonavir and fentanyl was investigated in eleven healthy volunteers in a randomized crossover study. Subjects received oral ritonavir or placebo for 3 days. The ritonavir dose was 200 mg tid on Day 1 and 300 mg tid on Day 2 followed by one morning dose of 300 mg on Day 3. On Day 2, fentanyl was given as a single IV dose at 5 mcg/kg two hours after the afternoon dose of oral ritonavir or placebo. Naloxone was administered to counteract the side effects of fentanyl. The results suggested that ritonavir might decrease the clearance of fentanyl by 67%, resulting in a 174% (range 52%-420%) increase in fentanyl AUC_{0-inf}. Coadministration of ritonavir in patients receiving *FENTORA* has not been studied; however, an increase in fentanyl AUC is expected. (See **DOSAGE AND ADMINISTRATION** and **PRECAUTIONS**.)

CLINICAL TRIALS

Breakthrough Pain:

The efficacy of *FENTORA* was demonstrated in a double-blind, placebo-controlled, cross-over study in opioid tolerant patients with cancer and breakthrough pain. Patients considered opioid tolerant were those who were taking at least 60 mg of oral morphine/day, at least 25 mcg of transdermal fentanyl/hour, at least 30 mg of oxycodone daily, at least 8 mg of oral hydromorphone daily or an equianalgesic dose of another opioid for a week or longer.

In this trial, patients were titrated in an open-label manner to a successful dose of *FENTORA*. A successful dose was defined as the dose in which a patient obtained adequate analgesia with tolerable side effects. Patients who identified a successful dose were randomized to a sequence of 10 treatments with 7 being the successful dose of *FENTORA* and 3 being placebo. Patients used one tablet (either *FENTORA* or Placebo) per breakthrough pain episode.

Patients assessed pain intensity on a scale that rated the pain as 0=none to 10=worst possible pain. With each episode of breakthrough pain, pain intensity was assessed first and then treatment was administered. Pain intensity (0-10) was measured at 15, 30, 45 and 60 minutes after the start of administration. The sum of differences in pain intensity scores at 15 and 30 minutes from baseline ($SPID_{30}$) was the primary efficacy measure.

Sixty five percent of patients who entered the study achieved a successful dose during the titration phase. The distribution of successful doses is shown in Table 4. The median dose was 400 mcg.

Table 4. Successful Dose of *FENTORA* Following Initial Titration

FENTORA Dose	(N=80) n(%)
100 mcg	13 (16)
200 mcg	11 (14)
400 mcg	21 (26)
600 mcg	10 (13)
800 mcg	25 (31)

The LS mean (SE) $SPID_{30}$ for *FENTORA*-treated episodes was 3.0 (0.12) while for placebo-treated episodes it was 1.8 (0.18) (p<0.0001).

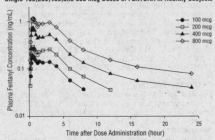

Figure 3. Mean Pain Intensity Difference (PID) at Each Time Point During the Double-Blind Treatment Period

*p<0.01 *FENTORA* versus placebo, in favor of *FENTORA*, by one-sample Wilcoxon signed rank test
†p<0.0001 *FENTORA* versus placebo, in favor of *FENTORA*, by one-sample Wilcoxon signed rank test
PID=pain intensity difference; *FENTORA* fentanyl; SEM=standard error of the mean

INDICATIONS AND USAGE

(See **BOXED WARNING and CONTRAINDICATIONS**.)
FENTORA is indicated only for the management of breakthrough pain in patients with cancer who are **already receiving and who are tolerant to around-the-clock opioid therapy for their underlying persistent cancer pain.** Patients considered opioid tolerant are those who are taking around-the-clock medicine consisting of at least 60 mg of oral morphine daily, at least 25 mcg of transdermal fentanyl/hour, at least 30 mg of oxycodone daily, at least 8 mg of oral hydromorphone daily or an equianalgesic dose of another opioid daily for a week or longer.

This product **must not** be used in opioid non-tolerant patients because life-threatening hypoventilation and death could occur at any dose in patients not on a chronic regimen of opioids. For this reason, *FENTORA* is contraindicated in the management of acute or postoperative pain.

FENTORA is intended to be used only in the care of opioid tolerant cancer patients and only by healthcare professionals who are knowledgeable of and skilled in the use of Schedule II opioids to treat cancer pain.

CONTRAINDICATIONS

FENTORA is contraindicated in opioid non-tolerant patients. *FENTORA* is contraindicated in the management of acute or postoperative pain including headache/migraine. Life-threatening respiratory depression and death could occur at any dose in opioid non-tolerant patients.

FENTORA is contraindicated in patients with known intolerance or hypersensitivity to any of its components or the drug fentanyl.

WARNINGS

See BOXED WARNING

When prescribing, DO NOT convert a patient from Actiq to *FENTORA* without following the instructions found in the prescribing information as Actiq and *FENTORA* are not equivalent on a microgram per microgram basis. *FENTORA* is NOT a generic version of Actiq.

When dispensing, DO NOT substitute a *FENTORA* prescription for an Actiq prescription under any circumstances. *FENTORA* and Actiq are not equivalent. Substantial differences exist in the pharmacokinetic profile of *FENTORA* compared to other fentanyl products including Actiq that result in clinically important differences in the rate and extent of absorption of fentanyl. **As a result of these differences, the substitution of the same dose of *FENTORA* for the same dose of Actiq or any other fentanyl product may result in a fatal overdose.**

There are no safe conversion directions available for patients on any other fentanyl products. (Note: This includes oral, transdermal, or parenteral formulations of fentanyl.) Therefore, for opioid tolerant patients, the initial dose of *FENTORA* should be 100 mcg. Each patient should be individually titrated to provide adequate analgesia while minimizing side effects. (See **DOSAGE AND ADMINISTRATION**.)

Use with CNS Depressants

The concomitant use of other CNS depressants, including other opioids, sedatives or hypnotics, general anesthetics, phenothiazines, tranquilizers, skeletal muscle relaxants, sedating antihistamines, potent inhibitors of cytochrome P450 3A4 isoform (e.g., erythromycin, ketoconazole, and certain protease inhibitors), and alcoholic beverages may produce increased depressant effects. Hypoventilation, hypotension, and profound sedation may occur.

FENTORA is not recommended for use in patients who have received MAO inhibitors within 14 days, because severe and unpredictable potentiation by MAO inhibitors has been reported with opioid analgesics.

Pediatric Use: The safety and efficacy of *FENTORA* have not been established in pediatric patients below the age of 18 years.

Patients and their caregivers must be instructed that *FENTORA* **contains a medicine in an amount which can be fatal to a child.** Patients and their caregivers must be instructed to keep tablets out of the reach of children. (See **SAFETY AND HANDLING, PRECAUTIONS,** and **MEDICATION GUIDE** for specific patient instructions.)

Drug Abuse, Addiction and Diversion of Opioids

FENTORA contains fentanyl, a mu-opioid agonist and a Schedule II controlled substance with high potential for abuse similar to hydromorphone, methadone, morphine, oxycodone, and oxymorphone. Fentanyl can be abused and is subject to misuse, and criminal diversion.

Concerns about abuse, addiction, and diversion should not prevent the proper management of pain. However, all patients treated with opioids require careful monitoring for signs of abuse and addiction, since use of opioid analgesic products carries the risk of addiction even under appropriate medical use.

Addiction is a primary, chronic, neurobiologic disease, with genetic, psychosocial, and environmental factors influencing its development and manifestations. It is characterized by behaviors that include one or more of the following: impaired control over drug use, compulsive use, continued use despite harm, and craving. Drug addiction is a treatable disease, utilizing a multidisciplinary approach, but relapse is common.

"Drug-seeking" behavior is very common in addicts and drug abusers.

Abuse and addiction are separate and distinct from physical dependence and tolerance. Physicians should be aware that addiction may not be accompanied by concurrent tolerance and symptoms of physical dependence in all addicts. In addition, abuse of opioids can occur in the absence of addiction and is characterized by misuse for non-medical purposes, often in combination with other psychoactive substances. Since *FENTORA* tablets may be diverted for non-medical use, careful record keeping of prescribing information, including quantity, frequency, and renewal requests is strongly advised.

Proper assessment of patients, proper prescribing practices, periodic re-evaluation of therapy, and proper dispensing and storage are appropriate measures that help to limit abuse of opioid drugs.

FENTORA should be handled appropriately to minimize the risk of diversion, including restriction of access and accounting procedures as appropriate to the clinical setting and as required by law.

Healthcare professionals should contact their State Professional Licensing Board, or State Controlled Substances Authority for information on how to prevent and detect abuse or diversion of this product.

Physical Dependence and Withdrawal

The administration of *FENTORA* should be guided by the response of the patient. Physical dependence, per se, is not ordinarily a concern when one is treating a patient with cancer and chronic pain, and fear of tolerance and physical dependence should not deter using doses that adequately relieve the pain.

Opioid analgesics may cause physical dependence. Physical dependence results in withdrawal symptoms in patients who abruptly discontinue the drug. Withdrawal also may be precipitated through the administration of drugs with opioid antagonist activity, e.g., naloxone, nalmefene, or mixed agonist/antagonist analgesics (pentazocine, butorphanol, buprenorphine, nalbuphine).

Physical dependence usually does not occur to a clinically significant degree until after several weeks of continued opioid usage. Tolerance, in which increasingly larger doses are required in order to produce the same degree of analgesia, is initially manifested by a shortened duration of analgesic effect, and subsequently, by decreases in the intensity of analgesia.

Respiratory Depression

Respiratory depression is the chief hazard of opioid agonists, including fentanyl, the active ingredient in *FENTORA*. Respiratory depression is more likely to occur in patients with underlying respiratory disorders and elderly or debilitated patients, usually following large initial doses in opioid non-tolerant patients, or when opioids are given in conjunction with other drugs that depress respiration.

Respiratory depression from opioids is manifested by a reduced urge to breathe and a decreased rate of respiration, often associated with the "sighing" pattern of breathing (deep breaths separated by abnormally long pauses). Carbon dioxide retention from opioid-induced respiratory depression can exacerbate the sedating effects of opioids. This makes overdoses involving drugs with sedative properties and opioids especially dangerous.

Table 5.
Adverse Events Which Occurred During Titration at a Frequency of ≥5%

System Organ Class MeDRA preferred term, n (%)	100 mcg (N=45)	200 mcg (N=34)	400 mcg (N=53)	600 mcg (N=56)	800 mcg (N=113)	Total (N=304)*
Gastrointestinal disorders						
Nausea	4 (9)	5 (15)	10 (19)	13 (23)	18 (16)	50 (17)
Vomiting	0	2 (6)	2 (4)	7 (13)	3 (3)	14 (5)
General disorders and administration site conditions						
Fatigue	3 (7)	1 (3)	9 (17)	1 (2)	5 (4)	19 (6)
Nervous system disorders						
Dizziness	5 (11)	2 (6)	12 (23)	18 (32)	21 (19)	58 (19)
Somnolence	2 (4)	2 (6)	6 (12)	7 (13)	3 (3)	20 (7)
Headache	1 (2)	3 (9)	4 (8)	8 (14)	10 (9)	26 (9)

* Three hundred and two (302) patients were included in the safety analysis.

PRECAUTIONS

General

Opioid analgesics impair the mental and/or physical ability required for the performance of potentially dangerous tasks (e.g., driving a car or operating machinery). Patients taking *FENTORA* should be warned of these dangers and should be counseled accordingly.

The use of concomitant CNS active drugs requires special patient care and observation. (See **WARNINGS**.)

Chronic Pulmonary Disease

Because potent opioids can cause respiratory depression, *FENTORA* should be titrated with caution in patients with chronic obstructive pulmonary disease or pre-existing medical conditions predisposing them to respiratory depression. In such patients, even normal therapeutic doses of *FENTORA* may further decrease respiratory drive to the point of respiratory failure.

Head Injuries and Increased Intracranial Pressure

FENTORA should only be administered with extreme caution in patients who may be particularly susceptible to the intracranial effects of CO_2 retention such as those with evidence of increased intracranial pressure or impaired consciousness. Opioids may obscure the clinical course of a patient with a head injury and should be used only if clinically warranted.

Application Site Reactions

In clinical trials, 10% of all patients exposed to *FENTORA* reported application site reactions. These reactions ranged from paresthesia to ulceration and bleeding. Application site reactions occurring in ≥1% of patients were pain (4%), ulcer (3%), and irritation (3%). Application site reactions tended to occur early in treatment, were self-limited and only resulted in treatment discontinuation for 2% of patients.

Cardiac Disease

Intravenous fentanyl may produce bradycardia. Therefore, *FENTORA* should be used with caution in patients with bradyarrhythmias.

Hepatic or Renal Disease

Insufficient information exists to make recommendations regarding the use of *FENTORA* in patients with impaired renal or hepatic function. Fentanyl is metabolized primarily via human cytochrome P450 3A4 isoenzyme system and mostly eliminated in urine. If the drug is used in these patients, it should be used with caution because of the hepatic metabolism and renal excretion of fentanyl.

Information for Patients and Caregivers

1. **Patients and their caregivers must be instructed that children, especially small children, exposed to** *FENTORA* **are at high risk of FATAL RESPIRATORY DEPRESSION.** Patients and their caregivers must be instructed to keep *FENTORA* tablets out of the reach of children. (See **SAFETY AND HANDLING, WARNINGS,** and **MEDICATION GUIDE** for specific patient instructions.)

2. Patients and their caregivers must be provided a Medication Guide each time *FENTORA* is dispensed because new information may be available.

3. Patients must be instructed not to take *FENTORA* for acute pain, postoperative pain, pain from injuries, headache, migraine or any other short term pain, even if they have taken other opioid analgesics for these conditions.

4. Patients must be instructed on the meaning of opioid tolerance and that *FENTORA* is only to be used as a supplemental pain medication for patients with pain requiring around-the-clock opioids, who have developed tolerance to the opioid medication, and who need additional opioid treatment of breakthrough pain episodes.

5. Patients must be instructed that, if they are not taking an opioid medication on a scheduled basis (around-the-clock), they should not take *FENTORA*.

6. Patients should be instructed that the titration phase is the only period in which they may take more than ONE tablet to achieve a desired dose (e.g., two 100 mcg tablets for a 200 mcg dose).

7. Patients must be instructed that, if the breakthrough pain episode is not relieved after 30 minutes, they may take ONLY ONE ADDITIONAL DOSE OF *FENTORA* US-

ING THE SAME STRENGTH FOR THAT EPISODE. Thus, patients should take a maximum of two doses of *FENTORA* for any breakthrough pain episode.

8. Patients must be instructed that they MUST wait at least 4 hours before treating another episode of breakthrough pain with *FENTORA*.

9. Patients must be instructed NOT to share *FENTORA* and that sharing *FENTORA* with anyone else could result in the other individual's death due to overdose.

10. Patients must be aware that *FENTORA* contains fentanyl which is a strong pain medication similar to hydromorphone, methadone, morphine, oxycodone, and oxymorphone.

11. Patients must be instructed that the active ingredient in *FENTORA*, fentanyl, is a drug that some people abuse. *FENTORA* should be taken only by the patient it was prescribed for, and it should be protected from theft or misuse in the work or home environment.

12. Patients should be instructed that *FENTORA* tablets are not to be swallowed whole; this will reduce the effectiveness of the medication. Tablets are to be placed between the cheek and gum above a molar tooth and allowed to dissolve. After 30 minutes if remnants of the tablet still remain, patients may swallow it with a glass of water.

13. Patients must be cautioned to talk to their doctor if breakthrough pain is not alleviated or worsens after taking *FENTORA*.

14. Patients must be instructed to use *FENTORA* exactly as prescribed by their doctor and not to take *FENTORA* more often than prescribed.

15. Patients must be cautioned that *FENTORA* can affect a person's ability to perform activities that require a high level of attention (such as driving or using heavy machinery). Patients taking *FENTORA* should be warned of these dangers and counseled accordingly.

16. Patients must be warned to not combine *FENTORA* with alcohol, sleep aids, or tranquilizers except by the orders of the prescribing physician, because dangerous additive effects may occur, resulting in serious injury or death.

17. Female patients must be informed that if they become pregnant or plan to become pregnant during treatment with *FENTORA*, they should ask their doctor about the effects that *FENTORA* (or any medicine) may have on them and their unborn children.

18. Patients and caregivers must be advised that if they have been receiving treatment with *FENTORA* and the medicine is no longer needed they should flush any remaining product down the toilet, and if they then need further assistance, contact Cephalon at 1-800-896-5855.

Disposal of Unopened *FENTORA* Blister Packages When No Longer Needed

Patients and members of their household must be advised to dispose of any unopened blister packages remaining from a prescription as soon as they are no longer needed.

To dispose of unused *FENTORA*, remove *FENTORA* tablets from blister packages and flush down the toilet. Do not flush the *FENTORA* blister packages or cartons down the toilet. (See **SAFETY AND HANDLING**.)

Detailed instructions for the proper storage, administration, disposal, and important instructions for managing an overdose of *FENTORA* are provided in the *FENTORA* Medication Guide. Patients should be encouraged to read this information in its entirety and be given an opportunity to have their questions answered.

In the event that a caregiver requires additional assistance in disposing of excess unusable tablets that remain in the home after a patient has expired, they should be instructed to call the Cephalon toll-free number (1-800-896-5855) or seek assistance from their local DEA office.

Laboratory Tests

The effects of *FENTORA* on laboratory tests have not been evaluated.

Continued on next page

Fentora—Cont.

Drug Interactions
See **WARNINGS.**

Fentanyl is metabolized mainly via the human cytochrome P450 3A4 isoenzyme system (CYP3A4); therefore potential interactions may occur when *FENTORA* is given concurrently with agents that affect CYP3A4 activity. The concomitant use of *FENTORA* with strong CYP3A4 inhibitors (e.g., ritonavir, ketoconazole, itraconazole, troleandomycin, clarithromycin, nelfinavir, and nefazadone) or moderate CYP3A4 inhibitors (e.g., amprenavir, aprepitant, diltiazem, erythromycin, fluconazole, fosamprenavir, and verapamil) may result in increased fentanyl plasma concentrations, potentially causing serious adverse drug effects including fatal respiratory depression. Patients receiving *FENTORA* concomitantly with moderate or strong CYP3A4 inhibitors should be carefully monitored for an extended period of time. Dosage increase should be done conservatively. (See **PHARMACOKINETICS, Drug Interactions** and **DOSAGE AND ADMINISTRATION.**)

Grapefruit and grapefruit juice decrease CYP3A4 activity, increasing blood concentrations of fentanyl, thus should be avoided.

Drugs that induce cytochrome P450 3A4 activity may have the opposite effects.

Concomitant use of *FENTORA* with an MAO inhibitor, or within 14 days of discontinuation, is not recommended.

Carcinogenesis, Mutagenesis, and Impairment of Fertility
Long-term studies in animals have not been performed to evaluate the carcinogenic potential of fentanyl.

Fentanyl citrate was not mutagenic in the *in vitro* Ames reverse mutation assay in *S. tymphimurium* or *E. coli*, or the mouse lymphoma mutagenesis assay. Fentanyl citrate was not clastogenic in the *in vivo* mouse micronucleus assay.

Fentanyl impairs fertility in rats at doses of 30 mcg/kg IV and 160 mcg/kg SC. Conversion to human equivalent doses indicates this is within the range of the human recommended dosing for *FENTORA*.

Pregnancy - Category C
There are no adequate and well-controlled studies in pregnant women. *FENTORA* should be used during pregnancy only if the potential benefit justifies the potential risk to the fetus. No epidemiological studies of congenital anomalies in infants born to women treated with fentanyl during pregnancy have been reported.

Chronic maternal treatment with fentanyl during pregnancy has been associated with transient respiratory depression, behavioral changes, or seizures characteristic of neonatal abstinence syndrome in newborn infants. Symptoms of neonatal respiratory or neurological depression were no more frequent than expected in most studies of infants born to women treated acutely during labor with intravenous or epidural fentanyl. Transient neonatal muscular rigidity has been observed in infants whose mothers were treated with intravenous fentanyl.

Fentanyl is embryocidal as evidenced by increased resorptions in pregnant rats at doses of 30 mcg/kg IV or 160 mcg/kg SC. Conversion to human equivalent doses indicates this is within the range of the human recommended dosing for *FENTORA*.

Fentanyl citrate was not teratogenic when administered to pregnant animals. Published studies demonstrated that administration of fentanyl (10, 100, or 500 mcg/kg/day) to pregnant rats from day 7 to 21, of their 21 day gestation, via implanted microosmotic minipumps was not teratogenic (the high dose was approximately 3-times the human dose of 1600 mcg per pain episode on a mg/m² basis). Intravenous administration of fentanyl (10 or 30 mcg/kg) to pregnant female rats from gestation day 6 to 18, was embryo or fetal toxic, and caused a slightly increased mean delivery time in the 30 mcg/kg/day group, but was not teratogenic.

Labor and Delivery
Fentanyl readily passes across the placenta to the fetus; therefore *FENTORA* is not recommended for analgesia during labor and delivery.

Nursing Mothers
Fentanyl is excreted in human milk; therefore *FENTORA* should not be used in nursing women because of the possibility of sedation and/or respiratory depression in their infants. Symptoms of opioid withdrawal may occur in infants at the cessation of nursing by women using *FENTORA*.

Pediatric Use
See **WARNINGS.**

Geriatric Use
Of the 304 patients with cancer in clinical studies of *FENTORA*, 69 (23%) were 65 years of age and older.

Patients over the age of 65 years tended to titrate to slightly lower doses than younger patients.

Patients over the age of 65 years reported a slightly higher frequency for some adverse events specifically vomiting, constipation, and abdominal pain. Therefore, caution should be exercised in individually titrating *FENTORA* in elderly patients to provide adequate efficacy while minimizing risk.

ADVERSE REACTIONS
Pre-Marketing Clinical Trial Experience
The safety of *FENTORA* has been evaluated in 304 opioid tolerant cancer patients with breakthrough pain. The average duration of therapy was 76 days with some patients being treated for over 12 months.

The most commonly observed adverse events seen with *FENTORA* are typical of opioid side effects. Opioid side effects should be expected and managed accordingly.

Table 6.
Adverse Events Which Occurred During Long-Term Treatment at a Frequency of ≥5%

System Organ Class MeDRA preferred term, n (%)	100 mcg (N=19)	200 mcg (N=31)	400 mcg (N=44)	600 mcg (N=48)	800 mcg (N=58)	Total (N=200)
Blood and lymphatic system disorders						
Anemia	6 (32)	4 (13)	4 (9)	5 (10)	7 (13)	26 (13)
Neutropenia	0	2 (6)	1 (2)	4 (8)	4 (7)	11 (6)
Gastrointestinal disorders						
Nausea	8 (42)	5 (16)	14 (32)	13 (27)	17 (31)	57 (29)
Vomiting	7 (37)	5 (16)	9 (20)	8 (17)	11 (20)	40 (20)
Constipation	5 (26)	4 (13)	5 (11)	4 (8)	6 (11)	24 (12)
Diarrhea	3 (16)	0	4 (9)	3 (6)	5 (9)	15 (8)
Abdominal pain	2 (11)	1 (3)	4 (9)	7 (15)	4 (7)	18 (9)
General disorders and administration site conditions						
Edema peripheral	6 (32)	5 (16)	4 (9)	5 (10)	3 (5)	23 (12)
Asthenia	3 (16)	5 (16)	2 (5)	3 (6)	8 (15)	21 (11)
Fatigue	3 (16)	3 (10)	9 (20)	9 (19)	8 (15)	32 (16)
Infections and infestations						
Pneumonia	1 (5)	5 (16)	1 (2)	1 (2)	4 (7)	12 (6)
Investigations						
Weight decreased	1 (5)	1 (3)	3 (7)	2 (4)	6 (11)	13 (7)
Metabolism and nutrition disorders						
Dehydration	4 (21)	0	4 (9)	6 (13)	7 (13)	21 (11)
Anorexia	1 (5)	2 (6)	4 (9)	3 (6)	6 (11)	16 (8)
Hypokalemia	0	2 (6)	0	1 (2)	8 (15)	11 (6)
Musculoskeletal and connective tissue disorders						
Back pain	2 (11)	0	2 (5)	3 (6)	2 (4)	9 (5)
Arthralgia	0	1 (3)	3 (7)	4 (8)	3 (5)	11 (6)
Neoplasms benign, malignant and unspecified (including cysts and polyps)						
Cancer pain	3 (16)	1 (3)	3 (7)	2 (4)	1 (2)	10 (5)
Nervous system disorders						
Dizziness	5 (26)	3 (10)	5 (11)	6 (13)	6 (11)	25 (13)
Headache	2 (11)	1 (3)	4 (9)	5 (10)	8 (15)	20 (10)
Somnolence	0	1 (3)	4 (9)	4 (8)	8 (15)	17 (9)
Psychiatric disorders						
Confusional state	3 (16)	1 (3)	2 (5)	3 (6)	5 (9)	14 (7)
Depression	2 (11)	1 (3)	4 (9)	3 (6)	5 (9)	15 (8)
Insomnia	2 (11)	1 (3)	3 (7)	2 (4)	4 (7)	12 (6)
Respiratory, thoracic, and mediastinal disorders						
Cough	1 (5)	1 (3)	2 (5)	4 (8)	5 (9)	13 (7)
Dyspnea	1 (5)	6 (19)	0	7 (15)	4 (7)	18 (9)

The clinical trials of *FENTORA* were designed to evaluate safety and efficacy in treating patients with cancer and breakthrough pain; all patients were taking concomitant opioids, such as sustained-release morphine, sustained-release oxycodone or transdermal fentanyl, for their persistent pain.

The adverse event data presented here reflect the actual percentage of patients experiencing each adverse effect among patients who received *FENTORA* for breakthrough pain along with a concomitant opioid for persistent pain. There has been no attempt to correct for concomitant use of other opioids, duration of *FENTORA* therapy or cancer-related symptoms.

Table 5 lists, by maximum dose received, adverse events with an overall frequency of 5% or greater within the total population that occurred during titration. The ability to assign a dose-response relationship to these adverse events is limited by the titration schemes used in these studies.
[See table 5 at top of previous page]

Table 6 lists, by successful dose, adverse events with an overall frequency of ≥ 5% within the total population that occurred after a successful dose had been determined.
[See table 6 above]

In addition, a small number of patients (n=11) with Grade 1 mucositis were included in clinical trials designed to support the safety of *FENTORA*. There was no evidence of excess toxicity in this subset of patients.

The duration of exposure to *FENTORA* varied greatly, and included open-label and double-blind studies. The frequencies listed below represent the ≥1% of patients from three clinical trials (titration and post-titration periods combined) who experienced that event while receiving *FENTORA*. Events are classified by system organ class.

Adverse Events (≥1%)

Blood and Lymphatic System Disorders: Anemia, Neutropenia, Thrombocytopenia, Leukopenia

Cardiac Disorders: Tachycardia

Gastrointestinal Disorders: Nausea, Vomiting, Constipation, Abdominal Pain, Diarrhea, Stomatitis, Dry Mouth, Dyspepsia, Upper Abdominal Pain, Abdominal Distension, Dysphagia, Gingival Pain, Stomach Discomfort, Gastroesophageal Reflux Disease, Glossodynia, Mouth Ulceration

General Disorders and Administration Site Conditions: Fatigue, Edema Peripheral, Asthenia, Pyrexia, Application Site Pain, Application Site Ulcer, Chest Pain, Chills, Application Site Irritation, Edema, Mucosal Inflammation, Pain

Hepatobiliary Disorders: Jaundice

Infections and Infestations: Pneumonia, Oral Candidiasis, Urinary Tract Infection, Cellulitis, Nasopharyngitis, Sinusitis, Upper Respiratory Tract Infection, Influenza, Tooth Abscess

Injury, Poisoning and Procedural Complications: Fall, Spinal Compression Fracture

Investigations: Decreased Weight, Decreased Hemoglobin, Increased Blood Glucose, Decreased Hematocrit, Decreased Platelet Count
Metabolism and Nutrition Disorders: Dehydration, Anorexia, Hypokalemia, Decreased Appetite, Hypoalbuminemia, Hypercalcemia, Hypomagnesemia, Hyponatremia, Reduced Oral Intake
Musculoskeletal and Connective Tissue Disorders: Arthralgia, Back Pain, Pain in Extremity, Myalgia, Chest Wall Pain, Muscle Spasms, Neck Pain, Shoulder Pain
Nervous System Disorders: Dizziness, Headache, Somnolence, Hypoesthesia, Dysgeusia, Lethargy, Peripheral Neuropathy, Paresthesia, Balance Disorder, Migraine, Neuropathy
Psychiatric Disorders: Confusional State, Depression, Insomnia, Anxiety, Disorientation, Euphoric Mood, Hallucination, Nervousness
Renal and Urinary Disorders: Renal Failure
Respiratory, Thoracic and Mediastinal Disorders: Dyspnea, Cough, Pharyngolaryngeal Pain, Exertional Dyspnea, Pleural Effusion, Decreased Breathing Sounds, Wheezing
Skin and Subcutaneous Tissue Disorders: Pruritus, Rash, Hyperhidrosis, Cold Sweat
Vascular Disorders: Hypertension, Hypotension, Pallor, Deep Vein Thrombosis

OVERDOSAGE

Clinical Presentation

The manifestations of *FENTORA* overdosage are expected to be similar in nature to intravenous fentanyl and other opioids, and are an extension of its pharmacological actions with the most serious significant effect being hypoventilation. (See **CLINICAL PHARMACOLOGY**.)

General

Immediate management of opioid overdose includes removal of the *FENTORA* tablet, if still in the mouth, ensuring a patent airway, physical and verbal stimulation of the patient, and assessment of level of consciousness, as well as ventilatory and circulatory status.

Treatment of Overdosage in the Opioid Non-Tolerant Person

Ventilatory support should be provided, intravenous access obtained, and naloxone or other opioid antagonists should be employed as clinically indicated. The duration of respiratory depression following overdose may be longer than the effects of the opioid antagonist's action (e.g., the half-life of naloxone ranges from 30 to 81 minutes) and repeated administration may be necessary. Consult the package insert of the individual opioid antagonist for details about such use.

Treatment of Overdose in Opioid-Tolerant Patients

Ventilatory support should be provided and intravenous access obtained as clinically indicated. Judicious use of naloxone or another opioid antagonist may be warranted in some instances, but it is associated with the risk of precipitating an acute withdrawal syndrome.

General Considerations for Overdose

Management of severe *FENTORA* overdose includes: securing a patent airway, assisting or controlling ventilation, establishing intravenous access, and GI decontamination by lavage and/or activated charcoal, once the patient's airway is secure. In the presence of hypoventilation or apnea, ventilation should be assisted or controlled and oxygen administered as indicated.

Patients with overdose should be carefully observed and appropriately managed until their clinical condition is well controlled.

Although muscle rigidity interfering with respiration has not been seen following the use of *FENTORA*, this is possible with fentanyl and other opioids. If it occurs, it should be managed by the use of assisted or controlled ventilation, by an opioid antagonist, and as a final alternative, by a neuromuscular blocking agent.

DOSAGE AND ADMINISTRATION

Physicians should individualize treatment using a progressive plan of pain management. Healthcare professionals should follow appropriate pain management principles of careful assessment and ongoing monitoring. (See **BOXED WARNING** and **Dosing.**)

It is important to minimize the number of strengths available to patients at any time to prevent confusion and possible overdose.

Dosing

1. Initial Dose

a. For opioid-tolerant patients **not** being converted from Actiq, the initial dose of *FENTORA* is **always** 100 mcg.
b. For patients being converted from Actiq, prescribers must use the Initial Dosing Recommendations table below (Table 7). The doses of *FENTORA* in this table are starting doses and not intended to represent equianalgesic doses to Actiq. Patients must be instructed to stop the use of Actiq and dispose of any remaining units.

Table 7. Initial Dosing Recommendations for Patients on Actiq

Current Actiq Dose (mcg)	Initial *FENTORA* Dose (mcg)
200	100 mcg tablet
400	100 mcg tablet
600	200 mcg tablet
800	200 mcg tablet
1200	2 × 200 mcg tablets
1600	2 × 200 mcg tablets

c. For patients converting from Actiq doses equal to or greater than 600 mcg, titration should be initiated with the 200 mcg *FENTORA* tablet and should proceed using multiples of this tablet strength.
d. In cases where the breakthrough pain episode is not relieved after 30 minutes, patients may take **ONLY ONE** additional dose using the same strength for that episode. Thus patients should take a maximum of two doses of *FENTORA* for any episode of breakthrough pain.
e. Patients MUST wait **at least 4 hours** before treating another episode of breakthrough pain with *FENTORA*.

2. Titration

a. From an initial dose, patients should be closely followed by the prescriber and the dosage strength changed until the patient reaches a dose that provides adequate analgesia with tolerable side effects. Patients should record their use of *FENTORA* over several episodes of breakthrough pain and discuss their experience with their physician to determine if a dosage adjustment is warranted.
b. Patients whose initial dose is 100 mcg and who need to titrate to a higher dose, can be instructed to use two 100-mcg tablets (one on each side of the mouth in the buccal cavity) with their next breakthrough pain episode. If this dosage is not successful, the patient may be instructed to place two 100-mcg tablets on each side of the mouth in the buccal cavity (total of four 100-mcg tablets). Titrate using multiples of the 200-mcg *FENTORA* tablet for doses above 400 mcg (600 mcg and 800 mcg). Note: Do not use more than 4 tablets simultaneously.
c. In cases where the breakthrough pain episode is not relieved after 30 minutes, patients may take **ONLY ONE** additional dose of the same strength for that episode. Thus patients should take a maximum of two doses of *FENTORA* for any breakthrough pain episode. During titration, one **dose** of *FENTORA* may include administration of 1 to 4 tablets of the same dosage strength (100 mcg or 200 mcg).
d. Patients MUST wait **at least 4 hours** before treating another episode of breakthrough pain with *FENTORA*. To reduce the risk of overdosing during titration, patients should have only one strength of *FENTORA* tablets available at any one time.
e. Patients should be strongly encouraged to use all of their *FENTORA* tablets of one strength prior to being prescribed the next strength. If this is not practical, unused *FENTORA* should be disposed of safely. (See **DISPOSAL OF *FENTORA*.**) Dispose of any unopened *FENTORA* tablets remaining from a prescription as soon as they are no longer needed.

3. Maintenance Dosing

a. Once titrated to an effective dose, patients should generally use **only ONE** *FENTORA* tablet of the appropriate strength per breakthrough pain episode.
b. On occasion when the breakthrough pain episode is not relieved after 30 minutes, patients may take **ONLY ONE** additional dose using the same strength for that episode.
c. Patients MUST wait **at least 4 hours** before treating another episode of breakthrough pain with *FENTORA*.
d. Dosage adjustment of *FENTORA* may be required in some patients in order to continue to provide adequate relief of breakthrough pain.

Generally, the *FENTORA* dose should be increased only when a single administration of the current dose fails to adequately treat the breakthrough pain episode for several consecutive episodes.

If the patient experiences greater than four breakthrough pain episodes per day, the dose of the maintenance (around-the-clock) opioid used for persistent pain should be reevaluated.

Patients with hepatic and/or renal impairment

Caution should be exercised for patients with hepatic and/or renal impairment, and the lowest possible dose should be used in these patients. (See **PRECAUTIONS.**)

Patients receiving CYP3A4 inhibitors

Particular caution should be exercised for patients receiving CYP3A4 inhibitors, and the lowest possible dose should be used in these patients. (See **PRECAUTIONS.**)

Patients with mucositis

No dose adjustment appears necessary in patients with Grade 1 mucositis. The safety and efficacy of *FENTORA* when used in patients with mucositis more severe than Grade 1 have not been studied.

Opening the Blister Package

1. Patients should be instructed not to open the blister until ready to administer *FENTORA*.
2. A single blister unit should be separated from the blister card by bending and tearing apart at the perforations.
3. The blister unit should then be bent along the line where indicated.
4. The blister backing should then be peeled back to expose the tablet. **Patients should NOT attempt to push the tablet through the blister as this may cause damage to the tablet.**
5. The tablet should not be stored once it has been removed from the blister package as the tablet integrity may be compromised, and more importantly, because this increases the risk of accidental exposure to the tablet.

Tablet Administration

Once the tablet is removed from the blister unit, the patient should **immediately** place the entire *FENTORA* tablet in the buccal cavity (above a rear molar, between the upper cheek and gum). **Patients should not split the tablet.**

The *FENTORA* tablet should not be sucked, chewed or swallowed, as this will result in lower plasma concentrations than when taken as directed.

The *FENTORA* tablet should be left between the cheek and gum until it has disintegrated, which usually takes approximately 14-25 minutes.

After 30 minutes, if remnants from the *FENTORA* tablet remain, they may be swallowed with a glass of water.

It is recommended that patients alternate sides of the mouth when administering subsequent doses of *FENTORA*.

SAFETY AND HANDLING

FENTORA is supplied in individually sealed, child-resistant blister packages. The amount of fentanyl contained in *FENTORA* can be fatal to a child. **Patients and their caregivers must be instructed to keep *FENTORA* out of the reach of children.** (See **BOXED WARNING, WARNINGS, PRECAUTIONS,** and **MEDICATION GUIDE.**)

Store at 20-25°C (68-77°F) with excursions permitted between 15° and 30°C (59° to 86°F) until ready to use. (See USP Controlled Room Temperature.)

FENTORA should be protected from freezing and moisture. Do not use if the blister package has been tampered with.

DISPOSAL OF FENTORA

Patients and members of their household must be advised to dispose of any tablets remaining from a prescription as soon as they are no longer needed. Information is available in the **Information for Patients and Caregivers** and in the Medication Guide. If additional assistance is required, referral to the Cephalon 800# (1-800-896-5855) should be made.

To dispose of unused *FENTORA*, remove *FENTORA* tablets from blister packages and flush down the toilet. Do not flush *FENTORA* blister packages or cartons down the toilet. If you need additional assistance with disposal of *FENTORA*, call Cephalon, Inc., at 1-800-896-5855.

HOW SUPPLIED

Each carton contains 7 blister cards with 4 white tablets in each card. The blisters are child-resistant, encased in peelable foil, and provide protection from moisture. Each tablet is debossed on one side with [C], and the other side of each dosage strength is uniquely identified by the debossing on the tablet as described in the table below. The dosage strength of each tablet is marked on the tablet, the blister package and the carton. See blister package and carton for product information.

Dosage Strength (fentanyl base)	Debossing	Carton/ Blister Package Color	NDC Number
100 mcg	1	Blue	NDC 63459-541-28
200 mcg	2	Orange	NDC 63459-542-28
300 mcg	3	Gray	NDC 63459-543-28
400 mcg	4	Sage green	NDC 63459-544-28
600 mcg	6	Magenta (pink)	NDC 63459-546-28
800 mcg	8	Yellow	NDC 63459-548-28

Note: Carton/blister package colors are a secondary aid in product identification. Please be sure to confirm the printed dosage before dispensing.

Rx only.
DEA order form required. A Schedule CII narcotic.
Manufactured for:
Cephalon, Inc.
Frazer, PA 19355
By:
CIMA LABS, INC.
10000 Valley View Road
Eden Prairie, MN 55344
and
Cephalon, Inc.
4745 Wiley Post Way
Salt Lake City, UT 84116
U. S. Patent Nos. 6,200,604 and 6,974,590
Printed in USA
Label code 074000107.03
October 2007
©2006, 2007 Cephalon, Inc. All rights reserved.
FENT218

Continued on next page

VIVITROL® ℞

[vĭ-vĭ-trōl]

(naltrexone for extended-release injectable suspension) 380 mg/vial

Prescribing information for this product, which appears on pages 972–976 of the 2008 PDR, has been completely revised as follows. Please write "See Supplement A" next to the product heading.

DESCRIPTION

VIVITROL® (naltrexone for extended-release injectable suspension) is supplied as a microsphere formulation of naltrexone for suspension, to be administered by intramuscular injection. Naltrexone is an opioid antagonist with little, if any, opioid agonist activity.

Naltrexone is designated chemically as morphinan-6-one, 17-(cyclopropylmethyl)-4,5-epoxy-3,14-dihydroxy-(5α) (CAS Registry # 16590-41-3). The molecular formula is $C_{20}H_{23}NO_4$ and its molecular weight is 341.41 in the anhydrous form (i.e., < 1% maximum water content). The structural formula is:

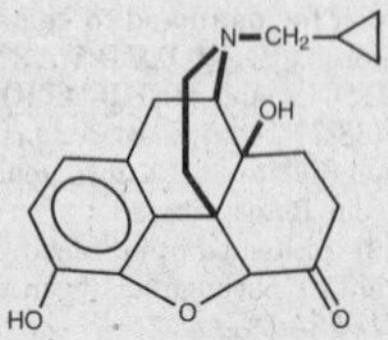

Naltrexone base anhydrous is an off-white to a light tan powder with a melting point of 168-170° C (334-338° F). It is insoluble in water and is soluble in ethanol.

VIVITROL is provided as a carton containing a vial each of VIVITROL microspheres and diluent, one 5-mL syringe, one ½-inch 20-gauge preparation needle, and two 1½-inch 20-gauge administration needles with safety device.

VIVITROL microspheres consist of a sterile, off-white to light tan powder that is available in a dosage strength of 380-mg naltrexone per vial. Naltrexone is incorporated in 75:25 polylactide-co-glycolide (PLG) at a concentration of 337 mg of naltrexone per gram of microspheres.

The diluent is a clear, colorless solution. The composition of the diluent includes carboxymethylcellulose sodium salt, polysorbate 20, sodium chloride, and water for injection. The microspheres must be suspended in the diluent prior to injection.

CLINICAL PHARMACOLOGY

Pharmacodynamics

Mechanism of Action

Naltrexone is an opioid antagonist with highest affinity for the mu opioid receptor. Naltrexone has few, if any, intrinsic actions besides its opioid blocking properties. However, it does produce some pupillary constriction, by an unknown mechanism.

The administration of VIVITROL is not associated with the development of tolerance or dependence. In subjects physically dependent on opioids, VIVITROL will precipitate withdrawal symptomatology.

Occupation of opioid receptors by naltrexone may block the effects of endogenous opioid peptides. The neurobiological mechanisms responsible for the reduction in alcohol consumption observed in alcohol-dependent patients treated with naltrexone are not entirely understood. However, involvement of the endogenous opioid system is suggested by preclinical data.

Naltrexone blocks the effects of opioids by competitive binding at opioid receptors. This makes the blockade produced potentially surmountable, but overcoming full naltrexone blockade by administration of opioids may result in non-opioid receptor-mediated symptoms such as histamine release.

VIVITROL is not aversive therapy and does not cause a disulfiram-like reaction either as a result of opiate use or ethanol ingestion.

Pharmacokinetics

Absorption

VIVITROL is an extended-release, microsphere formulation of naltrexone designed to be administered by intramuscular (IM) gluteal injection every 4 weeks or once a month. After IM injection, the naltrexone plasma concentration time profile is characterized by a transient initial peak, which occurs approximately 2 hours after injection, followed by a second peak observed approximately 2-3 days later. Beginning approximately 14 days after dosing, concentrations slowly decline, with measurable levels for greater than 1 month.

Maximum plasma concentration (C_{max}) and area under the curve (AUC) for naltrexone and 6β-naltrexol (the major metabolite) following VIVITROL administration are dose proportional. Compared to daily oral dosing with naltrexone 50 mg over 28 days, total naltrexone exposure is 3 to 4-fold higher following administration of a single dose of VIVITROL 380 mg. Steady state is reached at the end of the dosing interval following the first injection. There is minimal accumulation (<15%) of naltrexone or 6β-naltrexol upon repeat administration of VIVITROL.

Distribution

In vitro data demonstrate that naltrexone plasma protein binding is low (21%).

Metabolism

Naltrexone is extensively metabolized in humans. Production of the primary metabolite, 6β-naltrexol, is mediated by dihydrodiol dehydrogenase, a cytosolic family of enzymes. The cytochrome P450 system is not involved in naltrexone metabolism. Two other minor metabolites are 2-hydroxy-3-methoxy-6β-naltrexol and 2-hydroxy-3-methoxy-naltrexone. Naltrexone and its metabolites are also conjugated to form glucuronide products.

Significantly less 6β-naltrexol is generated following IM administration of VIVITROL compared to administration of oral naltrexone due to a reduction in first-pass hepatic metabolism.

Elimination

Elimination of naltrexone and its metabolites occurs primarily via urine, with minimal excretion of unchanged naltrexone.

The elimination half life of naltrexone following VIVITROL administration is 5 to 10 days and is dependent on the erosion of the polymer. The elimination half life of 6β-naltrexol following VIVITROL administration is 5 to 10 days.

Special Populations

Hepatic Impairment: The pharmacokinetics of VIVITROL are not altered in subjects with mild to moderate hepatic impairment (Groups A and B of the Child-Pugh classification). Dose adjustment is not required in subjects with mild or moderate hepatic impairment. VIVITROL pharmacokinetics were not evaluated in subjects with severe hepatic impairment **(see PRECAUTIONS)**.

Renal Impairment: A population pharmacokinetic analysis indicated mild renal insufficiency (creatinine clearance of 50-80 mL/min) had little or no influence on VIVITROL pharmacokinetics and that no dosage adjustment is necessary **(see PRECAUTIONS)**. VIVITROL pharmacokinetics have not been evaluated in subjects with moderate and severe renal insufficiency **(see PRECAUTIONS)**.

Gender: In a study in healthy subjects (n=18 females and 18 males), gender did not influence the pharmacokinetics of VIVITROL.

Age: The pharmacokinetics of VIVITROL have not been evaluated in the geriatric population.

Race: The effect of race on the pharmacokinetics of VIVITROL has not been studied.

Pediatrics: The pharmacokinetics of VIVITROL have not been evaluated in a pediatric population.

Drug-Drug Interactions

Clinical drug interaction studies with VIVITROL have not been performed.

Naltrexone antagonizes the effects of opioid-containing medicines, such as cough and cold remedies, antidiarrheal preparations and opioid analgesics **(see PRECAUTIONS)**.

CLINICAL STUDIES

The efficacy of VIVITROL in the treatment of alcohol dependence was evaluated in a 24-week, placebo-controlled, multi-center, double-blind, randomized trial of alcohol dependent (DSM-IV criteria) outpatients. Subjects were treated with an injection every 4 weeks of VIVITROL 190 mg, VIVITROL 380 mg or placebo. Oral naltrexone was not administered prior to the initial or subsequent injections of study medication. Psychosocial support was provided to all subjects in addition to medication.

Subjects treated with VIVITROL 380 mg demonstrated a greater reduction in days of heavy drinking than those treated with placebo. Heavy drinking was defined as self-report of 5 or more standard drinks consumed on a given day for male patients and 4 or more drinks for female patients. Among the subset of patients (n=53, 8% of the total study population) who abstained completely from drinking during the week prior to the first dose of medication, compared with placebo-treated patients, those treated with VIVITROL 380 mg had greater reductions in the number of drinking days and the number of heavy drinking days. In this subset, patients treated with VIVITROL were also more likely than placebo-treated patients to maintain complete abstinence throughout treatment. The same treatment effects were not evident among the subset of patients (n=571, 92% of the total study population) who were actively drinking at the time of treatment initiation.

INDICATIONS AND USAGE

VIVITROL is indicated for the treatment of alcohol dependence in patients who are able to abstain from alcohol in an outpatient setting prior to initiation of treatment with VIVITROL.

Patients should not be actively drinking at the time of initial VIVITROL administration.

Treatment with VIVITROL should be part of a comprehensive management program that includes psychosocial support.

CONTRAINDICATIONS

VIVITROL is contraindicated in:

- Patients receiving opioid analgesics **(see PRECAUTIONS)**.
- Patients with current physiologic opioid dependence **(see WARNINGS)**.
- Patients in acute opiate withdrawal **(see WARNINGS)**.
- Any individual who has failed the naloxone challenge test or has a positive urine screen for opioids.
- Patients who have previously exhibited hypersensitivity to naltrexone, PLG, carboxymethylcellulose, or any other components of the diluent.

WARNINGS

Hepatotoxicity

> Naltrexone has the capacity to cause hepatocellular injury when given in excessive doses.
> Naltrexone is contraindicated in acute hepatitis or liver failure, and its use in patients with active liver disease must be carefully considered in light of its hepatotoxic effects.
> The margin of separation between the apparently safe dose of naltrexone and the dose causing hepatic injury appears to be only five-fold or less. VIVITROL does not appear to be a hepatotoxin at the recommended doses.
> Patients should be warned of the risk of hepatic injury and advised to seek medical attention if they experience symptoms of acute hepatitis. Use of VIVITROL should be discontinued in the event of symptoms and/or signs of acute hepatitis.

Eosinophilic pneumonia

In clinical trials with VIVITROL, there was one diagnosed case and one suspected case of eosinophilic pneumonia. Both cases required hospitalization, and resolved after treatment with antibiotics and corticosteroids. Should a person receiving VIVITROL develop progressive dyspnea and hypoxemia, the diagnosis of eosinophilic pneumonia should be considered **(see ADVERSE REACTIONS)**. Patients should be warned of the risk of eosinophilic pneumonia, and advised to seek medical attention should they develop symptoms of pneumonia. Clinicians should consider the possibility of eosinophilic pneumonia in patients who do not respond to antibiotics.

Unintended Precipitation of Opioid Withdrawal

To prevent occurrence of an acute abstinence syndrome (withdrawal) in patients dependent on opioids, or exacerbation of a pre-existing subclinical abstinence syndrome, patients must be opioid-free for a minimum of 7-10 days before starting VIVITROL treatment. Since the absence of an opioid drug in the urine is often not sufficient proof that a patient is opioid-free, a naloxone challenge test should be employed if the prescribing physician feels there is a risk of precipitating a withdrawal reaction following administration of VIVITROL.

Opioid Overdose Following an Attempt to Overcome Opiate Blockade

VIVITROL is not indicated for the purpose of opioid blockade or the treatment of opiate dependence. Although VIVITROL is a potent antagonist with a prolonged pharmacological effect, the blockade produced by VIVITROL is surmountable. This poses a potential risk to individuals who attempt, on their own, to overcome the blockade by administering large amounts of exogenous opioids. Indeed, any attempt by a patient to overcome the antagonism by taking opioids is very dangerous and may lead to fatal overdose. Injury may arise because the plasma concentration of exogenous opioids attained immediately following their acute administration may be sufficient to overcome the competitive receptor blockade. As a consequence, the patient may be in immediate danger of suffering life-endangering opioid intoxication (e.g., respiratory arrest, circulatory collapse). Patients should be told of the serious consequences of trying to overcome the opioid blockade **(see INFORMATION FOR PATIENTS)**.

There is also the possibility that a patient who had been treated with VIVITROL will respond to lower doses of opioids than previously used. This could result in potentially life-threatening opioid intoxication (respiratory compromise or arrest, circulatory collapse, etc.). Patients should be aware that they may be more sensitive to lower doses of opioids after VIVITROL treatment is discontinued **(see INFORMATION FOR PATIENTS)**.

PRECAUTIONS

General

When Reversal of VIVITROL Blockade Is Required for Pain Management

In an emergency situation in patients receiving VIVITROL, a suggested plan for pain management is regional analgesia, conscious sedation with a benzodiazepine, and use of non-opioid analgesics or general anesthesia.

In a situation requiring opioid analgesia, the amount of opioid required may be greater than usual, and the resulting respiratory depression may be deeper and more prolonged.

A rapidly acting opioid analgesic which minimizes the duration of respiratory depression is preferred. The amount of analgesic administered should be titrated to the needs of the patient. Non-receptor mediated actions may occur and should be expected (e.g., facial swelling, itching, generalized erythema, or bronchoconstriction), presumably due to histamine release.

Irrespective of the drug chosen to reverse VIVITROL blockade, the patient should be monitored closely by appropriately trained personnel in a setting equipped and staffed for cardiopulmonary resuscitation.

Depression and Suicidality

In controlled clinical trials of VIVITROL, adverse events of a suicidal nature (suicidal ideation, suicide attempts, completed suicides) were infrequent overall, but were more common in patients treated with VIVITROL than in patients treated with placebo (1% vs. 0). In some cases, the suicidal thoughts or behavior occurred after study discontinuation, but were in the context of an episode of depression which began while the patient was on study drug. Two completed suicides occurred, both involving patients treated with VIVITROL.

Depression-related events associated with premature discontinuation of study drug were also more common in patients treated with VIVITROL (~1%) than in placebo-treated patients (0).

In the 24-week, placebo-controlled pivotal trial, adverse events involving depressed mood were reported by 10% of patients treated with VIVITROL 380 mg, as compared to 5% of patients treated with placebo injections.

Alcohol dependent patients, including those taking VIVITROL, should be monitored for the development of depression or suicidal thinking. Families and caregivers of patients being treated with VIVITROL should be alerted to the need to monitor patients for the emergence of symptoms of depression or suicidality, and to report such symptoms to the patient's healthcare provider.

Injection Site Reactions
VIVITROL injections may be followed by pain, tenderness, induration, or pruritus. In the clinical trials, one patient developed an area of induration that continued to enlarge after 4 weeks, with subsequent development of necrotic tissue that required surgical excision. Patients should be informed that any concerning injection site reactions should be brought to the attention of the physician (see INFORMATION FOR PATIENTS).

Renal Impairment
VIVITROL pharmacokinetics have not been evaluated in subjects with moderate and severe renal insufficiency. Because naltrexone and its primary metabolite are excreted primarily in the urine, caution is recommended in administering VIVITROL to patients with moderate to severe renal impairment.

Alcohol Withdrawal
Use of VIVITROL does not eliminate nor diminish alcohol withdrawal symptoms.

Intramuscular injections
As with any intramuscular injection, VIVITROL should be administered with caution to patients with thrombocytopenia or any coagulation disorder (e.g., hemophilia and severe hepatic failure).

Information for Patients
Physicians should discuss the following issues with patients for whom they prescribe VIVITROL:

- Patients should be advised to carry documentation to alert medical personnel to the fact that they are taking VIVITROL (naltrexone for extended-release injectable suspension). This will help to ensure that the patients obtain adequate medical treatment in an emergency.
- Patients should be advised that administration of large doses of heroin or any other opioid while on VIVITROL may lead to serious injury, coma, or death.
- Patients should be advised that because VIVITROL can block the effects of opiates and opiate-like drugs, patients will not perceive any effect if they attempt to self-administer heroin or any other opioid drug in small doses while on VIVITROL. Also, patients on VIVITROL may not experience the same effects from opioid containing analgesic, antidiarrheal, or antitussive medications.
- Patients should be advised that if they previously used opioids, they may be more sensitive to lower doses of opioids after VIVITROL treatment is discontinued.
- Patients should be advised that VIVITROL may cause liver injury in people who develop liver disease from other causes. Patients should immediately notify their physician if they develop symptoms and/or signs of liver disease.
- Patients should be advised that VIVITROL may cause an allergic pneumonia. Patients should immediately notify their physician if they develop signs and symptoms of pneumonia, including dyspnea, coughing or wheezing.
- Patients should be advised that a reaction at the site of VIVITROL injection may occur. Reactions include pain, tenderness, induration, and pruritus. Rarely, serious injection site reactions may occur. Patients should be advised to seek medical attention for worsening skin reactions, particularly if the reaction does not improve one month following the injection.
- Patients should be advised that they may experience nausea following the initial injection of VIVITROL. These episodes of nausea tend to be mild and subside within a few days post-injection. Patients are less likely to experience nausea in subsequent injections.
- Patients should be advised that because VIVITROL is an intramuscular injection and not an implanted device, once VIVITROL is injected, it is not possible to remove it from the body.
- Patients should be advised that VIVITROL has been shown to treat alcohol dependence only when used as part of a treatment program that includes counseling and support.
- Patients should be advised to notify their physician if they:
  - become pregnant or intend to become pregnant during treatment with VIVITROL.
  - are breast-feeding.
  - experience respiratory symptoms such as dyspnea, coughing, or wheezing when taking VIVITROL.
  - experience significant pain or redness at the site of injection, particularly if the reaction does not improve one month following the injection.
  - experience other unusual or significant side effects while on VIVITROL therapy.

Drug Interactions
Patients taking VIVITROL may not benefit from opioid-containing medicines (see PRECAUTIONS, Pain Management).

Because naltrexone is not a substrate for CYP drug metabolizing enzymes, inducers or inhibitors of these enzymes are unlikely to change the clearance of VIVITROL. No clinical drug interaction studies have been performed with VIVITROL to evaluate drug interactions, therefore prescribers should weigh the risks and benefits of concomitant drug use.

The safety profile of patients treated with VIVITROL concomitantly with antidepressants was similar to that of patients taking VIVITROL without antidepressants.

Carcinogenesis, mutagenesis, impairment of fertility
Carcinogenicity studies have not been conducted with VIVITROL.

Carcinogenicity studies of oral naltrexone hydrochloride (administered via the diet) have been conducted in rats and mice. In rats, there were small increases in the numbers of testicular mesotheliomas in males and tumors of vascular origin in males and females. The clinical significance of these findings is not known.

Naltrexone was negative in the following in vitro genotoxicity studies: bacterial reverse mutation assay (Ames test), the heritable translocation assay, CHO cell sister chromatid exchange assay, and the mouse lymphoma gene mutation assay. Naltrexone was also negative in an in vivo mouse micronucleus assay. In contrast, naltrexone tested positive in the following assays: Drosophila recessive lethal frequency assay, non-specific DNA damage in repair tests with *E. coli* and WI-38 cells, and urinalysis for methylated histidine residues.

Naltrexone given orally caused a significant increase in pseudopregnancy and a decrease in pregnancy rates in rats at 100 mg/kg/day (600 mg/m^2/day). There was no effect on male fertility at this dose level. The relevance of these observations to human fertility is not known.

Pregnancy Category C
Reproduction and developmental studies have not been conducted for VIVITROL. Studies with naltrexone administered via the oral route have been conducted in pregnant rats and rabbits.

Teratogenic Effects: Oral naltrexone has been shown to increase the incidence of early fetal loss in rats administered ≥ 30 mg/kg/day (180 mg/m^2/day) and rabbits administered ≥ 60 mg/kg/day (720 mg/m^2/day).

There are no adequate and well-controlled studies of either naltrexone or VIVITROL in pregnant women. VIVITROL should be used during pregnancy only if the potential benefit justifies the potential risk to the fetus.

Labor and Delivery
The potential effect of VIVITROL on duration of labor and delivery in humans is unknown.

Nursing Mothers
Transfer of naltrexone and 6β-naltrexol into human milk has been reported with oral naltrexone. Because of the potential for tumorigenicity shown for naltrexone in animal studies, and because of the potential for serious adverse reactions in nursing infants from VIVITROL, a decision should be made whether to discontinue nursing or to discontinue the drug, taking into account the importance of the drug to the mother.

Pediatric Use
The safety and efficacy of VIVITROL have not been established in the pediatric population.

Geriatric Use
In trials of alcohol dependent subjects, 2.6% (n=26) of subjects were >65 years of age, and one patient was >75 years of age. Clinical studies of VIVITROL did not include sufficient numbers of subjects age 65 and over to determine whether they respond differently from younger subjects.

ADVERSE REACTIONS

In all controlled and uncontrolled trials during the premarketing development of VIVITROL, more than 900 patients with alcohol and/or opioid dependence have been treated with VIVITROL. Approximately 400 patients have been treated for 6 months or more, and 230 for 1 year or longer.

Adverse Events Leading to Discontinuation of Treatment
In controlled trials of 6 months or less, 9% of patients treated with VIVITROL discontinued treatment due to an adverse event, as compared to 7% of the patients treated with placebo. Adverse events in the VIVITROL 380-mg group that led to more dropouts were injection site reactions (3%), nausea (2%), pregnancy (1%), headache (1%), and suicide-related events (0.3%). In the placebo group, 1% of patients withdrew due to injection site reactions, and 0% of patients withdrew due to the other adverse events.

Common Adverse Events (by body system and preferred term/high level group term) in ≥ 5% of Patients Treated with VIVITROL

Body system	Adverse Event/Preferred Term	Placebo N = 214		Naltrexone for extended-release injectable suspension							
				400 mg N = 25		380 mg N = 205		190 mg N = 210		All N = 440	
		N	%	N	%	N	%	N	%	N	%
Gastrointestinal disorders	Nausea	24	11	8	32	68	33	53	25	129	29
	Vomiting NOS	12	6	3	12	28	14	22	10	53	12
	Diarrhea[1]	21	10	3	12	27	13	27	13	57	13
	Abdominal pain[2]	17	8	4	16	23	11	23	11	50	11
	Dry mouth	9	4	6	24	10	5	8	4	24	5
Infections and infestations	Upper respiratory tract infection–Other[3]	28	13	0	0	27	13	25	12	52	12
	Pharyngitis[4]	23	11	0	0	22	11	35	17	57	13
Psychiatric disorders	Insomnia, sleep disorders	25	12	2	8	29	14	27	13	58	13
	Anxiety[5]	17	8	2	8	24	12	16	8	42	10
	Depression	9	4	0	0	17	8	7	3	24	5
General disorders and administration site conditions	Any ISR	106	50	22	88	142	69	121	58	285	65
	Injection site tenderness	83	39	18	72	92	45	89	42	199	45
	Injection site induration	18	8	7	28	71	35	52	25	130	30
	Injection site pain	16	7	0	0	34	17	22	10	56	13
	Other ISR (primarily nodules, swelling)	8	4	8	32	30	15	16	8	54	12
	Injection site pruritus	0	0	0	0	21	10	13	6	34	8
	Injection site ecchymosis	11	5	0	0	14	7	9	4	23	5
	Asthenic conditions[6]	26	12	3	12	47	23	40	19	90	20
Musculoskeletal and connective tissue disorders	Arthralgia, arthritis, joint stiffness	11	5	1	4	24	12	12	6	37	9
	Back pain, back stiffness	10	5	1	4	12	6	14	7	27	6
	Muscle cramps[7]	3	1	0	0	16	8	5	2	21	5

(Table continued on next page)

Vivitrol—Cont.

Common Adverse Events

The table lists all adverse events, regardless of causality, occurring in ≥5% of patients with alcohol dependence, for which the incidence was greater in the combined VIVITROL group than in the placebo group. A majority of patients treated with VIVITROL in clinical studies had adverse events with a maximum intensity of "mild" or "moderate."

Post-marketing Reports

Reports From Other Intramuscular Drug Products Containing Polylactide-co-glycolide (PLG) Microspheres – Not With VIVITROL

Retinal Artery Occlusion

Retinal artery occlusion after injection with another drug product containing polylactide-co-glycolide (PLG) microspheres has been reported very rarely during post-marketing surveillance. This event has been reported in the presence of abnormal arteriovenous anastamosis. No cases of retinal artery occlusion have been reported during VIVITROL clinical trials or post-marketing surveillance. VIVITROL should be administered by intramuscular (IM) injection into the gluteal muscle, and care must be taken to avoid inadvertent injection into a blood vessel (**see DOSAGE AND ADMINISTRATION**).

[See table on previous page and above]

Laboratory Tests

In clinical trials, subjects on VIVITROL had increases in eosinophil counts relative to subjects on placebo. With continued use of VIVITROL, eosinophil counts returned to normal over a period of several months.

VIVITROL 380-mg was associated with a decrease in platelet count. Patients treated with high dose VIVITROL experienced a mean maximal decrease in platelet count of $17.8 \times 10^3/\mu L$, compared to $2.6 \times 10^3/\mu L$ in placebo patients. In randomized controlled trials, VIVITROL was not associated with an increase in bleeding related adverse events.

In short-term, controlled trials, the incidence of AST elevations associated with VIVITROL treatment was similar to that observed with oral naltrexone treatment (1.5% each) and slightly higher than observed with placebo treatment (0.9%).

In short-term controlled trials, more patients treated with Vivitrol 380 mg (11%) and oral naltrexone (17%) shifted from normal creatinine phosphokinase (CPK) levels before treatment to abnormal CPK levels at the end of the trials, compared to placebo patients (8%). In open-label trials, 16% of patients dosed for more than 6 months had increases in CPK. For both the oral naltrexone and Vivitrol 380-mg groups, CPK abnormalities were most frequently in the range of 1-2 × ULN. However, there were reports of CPK abnormalities as high as 4 × ULN for the oral naltrexone group, and 35 × ULN for the Vivitrol 380-mg group. Overall, there were no differences between the placebo and naltrexone (oral or injectable) groups with respect to the proportions of patients with a CPK value at least three times the upper limit of normal. No factors other than naltrexone exposure were associated with the CPK elevations.

VIVITROL may be cross-reactive with certain immunoassay methods for the detection of drugs of abuse (specifically opioids) in urine. For further information, reference to the specific immunoassay instructions is recommended.

Other Events Observed During the Premarketing Evaluation of VIVITROL

The following is a list of preferred terms that reflect events reported by alcohol and/or opiate dependent subjects treated with VIVITROL in controlled trials. The listing does not include those events already listed in the previous tables or elsewhere in labeling, those events for which a drug cause was remote, those events which were so general as to be uninformative, and those events reported only once which did not have a substantial probability of being acutely life-threatening.

Gastrointestinal Disorders—constipation, toothache, flatulence, gastroesophageal reflux disease, hemorrhoids, colitis, gastrointestinal hemorrhage, paralytic ileus, perirectal abscess

Infections and Infestations—influenza, bronchitis, urinary tract infection, gastroenteritis, tooth abscess, pneumonia, cellulitis

General Disorders and Administration Site Conditions—pyrexia, lethargy, rigors, chest pain, chest tightness, weight decreased

Psychiatric Disorders—irritability, libido decreased, abnormal dreams, alcohol withdrawal syndrome, agitation, euphoric mood, delirium

Nervous System Disorders—dysgeusia, disturbance in attention, migraine, mental impairment, convulsions, ischemic stroke, cerebral arterial aneurysm

Musculoskeletal and Connective Tissue Disorders—pain in limb, muscle spasms, joint stiffness

Skin and Subcutaneous Tissue Disorders—sweating increased, night sweats, pruritus

Respiratory, Thoracic, and Mediastinal Disorders—pharyngolaryngeal pain, dyspnea, sinus congestion, chronic obstructive airways disease

Metabolism and Nutrition Disorders—appetite increased, heat exhaustion, dehydration, hypercholesterolemia

Vascular Disorders—hypertension, hot flushes, deep venous thrombosis, pulmonary embolism

Eye Disorders—conjunctivitis

Common Adverse Events (by body system and preferred term/high level group term) in ≥ 5% of Patients Treated with VIVITROL (cont.)

Body system	Adverse Event/Preferred Term	Placebo		Naltrexone for extended-release injectable suspension							
		N = 214		400 mg N = 25		380 mg N = 205		190 mg N = 210		All N = 440	
		N	%	N	%	N	%	N	%	N	%
Skin and subcutaneous tissue disorders	Rash[8]	8	4	3	12	12	6	10	5	25	6
Nervous system disorders	Headache[9]	39	18	9	36	51	25	34	16	94	21
	Dizziness, syncope	9	4	4	16	27	13	27	13	58	13
	Somnolence, sedation	2	1	3	12	8	4	9	4	20	5
Metabolism and nutrition disorders	Anorexia, appetite, decreased NOS, appetite disorder NOS	6	3	5	20	30	14	13	6	48	11

[1] Includes the preferred terms: diarrhea NOS; frequent bowel movements; gastrointestinal upset; loose stools
[2] Includes the preferred terms: abdominal pain NOS; abdominal pain upper; stomach discomfort; abdominal pain lower
[3] Includes the preferred terms: upper respiratory tract infection NOS; laryngitis NOS; sinusitis NOS
[4] Includes the preferred terms: nasopharyngitis; pharyngitis streptococcal; pharyngitis NOS
[5] Includes the preferred terms: anxiety NEC; anxiety aggravated; agitation; obsessive compulsive disorder; panic attack; nervousness; post-traumatic stress
[6] Includes the preferred terms: malaise; fatigue (these two comprise the majority of cases); lethargy; sluggishness
[7] Includes the preferred terms: muscle cramps; spasms; tightness; twitching; stiffness; rigidity
[8] Includes the preferred terms: rash NOS; rash papular; heat rash
[9] Includes the preferred terms: headache NOS; sinus headache; migraine; frequent headaches

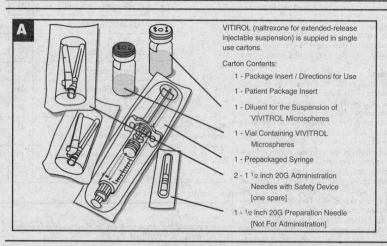

VITIROL (naltrexone for extended-release injectable suspension) is supplied in single use cartons.

Carton Contents:

1 - Package Insert / Directions for Use

1 - Patient Package Insert

1 - Diluent for the Suspension of VIVITROL Microspheres

1 - Vial Containing VIVITROL Microspheres

1 - Prepackaged Syringe

2 - 1 ½ inch 20G Administration Needles with Safety Device [one spare]

1 - ½ inch 20G Preparation Needle [Not For Administration]

Blood and Lymphatic System Disorders—lymphadenopathy (including cervical adenitis), white blood cell count increased

Cardiac Disorders—palpitations, atrial fibrillation, myocardial infarction, angina pectoris, angina unstable, cardiac failure congestive, coronary artery atherosclerosis

Immune System Disorders—seasonal allergy, hypersensitivity reaction (including angioneurotic edema and urticaria)

Pregnancy, Puerperium, and Perinatal Conditions—abortion missed

Hepatobiliary Disorders—cholelithiasis, aspartate aminotransferase increased, alanine aminotransferase increased, cholecystitis acute

DRUG ABUSE AND DEPENDENCE

Controlled Substance Class

VIVITROL is not a controlled substance.

Physical and Psychological Dependence

Naltrexone, the active ingredient in VIVITROL, is a pure opioid antagonist that does not lead to physical or psychological dependence. Tolerance to the opioid antagonist effect is not known to occur.

OVERDOSAGE

There is limited experience with overdose of VIVITROL. Single doses up to 784 mg were administered to 5 healthy subjects. There were no serious or severe adverse events. The most common effects were injection site reactions, nausea, abdominal pain, somnolence, and dizziness. There were no significant increases in hepatic enzymes.

In the event of an overdose, appropriate supportive treatment should be initiated.

DOSAGE AND ADMINISTRATION

VIVITROL must be administered by a health care professional.

The recommended dose of VIVITROL is 380 mg delivered intramuscularly every 4 weeks or once a month. The injection should be administered by a health care professional as an intramuscular (IM) gluteal injection, alternating buttocks, using the carton components provided (**see HOW SUPPLIED**). VIVITROL must not be administered intravenously.

If a patient misses a dose, he/she should be instructed to receive the next dose as soon as possible.

Pretreatment with oral naltrexone is not required before using VIVITROL.

Reinitiation of Treatment in Patients Previously Discontinued

There are no data to specifically address reinitiation of treatment.

Switching From Oral Naltrexone for Alcohol Dependence

There are no systematically collected data that specifically address the switch from oral naltrexone to VIVITROL.

Preparation of Dose

VIVITROL must be suspended **only** in the diluent supplied in the carton and must be administered with the needle supplied in the carton. All components (i.e., the microspheres, diluent, preparation needle, and an administration needle with safety device) are required for administration. A spare administration needle is provided in case of clogging. Do not substitute any other components for the components of the carton.

HOW SUPPLIED

VIVITROL (naltrexone for extended-release injectable suspension) is supplied in single use cartons. Each carton contains one 380 mg vial of VIVITROL microspheres, one vial containing 4 mL (to deliver 3.4 mL) Diluent for the suspension of VIVITROL, one 5-mL prepackaged syringe, one 20-gauge ½-inch needle, and two 20-gauge 1½-inch needles with safety device: NDC 63459-300-42.

Storage and Handling

The entire dose pack should be stored in the refrigerator (2-8°C, 36-46°F). Unrefrigerated, VIVITROL can be stored at temperatures not exceeding 25°C (77°F) for no more than 7 days prior to administration. Do not expose the product to temperatures above 25°C (77°F). VIVITROL should not be frozen.

Parenteral products should be visually inspected for particulate matter and discoloration prior to administration whenever solution and container permit. A properly mixed suspension will be milky white, will not contain clumps, and will move freely down the wall of the vial.

Keep out of Reach of Children.

US Patent Nos. 5,650,173; 5,654,008; 5,792,477; 5,916,598; 6,110,503; 6,194,006; 6,264,987; 6,331,317; 6,379,703; 6,379,704; 6,395,304; 6,403,114; 6,495,164; 6,495,166;

6,534,092; 6,537,586; 6,540,393; 6,596,316; 6,667,061; 6,705,757; 6,713,090; 6,861,016; 6,939,033

Directions for Use:

To ensure proper dosing, it is important that you follow the preparation and administration instructions outlined in this document.

[See figure A at top of previous page]

THE CARTON SHOULD NOT BE EXPOSED TO TEMPERATURES EXCEEDING 25 °C (77 °F).

VIVITROL must be suspended only in the diluent supplied in the carton, and must be administered with the needle supplied in the carton. Do not make any substitutions for components of the carton.

Product to be prepared and administered by a healthcare professional.

Do not substitute carton components.

Keep out of reach of children.

Prepare and administer the VIVITROL suspension using aseptic technique.

The entire carton should be stored in the refrigerator (2-8 °C, 36-46 °F). Unrefrigerated, VIVITROL Microspheres can be stored at temperatures not exceeding 25 °C (77 °F) for no more than 7 days prior to administration. Do not expose unrefrigerated product to temperatures above 25 °C (77 °F). VIVITROL should not be frozen.

Parenteral products should be visually inspected for particulate matter and discoloration prior to administration whenever solution and container permit.

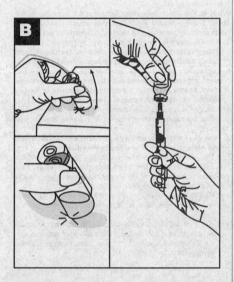

1. **Remove the carton from refrigeration. Prior to preparation, allow drug to reach room temperature (approximately 45 minutes).**

2. To ease mixing, firmly tap the vial on a hard surface, ensuring the powder moves freely. (see Figure B)

3. Remove flip-off caps from both vials. DO NOT USE IF FLIP-OFF CAPS ARE BROKEN OR MISSING.

4. Wipe the vial tops with an alcohol swab.

5. Place the ½ inch preparation needle on the syringe and withdraw 3.4 mL of the diluent from the diluent vial. Some diluent will remain in the diluent vial. (see Figure B)

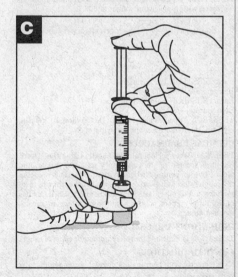

Inject the 3.4 mL of diluent into the VIVITROL Microsphere vial. (see Figure C)

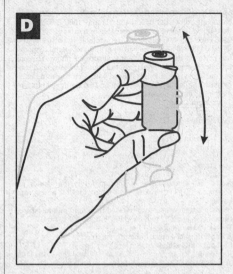

Mix the powder and diluent by **vigorously** shaking the vial for approximately 1 minute. (see Figure D) Ensure that the dose is thoroughly suspended prior to proceeding to Step E. A PROPERLY MIXED SUSPENSION WILL BE MILKY WHITE, WILL NOT CONTAIN CLUMPS, AND WILL MOVE FREELY DOWN THE WALLS OF THE VIAL

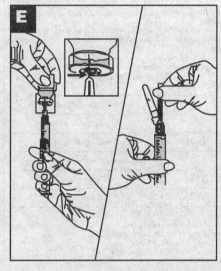

1. Immediately after suspension, withdraw 4.2 mL of the suspension into the syringe using the same preparation needle.

2. Remove the preparation needle and replace with a 1½ inch administration needle for immediate use. (see Figure E)

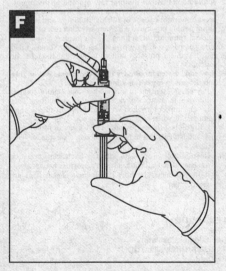

Prior to injecting, tap the syringe to release any air bubbles, then push gently on the plunger until **4 mL** of the suspension remains in the syringe. (see Figure F)

THE SUSPENSION IS NOW READY FOR IMMEDIATE ADMINISTRATION.

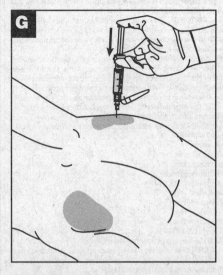

1. Administer the suspension by deep intramuscular (IM) injection into a gluteal muscle, alternating buttocks per injection. Remember to aspirate for blood before injection. (see Figure G)

2. Inject the suspension in a smooth and continuous motion.

3. If blood aspirates or the needle clogs, do not inject. Change to the spare needle provided in the carton and administer into an adjacent site in the same gluteal region, again aspirating for blood before injection.

VIVITROL must NOT be given intravenously.

After the injection is administered, cover the needle by pressing the safety sheath against a hard surface using a one-handed motion away from self and others. (see Figure H)

Activation of the safety sheath may cause minimum splatter of fluid that may remain on the needle after injection.

DISPOSE OF USED AND UNUSED ITEMS IN PROPER WASTE CONTAINERS

FREQUENTLY ASKED QUESTIONS:

1. Can I prepare the suspension prior to my patient's arrival?

No. You may remove the carton from the refrigerator prior to the patient's arrival, but once the diluent is added to the VIVITROL Microspheres, the dose should be mixed and the suspension administered immediately. It is very important to use proper aseptic technique when preparing the suspension.

2. How much time do I have between preparing and administering the dose?

It is recommended that the suspension be administered **immediately** once the product has been suspended and transferred into the syringe. If a few minutes' delay occurs after suspension but before transfer into the syringe (Figure D), the vial can be inverted a few times to resuspend and then transferred into the syringe for immediate use.

3. Can I use needles other than those provided in the carton?

The needles in the carton are specially designed for administration of VIVITROL. Do not make any substitutions for components of the carton.

Continued on next page

Vivitrol—Cont.

4. The suspension is milky white upon mixing with the diluent. Is this normal?
Yes. VIVITROL Microspheres will form a milky white suspension when mixed with the provided diluent.

5. What if a needle clog occurs during administration of the product?
If a clog occurs during administration, the needle should be withdrawn from the patient, capped with the attached safety device, and replaced with the spare administration needle provided. Gently push on the plunger until a bead of the suspension appears at the tip of the needle. The remainder of the suspension should then be administered into an adjacent site in the same gluteal region.
For additional information, visit www.vivitrol.com or call **1-800-848-4876**
Alkermes.
Manufactured by:
Alkermes, Inc.
88 Sidney Street
Cambridge, MA 02139
Cephalon
Marketed by:
Cephalon, Inc.
41 Moores Road
Frazer, PA 19355
©2007 Alkermes. All rights reserved.
ALKERMES® is a registered trademark of Alkermes, Inc.
VIVITROL® is a registered trademark of Cephalon, Inc.
Manufactured by: Alkermes, Inc.
Marketed by: Cephalon, Inc.
Printed in U.S.A.
REV MAY 2007

Forest Pharmaceuticals, Inc. (Subsidiary of Forest Laboratories, Inc.)
13600 SHORELINE DRIVE
ST. LOUIS, MO 63045

Direct Inquiries to:
Professional Affairs Department
13600 Shoreline Drive
St. Louis, MO 63045
(800) 678-1605

ARMOUR® THYROID ℞
[ar-mor thī 'roid]
(thyroid tablets, USP)
Rx only

Prescribing information for this product, which appears on page 1159 of the 2008 PDR, has been completely revised as follows. Please write "See Supplement A" next to the product heading.

DESCRIPTION
Armour® Thyroid (thyroid tablets, USP) for oral use is a natural preparation derived from porcine thyroid glands and has a strong, characteristic odor. (T3 liothyronine is approximately four times as potent as T4 levothyroxine on a microgram for microgram basis.) They provide 38 mcg levothyroxine (T4) and 9 mcg liothyronine (T3) per grain of thyroid. The inactive ingredients are calcium stearate, dextrose, microcrystalline cellulose, sodium starch glycolate and opadry white.
STRUCTURAL FORMULAS

liothyronine (T3)

levothyroxine (T4)

HOW SUPPLIED
Armour Thyroid tablets (thyroid tablets, USP) are supplied as follows: 15 mg (1/4 gr) are available in bottles of 100 (NDC 0456-0457-01). 30 mg (1/2 gr) are available in bottles of 100 (NDC 0456-0458-01), 1000 (NDC 0456-0458-00), containers of 50,000 (NDC 0456-0458-69) and unit dose cartons of 100 (NDC 0456-0458-63). 60 mg (1 gr) are available in bottles of 100 (NDC 0456-0459-01), 1000 (NDC 0456-0459-00), 5000 (NDC 0456-0459-51), containers of 50,000 (NDC 0456-0459-69) and unit dose cartons of 100 (NDC 0456-0459-63). 90 mg (1 1/2 gr) are available in bottles of 100 (NDC 0456-0460-01). 120 mg (2 gr) are available in bottles of 100 (NDC 0456-0461-01), 1000 (NDC 0456-0461-00), containers of 50,000 (NDC 0456-0461-69) and unit dose cartons

of 100 (NDC 0456-0461-63). 180 mg (3 gr) are available in bottles of 100 (NDC 0456-0462-01) and 1000 (NDC 0456-0462-00). 240 mg (4 gr) are available in bottles of 100 (NDC 0456-0463-01). 300 mg (5 gr) are available in bottles of 100 (NDC 0456-0464-01). The bottles of 100 are special dispensing bottles with child-resistant closures. Armour Thyroid tablets are evenly colored, light tan, round tablets, with convex surfaces. One side is debossed with a mortar and pestle beneath the letter "A" on the top and strength code letters on the bottom as defined below

Strength Code

1/4 grain	TC
1/2 grain	TD
1 grain	TE
1 1/2 grain	TJ
2 grain	TF
3 grain	TG (bisected)
4 grain	TH
5 grain	TI (bisected)

Note: (T3 liothyronine is approximately four times as potent as T4 levothyroxine on a microgram for microgram basis.)
Store in a tight container protected from light and moisture.
Store between 15°C and 30°C (59°F and 86°F).
Forest Pharmaceuticals, Inc.
A Subsidiary of Forest Laboratories, Inc.
St. Louis, MO 63045
Rev. 04/06   11841102
® 2006 Forest Laboratories, Inc.

CELEXA® ℞
[sĕ-lĕk-să]
(citalopram hydrobromide)
Tablets/Oral Solution
Rx Only

Prescribing information for this product, which appears on pages 1161–1166 of the 2008 PDR, has been revised as follows. Please write "See Supplement A" next to the product heading.
In the WARNINGS section, under the subsection Clinical Worsening and Suicide Risk Table 1 has been revised as follows:

Age Range	Drug-Placebo Difference in Number of Cases of Suicidality per 1000 Patients Treated
	Increases Compared to Placebo
<18	14 additional cases
18-24	5 additional cases
	Decreases Compared to Placebo
25-64	1 fewer case
≥65	6 fewer cases

Forest Pharmaceuticals, Inc.
Subsidiary of Forest Laboratories, Inc.
St. Louis, MO 63045 USA
Licensed from H. Lundbeck A/S
Rev. 07/07
© 2007 Forest Laboratories, Inc.
MG #13940(25)
In the Medication Guide section, the second paragraph has been revised as follows:
What is the most important information I should know about antidepressant medicines, depression and other serious mental illnesses, and suicidal thoughts or actions?
1. **Antidepressant medicines may increase suicidal thoughts or actions in some children, teenagers, and young adults within the first few months of treatment.**
2. **Depression and other serious mental illnesses are the most important causes of suicidal thoughts and actions. Some people may have a particularly high risk of having suicidal thoughts or actions. These include people who have (or have a family history of) bipolar illness (also called manic-depressive illness) or suicidal thoughts or actions.**
3. **How can I watch for and try to prevent suicidal thoughts and actions in myself or a family member?**
   - Pay close attention to any changes, especially sudden changes, in mood, behaviors, thoughts, or feelings. This is very important when an antidepressant medicine is started or when the dose is changed.
   - Call the healthcare provider right away to report new or sudden changes in mood, behavior, thoughts, or feelings.
   - Keep all follow-up visits with the healthcare provider as scheduled. Call the healthcare provider between visits as needed, especially if you have concerns about symptoms.

LEXAPRO® ℞
[lĕks'ă-prŏ]
(escitalopram oxalate)
TABLETS/ORAL SOLUTION
Rx Only

Prescribing information for this product, which appears on pages 1175–1181 of the 2008 PDR, has been completely revised as follows. Please write "See Supplement A" next to the product heading.

In the WARNINGS section, under the subsection Clinical Worsening and Suicide Risk Table 1 has been revised as follows:

TABLE 1

Age Range	Drug-Placebo Difference in Number of Cases of Suicidality per 1000 Patients Treated
	Increases Compared to Placebo
<18	14 additional cases
18-24	5 additional cases
	Decreases Compared to Placebo
25-64	1 fewer case
≥65	6 fewer cases

Forest Pharmaceuticals, Inc.
Subsidiary of Forest Laboratories, Inc.
St. Louis, MO 63045 USA
Licensed from H. Lundbeck A/S
Rev. 07/07
© 2007 Forest Laboratories, Inc.
In the Medication Guide section, the second paragraph has been revised as follows:
What is the most important information I should know about antidepressant medicines, depression and other serious mental illnesses, and suicidal thoughts or actions?
1. **Antidepressant medicines may increase suicidal thoughts or actions in some children, teenagers, and young adults within the first few months of treatment.**
2. **Depression and other serious mental illnesses are the most important causes of suicidal thoughts and actions. Some people may have a particularly high risk of having suicidal thoughts or actions. These include people who have (or have a family history of) bipolar illness (also called manic-depressive illness) or suicidal thoughts or actions.**
3. **How can I watch for and try to prevent suicidal thoughts and actions in myself or a family member?**
   - Pay close attention to any changes, especially sudden changes, in mood, behaviors, thoughts, or feelings. This is very important when an antidepressant medicine is started or when the dose is changed.
   - Call the healthcare provider right away to report new or sudden changes in mood, behavior, thoughts, or feelings.
   - Keep all follow-up visits with the healthcare provider as scheduled. Call the healthcare provider between visits as needed, especially if you have concerns about symptoms.

TESSALON® ℞
(benzonatate, USP)
100 mg Perles
200 mg Capsules
Rx only

Prescribing information for this product, which appears on page 1185 of the 2008 PDR, has been completely revised as follows. Please write "See Supplement A" next to the product heading.

DESCRIPTION
TESSALON, a non-narcotic oral antitussive agent, is 2, 5, 8, 11, 14, 17, 20, 23, 26-nonaoxaoctacosan-28-yl p-(butylamino) benzoate; with a molecular weight of 603.7.

$CH_3(CH_2)_2CH_2NH-\langle\bigcirc\rangle-COOCH_2CH_2(OCH_2CH_2)_nOCH_3$

$C_{30}H_{53}NO_{11}$

Each TESSALON Perle contains:
Benzonatate, USP 100 mg
Each TESSALON Capsule contains:
Benzonatate, USP 200 mg
TESSALON Capsules also contain: D&C Yellow 10, gelatin, glycerin, methylparaben and propylparaben.

CLINICAL PHARMACOLOGY
TESSALON acts peripherally by anesthetizing the stretch receptors located in the respiratory passages, lungs, and pleura by dampening their activity and thereby reducing the cough reflex at its source. It begins to act within 15 to 20 minutes and its effect lasts for 3 to 8 hours. TESSALON has no inhibitory effect on the respiratory center in recommended dosage.

INDICATIONS AND USAGE
TESSALON is indicated for the symptomatic relief of cough.

CONTRAINDICATIONS
Hypersensitivity to benzonatate or related compounds.

WARNINGS
Severe hypersensitivity reactions (including bronchospasm, laryngospasm and cardiovascular collapse) have been reported which are possibly related to local anesthesia from

sucking or chewing the capsule instead of swallowing it. Severe reactions have required intervention with vasopressor agents and supportive measures.
Isolated instances of bizarre behavior, including mental confusion and visual hallucinations, have also been reported in patients taking TESSALON in combination with other prescribed drugs.

PRECAUTIONS

Benzonatate is chemically related to anesthetic agents of the para-amino-benzoic acid class (e.g. procaine; tetracaine) and has been associated with adverse CNS effects possibly related to a prior sensitivity to related agents or interaction with concomitant medication.
Information for patients: Release of TESSALON from the capsule in the mouth can produce a temporary local anesthesia of the oral mucosa and choking could occur. Therefore, the capsules should be swallowed without chewing.
Usage in Pregnancy: Pregnancy Category C. Animal reproduction studies have not been conducted with TESSALON. It is also not known whether TESSALON can cause fetal harm when administered to a pregnant woman or can affect reproduction capacity. TESSALON should be given to a pregnant woman only if clearly needed.
Nursing mothers: It is not known whether this drug is excreted in human milk. Because many drugs are excreted in human milk caution should be exercised when TESSALON is administered to a nursing woman.
Carcinogenesis, mutagenesis, impairment of fertility: Carcinogenicity, mutagenicity, and reproduction studies have not been conducted with TESSALON.
Pediatric Use: Safety and effectiveness in children below the age of 10 have not been established.

ADVERSE REACTIONS

Potential Adverse Reactions to TESSALON may include:
Hypersensitivity reactions including bronchospasm, laryngospasm, cardiovascular collapse possibly related to local anesthesia from chewing or sucking the capsule.
CNS: sedation; headache; dizziness; mental confusion; visual hallucinations.
GI: constipation, nausea; GI upset.
Dermatologic: pruritus; skin eruptions.
Other: nasal congestion; sensation of burning in the eyes; vague "chilly" sensation; numbness of the chest; hypersensitivity.
Rare instances of deliberate or accidental overdose have resulted in death.

OVERDOSAGE

Overdose may result in death.
The drug is chemically related to tetracaine and other topical anesthetics and shares various aspects of their pharmacology and toxicology. Drugs of this type are generally well absorbed after ingestion.
Signs and Symptoms:
If capsules are chewed or dissolved in the mouth, oropharyngeal anesthesia will develop rapidly. CNS stimulation may cause restlessness and tremors which may proceed to chronic convulsions followed by profound CNS depression.
Treatment:
Evacuate gastric contents and administer copious amounts of activated charcoal slurry. Even in the conscious patient, cough and gag reflexes may be so depressed as to necessitate special attention to protection against aspiration of gastric contents and orally administered materials. Convulsions should be treated with a short-acting barbiturate given intravenously and carefully titrated for the smallest effective dosage. Intensive support of respiration and cardiovascular-renal function is an essential feature of the treatment of severe intoxication from overdosage.
Do not use CNS stimulants.

DOSAGE AND ADMINISTRATION

Adults and Children over 10: Usual dose is one 100 mg or 200 mg capsule t.i.d. as required. If necessary, up to 600 mg daily may be given.

HOW SUPPLIED

Perles, 100 mg (yellow);
bottles of 100
NDC 0456-0688-01
Imprint: T.
Perles, 100 mg (yellow);
bottles of 500
NDC 0456-0688-02
Imprint: T
Capsules, 200 mg (yellow);
bottles of 100
NDC 0456-0698-01
Imprint: 0698.
Store at 25°C (77°F); excursions permitted to 15-30°C (59-86°F) [see USP Controlled Room Temperature].
Rev. 07/07
MG #14183(06)
Mfd by
Catalent Pharma Solutions
St. Petersburg, Florida 33716
FOREST PHARMACEUTICALS, INC.
SUBSIDIARY OF FOREST LABORATORIES, INC.
ST. LOUIS, MO 63045 USA

THYROLAR® TABLETS ℞

[*thī-rō-lär*]
(Liotrix Tablets)
Rx only

Prescribing information for this product, which appears on pages 1185–1187 of the 2008 PDR, has been completely revised as follows. Please write "See Supplement A" next to the product heading.
The DESCRIPTION *section was revised as follows:*

DESCRIPTION

Thyrolar Tablets (Liotrix Tablets, USP) contain triiodothyronine (T3 liothyronine) sodium and tetraiodothyronine (T4 levothyroxine) sodium in the amounts listed in the "How Supplied" section. (T3 liothyronine sodium is approximately four times as potent as T4 thyroxine on a microgram for microgram basis.)
The inactive ingredients are calcium phosphate, colloidal silicon dioxide, corn starch, lactose, and magnesium stearate. The tablets also contain the following dyes: Thyrolar 1/4 - FD&C Blue #1 and FD&C Red #40; Thyrolar 1/2 - FD&C Red #40 and D&C Yellow #10; Thyrolar 1 - FD&C Red #40; Thyrolar 2 - FD&C Blue #1, FD&C Red #40, and D&C Yellow #10; Thyrolar 3 - FD&C Red #40 and D&C Yellow #10.
STRUCTURAL FORMULAS

Liothyronine (T_3) Sodium

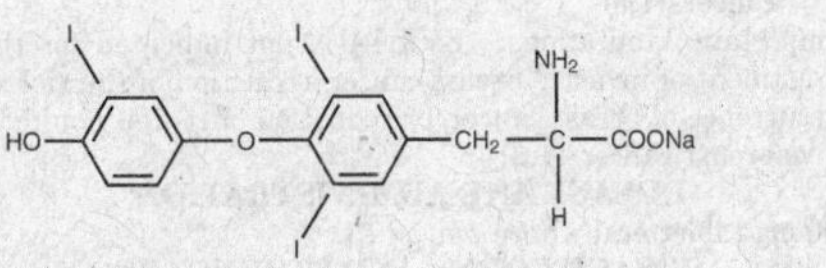

Levothyroxine (T_4) Sodium

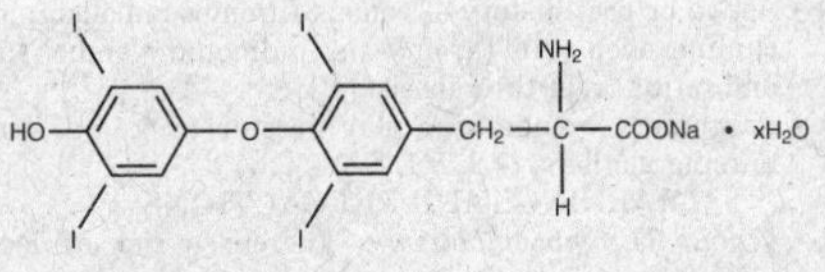

The ADVERSE REACTIONS *section was revised as follows:*

ADVERSE REACTIONS

During postmarketing surveillance, the following events have been observed to have occured in patients administered Thyrolar: fatigue, sluggishness, increase in weight, alopecia, palpitations, dry skin, urticaria, headache, hyperhidrosis, pruritus, asthenia, increased blood pressure, arthralgia, myalgia, tremor, hypothyroidism, increase in TSH, decrease in TSH, nausea, chest pain, hypersensitivity, keratoconjunctivitis sicca, increased heart rate, irregular heart rate, anxiety, depression, and insomnia.
Adverse reactions other than those indicative of hyperthyroidism because of therapeutic overdosage, either initially or during the maintenance period, are rare (See OVERDOSAGE).

The OVERDOSAGE *section was revised as follows:*

OVERDOSAGE

Signs and Symptoms—Excessive doses of thyroid result in a hypermetabolic state resembling in every respect the condition of endogenous origin. The condition may be self-induced.
Treatment of Overdosage—Dosage should be reduced or therapy temporarily discontinued if signs and symptoms of overdosage appear.
Treatment may be reinstituted at a lower dosage. In normal individuals, normal hypothalamic-pituitary-thyroid axis function is restored in 6 to 8 weeks after thyroid suppression.
Treatment of acute massive thyroid hormone overdosage is aimed at reducing gastrointestinal absorption of the drugs and counteracting central and peripheral effects, mainly those of increased sympathetic activity. Vomiting may be induced initially if further gastrointestinal absorption can reasonably be prevented and barring contraindications such as coma, convulsions, or loss of the gagging reflex. Treatment is symptomatic and supportive. Oxygen may be administered and ventilation maintained. Cardiac glycosides may be indicated if congestive heart failure develops. Measures to control fever, hypoglycemia, or fluid loss should be instituted if needed. Antiadrenergic agents, particularly propranolol, have been used advantageously in the treatment of increased sympathetic activity. Propranolol may be administered intravenously at a dosage of 1 to 3 mg over a 10 minute period or orally, 80 to 160 mg/day, initially, especially when no contraindications exist for its use.

The DOSAGE AND ADMINISTRATION *section was revised as follows:*

DOSAGE AND ADMINISTRATION

The dosage of Thyrolar Tablets (Liotrix Tablets, USP) is determined by the indication and must in every case be individualized according to patient response and laboratory findings.
Thyroid hormones are given orally. In acute, emergency conditions, injectable sodium levothyroxine may be given intravenously when oral administration is not feasible or desirable, as in the treatment of myxedema coma, or during total parenteral nutrition. Intramuscular administration is not advisable because of reported poor absorption.
Hypothyroidism—Therapy is usually instituted using low doses with increments which depend on the cardiovascular status of the patient. The usual starting dose is one tablet of Thyrolar ½ with increments of one tablet of Thyrolar ¼ every 2 to 3 weeks. A lower starting dosage, one tablet of Thyrolar ¼/day, is recommended in patients with long-standing myxedema, particularly if cardiovascular impairment is suspected, in which case extreme caution is recommended. The appearance of angina is an indication for a reduction in dosage. Most patients require one tablet of Thyrolar 1 to one tablet of Thyrolar 2 per day. Failure to respond to doses of one tablet of Thyrolar 3 suggests lack of compliance or malabsorption. Maintenance dosages of one tablet of Thyrolar 1 to one tablet of Thyrolar 2 per day usually result in normal serum levothyroxine (T4) and triiodothyronine (T3) levels. Adequate therapy usually results in normal TSH and T4 levels after 2 to 3 weeks of therapy.
Readjustment of thyroid hormone dosage should be made within the first four weeks of therapy, after proper clinical and laboratory evaluations, including serum levels of T4, bound and free, and TSH.
T3 may be used in preference to levothyroxine (T4) during radio-isotope scanning procedures, since induction of hypothyroidism in those cases is more abrupt and can be of shorter duration. It may also be preferred when impairment of peripheral conversion of T4 and T3 is suspected.
Myxedema Coma—Myxedema coma is usually precipitated in the hypothyroid patient of long-standing by intercurrent illness or drugs such as sedatives and anesthetics and should be considered a medical emergency. Therapy should be directed at the correction of electrolyte disturbances and possible infection besides the administration of thyroid hormones. Corticosteroids should be administered routinely. T4 and T3 may be administered via a nasogastric tube but the preferred route of administration of both hormones is intravenous. Sodium levothyroxine (T4) is given at a starting dose of 400 mcg (100 mcg/mL) given rapidly, and is usually well tolerated, even in the elderly. This initial dose is followed by daily supplements of 100 to 200 mcg given IV. Normal T4 levels are achieved in 24 hours followed in 3 days by threefold elevation of T3. Oral therapy with thyroid hormone would be resumed as soon as the clinical situation has been stabilized and the patient is able to take oral medication.
Thyroid Cancer—Exogenous thyroid hormone may produce regression of metastases from follicular and papillary carcinoma of the thyroid and is used as ancillary therapy of these conditions with radioactive iodine. TSH should be suppressed to low or undetectable levels. Therefore, larger amounts of thyroid hormone than those used for replacement therapy are required. Medullary carcinoma of the thyroid is usually unresponsive to this therapy.
Thyroid Suppression Therapy—Administration of thyroid hormone in doses higher than those produced physiologically by the gland results in suppression of the production of endogenous hormone. This is the basis for the thyroid suppression test and is used as an aid in the diagnosis of patients with signs of mild hyperthyroidism in whom baseline laboratory tests appear normal, or to demonstrate thyroid gland autonomy in patients with Grave's ophthalmopathy. 131I uptake is determined before and after the administration of the exogenous hormone. A fifty percent or greater suppression of uptake indicates a normal thyroid-pituitary axis and thus rules out thyroid gland autonomy.
For adults, the usual suppressive dose of levothyroxine (T4) is 1.56 mcg/kg of body weight per day given for 7 to 10 days. These doses usually yield normal serum T4 and T3 levels and lack of response to TSH.
Thyroid hormones should be administered cautiously to patients in whom there is strong suspicion of thyroid gland autonomy, in view of the fact that the exogenous hormone effects will be additive to the endogenous source.
Pediatric Dosage—Pediatric dosage should follow the recommendations summarized in Table 1. In infants with congenital hypothyroidism, therapy with full doses should be instituted as soon as the diagnosis has been made.

Table 1 Recommended Pediatric Dosage for Congenital Hypothyroidism Dose per day in mcg

Age	T3/T4	to	T3/T4
0-6 mos	3.1/12.5	to	6.25/25

Continued on next page

Name	Composition (T3/T4 per tablet)	Color	Armacode®	NDC
Thyrolar-1/4	3.1 mcg/ 12.5 mcg	Violet/White	YC	0456-0040-01
Thyrolar-1/2	6.25 mcg/ 25 mcg	Peach/White	YD	0456-0045-01
Thyrolar-1	12.5 mcg/ 50 mcg	Pink/White	YE	0456-0050-01
Thyrolar-2	25 mcg/ 100 mcg	Green/White	YF	0456-0055-01
Thyrolar-3	37.5 mcg/ 150 mcg	Yellow/White	YH	0456-0060-01

Thyrolar—Cont.

6-12 mos	6.25/25	to	9.35/37.5
1-5 yrs	9.35/37.5	to	12.5/50
6-12 yrs	12.5/50	to	18.75/75
Over 12 yrs		over	18.75/75

The HOW SUPPLIED section was revised as follows:

HOW SUPPLIED

Thyrolar Tablets (Liotrix Tablets, USP) are available in five potencies coded as follows:
[See table at bottom of previous page.]
Supplied in bottles of 100, two-layered compressed tablets. Tablets should be stored at cold temperature, between 36°F and 46°F (2°C and 8°C) in a tight, light-resistant container. Note: (T3 liothyronine sodium is approximately four times as potent as T4 thyroxine on a microgram for microgram basis.)
FOREST PHARMACEUTICALS, INC.
A Subsidiary of Forest Laboratories, Inc.
St. Louis, MO 63045
Rev. 04/05
RMC #1436
© 2005 Forest Laboratories, Inc.

TIAZAC® Rx
(diltiazem hydrochloride)
Extended Release Capsules USP
Drug Release Test 6
Rx Only

Prescribing information for this product, which appears on pages 1187–1189 of the 2008 PDR, has been revised as follows. Please write "See Supplement A" next to the product heading.
The following paragraph was added under the PRECAUTIONS section, after the subsection Beta Blockers:
Buspirone. In nine healthy subjects, diltiazem significantly increased the mean buspirone AUC 5.5 fold and Cmax 4.1 fold compared to placebo. The T½ and Tmax of buspirone were not significantly affected by diltiazem. Enhanced effects and increased toxicity of buspirone may be possible during concomitant administration with diltiazem. Subsequent dose adjustments may be necessary during co-administration, and should be based on clinical assessment.
The following paragraph was added under the PRECAUTIONS section, after the subsection Digitalis:
Quinidine. Diltiazem significantly increases the AUC(0→∞) of quinidine by 51%, T½ by 36%, and decreases its CLoral by 33%. Monitoring for quinidine adverse effects may be warranted and the dose adjusted accordingly.
Manufactured by:
Biovail Corporation
Mississauga, Ontario CANADA L5N 8M5
Manufactured for:
Forest Pharmaceuticals, Inc.
Subsidiary of Forest Laboratories, Inc.
St. Louis, Missouri 63045
Rev. 04/06
LB0001-09

Eli Lilly and Company
LILLY CORPORATE CENTER
INDIANAPOLIS, IN 46285

Direct Inquiries to:
Lilly Corporate Center
Indianapolis, IN 46285
(317) 276-2000
www.lilly.com
For Medical Information Contact:
Lilly Research Laboratories
Lilly Corporate Center
Indianapolis, IN 46285
(800) 545-5979

EVISTA® Rx
[ē-vis-tǎ]
(raloxifene hydrochloride)
Tablets for Oral use

Prescribing information for this product, which appears on pages 1798–1803 of the 2008 PDR, has been completely revised as follows. Please write "See Supplement A" next to the product heading.
HIGHLIGHTS OF PRESCRIBING INFORMATION
These highlights do not include all the information needed to use Evista safely and effectively. See full prescribing information for Evista.
Evista (raloxifene hydrochloride) Tablet for Oral use
Initial U.S. Approval: 1997

> **WARNING: INCREASED RISK OF VENOUS THROM-BOEMBOLISM AND DEATH FROM STROKE**
> *See full prescribing information for complete boxed warning.*

> • Increased risk of deep vein thrombosis and pulmonary embolism have been reported with EVISTA (5.1). Women with active or past history of venous thromboembolism should not take EVISTA (4.1).
> • Increased risk of death due to stroke occurred in a trial in postmenopausal women with documented coronary heart disease or at increased risk for major coronary events. Consider risk-benefit balance in women at risk for stroke (5.2, 14.5).

RECENT MAJOR CHANGES

Boxed Warning	9/2007
Indications and Usage, Invasive Breast Cancer Risk Reduction (1)	9/2007
Warnings and Precautions, Death Due to Stroke (5.2)	7/2007
Warnings and Precautions, Cardiovascular Disease (5.3)	7/2007
Warnings and Precautions, Renal Impairment (5.8)	7/2007

INDICATIONS AND USAGE
EVISTA® is an estrogen agonist/antagonist indicated for:
• Treatment and prevention of osteoporosis in postmenopausal women. (1.1)
• Reduction in risk of invasive breast cancer in postmenopausal women with osteoporosis. (1.2)
• Reduction in risk of invasive breast cancer in postmenopausal women at high risk for invasive breast cancer. (1.3)
Important Limitations: EVISTA is not indicated for the treatment of invasive breast cancer, reduction of the risk of recurrence of breast cancer, or reduction of risk of noninvasive breast cancer. (1.3)

DOSAGE AND ADMINISTRATION
60 mg tablet orally once daily. (2.1)
DOSAGE FORMS AND STRENGTHS
Tablets (not scored): 60 mg (3)
CONTRAINDICATIONS
• Active or past history of venous thromboembolism, including deep vein thrombosis, pulmonary embolism, and retinal vein thrombosis. (4.1)
• Pregnancy, women who may become pregnant, and nursing mothers. (4.2, 8.1, 8.3)
WARNINGS AND PRECAUTIONS
• *Venous Thromboembolism:* Increased risk of deep vein thrombosis, pulmonary embolism, and retinal vein thrombosis. Discontinue use 72 hours prior to and during prolonged immobilization. (5.1, 6.1)
• *Death Due to Stroke:* Increased risk of death due to stroke occurred in a trial in postmenopausal women with documented coronary heart disease or at increased risk for major coronary events. No increased risk of stroke was seen in this trial. Consider risk-benefit balance in women at risk for stroke. (5.2, 14.5)
• *Cardiovascular Disease:* EVISTA should not be used for the primary or secondary prevention of cardiovascular disease. (5.3, 14.5)
• *Premenopausal Women:* Use is not recommended. (5.4)
• *Hepatic Impairment:* Use with caution. (5.5)
• *Concomitant Use with Systemic Estrogens:* Not recommended. (5.6)
• *Hypertriglyceridemia:* If previous treatment with estrogen resulted in hypertriglyceridemia, monitor serum triglycerides. (5.7)
ADVERSE REACTIONS
*Adverse reactions (>2% and more common than with placebo) include: hot flashes, leg cramps, peripheral edema, flu syndrome, arthralgia, sweating. (6.1)
To report SUSPECTED ADVERSE REACTIONS, contact Eli Lilly and Company at 1-800-545-5979 or FDA at 1-800-FDA-1088 or www.fda.gov/medwatch
DRUG INTERACTIONS
• *Cholestyramine:* Use with EVISTA is not recommended. Reduces the absorption and enterohepatic cycling of raloxifene. (7.1, 12.3)
• *Warfarin:* Monitor prothrombin time when starting or stopping EVISTA. (7.2, 12.3)
• *Highly Protein-Bound Drugs:* Use with EVISTA with caution. Highly protein-bound drugs include diazepam, diazoxide, and lidocaine. EVISTA is more than 95% bound to plasma proteins. (7.3, 12.3)
USE IN SPECIFIC POPULATIONS
• *Pediatric Use:* Safety and effectiveness not established. (8.4)
See 17 for PATIENT COUNSELING INFORMATION and the FDA-approved Medication Guide

Revised: 10/2007

FULL PRESCRIBING INFORMATION: CONTENTS*
WARNING: INCREASED RISK OF VENOUS THROMBOEMBOLISM AND DEATH FROM STROKE

* Sections or subsections omitted from the full prescribing information are not listed.

FULL PRESCRIBING INFORMATION

> **WARNING: INCREASED RISK OF VENOUS THROMBOEMBOLISM AND DEATH FROM STROKE**
>
> • Increased risk of deep vein thrombosis and pulmonary embolism have been reported with EVISTA *(5.1)*. Women with active or past history of venous thromboembolism should not take EVISTA *(4.1)*.
> • Increased risk of death due to stroke occurred in a trial in postmenopausal women with documented coronary heart disease or at increased risk for major coronary events. Consider risk-benefit balance in women at risk for stroke *(5.2, 14.5)*.

1 INDICATIONS AND USAGE
1.1 Treatment and Prevention of Osteoporosis in Postmenopausal Women
EVISTA is indicated for the treatment and prevention of osteoporosis in postmenopausal women *[see Clinical Studies (14.1, 14.2)]*.
1.2 Reduction in the Risk of Invasive Breast Cancer in Postmenopausal Women with Osteoporosis
EVISTA is indicated for the reduction in risk of invasive breast cancer in postmenopausal women with osteoporosis *[see Clinical Studies (14.3)]*.
1.3 Reduction in the Risk of Invasive Breast Cancer in Postmenopausal Women at High Risk of Invasive Breast Cancer
EVISTA is indicated for the reduction in risk of invasive breast cancer in postmenopausal women at high risk of invasive breast cancer *[see Clinical Studies (14.4)]*.
The effect in the reduction in the incidence of breast cancer was shown in a study of postmenopausal women at high risk for breast cancer with a 5-year planned duration with a median follow-up of 4.3 years *[see Clinical Studies (14.4)]*.

Twenty-seven percent of the participants received drug for 5 years. The long-term effects and the recommended length of treatment are not known.

High risk of breast cancer is defined as at least one breast biopsy showing lobular carcinoma in situ (LCIS) or atypical hyperplasia, one or more first-degree relatives with breast cancer, or a 5-year predicted risk of breast cancer ≥1.66% (based on the modified Gail model). Among the factors included in the modified Gail model are the following: current age, number of first-degree relatives with breast cancer, number of breast biopsies, age at menarche, nulliparity or age of first live birth. Healthcare professionals can obtain a Gail Model Risk Assessment Tool by dialing 1-800-545-5979. Currently, no single clinical finding or test result can quantify risk of breast cancer with certainty.

After an assessment of the risk of developing breast cancer, the decision regarding therapy with EVISTA should be based upon an individual assessment of the benefits and risks.

EVISTA does not eliminate the risk of breast cancer. Patients should have breast exams and mammograms before starting EVISTA and should continue regular breast exams and mammograms in keeping with good medical practice after beginning treatment with EVISTA.

Important Limitations of Use for Breast Cancer Risk Reduction

- There are no data available regarding the effect of EVISTA on invasive breast cancer incidence in women with inherited mutations (BRCA1, BRCA2) to be able to make specific recommendations on the effectiveness of EVISTA.
- EVISTA is not indicated for the treatment of invasive breast cancer or reduction of the risk of recurrence.
- EVISTA is not indicated for the reduction in the risk of noninvasive breast cancer.

2 DOSAGE AND ADMINISTRATION
2.1 Recommended Dosing
The recommended dosage is one 60 mg EVISTA tablet daily, which may be administered any time of day without regard to meals [see Clinical Pharmacology (12.3)].

For the indications in risk of invasive breast cancer the optimum duration of treatment is not known [see Clinical Studies (14.3, 14.4)].

2.2 Recommendations for Calcium and Vitamin D Supplementation
For either osteoporosis treatment or prevention, supplemental calcium and/or vitamin D should be added to the diet if daily intake is inadequate. Postmenopausal women require an average of 1500 mg/day of elemental calcium. Total daily intake of calcium above 1500 mg has not demonstrated additional bone benefits while daily intake above 2000 mg has been associated with increased risk of adverse effects, including hypercalcemia and kidney stones. The recommended intake of vitamin D is 400-800 IU daily. Patients at increased risk for vitamin D insufficiency (e.g., over the age of 70 years, nursing home bound, or chronically ill) may need additional vitamin D supplements. Patients with gastrointestinal malabsorption syndromes may require higher doses of vitamin D supplementation and measurement of 25-hydroxyvitamin D should be considered.

3 DOSAGE FORMS AND STRENGTHS
60 mg, white, elliptical, film-coated tablets (not scored). They are imprinted on one side with LILLY and the tablet code 4165 in edible blue ink.

4 CONTRAINDICATIONS
4.1 Venous Thromboembolism
EVISTA is contraindicated in women with active or past history of venous thromboembolism (VTE), including deep vein thrombosis, pulmonary embolism, and retinal vein thrombosis [see Warnings and Precautions (5.1)].

4.2 Pregnancy, Women Who May Become Pregnant, and Nursing Mothers
EVISTA is contraindicated in pregnancy, in women who may become pregnant, and in nursing mothers [see Use in Specific Populations (8.1, 8.3)]. EVISTA may cause fetal harm when administered to a pregnant woman. If this drug is used during pregnancy, or if the patient becomes pregnant while taking this drug, the patient should be apprised of the potential hazard to the fetus.

In rabbit studies, abortion and a low rate of fetal heart anomalies (ventricular septal defects) occurred in rabbits at doses ≥0.1 mg/kg (≥0.04 times the human dose based on surface area, mg/m²), and hydrocephaly was observed in fetuses at doses ≥10 mg/kg (≥4 times the human dose based on surface area, mg/m²). In rat studies, retardation of fetal development and developmental abnormalities (wavy ribs, kidney cavitation) occurred at doses ≥1 mg/kg (≥0.2 times the human dose based on surface area, mg/m²). Treatment of rats at doses of 0.1 to 10 mg/kg (0.02 to 1.6 times the human dose based on surface area, mg/m²) during gestation and lactation produced effects that included delayed and disrupted parturition; decreased neonatal survival and altered physical development; sex- and age-specific reductions in growth and changes in pituitary hormone content; and decreased lymphoid compartment size in offspring. At 10 mg/kg, raloxifene disrupted parturition, which resulted in maternal and progeny death and morbidity. Effects in adult offspring (4 months of age) included uterine hypoplasia and reduced fertility; however, no ovarian or vaginal pathology was observed.

Table 1: Adverse Reactions Occurring in Placebo–Controlled Osteoporosis Clinical Trials at a Frequency ≥2.0% and in More EVISTA-Treated (60 mg Once Daily) Women than Placebo–Treated Women*

| | Treatment | | Prevention | |
	EVISTA N=2557 %	Placebo N=2576 %	EVISTA N=581 %	Placebo N=584 %
Body as a Whole				
Infection	A	A	15.1	14.6
Flu Syndrome	13.5	11.4	14.6	13.5
Headache	9.2	8.5	A	A
Leg Cramps	7.0	3.7	5.9	1.9
Chest Pain	A	A	4.0	3.6
Fever	3.9	3.8	3.1	2.6
Cardiovascular System				
Hot Flashes	9.7	6.4	24.6	18.3
Migraine	A	A	2.4	2.1
Syncope	2.3	2.1	B	B
Varicose Vein	2.2	1.5	A	A
Digestive System				
Nausea	8.3	7.8	8.8	8.6
Diarrhea	7.2	6.9	A	A
Dyspepsia	A	A	5.9	5.8
Vomiting	4.8	4.3	3.4	3.3
Flatulence	A	A	3.1	2.4
Gastrointestinal Disorder	A	A	3.3	2.1
Gastroenteritis	B	B	2.6	2.1
Metabolic and Nutritional				
Weight Gain	A	A	8.8	6.8
Peripheral Edema	5.2	4.4	3.3	1.9
Musculoskeletal System				
Arthralgia	15.5	14.0	10.7	10.1
Myalgia	A	A	7.7	6.2
Arthritis	A	A	4.0	3.6
Tendon Disorder	3.6	3.1	A	A
Nervous System				
Depression	A	A	6.4	6.0
Insomnia	A	A	5.5	4.3
Vertigo	4.1	3.7	A	A
Neuralgia	2.4	1.9	B	B
Hypesthesia	2.1	2.0	B	B
Respiratory System				
Sinusitis	7.9	7.5	10.3	6.5
Rhinitis	10.2	10.1	A	A
Bronchitis	9.5	8.6	A	A
Pharyngitis	5.3	5.1	7.6	7.2
Cough Increased	9.3	9.2	6.0	5.7
Pneumonia	A	A	2.6	1.5
Laryngitis	B	B	2.2	1.4
Skin and Appendages				
Rash	A	A	5.5	3.8
Sweating	2.5	2.0	3.1	1.7
Special Senses				
Conjunctivitis	2.2	1.7	A	A
Urogenital System				
Vaginitis	A	A	4.3	3.6
Urinary Tract Infection	A	A	4.0	3.9
Cystitis	4.6	4.5	3.3	3.1
Leukorrhea	A	A	3.3	1.7
Uterine Disorder†,‡	3.3	2.3	A	A
Endometrial Disorder†	B	B	3.1	1.9
Vaginal Hemorrhage	2.5	2.4	A	A
Urinary Tract Disorder	2.5	2.1	A	A

* A: Placebo incidence greater than or equal to EVISTA incidence; B: Less than 2% incidence and more frequent with EVISTA.
† Includes only patients with an intact uterus: Prevention Trials: EVISTA, n=354, Placebo, n=364; Treatment Trial: EVISTA, n=1948, Placebo, n=1999.
‡ Actual terms most frequently referred to endometrial fluid.

5 WARNINGS AND PRECAUTIONS
5.1 Venous Thromboembolism
In clinical trials, EVISTA-treated women had an increased risk of venous thromboembolism (deep vein thrombosis and pulmonary embolism). Other venous thromboembolic events also could occur. A less serious event, superficial thrombophlebitis, also has been reported more frequently with EVISTA than with placebo. The greatest risk for deep vein thrombosis and pulmonary embolism occurs during the first 4 months of treatment, and the magnitude of risk appears to be similar to the reported risk associated with use of hormone therapy. Because immobilization increases the risk for venous thromboembolic events independent of therapy, EVISTA should be discontinued at least 72 hours prior to and during prolonged immobilization (e.g., post-surgical recovery, prolonged bed rest), and EVISTA therapy should be resumed only after the patient is fully ambulatory. In addition, women taking EVISTA should be advised to move about periodically during prolonged travel. The risk-benefit balance should be considered in women at risk of thromboembolic disease for other reasons, such as congestive heart failure, superficial thrombophlebitis, and active malignancy [see Contraindications (4.1) and Adverse Reactions (6.1)].

5.2 Death Due to Stroke
In a clinical trial of postmenopausal women with documented coronary heart disease or at increased risk for coronary events, an increased risk of death due to stroke was observed after treatment with EVISTA. During an average follow-up of 5.6 years, 59 (1.2%) EVISTA-treated women died due to a stroke compared to 39 (0.8%) placebo-treated women (22 versus 15 per 10,000 women-years; hazard ratio 1.49; 95% confidence interval, 1.00-2.24; p=0.0499). There was no statistically significant difference between treatment groups in the incidence of stroke (249 in EVISTA [4.9%] versus 224 placebo [4.4%]). EVISTA had no significant effect on all-cause mortality. The risk-benefit balance should be considered in women at risk for stroke, such as prior stroke or transient ischemic attack (TIA), atrial fibrillation, hypertension, or cigarette smoking [see Clinical Studies (14.5)].

5.3 Cardiovascular Disease
EVISTA should not be used for the primary or secondary prevention of cardiovascular disease. In a clinical trial of postmenopausal women with documented coronary heart disease or at increased risk for coronary events, no cardiovascular benefit was demonstrated after treatment with raloxifene for 5 years [see Clinical Studies (14.5)].

5.4 Premenopausal Use
There is no indication for premenopausal use of EVISTA. Safety of EVISTA in premenopausal women has not been established and its use is not recommended.

5.5 Hepatic Impairment
EVISTA should be used with caution in patients with hepatic impairment. Safety and efficacy have not been established in patients with hepatic impairment [see Clinical Pharmacology (12.3)].

5.6 Concomitant Estrogen Therapy
The safety of concomitant use of EVISTA with systemic estrogens has not been established and its use is not recommended.

Continued on next page

This product information was prepared in March 2008. Current information on products of Eli Lilly and Company may be obtained by calling 1-800-545-5979.

Evista—Cont.

5.7 History of Hypertriglyceridemia when Treated with Estrogens
Limited clinical data suggest that some women with a history of marked hypertriglyceridemia (>5.6 mmol/L or >500 mg/dL) in response to treatment with oral estrogen or estrogen plus progestin may develop increased levels of triglycerides when treated with EVISTA. Women with this medical history should have serum triglycerides monitored when taking EVISTA.

5.8 Renal Impairment
EVISTA should be used with caution in patients with moderate or severe renal impairment. Safety and efficacy have not been established in patients with moderate or severe renal impairment *[see Clinical Pharmacology (12.3)]*.

5.9 History of Breast Cancer
EVISTA has not been adequately studied in women with a prior history of breast cancer.

5.10 Use in Men
There is no indication for the use of EVISTA in men. EVISTA has not been adequately studied in men and its use is not recommended.

5.11 Unexplained Uterine Bleeding
Any unexplained uterine bleeding should be investigated as clinically indicated. EVISTA-treated and placebo-treated groups had similar incidences of endometrial proliferation *[see Clinical Studies (14.1, 14.2)]*.

5.12 Breast Abnormalities
Any unexplained breast abnormality occurring during EVISTA therapy should be investigated. EVISTA does not eliminate the risk of breast cancer *[see Clinical Studies (14.4)]*.

6 ADVERSE REACTIONS

6.1 Clinical Trials Experience
Because clinical studies are conducted under widely varying conditions, adverse reaction rates observed in the clinical trials of a drug cannot be directly compared to rates in the clinical trials of another drug and may not reflect the rates observed in practice.
The data described below reflect exposure to EVISTA in 8429 patients who were enrolled in placebo-controlled trials, including 6666 exposed for 1 year and 5685 for at least 3 years.
Osteoporosis Treatment Clinical Trial (MORE) — The safety of raloxifene in the treatment of osteoporosis was assessed in a large (7705 patients) multinational, placebo-controlled trial. Duration of treatment was 36 months, and 5129 postmenopausal women were exposed to raloxifene (2557 received 60 mg/day, and 2572 received 120 mg/day). The incidence of all-cause mortality was similar among groups: 23 (0.9%) placebo, 13 (0.5%) EVISTA-treated (raloxifene 60 mg), and 28 (1.1%) raloxifene 120 mg women died. Therapy was discontinued due to an adverse reaction in 10.9% of EVISTA-treated women and 8.8% of placebo-treated women.
Venous Thromboembolism: The most serious adverse reaction related to EVISTA was VTE (deep venous thrombosis, pulmonary embolism, and retinal vein thrombosis). During an average of study-drug exposure of 2.6 years, VTE occurred in about 1 out of 100 patients treated with EVISTA. Twenty-six EVISTA-treated women had a VTE compared to 11 placebo-treated women, the hazard ratio was 2.4 (95% confidence interval, 1.2, 4.5), and the highest VTE risk was during the initial months of treatment.
Common adverse reactions considered to be related to EVISTA therapy were hot flashes and leg cramps. Hot flashes occurred in about one in 10 patients on EVISTA and were most commonly reported during the first 6 months of treatment and were not different from placebo thereafter. Leg cramps occurred in about one in 14 patients on EVISTA.
Placebo-Controlled Osteoporosis Prevention Clinical Trials — The safety of raloxifene has been assessed primarily in 12 Phase 2 and Phase 3 studies with placebo, estrogen, and estrogen-progestin therapy control groups. The duration of treatment ranged from 2 to 30 months, and 2036 women were exposed to raloxifene (371 patients received 10 to 50 mg/day, 828 received 60 mg/day, and 837 received from 120 to 600 mg/day).
Therapy was discontinued due to an adverse reaction in 11.4% of 581 EVISTA-treated women and 12.2% of 584 placebo-treated women. Discontinuation rates due to hot flashes did not differ significantly between EVISTA and placebo groups (1.7% and 2.2%, respectively).
Common adverse reactions considered to be drug-related were hot flashes and leg cramps. Hot flashes occurred in about one in four patients on EVISTA versus about one in six on placebo. The first occurrence of hot flashes was most commonly reported during the first 6 months of treatment.
Table 1 lists adverse reactions occurring in either the osteoporosis treatment or in five prevention placebo-controlled clinical trials at a frequency ≥2.0% in either group and in more EVISTA-treated women than in placebo-treated women. Adverse reactions are shown without attribution of causality. The majority of adverse reactions occurring during the studies were mild and generally did not require discontinuation of therapy.
[See table 1 at top of previous page]
Comparison of EVISTA and Hormone Therapy — EVISTA was compared with estrogen-progestin therapy in three clinical trials for prevention of osteoporosis. Table 2 shows adverse reactions occurring more frequently in one treatment group and at an incidence ≥2.0% in any group. Adverse reactions are shown without attribution of causality.
[See table 2 above]

Table 2: Adverse Reactions Reported in the Clinical Trials for Osteoporosis Prevention with EVISTA (60 mg Once Daily) and Continuous Combined or Cyclic Estrogen Plus Progestin (Hormone Therapy) at an Incidence ≥2.0% in any Treatment Group*

	EVISTA (N=317) %	Hormone Therapy–Continuous Combined† (N=96) %	Hormone Therapy–Cyclic‡ (N=219) %
Urogenital			
Breast Pain	4.4	37.5	29.7
Vaginal Bleeding§	6.2	64.2	88.5
Digestive			
Flatulence	1.6	12.5	6.4
Cardiovascular			
Hot Flashes	28.7	3.1	5.9
Body as a Whole			
Infection	11.0	0	6.8
Abdominal Pain	6.6	10.4	18.7
Chest Pain	2.8	0	0.5

* These data are from both blinded and open-label studies.
† Continuous Combined Hormone Therapy = 0.625 mg conjugated estrogens plus 2.5 mg medroxyprogesterone acetate.
‡ Cyclic Hormone Therapy = 0.625 mg conjugated estrogens for 28 days with concomitant 5 mg medroxyprogesterone acetate or 0.15 mg norgestrel on Days 1 through 14 or 17 through 28.
§ Includes only patients with an intact uterus: EVISTA, n=290; Hormone Therapy–Continuous Combined, n=67; Hormone Therapy–Cyclic, n=217.

Breast Pain — Across all placebo-controlled trials, EVISTA was indistinguishable from placebo with regard to frequency and severity of breast pain and tenderness. EVISTA was associated with less breast pain and tenderness than reported by women receiving estrogens with or without added progestin.
Gynecologic Cancers — EVISTA-treated and placebo-treated groups had similar incidences of endometrial cancer and ovarian cancer.
Placebo-Controlled Trial of Postmenopausal Women at Increased Risk for Major Coronary Events (RUTH) — The safety of EVISTA (60 mg once daily) was assessed in a placebo-controlled multinational trial of 10,101 postmenopausal women (age range 55-92) with documented coronary heart disease (CHD) or multiple CHD risk factors. Median study drug exposure was 5.1 years for both treatment groups *[see Clinical Studies (14.3)]*. Therapy was discontinued due to an adverse reaction in 25% of 5044 EVISTA-treated women and 24% of 5057 placebo-treated women. The incidence per year of all-cause mortality was similar between the raloxifene (2.07%) and placebo (2.25%) groups.
Adverse reactions reported more frequently in EVISTA-treated women than in placebo-treated women included peripheral edema (14.1% raloxifene versus 11.7% placebo), muscle spasms/leg cramps (12.1% raloxifene versus 8.3% placebo), hot flashes (7.8% raloxifene versus 4.7% placebo), venous thromboembolic events (2.0% raloxifene versus 1.4% placebo), and cholelithiasis (3.3% raloxifene versus 2.6% placebo) *[see Clinical Studies (14.3, 14.5)]*.
Tamoxifen-Controlled Trial of Postmenopausal Women at Increased Risk for Invasive Breast Cancer (STAR) — The safety of EVISTA 60 mg/day versus tamoxifen 20 mg/day over 5 years was assessed in 19,747 postmenopausal women (age range 35-83 years) in a randomized, double-blind trial. As of 31 December 2005, the median follow-up was 4.3 years. The safety profile of raloxifene was similar to that in the placebo-controlled raloxifene trials *[see Clinical Studies (14.4)]*.

6.2 Postmarketing Experience
Because these reactions are reported voluntarily from a population of uncertain size, it is not always possible to reliably estimate their frequency or establish a causal relationship to drug exposure.
Adverse reactions reported very rarely since market introduction include retinal vein occlusion, stroke, and death associated with venous thromboembolism (VTE).

7 DRUG INTERACTIONS

7.1 Cholestyramine
Concomitant administration of cholestyramine with EVISTA is not recommended. Although not specifically studied, it is anticipated that other anion exchange resins would have a similar effect. EVISTA should not be coadministered with other anion exchange resins *[see Clinical Pharmacology (12.3)]*.

7.2 Warfarin
If EVISTA is given concomitantly with warfarin or other warfarin derivatives, prothrombin time should be monitored more closely when starting or stopping therapy with EVISTA *[see Clinical Pharmacology (12.3)]*.

7.3 Other Highly Protein-Bound Drugs
EVISTA should be used with caution with certain other highly protein-bound drugs such as diazepam, diazoxide, and lidocaine. Although not examined, EVISTA might affect the protein binding of other drugs. Raloxifene is more than 95% bound to plasma proteins *[see Clinical Pharmacology (12.3)]*.

7.4 Systemic Estrogens
The safety of concomitant use of EVISTA with systemic estrogens has not been established and its use is not recommended.

7.5 Other Concomitant Medications
EVISTA can be concomitantly administered with ampicillin, amoxicillin, antacids, corticosteroids, and digoxin *[see Clinical Pharmacology (12.3)]*.
The concomitant use of EVISTA and lipid-lowering agents has not been studied.

8 USE IN SPECIFIC POPULATIONS

8.1 Pregnancy
Pregnancy Category X. EVISTA should not be used in women who are or may become pregnant *[see Contraindications (4.2)]*.

8.3 Nursing Mothers
EVISTA should not be used by lactating women *[see Contraindications (4.2)]*. It is not known whether this drug is excreted in human milk. Because many drugs are excreted in human milk, caution should be exercised when raloxifene is administered to a nursing woman.

8.4 Pediatric Use
Safety and effectiveness in pediatric patients have not been established.

8.5 Geriatric Use
Of the total number of patients in placebo-controlled clinical studies of EVISTA, 61% were 65 and over, while 15.5% were 75 and over. No overall differences in safety or effectiveness were observed between these subjects and younger subjects, and other reported clinical experience has not identified differences in responses between the elderly and younger patients, but greater sensitivity of some older individuals cannot be ruled out. Based on clinical trials, there is no need for dose adjustment for geriatric patients *[see Clinical Pharmacology (12.3)]*.

8.6 Renal Impairment
EVISTA should be used with caution in patients with moderate or severe renal impairment *[see Warnings and Precautions (5.8) and Clinical Pharmacology (12.3)]*.

8.7 Hepatic Impairment
EVISTA should be used with caution in patients with hepatic impairment *[see Warnings and Precautions (5.5) and Clinical Pharmacology (12.3)]*.

10 OVERDOSAGE

In an 8-week study of 63 postmenopausal women, a dose of raloxifene HCl 600 mg/day was safely tolerated. In clinical trials, no raloxifene overdose has been reported.
In postmarketing spontaneous reports, raloxifene overdose has been reported very rarely (less than 1 out of 10,000 [<0.01%] patients treated). The highest overdose has been approximately 1.5 grams. No fatalities associated with raloxifene overdose have been reported. Adverse reactions were reported in approximately half of the adults who took ≥180 mg raloxifene and included leg cramps and dizziness. Two 18-month-old children each ingested raloxifene 180 mg. In these two children, symptoms reported included ataxia, dizziness, vomiting, rash, diarrhea, tremor, and flushing, as well as elevation in alkaline phosphatase.
There is no specific antidote for raloxifene.
No mortality was seen after a single oral dose in rats or mice at 5000 mg/kg (810 times the human dose for rats and 405 times the human dose for mice based on surface area, mg/m^2) or in monkeys at 1000 mg/kg (80 times the AUC in humans).

11 DESCRIPTION

EVISTA (raloxifene hydrochloride) is an estrogen agonist/antagonist, commonly referred to as a selective estrogen receptor modulator (SERM) that belongs to the benzothiophene class of compounds. The chemical structure is:

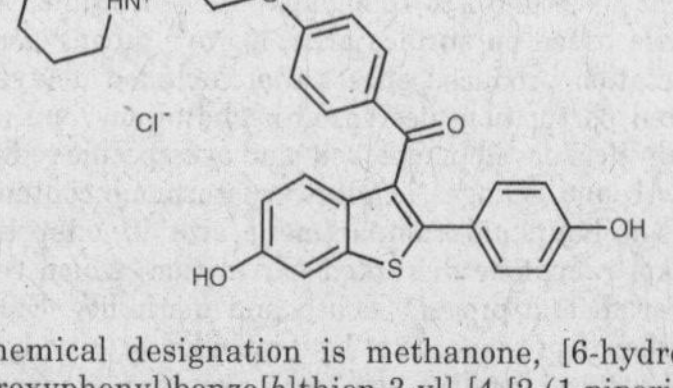

The chemical designation is methanone, [6-hydroxy-2-(4-hydroxyphenyl)benzo[b]thien-3-yl]-[4-[2-(1-piperidinyl) ethoxy]phenyl]-, hydrochloride. Raloxifene hydrochloride

(HCl) has the empirical formula $C_{28}H_{27}NO_4S•HCl$, which corresponds to a molecular weight of 510.05. Raloxifene HCl is an off-white to pale-yellow solid that is very slightly soluble in water.

EVISTA is supplied in a tablet dosage form for oral administration. Each EVISTA tablet contains 60 mg of raloxifene HCl, which is the molar equivalent of 55.71 mg of free base. Inactive ingredients include anhydrous lactose, carnauba wax, crospovidone, FD&C Blue No. 2 aluminum lake, hypromellose, lactose monohydrate, magnesium stearate, modified pharmaceutical glaze, polyethylene glycol, polysorbate 80, povidone, propylene glycol, and titanium dioxide.

12 CLINICAL PHARMACOLOGY

12.1 Mechanism of Action

Raloxifene is an estrogen agonist/antagonist, commonly referred to as a selective estrogen receptor modulator (SERM). The biological actions of raloxifene are largely mediated through binding to estrogen receptors. This binding results in activation of estrogenic pathways in some tissues (agonism) and blockade of estrogenic pathways in others (antagonism). The agonistic or antagonistic action of raloxifene depends on the extent of recruitment of coactivators and corepressors to estrogen receptor (ER) target gene promotors.

Raloxifene appears to act as an estrogen agonist in bone. It decreases bone resorption and bone turnover, increases bone mineral density (BMD) and decreases fracture incidence. Preclinical data demonstrate that raloxifene is an estrogen antagonist in uterine and breast tissues. These results are consistent with findings in clinical trials, which suggest that EVISTA lacks estrogen-like effects on the uterus and breast tissue.

12.2 Pharmacodynamics

Decreases in estrogen levels after oophorectomy or menopause lead to increases in bone resorption and accelerated bone loss. Bone is initially lost rapidly because the compensatory increase in bone formation is inadequate to offset resorptive losses. In addition to loss of estrogen, this imbalance between resorption and formation may be due to age-related impairment of osteoblasts or their precursors. In some women, these changes will eventually lead to decreased bone mass, osteoporosis, and increased risk for fractures, particularly of the spine, hip, and wrist. Vertebral fractures are the most common type of osteoporotic fracture in postmenopausal women.

In both the osteoporosis treatment and prevention trials, EVISTA therapy resulted in consistent, statistically significant suppression of bone resorption and bone formation, as reflected by changes in serum and urine markers of bone turnover (e.g., bone-specific alkaline phosphatase, osteocalcin, and collagen breakdown products). The suppression of bone turnover markers was evident by 3 months and persisted throughout the 36-month and 24-month observation periods.

In a 31-week, open-label, radiocalcium kinetics study, 33 early postmenopausal women were randomized to treatment with once-daily EVISTA 60 mg, cyclic estrogen/progestin (0.625 mg conjugated estrogens daily with 5 mg medroxyprogesterone acetate daily for the first 2 weeks of each month [hormone therapy]), or no treatment. Treatment with either EVISTA or hormone therapy was associated with reduced bone resorption and a positive shift in calcium balance (-82 mg Ca/day and +60 mg Ca/day, respectively, for EVISTA and -162 mg Ca/day and +91 mg Ca/day, respectively, for hormone therapy).

There were small decreases in serum total calcium, inorganic phosphate, total protein, and albumin, which were generally of lesser magnitude than decreases observed during estrogen or hormone therapy. Platelet count was also decreased slightly and was not different from estrogen therapy.

12.3 Pharmacokinetics

The disposition of raloxifene has been evaluated in more than 3000 postmenopausal women in selected raloxifene osteoporosis treatment and prevention clinical trials, using a population approach. Pharmacokinetic data also were obtained in conventional pharmacology studies in 292 postmenopausal women. Raloxifene exhibits high within-subject variability (approximately 30% coefficient of variation) of most pharmacokinetic parameters. Table 3 summarizes the pharmacokinetic parameters of raloxifene.

Absorption — Raloxifene is absorbed rapidly after oral administration. Approximately 60% of an oral dose is absorbed, but presystemic glucuronide conjugation is extensive. Absolute bioavailability of raloxifene is 2%. The time to reach average maximum plasma concentration and bioavailability are functions of systemic interconversion and enterohepatic cycling of raloxifene and its glucuronide metabolites.

Administration of raloxifene HCl with a standardized, high-fat meal increases the absorption of raloxifene (C_{max} 28% and AUC 16%), but does not lead to clinically meaningful changes in systemic exposure. EVISTA can be administered without regard to meals.

Distribution — Following oral administration of single doses ranging from 30 to 150 mg of raloxifene HCl, the apparent volume of distribution is 2348 L/kg and is not dose dependent.

Raloxifene and the monoglucuronide conjugates are highly (95%) bound to plasma proteins. Raloxifene binds to both albumin and α1-acid glycoprotein, but not to sex-steroid binding globulin.

Metabolism — Biotransformation and disposition of raloxifene in humans have been determined following oral administration of ^{14}C-labeled raloxifene. Raloxifene undergoes extensive first-pass metabolism to the glucuronide conjugates: raloxifene-4'-glucuronide, raloxifene-6-glucuronide, and raloxifene-6, 4'-diglucuronide. No other metabolites have been detected, providing strong evidence that raloxifene is not metabolized by cytochrome P450 pathways. Unconjugated raloxifene comprises less than 1% of the total radiolabeled material in plasma. The terminal log-linear portions of the plasma concentration curves for raloxifene and the glucuronides are generally parallel. This is consistent with interconversion of raloxifene and the glucuronide metabolites.

Following intravenous administration, raloxifene is cleared at a rate approximating hepatic blood flow. Apparent oral clearance is 44.1 L/kg•hr. Raloxifene and its glucuronide conjugates are interconverted by reversible systemic metabolism and enterohepatic cycling, thereby prolonging its plasma elimination half-life to 27.7 hours after oral dosing. Results from single oral doses of raloxifene predict multiple-dose pharmacokinetics. Following chronic dosing, clearance ranges from 40 to 60 L/kg•hr. Increasing doses of raloxifene HCl (ranging from 30 to 150 mg) result in slightly less than a proportional increase in the area under the plasma time concentration curve (AUC).

Excretion — Raloxifene is primarily excreted in feces, and less than 0.2% is excreted unchanged in urine. Less than 6% of the raloxifene dose is eliminated in urine as glucuronide conjugates.

[See table 3 above]

Table 3: Summary of Raloxifene Pharmacokinetic Parameters in the Healthy Postmenopausal Woman

	C_{max}*,† (ng/mL)/ (mg/kg)	$t_{½}$(hr)*	$AUC_{0-\infty}$*,† (ng•hr/mL)/ (mg/kg)	CL/F* (L/kg•hr)	V/F* (L/kg)
Single Dose					
Mean	0.50	27.7	27.2	44.1	2348
CV* (%)	52	10.7 to 273‡	44	46	52
Multiple Dose					
Mean	1.36	32.5	24.2	47.4	2853
CV* (%)	37	15.8 to 86.6‡	36	41	56

* Abbreviations: C_{max}= maximum plasma concentration, $t_{½}$= half-life, AUC = area under the curve, CL = clearance, V = volume of distribution, F = bioavailability, CV= coefficient of variation.
† Data normalized for dose in mg and body weight in kg.
‡ Range of observed half-life.

Special Populations

Pediatric — The pharmacokinetics of raloxifene has not been evaluated in a pediatric population *[see Use in Specific Populations (8.4)]*.

Geriatric — No differences in raloxifene pharmacokinetics were detected with regard to age (range 42 to 84 years) *[see Use in Specific Populations (8.5)]*.

Gender — Total extent of exposure and oral clearance, normalized for lean body weight, are not significantly different between age-matched female and male volunteers.

Race — Pharmacokinetic differences due to race have been studied in 1712 women, including 97.5% White, 1.0% Asian, 0.7% Hispanic, and 0.5% Black in the osteoporosis treatment trial and in 1053 women, including 93.5% White, 4.3% Hispanic, 1.2% Asian, and 0.5% Black in the osteoporosis prevention trials. There were no discernible differences in raloxifene plasma concentrations among these groups; however, the influence of race cannot be conclusively determined.

Renal Impairment — In the osteoporosis treatment and prevention trials, raloxifene concentrations in women with mild renal impairment are similar to women with normal creatinine clearance. When a single dose of 120 mg raloxifene HCl was administered to 10 renally impaired males [7 moderate impairment (CrCl = 31–50 mL/min); 3 severe impairment (CrCl ≤30 mL/min)] and to 10 healthy males (CrCl >80 mL/min), plasma raloxifene concentrations were 122% ($AUC_{0-\infty}$) higher in renally impaired patients than those of healthy volunteers. Raloxifene should be used with caution in patients with moderate or severe renal impairment *[see Warnings and Precautions (5.8) and Use in Specific Populations (8.6)]*.

Hepatic Impairment — The disposition of raloxifene was compared in 9 patients with mild (Child-Pugh Class A) hepatic impairment (total bilirubin ranging from 0.6 to 2 mg/dL) to 8 subjects with normal hepatic function following a single dose of 60 mg raloxifene HCl. Apparent clearance of raloxifene was reduced 56% and the half-life of raloxifene was not altered in patients with mild hepatic impairment. Plasma raloxifene concentrations were approximately 150% higher than those in healthy volunteers and correlated with total bilirubin concentrations. The pharmacokinetics of raloxifene has not been studied in patients with moderate or severe hepatic impairment. Raloxifene should be used with caution in patients with hepatic impairment *[see Warnings and Precautions (5.5) and Use in Specific Populations (8.7)]*.

Drug Interactions

Cholestyramine — Cholestyramine, an anion exchange resin, causes a 60% reduction in the absorption and enterohepatic cycling of raloxifene after a single dose. Although not specifically studied, it is anticipated that other anion exchange resins would have a similar effect *[see Drug Interactions (7.1)]*.

Warfarin — In vitro, raloxifene did not interact with the binding of warfarin. The concomitant administration of EVISTA and warfarin, a coumarin derivative, has been assessed in a single-dose study. In this study, raloxifene had no effect on the pharmacokinetics of warfarin. However, a 10% decrease in prothrombin time was observed in the single-dose study. In the osteoporosis treatment trial, there were no clinically relevant effects of warfarin co-administration on plasma concentrations of raloxifene *[see Drug Interactions (7.2)]*.

Other Highly Protein-Bound Drugs — In the osteoporosis treatment trial, there were no clinically relevant effects of co-administration of other highly protein-bound drugs (e.g., gemfibrozil) on plasma concentrations of raloxifene. In vitro, raloxifene did not interact with the binding of phenytoin, tamoxifen, or warfarin (*see* above) *[see Drug Interactions (7.3)]*.

Ampicillin and Amoxicillin — Peak concentrations of raloxifene and the overall extent of absorption are reduced 28% and 14%, respectively, with co-administration of ampicillin. These reductions are consistent with decreased enterohepatic cycling associated with antibiotic reduction of enteric bacteria. However, the systemic exposure and the elimination rate of raloxifene were not affected. In the osteoporosis treatment trial, co-administration of amoxicillin had no discernible differences in plasma raloxifene concentrations *[see Drug Interactions (7.5)]*.

Antacids — Concomitant administration of calcium carbonate or aluminum and magnesium hydroxide-containing antacids does not affect the systemic exposure of raloxifene *[see Drug Interactions (7.5)]*.

Corticosteroids — The chronic administration of raloxifene in postmenopausal women has no effect on the pharmacokinetics of methylprednisolone given as a single oral dose *[see Drug Interactions (7.5)]*.

Digoxin — Raloxifene has no effect on the pharmacokinetics of digoxin *[see Drug Interactions (7.5)]*.

Cyclosporine — Concomitant administration of EVISTA with cyclosporine has not been studied.

Lipid-Lowering Agents — Concomitant administration of EVISTA with lipid-lowering agents has not been studied.

13 NONCLINICAL TOXICOLOGY

13.1 Carcinogenesis, Mutagenesis, Impairment of Fertility

Carcinogenesis — In a 21-month carcinogenicity study in mice, there was an increased incidence of ovarian tumors in female animals given 9 to 242 mg/kg, which included benign and malignant tumors of granulosa/theca cell origin and benign tumors of epithelial cell origin. Systemic exposure (AUC) of raloxifene in this group was 0.3 to 34 times that in postmenopausal women administered a 60 mg dose. There was also an increased incidence of testicular interstitial cell tumors and prostatic adenomas and adenocarcinomas in male mice given 41 or 210 mg/kg (4.7 or 24 times the AUC in humans) and prostatic leiomyoblastoma in male mice given 210 mg/kg.

In a 2-year carcinogenicity study in rats, an increased incidence in ovarian tumors of granulosa/theca cell origin was observed in female rats given 279 mg/kg (approximately 400 times the AUC in humans). The female rodents in these studies were treated during their reproductive lives when their ovaries were functional and responsive to hormonal stimulation.

Mutagenesis — Raloxifene HCl was not genotoxic in any of the following test systems: the Ames test for bacterial mutagenesis with and without metabolic activation, the unscheduled DNA synthesis assay in rat hepatocytes, the mouse lymphoma assay for mammalian cell mutation, the chromosomal aberration assay in Chinese hamster ovary cells, the in vivo sister chromatid exchange assay in Chinese hamsters, and the in vivo micronucleus test in mice.

Impairment of Fertility — When male and female rats were given daily doses ≥5 mg/kg (≥0.8 times the human dose based on surface area, mg/m^2) prior to and during mating, no pregnancies occurred. In male rats, daily doses up to 100 mg/kg (16 times the human dose based on surface area, mg/m^2) for at least 2 weeks did not affect sperm production or quality or reproductive performance. In female rats, at doses of 0.1 to 10 mg/kg/day (0.02 to 1.6 times the human dose based on surface area, mg/m^2), raloxifene disrupted es-

Continued on next page

This product information was prepared in March 2008. Current information on products of Eli Lilly and Company may be obtained by calling 1-800-545-5979.

Table 4: Effect of EVISTA on Risk of Vertebral Fractures

	Number of Patients		Absolute Risk Reduction (ARR)	Relative Risk Reduction (95% CI)
	EVISTA	Placebo		
Fractures diagnosed radiographically				
Patients with no baseline fracture*	n=1401	n=1457		
Number (%) of patients with ≥1 new vertebral fracture	27 (1.9%)	62 (4.3%)	2.4%	55% (29%, 71%)
Patients with ≥1 baseline fracture*	n=858	n=835		
Number (%) of patients with ≥1 new vertebral fracture	121 (14.1%)	169 (20.2%)	6.1%	30% (14%, 44%)
Symptomatic vertebral fractures				
All randomized patients	n=2557	n=2576		
Number (%) of patients with ≥1 new clinical (painful) vertebral fracture	47 (1.8%)	81 (3.1%)	1.3%	41% (17%, 59%)

*Includes all patients with baseline and at least one follow-up radiograph.

Evista—Cont.

trous cycles and inhibited ovulation. These effects of raloxifene were reversible. In another study in rats in which raloxifene was given during the preimplantation period at doses ≥0.1 mg/kg (≥0.02 times the human dose based on surface area, mg/m²), raloxifene delayed and disrupted embryo implantation, resulting in prolonged gestation and reduced litter size. The reproductive and developmental effects observed in animals are consistent with the estrogen receptor activity of raloxifene.

13.2 Animal Toxicology and/or Pharmacology

The skeletal effects of raloxifene treatment were assessed in ovariectomized rats and monkeys. In rats, raloxifene prevented increased bone resorption and bone loss after ovariectomy. There were positive effects of raloxifene on bone strength, but the effects varied with time. Cynomolgus monkeys were treated with raloxifene or conjugated estrogens for 2 years. In terms of bone cycles, this is equivalent to approximately 6 years in humans. Raloxifene and estrogen suppressed bone turnover and increased BMD in the lumbar spine and in the central cancellous bone of the proximal tibia. In this animal model, there was a positive correlation between vertebral compressive breaking force and BMD of the lumbar spine.

Histologic examination of bone from rats and monkeys treated with raloxifene showed no evidence of woven bone, marrow fibrosis, or mineralization defects.

These results are consistent with data from human studies of radiocalcium kinetics and markers of bone metabolism, and are consistent with the action of EVISTA as a skeletal antiresorptive agent.

14 CLINICAL STUDIES

14.1 Treatment of Postmenopausal Osteoporosis

Effect on Fracture Incidence

The effects of EVISTA on fracture incidence and BMD in postmenopausal women with osteoporosis were examined at 3 years in a large randomized, placebo-controlled, double-blind, multinational osteoporosis treatment trial (MORE). All vertebral fractures were diagnosed radiographically; some of these fractures also were associated with symptoms (i.e., clinical fractures). The study population consisted of 7705 postmenopausal women with osteoporosis as defined by: a) low BMD (vertebral or hip BMD at least 2.5 standard deviations below the mean value for healthy young women) without baseline vertebral fractures or b) one or more baseline vertebral fractures. Women enrolled in this study had a median age of 67 years (range 31 to 80) and a median time since menopause of 19 years.

Effect on Bone Mineral Density

EVISTA, 60 mg administered once daily, increased spine and hip BMD by 2 to 3%. EVISTA decreased the incidence of the first vertebral fracture from 4.3% for placebo to 1.9% for EVISTA (relative risk reduction = 55%) and subsequent vertebral fractures from 20.2% for placebo to 14.1% for EVISTA (relative risk reduction = 30%) (see Table 4). All women in the study received calcium (500 mg/day) and vitamin D (400 to 600 IU/day). EVISTA reduced the incidence of vertebral fractures whether or not patients had a vertebral fracture upon study entry. The decrease in incidence of vertebral fracture was greater than could be accounted for by increase in BMD alone.

[See table 4 above]

The mean percentage change in BMD from baseline for EVISTA was statistically significantly greater than for placebo at each skeletal site (see Table 5).

Table 5: EVISTA- (60 mg Once Daily) Related Increases in BMD* for the Osteoporosis Treatment Study Expressed as Mean Percentage Increase vs. Placebo[†,‡]

	Time		
	12 Months	24 Months	36 Months
Site	%	%	%
Lumbar Spine	2.0	2.6	2.6
Femoral Neck	1.3	1.9	2.1
Ultradistal Radius	ND§	2.2	ND§
Distal Radius	ND§	0.9	ND§
Total Body	ND§	1.1	ND§

* Note: all BMD increases were significant (p<0.001).

† Intent-to-treat analysis; last observation carried forward.

‡ All patients received calcium and vitamin D.

§ ND = not done (total body and radius BMD were measured only at 24 months).

Discontinuation from the study was required when excessive bone loss or multiple incident vertebral fractures occurred. Such discontinuation was statistically significantly more frequent in the placebo group (3.7%) than in the EVISTA group (1.1%).

Bone Histology

Bone biopsies for qualitative and quantitative histomorphometry were obtained at baseline and after 2 years of treatment. There were 56 paired biopsies evaluable for all indices. In EVISTA-treated patients, there were statistically significant decreases in bone formation rate per tissue volume, consistent with a reduction in bone turnover. Normal bone quality was maintained; specifically, there was no evidence of osteomalacia, marrow fibrosis, cellular toxicity, or woven bone after 2 years of treatment.

Effect on Endometrium

Endometrial thickness was evaluated annually in a subset of the study population (1781 patients) for 3 years. Placebo-treated women had a 0.27 mm mean decrease from baseline in endometrial thickness over 3 years, whereas the EVISTA-treated women had a 0.06 mm mean increase. Patients in the osteoporosis treatment study were not screened at baseline or excluded for pre-existing endometrial or uterine disease. This study was not specifically designed to detect endometrial polyps. Over the 36 months of the study, clinically or histologically benign endometrial polyps were reported in 17 of 1999 placebo-treated women, 37 of 1948 EVISTA-treated women, and in 31 of 2010 women treated with raloxifene HCl 120 mg/day. There was no difference between EVISTA- and placebo-treated women in the incidences of endometrial carcinoma, vaginal bleeding, or vaginal discharge.

14.2 Prevention of Postmenopausal Osteoporosis

The effects of EVISTA on BMD in postmenopausal women were examined in three randomized, placebo-controlled, double-blind osteoporosis prevention trials: (1) a North American trial enrolled 544 women; (2) a European trial, 601 women; and (3) an international trial, 619 women who had undergone hysterectomy. In these trials, all women received calcium supplementation (400 to 600 mg/day). Women enrolled in these trials had a median age of 54 years and a median time since menopause of 5 years (less than 1 year up to 15 years postmenopause). The majority of the women were White (93.5%). Women were included if they had spine BMD between 2.5 standard deviations below and 2 standard deviations above the mean value for healthy young women. The mean T scores (number of standard deviations above or below the mean in healthy young women) for the three trials ranged from -1.01 to -0.74 for spine BMD and included women both with normal and low BMD. EVISTA, 60 mg administered once daily, produced increases in bone mass versus calcium supplementation alone, as reflected by dual-energy x-ray absorptiometric (DXA) measurements of hip, spine, and total body BMD.

Effect on Bone Mineral Density

Compared with placebo, the increases in BMD for each of the three studies were statistically significant at 12 months and were maintained at 24 months (see Table 6). The placebo groups lost approximately 1% of BMD over 24 months.

Table 6: EVISTA- (60 mg Once Daily) Related Increases in BMD* for the Three Osteoporosis Prevention Studies Expressed as Mean Percentage Increase vs. Placebo[†] at 24 Months[‡]

	Study		
	NA§	EU§	INT[§,¶]
Site	%	%	%
Total Hip	2.0	2.4	1.3
Femoral Neck	2.1	2.5	1.6
Trochanter	2.2	2.7	1.3
Intertrochanter	2.3	2.4	1.3
Lumbar Spine	2.0	2.4	1.8

* Note: all BMD increases were significant (p≤0.001).

† All patients received calcium.

‡ Intent-to-treat analysis; last observation carried forward.

§ Abbreviations: NA = North American, EU = European, INT = International.

¶ All women in the study had previously undergone hysterectomy.

EVISTA also increased BMD compared with placebo in the total body by 1.3% to 2.0% and in Ward's Triangle (hip) by 3.1% to 4.0%. The effects of EVISTA on forearm BMD were inconsistent between studies. In Study EU, EVISTA prevented bone loss at the ultradistal radius, whereas in Study NA, it did not (see Figure 1).

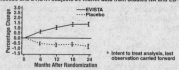

Total hip mean percentage change from baseline
All placebo and EVISTA subjects 24-month data from Studies NA and EU[a]

[a] Intent to treat analysis, last observation carried forward

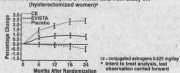

Total hip mean percentage change from baseline
All placebo, EVISTA, and CE subjects 24-month data from Study INT (hysterectomized women)

CE = conjugated estrogens 0.625 mg/day
[a] Intent to treat analysis, last observation carried forward

Figure 1: Total hip bone mineral density mean percentage change from baseline

Effect on Endometrium

In placebo-controlled osteoporosis prevention trials, endometrial thickness was evaluated every 6 months (for 24 months) by transvaginal ultrasonography (TVU). A total of 2978 TVU measurements were collected from 831 women in all dose groups. Placebo-treated women had a 0.04 mm mean increase from baseline in endometrial thickness over 2 years, whereas the EVISTA-treated women had a 0.09 mm mean increase. Endometrial thickness measurements in raloxifene-treated women were indistinguishable from placebo. There were no differences between the raloxifene and placebo groups with respect to the incidence of reported vaginal bleeding.

14.3 Reduction in Risk of Invasive Breast Cancer in Postmenopausal Women with Osteoporosis

MORE Trial

The effect of EVISTA on the incidence of breast cancer was assessed as a secondary safety endpoint in a randomized, placebo-controlled, double-blind, multinational osteoporosis treatment trial in postmenopausal women [see Clinical Studies (14.1)]. After 4 years, EVISTA, 60 mg administered once daily, reduced the incidence of all breast cancers by 62%, compared with placebo (HR 0.38, 95% CI 0.22-0.67). EVISTA reduced the incidence of invasive breast cancer by 71%, compared with placebo (ARR 3.1 per 1000 women-years); this was primarily due to an 80% reduction in the incidence of ER-positive invasive breast cancer in the EVISTA group compared with placebo. Table 7 presents efficacy and selected safety outcomes.

CORE Trial

The effect of EVISTA on the incidence of invasive breast cancer was evaluated for 4 additional years in a follow-up study conducted in a subset of postmenopausal women originally enrolled in the MORE osteoporosis treatment trial. Women were not re-randomized; the treatment assignment from the osteoporosis treatment trial was carried forward to this study. EVISTA, 60 mg administered once daily, reduced the incidence of invasive breast cancer by 56%, compared with placebo (ARR 3.0 per 1000 women-years); this was primarily due to a 63% reduction in the incidence of ER-positive invasive breast cancer in the EVISTA group compared with placebo. There was no reduction in the incidence of ER-negative breast cancer. In the osteoporosis treatment trial and the follow-up study, there was no difference in incidence of noninvasive breast cancer between the EVISTA and placebo groups. Table 7 presents efficacy and selected safety outcomes.

In a subset of postmenopausal women followed for up to 8 years from randomization in MORE to the end of CORE, EVISTA, 60 mg administered once daily, reduced the incidence of invasive breast cancer by 60% in women assigned EVISTA (N=1355) compared with placebo (N=1286) (HR 0.40, 95% CI 0.21, 0.77; ARR 1.95 per 1000 women-years); this was primarily due to a 65% reduction in the incidence of ER-positive invasive breast cancer in the EVISTA group compared with placebo.

[See table 7 at top of next page]

RUTH Trial

The effect of EVISTA on the incidence of invasive breast cancer was assessed in a randomized, placebo-controlled, double-blind, multinational study in 10,101 postmenopausal women at increased risk of coronary events. Women in this study had a median age of 67.6 years (range 55-92) and were followed for a median of 5.6 years (range 0.01-7.1). Eighty-four percent were White, 9.8% of women reported a first-degree relative with a history of breast cancer, and 41.4% of the women had a 5-year predicted risk of invasive breast cancer ≥1.66%, based on the modified Gail model.

EVISTA, 60 mg administered once daily, reduced the incidence of invasive breast cancer by 44% compared with placebo [absolute risk reduction (ARR) 1.2 per 1000 women-years]; this was primarily due to a 55% reduction in estrogen receptor (ER)-positive invasive breast cancer in the EVISTA group compared with placebo (ARR 1.2 per 1000 women-years). There was no reduction in ER-negative invasive breast cancer. Table 8 presents efficacy and selected safety outcomes.

[See table 8 above]

The effect of EVISTA in reducing the incidence of invasive breast cancer was consistent among women above or below age 65 or with a 5-year predicted invasive breast cancer risk, based on the modified Gail model, <1.66%, or ≥1.66%.

14.4 Reduction in Risk of Invasive Breast Cancer in Postmenopausal Women at High Risk of Invasive Breast Cancer

STAR Trial

The effects of EVISTA 60 mg/day versus tamoxifen 20 mg/day over 5 years on reducing the incidence of invasive breast cancer were assessed in 19,747 postmenopausal women in a randomized, double-blind trial conducted in North America by the National Surgical Adjuvant Breast and Bowel Project and sponsored by the National Cancer Institute. Women in this study had a mean age of 58.5 years (range 35-83), a mean 5-year predicted invasive breast cancer risk of 4.03% (range 1.66-23.61%), and 9.1% had a history of lobular carcinoma in situ (LCIS). More than 93% of participants were White. As of 31 December 2005, the median time of follow-up was 4.3 years (range 0.07-6.50 years). EVISTA was not superior to tamoxifen in reducing the incidence of invasive breast cancer. The observed incidence rates of invasive breast cancer were EVISTA 4.4 and tamoxifen 4.3 per 1000 women per year. The results from a noninferiority analysis are consistent with EVISTA potentially losing up to 35% of the tamoxifen effect on reduction of invasive breast cancer. The effect of each treatment on invasive breast cancer was consistent when women were compared by baseline age, history of LCIS, history of atypical hyperplasia, 5-year predicted risk of breast cancer by the modified Gail model, or the number of relatives with a history of breast cancer. Fewer noninvasive breast cancers occurred in the tamoxifen group compared to the EVISTA group. Table 9 presents efficacy and selected safety outcomes.

[See table 9 at top of next page]

14.5 Effects on Cardiovascular Disease

In a randomized, placebo-controlled, double-blind, multinational clinical trial (RUTH) of 10,101 postmenopausal women with documented coronary heart disease or at increased risk for coronary events, no cardiovascular benefit was demonstrated after treatment with EVISTA 60 mg once daily for a median follow-up of 5.6 years. No significant increase or decrease was observed for coronary events (death from coronary causes, nonfatal myocardial infarction, or hospitalization for an acute coronary syndrome). An increased risk of death due to stroke after treatment with EVISTA was observed: 59 (1.2%) EVISTA-treated women died due to a stroke compared to 39 (0.8%) placebo-treated women (2.2 versus 1.5 per 1000 women-years; hazard ratio 1.49; 95% confidence interval, 1.00-2.24; p=0.0499). The incidence of stroke did not differ significantly between treatment groups (249 with EVISTA [4.9%] versus 224 with placebo [4.4%]; hazard ratio 1.10; 95% confidence interval 0.92-1.32; p=0.30; 9.5 versus 8.6 per 1000 women-years) *[see Warnings and Precautions (5.2, 5.3)]*.

16 HOW SUPPLIED/STORAGE AND HANDLING

16.1 How Supplied

EVISTA 60 mg tablets are white, elliptical, and film coated. They are imprinted on one side with LILLY and the tablet code 4165 in edible blue ink. They are available as follows:

Bottle (count)	NDC Number
30 (unit of use)	NDC 0002–4165–30
100 (unit of use)	NDC 0002–4165–02
2000	NDC 0002–4165–07

Table 7: EVISTA (60 mg Once Daily) vs. Placebo on Outcomes in Postmenopausal Women with Osteoporosis

Outcomes	MORE 4 years: Placebo (N=2576) n	IR†	EVISTA (N=2557) n	IR†	HR (95% CI)†	CORE* 4 years: Placebo (N=1286) n	IR†	EVISTA (N=2725) n	IR†	HR (95% CI)†
Invasive‡ breast cancer	38	4.36	11	1.26	0.29 (0.15, 0.56)§	20	5.41	19	2.43	0.44 (0.24, 0.83)§
ER†,‡ positive	29	3.33	6	0.69	0.20 (0.08, 0.49)	15	4.05	12	1.54	0.37 (0.17, 0.79)
ER†,‡ negative	4	0.46	5	0.57	1.23 (0.33, 4.60)	3	0.81	6	0.77	0.95 (0.24, 3.79)
ER†,‡ unknown	5	0.57	0	0.00	N/A†	2	0.54	1	0.13	N/A†
Noninvasive‡,¶ breast cancer	5	0.57	3	0.34	0.59 (0.14, 2.47)	2	0.54	5	0.64	1.18 (0.23, 6.07)
Clinical vertebral fractures	107	12.27	62	7.08	0.57 (0.42, 0.78)	N/A†	N/A†	N/A†	N/A†	N/A†
Death	36	4.13	23	2.63	0.63 (0.38, 1.07)	29	7.76	47	5.99	0.77 (0.49, 1.23)
Death due to stroke	6	0.69	3	0.34	0.49 (0.12, 1.98)	1	0.27	6	0.76	2.87 (0.35, 23.80)
Stroke	56	6.42	43	4.91	0.76 (0.51, 1.14)	14	3.75	49	6.24	1.67 (0.92, 3.03)
Deep vein thrombosis	8	0.92	20	2.28	2.50 (1.10, 5.68)	4	1.07	17	2.17	2.03 (0.68, 6.03)
Pulmonary embolism	4	0.46	11	1.26	2.76 (0.88, 8.67)	0	0.00	9	1.15	N/A†
Endometrial and uterine cancer#	5	0.74	5	0.74	1.01 (0.29, 3.49)	3	1.02	4	0.65	0.64 (0.14, 2.85)
Ovarian cancer	6	0.69	3	0.34	0.49 (0.12, 1.95)	2	0.54	2	0.25	0.47 (0.07, 3.36)
Hot flashes	151	17.31	237	27.06	1.61 (1.31, 1.97)	11	2.94	26	3.31	1.12 (0.55, 2.27)
Peripheral edema	134	15.36	164	18.73	1.23 (0.98, 1.54)	30	8.03	61	7.77	0.96 (0.62, 1.49)
Cholelithiasis	45	5.16	53	6.05	1.18 (0.79, 1.75)	12	3.21	35	4.46	1.39 (0.72, 2.67)

* CORE was a follow-up study conducted in a subset of 4011 postmenopausal women who originally enrolled in MORE. Women were not re-randomized; the treatment assignment from MORE was carried forward to this study. At CORE enrollment, the EVISTA group included 2725 total patients with 1355 patients who were originally assigned to raloxifene 60 mg once daily and 1370 patients who were originally assigned to raloxifene 120 mg at MORE randomization.
† Abbreviations: CI = confidence interval; ER = estrogen receptor; HR = hazard ratio; IR = annual incidence rate per 1000 women; N/A = not applicable.
‡ Included 1274 patients in placebo and 2716 patients in EVISTA who were not diagnosed with breast cancer prior to CORE enrollment.
§ p<0.05, obtained from the log-rank test, and not adjusted for multiple comparisons in MORE.
¶ All cases were ductal carcinoma in situ.
\# Only patients with an intact uterus were included (MORE: placebo = 1999, EVISTA = 1950; CORE: placebo = 1008, EVISTA = 2138).

Table 8: EVISTA (60 mg Once Daily) vs. Placebo on Outcomes in Postmenopausal Women at Increased Risk for Major Coronary Events

Outcomes	Placebo* (N=5057) n	IR†	EVISTA* (N=5044) n	IR†	HR (95% CI)†
Invasive breast cancer	70	2.66	40	1.50	0.56 (0.38, 0.83)‡
ER† positive	55	2.09	25	0.94	0.45 (0.28, 0.72)
ER† negative	9	0.34	13	0.49	1.44 (0.61, 3.36)
ER† unknown	6	0.23	2	0.07	0.33 (0.07, 1.63)
Noninvasive§ breast cancer	5	0.19	11	0.41	2.17 (0.75, 6.24)
Clinical vertebral fractures	97	3.70	64	2.40	0.65 (0.47, 0.89)
Death	595	22.45	554	20.68	0.92 (0.82, 1.03)
Death due to stroke	39	1.47	59	2.20	1.49 (1.00, 2.24)
Stroke	224	8.60	249	9.46	1.10 (0.92, 1.32)
Deep vein thrombosis	47	1.78	65	2.44	1.37 (0.94, 1.99)
Pulmonary embolism	24	0.91	36	1.35	1.49 (0.89, 2.49)
Endometrial and uterine cancer¶	17	0.83	21	1.01	1.21 (0.64-2.30)
Ovarian cancer#	10	0.41	17	0.70	1.69 (0.78, 3.70)
Hot flashes	241	9.09	397	14.82	1.68 (1.43, 1.97)
Peripheral edema	583	22.00	706	26.36	1.22 (1.09, 1.36)
Cholelithiasisᵇ	131	6.20	168	7.83	1.26 (1.01, 1.59)

* Note: There were a total of 76 breast cancer cases in the placebo group and 52 in the EVISTA group. For two cases, one in each treatment group, invasive status was unknown.
† Abbreviations: CI = confidence interval; ER = estrogen receptor; HR = hazard ratio; IR = annual incidence rate per 1000 women.
‡ p<0.05, obtained from the log-rank test, after adjusting for the co-primary endpoint of major coronary events.
§ All cases were ductal carcinoma in situ.
¶ Only patients with an intact uterus were included (placebo = 3882, EVISTA = 3900).
\# Only patients with at least one ovary were included (placebo = 4606, EVISTA = 4559).
Þ Only patients with an intact gallbladder at baseline were included (placebo = 4111, EVISTA = 4144).

16.2 Storage and Handling

Store at controlled room temperature, 20° to 25°C (68° to 77°F) [*see* USP]. The USP defines controlled room temperature as a temperature maintained thermostatically that encompasses the usual and customary working environment of 20° to 25°C (68° to 77°F); that results in a mean kinetic temperature calculated to be not more than 25°C; and that allows for excursions between 15° and 30°C (59° and 86°F) that are experienced in pharmacies, hospitals, and warehouses.

17 PATIENT COUNSELING INFORMATION

See FDA-approved Medication Guide.

Physicians should instruct their patients to read the Medication Guide before starting therapy with EVISTA and to reread it each time the prescription is renewed.

17.1 Osteoporosis Recommendations, Including Calcium and Vitamin D Supplementation

For osteoporosis treatment or prevention, patients should be instructed to take supplemental calcium and/or vitamin D if intake is inadequate. Patients at increased risk for vitamin D insufficiency (e.g., over the age of 70 years, nursing home bound, chronically ill, or with gastrointestinal malabsorption syndromes) should be instructed to take additional vitamin D if needed. Weight-bearing exercises should be considered along with the modification of certain behavioral factors, such as cigarette smoking and/or excessive alcohol consumption, if these factors exist.

17.2 Patient Immobilization

EVISTA should be discontinued at least 72 hours prior to and during prolonged immobilization (e.g., post-surgical recovery, prolonged bed rest), and patients should be advised to avoid prolonged restrictions of movement during travel because of the increased risk of venous thromboembolic events *[see Warnings and Precautions (5.1)]*.

17.3 Hot Flashes or Flushes

EVISTA may increase the incidence of hot flashes and is not effective in reducing hot flashes or flushes associated with estrogen deficiency. In some asymptomatic patients, hot flashes may occur upon beginning EVISTA therapy.

17.4 Reduction in Risk of Invasive Breast Cancer in Postmenopausal Women with Osteoporosis or at High Risk of Invasive Breast Cancer

Use of EVISTA is associated with the reduction of the risk of invasive breast cancer in postmenopausal women. EVISTA has not been shown to reduce the risk of noninvasive breast cancer. When considering treatment, physicians need to discuss the potential benefits and risks of EVISTA treatment with the patient.

EVISTA is not indicated for the treatment of invasive breast cancer or reduction of the risk of recurrence.

Patients should have breast exams and mammograms before starting EVISTA and should continue regular breast exams and mammograms in keeping with good medical practice after beginning treatment with EVISTA.

Literature revised September 13, 2007

Eli Lilly and Company, Indianapolis, IN 46285, USA

PV 3088 AMP

Medication Guide

EVISTA® (É-VISS-tah)

(raloxifene hydrochloride)

Tablets for Oral Use

Read the Medication Guide that comes with EVISTA before you start taking it and each time you refill your prescription. The information may have changed. This Medication Guide does not take the place of talking with your doctor

Continued on next page

This product information was prepared in March 2008. Current information on products of Eli Lilly and Company may be obtained by calling 1-800-545-5979.

Evista—Cont.

about your medical condition or treatment. Talk with your doctor about EVISTA when you start taking it and at regular checkups.

What is the most important information I should know about EVISTA?

Serious and life-threatening side effects can occur while taking EVISTA. These include blood clots and dying from stroke:

- Increased risk of blood clots in the legs (deep vein thrombosis) and lungs (pulmonary embolism) have been reported with EVISTA. Women who have or have had blood clots in the legs, lungs, or eyes should not take EVISTA.
- Women who have had a heart attack or are at risk for a heart attack may have an increased risk of dying from stroke when taking EVISTA.

1. Before starting EVISTA, tell your doctor if you have had blood clots in your legs, lungs, or eyes, a stroke, mini-stroke (transient ischemic attack), or have an irregular heartbeat.
2. Stop taking EVISTA and call your doctor if you have:
   - leg pain or a feeling of warmth in the lower leg (calf).
   - swelling of the legs, hands, or feet.
   - sudden chest pain, shortness of breath, or coughing up blood.
   - sudden change in your vision, such as loss of vision or blurred vision.
3. Being still for a long time (such as sitting still during a long car or airplane trip or being in bed after surgery) can increase your risk of blood clots. (See **"What should I avoid if I am taking EVISTA?"**)

What is EVISTA?

EVISTA is a type of prescription medicine called a Selective Estrogen Receptor Modulator (SERM). EVISTA is for women after menopause, and has more than one use:

- **Osteoporosis:** EVISTA treats and prevents osteoporosis by helping make your bones stronger and less likely to break.
- **Invasive Breast Cancer:** If you have osteoporosis or are at high risk for breast cancer, EVISTA can be used to lower your chance of getting invasive breast cancer. EVISTA will not totally get rid of your chance of getting breast cancer. Your doctor can estimate your risk of breast cancer by asking you about risk factors, including:
  - your age (getting older).
  - family history of breast cancer in your mother, sister, or daughter.
  - a history of any breast biopsy, especially an abnormal biopsy.

You and your doctor should talk about whether the possible benefit of EVISTA in lowering your chance of getting invasive breast cancer is greater than its possible risks.

EVISTA is not for use in premenopausal women (women who have not passed menopause).

Who should not take EVISTA?

Do not take EVISTA if you:

- have or have had blood clots in your legs, lungs, or eyes. Taking EVISTA may increase the risk of getting blood clots.
- are pregnant or could become pregnant. EVISTA could harm your unborn child.
- are nursing a baby. It is not known if EVISTA passes into breast milk or what effect it might have on the baby.

What should I tell my doctor before taking EVISTA?

EVISTA may not be right for you. Before taking EVISTA, tell your doctor about all your medical conditions, including if you:

- have had blood clots in your legs, lungs, or eyes, a stroke, mini-stroke (TIA/transient ischemic attack), or a type of irregular heartbeat (atrial fibrillation).
- have had breast cancer. EVISTA has not been fully studied in women who have a history of breast cancer.
- have liver or kidney problems.
- have taken estrogen in the past and had a high increase of triglycerides (a kind of fat in the blood).
- are pregnant, planning to become pregnant, or breast-feeding (see **"Who should not take EVISTA?"**).

Tell your doctor about all medicines you take, including prescription and non-prescription medicines, vitamins, and herbal supplements. Know the medicines you take. Keep a list of them and show it to your doctor and pharmacist each time you get a new medicine. Especially tell your doctor if you take*:

- warfarin (Coumadin®, Jantoven®)
  If you are taking warfarin or other coumarin blood thinners, your doctor may need to do a blood test when you first start or if you need to stop taking EVISTA. Names for this test include "prothrombin time," "pro-time," or "INR." Your doctor may need to adjust the dose of your warfarin or other coumarin blood thinner.
- cholestyramine
- estrogens

EVISTA should not be taken with cholestyramine or estrogens.

How should I take EVISTA?

- Take EVISTA exactly how your doctor tells you to.
- Keep taking EVISTA for as long as your doctor prescribes it for you. It is not known how long you should

keep taking EVISTA to lower your chance of getting invasive breast cancers.

- It is important to get your refills on time so you do not run out of the medicine.
- Take one EVISTA tablet each day.
- Take EVISTA at any time of the day, with or without food.
- To help you remember to take EVISTA, it may be best to take it at about the same time each day.
- Calcium and vitamin D may be taken at the same time as EVISTA. It is important to take calcium and vitamin D, as directed by your physician, to prevent or treat osteoporosis.
- If you miss a dose, take it as soon as you remember. However, if it is almost time for your next dose, skip the missed dose and take only your next regularly scheduled dose. Do not take two doses at the same time.

What should I avoid while taking EVISTA?

- Being still for a long time (such as during long trips or being in bed after surgery) can increase the risk of blood clots. EVISTA may add to this risk. If you will need to be still for a long time, talk with your doctor about ways to reduce the risk of blood clots. On long trips, move around periodically. Stop taking EVISTA at least 3 days before a planned surgery or before you plan on being still for a long time. You should start taking EVISTA again when you return to your normal activities.
- Some medicines should not be taken with EVISTA (see "What should I tell my doctor before taking EVISTA?").

What are the possible side effects of EVISTA?

Serious and life-threatening side effects can occur while taking EVISTA. These include blood clots and dying from stroke:

- Increased risk of blood clots in the legs (deep vein thrombosis) and lungs (pulmonary embolism) have been reported with EVISTA. Women who have or have had blood clots in the legs, lungs, or eyes should not take EVISTA.
- Women who have had a heart attack or are at risk for a heart attack may have an increased risk of dying from stroke when taking EVISTA.

See **"What is the most important information I should know about EVISTA?"**

The most common side effects of EVISTA are hot flashes, leg cramps, swelling of the feet, ankles, and legs, flu syndrome, joint pain, and sweating. Hot flashes are more common during the first 6 months after starting treatment.

These are not all the side effects of EVISTA. Tell your doctor about any side effect that bothers you or that does not go away. If you have any problems or questions that concern you while taking EVISTA, ask your doctor or pharmacist for more information.

What else should I know about EVISTA?

- Do not use EVISTA to prevent heart disease, heart attack, or strokes.
- To get the calcium and vitamin D you need, your doctor may advise you to change your diet and/or take supplemental calcium and vitamin D. Your doctor may suggest other ways to help treat or prevent osteoporosis, in addition to taking EVISTA and getting the calcium and vitamin D you need. These may include regular exercise, stopping smoking, and drinking less alcohol.
- Women who have hot flashes can take EVISTA. EVISTA does not treat hot flashes, and it may cause hot

flashes in some women. (See **"What are the possible side effects of EVISTA?"**)

- EVISTA has not been found to cause breast tenderness or enlargement. If you notice any changes in your breasts, call your doctor to find out the cause. Before starting and while taking EVISTA you should have breast exams and mammograms, as directed by your doctor. Because EVISTA does not eliminate the chance of developing breast cancers, you need these examinations to find any breast cancers as early as possible.
- EVISTA should not cause spotting or menstrual-type bleeding. If you have any vaginal bleeding, call your doctor to find out the cause. EVISTA has not been found to increase the risk for cancer of the lining of the uterus.
- Women in clinical trials have taken EVISTA for up to eight years.

How should I store EVISTA?

- Store EVISTA at 68°F to 77°F (20°C-25°C).
- **Keep EVISTA and all medicines out of the reach of children.**

General Information about the safe and effective use of EVISTA

Medicines are sometimes prescribed for purposes other than those listed in a Medication Guide. Do not use EVISTA for a condition for which it was not prescribed. Do not give your EVISTA to other people, even if they have the same symptoms you have. It may harm them.

This Medication Guide is a summary of the most important information about EVISTA. If you would like more information about EVISTA, talk with your doctor. You can ask your doctor or pharmacist for information about EVISTA that is written for health professionals. For more information, call 1-800-545-5979 (toll-free) or go to the following website: www.evista.com.

What are the ingredients in EVISTA?

Active Ingredient: raloxifene hydrochloride

Inactive Ingredients: anhydrous lactose, carnauba wax, crospovidone, FD&C Blue No. 2 aluminum lake, hypromellose, lactose monohydrate, magnesium stearate, modified pharmaceutical glaze, polyethylene glycol, polysorbate 80, povidone, propylene glycol, and titanium dioxide.

This Medication Guide has been approved by the U.S. Food and Drug Administration.

*The brands listed are trademarks of their respective owners and are not trademarks of Eli Lilly and Company. The makers of these brands are not affiliated with and do not endorse Eli Lilly and Company or its products.

Medication Guide issued September 13, 2007

Eli Lilly and Company, Indianapolis, IN 46285, USA

Copyright © 1997, 2007, Eli Lilly and Company. All rights reserved.

PV 3124 AMP

Table 9: EVISTA (60 mg Once Daily) vs. Tamoxifen (20 mg Once Daily) on Outcomes in Postmenopausal Women at Increased Risk for Invasive Breast Cancer

Outcomes	EVISTA (N=9751)		Tamoxifen (N=9736)		RR (95% CI)*
	n	IR*	n	IR*	
Invasive breast cancer	173	4.40	168	4.30	1.02 (0.82, 1.27)
ER* positive	115	2.93	120	3.07	0.95 (0.73, 1.24)
ER* negative	52	1.32	46	1.18	1.12 (0.74, 1.71)
ER* unknown	6	0.15	2	0.05	2.98 (0.53, 30.21)
Noninvasive breast cancer†	83	2.12	60	1.54	1.38 (0.98, 1.95)
DCIS*	47	1.20	32	0.82	1.46 (0.91, 2.37)
LCIS*	29	0.74	23	0.59	1.26 (0.70, 2.27)
Uterine cancer‡	23	1.21	37	1.99	0.61 (0.34, 1.05)
Endometrial hyperplasia‡	17	0.90	100	5.42	0.17 (0.09, 0.28)
Hysterectomy‡	92	4.84	246	13.25	0.37 (0.28, 0.47)
Ovarian cancer§	18	0.66	14	0.52	1.27 (0.60, 2.76)
Ischemic heart disease¶	138	3.50	125	3.19	1.10 (0.86, 1.41)
Stroke	54	1.36	56	1.42	0.96 (0.65, 1.42)
Deep vein thrombosis	67	1.69	92	2.35	0.72 (0.52, 1.00)
Pulmonary embolism	38	0.96	58	1.47	0.65 (0.42, 1.00)
Clinical vertebral fractures	58	1.46	58	1.47	0.99 (0.68, 1.46)
Cataracts#	343	10.34	435	13.19	0.78 (0.68, 0.91)
Cataract surgery#	240	7.17	295	8.85	0.81 (0.68, 0.96)
Death	104	2.62	109	2.76	0.95 (0.72, 1.25)
Edemaᵇ	741	18.66	664	16.83	1.11 (1.00, 1.23)
Hot flashes	6748	169.91	7170	181.71	0.94 (0.90, 0.97)

* Abbreviations: CI = confidence interval; DCIS = ductal carcinoma in situ; ER = estrogen receptor; IR = annual incidence rate per 1000 women; LCIS = lobular carcinoma in situ; RR = risk ratio for women in the EVISTA group compared with those in the tamoxifen group.

† Of the 60 noninvasive breast cases in the tamoxifen group, 5 were mixed types. Of the 83 noninvasive breast cancers in the raloxifene group, 7 were mixed types.

‡ Only patients with an intact uterus at baseline were included (tamoxifen = 4739, EVISTA = 4715).

§ Only patients with at least one intact ovary at baseline were included (tamoxifen = 6813, EVISTA = 6787).

¶ Defined as myocardial infarction, severe angina, or acute ischemic syndromes.

Only patients who were free of cataracts at baseline were included (tamoxifen = 8342; EVISTA = 8333).

Þ Peripheral edema events are included in the term edema.

SYMBYAX®

[sim-bee-ax]

(olanzapine and fluoxetine hydrochloride) Capsule

℞

Prescribing information for this product, which appears on pages 1855-1863 of the 2008 PDR, has been completely revised as follows. Please write "See Supplement A" next to the product heading.

WARNING

Suicidality and Antidepressant Drugs—Antidepressants increased the risk compared to placebo of suicidal thinking and behavior (suicidality) in children, adolescents, and young adults in short-term studies of major depressive disorder (MDD) and other psychiatric disorders. Anyone considering the use of SYMBYAX or any other antidepressant in a child, adolescent, or young adult must balance this risk with the clinical need. Short-term studies did not show an increase in the risk of suicidality with antidepressants compared to placebo in adults beyond age 24; there was a reduction in risk with antidepressants compared to placebo in adults aged 65 and older. Depression and certain other psychiatric disorders are themselves associated with increases in the risk of suicide. Patients of all ages who are started on antidepressant therapy should be monitored appropriately and observed closely for clinical worsening, suicidality, or unusual changes in behavior. Families and caregivers should be advised of the need for close observation and communication with the prescriber. SYMBYAX is not approved for use in pediatric patients. *(See* WARNINGS, Clinical Worsening and Suicide Risk, PRECAUTIONS, Information for Patients, *and* PRECAUTIONS, Pediatric Use.)

Increased Mortality in Elderly Patients with Dementia-Related Psychosis—Elderly patients with dementia-related psychosis treated with atypical antipsychotic drugs are at an increased risk of death compared to placebo. Analyses of seventeen placebo-controlled trials (modal duration of 10 weeks) in these patients revealed a risk of death in the drug-treated patients of between 1.6 to 1.7 times that seen in placebo-treated patients. Over the course of a typical 10-week controlled trial, the rate of death in drug-treated patients was about 4.5%, compared to a rate of about 2.6% in the placebo group. Although the causes of death were varied, most of the deaths appeared to be either cardiovascular (e.g., heart failure, sudden death) or infectious (e.g., pneumonia) in nature. SYMBYAX (olanzapine and fluoxetine HCl) is not approved for the treatment of patients with dementia-related psychosis *(see* WARNINGS).

DESCRIPTION

SYMBYAX® (olanzapine and fluoxetine HCl capsules) combines 2 psychotropic agents, olanzapine (the active ingredient in Zyprexa®, and Zyprexa Zydis®) and fluoxetine hydrochloride (the active ingredient in Prozac®, Prozac Weekly™, and Sarafem®).

Olanzapine belongs to the thienobenzodiazepine class. The chemical designation is 2-methyl-4-(4-methyl-1-piperazinyl)-10*H*-thieno[2,3-*b*] [1,5]benzodiazepine. The molecular formula is $C_{17}H_{20}N_4S$, which corresponds to a molecular weight of 312.44.

Fluoxetine hydrochloride is a selective serotonin reuptake inhibitor (SSRI). The chemical designation is (±)-N-methyl-3-phenyl-3-[(α,α,α-trifluoro-*p*-tolyl)oxy]propylamine hydrochloride. The molecular formula is $C_{17}H_{18}F_3NO \cdot HCl$, which corresponds to a molecular weight of 345.79.

The chemical structures are:

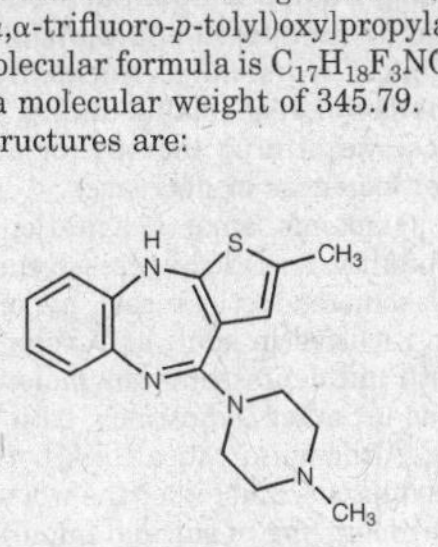

olanzapine

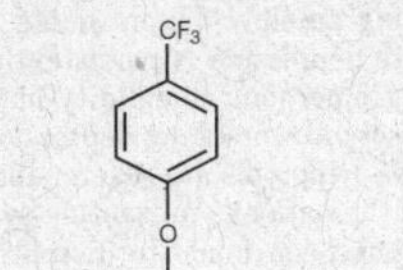

fluoxetine hydrochloride

Olanzapine is a yellow crystalline solid, which is practically insoluble in water.

Fluoxetine hydrochloride is a white to off-white crystalline solid with a solubility of 14 mg/mL in water.

SYMBYAX capsules are available for oral administration in the following strength combinations:

[See table above]

	3 mg/25 mg	6 mg/25 mg	6 mg/50 mg	12 mg/25 mg	12 mg/50 mg
olanzapine equivalent	3	6	6	12	12
fluoxetine base equivalent	25	25	50	25	50

Each capsule also contains pregelatinized starch, gelatin, dimethicone, titanium dioxide, sodium lauryl sulfate, edible black ink, red iron oxide, yellow iron oxide, and/or black iron oxide.

CLINICAL PHARMACOLOGY

Pharmacodynamics

Although the exact mechanism of SYMBYAX is unknown, it has been proposed that the activation of 3 monoaminergic neural systems (serotonin, norepinephrine, and dopamine) is responsible for its enhanced antidepressant effect. This is supported by animal studies in which the olanzapine/fluoxetine combination has been shown to produce synergistic increases in norepinephrine and dopamine release in the prefrontal cortex compared with either component alone, as well as increases in serotonin.

Olanzapine is a psychotropic agent with high affinity binding to the following receptors: serotonin $5HT_{2A/2C}$, $5HT_6$, (K_i=4, 11, and 5 nM, respectively), dopamine D_{1-4} (K_i=11 to 31 nM), histamine H_1 (K_i=7 nM), and adrenergic α_1 receptors (K_i=19 nM). Olanzapine is an antagonist with moderate affinity binding for serotonin $5HT_3$ (K_i=57 nM) and muscarinic M_{1-5} (K_i=73, 96, 132, 32, and 48 nM, respectively). Olanzapine binds weakly to $GABA_A$, BZD, and β-adrenergic receptors (K_i>10 µM). Fluoxetine is an inhibitor of the serotonin transporter and is a weak inhibitor of the norepinephrine and dopamine transporters.

Antagonism at receptors other than dopamine and $5HT_2$ may explain some of the other therapeutic and side effects of olanzapine. Olanzapine's antagonism of muscarinic M_{1-5} receptors may explain its anticholinergic-like effects. The antagonism of histamine H_1 receptors by olanzapine may explain the somnolence observed with this drug. The antagonism of α_1 -adrenergic receptors by olanzapine may explain the orthostatic hypotension observed with this drug. Fluoxetine has relatively low affinity for muscarinic, α_1-adrenergic, and histamine H_1 receptors.

Pharmacokinetics

Fluoxetine (administered as a 60-mg single dose or 60 mg daily for 8 days) caused a small increase in the mean maximum concentration of olanzapine (16%) following a 5-mg dose, an increase in the mean area under the curve (17%) and a small decrease in mean apparent clearance of olanzapine (16%). In another study, a similar decrease in apparent clearance of olanzapine of 14% was observed following olanzapine doses of 6 or 12 mg with concomitant fluoxetine doses of 25 mg or more. The decrease in clearance reflects an increase in bioavailability. The terminal half-life is not affected, and therefore the time to reach steady state should not be altered. The overall steady-state plasma concentrations of olanzapine and fluoxetine when given as the combination in the therapeutic dose ranges were comparable with those typically attained with each of the monotherapies. The small change in olanzapine clearance, observed in both studies, likely reflects the inhibition of a minor metabolic pathway for olanzapine via CYP2D6 by fluoxetine, a potent CYP2D6 inhibitor, and was not deemed clinically significant. Therefore, the pharmacokinetics of the individual components is expected to reasonably characterize the overall pharmacokinetics of the combination.

Absorption and Bioavailability

SYMBYAX—Following a single oral 12-mg/50-mg dose of SYMBYAX, peak plasma concentrations of olanzapine and fluoxetine occur at approximately 4 and 6 hours, respectively. The effect of food on the absorption and bioavailability of SYMBYAX has not been evaluated. The bioavailability of olanzapine given as Zyprexa, and the bioavailability of fluoxetine given as Prozac were not affected by food. It is unlikely that there would be a significant food effect on the bioavailability of SYMBYAX.

Olanzapine—Olanzapine is well absorbed and reaches peak concentration approximately 6 hours following an oral dose. Food does not affect the rate or extent of olanzapine absorption when olanzapine is given as Zyprexa. It is eliminated extensively by first pass metabolism, with approximately 40% of the dose metabolized before reaching the systemic circulation.

Fluoxetine—Following a single oral 40-mg dose, peak plasma concentrations of fluoxetine from 15 to 55 ng/mL are observed after 6 to 8 hours. Food does not appear to affect the systemic bioavailability of fluoxetine given as Prozac, although it may delay its absorption by 1 to 2 hours, which is probably not clinically significant.

Distribution

SYMBYAX—The in vitro binding to human plasma proteins of the olanzapine/fluoxetine combination is similar to the binding of the individual components.

Olanzapine—Olanzapine is extensively distributed throughout the body, with a volume of distribution of approximately 1000 L. It is 93% bound to plasma proteins over the concentration range of 7 to 1100 ng/mL, binding primarily to albumin and α_1-acid glycoprotein.

Fluoxetine—Over the concentration range from 200 to 1000 ng/mL, approximately 94.5% of fluoxetine is bound in vitro to human serum proteins, including albumin and α_1-glycoprotein. The interaction between fluoxetine and other highly protein-bound drugs has not been fully evaluated (*see* **PRECAUTIONS, Drugs tightly bound to plasma proteins**).

Metabolism and Elimination

SYMBYAX—SYMBYAX therapy yielded steady-state concentrations of norfluoxetine similar to those seen with fluoxetine in the therapeutic dose range.

Olanzapine—Olanzapine displays linear pharmacokinetics over the clinical dosing range. Its half-life ranges from 21 to 54 hours (5th to 95th percentile; mean of 30 hr), and apparent plasma clearance ranges from 12 to 47 L/hr (5th to 95th percentile; mean of 25 L/hr). Administration of olanzapine once daily leads to steady-state concentrations in about 1 week that are approximately twice the concentrations after single doses. Plasma concentrations, half-life, and clearance of olanzapine may vary between individuals on the basis of smoking status, gender, and age (*see* **Special Populations**).

Following a single oral dose of ^{14}C-labeled olanzapine, 7% of the dose of olanzapine was recovered in the urine as unchanged drug, indicating that olanzapine is highly metabolized. Approximately 57% and 30% of the dose was recovered in the urine and feces, respectively. In the plasma, olanzapine accounted for only 12% of the AUC for total radioactivity, indicating significant exposure to metabolites. After multiple dosing, the major circulating metabolites were the 10-N-glucuronide, present at steady state at 44% of the concentration of olanzapine, and 4′-N-desmethyl olanzapine, present at steady state at 31% of the concentration of olanzapine. Both metabolites lack pharmacological activity at the concentrations observed.

Direct glucuronidation and CYP450-mediated oxidation are the primary metabolic pathways for olanzapine. In vitro studies suggest that CYP1A2, CYP2D6, and the flavin-containing monooxygenase system are involved in olanzapine oxidation. CYP2D6-mediated oxidation appears to be a minor metabolic pathway in vivo, because the clearance of olanzapine is not reduced in subjects who are deficient in this enzyme.

Fluoxetine—Fluoxetine is a racemic mixture (50/50) of *R*-fluoxetine and *S*-fluoxetine enantiomers. In animal models, both enantiomers are specific and potent serotonin uptake inhibitors with essentially equivalent pharmacologic activity. The *S*-fluoxetine enantiomer is eliminated more slowly and is the predominant enantiomer present in plasma at steady state.

Fluoxetine is extensively metabolized in the liver to its only identified active metabolite, norfluoxetine, via the CYP2D6 pathway. A number of unidentified metabolites exist.

In animal models, *S*-norfluoxetine is a potent and selective inhibitor of serotonin uptake and has activity essentially equivalent to *R*- or *S*-fluoxetine. *R*-norfluoxetine is significantly less potent than the parent drug in the inhibition of serotonin uptake. The primary route of elimination appears to be hepatic metabolism to inactive metabolites excreted by the kidney.

Clinical Issues Related to Metabolism and Elimination—The complexity of the metabolism of fluoxetine has several consequences that may potentially affect the clinical use of SYMBYAX.

Variability in metabolism—A subset (about 7%) of the population has reduced activity of the drug metabolizing enzyme CYP2D6. Such individuals are referred to as "poor metabolizers" of drugs such as debrisoquin, dextromethorphan, and the tricyclic antidepressants (TCAs). In a study involving labeled and unlabeled enantiomers administered as a racemate, these individuals metabolized *S*-fluoxetine at a slower rate and thus achieved higher concentrations of *S*-fluoxetine. Consequently, concentrations of *S*-norfluoxetine at steady state were lower. The metabolism of *R*-fluoxetine in these poor metabolizers appears normal. When compared with normal metabolizers, the total sum at steady state of the plasma concentrations of the 4 enantiomers was not significantly greater among poor metabolizers. Thus, the net pharmacodynamic activities were essentially the same. Alternative nonsaturable pathways (non-CYP2D6) also contribute to the metabolism of fluoxetine. This explains how fluoxetine achieves a steady-state concentration rather than increasing without limit.

Because the metabolism of fluoxetine, like that of a number of other compounds including TCAs and other selective serotonin antidepressants, involves the CYP2D6 system, concomitant therapy with drugs also metabolized by this enzyme system (such as the TCAs) may lead to drug interactions (*see* **PRECAUTIONS, Drug Interactions**).

Accumulation and slow elimination—The relatively slow elimination of fluoxetine (elimination half-life of 1 to 3 days after acute administration and 4 to 6 days after chronic administration) and its active metabolite, norfluoxetine (elimination half-life of 4 to 16 days after acute and chronic administration), leads to significant accumulation of these active species in chronic use and delayed attainment of steady state, even when a fixed dose is used. After 30 days of dosing at 40 mg/day, plasma concentrations of fluoxetine in the range of 91 to 302 ng/mL and norfluoxetine in the range of 72 to 258 ng/mL have been observed. Plasma concentrations of fluoxetine were higher than those predicted by single-dose studies, because the metabolism of fluoxetine is not proportional to dose. However, norfluoxetine appears to have linear pharmacokinetics. Its mean terminal half-life after a single dose was 8.6 days and after multiple dosing was 9.3 days. Steady-state levels after prolonged dosing are similar to levels seen at 4 to 5 weeks.

Continued on next page

This product information was prepared in March 2008. Current information on products of Eli Lilly and Company may be obtained by calling 1-800-545-5979.

Symbyax—Cont.

The long elimination half–lives of fluoxetine and norfluoxetine assure that, even when dosing is stopped, active drug substance will persist in the body for weeks (primarily depending on individual patient characteristics, previous dosing regimen, and length of previous therapy at discontinuation). This is of potential consequence when drug discontinuation is required or when drugs are prescribed that might interact with fluoxetine and norfluoxetine following the discontinuation of fluoxetine.

Special Populations

Geriatric

Based on the individual pharmacokinetic profiles of olanzapine and fluoxetine, the pharmacokinetics of SYMBYAX may be altered in geriatric patients. Caution should be used in dosing the elderly, especially if there are other factors that might additively influence drug metabolism and/or pharmacodynamic sensitivity.

In a study involving 24 healthy subjects, the mean elimination half–life of olanzapine was about 1.5 times greater in elderly subjects (>65 years of age) than in non–elderly subjects (≤65 years of age).

The disposition of single doses of fluoxetine in healthy elderly subjects (>65 years of age) did not differ significantly from that in younger normal subjects. However, given the long half–life and nonlinear disposition of the drug, a single–dose study is not adequate to rule out the possibility of altered pharmacokinetics in the elderly, particularly if they have systemic illness or are receiving multiple drugs for concomitant diseases. The effects of age upon the metabolism of fluoxetine have been investigated in 260 elderly but otherwise healthy depressed patients (≥60 years of age) who received 20 mg fluoxetine for 6 weeks. Combined fluoxetine plus norfluoxetine plasma concentrations were 209.3 ± 85.7 ng/mL at the end of 6 weeks. No unusual age–associated pattern of adverse events was observed in those elderly patients.

Renal Impairment

The pharmacokinetics of SYMBYAX has not been studied in patients with renal impairment. However, olanzapine and fluoxetine individual pharmacokinetics do not differ significantly in patients with renal impairment. SYMBYAX dosing adjustment based upon renal impairment is not routinely required.

Because olanzapine is highly metabolized before excretion and only 7% of the drug is excreted unchanged, renal dysfunction alone is unlikely to have a major impact on the pharmacokinetics of olanzapine. The pharmacokinetic characteristics of olanzapine were similar in patients with severe renal impairment and normal subjects, indicating that dosage adjustment based upon the degree of renal impairment is not required. In addition, olanzapine is not removed by dialysis. The effect of renal impairment on olanzapine metabolite elimination has not been studied.

In depressed patients on dialysis (N=12), fluoxetine administered as 20 mg once daily for 2 months produced steady-state fluoxetine and norfluoxetine plasma concentrations comparable with those seen in patients with normal renal function. While the possibility exists that renally excreted metabolites of fluoxetine may accumulate to higher levels in patients with severe renal dysfunction, use of a lower or less frequent dose is not routinely necessary in renally impaired patients.

Hepatic Impairment

Based on the individual pharmacokinetic profiles of olanzapine and fluoxetine, the pharmacokinetics of SYMBYAX may be altered in patients with hepatic impairment. The lowest starting dose should be considered for patients with hepatic impairment (see PRECAUTIONS, Use in Patients with Concomitant Illness and DOSAGE AND ADMINISTRATION, Special Populations).

Although the presence of hepatic impairment may be expected to reduce the clearance of olanzapine, a study of the effect of impaired liver function in subjects (N=6) with clinically significant cirrhosis (Childs–Pugh Classification A and B) revealed little effect on the pharmacokinetics of olanzapine.

As might be predicted from its primary site of metabolism, liver impairment can affect the elimination of fluoxetine. The elimination half–life of fluoxetine was prolonged in a study of cirrhotic patients, with a mean of 7.6 days compared with the range of 2 to 3 days seen in subjects without liver disease; norfluoxetine elimination was also delayed, with a mean duration of 12 days for cirrhotic patients compared with the range of 7 to 9 days in normal subjects.

Gender

Clearance of olanzapine is approximately 30% lower in women than in men. There were, however, no apparent differences between men and women in effectiveness or adverse effects. Dosage modifications based on gender should not be needed.

Smoking Status

Olanzapine clearance is about 40% higher in smokers than in nonsmokers, although dosage modifications are not routinely required.

Race

No SYMBYAX pharmacokinetic study was conducted to investigate the effects of race. In vivo studies have shown that exposures to olanzapine are similar among Japanese, Chinese and Caucasians, especially after normalization for body weight differences. Dosage modifications for race, therefore, are not routinely required.

Combined Effects

The combined effects of age, smoking, and gender could lead to substantial pharmacokinetic differences in populations. The clearance of olanzapine in young smoking males, for example, may be 3 times higher than that in elderly nonsmoking females. SYMBYAX dosing modification may be necessary in patients who exhibit a combination of factors that may result in slower metabolism of the olanzapine component (see DOSAGE AND ADMINISTRATION, Special Populations).

CLINICAL STUDIES

The efficacy of SYMBYAX for the treatment of depressive episodes associated with bipolar disorder was established in 2 identically designed, 8–week, randomized, double-blind, controlled studies of patients who met Diagnostic and Statistical Manual 4th edition (DSM–IV) criteria for Bipolar I Disorder, Depressed utilizing flexible dosing of SYMBYAX (6/25, 6/50, or 12/50 mg/day), olanzapine (5 to 20 mg/day), and placebo. These studies included patients (≥18 years of age) with or without psychotic symptoms and with or without a rapid cycling course.

The primary rating instrument used to assess depressive symptoms in these studies was the Montgomery–Asberg Depression Rating Scale (MADRS), a 10–item clinician-rated scale with total scores ranging from 0 to 60. The primary outcome measure of these studies was the change from baseline to endpoint in the MADRS total score. In both studies, SYMBYAX was statistically significantly superior to both olanzapine monotherapy and placebo in reduction of the MADRS total score. The results of the studies are summarized below (Table 1).

**Table 1: MADRS Total Score
Mean Change from Baseline to Endpoint**

	Treatment Group	Baseline Mean	Change to Endpoint Mean*
Study 1	SYMBYAX (N=40)	30	−16[†]
	Olanzapine (N=182)	32	−12
	Placebo (N=181)	31	−10
Study 2	SYMBYAX (N=42)	32	−18[†]
	Olanzapine (N=169)	33	−14
	Placebo (N=174)	31	−9

* Negative number denotes improvement from baseline.
[†] Statistically significant compared to both olanzapine and placebo.

INDICATIONS AND USAGE

SYMBYAX is indicated for the treatment of depressive episodes associated with bipolar disorder. The efficacy of SYMBYAX was established in 2 identically designed, 8–week, randomized, double–blind clinical studies.

Unlike with unipolar depression, there are no established guidelines for the length of time patients with bipolar disorder experiencing a major depressive episode should be treated with agents containing antidepressant drugs.

The effectiveness of SYMBYAX for maintaining antidepressant response in this patient population beyond 8 weeks has not been established in controlled clinical studies. Physicians who elect to use SYMBYAX for extended periods should periodically reevaluate the benefits and long–term risks of the drug for the individual patient.

CONTRAINDICATIONS

Hypersensitivity—SYMBYAX is contraindicated in patients with a known hypersensitivity to the product or any component of the product.

Monoamine Oxidase Inhibitors (MAOI)—There have been reports of serious, sometimes fatal reactions (including hyperthermia, rigidity, myoclonus, autonomic instability with possible rapid fluctuations of vital signs, and mental status changes that include extreme agitation progressing to delirium and coma) in patients receiving fluoxetine in combination with an MAOI, and in patients who have recently discontinued fluoxetine and are then started on an MAOI. Some cases presented with features resembling neuroleptic malignant syndrome. Therefore, SYMBYAX should not be used in combination with an MAOI, or within a minimum of 14 days of discontinuing therapy with an MAOI. Since fluoxetine and its major metabolite have very long elimination half–lives, at least 5 weeks [perhaps longer, especially if fluoxetine has been prescribed chronically and/or at higher doses (see CLINICAL PHARMACOLOGY, Accumulation and slow elimination)] should be allowed after stopping SYMBYAX before starting an MAOI.

Pimozide—Concomitant use in patients taking pimozide is contraindicated (see PRECAUTIONS).

Thioridazine—Thioridazine should not be administered with SYMBYAX or administered within a minimum of 5 weeks after discontinuation of SYMBYAX (see WARNINGS, Thioridazine).

WARNINGS

Clinical Worsening and Suicide Risk—Patients with major depressive disorder (MDD), both adult and pediatric, may experience worsening of their depression and/or the emergence of suicidal ideation and behavior (suicidality) or unusual changes in behavior, whether or not they are taking antidepressant medications, and this risk may persist until significant remission occurs. Suicide is a known risk of depression and certain other psychiatric disorders, and these disorders themselves are the strongest predictors of suicide. There has been a long–standing concern, however, that antidepressants may have a role in inducing worsening of depression and the emergence of suicidality in certain patients during the early phases of treatment. Pooled analyses of short–term placebo–controlled trials of antidepressant drugs (SSRIs and others) showed that these drugs increase the risk of suicidal thinking and behavior (suicidality) in children, adolescents, and young adults (ages 18–24) with major depressive disorder (MDD) and other psychiatric disorders. Short–term studies did not show an increase in the risk of suicidality with antidepressants compared to placebo in adults beyond age 24; there was a reduction with antidepressants compared to placebo in adults aged 65 and older. The pooled analyses of placebo–controlled trials in children and adolescents with MDD, obsessive compulsive disorder (OCD), or other psychiatric disorders included a total of 24 short–term trials of 9 antidepressant drugs in over 4400 patients. The pooled analyses of placebo-controlled trials in adults with MDD or other psychiatric disorders included a total of 295 short–term trials (median duration of 2 months) of 11 antidepressant drugs in over 77,000 patients. There was considerable variation in risk of suicidality among drugs, but a tendency toward an increase in the younger patients for almost all drugs studied. There were differences in absolute risk of suicidality across the different indications, with the highest incidence in MDD. The risk differences (drug versus placebo), however, were relatively stable within age strata and across indications. These risk differences (drug–placebo difference in the number of cases of suicidality per 1000 patients treated) are provided in Table 2.

Table 2

Age Range	Drug-Placebo Difference in Number of Cases of Suicidality per 1000 Patients Treated
	Increases Compared to Placebo
<18	14 additional cases
18–24	5 additional cases
	Decreases Compared to Placebo
25–64	1 fewer case
≥65	6 fewer cases

No suicides occurred in any of the pediatric trials. There were suicides in the adult trials, but the number was not sufficient to reach any conclusion about drug effect on suicide.

It is unknown whether the suicidality risk extends to longer–term use, i.e., beyond several months. However, there is substantial evidence from placebo-controlled maintenance trials in adults with depression that the use of antidepressants can delay the recurrence of depression.

All patients being treated with antidepressants for any indication should be monitored appropriately and observed closely for clinical worsening, suicidality, and unusual changes in behavior, especially during the initial few months of a course of drug therapy, or at times of dose changes, either increases or decreases.

The following symptoms, anxiety, agitation, panic attacks, insomnia, irritability, hostility, aggressiveness, impulsivity, akathisia (psychomotor restlessness), hypomania, and mania, have been reported in adult and pediatric patients being treated with antidepressants for major depressive disorder as well as for other indications, both psychiatric and nonpsychiatric. Although a causal link between the emergence of such symptoms and either the worsening of depression and/or the emergence of suicidal impulses has not been established, there is concern that such symptoms may represent precursors to emerging suicidality.

Consideration should be given to changing the therapeutic regimen, including possibly discontinuing the medication, in patients whose depression is persistently worse, or who are experiencing emergent suicidality or symptoms that might be precursors to worsening depression or suicidality, especially if these symptoms are severe, abrupt in onset, or were not part of the patient's presenting symptoms.

If the decision has been made to discontinue treatment, medication should be tapered, as rapidly as is feasible, but with recognition that abrupt discontinuation can be associated with certain symptoms (see PRECAUTIONS and DOSAGE AND ADMINISTRATION, Discontinuation of Treatment with SYMBYAX, for a description of the risks of discontinuation of SYMBYAX).

Families and caregivers of patients being treated with antidepressants for major depressive disorder or other indications, both psychiatric and nonpsychiatric, should be alerted about the need to monitor patients for the emergence of agitation, irritability, unusual changes in behavior, and the other symptoms described above, as well as the emergence of suicidality, and to report such symptoms immediately to health care providers. Such monitoring should include daily observation by families and caregivers. Prescriptions for SYMBYAX should be written for the smallest quantity of capsules consistent with good patient management, in order to reduce the risk of overdose.

It should be noted that SYMBYAX is not approved for use in treating any indications in the pediatric population.

Screening Patients for Bipolar Disorder—A major depressive episode may be the initial presentation of bipolar disorder. It is generally believed (though not established in controlled trials) that treating such an episode with an antidepressant alone may increase the likelihood of precipitation of a mixed/manic episode in patients at risk for bipolar disorder. Whether any of the symptoms described above represent such a conversion is unknown. However, prior to initiating treatment with an antidepressant, patients with depressive symptoms should be adequately screened to determine if they are at risk for bipolar disorder; such screening should include a detailed psychiatric history, including a family history of suicide, bipolar disorder, and depression. It should be noted that SYMBYAX is approved for use in treating bipolar depression.

Increased Mortality in Elderly Patients with Dementia–Related Psychosis—Elderly patients with dementia–related psychosis treated with atypical antipsychotic drugs are at an increased risk of death compared to placebo. SYMBYAX (olanzapine and fluoxetine HCl) is not approved for the treatment of patients with dementia–related psychosis (*see* BOX WARNING).

In olanzapine placebo–controlled clinical trials of elderly patients with dementia–related psychosis, the incidence of death in olanzapine–treated patients was significantly greater than placebo–treated patients (3.5% vs 1.5%, respectively).

Cerebrovascular Adverse Events (CVAE), Including Stroke, in Elderly Patients with Dementia–Related Psychosis—Cerebrovascular adverse events (e.g., stroke, transient ischemic attack), including fatalities, were reported in patients in trials of olanzapine in elderly patients with dementia–related psychosis. In placebo–controlled trials, there was a significantly higher incidence of cerebrovascular adverse events in patients treated with olanzapine compared to patients treated with placebo. Olanzapine is not approved for the treatment of patients with dementia–related psychosis.

Hyperglycemia—Hyperglycemia, in some cases extreme and associated with ketoacidosis or hyperosmolar coma or death, has been reported in patients treated with atypical antipsychotics, including olanzapine alone, as well as olanzapine taken concomitantly with fluoxetine. Assessment of the relationship between atypical antipsychotic use and glucose abnormalities is complicated by the possibility of an increased background risk of diabetes mellitus in patients with schizophrenia and the increasing incidence of diabetes mellitus in the general population. Given these confounders, the relationship between atypical antipsychotic use and hyperglycemia–related adverse events is not completely understood. However, epidemiological studies suggest an increased risk of treatment–emergent hyperglycemia–related adverse events in patients treated with the atypical antipsychotics. While relative risk estimates are inconsistent, the association between atypical antipsychotics and increases in glucose levels appears to fall on a continuum and olanzapine appears to have a greater association than some other atypical antipsychotics.

Mean increases in blood glucose have been observed in patients treated (median exposure of 9.2 months) with olanzapine in phase 1 of the Clinical Antipsychotic Trials of Intervention Effectiveness (CATIE). The mean increase of serum glucose (fasting and nonfasting samples) from baseline to the average of the two highest serum concentrations was 15.0 mg/dL.

In an analysis of 7 controlled clinical studies, 2 of which were placebo-controlled, with treatment duration up to 12 weeks, SYMBYAX was associated with a statistically significantly greater mean change in random glucose compared to placebo (8.65 mg/dL versus – 3.86 mg/dL). In patients with baseline normal random glucose levels (<140 mg/dL), 2.3% of those treated with SYMBYAX were found to have high glucose levels (≥200 mg/dL) during SYMBYAX treatment and were statistically significantly different compared to 0.3% of those treated with placebo. In patients with baseline borderline random glucose levels (≥140 mg/dL and <200 mg/dL), 34.1% of those treated with SYMBYAX were found to have high glucose levels (≥200 mg/dL) during SYMBYAX treatment and were statistically significantly different compared to 3.6% of those treated with placebo. The difference in mean changes between SYMBYAX and placebo was greater in patients with evidence of glucose dysregulation at baseline (including those patients diagnosed with diabetes mellitus or related adverse events, patients treated with anti-diabetic agents, patients with a baseline random glucose level ≥200 mg/dL, or a baseline fasting glucose level ≥126 mg/dL). These patients had a greater mean increase in HbA$_{1c}$.

Controlled fasting glucose data is limited for SYMBYAX; however, in an analysis of 5 placebo–controlled olanzapine monotherapy studies with treatment duration up to 12 weeks, olanzapine was associated with a greater mean change in fasting glucose levels compared to placebo (2.76 mg/dL vs 0.17 mg/dL).

Olanzapine Monotherapy in Adolescents—The safety and efficacy of olanzapine and olanzapine and fluoxetine in combination have not been established in patients under the age of 18 years. In an analysis of 3 placebo–controlled olanzapine monotherapy studies of adolescent patients, including those with schizophrenia (6 weeks) or bipolar disorder (manic or mixed episodes) (3 weeks), olanzapine was associated with a statistically significantly greater mean change in fasting glucose levels compared to placebo (2.68 mg/dL versus −2.59 mg/dL). In patients with baseline normal fasting glucose levels (<100 mg/dL), zero out of 124 (0%) of those treated with olanzapine were found to have high glucose levels (≥126 mg/dL) during olanzapine treat-

ment versus 1 out of 53 (1.9%) of those treated with placebo. In patients with baseline borderline fasting glucose levels (≥100 mg/dL and <126 mg/dL), 2 out of 14 (14.3%) of those treated with olanzapine were found to have high glucose levels (≥126 mg/dL) during olanzapine treatment versus zero out of 13 (0%) of those treated with placebo.

Physicians should consider the risks and benefits when prescribing SYMBYAX to patients with an established diagnosis of diabetes mellitus, or having borderline increased blood glucose level (fasting 100–126 mg/dL, nonfasting 140–200 mg/dL). Patients taking SYMBYAX should be monitored regularly for worsening of glucose control. Patients with risk factors for diabetes mellitus (e.g., obesity, family history of diabetes) who are starting treatment with atypical antipsychotics should undergo fasting blood glucose testing at the beginning of treatment and periodically during treatment. Any patient treated with atypical antipsychotics should be monitored for symptoms of hyperglycemia including polydipsia, polyuria, polyphagia, and weakness. Patients who develop symptoms of hyperglycemia during treatment with atypical antipsychotics should undergo fasting blood glucose testing. In some cases, hyperglycemia has resolved when the atypical antipsychotic was discontinued; however, some patients required continuation of anti–diabetic treatment despite discontinuation of the suspect drug.

Hyperlipidemia—Undesirable alterations in lipids have been observed with SYMBYAX use. Clinical monitoring, including baseline and follow-up lipid evaluations in patients using SYMBYAX, is advised.

Significant, and sometimes very high (>500 mg/dL), elevations in triglyceride levels have been observed with SYMBYAX use. Significant increases in total cholesterol have also been seen with SYMBYAX use.

Controlled fasting lipid data is limited for SYMBYAX.

In an analysis of 7 controlled clinical studies, 2 of which were placebo-controlled, with treatment duration up to 12 weeks, SYMBYAX–treated patients had an increase from baseline in mean random total cholesterol of 12.1 mg/dL compared to a statistically significantly different increase from baseline in mean random total cholesterol of 4.8 mg/dL for olanzapine–treated patients and a decrease in mean random total cholesterol of 5.5 mg/dL for placebo-treated patients. Table 3 shows categorical changes in nonfasting lipid values.

[See table 3 above]

Controlled fasting lipid data is limited for SYMBYAX; however, in an analysis of 5 placebo–controlled olanzapine monotherapy studies with treatment duration up to 12 weeks, olanzapine–treated patients had statistically significant increases from baseline in mean fasting total cholesterol, LDL cholesterol, and triglycerides of 5.3 mg/dL, 3.0 mg/dL, and 20.8 mg/dL respectively compared to decreases from baseline in mean fasting total cholesterol, LDL cholesterol, and triglycerides of 6.1 mg/dL, 4.3 mg/dL, and 10.7 mg/dL for placebo–treated patients. For fasting HDL cholesterol, no statistically significant differences were ob-

served between olanzapine–treated patients and placebo–treated patients. Mean increases in fasting lipid values (total cholesterol, LDL cholesterol, and triglycerides) were greater in patients without evidence of lipid dysregulation at baseline, where lipid dysregulation was defined as patients diagnosed with dyslipidemia or related adverse events, patients treated with lipid lowering agents, patients with high baseline lipid levels. Table 4 shows categorical changes in fasting lipid values.

[See table 4 above]

In phase 1 of the Clinical Antipsychotic Trials of Intervention Effectiveness (CATIE), over a median exposure of 9.2 months, the mean increase in triglycerides in patients taking olanzapine was 40.5 mg/dL. In phase 1 of CATIE, the median increase in total cholesterol was 9.4 mg/dL.

Olanzapine Monotherapy in Adolescents—The safety and efficacy of olanzapine and olanzapine and fluoxetine in combination have not been established in patients under the age of 18 years. In an analysis of 3 placebo–controlled olanzapine monotherapy studies of adolescent patients, including those with schizophrenia (6 weeks) or bipolar disorder (manic or mixed episodes) (3 weeks), for fasting HDL cholesterol, no statistically significant differences were observed between olanzapine–treated patients and placebo–treated patients. Table 5 shows categorical changes in fasting lipid values in adolescent patients.

[See table 5 at top of next page]

Weight Gain—Potential consequences of weight gain should be considered prior to starting SYMBYAX. Patients receiving SYMBYAX should receive regular monitoring of weight. In an analysis of 7 controlled clinical studies, 2 of which were placebo-controlled, the mean weight increase for SYMBYAX–treated patients was statistically significantly greater than placebo-treated patients (4 kg vs −0.3 kg). Twenty-two percent of SYMBYAX–treated patients gained at least 7% of their baseline weight, with a median exposure of 6 weeks. This was statistically significantly greater than in placebo-treated patients (1.8%). Approximately three percent of SYMBYAX–treated patients gained at least 15% of their baseline weight, with a median exposure of 8 weeks. This was statistically significantly greater than in placebo-treated patients (0%). Clinically significant weight gain was observed across all baseline Body Mass Index (BMI) categories. Discontinuation due to weight gain occurred in 2.5% of SYMBYAX–treated patients and zero placebo-treated patients.

Table 6 includes data on weight gain with olanzapine pooled from 68 clinical trials. The data in each column represent data for those patients who completed treatment periods of the durations specified.

Continued on next page

This product information was prepared in March 2008. Current information on products of Eli Lilly and Company may be obtained by calling 1-800-545-5979.

Table 3: Changes in Nonfasting Lipids Values from Controlled Clinical Studies with Treatment Duration up to 12 Weeks

Laboratory Analyte	Category Change from Baseline	Treatment Arm	N	Patients
	Increase by ≥50 mg/dL	OFC	174	67.8%
		Olanzapine	172	72.7%
Nonfasting Triglycerides	Normal to High (<150 mg/dL to ≥500 mg/dL)	OFC	57	0%
		Olanzapine	58	0%
	Borderline to High (≥150 mg/dL and <500 mg/dL to ≥500 mg/dL)	OFC	106	15.1%
		Olanzapine	103	8.7%
	Increase by ≥40 mg/dL	OFC	685	35%*†
		Olanzapine	749	22.7%
		Placebo	390	9%
Nonfasting Total Cholesterol	Normal to High (<200 mg/dL to ≥240 mg/dL)	OFC	256	8.2%*†
		Olanzapine	279	2.9%
		Placebo	175	1.7%
	Borderline to High (≥200 mg/dL and <240 mg/dL to ≥240 mg/dL)	OFC	213	36.2%*†
		Olanzapine	261	27.6%
		Placebo	111	9.9%

* Statistically significant compared to olanzapine.
† Statistically significant compared to placebo.

Table 4: Changes in Fasting Lipids Values from Adult Placebo-Controlled Olanzapine Monotherapy Studies with Treatment Duration up to 12 Weeks

Laboratory Analyte	Category Change from Baseline	Treatment Arm	N	Patients
	Increase by ≥50 mg/dL	Olanzapine	745	39.6%*
		Placebo	402	26.1%
Fasting Triglycerides	Normal to High (<150 mg/dL to ≥200 mg/dL)	Olanzapine	457	9.2%*
		Placebo	251	4.4%
	Borderline to High (≥150 mg/dL and <200 mg/dL to ≥200 mg/dL)	Olanzapine	135	39.3%*
		Placebo	65	20.0%
	Increase by ≥40 mg/dL	Olanzapine	745	21.6%*
		Placebo	402	9.5%
Fasting Total Cholesterol	Normal to High (<200 mg/dL to ≥240 mg/dL)	Olanzapine	392	2.8%
		Placebo	207	2.4%
	Borderline to High (≥200 mg/dL and <240 mg/dL to ≥240 mg/dL)	Olanzapine	222	23.0%*
		Placebo	112	12.5%
	Increase by ≥30 mg/dL	Olanzapine	536	23.7%*
		Placebo	304	14.1%
Fasting LDL Cholesterol	Normal to High (<100 mg/dL to ≥160 mg/dL)	Olanzapine	154	0%
		Placebo	82	1.2%
	Borderline to High (≥100 mg/dL and ≥160 mg/dL to ≥160 mg/dL)	Olanzapine	302	10.6%
		Placebo	173	8.1%

*Statistically significant compared to placebo.

Symbyax—Cont.

[See table 6 at right]

During long-term continuation therapy with olanzapine monotherapy (238 median days of exposure), 56% of olanzapine patients met the criterion for having gained greater than 7% of their baseline weight. Average weight gain during long-term therapy was 5.4 kg.

Olanzapine Monotherapy in Adolescents—The safety and efficacy of olanzapine and olanzapine and fluoxetine in combination have not been established in patients under the age of 18 years. In an analysis of 4 placebo-controlled olanzapine monotherapy studies of adolescent patients (ages 13 to 17 years), including those with schizophrenia (6 weeks) or bipolar disorder (manic or mixed episodes) (3 weeks), olanzapine-treated patients gained an average of 4.6 kg, which was statistically significantly different compared to an average of 0.3 kg in placebo-treated patients, with a median exposure of 3 weeks; 40.6% of olanzapine-treated patients gained at least 7% of their baseline body weight, which was statistically significantly different compared to 9.8% of placebo-treated patients, with a median exposure of 4 weeks; 7.1% of olanzapine-treated patients gained at least 15% of their baseline weight, compared to 2.7% of placebo-treated patients, with a median exposure of 19 weeks. Clinically significant weight gain was observed across all baseline Body Mass Index (BMI) categories, but mean changes in weight were greater in adolescents with BMI categories above normal at baseline. Discontinuation due to weight gain occurred in 1% of olanzapine-treated patients, compared to zero placebo-treated patients.

During long-term continuation therapy with olanzapine, 65% of olanzapine-treated patients met the criterion for having gained greater than 7% of their baseline weight. Average weight gain during long-term therapy was 7.4 kg.

Orthostatic Hypotension—SYMBYAX may induce orthostatic hypotension associated with dizziness, tachycardia, bradycardia, and in some patients, syncope, especially during the initial dose-titration period.

In the bipolar depression studies, statistically significantly more orthostatic changes occurred with the SYMBYAX group compared to placebo and olanzapine groups. Orthostatic systolic blood pressure decrease of at least 30 mm Hg occurred in 7.3% (6/82), 1.4% (5/346), and 1.4% (5/352) of the SYMBYAX, olanzapine and placebo groups, respectively.

Among the group of controlled clinical studies with SYMBYAX, an orthostatic systolic blood pressure decrease of ≥30 mm Hg occurred in 4% (21/512) of SYMBYAX-treated patients, 5% (10/204) of fluoxetine-treated patients, 2% (16/644) of olanzapine-treated patients, and 2% (8/445) of placebo-treated patients. In this group of studies, the incidence of syncope in SYMBYAX-treated patients was 0.4% (2/571) compared to placebo 0.2% (1/477).

In a clinical pharmacology study of SYMBYAX, three healthy subjects were discontinued from the trial after experiencing severe, but self-limited, hypotension and bradycardia that occurred 2 to 9 hours following a single 12-mg/50-mg dose of SYMBYAX. Reactions consisting of this combination of hypotension and bradycardia (and also accompanied by sinus pause) have been observed in at least three other healthy subjects treated with various formulations of olanzapine (one oral, two intramuscular). In controlled clinical studies, the incidence of patients with a ≥20 bpm decrease in orthostatic pulse concomitantly with a ≥20 mm Hg decrease in orthostatic systolic blood pressure was 0.4% (2/549) in the SYMBYAX group, 0.2% (1/455) in the placebo group, 0.8% (5/659) in the olanzapine group, and 0% (0/241) in the fluoxetine group.

SYMBYAX should be used with particular caution in patients with known cardiovascular disease (history of myocardial infarction or ischemia, heart failure, or conduction abnormalities), cerebrovascular disease, or conditions that would predispose patients to hypotension (dehydration, hypovolemia, and treatment with antihypertensive medications).

Allergic Events and Rash—In SYMBYAX premarketing controlled clinical studies, the overall incidence of rash or allergic events in SYMBYAX-treated patients [4.6% (26/571)] was similar to that of placebo [5.2% (25/477)]. The majority of the cases of rash and/or urticaria were mild; however, three patients discontinued (one due to rash, which was moderate in severity, and two due to allergic events, one of which included face edema).

In fluoxetine US clinical studies, 7% of 10,782 fluoxetine-treated patients developed various types of rashes and/or urticaria. Among the cases of rash and/or urticaria reported in premarketing clinical studies, almost a third were withdrawn from treatment because of the rash and/or systemic signs or symptoms associated with the rash. Clinical findings reported in association with rash include fever, leukocytosis, arthralgias, edema, carpal tunnel syndrome, respiratory distress, lymphadenopathy, proteinuria, and mild transaminase elevation. Most patients improved promptly with discontinuation of fluoxetine and/or adjunctive treatment with antihistamines or steroids, and all patients experiencing these events were reported to recover completely.

In fluoxetine premarketing clinical studies, 2 patients are known to have developed a serious cutaneous systemic illness. In neither patient was there an unequivocal diagnosis, but 1 was considered to have a leukocytoclastic vasculitis, and the other, a severe desquamating syndrome that was considered variously to be a vasculitis or erythema multiforme. Other patients have had systemic syndromes suggestive of serum sickness.

Table 5: Changes in Fasting Lipids Values from Adolescent Placebo-Controlled Olanzapine Monotherapy Studies

Laboratory Analyte	Category Change from Baseline	Treatment Arm	N	Patients
Fasting Triglycerides	Increase by ≥50 mg/dL	Olanzapine	138	37%*
		Placebo	66	15.2%
	Normal to High (<90 mg/dL to ≥130 mg/dL)	Olanzapine	67	26.9%
		Placebo	28	10.7%
	Borderline to High (≥90 mg/dL and <130 mg/dL to ≥130 mg/dL)	Olanzapine	37	59.5%
		Placebo	17	35.3%
Fasting Total Cholesterol	Increase by ≥40 mg/dL	Olanzapine	138	14.5%*
		Placebo	66	4.5%
	Normal to High (<170 mg/dL to ≥200 mg/dL)	Olanzapine	87	6.9%
		Placebo	43	2.3%
	Borderline to High (≥170 mg/dL and <200 mg/dL to ≥200 mg/dL)	Olanzapine	36	38.9%*
		Placebo	13	7.7%
Fasting LDL Cholesterol	Increase by ≥30 mg/dL	Olanzapine	137	17.5%
		Placebo	63	11.1%
	Normal to High (<110 mg/dL to ≥130 mg/dL)	Olanzapine	98	5.1%
		Placebo	44	4.5%
	Borderline to High (≥110 mg/dL and <130 mg/dL to ≥130 mg/dL)	Olanzapine	29	48.3%*
		Placebo	9	0%

*Statistically significant compared to placebo.

Table 6: Weight Gain with Olanzapine Use

Amount Gained kg (lb)	6 Weeks (N=2976) (%)	6 Months (N=1536) (%)	12 Months (N=778) (%)	24 Months (N=422) (%)
≤0	27	21	20	22
0–5 (0–11 lb)	57	34	25	22
5–10 (11–22 lb)	15	26	25	22
10–15 (22–33 lb)	2	12	16	18
>15 (>33 lb)	0	6	14	16

Since the introduction of fluoxetine, systemic events, possibly related to vasculitis, have developed in patients with rash. Although these events are rare, they may be serious, involving the lung, kidney, or liver. Death has been reported to occur in association with these systemic events.

Anaphylactoid events, including bronchospasm, angioedema, and urticaria alone and in combination, have been reported.

Pulmonary events, including inflammatory processes of varying histopathology and/or fibrosis, have been reported rarely. These events have occurred with dyspnea as the only preceding symptom.

Whether these systemic events and rash have a common underlying cause or are due to different etiologies or pathogenic processes is not known. Furthermore, a specific underlying immunologic basis for these events has not been identified. Upon the appearance of rash or of other possible allergic phenomena for which an alternative etiology cannot be identified, SYMBYAX should be discontinued.

Serotonin Syndrome—The development of a potentially life-threatening serotonin syndrome may occur with SNRIs and SSRIs, including SYMBYAX treatment, particularly with concomitant use of serotonergic drugs (including triptans) and with drugs which impair metabolism of serotonin (including MAOIs). Serotonin syndrome symptoms may include mental status changes (e.g., agitation, hallucinations, coma), autonomic instability (e.g., tachycardia, labile blood pressure, hyperthermia), neuromuscular aberrations (e.g., hyperreflexia, incoordination) and/or gastrointestinal symptoms (e.g., nausea, vomiting, diarrhea).

The concomitant use of SYMBYAX with MAOIs intended to treat depression is contraindicated (*see* **CONTRAINDICATIONS, Monoamine Oxidase Inhibitors (MAOI)** *and* **PRECAUTIONS, Drug Interactions**).

If concomitant treatment of SYMBYAX with a 5-hydroxytryptamine receptor agonist (triptan) is clinically warranted, careful observation of the patient is advised, particularly during treatment initiation and dose increases (*see* **PRECAUTIONS, Drug Interactions**).

The concomitant use of SYMBYAX with serotonin precursors (such as tryptophan) is not recommended (*see* **PRECAUTIONS, Drug Interactions**).

Neuroleptic Malignant Syndrome (NMS)—A potentially fatal symptom complex sometimes referred to as NMS has been reported in association with administration of antipsychotic drugs, including olanzapine. Clinical manifestations of NMS are hyperpyrexia, muscle rigidity, altered mental status, and evidence of autonomic instability (irregular pulse or blood pressure, tachycardia, diaphoresis, and cardiac dysrhythmia). Additional signs may include elevated creatinine phosphokinase, myoglobinuria (rhabdomyolysis), and acute renal failure.

The diagnostic evaluation of patients with this syndrome is complicated. In arriving at a diagnosis, it is important to exclude cases where the clinical presentation includes both serious medical illness (e.g., pneumonia, systemic infection, etc.) and untreated or inadequately treated extrapyramidal signs and symptoms (EPS). Other important considerations in the differential diagnosis include central anticholinergic toxicity, heat stroke, drug fever, and primary central nervous system pathology.

The management of NMS should include: 1) immediate discontinuation of antipsychotic drugs and other drugs not essential to concurrent therapy, 2) intensive symptomatic treatment and medical monitoring, and 3) treatment of any concomitant serious medical problems for which specific treatments are available. There is no general agreement about specific pharmacological treatment regimens for NMS.

If after recovering from NMS, a patient requires treatment with an antipsychotic, the patient should be carefully monitored, since recurrences of NMS have been reported.

Tardive Dyskinesia—A syndrome of potentially irreversible, involuntary, dyskinetic movements may develop in patients treated with antipsychotic drugs. Although the prevalence of the syndrome appears to be highest among the elderly, especially elderly women, it is impossible to rely upon prevalence estimates to predict, at the inception of antipsychotic treatment, which patients are likely to develop the syndrome. Whether antipsychotic drug products differ in their potential to cause tardive dyskinesia is unknown.

The risk of developing tardive dyskinesia and the likelihood that it will become irreversible are believed to increase as the duration of treatment and the total cumulative dose of antipsychotic drugs administered to the patient increase. However, the syndrome can develop, although much less commonly, after relatively brief treatment periods at low doses or may even arise after discontinuation of treatment. There is no known treatment for established cases of tardive dyskinesia, although the syndrome may remit, partially or completely, if antipsychotic treatment is withdrawn. Antipsychotic treatment itself, however, may suppress (or partially suppress) the signs and symptoms of the syndrome and thereby may possibly mask the underlying process. The effect that symptomatic suppression has upon the long-term course of the syndrome is unknown.

The incidence of dyskinetic movement in SYMBYAX-treated patients was infrequent. The mean score on the Abnormal Involuntary Movement Scale (AIMS) across clinical studies involving SYMBYAX-treated patients decreased from baseline. Nonetheless, SYMBYAX should be prescribed in a manner that is most likely to minimize the risk of tardive dyskinesia. If signs and symptoms of tardive dyskinesia appear in a patient on SYMBYAX, drug discontinuation should be considered. However, some patients may require treatment with SYMBYAX despite the presence of the syndrome. The need for continued treatment should be reassessed periodically.

Thioridazine—In a study of 19 healthy male subjects, which included 6 slow and 13 rapid hydroxylators of debrisoquin, a single 25-mg oral dose of thioridazine produced a 2.4-fold higher C_{max} and a 4.5-fold higher AUC for thioridazine in the slow hydroxylators compared with the rapid hydroxylators. The rate of debrisoquin hydroxylation is felt to depend on the level of CYP2D6 isozyme activity. Thus, this study suggests that drugs that inhibit CYP2D6, such as certain SSRIs, including fluoxetine, will produce elevated plasma levels of thioridazine (*see* **PRECAUTIONS**).

Thioridazine administration produces a dose-related prolongation of the QT_c interval, which is associated with serious ventricular arrhythmias, such as torsades de pointes-type arrhythmias and sudden death. This risk is expected to increase with fluoxetine-induced inhibition of thioridazine metabolism (*see* **CONTRAINDICATIONS, Thioridazine**).

PRECAUTIONS

General

Concomitant Use of Olanzapine and Fluoxetine Products—SYMBYAX contains the same active ingredients that are in Zyprexa and Zyprexa Zydis (olanzapine) and in Prozac, Prozac Weekly, and Sarafem (fluoxetine HCl). Caution should be exercised when prescribing these medications concomitantly with SYMBYAX.

Abnormal Bleeding—SSRIs and SNRIs, including fluoxetine, may increase the risk of bleeding events. Concomitant use of aspirin, nonsteroidal anti-inflammatory drugs, warfarin, and other anti-coagulants may add to this risk. Case reports and epidemiological studies (case-control and cohort design) have demonstrated an association between use of drugs that interfere with serotonin reuptake and the occurrence of gastrointestinal bleeding. Bleeding events related to SSRIs and SNRIs use have ranged from ecchymoses, hematomas, epistaxis, and petechiae to life-threatening hemorrhages.

Patients should be cautioned about the risk of bleeding associated with the concomitant use of SYMBYAX and NSAIDs, aspirin, or other drugs that affect coagulation (*see* **DRUG INTERACTIONS**).

Mania/Hypomania—In the two controlled bipolar depression studies there was no statistically significant difference in the incidence of manic events (manic reaction or manic depressive reaction) between SYMBYAX- and placebo-treated patients. In one of the studies, the incidence of manic events was (7% [3/43]) in SYMBYAX-treated patients compared to (3% [5/184]) in placebo-treated patients. In the other study, the incidence of manic events was (2% [1/43]) in SYMBYAX-treated patients compared to (8% [15/193]) in placebo-treated patients. This limited controlled trial experience of SYMBYAX in the treatment of bipolar depression makes it difficult to interpret these findings until additional data is obtained. Because of this and the cyclical nature of bipolar disorder, patients should be monitored closely for the development of symptoms of mania/hypomania during treatment with SYMBYAX.

Body Temperature Regulation—Disruption of the body's ability to reduce core body temperature has been attributed to antipsychotic drugs. Appropriate care is advised when prescribing SYMBYAX for patients who will be experiencing conditions which may contribute to an elevation in core body temperature (e.g., exercising strenuously, exposure to extreme heat, receiving concomitant medication with anticholinergic activity, or being subject to dehydration).

Cognitive and Motor Impairment —Somnolence was a commonly reported adverse event associated with SYMBYAX treatment, occurring at an incidence of 22% in SYMBYAX patients compared with 11% in placebo patients. Somnolence led to discontinuation in 2% (10/571) of patients in the premarketing controlled clinical studies.

As with any CNS-active drug, SYMBYAX has the potential to impair judgment, thinking, or motor skills. Patients should be cautioned about operating hazardous machinery, including automobiles, until they are reasonably certain that SYMBYAX therapy does not affect them adversely.

Discontinuation of Treatment with SYMBYAX

During marketing of fluoxetine, a component of SYMBYAX, and other SSRIs and SNRIs (serotonin and norepinephrine reuptake inhibitors), there have been spontaneous reports of adverse events occurring upon discontinuation of these drugs, particularly when abrupt, including the following: dysphoric mood, irritability, agitation, dizziness, sensory disturbances (e.g., paresthesias such as electric shock sensations), anxiety, confusion, headache, lethargy, emotional lability, insomnia, and hypomania. While these events are generally self-limiting, there have been reports of serious discontinuation symptoms. Patients should be monitored for these symptoms when discontinuing treatment with fluoxetine. A gradual reduction in the dose rather than abrupt cessation is recommended whenever possible. If intolerable symptoms occur following a decrease in the dose or upon discontinuation of treatment, then resuming the previously prescribed dose may be considered. Subsequently, the physician may continue decreasing the dose but at a more gradual rate. Plasma fluoxetine and norfluoxetine concentration decrease gradually at the conclusion of therapy, which may minimize the risk of discontinuation symptoms with this drug (*see* **DOSAGE AND ADMINISTRATION**).

Dysphagia—Esophageal dysmotility and aspiration have been associated with antipsychotic drug use. Aspiration pneumonia is a common cause of morbidity and mortality in patients with advanced Alzheimer's disease. Olanzapine and other antipsychotic drugs should be used cautiously in patients at risk for aspiration pneumonia.

Half-Life—Because of the long elimination half-lives of fluoxetine and its major active metabolite, changes in dose will not be fully reflected in plasma for several weeks, affecting both strategies for titration to final dose and withdrawal from treatment (*see* **CLINICAL PHARMACOLOGY, Accumulation and slow elimination**).

Hyperprolactinemia—As with other drugs that antagonize dopamine D_2 receptors, SYMBYAX elevates prolactin levels, and a modest elevation persists during administration; however, possibly associated clinical manifestations (e.g., galactorrhea and breast enlargement) were infrequently observed.

Tissue culture experiments indicate that approximately one-third of human breast cancers are prolactin dependent in vitro, a factor of potential importance if the prescription of these drugs is contemplated in a patient with previously detected breast cancer of this type. Although disturbances such as galactorrhea, amenorrhea, gynecomastia, and impotence have been reported with prolactin-elevating compounds, the clinical significance of elevated serum prolactin levels is unknown for most patients. As is common with compounds that increase prolactin release, an increase in mammary gland neoplasia was observed in the olanzapine carcinogenicity studies conducted in mice and rats (*see* **Carcinogenesis**). However, neither clinical studies nor epidemiologic studies have shown an association between chronic administration of this class of drugs and tumorigenesis in humans; the available evidence is considered too limited to be conclusive.

Hyponatremia—Hyponatremia may occur as a result of treatment with SSRIs and SNRIs, including SYMBYAX. In many cases, this hyponatremia appears to be the result of the syndrome of inappropriate antidiuretic hormone secretion (SIADH). Cases with serum sodium lower than 110 mmol/L have been reported and appeared to be reversible when Symbyax was discontinued. Elderly patients may be at greater risk of developing hyponatremia with SSRIs and SNRIs. Also, patients taking diuretics or who are otherwise volume depleted may be at greater risk (*see* **Geriatric Use**). Discontinuation of SYMBYAX should be considered in patients with symptomatic hyponatremia and appropriate medical intervention should be instituted.

Signs and symptoms of hyponatremia include headache, difficulty concentrating, memory impairment, confusion, weakness, and unsteadiness, which may lead to falls. More severe and/or acute cases have been associated with hallucination, syncope, seizure, coma, respiratory arrest, and death.

Seizures—Seizures occurred in 0.2% (4/2066) of SYMBYAX-treated patients during open-label premarketing clinical studies. No seizures occurred in the premarketing controlled SYMBYAX studies. Seizures have also been reported with both olanzapine and fluoxetine monotherapy. Therefore, SYMBYAX should be used cautiously in patients with a history of seizures or with conditions that potentially lower the seizure threshold. Conditions that lower the seizure threshold may be more prevalent in a population of ≥65 years of age.

Transaminase Elevations—As with olanzapine, asymptomatic elevations of hepatic transaminases [ALT (SGPT), AST (SGOT), and GGT] and alkaline phosphatase have been observed with SYMBYAX. In the SYMBYAX-controlled database, ALT (SGPT) elevations (≥3 times the upper limit of the normal range) were observed in 6.3% (31/495) of patients exposed to SYMBYAX compared with 0.5% (2/384) of the placebo patients and 4.5% (25/560) of olanzapine-treated patients. The difference between SYMBYAX and placebo was statistically significant. None of these 31 SYMBYAX-treated patients experienced jaundice and three had transient elevations >200 IU/L.

In olanzapine placebo-controlled studies, clinically significant ALT (SGPT) elevations (≥3 times the upper limit of the normal range) were observed in 2% (6/243) of patients exposed to olanzapine compared with 0% (0/115) of the placebo patients. None of these patients experienced jaundice. In 2 of these patients, liver enzymes decreased toward normal despite continued treatment, and in 2 others, enzymes decreased upon discontinuation of olanzapine. In the remaining 2 patients, 1, seropositive for hepatitis C, had persistent enzyme elevations for 4 months after discontinuation, and the other had insufficient follow-up to determine if enzymes normalized.

Within the larger olanzapine premarketing database of about 2400 patients with baseline SGPT ≤90 IU/L, the incidence of SGPT elevation to >200 IU/L was 2% (50/2381). Again, none of these patients experienced jaundice or other symptoms attributable to liver impairment and most had transient changes that tended to normalize while olanzapine treatment was continued. Among all 2500 patients in olanzapine clinical studies, approximately 1% (23/2500) discontinued treatment due to transaminase increases.

Rare postmarketing reports of hepatitis have been received. Very rare cases of cholestatic or mixed liver injury have also been reported in the postmarketing period.

Caution should be exercised in patients with signs and symptoms of hepatic impairment, in patients with pre-existing conditions associated with limited hepatic functional reserve, and in patients who are being treated with potentially hepatotoxic drugs. Periodic assessment of transaminases is recommended in patients with significant hepatic disease (*see* **Laboratory Tests**).

Use in Patients with Concomitant Illness

Clinical experience with SYMBYAX in patients with concomitant systemic illnesses is limited (*see* **CLINICAL PHARMACOLOGY, Renal Impairment** *and* **Hepatic Impairment**). The following precautions for the individual components may be applicable to SYMBYAX.

Olanzapine exhibits in vitro muscarinic receptor affinity. In premarketing clinical studies, SYMBYAX was associated with constipation, dry mouth, and tachycardia, all adverse events possibly related to cholinergic antagonism. Such adverse events were not often the basis for study discontinuations; SYMBYAX should be used with caution in patients with clinically significant prostatic hypertrophy, narrow angle glaucoma, a history of paralytic ileus, or related conditions.

In five placebo-controlled studies of olanzapine in elderly patients with dementia-related psychosis (n=1184), the following treatment-emergent adverse events were reported in olanzapine-treated patients at an incidence of at least 2% and significantly greater than placebo-treated patients: falls, somnolence, peripheral edema, abnormal gait, urinary incontinence, lethargy, increased weight, asthenia, pyrexia, pneumonia, dry mouth and visual hallucinations. The rate of discontinuation due to adverse events was significantly greater with olanzapine than placebo (13% vs 7%). Elderly patients with dementia-related psychosis treated with olanzapine are at an increased risk of death compared to placebo. Olanzapine is not approved for the treatment of patients with dementia-related psychosis. If the prescriber elects to treat elderly patients with dementia-related psychosis, vigilance should be exercised (*see* **BOX WARNING** *and* **WARNINGS**).

As with other CNS-active drugs, SYMBYAX should be used with caution in elderly patients with dementia. Olanzapine is not approved for the treatment of patients with dementia-related psychosis. If the prescriber elects to treat elderly patients with dementia-related psychosis, vigilance should be exercised (*see* **BOX WARNING** *and* **WARNINGS**).

SYMBYAX has not been evaluated or used to any appreciable extent in patients with a recent history of myocardial infarction or unstable heart disease. Patients with these diagnoses were excluded from clinical studies during the premarket testing.

Caution is advised when using SYMBYAX in cardiac patients and in patients with diseases or conditions that could affect hemodynamic responses (*see* **WARNINGS, Orthostatic Hypotension**).

In subjects with cirrhosis of the liver, the clearances of fluoxetine and its active metabolite, norfluoxetine, were decreased, thus increasing the elimination half-lives of these substances. A lower dose of the fluoxetine-component of SYMBYAX should be used in patients with cirrhosis. Caution is advised when using SYMBYAX in patients with diseases or conditions that could affect its metabolism (*see* **CLINICAL PHARMACOLOGY, Hepatic Impairment** *and* **DOSING AND ADMINISTRATION, Special Populations**).

Olanzapine and fluoxetine individual pharmacokinetics do not differ significantly in patients with renal impairment. SYMBYAX dosing adjustment based upon renal impairment is not routinely required (*see* **CLINICAL PHARMACOLOGY, Renal Impairment**).

Information for Patients

Prescribers or other health professionals should inform patients, their families, and their caregivers about the benefits and risks associated with treatment with SYMBYAX and should counsel them in its appropriate use. A patient Medication Guide about "Antidepressant Medicines, Depression and other Serious Mental Illness, and Suicidal Thoughts or Actions" is available for SYMBYAX. The prescriber or health professional should instruct patients, their families, and their caregivers to read the Medication Guide and should assist them in understanding its contents. Patients should be given the opportunity to discuss the contents of the Medication Guide and to obtain answers to any questions they may have. The complete text of the Medication Guide is reprinted at the end of this document.

Patients should be advised of the following issues and asked to alert their prescriber if these occur while taking SYMBYAX.

Clinical Worsening and Suicide Risk—Patients, their families, and their caregivers should be encouraged to be alert to the emergence of anxiety, agitation, panic attacks, insomnia, irritability, hostility, aggressiveness, impulsivity, akathisia (psychomotor restlessness), hypomania, mania, other unusual changes in behavior, worsening of depression, and suicidal ideation, especially early during antidepressant treatment and when the dose is adjusted up or down. Families and caregivers of patients should be advised to look for the emergence of such symptoms on a day-to-day basis, since changes may be abrupt. Such symptoms should be reported to the patient's prescriber or health professional, especially if they are severe, abrupt in onset, or were not part of the patient's presenting symptoms. Symptoms such as these may be associated with an increased risk for suicidal thinking and behavior and indicate a need for very close monitoring and possibly changes in the medication.

Hyperglycemia—Patients should be advised of the potential risk of hyperglycemia-related adverse events. Patients should be monitored regularly for worsening of glucose control.

Weight Gain—Patients should be counseled that SYMBYAX is associated with weight gain. Patients should have their weight monitored regularly.

Serotonin Syndrome—Patients should be cautioned about the risk of serotonin syndrome with the concomitant use of SYMBYAX and triptans, tramadol or other serotonergic agents.

Abnormal Bleeding—Patients should be cautioned about the concomitant use of SYMBYAX and NSAIDs, aspirin, warfarin, or other drugs that affect coagulation since the combined use of psychotropic drugs that interfere with serotonin reuptake and these agents has been associated with an increased risk of bleeding (*see* **PRECAUTIONS, Abnormal Bleeding**).

Alcohol—Patients should be advised to avoid alcohol while taking SYMBYAX.

Cognitive and Motor Impairment—As with any CNS-active drug, SYMBYAX has the potential to impair judgment, thinking, or motor skills. Patients should be cautioned about operating hazardous machinery, including automobiles, until they are reasonably certain that SYMBYAX therapy does not affect them adversely.

Concomitant Medication—Patients should be advised to inform their physician if they are taking Prozac®, Prozac Weekly™, Sarafem®, fluoxetine, Zyprexa®, or Zyprexa Zydis®. Patients should also be advised to inform their phy-

Continued on next page

This product information was prepared in March 2008. Current information on products of Eli Lilly and Company may be obtained by calling 1-800-545-5979.

Symbyax—Cont.

sicians if they are taking or plan to take any prescription or over–the–counter drugs, including herbal supplements, since there is a potential for interactions.

Heat Exposure and Dehydration—Patients should be advised regarding appropriate care in avoiding overheating and dehydration.

Nursing—Patients, if taking SYMBYAX, should be advised not to breast–feed.

Orthostatic Hypotension—Patients should be advised of the risk of orthostatic hypotension, especially during the period of initial dose titration and in association with the use of concomitant drugs that may potentiate the orthostatic effect of olanzapine, e.g., diazepam or alcohol (see **WARNINGS** and **Drug Interactions**).

Pregnancy—Patients should be advised to notify their physician if they become pregnant or intend to become pregnant during SYMBYAX therapy.

Rash—Patients should be advised to notify their physician if they develop a rash or hives while taking SYMBYAX.

Treatment Adherence—Patients should be advised to take SYMBYAX exactly as prescribed, and to continue taking SYMBYAX as prescribed even after their mood symptoms improve. Patients should be advised that they should not alter their dosing regimen, or stop taking SYMBYAX, without consulting their physician.

Patient information is printed at the end of this insert. Physicians should discuss this information with their patients and instruct them to read the Medication Guide before starting therapy with SYMBYAX and each time their prescription is refilled.

Laboratory Tests
Periodic assessment of transaminases is recommended in patients with significant hepatic disease (see **Transaminase Elevations**).

Drug Interactions
The risks of using SYMBYAX in combination with other drugs have not been extensively evaluated in systematic studies. The drug–drug interactions of the individual components are applicable to SYMBYAX. As with all drugs, the potential for interaction by a variety of mechanisms (e.g., pharmacodynamic, pharmacokinetic drug inhibition or enhancement, etc.) is a possibility. Caution is advised if the concomitant administration of SYMBYAX and other CNS–active drugs is required. In evaluating individual cases, consideration should be given to using lower initial doses of the concomitantly administered drugs, using conservative titration schedules, and monitoring of clinical status (see **CLINICAL PHARMACOLOGY, Accumulation and slow elimination**).

Antihypertensive agents—Because of the potential for olanzapine to induce hypotension, SYMBYAX may enhance the effects of certain antihypertensive agents (see **WARNINGS, Orthostatic Hypotension**).

Anti–Parkinsonian—The olanzapine component of SYMBYAX may antagonize the effects of levodopa and dopamine agonists.

Benzodiazepines—Multiple doses of olanzapine did not influence the pharmacokinetics of diazepam and its active metabolite N–desmethyldiazepam. However, the coadministration of diazepam with olanzapine potentiated the orthostatic hypotension observed with olanzapine.

When concurrently administered with fluoxetine, the half-life of diazepam may be prolonged in some patients (see **CLINICAL PHARMACOLOGY, Accumulation and slow elimination**). Coadministration of alprazolam and fluoxetine has resulted in increased alprazolam plasma concentrations and in further psychomotor performance decrement due to increased alprazolam levels.

Biperiden—Multiple doses of olanzapine did not influence the pharmacokinetics of biperiden.

Carbamazepine—Carbamazepine therapy (200 mg BID) causes an approximate 50% increase in the clearance of olanzapine. This increase is likely due to the fact that carbamazepine is a potent inducer of CYP1A2 activity. Higher daily doses of carbamazepine may cause an even greater increase in olanzapine clearance.

Patients on stable doses of carbamazepine have developed elevated plasma anticonvulsant concentrations and clinical anticonvulsant toxicity following initiation of concomitant fluoxetine treatment.

Clozapine—Elevation of blood levels of clozapine has been observed in patients receiving concomitant fluoxetine.

Electroconvulsive therapy (ECT)—There are no clinical studies establishing the benefit of the combined use of ECT and fluoxetine. There have been rare reports of prolonged seizures in patients on fluoxetine receiving ECT treatment (see **Seizures**).

Ethanol—Ethanol (45 mg/70 kg single dose) did not have an effect on olanzapine pharmacokinetics. The coadministration of ethanol with SYMBYAX may potentiate sedation and orthostatic hypotension.

Fluvoxamine—Fluvoxamine, a CYP1A2 inhibitor, decreases the clearance of olanzapine. This results in a mean increase in olanzapine C_{max} following fluvoxamine administration of 54% in female nonsmokers and 77% in male smokers. The mean increase in olanzapine AUC is 52% and 108%, respectively. Lower doses of the olanzapine component of SYMBYAX should be considered in patients receiving concomitant treatment with fluvoxamine.

Haloperidol—Elevation of blood levels of haloperidol has been observed in patients receiving concomitant fluoxetine.

Lithium—Multiple doses of olanzapine did not influence the pharmacokinetics of lithium.

There have been reports of both increased and decreased lithium levels when lithium was used concomitantly with fluoxetine. Cases of lithium toxicity and increased serotonergic effects have been reported. Lithium levels should be monitored in patients taking SYMBYAX concomitantly with lithium.

Monoamine oxidase inhibitors—See **CONTRAINDICATIONS**.

Phenytoin—Patients on stable doses of phenytoin have developed elevated plasma levels of phenytoin with clinical phenytoin toxicity following initiation of concomitant fluoxetine.

Pimozide—Clinical studies of pimozide with other antidepressants demonstrate an increase in drug interaction or QT_c prolongation. While a specific study with pimozide and fluoxetine has not been conducted, the potential for drug interactions or QT_c prolongation warrants restricting the concurrent use of pimozide and fluoxetine. Concomitant use of fluoxetine and pimozide is contraindicated (see **CONTRAINDICATIONS**).

Serotonergic drugs—Based on the mechanism of action of SNRIs and SSRIs, including SYMBYAX, and the potential for serotonin syndrome, caution is advised when SYMBYAX is coadministered with other drugs that may affect the serotonergic neurotransmitter systems, such as triptans, linezolid (an antibiotic which is a reversible non–selective MAOI), lithium, tramadol, or St. John's Wort (see **WARNINGS, Serotonin Syndrome**). The concomitant use of SYMBYAX with other SSRIs, SNRIs or tryptophan is not recommended (see **Tryptophan**).

Theophylline—Multiple doses of olanzapine did not affect the pharmacokinetics of theophylline or its metabolites.

Thioridazine—See **CONTRAINDICATIONS** and **WARNINGS, Thioridazine**.

Tricyclic antidepressants (TCAs)—Single doses of olanzapine did not affect the pharmacokinetics of imipramine or its active metabolite desipramine.

In two fluoxetine studies, previously stable plasma levels of imipramine and desipramine have increased >2–to 10–fold when fluoxetine has been administered in combination. This influence may persist for three weeks or longer after fluoxetine is discontinued. Thus, the dose of TCA may need to be reduced and plasma TCA concentrations may need to be monitored temporarily when SYMBYAX is coadministered or has been recently discontinued (see **Drugs metabolized by CYP2D6** and **CLINICAL PHARMACOLOGY, Accumulation and slow elimination**).

Triptans—There have been rare postmarketing reports of serotonin syndrome with use of an SSRI and a triptan. If concomitant treatment of SYMBYAX with a triptan is clinically warranted, careful observation of the patient is advised, particularly during treatment initiation and dose increases (see **WARNINGS, Serotonin Syndrome**).

Tryptophan—Five patients receiving fluoxetine in combination with tryptophan experienced adverse reactions, including agitation, restlessness, and gastrointestinal distress.

Valproate—In vitro studies using human liver microsomes determined that olanzapine has little potential to inhibit the major metabolic pathway, glucuronidation, of valproate. Further, valproate has little effect on the metabolism of olanzapine in vitro. Thus, a clinically significant pharmacokinetic interaction between olanzapine and valproate is unlikely.

Warfarin—Warfarin (20–mg single dose) did not affect olanzapine pharmacokinetics. Single doses of olanzapine did not affect the pharmacokinetics of warfarin.

Drugs that interfere with hemostasis (e.g., NSAIDs, Aspirin, Warfarin)—Serotonin release by platelets plays an important role in hemostasis. Epidemiological studies of the case–control and cohort design that have demonstrated an association between use of psychotropic drugs that interfere with serotonin reuptake and the occurrence of upper gastrointestinal bleeding have also shown that concurrent use of an NSAID or aspirin may potentiate this risk of bleeding (see **PRECAUTIONS, Abnormal Bleeding**). Altered anticoagulant effects, including increased bleeding, have been reported when SSRIs or SNRIs are coadministered with warfarin (see **PRECAUTIONS, Abnormal Bleeding**). Patients receiving warfarin therapy should be carefully monitored when SYMBYAX is initiated or discontinued.

Drugs metabolized by CYP2D6—In vitro studies utilizing human liver microsomes suggest that olanzapine has little potential to inhibit CYP2D6. Thus, olanzapine is unlikely to cause clinically important drug interactions mediated by this enzyme.

Fluoxetine inhibits the activity of CYP2D6, and may make individuals with normal CYP2D6 metabolic activity resemble a poor metabolizer. Coadministration of fluoxetine with other drugs that are metabolized by CYP2D6, including certain antidepressants (e.g., TCAs), antipsychotics (e.g., phenothiazines and most atypicals), and antiarrhythmics (e.g., propafenone, flecainide, and others) should be approached with caution. Therapy with medications that are predominantly metabolized by the CYP2D6 system and that have a relatively narrow therapeutic index should be initiated at the low end of the dose range if a patient is receiving fluoxetine concurrently or has taken it in the previous five weeks. If fluoxetine is added to the treatment regimen of a patient already receiving a drug metabolized by CYP2D6, the need for a decreased dose of the original medication should be considered. Drugs with a narrow therapeutic index represent the greatest concern (including but not limited to, flecainide, propafenone, vinblastine, and TCAs). Due

to the risk of serious ventricular arrhythmias and sudden death potentially associated with elevated thioridazine plasma levels, thioridazine should not be administered with fluoxetine or within a minimum of five weeks after fluoxetine has been discontinued (see **CONTRAINDICATIONS, Monoamine Oxidase Inhibitors (MAOI)** and **WARNINGS, Thioridazine**).

Drugs metabolized by CYP3A—In vitro studies utilizing human liver microsomes suggest that olanzapine has little potential to inhibit CYP3A. Thus, olanzapine is unlikely to cause clinically important drug interactions mediated by these enzymes.

In an in vivo interaction study involving the coadministration of fluoxetine with single doses of terfenadine (a CYP3A substrate), no increase in plasma terfenadine concentrations occurred with concomitant fluoxetine. In addition, in vitro studies have shown ketoconazole, a potent inhibitor of CYP3A activity, to be at least 100 times more potent than fluoxetine or norfluoxetine as an inhibitor of the metabolism of several substrates for this enzyme, including astemizole, cisapride, and midazolam. These data indicate that fluoxetine's extent of inhibition of CYP3A activity is not likely to be of clinical significance.

Effect of olanzapine on drugs metabolized by other CYP enzymes—In vitro studies utilizing human liver microsomes suggest that olanzapine has little potential to inhibit CYP1A2, CYP2C9, and CYP2C19. Thus, olanzapine is unlikely to cause clinically important drug interactions mediated by these enzymes.

The effect of other drugs on olanzapine—Fluoxetine, an inhibitor of CYP2D6, decreases olanzapine clearance a small amount (see **CLINICAL PHARMACOLOGY, Pharmacokinetics**). Agents that induce CYP1A2 or glucuronyl transferase enzymes, such as omeprazole and rifampin, may cause an increase in olanzapine clearance. Fluvoxamine, an inhibitor of CYP1A2, decreases olanzapine clearance (see **Drug Interactions, Fluvoxamine**). The effect of CYP1A2 inhibitors, such as fluvoxamine and some fluoroquinolone antibiotics, on SYMBYAX has not been evaluated. Although olanzapine is metabolized by multiple enzyme systems, induction or inhibition of a single enzyme may appreciably alter olanzapine clearance. Therefore, a dosage increase (for induction) or a dosage decrease (for inhibition) may need to be considered with specific drugs.

Drugs tightly bound to plasma proteins—The in vitro binding of SYMBYAX to human plasma proteins is similar to the individual components. The interaction between SYMBYAX and other highly protein–bound drugs has not been fully evaluated. Because fluoxetine is tightly bound to plasma protein, the administration of fluoxetine to a patient taking another drug that is tightly bound to protein (e.g., Coumadin, digitoxin) may cause a shift in plasma concentrations potentially resulting in an adverse effect. Conversely, adverse effects may result from displacement of protein–bound fluoxetine by other tightly bound drugs (see **CLINICAL PHARMACOLOGY, Distribution** and **PRECAUTIONS, Drug Interactions**).

Carcinogenesis, Mutagenesis, Impairment of Fertility
No carcinogenicity, mutagenicity, or fertility studies were conducted with SYMBYAX. The following data are based on findings in studies performed with the individual components.

Carcinogenesis
Olanzapine—Oral carcinogenicity studies were conducted in mice and rats. Olanzapine was administered to mice in two 78–week studies at doses of 3, 10, and 30/20 mg/kg/day [equivalent to 0.8 to 5 times the maximum recommended human daily dose (MRHD) on a mg/m² basis] and 0.25, 2, and 8 mg/kg/day (equivalent to 0.06 to 2 times the MRHD on a mg/m² basis). Rats were dosed for 2 years at doses of 0.25, 1, 2.5, and 4 mg/kg/day (males) and 0.25, 1, 4, and 8 mg/kg/day (females) (equivalent to 0.1 to 2 and 0.1 to 4 times the MRHD on a mg/m² basis, respectively). The incidence of liver hemangiomas and hemangiosarcomas was significantly increased in one mouse study in females dosed at 8 mg/kg/day (2 times the MRHD on a mg/m² basis). These tumors were not increased in another mouse study in females dosed at 10 or 30/20 mg/kg/day (2 to 5 times the MRHD on a mg/m² basis); in this study, there was a high incidence of early mortalities in males of the 30/20 mg/kg/day group. The incidence of mammary gland adenomas and adenocarcinomas was significantly increased in female mice dosed at ≥2 mg/kg/day and in female rats dosed at ≥4 mg/kg/day (0.5 and 2 times the MRHD on a mg/m² basis, respectively). Antipsychotic drugs have been shown to chronically elevate prolactin levels in rodents. Serum prolactin levels were not measured during the olanzapine carcinogenicity studies; however, measurements during subchronic toxicity studies showed that olanzapine elevated serum prolactin levels up to 4–fold in rats at the same doses used in the carcinogenicity study. An increase in mammary gland neoplasms has been found in rodents after chronic administration of other antipsychotic drugs and is considered to be prolactin–mediated. The relevance for human risk of the finding of prolactin–mediated endocrine tumors in rodents is unknown (see **PRECAUTIONS, Hyperprolactinemia**).

Fluoxetine—The dietary administration of fluoxetine to rats and mice for two years at doses of up to 10 and 12 mg/kg/day, respectively (approximately 1.2 and 0.7 times, respectively, the MRHD on a mg/m² basis), produced no evidence of carcinogenicity.

Mutagenesis
Olanzapine—No evidence of mutagenic potential for olanzapine was found in the Ames reverse mutation test, in

vivo micronucleus test in mice, the chromosomal aberration test in Chinese hamster ovary cells, unscheduled DNA synthesis test in rat hepatocytes, induction of forward mutation test in mouse lymphoma cells, or in vivo sister chromatid exchange test in bone marrow of Chinese hamsters.

Fluoxetine—Fluoxetine and norfluoxetine have been shown to have no genotoxic effects based on the following assays: bacterial mutation assay, DNA repair assay in cultured rat hepatocytes, mouse lymphoma assay, and in vivo sister chromatid exchange assay in Chinese hamster bone marrow cells.

Impairment of Fertility

SYMBYAX—Fertility studies were not conducted with SYMBYAX. However, in a repeat–dose rat toxicology study of three months duration, ovary weight was decreased in females treated with the low–dose [2 and 4 mg/kg/day (1 and 0.5 times the MRHD on a mg/m^2 basis), respectively] and high–dose [4 and 8 mg/kg/day (2 and 1 times the MRHD on a mg/m^2 basis), respectively] combinations of olanzapine and fluoxetine. Decreased ovary weight, and corpora luteal depletion and uterine atrophy were observed to a greater extent in the females receiving the high–dose combination than in females receiving either olanzapine or fluoxetine alone. In a 3–month repeat–dose dog toxicology study, reduced epididymal sperm and reduced testicular and prostate weights were observed with the high–dose combination of olanzapine and fluoxetine [5 and 5 mg/kg/day (9 and 2 times the MRHD on a mg/m^2 basis), respectively] and with olanzapine alone (5 mg/kg/day or 9 times the MRHD on a mg/m^2 basis).

Olanzapine—In a fertility and reproductive performance study in rats, male mating performance, but not fertility, was impaired at a dose of 22.4 mg/kg/day and female fertility was decreased at a dose of 3 mg/kg/day (11 and 1.5 times the MRHD on a mg/m^2 basis, respectively). Discontinuance of olanzapine treatment reversed the effects on male–mating performance. In female rats, the precoital period was increased and the mating index reduced at 5 mg/kg/day (2.5 times the MRHD on a mg/m^2 basis). Diestrous was prolonged and estrous was delayed at 1.1 mg/kg/day (0.6 times the MRHD on a mg/m^2 basis); therefore, olanzapine may produce a delay in ovulation.

Fluoxetine—Two fertility studies conducted in adult rats at doses of up to 7.5 and 12.5 mg/kg/day (approximately 0.9 and 1.5 times the MRHD on a mg/m^2 basis) indicated that fluoxetine had no adverse effects on fertility (see **Pediatric Use**).

Pregnancy—Pregnancy Category C

SYMBYAX

Embryo fetal development studies were conducted in rats and rabbits with olanzapine and fluoxetine in low–dose and high–dose combinations. In rats, the doses were: 2 and 4 mg/kg/day (low–dose) [1 and 0.5 times the MRHD on a mg/m^2 basis, respectively], and 4 and 8 mg/kg/day (high–dose) [2 and 1 times the MRHD on a mg/m^2 basis, respectively]. In rabbits, the doses were 4 and 4 mg/kg/day (low–dose) [4 and 1 times the MRHD on a mg/m^2 basis, respectively], and 8 and 8 mg/kg/day (high–dose) [9 and 2 times the MRHD on a mg/m^2 basis, respectively]. In these studies, olanzapine and fluoxetine were also administered alone at the high–doses (4 and 8 mg/kg/day, respectively, in the rat; 8 and 8 mg/kg/day, respectively, in the rabbit). In the rabbit, there was no evidence of teratogenicity; however, the high–dose combination produced decreases in fetal weight and retarded skeletal ossification in conjunction with maternal toxicity. Similarly, in the rat there was no evidence of teratogenicity; however, a decrease in fetal weight was observed with the high–dose combination.

In a pre– and postnatal study conducted in rats, olanzapine and fluoxetine were administered during pregnancy and throughout lactation in combination (low–dose: 2 and 4 mg/kg/day [1 and 0.5 times the MRHD on a mg/m^2 basis], respectively, high–dose: 4 and 8 mg/kg/day [2 and 1 times the MRHD on a mg/m^2 basis], respectively, and alone: 4 and 8 mg/kg/day [2 and 1 times the MRHD on a mg/m^2 basis], respectively). Administration of the high–dose combination resulted in a marked elevation in offspring mortality and growth retardation in comparison to the same doses of olanzapine and fluoxetine administered alone. These effects were not observed with the low–dose combination; however, there were a few cases of testicular degeneration and atrophy, depletion of epididymal sperm and infertility in the male progeny. The effects of the high–dose combination on postnatal endpoints could not be assessed due to high progeny mortality.

There are no adequate and well–controlled studies with SYMBYAX in pregnant women.

SYMBYAX should be used during pregnancy only if the potential benefit justifies the potential risk to the fetus.

Olanzapine

In reproduction studies in rats at doses up to 18 mg/kg/day and in rabbits at doses up to 30 mg/kg/day (9 and 30 times the MRHD on a mg/m^2 basis, respectively), no evidence of teratogenicity was observed. In a rat teratology study, early resorptions and increased numbers of nonviable fetuses were observed at a dose of 18 mg/kg/day (9 times the MRHD on a mg/m^2 basis). Gestation was prolonged at 10 mg/kg/day (5 times the MRHD on a mg/m^2 basis). In a rabbit teratology study, fetal toxicity (manifested as increased resorptions and decreased fetal weight) occurred at a maternally toxic

dose of 30 mg/kg/day (30 times the MRHD on a mg/m^2 basis).

Placental transfer of olanzapine occurs in rat pups.

There are no adequate and well–controlled clinical studies with olanzapine in pregnant women. Seven pregnancies were observed during premarketing clinical studies with olanzapine, including two resulting in normal births, one resulting in neonatal death due to a cardiovascular defect, three therapeutic abortions, and one spontaneous abortion.

Fluoxetine

In embryo fetal development studies in rats and rabbits, there was no evidence of teratogenicity following administration of up to 12.5 and 15 mg/kg/day, respectively (1.5 and 3.6 times the MRHD on a mg/m^2 basis, respectively) throughout organogenesis. However, in rat reproduction studies, an increase in stillborn pups, a decrease in pup weight, and an increase in pup deaths during the first 7 days postpartum occurred following maternal exposure to 12 mg/kg/day (1.5 times the MRHD on a mg/m^2 basis) during gestation or 7.5 mg/kg/day (0.9 times the MRHD on a mg/m^2 basis) during gestation and lactation. There was no evidence of developmental neurotoxicity in the surviving offspring of rats treated with 12 mg/kg/day during gestation. The no–effect dose for rat pup mortality was 5 mg/kg/day (0.6 times the MRHD on a mg/m^2 basis).

Nonteratogenic Effects—Neonates exposed to fluoxetine and other SSRIs or serotonin and norepinephrine reuptake inhibitors (SNRIs), late in the third trimester have developed complications requiring prolonged hospitalization, respiratory support, and tube feeding. Such complications can arise immediately upon delivery. Reported clinical findings have included respiratory distress, cyanosis, apnea, seizures, temperature instability, feeding difficulty, vomiting, hypoglycemia, hypotonia, hypertonia, hyperreflexia, tremor, jitteriness, irritability, and constant crying. These features are consistent with either a direct toxic effect of SSRIs and SNRIs or, possibly, a drug discontinuation syndrome. It should be noted that, in some cases, the clinical picture is consistent with serotonin syndrome (see **CONTRAINDICATIONS, Monoamine Oxidase Inhibitors**).

Infants exposed to SSRIs in late pregnancy may have an increased risk for persistent pulmonary hypertension of the newborn (PPHN). PPHN occurs in 1–2 per 1000 live births in the general population and is associated with substantial neonatal morbidity and mortality. In a retrospective case-control study of 377 women whose infants were born with PPHN and 836 women whose infants were born healthy, the risk for developing PPHN was approximately six–fold higher for infants exposed to SSRIs after the 20th week of gestation compared to infants who had not been exposed to antidepressants during pregnancy. There is currently no corroborative evidence regarding the risk for PPHN following exposure to SSRIs in pregnancy; this is the first study that has investigated the potential risk. The study did not include enough cases with exposure to individual SSRIs to determine if all SSRIs posed similar levels of PPHN risk.

When treating a pregnant woman with fluoxetine during the third trimester, the physician should carefully consider both the potential risks and benefits of treatment (see **DOSAGE AND ADMINISTRATION**). Physicians should note that in a prospective longitudinal study of 201 women with a history of major depression who were euthymic at the beginning of pregnancy, women who discontinued antidepressant medication during pregnancy were more likely to experience a relapse of major depression than women who continued antidepressant medication.

Labor and Delivery

SYMBYAX

The effect of SYMBYAX on labor and delivery in humans is unknown. Parturition in rats was not affected by SYMBYAX. SYMBYAX should be used during labor and delivery only if the potential benefit justifies the potential risk.

Olanzapine

Parturition in rats was not affected by olanzapine. The effect of olanzapine on labor and delivery in humans is unknown.

Fluoxetine

The effect of fluoxetine on labor and delivery in humans is unknown. Fluoxetine crosses the placenta; therefore, there is a possibility that fluoxetine may have adverse effects on the newborn.

Nursing Mothers

SYMBYAX

There are no adequate and well–controlled studies with SYMBYAX in nursing mothers or infants. No studies have been conducted to examine the excretion of olanzapine or fluoxetine in breast milk following SYMBYAX treatment. It is recommended that women not breast–feed when receiving SYMBYAX.

Olanzapine

In a study in lactating, healthy women, olanzapine was excreted in breast milk. Mean infant dose at steady state was estimated to be 1.8% of the maternal olanzapine dose.

Fluoxetine

Fluoxetine is excreted in human breast milk. In one breast milk sample, the concentration of fluoxetine plus norfluoxetine was 70.4 ng/mL. The concentration in the mother's plasma was 295.0 ng/mL. No adverse effects on the infant were reported. In another case, an infant nursed by a mother on fluoxetine developed crying, sleep disturbance,

vomiting, and watery stools. The infant's plasma drug levels were 340 ng/mL of fluoxetine and 208 ng/mL of norfluoxetine on the 2nd day of feeding.

Pediatric Use

Safety and effectiveness in the pediatric population have not been established (see **BOX WARNING** and **WARNINGS, Clinical Worsening and Suicide Risk**). Anyone considering the use of SYMBYAX in a child or adolescent must balance the potential risks with the clinical need.

Fluoxetine

Significant toxicity, including myotoxicity, long–term neurobehavioral and reproductive toxicity, and impaired bone development, has been observed following exposure of juvenile animals to fluoxetine. Some of these effects occurred at clinically relevant exposures.

In a study in which fluoxetine (3, 10, or 30 mg/kg) was orally administered to young rats from weaning (Postnatal Day 21) through adulthood (Day 90), male and female sexual development was delayed at all doses, and growth (body weight gain, femur length) was decreased during the dosing period in animals receiving the highest dose. At the end of the treatment period, serum levels of creatine kinase (marker of muscle damage) were increased at the intermediate and high doses, and abnormal muscle and reproductive organ histopathology (skeletal muscle degeneration and necrosis, testicular degeneration and necrosis, epididymal vacuolation and hypospermia) was observed at the high dose. When animals were evaluated after a recovery period (up to 11 weeks after cessation of dosing), neurobehavioral abnormalities (decreased reactivity at all doses and learning deficit at the high dose) and reproductive functional impairment (decreased mating at all doses and impaired fertility at the high dose) were seen; in addition, testicular and epididymal microscopic lesions and decreased sperm concentrations were found in the high dose group, indicating that the reproductive organ effects seen at the end of treatment were irreversible. The reversibility of fluoxetine-induced muscle damage was not assessed. Adverse effects similar to those observed in rats treated with fluoxetine during the juvenile period have not been reported after administration of fluoxetine to adult animals. Plasma exposures (AUC) to fluoxetine in juvenile rats receiving the low, intermediate, and high dose in this study were approximately 0.1–0.2, 1–2, and 5–10 times, respectively, the average exposure in pediatric patients receiving the maximum recommended dose (MRD) of 20 mg/day. Rat exposures to the major metabolite, norfluoxetine, were approximately 0.3–0.8, 1–8, and 3–20 times, respectively, pediatric exposure at the MRD.

A specific effect of fluoxetine on bone development has been reported in mice treated with fluoxetine during the juvenile period. When mice were treated with fluoxetine (5 or 20 mg/kg, intraperitoneal) for 4 weeks starting at 4 weeks of age, bone formation was reduced resulting in decreased bone mineral content and density. These doses did not affect overall growth (body weight gain or femoral length). The doses administered to juvenile mice in this study are approximately 0.5 and 2 times the MRD for pediatric patients on a body surface area (mg/m^2) basis.

In another mouse study, administration of fluoxetine (10 mg/kg intraperitoneal) during early postnatal development (Postnatal Days 4 to 21) produced abnormal emotional behaviors (decreased exploratory behavior in elevated plus–maze, increased shock avoidance latency) in adulthood (12 weeks of age). The dose used in this study is approximately equal to the pediatric MRD on a mg/m^2 basis. Because of the early dosing period in this study, the significance of these findings to the approved pediatric use in humans is uncertain.

Geriatric Use

SYMBYAX

Clinical studies of SYMBYAX did not include sufficient numbers of patients ≥65 years of age to determine whether they respond differently from younger patients. Other reported clinical experience has not identified differences in responses between the elderly and younger patients. In general, dose selection for an elderly patient should be cautious, usually starting at the low end of the dosing range, reflecting the greater frequency of decreased hepatic, renal, or cardiac function, and of concomitant disease or other drug therapy (see **DOSAGE AND ADMINISTRATION**).

Olanzapine

Of the 2500 patients in premarketing clinical studies with olanzapine, 11% (263 patients) were ≥65 years of age. In patients with schizophrenia, there was no indication of any different tolerability of olanzapine in the elderly compared with younger patients. Studies in patients with dementia–related psychosis have suggested that there may be a different tolerability profile in this population compared with younger patients with schizophrenia. In placebo–controlled studies of olanzapine in elderly patients with dementia–related psychosis, there was a significantly higher incidence of cerebrovascular adverse events (e.g., stroke, transient is-

Continued on next page

This product information was prepared in March 2008. Current information on products of Eli Lilly and Company may be obtained by calling 1-800-545-5979.

Symbyax—Cont.

chemic attack) in patients treated with olanzapine compared to patients treated with placebo. Olanzapine is not approved for the treatment of patients with dementia–related psychosis. If the prescriber elects to treat elderly patients with dementia–related psychosis, vigilance should be exercised (*see* **BOX WARNING, WARNINGS, PRECAUTIONS, Use in Patients with Concomitant Illness** *and* **DOSAGE AND ADMINISTRATION, Special Populations**).

As with other CNS–active drugs, olanzapine should be used with caution in elderly patients with dementia. Also, the presence of factors that might decrease pharmacokinetic clearance or increase the pharmacodynamic response to olanzapine should lead to consideration of a lower starting dose for any geriatric patient.

Fluoxetine

US fluoxetine clinical studies included 687 patients ≥65 years of age and 93 patients ≥75 years of age. No overall differences in safety or effectiveness were observed between these subjects and younger subjects, and other reported clinical experience has not identified differences in responses between the elderly and younger patients, but greater sensitivity of some older individuals cannot be ruled out. SSRIs and SNRIs, including SYMBYAX, have been associated with cases of clinically significant hyponatremia in elderly patients, who may be at greater risk for this adverse event (*see* **PRECAUTIONS, Hyponatremia**).

ADVERSE REACTIONS

The information below is derived from a premarketing clinical study database for SYMBYAX consisting of 2066 patients with various diagnoses with approximately 1061 patient–years of exposure. The conditions and duration of treatment with SYMBYAX varied greatly and included (in overlapping categories) open–label and double–blind phases of studies, inpatients and outpatients, fixed–dose and dose–titration studies, and short–term or long–term exposure.

Adverse events were recorded by clinical investigators using descriptive terminology of their own choosing. Consequently, it is not possible to provide a meaningful estimate of the proportion of individuals experiencing adverse events without first grouping similar types of events into a limited (i.e., reduced) number of standardized event categories.

In the tables and tabulations that follow, COSTART Dictionary terminology has been used to classify reported adverse events. The data in the tables represent the proportion of individuals who experienced, at least once, a treatment–emergent adverse event of the type listed. An event was considered treatment–emergent if it occurred for the first time or worsened while receiving therapy following baseline evaluation. It is possible that events reported during therapy were not necessarily related to drug exposure.

The prescriber should be aware that the figures in the tables and tabulations cannot be used to predict the incidence of side effects in the course of usual medical practice where patient characteristics and other factors differ from those that prevailed in the clinical studies. Similarly, the cited frequencies cannot be compared with figures obtained from other clinical investigations involving different treatments, uses, and investigators. The cited figures, however, do provide the prescribing clinician with some basis for estimating the relative contribution of drug and non–drug factors to the side effect incidence rate in the population studied.

Incidence in Controlled Clinical Studies

The following findings are based on the short–term, controlled premarketing studies in various diagnoses including bipolar depression.

Adverse events associated with discontinuation of treatment—Overall, 10% of the patients in the SYMBYAX group discontinued due to adverse events compared with 4.6% for placebo. Table 7 enumerates the adverse events leading to discontinuation associated with the use of SYMBYAX (incidence of at least 1% for SYMBYAX and greater than that for placebo). The bipolar depression column shows the incidence of adverse events with SYMBYAX in the bipolar depression studies and the "SYMBYAX–Controlled" column shows the incidence in the controlled SYMBYAX studies; the placebo column shows the incidence in the pooled controlled studies that included a placebo arm.

Table 7: Adverse Events Associated with Discontinuation*

Adverse Event	Percentage of Patients Reporting Event		
	SYMBYAX		Placebo
	Bipolar Depression (N=86)	SYMBYAX-Controlled (N=571)	(N=477)
Asthenia	0	1	0
Somnolence	0	2	0
Weight gain	0	2	0
Chest pain	1	0	0

*Table includes events associated with discontinuation of at least 1% and greater than placebo

Commonly observed adverse events in controlled clinical studies—The most commonly observed adverse events associated with the use of SYMBYAX (incidence of ≥5% and at least twice that for placebo in the SYMBYAX–controlled database) were: asthenia, edema, increased appetite, peripheral edema, pharyngitis, somnolence, thinking abnormal, tremor, and weight gain.

Adverse events occurring at an incidence of 2% or more in controlled clinical studies—Table 8 enumerates the treatment–emergent adverse events associated with the use of SYMBYAX (incidence of at least 2% for SYMBYAX and twice or more that for placebo).

Table 8: Treatment-Emergent Adverse Events: Incidence in Controlled Clinical Studies

Body System/ Adverse Event*	Percentage of Patients Reporting Event		
	SYMBYAX		Placebo
	Bipolar Depression (N=86)	SYMBYAX-Controlled (N=571)	(N=477)
Body as a Whole			
Asthenia	13	15	3
Accidental injury	5	3	2
Fever	4	3	1
Cardiovascular System			
Hypertension	2	2	1
Tachycardia	2	2	0
Digestive System			
Diarrhea	19	8	7
Dry mouth	16	11	6
Increased appetite	13	16	4
Tooth disorder	1	2	1
Metabolic and Nutritional Disorders			
Weight gain	17	21	3
Peripheral edema	4	8	1
Edema	0	5	0
Musculoskeletal System			
Joint disorder	1	2	1
Twitching	6	2	1
Arthralgia	5	3	1
Nervous System			
Somnolence	21	22	11
Tremor	9	8	3
Thinking abnormal	6	6	3
Libido decreased	4	2	1
Hyperkinesia	2	1	1
Personality disorder	2	1	1
Sleep disorder	2	1	1
Amnesia	1	3	0
Respiratory System			
Pharyngitis	4	6	3
Dyspnea	1	2	1
Special Senses			
Amblyopia	5	4	2
Ear pain	2	1	1
Otitis media	2	0	0
Speech disorder	0	2	0
Urogenital System			
Abnormal ejaculation†	7	2	1
Impotence†	4	2	1
Anorgasmia	3	1	0

* Included are events reported by at least 2% of patients taking SYMBYAX except the following events, which had an incidence on placebo ≥ SYMBYAX: abdominal pain, abnormal dreams, agitation, akathisia, anorexia, anxiety, apathy, back pain, chest pain, constipation, cough increased, depression, dizziness, dysmenorrhea (adjusted for gender), dyspepsia, flatulence, flu syndrome, headache, hypertonia, insomnia, manic reaction, myalgia, nausea, nervousness, pain, palpitation, paresthesia, rash, rhinitis, sinusitis, sweating, vomiting.

† Adjusted for gender.

Extrapyramidal Symptoms

Dystonia, Class Effect for Antipsychotics - Symptoms of dystonia, prolonged abnormal contractions of muscle groups, may occur in susceptible individuals during the first few days of treatment. Dystonic symptoms include: spasm of the neck muscles, sometimes progressing to tightness of the throat, swallowing difficulty, difficulty breathing, and/or protrusion of the tongue. While these symptoms can occur at low doses, the frequency and severity are greater with high potency and at higher doses of first generation antipsychotic drugs. In general, an elevated risk of acute dystonia may be observed in males and younger age groups receiving antipsychotics; however, events of dystonia have been reported infrequently (<1%) with the olanzapine and fluoxetine combination.

Additional Findings Observed in Clinical Studies

The following findings are based on clinical studies.

Effect on cardiac repolarization—The mean increase in QT_c interval for SYMBYAX–treated patients (4.9 msec) in clinical studies was significantly greater than that for placebo–treated (–0.9 msec) and olanzapine–treated (0.6 msec) patients, but was not significantly different from fluoxetine–treated (3.7 msec) patients. There were no differences between patients treated with SYMBYAX, placebo, olanzapine, or fluoxetine in the incidence of QT_c outliers (>500 msec).

Laboratory changes—In SYMBYAX clinical studies, SYMBYAX was associated with asymptomatic mean increases in alkaline phosphatase, cholesterol, GGT, and uric acid compared with placebo (*see* **PRECAUTIONS, Transaminase Elevations**).

SYMBYAX was associated with a slight decrease in hemoglobin that was statistically significantly greater than that seen with placebo, olanzapine, and fluoxetine.

An elevation in serum prolactin was observed with SYMBYAX. This elevation was not statistically different than that seen with olanzapine (*see* **PRECAUTIONS, Hyperprolactinemia**).

Sexual dysfunction—In the pool of controlled SYMBYAX studies, there were higher rates of the treatment–emergent adverse events decreased libido, anorgasmia, impotence and abnormal ejaculation in the SYMBYAX group than in the placebo group. One case of decreased libido led to discontinuation in the SYMBYAX group. In the controlled studies that contained a fluoxetine arm, the rates of decreased libido and abnormal ejaculation in the SYMBYAX group were less than the rates in the fluoxetine group. None of the differences were statistically significant.

Sexual dysfunction, including priapism, has been reported with all SSRIs. While it is difficult to know the precise risk of sexual dysfunction associated with the use of SSRIs, physicians should routinely inquire about such possible side effects.

Vital signs—Tachycardia, bradycardia, and orthostatic hypotension have occurred in SYMBYAX–treated patients (*see* **WARNINGS, Orthostatic Hypotension**). The mean pulse of SYMBYAX–treated patients was reduced by 1.6 beats/min.

Additional findings—In a single 8–week randomized, double–blind, fixed–dose, study comparing 10 (N=199), 20 (N=200) and 40 (N=200) mg/day of olanzapine in patients with schizophrenia or schizoaffective disorder, statistically significant differences among 3 dose groups were observed for the following safety outcomes: weight gain, prolactin elevation, fatigue and dizziness. Mean baseline to endpoint increase in weight (10 mg/day: 1.9 kg; 20 mg/day: 2.3 kg; 40 mg/day: 3 kg) was observed with significant differences between 10 vs 40 mg/day. Incidence of treatment–emergent prolactin elevation >24.2 ng/mL (female) or >18.77 ng/mL (male) at any time during the trial (10 mg/day: 31.2%; 20 mg/day: 42.7%; 40 mg/day: 61.1%) with significant differences between 10 vs 40 mg/day and 20 vs 40 mg/day; fatigue (10 mg/day: 1.5%; 20 mg/day: 2.1%; 40 mg/day: 6.6%) with significant differences between 10 vs 40 and 20 vs 40 mg/day; and dizziness (10 mg/day: 2.6%; 20 mg/day: 1.6%; 40 mg/day: 6.6%) with significant differences between 20 vs 40 mg, was observed.

Other Events Observed in Clinical Studies

Following is a list of all treatment–emergent adverse events reported at anytime by individuals taking SYMBYAX in clinical studies except (1) those listed in the body or footnotes of Tables 7 and 8 above or elsewhere in labeling, (2) those for which the COSTART terms were uninformative or misleading, (3) those events for which a causal relationship to SYMBYAX use was considered remote, and (4) events occurring in only 1 patient treated with SYMBYAX and which did not have a substantial probability of being acutely life–threatening.

Events are classified within body system categories using the following definitions: frequent adverse events are defined as those occurring on 1 or more occasions in at least 1/100 patients, infrequent adverse events are those occurring in 1/100 to 1/1000 patients, and rare events are those occurring in <1/1000 patients.

Body as a Whole—*Frequent:* chills, infection, neck pain, neck rigidity, photosensitivity reaction; *Infrequent:* cellulitis, cyst, hernia, intentional injury, intentional overdose, malaise, moniliasis, overdose, pelvic pain, suicide attempt; *Rare:* death, tolerance decreased.

Cardiovascular System—*Frequent:* migraine, vasodilatation; *Infrequent:* arrhythmia, bradycardia, cerebral ischemia, electrocardiogram abnormal, hypotension, QT–interval prolonged; *Rare:* angina pectoris, atrial arrhythmia, atrial fibrillation, bundle branch block, congestive heart failure, myocardial infarct, peripheral vascular disorder, T—wave inverted.

Digestive System—*Frequent:* increased salivation, thirst; *Infrequent:* cholelithiasis, colitis, eructation, esophagitis, gastritis, gastroenteritis, gingivitis, hepatomegaly, nausea and vomiting, peptic ulcer, periodontal abscess, stomatitis, tooth caries; *Rare:* aphthous stomatitis, fecal incontinence, gastrointestinal hemorrhage, gum hemorrhage, intestinal obstruction, liver fatty deposit, pancreatitis.

Endocrine System—*Infrequent:* hypothyroidism.

Hemic and Lymphatic System—*Frequent:* ecchymosis; *Infrequent:* anemia, leukocytosis, lymphadenopathy; *Rare:* coagulation disorder, leukopenia, purpura, thrombocythemia.

Metabolic and Nutritional—*Frequent:* generalized edema, weight loss; *Infrequent:* alcohol intolerance, dehydration, glycosuria, hyperlipemia, hypoglycemia, hypokalemia, obesity; *Rare:* acidosis, bilirubinemia, creatinine increased, gout, hyperkalemia, hypoglycemic reaction.

Musculoskeletal System—*Infrequent:* arthritis, bone disorder, generalized spasm, leg cramps, tendinous contracture, tenosynovitis; *Rare:* arthrosis, bursitis, myasthenia, myopathy, osteoporosis, rheumatoid arthritis.

Nervous System—*Infrequent:* abnormal gait, ataxia, buccoglossal syndrome, cogwheel rigidity, coma, confusion, depersonalization, dysarthria, emotional lability, euphoria, extrapyramidal syndrome, hostility, hypesthesia, hypokinesia, incoordination, movement disorder, myoclonus, neuralgia, neurosis, vertigo; *Rare:* acute brain syndrome, aphasia, dystonia, libido increased, subarachnoid hemorrhage, withdrawal syndrome.

Respiratory System—*Frequent:* bronchitis, lung disorder; *Infrequent:* apnea, asthma, epistaxis, hiccup, hyperventilation, laryngitis, pneumonia, voice alteration, yawn; *Rare:* emphysema, hemoptysis, laryngismus.
Skin and Appendages—*Infrequent:* acne, alopecia, contact dermatitis, dry skin, eczema, pruritis, psoriasis, skin discoloration, vesiculobullous rash; *Rare:* exfoliative dermatitis, maculopapular rash, seborrhea, skin ulcer.
Special Senses—*Frequent:* abnormal vision, taste perversion, tinnitus; *Infrequent:* abnormality of accommodation, conjunctivitis, deafness, diplopia, dry eyes, eye pain, miosis; *Rare:* eye hemorrhage.
Urogenital System—*Frequent:* breast pain, menorrhagia[1], urinary frequency, urinary incontinence, urinary tract infection; *Infrequent:* amenorrhea[1], breast enlargement, breast neoplasm, cystitis, dysuria, female lactation[1], fibrocystic breast[1], hematuria, hypomenorrhea[1], leukorrhea[1], menopause[1], metrorrhagia[1], oliguria, ovarian disorder[1], polyuria, urinary retention, urinary urgency, urination impaired, vaginal hemorrhage[1], vaginal moniliasis[1], vaginitis[1]; *Rare:* breast carcinoma, breast engorgement, endometrial disorder[1], gynecomastia[1], kidney calculus, uterine fibroids enlarged[1].

Other Events Observed with Olanzapine or Fluoxetine Monotherapy

The following adverse events were not observed in SYMBYAX–treated patients during premarketing clinical studies but have been reported with olanzapine or fluoxetine monotherapy: aplastic anemia, cholestatic jaundice, diabetic coma, dyskinesia, eosinophilic pneumonia, erythema multiforme, hepatitis, idiosyncratic hepatitis, jaundice, neutropenia, priapism, pulmonary embolism, rhabdomyolysis, serotonin syndrome, serum sickness–like reaction, sudden unexpected death, suicidal ideation, vasculitis, venous thromboembolic events (including pulmonary embolism and deep venous thrombosis), violent behaviors. Random cholesterol levels of ≥240 mg/dL and random triglyceride levels of ≥1000 mg/dL have been reported.

[1] Adjusted for gender.

DRUG ABUSE AND DEPENDENCE

Controlled Substance Class

SYMBYAX is not a controlled substance.

Physical and Psychological Dependence

SYMBYAX, as with fluoxetine and olanzapine, has not been systematically studied in humans for its potential for abuse, tolerance, or physical dependence. While the clinical studies did not reveal any tendency for any drug–seeking behavior, these observations were not systematic, and it is not possible to predict on the basis of this limited experience the extent to which a CNS–active drug will be misused, diverted, and/or abused once marketed. Consequently, physicians should carefully evaluate patients for history of drug abuse and follow such patients closely, observing them for signs of misuse or abuse of SYMBYAX (e.g., development of tolerance, incrementation of dose, drug–seeking behavior).

In studies in rats and rhesus monkeys designed to assess abuse and dependence potential, olanzapine alone was shown to have acute depressive CNS effects but little or no potential of abuse or physical dependence at oral doses up to 15 (rat) and 8 (monkey) times the MRHD (20 mg) on a mg/m^2 basis.

OVERDOSAGE

SYMBYAX

During premarketing clinical studies of the olanzapine/fluoxetine combination, overdose of both fluoxetine and olanzapine were reported in five study subjects. Four of the five subjects experienced loss of consciousness (3) or coma (1). No fatalities occurred.

Since the market introduction of olanzapine in October 1996, adverse event cases involving combination use of fluoxetine and olanzapine have been reported to Eli Lilly and Company. An overdose of combination therapy is defined as confirmed or suspected ingestion of a dose of olanzapine 20 mg or greater in combination with a dose of fluoxetine 80 mg or greater. As of 1 February 2002, 12 cases of combination therapy overdose were reported, most of which involved additional substances. Adverse events associated with these reports included somnolence; impaired consciousness (coma, lethargy); impaired neurologic function (ataxia, confusion, convulsions, dysarthria); arrhythmias; and fatality. Fatalities have been confounded by exposure to additional substances including alcohol, thioridazine, oxycodone, and propoxyphene.

Olanzapine

In postmarketing reports of overdose with olanzapine alone, symptoms have been reported in the majority of cases. In symptomatic patients, symptoms with ≥10% incidence included agitation/aggressiveness, dysarthria, tachycardia, various extrapyramidal symptoms, and reduced level of consciousness ranging from sedation to coma. Among less commonly reported symptoms were the following potentially medically serious events: aspiration, cardiopulmonary arrest, cardiac arrhythmias (such as supraventricular tachycardia as well as a patient that experienced sinus pause with spontaneous resumption of normal rhythm), delirium, possible neuroleptic malignant syndrome, respiratory depression/arrest, convulsion, hypertension, and hypotension. Eli Lilly and Company has received reports of fatality in association with overdose of olanzapine alone. In 1 case of death, the amount of acutely ingested olanzapine was reported to be possibly as low as 450 mg of oral olanzapine; however, in another case, a patient was reported to survive an acute olanzapine ingestion of approximately 2 g of oral olanzapine.

Fluoxetine

Worldwide exposure to fluoxetine is estimated to be over 38 million patients (circa 1999). Of the 1578 cases of overdose involving fluoxetine, alone or with other drugs, reported from this population, there were 195 deaths.

Among 633 adult patients who overdosed on fluoxetine alone, 34 resulted in a fatal outcome, 378 completely recovered, and 15 patients experienced sequelae after overdose, including abnormal accommodation, abnormal gait, confusion, unresponsiveness, nervousness, pulmonary dysfunction, vertigo, tremor, elevated blood pressure, impotence, movement disorder, and hypomania. The remaining 206 patients had an unknown outcome. The most common signs and symptoms associated with non–fatal overdose were seizures, somnolence, nausea, tachycardia, and vomiting. The largest known ingestion of fluoxetine in adult patients was 8 grams in a patient who took fluoxetine alone and who subsequently recovered. However, in an adult patient who took fluoxetine alone, an ingestion as low as 520 mg has been associated with lethal outcome, but causality has not been established.

Among pediatric patients (ages 3 months to 17 years), there were 156 cases of overdose involving fluoxetine alone or in combination with other drugs. Six patients died, 127 patients completely recovered, 1 patient experienced renal failure, and 22 patients had an unknown outcome. One of the 6 fatalities was a 9–year–old boy who had a history of OCD, Tourette's Syndrome with tics, attention deficit disorder, and fetal alcohol syndrome. He had been receiving 100 mg of fluoxetine daily for 6 months in addition to clonidine, methylphenidate, and promethazine. Mixed–drug ingestion or other methods of suicide complicated all 6 overdoses in children that resulted in fatalities. The largest ingestion in pediatric patients was 3 grams, which was non–lethal.

Other important adverse events reported with fluoxetine overdose (single or multiple drugs) included coma, delirium, ECG abnormalities (such as QT–interval prolongation and ventricular tachycardia, including torsades de pointes–type arrhythmias), hypotension, mania, neuroleptic malignant syndrome–like events, pyrexia, stupor, and syncope.

Management of Overdose

In managing overdose, the possibility of multiple drug involvement should be considered. In case of acute overdose, establish and maintain an airway and ensure adequate ventilation, which may include intubation. Induction of emesis is not recommended as the possibility of obtundation, seizures, or dystonic reactions of the head and neck following overdose may create a risk for aspiration. Gastric lavage (after intubation, if patient is unconscious) and administration of activated charcoal together with a laxative should be considered. Cardiovascular monitoring should commence immediately and should include continuous electrocardiographic monitoring to detect possible arrhythmias.

A specific precaution involves patients who are taking or have recently taken SYMBYAX and may have ingested excessive quantities of a TCA (tricyclic antidepressant). In such cases, accumulation of the parent TCA and/or an active metabolite may increase the possibility of serious sequelae and extend the time needed for close medical observation.

Due to the large volume of distribution of olanzapine and fluoxetine, forced diuresis, dialysis, hemoperfusion, and exchange transfusion are unlikely to be of benefit. No specific antidote for either fluoxetine or olanzapine overdose is known. Hypotension and circulatory collapse should be treated with appropriate measures such as intravenous fluids and/or sympathomimetic agents. Do not use epinephrine, dopamine, or other sympathomimetics with β–agonist activity, since beta stimulation may worsen hypotension in the setting of olanzapine–induced alpha blockade.

The physician should consider contacting a poison control center for additional information on the treatment of any overdose. Telephone numbers for certified poison control centers are listed in the *Physicians' Desk Reference (PDR).*

DOSAGE AND ADMINISTRATION

SYMBYAX should be administered once daily in the evening, generally beginning with the 6–mg/25–mg capsule. While food has no appreciable effect on the absorption of olanzapine and fluoxetine given individually, the effect of food on the absorption of SYMBYAX has not been studied. Dosage adjustments, if indicated, can be made according to efficacy and tolerability. Antidepressant efficacy was demonstrated with SYMBYAX in a dose range of olanzapine 6 to 12 mg and fluoxetine 25 to 50 mg (*see* **CLINICAL STUDIES**).

The safety of doses above 18 mg/75 mg has not been evaluated in clinical studies.

Special Populations

The starting dose of SYMBYAX 3 mg/25 mg–6 mg/25 mg should be used for patients with a predisposition to hypotensive reactions, patients with hepatic impairment, or patients who exhibit a combination of factors that may slow the metabolism of SYMBYAX (female gender, geriatric age, nonsmoking status) or those patients who may be pharmacodynamically sensitive to olanzapine. When indicated, dose escalation should be performed with caution in these patients. SYMBYAX has not been systematically studied in patients over 65 years of age or in patients <18 years of age (*see* **WARNINGS, Orthostatic Hypotension, PRECAUTIONS, Pediatric Use,** *and* **Geriatric Use,** *and* **CLINICAL PHARMACOLOGY, Pharmacokinetics**).

Treatment of Pregnant Women During the Third Trimester

Neonates exposed to fluoxetine, a component of SYMBYAX, and other SSRIs or SNRIs, late in the third trimester have developed complications requiring prolonged hospitalization, respiratory support, and tube feeding (*see* **PRECAUTIONS**). When treating pregnant women with fluoxetine during the third trimester, the physician should carefully consider the potential risks and benefits of treatment. The physician may consider tapering fluoxetine in the third trimester.

Discontinuation of Treatment with SYMBYAX

Symptoms associated with discontinuation of fluoxetine, a component of SYMBYAX, and other SSRIs and SNRIs, have been reported (*see* **PRECAUTIONS**). Patients should be monitored for these symptoms when discontinuing treatment. A gradual reduction in the dose rather than abrupt cessation is recommended whenever possible. If intolerable symptoms occur following a decrease in the dose or upon discontinuation of treatment, then resuming the previously prescribed dose may be considered. Subsequently, the physician may continue decreasing the dose but at a more gradual rate. Plasma fluoxetine and norfluoxetine concentration decrease gradually at the conclusion of therapy which may minimize the risk of discontinuation symptoms with this drug.

HOW SUPPLIED

SYMBYAX capsules are supplied in 3/25–, 6/25–, 6/50–, 12/25–, and 12/50–mg (mg equivalent olanzapine/mg equivalent fluoxetine[2]) strengths.
[See table above]

SYMBYAX	CAPSULE STRENGTH				
	3 mg/25 mg	6 mg/25 mg	6 mg/50 mg	12 mg/25 mg	12 mg/50 mg
Color	Peach & Light Yellow	Mustard Yellow & Light Yellow	Mustard Yellow & Light Grey	Red & Light Yellow	Red & Light Grey
Capsule No.	PU3230	PU3231	PU3233	PU3232	PU3234
Identification	Lilly 3230 3/25	Lilly 3231 6/25	Lilly 3233 6/50	Lilly 3232 12/25	Lilly 3234 12/50
NDC Codes					
Bottles 30	0002-3230-30	0002-3231-30	0002-3233-30	0002-3232-30	0002-3234-30
Bottles 100		0002-3231-02	0002-3233-02	0002-3232-02	0002-3234-02
Bottles 1000		0002-3231-04	0002-3233-04	0002-3232-04	0002-3234-04
Blisters ID* 100		0002-3231-33	0002-3233-33	0002-3232-33	0002-3234-33

*IDENTI–DOSE®, Unit Dose Medication, Lilly.

[2] Fluoxetine base equivalent.

Store at 25°C (77°F); excursions permitted to 15–30°C (59–86°F) [see USP Controlled Room Temperature].
Keep tightly closed and protect from moisture.
Literature revised March 19, 2008
Eli Lilly and Company
Indianapolis, IN 46285
www.SYMBYAX.com

PV 6231 AMP

Medication Guide

Antidepressant Medicines, Depression and other Serious Mental Illnesses, and Suicidal Thoughts or Actions

Read the Medication Guide that comes with your or your family member's antidepressant medicine. This Medication Guide is only about the risk of suicidal thoughts and actions with antidepressant medicines. **Talk to your, or your family member's, healthcare provider about:**

- all risks and benefits of treatment with antidepressant medicines
- all treatment choices for depression or other serious mental illness

What is the most important information I should know about antidepressant medicines, depression and other serious mental illnesses, and suicidal thoughts or actions?

1. **Antidepressant medicines may increase suicidal thoughts or actions in some children, teenagers, and young adults within the first few months of treatment.**
2. **Depression and other serious mental illnesses are the most important causes of suicidal thoughts and actions. Some people may have a particularly high risk**

Continued on next page

This product information was prepared in March 2008. Current information on products of Eli Lilly and Company may be obtained by calling 1-800-545-5979.

Symbyax—Cont.

of having suicidal thoughts or actions. These include people who have (or have a family history of) bipolar illness (also called manic-depressive illness) or suicidal thoughts or actions.

3. **How can I watch for and try to prevent suicidal thoughts and actions in myself or a family member?**
   - Pay close attention to any changes, especially sudden changes, in mood, behaviors, thoughts, or feelings. This is very important when an antidepressant medicine is started or when the dose is changed.
   - Call the healthcare provider right away to report new or sudden changes in mood, behavior, thoughts, or feelings.
   - Keep all follow-up visits with the healthcare provider as scheduled. Call the healthcare provider between visits as needed, especially if you have concerns about symptoms.

Call a healthcare provider right away if you or your family member has any of the following symptoms, especially if they are new, worse, or worry you:
- thoughts about suicide or dying
- attempts to commit suicide
- new or worse depression
- new or worse anxiety
- feeling very agitated or restless
- panic attacks
- trouble sleeping (insomnia)
- new or worse irritability
- acting aggressive, being angry, or violent
- acting on dangerous impulses
- an extreme increase in activity and talking (mania)
- other unusual changes in behavior or mood

What else do I need to know about antidepressant medicines?
- **Never stop an antidepressant medicine without first talking to a healthcare provider.** Stopping an antidepressant medicine suddenly can cause other symptoms.
- **Antidepressants are medicines used to treat depression and other illnesses.** It is important to discuss all the risks of treating depression and also the risks of not treating it. Patients and their families or other caregivers should discuss all treatment choices with the healthcare provider, not just the use of antidepressants.
- **Antidepressant medicines have other side effects.** Talk to the healthcare provider about the side effects of the medicine prescribed for you or your family member.
- **Antidepressant medicines can interact with other medicines.** Know all of the medicines that you or your family member takes. Keep a list of all medicines to show the healthcare provider. Do not start new medicines without first checking with your healthcare provider.
- **Not all antidepressant medicines prescribed for children are FDA approved for use in children.** Talk to your child's healthcare provider for more information.

This Medication Guide has been approved by the US Food and Drug Administration for all antidepressants.
Patient Information revised June 21, 2007

ZYPREXA® ℞
[*zī-prex-ah*]
(olanzapine)
Tablet

ZYPREXA® ZYDIS®
(olanzapine)
Tablet, Orally Disintegrating

ZYPREXA® IntraMuscular
(olanzapine)
Injection, Powder, For Solution
[Eli Lilly and Company]

Prescribing information for this product, which appears on pages 1866–1873 of the 2008 PDR, has been completely revised as follows. Please write "See Supplement A" next to the product heading.

> **WARNING**
>
> **Increased Mortality in Elderly Patients with Dementia-Related Psychosis—Elderly patients with dementia-related psychosis treated with atypical antipsychotic drugs are at an increased risk of death compared to placebo. Analyses of seventeen placebo-controlled trials (modal duration of 10 weeks) in these patients revealed a risk of death in the drug-treated patients of between 1.6 to 1.7 times that seen in placebo-treated patients. Over the course of a typical 10-week controlled trial, the rate of death in drug-treated patients was about 4.5%, compared to a rate of about 2.6% in the placebo group. Although the causes of death were varied, most of the deaths appeared to be either cardiovascular (e.g., heart failure, sudden death) or infectious (e.g., pneumonia) in nature. ZYPREXA (olanzapine) is not approved for the treatment of patients with dementia-related psychosis (*see* WARNINGS).**

DESCRIPTION

ZYPREXA (olanzapine) is a psychotropic agent that belongs to the thienobenzodiazepine class. The chemical designation is 2-methyl-4-(4-methyl-1-piperazinyl)-10*H*-thieno[2,3-*b*][1,5]benzodiazepine. The molecular formula is $C_{17}H_{20}N_4S$, which corresponds to a molecular weight of 312.44. The chemical structure is:

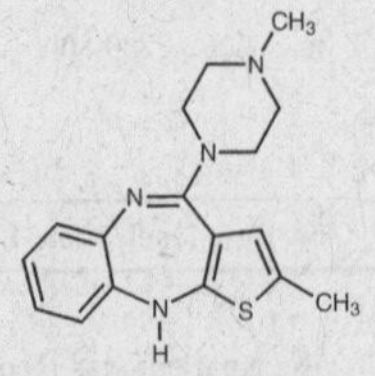

Olanzapine is a yellow crystalline solid, which is practically insoluble in water.

ZYPREXA tablets are intended for oral administration only.

Each tablet contains olanzapine equivalent to 2.5 mg (8 µmol), 5 mg (16 µmol), 7.5 mg (24 µmol), 10 mg (32 µmol), 15 mg (48 µmol), or 20 mg (64 µmol). Inactive ingredients are carnauba wax, crospovidone, hydroxypropyl cellulose, hypromellose, lactose, magnesium stearate, microcrystalline cellulose, and other inactive ingredients. The color coating contains Titanium Dioxide (all strengths), FD&C Blue No. 2 Aluminum Lake (15 mg), or Synthetic Red Iron Oxide (20 mg). The 2.5, 5, 7.5, and 10 mg tablets are imprinted with edible ink which contains FD&C Blue No. 2 Aluminum Lake.

ZYPREXA ZYDIS (olanzapine orally disintegrating tablets) is intended for oral administration only.

Each orally disintegrating tablet contains olanzapine equivalent to 5 mg (16 µmol), 10 mg (32 µmol), 15 mg (48 µmol) or 20 mg (64 µmol). It begins disintegrating in the mouth within seconds, allowing its contents to be subsequently swallowed with or without liquid. ZYPREXA ZYDIS (olanzapine orally disintegrating tablets) also contains the following inactive ingredients: gelatin, mannitol, aspartame, sodium methyl paraben and sodium propyl paraben.

ZYPREXA IntraMuscular (olanzapine for injection) is intended for intramuscular use only.

Each vial provides for the administration of 10 mg (32 µmol) olanzapine with inactive ingredients 50 mg lactose monohydrate and 3.5 mg tartaric acid. Hydrochloric acid and/or sodium hydroxide may have been added during manufacturing to adjust pH.

CLINICAL PHARMACOLOGY

Pharmacodynamics

Olanzapine is a selective monoaminergic antagonist with high affinity binding to the following receptors: serotonin $5HT_{2A/2C}$, $5HT_6$, (K_i=4, 11, and 5 nM, respectively), dopamine D_{1-4} (K_i=11–31 nM), histamine H_1 (K_i=7 nM), and adrenergic α_1 receptors (K_i=19 nM). Olanzapine is an antagonist with moderate affinity binding for serotonin $5HT_3$ (K_i=57 nM) and muscarinic M_{1-5} (K_i=73, 96, 132, 32, and 48 nM, respectively). Olanzapine binds weakly to $GABA_A$, BZD, and β adrenergic receptors (K_i>10 µM).

The mechanism of action of olanzapine, as with other drugs having efficacy in schizophrenia, is unknown. However, it has been proposed that this drug's efficacy in schizophrenia is mediated through a combination of dopamine and serotonin type 2 ($5HT_2$) antagonism. The mechanism of action of olanzapine in the treatment of acute manic episodes associated with Bipolar I Disorder is unknown.

Antagonism at receptors other than dopamine and $5HT_2$ may explain some of the other therapeutic and side effects of olanzapine. Olanzapine's antagonism of muscarinic M_{1-5} receptors may explain its anticholinergic-like effects. Olanzapine's antagonism of histamine H_1 receptors may explain the somnolence observed with this drug. Olanzapine's antagonism of adrenergic α_1 receptors may explain the orthostatic hypotension observed with this drug.

Pharmacokinetics

Oral Administration

Olanzapine is well absorbed and reaches peak concentrations in approximately 6 hours following an oral dose. It is eliminated extensively by first pass metabolism, with approximately 40% of the dose metabolized before reaching the systemic circulation. Food does not affect the rate or extent of olanzapine absorption. Pharmacokinetic studies showed that ZYPREXA tablets and ZYPREXA ZYDIS (olanzapine orally disintegrating tablets) dosage forms of olanzapine are bioequivalent.

Olanzapine displays linear kinetics over the clinical dosing range. Its half-life ranges from 21 to 54 hours (5th to 95th percentile; mean of 30 hr), and apparent plasma clearance ranges from 12 to 47 L/hr (5th to 95th percentile; mean of 25 L/hr).

Administration of olanzapine once daily leads to steady-state concentrations in about one week that are approximately twice the concentrations after single doses. Plasma concentrations, half-life, and clearance of olanzapine may vary between individuals on the basis of smoking status, gender, and age (*see* Special Populations).

Olanzapine is extensively distributed throughout the body, with a volume of distribution of approximately 1000 L. It is 93% bound to plasma proteins over the concentration range of 7 to 1100 ng/mL, binding primarily to albumin and α_1-acid glycoprotein.

Metabolism and Elimination—Following a single oral dose of ^{14}C labeled olanzapine, 7% of the dose of olanzapine was recovered in the urine as unchanged drug, indicating that olanzapine is highly metabolized. Approximately 57% and 30% of the dose was recovered in the urine and feces, respectively. In the plasma, olanzapine accounted for only 12% of the AUC for total radioactivity, indicating significant exposure to metabolites. After multiple dosing, the major circulating metabolites were the 10–N–glucuronide, present at steady state at 44% of the concentration of olanzapine, and 4′–N–desmethyl olanzapine, present at steady state at 31% of the concentration of olanzapine. Both metabolites lack pharmacological activity at the concentrations observed.

Direct glucuronidation and cytochrome P450 (CYP) mediated oxidation are the primary metabolic pathways for olanzapine. In vitro studies suggest that CYPs 1A2 and 2D6, and the flavin–containing monooxygenase system are involved in olanzapine oxidation. CYP2D6 mediated oxidation appears to be a minor metabolic pathway in vivo, because the clearance of olanzapine is not reduced in subjects who are deficient in this enzyme.

Intramuscular Administration

ZYPREXA IntraMuscular results in rapid absorption with peak plasma concentrations occurring within 15 to 45 minutes. Based upon a pharmacokinetic study in healthy volunteers, a 5 mg dose of intramuscular olanzapine for injection produces, on average, a maximum plasma concentration approximately 5 times higher than the maximum plasma concentration produced by a 5 mg dose of oral olanzapine. Area under the curve achieved after an intramuscular dose is similar to that achieved after oral administration of the same dose. The half-life observed after intramuscular administration is similar to that observed after oral dosing. The pharmacokinetics are linear over the clinical dosing range. Metabolic profiles after intramuscular administration are qualitatively similar to metabolic profiles after oral administration.

Special Populations

Renal Impairment

Because olanzapine is highly metabolized before excretion and only 7% of the drug is excreted unchanged, renal dysfunction alone is unlikely to have a major impact on the pharmacokinetics of olanzapine. The pharmacokinetic characteristics of olanzapine were similar in patients with severe renal impairment and normal subjects, indicating that dosage adjustment based upon the degree of renal impairment is not required. In addition, olanzapine is not removed by dialysis. The effect of renal impairment on metabolite elimination has not been studied.

Hepatic Impairment

Although the presence of hepatic impairment may be expected to reduce the clearance of olanzapine, a study of the effect of impaired liver function in subjects (n=6) with clinically significant (Childs Pugh Classification A and B) cirrhosis revealed little effect on the pharmacokinetics of olanzapine.

Age

In a study involving 24 healthy subjects, the mean elimination half-life of olanzapine was about 1.5 times greater in elderly (>65 years) than in non–elderly subjects (≤65 years). Caution should be used in dosing the elderly, especially if there are other factors that might additively influence drug metabolism and/or pharmacodynamic sensitivity (*see* DOSAGE AND ADMINISTRATION).

Gender

Clearance of olanzapine is approximately 30% lower in women than in men. There were, however, no apparent differences between men and women in effectiveness or adverse effects. Dosage modifications based on gender should not be needed.

Smoking Status

Olanzapine clearance is about 40% higher in smokers than in nonsmokers, although dosage modifications are not routinely recommended.

Race

In vivo studies have shown that exposures are similar among Japanese, Chinese and Caucasians, especially after normalization for body weight differences. Dosage modifications for race are, therefore, not recommended.

Combined Effects

The combined effects of age, smoking, and gender could lead to substantial pharmacokinetic differences in populations. The clearance in young smoking males, for example, may be 3 times higher than that in elderly nonsmoking females. Dosing modification may be necessary in patients who exhibit a combination of factors that may result in slower metabolism of olanzapine (*see* DOSAGE AND ADMINISTRATION).

For specific information about the pharmacology of lithium or valproate, refer to the CLINICAL PHARMACOLOGY section of the package inserts for these other products.

CLINICAL EFFICACY DATA

Schizophrenia

The efficacy of oral olanzapine in the treatment of schizophrenia was established in 2 short–term (6–week) controlled trials of inpatients who met DSM III–R criteria for schizophrenia. A single haloperidol arm was included as a comparative treatment in one of the two trials, but this trial did not compare these two drugs on the full range of clinically relevant doses for both.

Several instruments were used for assessing psychiatric signs and symptoms in these studies, among them the Brief Psychiatric Rating Scale (BPRS), a multi–item inventory of general psychopathology traditionally used to evaluate the effects of drug treatment in schizophrenia. The BPRS psychosis cluster (conceptual disorganization, hallucinatory behavior, suspiciousness, and unusual thought content) is considered a particularly useful subset for assessing actively psychotic schizophrenic patients. A second traditional assessment, the Clinical Global Impression (CGI), reflects the impression of a skilled observer, fully familiar with the manifestations of schizophrenia, about the overall clinical state of the patient. In addition, two more recently developed scales were employed; these included the 30–item Positive and Negative Symptoms Scale (PANSS), in which are embedded the 18 items of the BPRS, and the Scale for Assessing Negative Symptoms (SANS). The trial summaries below focus on the following outcomes: PANSS total and/or BPRS total; BPRS psychosis cluster; PANSS negative subscale or SANS; and CGI Severity. The results of the trials follow:

(1) In a 6–week, placebo–controlled trial (n=149) involving two fixed olanzapine doses of 1 and 10 mg/day (once daily schedule), olanzapine, at 10 mg/day (but not at 1 mg/day), was superior to placebo on the PANSS total score (also on the extracted BPRS total), on the BPRS psychosis cluster, on the PANSS Negative subscale, and on CGI Severity.

(2) In a 6–week, placebo–controlled trial (n=253) involving 3 fixed dose ranges of olanzapine (5 ± 2.5 mg/day, 10 ± 2.5 mg/day, and 15 ± 2.5 mg/day) on a once daily schedule, the two highest olanzapine dose groups (actual mean doses of 12 and 16 mg/day, respectively) were superior to placebo on BPRS total score, BPRS psychosis cluster, and CGI severity score; the highest olanzapine dose group was superior to placebo on the SANS. There was no clear advantage for the high dose group over the medium dose group.

Examination of population subsets (race and gender) did not reveal any differential responsiveness on the basis of these subgroupings.

In a longer–term trial, adult outpatients (n=326) who predominantly met DSM–IV criteria for schizophrenia and who remained stable on olanzapine during open label treatment for at least 8 weeks were randomized to continuation on their current olanzapine doses (ranging from 10 to 20 mg/day) or to placebo. The follow–up period to observe patients for relapse, defined in terms of increases in BPRS positive symptoms or hospitalization, was planned for 12 months, however, criteria were met for stopping the trial early due to an excess of placebo relapses compared to olanzapine relapses, and olanzapine was superior to placebo on time to relapse, the primary outcome for this study. Thus, olanzapine was more effective than placebo at maintaining efficacy in patients stabilized for approximately 8 weeks and followed for an observation period of up to 8 months.

Bipolar Disorder
Monotherapy—The efficacy of oral olanzapine in the treatment of acute manic or mixed episodes was established in 2 short–term (one 3–week and one 4–week) placebo–controlled trials in patients who met the DSM–IV criteria for Bipolar I Disorder with manic or mixed episodes. These trials included patients with or without psychotic features and with or without a rapid–cycling course.

The primary rating instrument used for assessing manic symptoms in these trials was the Young Mania Rating Scale (Y–MRS), an 11–item clinician–rated scale traditionally used to assess the degree of manic symptomatology (irritability, disruptive/aggressive behavior, sleep, elevated mood, speech, increased activity, sexual interest, language/thought disorder, thought content, appearance, and insight) in a range from 0 (no manic features) to 60 (maximum score). The primary outcome in these trials was change from baseline in the Y–MRS total score. The results of the trials follow:

(1) In one 3–week placebo–controlled trial (n=67) which involved a dose range of olanzapine (5–20 mg/day, once daily, starting at 10 mg/day), olanzapine was superior to placebo in the reduction of Y–MRS total score. In an identically designed trial conducted simultaneously with the first trial, olanzapine demonstrated a similar treatment difference, but possibly due to sample size and site variability, was not shown to be superior to placebo on this outcome.

(2) In a 4–week placebo–controlled trial (n=115) which involved a dose range of olanzapine (5–20 mg/day, once daily, starting at 15 mg/day), olanzapine was superior to placebo in the reduction of Y–MRS total score.

(3) In another trial, 361 patients meeting DSM–IV criteria for a manic or mixed episode of bipolar disorder who had responded during an initial open–label treatment phase for about two weeks, on average, to olanzapine 5 to 20 mg/day were randomized to either continuation of olanzapine at their same dose (n=225) or to placebo (n=136), for observation of relapse. Approximately 50% of the patients had discontinued from the olanzapine group by day 59 and 50% of the placebo group had discontinued by day 23 of double–blind treatment. Response during the open–label phase was defined by having a decrease of the Y–MRS total score to ≤12 and HAM–D 21 to ≤8. Relapse during the double–blind phase was defined as an increase of the Y–MRS or HAM–D 21 total score to ≥15, or being hospitalized for either mania or depression. In the randomized phase, patients receiving continued olanzapine experienced a significantly longer time to relapse.

Combination Therapy—The efficacy of oral olanzapine with concomitant lithium or valproate in the treatment of acute manic episodes was established in two controlled trials in patients who met the DSM–IV criteria for Bipolar I Disorder with manic or mixed episodes. These trials included patients with or without psychotic features and with or without a rapid–cycling course. The results of the trials follow:

(1) In one 6–week placebo–controlled combination trial, 175 outpatients on lithium or valproate therapy with inadequately controlled manic or mixed symptoms (Y–MRS ≥16) were randomized to receive either olanzapine or placebo, in combination with their original therapy. Olanzapine (in a dose range of 5–20 mg/day, once daily, starting at 10 mg/day) combined with lithium or valproate (in a therapeutic range of 0.6 mEq/L to 1.2 mEq/L or 50 µg/mL to 125 µg/mL, respectively) was superior to lithium or valproate alone in the reduction of Y–MRS total score.

(2) In a second 6–week placebo–controlled combination trial, 169 outpatients on lithium or valproate therapy with inadequately controlled manic or mixed symptoms (Y–MRS ≥16) were randomized to receive either olanzapine or placebo, in combination with their original therapy. Olanzapine (in a dose range of 5–20 mg/day, once daily, starting at 10 mg/day) combined with lithium or valproate (in a therapeutic range of 0.6 mEq/L to 1.2 mEq/L or 50 µg/mL to 125 µg/mL, respectively) was superior to lithium or valproate alone in the reduction of Y–MRS total score.

Agitation Associated with Schizophrenia and Bipolar I Mania
The efficacy of intramuscular olanzapine for injection for the treatment of agitation was established in 3 short–term (24 hours of IM treatment) placebo–controlled trials in agitated inpatients from two diagnostic groups: schizophrenia and Bipolar I Disorder (manic or mixed episodes). Each of the trials included a single active comparator treatment arm of either haloperidol injection (schizophrenia studies) or lorazepam injection (bipolar mania study). Patients enrolled in the trials needed to be: (1) judged by the clinical investigators as clinically agitated and clinically appropriate candidates for treatment with intramuscular medication, and (2) exhibiting a level of agitation that met or exceeded a threshold score of ≥14 on the five items comprising the Positive and Negative Syndrome Scale (PANSS) Excited Component (i.e., poor impulse control, tension, hostility, uncooperativeness and excitement items) with at least one individual item score ≥4 using a 1–7 scoring system (1=absent, 4=moderate, 7=extreme). In the studies, the mean baseline PANSS Excited Component score was 18.4, with scores ranging from 13 to 32 (out of a maximum score of 35), thus suggesting predominantly moderate levels of agitation with some patients experiencing mild or severe levels of agitation. The primary efficacy measure used for assessing agitation signs and symptoms in these trials was the change from baseline in the PANSS Excited Component at 2 hours post–injection. Patients could receive up to three injections during the 24 hour IM treatment periods; however, patients could not receive the second injection until after the initial 2 hour period when the primary efficacy measure was assessed. The results of the trials follow:

(1) In a placebo–controlled trial in agitated inpatients meeting DSM–IV criteria for schizophrenia (n=270), four fixed intramuscular olanzapine for injection doses of 2.5 mg, 5 mg, 7.5 mg and 10 mg were evaluated. All doses were statistically superior to placebo on the PANSS Excited Component at 2 hours post–injection. However, the effect was larger and more consistent for the three highest doses. There were no significant pairwise differences for the 7.5 and 10 mg doses over the 5 mg dose.

(2) In a second placebo–controlled trial in agitated inpatients meeting DSM–IV criteria for schizophrenia (n=311), one fixed intramuscular olanzapine for injection dose of 10 mg was evaluated. Olanzapine for injection was statistically superior to placebo on the PANSS Excited Component at 2 hours post–injection.

(3) In a placebo–controlled trial in agitated inpatients meeting DSM–IV criteria for Bipolar I Disorder (and currently displaying an acute manic or mixed episode with or without psychotic features) (n=201), one fixed intramuscular olanzapine for injection dose of 10 mg was evaluated. Olanzapine for injection was statistically superior to placebo on the PANSS Excited Component at 2 hours post–injection.

Examination of population subsets (age, race, and gender) did not reveal any differential responsiveness on the basis of these subgroupings.

INDICATIONS AND USAGE
Schizophrenia
Oral ZYPREXA is indicated for the treatment of schizophrenia.

The efficacy of ZYPREXA was established in short–term (6–week) controlled trials of schizophrenic inpatients (see CLINICAL EFFICACY DATA).

The effectiveness of oral ZYPREXA at maintaining a treatment response in schizophrenic patients who had been stable on ZYPREXA for approximately 8 weeks and were then followed for a period of up to 8 months has been demonstrated in a placebo–controlled trial (see CLINICAL EFFICACY DATA). Nevertheless, the physician who elects to use ZYPREXA for extended periods should periodically re–evaluate the long–term usefulness of the drug for the individual patient (see DOSAGE AND ADMINISTRATION).

Bipolar Disorder
Acute Monotherapy—Oral ZYPREXA is indicated for the treatment of acute mixed or manic episodes associated with Bipolar I Disorder.

The efficacy of ZYPREXA was established in two placebo–controlled trials (one 3–week and one 4–week) with patients meeting DSM–IV criteria for Bipolar I Disorder who currently displayed an acute manic or mixed episode with or without psychotic features (see CLINICAL EFFICACY DATA).

Maintenance Monotherapy—The benefit of maintaining bipolar patients on monotherapy with oral ZYPREXA after achieving a responder status for an average duration of two weeks was demonstrated in a controlled trial (see CLINICAL EFFICACY DATA). The physician who elects to use ZYPREXA for extended periods should periodically re–evaluate the long–term usefulness of the drug for the individual patient (see DOSAGE AND ADMINISTRATION).

Combination Therapy—The combination of oral ZYPREXA with lithium or valproate is indicated for the short–term treatment of acute mixed or manic episodes associated with Bipolar I Disorder.

The efficacy of ZYPREXA in combination with lithium or valproate was established in two placebo–controlled (6–week) trials with patients meeting DSM–IV criteria for Bipolar I Disorder who currently displayed an acute manic or mixed episode with or without psychotic features (see CLINICAL EFFICACY DATA).

Agitation Associated with Schizophrenia and Bipolar I Mania
ZYPREXA IntraMuscular is indicated for the treatment of agitation associated with schizophrenia and bipolar I mania. "Psychomotor agitation" is defined in DSM–IV as "excessive motor activity associated with a feeling of inner tension." Patients experiencing agitation often manifest behaviors that interfere with their diagnosis and care, e.g., threatening behaviors, escalating or urgently distressing behavior, or self–exhausting behavior, leading clinicians to the use of intramuscular antipsychotic medications to achieve immediate control of the agitation.

The efficacy of ZYPREXA IntraMuscular for the treatment of agitation associated with schizophrenia and bipolar I mania was established in 3 short–term (24 hours) placebo–controlled trials in agitated inpatients with schizophrenia or Bipolar I Disorder (manic or mixed episodes) (see CLINICAL EFFICACY DATA).

CONTRAINDICATIONS
ZYPREXA is contraindicated in patients with a known hypersensitivity to the product.

For specific information about the contraindications of lithium or valproate, refer to the CONTRAINDICATIONS section of the package inserts for these other products.

WARNINGS
Increased Mortality in Elderly Patients with Dementia–Related Psychosis—Elderly patients with dementia–related psychosis treated with atypical antipsychotic drugs are at an increased risk of death compared to placebo. ZYPREXA is not approved for the treatment of patients with dementia–related psychosis (see BOX WARNING).

In placebo–controlled clinical trials of elderly patients with dementia–related psychosis, the incidence of death in olanzapine–treated patients was significantly greater than placebo–treated patients (3.5% vs 1.5%, respectively).

Cerebrovascular Adverse Events, Including Stroke, in Elderly Patients with Dementia–Related Psychosis—Cerebrovascular adverse events (e.g., stroke, transient ischemic attack), including fatalities, were reported in patients in trials of olanzapine in elderly patients with dementia–related psychosis. In placebo–controlled trials, there was a significantly higher incidence of cerebrovascular adverse events in patients treated with olanzapine compared to patients treated with placebo. Olanzapine is not approved for the treatment of patients with dementia–related psychosis.

Hyperglycemia—Hyperglycemia, in some cases extreme and associated with ketoacidosis or hyperosmolar coma or death, has been reported in patients treated with atypical antipsychotics including olanzapine. Assessment of the relationship between atypical antipsychotic use and glucose abnormalities is complicated by the possibility of an increased background risk of diabetes mellitus in patients with schizophrenia and the increasing incidence of diabetes mellitus in the general population. Given these confounders, the relationship between atypical antipsychotic use and hyperglycemia–related adverse events is not completely understood. However, epidemiological studies suggest an increased risk of treatment–emergent hyperglycemia–related adverse events in patients treated with the atypical antipsychotics. While relative risk estimates are inconsistent, the association between atypical antipsychotics and increases in glucose levels appears to fall on a continuum and olanzapine appears to have a greater association than some other atypical antipsychotics.

Mean increases in blood glucose have been observed in patients treated (median exposure of 9.2 months) with olanzapine in phase 1 of the Clinical Antipsychotic Trials of Intervention Effectiveness (CATIE). The mean increase of serum glucose (fasting and nonfasting samples) from baseline to the average of the two highest serum concentrations was 15.0 mg/dL.

Olanzapine Monotherapy in Adults— In an analysis of 5 placebo–controlled adult olanzapine monotherapy studies with treatment duration up to 12 weeks, olanzapine was associated with a greater mean change in fasting glucose levels compared to placebo (2.76 mg/dL versus 0.17 mg/dL). The difference in mean changes between olanzapine and placebo was greater in patients with evidence of glucose

Continued on next page

This product information was prepared in March 2008. Current information on products of Eli Lilly and Company may be obtained by calling 1-800-545-5979.

Zyprexa—Cont.

dysregulation at baseline (patients diagnosed with diabetes mellitus or related adverse events, patients treated with anti–diabetic agents, patients with a baseline random glucose level ≥200 mg/dL, and/or a baseline fasting glucose level ≥126 mg/dL). These patients had a statistically significantly greater mean increase in HbA_{1c} compared to placebo. In patients with baseline normal fasting glucose levels (<100 mg/dL), 2.2% (N=543) of those treated with olanzapine were found to have high glucose levels (≥126 mg/dL) during olanzapine treatment versus 3.4% (N=293) of those treated with placebo. In patients with baseline borderline fasting glucose levels (≥100 mg/dL and <126 mg/dL), 17.4% (N=178) of those treated with olanzapine were found to have high glucose levels (≥126 mg/dL) during olanzapine treatment versus 11.5% (N=96) of those treated with placebo.

Olanzapine Monotherapy in Adolescents— The safety and efficacy of olanzapine have not been established in patients under the age of 18 years. In an analysis of 3 placebo–controlled olanzapine monotherapy studies of adolescent patients, including those with schizophrenia (6 weeks) or bipolar disorder (manic or mixed episodes) (3 weeks), olanzapine was associated with a statistically significantly greater mean change in fasting glucose levels compared to placebo (2.68 mg/dL versus –2.59 mg/dL). In patients with baseline normal fasting glucose levels (<100 mg/dL), zero out of 124 (0%) of those treated with olanzapine were found to have high glucose levels (≥126 mg/dL) during olanzapine treatment versus 1 out of 53 (1.9%) of those treated with placebo. In patients with baseline borderline fasting glucose levels (≥100 mg/dL and <126 mg/dL), 2 out of 14 (14.3%) of those treated with olanzapine were found to have high glucose levels (≥126 mg/dL) during olanzapine treatment versus zero out of 13 (0%) of those treated with placebo.

Physicians should consider the risks and benefits when prescribing olanzapine to patients with an established diagnosis of diabetes mellitus, or having borderline increased blood glucose level (fasting 100–126 mg/dL, non–fasting 140–200 mg/dL). Patients taking olanzapine should be monitored regularly for worsening of glucose control. Patients with risk factors for diabetes mellitus (e.g., obesity, family history of diabetes) who are starting treatment with atypical antipsychotics should undergo fasting blood glucose testing at the beginning of treatment and periodically during treatment. Any patient treated with atypical antipsychotics should be monitored for symptoms of hyperglycemia including polydipsia, polyuria, polyphagia, and weakness. Patients who develop symptoms of hyperglycemia during treatment with atypical antipsychotics should undergo fasting blood glucose testing. In some cases, hyperglycemia has resolved when the atypical antipsychotic was discontinued; however, some patients required continuation of anti–diabetic treatment despite discontinuation of the suspect drug.

Hyperlipidemia—Undesirable alterations in lipids have been observed with olanzapine use. Clinical monitoring, including baseline and follow–up lipid evaluations in patients using olanzapine, is advised.

Significant, and sometimes very high (>500 mg/dL), elevations in triglyceride levels have been observed with olanzapine use. Modest mean increases in total cholesterol have also been seen with olanzapine use.

Olanzapine Monotherapy in Adults— In an analysis of 5 placebo–controlled olanzapine monotherapy studies with treatment duration up to 12 weeks, olanzapine–treated patients had statistically significant increases from baseline in mean fasting total cholesterol, LDL cholesterol, and triglycerides of 5.3 mg/dL, 3.0 mg/dL, and 20.8 mg/dL respectively compared to decreases from baseline in mean fasting total cholesterol, LDL cholesterol, and triglycerides of 6.1 mg/dL, 4.3 mg/dL, and 10.7 mg/dL for placebo–treated patients. For fasting HDL cholesterol, no statistically significant differences were observed between olanzapine–treated patients and placebo–treated patients. Mean increases in fasting lipid values (total cholesterol, LDL cholesterol, and triglycerides) were greater in patients without evidence of lipid dysregulation at baseline, where lipid dysregulation was defined as patients diagnosed with dyslipidemia or related adverse events, patients treated with lipid lowering agents, or patients with high baseline lipid levels. Table 1 shows categorical changes in fasting lipid values.

[See table 1 above]

In phase 1 of the Clinical Antipsychotic Trials of Intervention Effectiveness (CATIE), over a median exposure of 9.2 months, the mean increase in triglycerides in patients taking olanzapine was 40.5 mg/dL. In phase 1 of CATIE, the mean increase in total cholesterol was 9.4 mg/dL.

Olanzapine Monotherapy in Adolescents—The safety and efficacy of olanzapine have not been established in patients under the age of 18 years. In an analysis of 3 placebo–controlled olanzapine monotherapy studies of adolescent patients, including those with schizophrenia (6 weeks) or bipolar disorder (manic or mixed episodes) (3 weeks), for fasting HDL cholesterol, no statistically significant differences were observed between olanzapine–treated patients and placebo–treated patients. Table 2 shows categorical changes in fasting lipid values in adolescent patients.

[See table 2 above]

Weight Gain—Potential consequences of weight gain should be considered prior to starting olanzapine. Patients receiving olanzapine should receive regular monitoring of weight.

Table 1 Changes in Fasting Lipids Values from Adult Placebo–Controlled Olanzapine Monotherapy Studies with Treatment Duration up to 12 Weeks

Laboratory Analyte	Category Change from Baseline	Treatment Arm	N	Patients
	Increase by ≥50 mg/dL	Olanzapine	745	39.6%*
		Placebo	402	26.1%
Fasting Triglycerides	Normal to High	Olanzapine	457	9.2%*
	(<150 mg/dL to ≥200 mg/dL)	Placebo	251	4.4%
	Borderline to High	Olanzapine	135	39.3%*
	(≥150 mg/dL and <200 mg/dL to ≥200 mg/dL)	Placebo	65	20.0%
	Increase by ≥40 mg/dL	Olanzapine	745	21.6%*
		Placebo	402	9.5%
Fasting Total Cholesterol	Normal to High	Olanzapine	392	2.8%
	(<200 mg/dL to ≥240 mg/dL)	Placebo	207	2.4%
	Borderline to High	Olanzapine	222	23.0%*
	(≥200 mg/dL and <240 mg/dL to ≥240 mg/dL)	Placebo	112	12.5%
	Increase by ≥30 mg/dL	Olanzapine	536	23.7%*
		Placebo	304	14.1%
Fasting LDL Cholesterol	Normal to High	Olanzapine	154	0%
	(<100 mg/dL to ≥160 mg/dL)	Placebo	82	1.2%
	Borderline to High	Olanzapine	302	10.6%
	(≥100 mg/dL and <160 mg/dL to ≥160 mg/dL)	Placebo	173	8.1%

*Statistically significant compared to placebo.

Table 2 Changes in Fasting Lipids Values from Adolescent Placebo–Controlled Olanzapine Monotherapy Studies

Laboratory Analyte	Category Change from Baseline	Treatment Arm	N	Patients
	Increase by ≥50 mg/dL	Olanzapine	138	37.0%*
		Placebo	66	15.2%
Fasting Triglycerides	Normal to High	Olanzapine	67	26.9%
	(<90 mg/dL to >130 mg/dL)	Placebo	28	10.7%
	Borderline to High	Olanzapine	37	59.5%
	(≥90 mg/dL and ≤130 mg/dL to >130 mg/dL)	Placebo	17	35.3%
	Increase by ≥40 mg/dL	Olanzapine	138	14.5%*
		Placebo	66	4.5%
Fasting Total Cholesterol	Normal to High	Olanzapine	87	6.9%
	(<170 mg/dL to ≥200 mg/dL)	Placebo	43	2.3%
	Borderline to High	Olanzapine	36	38.9%*
	(≥170 mg/dL and <200 mg/dL to ≥240 mg/dL)	Placebo	13	7.7%
	Increase by ≥30 mg/dL	Olanzapine	137	17.5%
		Placebo	63	11.1%
Fasting LDL Cholesterol	Normal to High	Olanzapine	98	5.1%
	(<110 mg/dL to ≥130 mg/dL)	Placebo	44	4.5%
	Borderline to High	Olanzapine	29	48.3%*
	(≥110 mg/dL and <130 mg/dL to ≥130 mg/dL)	Placebo	9	0%

*Statistically significant compared to placebo.

Olanzapine Monotherapy in Adults—In an analysis of 13 placebo–controlled olanzapine monotherapy studies, olanzapine–treated patients gained an average of 2.6 kg, which was statistically significantly different compared to an average 0.3 kg weight loss in placebo–treated patients with a median exposure of 6 weeks; 22.2% of olanzapine–treated patients gained at least 7% of their baseline weight, which was statistically significantly different compared to 3% of placebo–treated patients, with a median exposure of 8 weeks; 4.2% of olanzapine–treated patients gained at least 15% of their baseline weight, which was statistically significantly different compared to 0.3% of placebo–treated patients, with a median exposure of 12 weeks. Clinically significant weight gain was observed across all baseline Body Mass Index (BMI) categories. Discontinuation due to weight gain occurred in 0.2% of olanzapine–treated patients and in zero placebo–treated patients.

During long–term continuation therapy with olanzapine (238 median days of exposure), 56% of olanzapine patients met the criterion for having gained greater than 7% of their baseline weight. Average weight gain during long–term therapy was 5.4 kg.

Table 3 includes data on weight gain with olanzapine pooled from 68 clinical trials. The data in each column represent data for those patients who completed treatment periods of the durations specified.

Table 3 Weight Gain with Olanzapine Use

Amount Gained kg (lb)	6 Weeks (N=2976) (%)	6 Months (N=1536) (%)	12 Months (N=778) (%)	24 Months (N=422) (%)
≤0	27	21	20	22
0–5 (0–11 lb)	57	34	25	22
5–10 (11–22 lb)	15	26	25	22
10–15 (22–33 lb)	2	12	16	18
>15 (>33 lb)	0	6	14	16

Olanzapine Monotherapy in Adolescents—The safety and efficacy of olanzapine have not been established in patients under the age of 18 years. In an analysis of 4 placebo–controlled olanzapine monotherapy studies of adolescent patients (ages 13 to 17 years), including those with schizophrenia (6 weeks) or bipolar disorder (manic or mixed episodes) (3 weeks), olanzapine–treated patients gained an average of 4.6 kg, which was statistically significantly different compared to an average of 0.3 kg in placebo–treated patients, with a median exposure of 3 weeks; 40.6% of olanzapine–treated patients gained at least 7% of their baseline body weight, which was statistically significantly different compared to 9.8% of placebo–treated patients, with a median exposure of 4 weeks; 7.1% of olanzapine–treated patients gained at least 15% of their baseline weight, compared to 2.7% of placebo–treated patients, with a median exposure of 19 weeks. Clinically significant weight gain was observed across all baseline Body Mass Index (BMI) categories, but mean changes in weight were greater in adolescents with BMI categories above normal at baseline. Discontinuation due to weight gain occurred in 1% of olanzapine–treated patients, compared to zero placebo–treated patients.

During long–term continuation therapy with olanzapine, 65% of olanzapine–treated patients met the criterion for having gained greater than 7% of their baseline weight. Average weight gain during long–term therapy was 7.4 kg.

Neuroleptic Malignant Syndrome (NMS)—A potentially fatal symptom complex sometimes referred to as Neuroleptic Malignant Syndrome (NMS) has been reported in association with administration of antipsychotic drugs, including olanzapine. Clinical manifestations of NMS are hyperpyrexia, muscle rigidity, altered mental status and evidence of autonomic instability (irregular pulse or blood pressure, tachycardia, diaphoresis and cardiac dysrhythmia). Additional signs may include elevated creatinine phosphokinase, myoglobinuria (rhabdomyolysis), and acute renal failure.

The diagnostic evaluation of patients with this syndrome is complicated. In arriving at a diagnosis, it is important to exclude cases where the clinical presentation includes both serious medical illness (e.g., pneumonia, systemic infection, etc.) and untreated or inadequately treated extrapyramidal signs and symptoms (EPS). Other important considerations in the differential diagnosis include central anticholinergic toxicity, heat stroke, drug fever, and primary central nervous system pathology.

The management of NMS should include: 1) immediate discontinuation of antipsychotic drugs and other drugs not essential to concurrent therapy; 2) intensive symptomatic treatment and medical monitoring; and 3) treatment of any concomitant serious medical problems for which specific treatments are available. There is no general agreement about specific pharmacological treatment regimens for NMS.

If a patient requires antipsychotic drug treatment after recovery from NMS, the potential reintroduction of drug therapy should be carefully considered. The patient should be carefully monitored, since recurrences of NMS have been reported.

Tardive Dyskinesia—A syndrome of potentially irreversible, involuntary, dyskinetic movements may develop in patients treated with antipsychotic drugs. Although the prevalence of the syndrome appears to be highest among the elderly, especially elderly women, it is impossible to rely upon prevalence estimates to predict, at the inception of antipsychotic treatment, which patients are likely to develop the syndrome. Whether antipsychotic drug products differ in their potential to cause tardive dyskinesia is unknown.

The risk of developing tardive dyskinesia and the likelihood that it will become irreversible are believed to increase as the duration of treatment and the total cumulative dose of antipsychotic drugs administered to the patient increase. However, the syndrome can develop, although much less commonly, after relatively brief treatment periods at low doses.

There is no known treatment for established cases of tardive dyskinesia, although the syndrome may remit, partially or completely, if antipsychotic treatment is withdrawn. Antipsychotic treatment, itself, however, may suppress (or partially suppress) the signs and symptoms of the syndrome and thereby may possibly mask the underlying process. The effect that symptomatic suppression has upon the long–term course of the syndrome is unknown.

Given these considerations, olanzapine should be prescribed in a manner that is most likely to minimize the occurrence of tardive dyskinesia. Chronic antipsychotic treatment should generally be reserved for patients (1) who suffer from a chronic illness that is known to respond to antipsychotic drugs, and (2) for whom alternative, equally effective, but potentially less harmful treatments are not available or appropriate. In patients who do require chronic treatment, the smallest dose and the shortest duration of treatment producing a satisfactory clinical response should be sought. The need for continued treatment should be reassessed periodically.

If signs and symptoms of tardive dyskinesia appear in a patient on olanzapine, drug discontinuation should be considered. However, some patients may require treatment with olanzapine despite the presence of the syndrome.

For specific information about the warnings of lithium or valproate, refer to the WARNINGS section of the package inserts for these other products.

PRECAUTIONS

General

Hemodynamic Effects—Olanzapine may induce orthostatic hypotension associated with dizziness, tachycardia, and in some patients, syncope, especially during the initial dose-titration period, probably reflecting its α_1–adrenergic antagonistic properties. Hypotension, bradycardia with or without hypotension, tachycardia, and syncope were also reported during the clinical trials with intramuscular olanzapine for injection. In an open–label clinical pharmacology study in non–agitated patients with schizophrenia in which the safety and tolerability of intramuscular olanzapine were evaluated under a maximal dosing regimen (three 10 mg doses administered 4 hours apart), approximately one–third of these patients experienced a significant orthostatic decrease in systolic blood pressure (i.e., decrease ≥30 mmHg) (see DOSAGE AND ADMINISTRATION). Syncope was reported in 0.6% (15/2500) of olanzapine–treated patients in phase 2–3 oral olanzapine studies and in 0.3% (2/722) of olanzapine–treated patients with agitation in the intramuscular olanzapine for injection studies. Three normal volunteers in phase 1 studies with intramuscular olanzapine experienced hypotension, bradycardia, and sinus pauses of up to 6 seconds that spontaneously resolved (in 2 cases the events occurred on intramuscular olanzapine, and in 1 case, on oral olanzapine). The risk for this sequence of hypotension, bradycardia, and sinus pause may be greater in nonpsychiatric patients compared to psychiatric patients who are possibly more adapted to certain effects of psychotropic drugs.

For oral olanzapine therapy, the risk of orthostatic hypotension and syncope may be minimized by initiating therapy with 5 mg QD (see DOSAGE AND ADMINISTRATION). A more gradual titration to the target dose should be considered if hypotension occurs.

For intramuscular olanzapine for injection therapy, patients should remain recumbent if drowsy or dizzy after injection until examination has indicated that they are not experiencing postural hypotension, bradycardia, and/or hypoventilation.

Olanzapine should be used with particular caution in patients with known cardiovascular disease (history of myocardial infarction or ischemia, heart failure, or conduction abnormalities), cerebrovascular disease, and conditions which would predispose patients to hypotension (dehydration, hypovolemia, and treatment with antihypertensive medications) where the occurrence of syncope, or hypotension and/or bradycardia might put the patient at increased medical risk.

Caution is necessary in patients who receive treatment with other drugs having effects that can induce hypotension, bradycardia, respiratory or central nervous system depression (see Drug Interactions). Concomitant administration of intramuscular olanzapine and parenteral benzodiazepine has not been studied and is therefore not recommended. If use of intramuscular olanzapine in combination with parenteral benzodiazepines is considered, careful evaluation of clinical status for excessive sedation and cardiorespiratory depression is recommended.

Seizures—During premarketing testing, seizures occurred in 0.9% (22/2500) of olanzapine–treated patients. There

were confounding factors that may have contributed to the occurrence of seizures in many of these cases. Olanzapine should be used cautiously in patients with a history of seizures or with conditions that potentially lower the seizure threshold, e.g., Alzheimer's dementia. Conditions that lower the seizure threshold may be more prevalent in a population of 65 years or older.

Hyperprolactinemia—As with other drugs that antagonize dopamine D_2 receptors, olanzapine elevates prolactin levels, and a modest elevation persists during chronic administration. Tissue culture experiments indicate that approximately one–third of human breast cancers are prolactin dependent in vitro, a factor of potential importance if the prescription of these drugs is contemplated in a patient with previously detected breast cancer of this type. Although disturbances such as galactorrhea, amenorrhea, gynecomastia, and impotence have been reported with prolactin–elevating compounds, the clinical significance of elevated serum prolactin levels is unknown for most patients. As is common with compounds which increase prolactin release, an increase in mammary gland neoplasia was observed in the olanzapine carcinogenicity studies conducted in mice and rats (see Carcinogenesis). However, neither clinical studies nor epidemiologic studies have shown an association between chronic administration of this class of drugs and tumorigenesis in humans; the available evidence is considered too limited to be conclusive.

Transaminase Elevations—In placebo–controlled studies, clinically significant ALT (SGPT) elevations (≥3 times the upper limit of the normal range) were observed in 2% (6/243) of patients exposed to olanzapine compared to none (0/115) of the placebo patients. None of these patients experienced jaundice. In two of these patients, liver enzymes decreased toward normal despite continued treatment and in two others, enzymes decreased upon discontinuation of olanzapine. In the remaining two patients, one, seropositive for hepatitis C, had persistent enzyme elevation for four months after discontinuation, and the other had insufficient follow–up to determine if enzymes normalized.

Within the larger premarketing database of about 2400 patients with baseline SGPT ≤90 IU/L, the incidence of SGPT elevation to >200 IU/L was 2% (50/2381). Again, none of these patients experienced jaundice or other symptoms attributable to liver impairment and most had transient changes that tended to normalize while olanzapine treatment was continued.

Among 2500 patients in oral olanzapine clinical trials, about 1% (23/2500) discontinued treatment due to transaminase increases.

Rare postmarketing reports of hepatitis have been received. Very rare cases of cholestatic or mixed liver injury have also been reported in the postmarketing period.

Caution should be exercised in patients with signs and symptoms of hepatic impairment, in patients with pre-existing conditions associated with limited hepatic functional reserve, and in patients who are being treated with potentially hepatotoxic drugs. Periodic assessment of transaminases is recommended in patients with significant hepatic disease (see Laboratory Tests).

Potential for Cognitive and Motor Impairment—Somnolence was a commonly reported adverse event associated with olanzapine treatment, occurring at an incidence of 26% in olanzapine patients compared to 15% in placebo patients. This adverse event was also dose related. Somnolence led to discontinuation in 0.4% (9/2500) of patients in the premarketing database.

Since olanzapine has the potential to impair judgment, thinking, or motor skills, patients should be cautioned about operating hazardous machinery, including automobiles, until they are reasonably certain that olanzapine therapy does not affect them adversely.

Body Temperature Regulation—Disruption of the body's ability to reduce core body temperature has been attributed to antipsychotic agents. Appropriate care is advised when prescribing olanzapine for patients who will be experiencing conditions which may contribute to an elevation in core body temperature, e.g., exercising strenuously, exposure to extreme heat, receiving concomitant medication with anticholinergic activity, or being subject to dehydration.

Dysphagia—Esophageal dysmotility and aspiration have been associated with antipsychotic drug use. Aspiration pneumonia is a common cause of morbidity and mortality in patients with advanced Alzheimer's disease. Olanzapine and other antipsychotic drugs should be used cautiously in patients at risk for aspiration pneumonia.

Suicide—The possibility of a suicide attempt is inherent in schizophrenia and in bipolar disorder, and close supervision of high–risk patients should accompany drug therapy. Prescriptions for olanzapine should be written for the smallest quantity of tablets consistent with good patient management, in order to reduce the risk of overdose.

Use in Patients with Concomitant Illness—Clinical experience with olanzapine in patients with certain concomitant systemic illnesses (see Renal Impairment and Hepatic Impairment under CLINICAL PHARMACOLOGY, Special Populations) is limited.

Olanzapine exhibits in vitro muscarinic receptor affinity. In premarketing clinical trials with olanzapine, olanzapine was associated with constipation, dry mouth, and tachycardia, all adverse events possibly related to cholinergic antagonism. Such adverse events were not often the basis for

discontinuations from olanzapine, but olanzapine should be used with caution in patients with clinically significant prostatic hypertrophy, narrow angle glaucoma, or a history of paralytic ileus.

In five placebo–controlled studies of olanzapine in elderly patients with dementia–related psychosis (n=1184), the following treatment–emergent adverse events were reported in olanzapine–treated patients at an incidence of at least 2% and significantly greater than placebo–treated patients: falls, somnolence, peripheral edema, abnormal gait, urinary incontinence, lethargy, increased weight, asthenia, pyrexia, pneumonia, dry mouth and visual hallucinations. The rate of discontinuation due to adverse events was significantly greater with olanzapine than placebo (13% vs 7%). Elderly patients with dementia–related psychosis treated with olanzapine are at an increased risk of death compared to placebo. Olanzapine is not approved for the treatment of patients with dementia–related psychosis. If the prescriber elects to treat elderly patients with dementia–related psychosis, vigilance should be exercised (see BOX WARNING and WARNINGS).

Olanzapine has not been evaluated or used to any appreciable extent in patients with a recent history of myocardial infarction or unstable heart disease. Patients with these diagnoses were excluded from premarketing clinical studies. Because of the risk of orthostatic hypotension with olanzapine, caution should be observed in cardiac patients (see Hemodynamic Effects).

For specific information about the precautions of lithium or valproate, refer to the PRECAUTIONS section of the package inserts for these other products.

Information for Patients

Physicians are advised to discuss the following issues with patients for whom they prescribe olanzapine:

Hyperglycemia—Patients should be advised of the potential risk of hyperglycemia–related adverse events. Patients should be monitored regularly for worsening of glucose control.

Weight Gain—Patients should be counseled that olanzapine is associated with weight gain. Patients should have their weight monitored regularly.

Orthostatic Hypotension—Patients should be advised of the risk of orthostatic hypotension, especially during the period of initial dose titration and in association with the use of concomitant drugs that may potentiate the orthostatic effect of olanzapine, e.g., diazepam or alcohol (see Drug Interactions).

Interference with Cognitive and Motor Performance—Because olanzapine has the potential to impair judgment, thinking, or motor skills, patients should be cautioned about operating hazardous machinery, including automobiles, until they are reasonably certain that olanzapine therapy does not affect them adversely.

Pregnancy—Patients should be advised to notify their physician if they become pregnant or intend to become pregnant during therapy with olanzapine.

Nursing—Patients should be advised not to breast–feed an infant if they are taking olanzapine.

Concomitant Medication—Patients should be advised to inform their physicians if they are taking, or plan to take, any prescription or over–the–counter drugs, since there is a potential for interactions.

Alcohol—Patients should be advised to avoid alcohol while taking olanzapine.

Heat Exposure and Dehydration—Patients should be advised regarding appropriate care in avoiding overheating and dehydration.

Phenylketonurics—ZYPREXA ZYDIS (olanzapine orally disintegrating tablets) contains phenylalanine (0.34, 0.45, 0.67, or 0.90 mg per 5, 10, 15, or 20 mg tablet, respectively).

Laboratory Tests

Periodic assessment of transaminases is recommended in patients with significant hepatic disease (see Transaminase Elevations).

Drug Interactions

The risks of using olanzapine in combination with other drugs have not been extensively evaluated in systematic studies. Given the primary CNS effects of olanzapine, caution should be used when olanzapine is taken in combination with other centrally acting drugs and alcohol.

Because of its potential for inducing hypotension, olanzapine may enhance the effects of certain antihypertensive agents.

Olanzapine may antagonize the effects of levodopa and dopamine agonists.

The Effect of Other Drugs on Olanzapine—Agents that induce CYP1A2 or glucuronyl transferase enzymes, such as omeprazole and rifampin, may cause an increase in olanzapine clearance. Inhibitors of CYP1A2 could potentially inhibit olanzapine clearance. Although olanzapine is metabolized by multiple enzyme systems, induction or inhibition of a single enzyme may appreciably alter olanzapine clearance. Therefore, a dosage increase (for induction) or a dosage decrease (for inhibition) may need to be considered with specific drugs.

Continued on next page

This product information was prepared in March 2008. Current information on products of Eli Lilly and Company may be obtained by calling 1-800-545-5979.

Zyprexa—Cont.

Charcoal—The administration of activated charcoal (1 g) reduced the Cmax and AUC of oral olanzapine by about 60%. As peak olanzapine levels are not typically obtained until about 6 hours after dosing, charcoal may be a useful treatment for olanzapine overdose.

Cimetidine and Antacids—Single doses of cimetidine (800 mg) or aluminum– and magnesium–containing antacids did not affect the oral bioavailability of olanzapine.

Carbamazepine—Carbamazepine therapy (200 mg bid) causes an approximately 50% increase in the clearance of olanzapine. This increase is likely due to the fact that carbamazepine is a potent inducer of CYP1A2 activity. Higher daily doses of carbamazepine may cause an even greater increase in olanzapine clearance.

Ethanol— Ethanol (45 mg/70 kg single dose) did not have an effect on olanzapine pharmacokinetics.

Fluoxetine—Fluoxetine (60 mg single dose or 60 mg daily for 8 days) causes a small (mean 16%) increase in the maximum concentration of olanzapine and a small (mean 16%) decrease in olanzapine clearance. The magnitude of the impact of this factor is small in comparison to the overall variability between individuals, and therefore dose modification is not routinely recommended.

Fluvoxamine—Fluvoxamine, a CYP1A2 inhibitor, decreases the clearance of olanzapine. This results in a mean increase in olanzapine Cmax following fluvoxamine of 54% in female nonsmokers and 77% in male smokers. The mean increase in olanzapine AUC is 52% and 108%, respectively. Lower doses of olanzapine should be considered in patients receiving concomitant treatment with fluvoxamine.

Warfarin—Warfarin (20 mg single dose) did not affect olanzapine pharmacokinetics.

Effect of Olanzapine on Other Drugs—In vitro studies utilizing human liver microsomes suggest that olanzapine has little potential to inhibit CYP1A2, CYP2C9, CYP2C19, CYP2D6, and CYP3A. Thus, olanzapine is unlikely to cause clinically important drug interactions mediated by these enzymes.

Lithium—Multiple doses of olanzapine (10 mg for 8 days) did not influence the kinetics of lithium. Therefore, concomitant olanzapine administration does not require dosage adjustment of lithium.

Valproate—Studies in vitro using human liver microsomes determined that olanzapine has little potential to inhibit the major metabolic pathway, glucuronidation, of valproate. Further, valproate has little effect on the metabolism of olanzapine in vitro. In vivo administration of olanzapine (10 mg daily for 2 weeks) did not affect the steady state plasma concentrations of valproate. Therefore, concomitant olanzapine administration does not require dosage adjustment of valproate.

Single doses of olanzapine did not affect the pharmacokinetics of imipramine or its active metabolite desipramine, and warfarin. Multiple doses of olanzapine did not influence the kinetics of diazepam and its active metabolite N–desmethyldiazepam, ethanol, or biperiden. However, the co–administration of either diazepam or ethanol with olanzapine potentiated the orthostatic hypotension observed with olanzapine. Multiple doses of olanzapine did not affect the pharmacokinetics of theophylline or its metabolites.

Lorazepam—Administration of intramuscular lorazepam (2 mg) 1 hour after intramuscular olanzapine for injection (5 mg) did not significantly affect the pharmacokinetics of olanzapine, unconjugated lorazepam, or total lorazepam. However, this co–administration of intramuscular lorazepam and intramuscular olanzapine for injection added to the somnolence observed with either drug alone (see Hemodynamic Effects).

Carcinogenesis, Mutagenesis, Impairment of Fertility

Carcinogenesis—Oral carcinogenicity studies were conducted in mice and rats. Olanzapine was administered to mice in two 78–week studies at doses of 3, 10, 30/20 mg/kg/day (equivalent to 0.8–5 times the maximum recommended human daily oral dose on a mg/m² basis) and 0.25, 2, 8 mg/kg/day (equivalent to 0.06–2 times the maximum recommended human daily oral dose on a mg/m² basis). Rats were dosed for 2 years at doses of 0.25, 1, 2.5, 4 mg/kg/day (males) and 0.25, 1, 4, 8 mg/kg/day (females) (equivalent to 0.13–2 and 0.13–4 times the maximum recommended human daily oral dose on a mg/m² basis, respectively). The incidence of liver hemangiomas and hemangiosarcomas was significantly increased in one mouse study in female mice dosed at 8 mg/kg/day (2 times the maximum recommended human daily oral dose on a mg/m² basis). These tumors were not increased in another mouse study in females dosed at 10 or 30/20 mg/kg/day (2–5 times the maximum recommended human daily oral dose on a mg/m² basis); in this study, there was a high incidence of early mortalities in males of the 30/20 mg/kg/day group. The incidence of mammary gland adenomas and adenocarcinomas was significantly increased in female mice dosed at ≥2 mg/kg/day and in female rats dosed at ≥4 mg/kg/day (0.5 and 2 times the maximum recommended human daily oral dose on a mg/m² basis, respectively). Antipsychotic drugs have been shown to chronically elevate prolactin levels in rodents. Serum prolactin levels were not measured during the olanzapine carcinogenicity studies; however, measurements during subchronic toxicity studies showed that olanzapine elevated serum prolactin levels up to 4–fold in rats at the same doses used in the carcinogenicity study. An increase in mammary gland neoplasms has been found in rodents after chronic administration of other antipsychotic drugs and is considered to be prolactin mediated. The relevance for human risk of the finding of prolactin mediated endocrine tumors in rodents is unknown (see Hyperprolactinemia under PRECAUTIONS, General).

Mutagenesis—No evidence of mutagenic potential for olanzapine was found in the Ames reverse mutation test, in vivo micronucleus test in mice, the chromosomal aberration test in Chinese hamster ovary cells, unscheduled DNA synthesis test in rat hepatocytes, induction of forward mutation test in mouse lymphoma cells, or in vivo sister chromatid exchange test in bone marrow of Chinese hamsters.

Impairment of Fertility—In an oral fertility and reproductive performance study in rats, male mating performance, but not fertility, was impaired at a dose of 22.4 mg/kg/day and female fertility was decreased at a dose of 3 mg/kg/day (11 and 1.5 times the maximum recommended human daily oral dose on a mg/m² basis, respectively). Discontinuance of olanzapine treatment reversed the effects on male mating performance. In female rats, the precoital period was increased and the mating index reduced at 5 mg/kg/day (2.5 times the maximum recommended human daily oral dose on a mg/m² basis). Diestrous was prolonged and estrous delayed at 1.1 mg/kg/day (0.6 times the maximum recommended human daily oral dose on a mg/m² basis); therefore olanzapine may produce a delay in ovulation.

Pregnancy

Pregnancy Category C

In oral reproduction studies in rats at doses up to 18 mg/kg/day and in rabbits at doses up to 30 mg/kg/day (9 and 30 times the maximum recommended human daily oral dose on a mg/m² basis, respectively) no evidence of teratogenicity was observed. In an oral rat teratology study, early resorptions and increased numbers of nonviable fetuses were observed at a dose of 18 mg/kg/day (9 times the maximum recommended human daily oral dose on a mg/m² basis). Gestation was prolonged at 10 mg/kg/day (5 times the maximum recommended human daily oral dose on a mg/m² basis). In an oral rabbit teratology study, fetal toxicity (manifested as increased resorptions and decreased fetal weight) occurred at a maternally toxic dose of 30 mg/kg/day (30 times the maximum recommended human daily oral dose on a mg/m² basis).

Placental transfer of olanzapine occurs in rat pups.

There are no adequate and well–controlled trials with olanzapine in pregnant females. Seven pregnancies were observed during clinical trials with olanzapine, including 2 resulting in normal births, 1 resulting in neonatal death due to a cardiovascular defect, 3 therapeutic abortions, and 1 spontaneous abortion. Because animal reproduction studies are not always predictive of human response, this drug should be used during pregnancy only if the potential benefit justifies the potential risk to the fetus.

Labor and Delivery

Parturition in rats was not affected by olanzapine. The effect of olanzapine on labor and delivery in humans is unknown.

Nursing Mothers

In a study in lactating, healthy women, olanzapine was excreted in breast milk. Mean infant dose at steady state was estimated to be 1.8% of the maternal olanzapine dose. It is recommended that women receiving olanzapine should not breast–feed.

Pediatric Use

Safety and effectiveness in pediatric patients have not been established.

Geriatric Use

Of the 2500 patients in premarketing clinical studies with oral olanzapine, 11% (263) were 65 years of age or over. In patients with schizophrenia, there was no indication of any different tolerability of olanzapine in the elderly compared to younger patients. Studies in elderly patients with dementia–related psychosis have suggested that there may be a different tolerability profile in this population compared to younger patients with schizophrenia. Elderly patients with dementia–related psychosis treated with olanzapine are at an increased risk of death compared to placebo. Olanzapine is not approved for the treatment of patients with dementia–related psychosis. If the prescriber elects to treat elderly patients with dementia–related psychosis, vigilance should be exercised. Also, the presence of factors that might decrease pharmacokinetic clearance or increase the pharmacodynamic response to olanzapine should lead to consideration of a lower starting dose for any geriatric patient (see BOX WARNING, WARNINGS, PRECAUTIONS, and DOSAGE AND ADMINISTRATION).

ADVERSE REACTIONS

The information below is derived from a clinical trial database for olanzapine consisting of 8661 patients with approximately 4165 patient–years of exposure to oral olanzapine and 722 patients with exposure to intramuscular olanzapine for injection. This database includes: (1) 2500 patients who participated in multiple–dose oral olanzapine premarketing trials in schizophrenia and Alzheimer's disease representing approximately 1122 patient–years of exposure as of February 14, 1995; (2) 182 patients who participated in oral olanzapine premarketing bipolar mania trials representing approximately 66 patient–years of exposure; (3) 191 patients who participated in an oral olanzapine trial of patients having various psychiatric symptoms in association with Alzheimer's disease representing approximately 29 patient–years of exposure; (4) 5788 patients from 88 additional oral olanzapine clinical trials as of December 31, 2001; and (5) 722 patients who participated in intramuscular olanzapine for injection premarketing trials in agitated patients with schizophrenia, Bipolar I Disorder (manic or mixed episodes), or dementia. In addition, information from the premarketing 6–week clinical study database for olanzapine in combination with lithium or valproate, consisting of 224 patients who participated in bipolar mania trials with approximately 22 patient–years of exposure, is included below.

The conditions and duration of treatment with olanzapine varied greatly and included (in overlapping categories) open–label and double–blind phases of studies, inpatients and outpatients, fixed–dose and dose–titration studies, and short–term or longer–term exposure. Adverse reactions were assessed by collecting adverse events, results of physical examinations, vital signs, weights, laboratory analytes, ECGs, chest x–rays, and results of ophthalmologic examinations.

Certain portions of the discussion below relating to objective or numeric safety parameters, namely, dose–dependent adverse events, vital sign changes, weight gain, laboratory changes, and ECG changes are derived from studies in patients with schizophrenia and have not been duplicated for bipolar mania or agitation. However, this information is also generally applicable to bipolar mania and agitation.

Adverse events during exposure were obtained by spontaneous report and recorded by clinical investigators using terminology of their own choosing. Consequently, it is not possible to provide a meaningful estimate of the proportion of individuals experiencing adverse events without first grouping similar types of events into a smaller number of standardized event categories. In the tables and tabulations that follow, standard COSTART dictionary terminology has been used initially to classify reported adverse events.

The stated frequencies of adverse events represent the proportion of individuals who experienced, at least once, a treatment–emergent adverse event of the type listed. An event was considered treatment emergent if it occurred for the first time or worsened while receiving therapy following baseline evaluation. The reported events do not include those event terms that were so general as to be uninformative. Events listed elsewhere in labeling may not be repeated below. It is important to emphasize that, although the events occurred during treatment with olanzapine, they were not necessarily caused by it. The entire label should be read to gain a complete understanding of the safety profile of olanzapine.

The prescriber should be aware that the figures in the tables and tabulations cannot be used to predict the incidence of side effects in the course of usual medical practice where patient characteristics and other factors differ from those that prevailed in the clinical trials. Similarly, the cited frequencies cannot be compared with figures obtained from other clinical investigations involving different treatments, uses, and investigators. The cited figures, however, do provide the prescribing physician with some basis for estimating the relative contribution of drug and nondrug factors to the adverse event incidence in the population studied.

Incidence of Adverse Events in Short-Term, Placebo-Controlled and Combination Trials

The following findings are based on premarketing trials of (1) oral olanzapine for schizophrenia, bipolar mania, a subsequent trial of patients having various psychiatric symptoms in association with Alzheimer's disease, and premarketing combination trials, and (2) intramuscular olanzapine for injection in agitated patients with schizophrenia or bipolar mania.

Adverse Events Associated with Discontinuation of Treatment in Short-Term, Placebo-Controlled Trials

Schizophrenia—Overall, there was no difference in the incidence of discontinuation due to adverse events (5% for oral olanzapine vs 6% for placebo). However, discontinuations due to increases in SGPT were considered to be drug related (2% for oral olanzapine vs 0% for placebo) (see PRECAUTIONS).

Bipolar Mania Monotherapy—Overall, there was no difference in the incidence of discontinuation due to adverse events (2% for oral olanzapine vs 2% for placebo).

Agitation—Overall, there was no difference in the incidence of discontinuation due to adverse events (0.4% for intramuscular olanzapine for injection vs 0% for placebo).

Adverse Events Associated with Discontinuation of Treatment in Short-Term Combination Trials

Bipolar Mania Combination Therapy—In a study of patients who were already tolerating either lithium or valproate as monotherapy, discontinuation rates due to adverse events were 11% for the combination of oral olanzapine with lithium or valproate compared to 2% for patients who remained on lithium or valproate monotherapy. Discontinuations with the combination of oral olanzapine and lithium or valproate that occurred in more than 1 patient were: somnolence (3%), weight gain (1%), and peripheral edema (1%).

Commonly Observed Adverse Events in Short-Term, Placebo-Controlled Trials

The most commonly observed adverse events associated with the use of oral olanzapine (incidence of 5% or greater) and not observed at an equivalent incidence among placebo–treated patients (olanzapine incidence at least twice that for placebo) were:

Common Treatment–Emergent Adverse Events Associated with the Use of Oral Olanzapine in 6-Week Trials — SCHIZOPHRENIA

	Percentage of Patients Reporting Event	
Adverse Event	Olanzapine (N=248)	Placebo (N=118)
Postural hypotension	5	2
Constipation	9	3
Weight gain	6	1
Dizziness	11	4
Personality disorder*	8	4
Akathisia	5	1

*Personality disorder is the COSTART term for designating non–aggressive objectionable behavior.

Common Treatment–Emergent Adverse Events Associated with the Use of Oral Olanzapine in 3–Week and 4–Week Trials — BIPOLAR MANIA

	Percentage of Patients Reporting Event	
Adverse Event	Olanzapine (N=125)	Placebo (N=129)
Asthenia	15	6
Dry mouth	22	7
Constipation	11	5
Dyspepsia	11	5
Increased appetite	6	3
Somnolence	35	13
Dizziness	18	6
Tremor	6	3

There was one adverse event (somnolence) observed at an incidence of 5% or greater among intramuscular olanzapine for injection–treated patients and not observed at an equivalent incidence among placebo–treated patients (olanzapine incidence at least twice that for placebo) during the placebo–controlled premarketing studies. The incidence of somnolence during the 24 hour IM treatment period in clinical trials in agitated patients with schizophrenia or bipolar mania was 6% for intramuscular olanzapine for injection and 3% for placebo.

Adverse Events Occurring at an Incidence of 2% or More Among Oral Olanzapine–Treated Patients in Short-Term, Placebo-Controlled Trials

Table 4 enumerates the incidence, rounded to the nearest percent, of treatment–emergent adverse events that occurred in 2% or more of patients treated with oral olanzapine (doses ≥2.5 mg/day) and with incidence greater than placebo who participated in the acute phase of placebo–controlled trials.

Table 4 Treatment–Emergent Adverse Events: Incidence in Short–Term, Placebo–Controlled Clinical Trials* with Oral Olanzapine

	Percentage of Patients Reporting Event	
Body System/Adverse Event	Olanzapine (N=532)	Placebo (N=294)
Body as a Whole		
Accidental injury	12	8
Asthenia	10	9
Fever	6	2
Back pain	5	2
Chest pain	3	1
Cardiovascular System		
Postural hypotension	3	1
Tachycardia	3	1
Hypertension	2	1
Digestive System		
Dry mouth	9	5
Constipation	9	4
Dyspepsia	7	5
Vomiting	4	3
Increased appetite	3	2
Hemic and Lymphatic System		
Ecchymosis	5	3
Metabolic and Nutritional Disorders		
Weight gain	5	3
Peripheral edema	3	1
Musculoskeletal System		
Extremity pain (other than joint)	5	3
Joint pain	5	3
Nervous System		
Somnolence	29	13
Insomnia	12	11
Dizziness	11	4
Abnormal gait	6	1
Tremor	4	3
Akathisia	3	2
Hypertonia	3	2
Articulation impairment	2	1
Respiratory System		
Rhinitis	7	6
Cough increased	6	3
Pharyngitis	4	3
Special Senses		
Amblyopia	3	2

Urogenital System

Urinary incontinence	2	1
Urinary tract infection	2	1

*Events reported by at least 2% of patients treated with olanzapine, except the following events which had an incidence equal to or less than placebo: abdominal pain, agitation, anorexia, anxiety, apathy, confusion, depression, diarrhea, dysmenorrhea (denominator used was for females only [olanzapine, N=201; placebo, N=114]), hallucinations, headache, hostility, hyperkinesia, myalgia, nausea, nervousness, paranoid reaction, personality disorder (COSTART term for designating non–aggressive objectionable behavior), rash, thinking abnormal, weight loss.

Commonly Observed Adverse Events in Short-Term Combination Trials

In the bipolar mania combination placebo–controlled trials, the most commonly observed adverse events associated with the combination of olanzapine and lithium or valproate (incidence of ≥5% and at least twice placebo) were:

Common Treatment–Emergent Adverse Events Associated with the Use of Oral Olanzapine in 6–Week Combination Trials — BIPOLAR MANIA

	Percentage of Patients Reporting Event	
Adverse Event	Olanzapine with lithium or valproate (N=229)	Placebo with lithium or valproate (N=115)
Dry mouth	32	9
Weight gain	26	7
Increased appetite	24	8
Dizziness	14	7
Back pain	8	4
Constipation	8	4
Speech disorder	7	1
Increased salivation	6	2
Amnesia	5	2
Paresthesia	5	2

Adverse Events Occurring at an Incidence of 2% or More Among Oral Olanzapine–Treated Patients in Short-Term Combination Trials

Table 5 enumerates the incidence, rounded to the nearest percent, of treatment–emergent adverse events that occurred in 2% or more of patients treated with the combination of olanzapine (doses ≥5 mg/day) and lithium or valproate and with incidence greater than lithium or valproate alone who participated in the acute phase of placebo–controlled combination trials.

Table 5 Treatment-Emergent Adverse Events: Incidence in Short–Term, Placebo-Controlled Combination Clinical Trials* with Oral Olanzapine

	Percentage of Patients Reporting Event	
Body System/Adverse Event	Olanzapine with lithium or valproate (N=229)	Placebo with lithium or valproate (N=115)
Body as a Whole		
Asthenia	18	13
Back pain	8	4
Accidental injury	4	2
Chest pain	3	2
Cardiovascular System		
Hypertension	2	1
Digestive System		
Dry mouth	32	9
Increased appetite	24	8
Thirst	10	6
Constipation	8	4
Increased salivation	6	2
Metabolic and Nutritional Disorders		
Weight gain	26	7
Peripheral edema	6	4
Edema	2	1
Nervous System		
Somnolence	52	27
Tremor	23	13
Depression	18	17
Dizziness	14	7
Speech disorder	7	1
Amnesia	5	2
Paresthesia	5	2
Apathy	4	3
Confusion	4	1
Euphoria	3	2
Incoordination	2	0
Respiratory System		
Pharyngitis	4	1
Dyspnea	3	1
Skin and Appendages		
Sweating	3	1
Acne	2	0

Dry skin	2	0
Special Senses		
Amblyopia	9	5
Abnormal vision	2	0
Urogenital System		
Dysmenorrhea[†]	2	0
Vaginitis[†]	2	0

* Events reported by at least 2% of patients treated with olanzapine, except the following events which had an incidence equal to or less than placebo: abdominal pain, abnormal dreams, abnormal ejaculation, agitation, akathisia, anorexia, anxiety, arthralgia, cough increased, diarrhea, dyspepsia, emotional lability, fever, flatulence, flu syndrome, headache, hostility, insomnia, libido decreased, libido increased, menstrual disorder (denominator used was for females only [olanzapine, N=128; placebo, N=51]), myalgia, nausea, nervousness, pain, paranoid reaction, personality disorder, rash, rhinitis, sleep disorder, thinking abnormal, vomiting.
[†] Denominator used was for females only (olanzapine, N=128; placebo, N=51).

For specific information about the adverse reactions observed with lithium or valproate, refer to the ADVERSE REACTIONS section of the package inserts for these other products.

Adverse Events Occurring at an Incidence of 1% or More Among Intramuscular Olanzapine for Injection-Treated Patients in Short-Term, Placebo-Controlled Trials

Table 6 enumerates the incidence, rounded to the nearest percent, of treatment–emergent adverse events that occurred in 1% or more of patients treated with intramuscular olanzapine for injection (dose range of 2.5–10 mg/injection) and with incidence greater than placebo who participated in the short–term, placebo–controlled trials in agitated patients with schizophrenia or bipolar mania.

Table 6 Treatment–Emergent Adverse Events: Incidence in Short–Term (24 Hour), Placebo–Controlled Clinical Trials with Intramuscular Olanzapine for Injection in Agitated Patients with Schizophrenia or Bipolar Mania*

	Percentage of Patients Reporting Event	
Body System/Adverse Event	Olanzapine (N=415)	Placebo (N=150)
Body as a Whole		
Asthenia	2	1
Cardiovascular System		
Hypotension	2	0
Postural hypotension	1	0
Nervous System		
Somnolence	6	3
Dizziness	4	2
Tremor	1	0

*Events reported by at least 1% of patients treated with olanzapine for injection, except the following events which had an incidence equal to or less than placebo: agitation, anxiety, dry mouth, headache, hypertension, insomnia, nervousness.

Dose Dependency of Adverse Events in Short-Term, Placebo-Controlled Trials

Extrapyramidal Symptoms—The following table enumerates the percentage of patients with treatment–emergent extrapyramidal symptoms as assessed by categorical analyses of formal rating scales during acute therapy in a controlled clinical trial comparing oral olanzapine at 3 fixed doses with placebo in the treatment of schizophrenia.

[See first table at top of next page]

The following table enumerates the percentage of patients with treatment–emergent extrapyramidal symptoms as assessed by spontaneously reported adverse events during acute therapy in the same controlled clinical trial comparing olanzapine at 3 fixed doses with placebo in the treatment of schizophrenia.

[See second table at top of next page]

The following table enumerates the percentage of patients with treatment–emergent extrapyramidal symptoms as assessed by categorical analyses of formal rating scales during controlled clinical trials comparing fixed doses of intramuscular olanzapine for injection with placebo in agitation. Patients in each dose group could receive up to three injections during the trials (see CLINICAL EFFICACY DATA). Patient assessments were conducted during the 24 hours following the initial dose of intramuscular olanzapine for injection. There were no statistically significant differences from placebo.

[See third table at top of next page]

The following table enumerates the percentage of patients with treatment–emergent extrapyramidal symptoms as assessed by spontaneously reported adverse events in the same controlled clinical trial comparing fixed doses of intra-

Continued on next page

This product information was prepared in March 2008. Current information on products of Eli Lilly and Company may be obtained by calling 1-800-545-5979.

Zyprexa—Cont.

muscular olanzapine for injection with placebo in agitated patients with schizophrenia. There were no statistically significant differences from placebo.
[See fourth table above]

Dystonia, Class Effect - Symptoms of dystonia, prolonged abnormal contractions of muscle groups, may occur in susceptible individuals during the first few days of treatment. Dystonic symptoms include: spasm of the neck muscles, sometimes progressing to tightness of the throat, swallowing difficulty, difficulty breathing, and/or protrusion of the tongue. While these symptoms can occur at low doses, the frequency and severity are greater with high potency and at higher doses of first generation antipsychotic drugs. In general, an elevated risk of acute dystonia may be observed in males and younger age groups receiving antipsychotics; however, events of dystonia have been reported infrequently (<1%) with olanzapine use.

Other Adverse Events—The following table addresses dose relatedness for other adverse events using data from a schizophrenia trial involving fixed dosage ranges of oral olanzapine. It enumerates the percentage of patients with treatment–emergent adverse events for the three fixed–dose range groups and placebo. The data were analyzed using the Cochran–Armitage test, excluding the placebo group, and the table includes only those adverse events for which there was a statistically significant trend.
[See table at top of next page]

Additional Findings

In a single 8–week randomized, double–blind, fixed–dose study comparing 10 (N=199), 20 (N=200) and 40 (N=200) mg/day of olanzapine in patients with schizophrenia or schizoaffective disorder, statistically significant differences among 3 dose groups were observed for the following safety outcomes: weight gain, prolactin elevation, fatigue and dizziness. Mean baseline to endpoint increase in weight (10 mg/day: 1.9 kg; 20 mg/day: 2.3 kg; 40 mg/day: 3 kg) was observed with significant differences between 10 vs 40 mg/day. Incidence of treatment–emergent prolactin elevation >24.2 ng/mL (female) or >18.77 ng/mL (male) at any time during the trial (10 mg/day: 31.2%; 20 mg/day: 42.7%; 40 mg/day: 61.1%) with significant differences between 10 vs 40 mg/day and 20 vs 40 mg/day; fatigue (10 mg/day: 1.5%; 20 mg/day: 2.1%; 40 mg/day: 6.6%) with significant differences between 10 vs 40 and 20 vs 40 mg/day; and dizziness (10 mg/day: 2.6%; 20 mg/day: 1.6%; 40 mg/day: 6.6%) with significant differences between 20 vs 40 mg, was observed.

Additional Findings Observed in Clinical Trials

The following findings are based on clinical trials.

Vital Sign Changes—Oral olanzapine was associated with orthostatic hypotension and tachycardia in clinical trials. Intramuscular olanzapine for injection was associated with bradycardia, hypotension, and tachycardia in clinical trials (*see* PRECAUTIONS).

Laboratory Changes —An assessment of the premarketing experience for olanzapine revealed an association with asymptomatic increases in SGPT, SGOT, and GGT (*see* PRECAUTIONS). Olanzapine administration was also associated with increases in serum prolactin (*see* PRECAUTIONS), with an asymptomatic elevation of the eosinophil count in 0.3% of patients, and with an increase in CPK.

Given the concern about neutropenia associated with other psychotropic compounds and the finding of leukopenia associated with the administration of olanzapine in several animal models (*see* ANIMAL TOXICOLOGY), careful attention was given to examination of hematologic parameters in premarketing studies with olanzapine. There was no indication of a risk of clinically significant neutropenia associated with olanzapine treatment in the premarketing database for this drug.

ECG Changes—Between–group comparisons for pooled placebo–controlled trials revealed no statistically significant olanzapine/placebo differences in the proportions of patients experiencing potentially important changes in ECG parameters, including QT, QTc, and PR intervals. Olanzapine use was associated with a mean increase in heart rate of 2.4 beats per minute compared to no change among placebo patients. This slight tendency to tachycardia may be related to olanzapine's potential for inducing orthostatic changes (*see* PRECAUTIONS).

Other Adverse Events Observed During the Clinical Trial Evaluation of Olanzapine

Following is a list of terms that reflect treatment–emergent adverse events reported by patients treated with oral olanzapine (at multiple doses ≥1 mg/day) in clinical trials (8661 patients, 4165 patient–years of exposure). This listing may not include those events already listed in previous tables or elsewhere in labeling, those events for which a drug cause was remote, those event terms which were so general as to be uninformative, and those events reported only once or twice which did not have a substantial probability of being acutely life–threatening.

Events are further categorized by body system and listed in order of decreasing frequency according to the following definitions: frequent adverse events are those occurring in at least 1/100 patients (only those not already listed in the tabulated results from placebo–controlled trials appear in this listing); infrequent adverse events are those occurring in 1/100 to 1/1000 patients; rare events are those occurring in fewer than 1/1000 patients.

Body as a Whole—*Frequent:* dental pain and flu syndrome; *Infrequent:* abdomen enlarged, chills, face edema, intentional injury, malaise, moniliasis, neck pain, neck rigidity, pelvic pain, photosensitivity reaction, and suicide attempt; *Rare:* chills and fever, hangover effect, and sudden death.

Cardiovascular System—*Frequent:* hypotension; *Infrequent:* atrial fibrillation, bradycardia, cerebrovascular accident, congestive heart failure, heart arrest, hemorrhage, migraine, pallor, palpitation, vasodilatation, and ventricular extrasystoles; *Rare:* arteritis, heart failure, and pulmonary embolus.

Digestive System—*Frequent:* flatulence, increased salivation, and thirst; *Infrequent:* dysphagia, esophagitis, fecal impaction, fecal incontinence, gastritis, gastroenteritis, gingivitis, hepatitis, melena, mouth ulceration, nausea and vomiting, oral moniliasis, periodontal abscess, rectal hemorrhage, stomatitis, tongue edema, and tooth caries; *Rare:* aphthous stomatitis, enteritis, eructation, esophageal ulcer, glossitis, ileus, intestinal obstruction, liver fatty deposit, and tongue discoloration.

Endocrine System—*Infrequent:* diabetes mellitus; *Rare:* diabetic acidosis and goiter.

Hemic and Lymphatic System—*Infrequent:* anemia, cyanosis, leukocytosis, leukopenia, lymphadenopathy, and thrombocytopenia; *Rare:* normocytic anemia and thrombocythemia.

Metabolic and Nutritional Disorders—*Infrequent:* acidosis, alkaline phosphatase increased, bilirubinemia, dehydration, hypercholesteremia, hyperglycemia, hyperlipemia, hyperuricemia, hypoglycemia, hypokalemia, hyponatremia, lower extremity edema, and upper extremity edema; *Rare:* gout, hyperkalemia, hypernatremia, hypoproteinemia, ketosis, and water intoxication.

Musculoskeletal System—*Frequent:* joint stiffness and twitching; *Infrequent:* arthritis, arthrosis, leg cramps, and myasthenia; *Rare:* bone pain, bursitis, myopathy, osteoporosis, and rheumatoid arthritis.

Nervous System—*Frequent:* abnormal dreams, amnesia, delusions, emotional lability, euphoria, manic reaction, paresthesia, and schizophrenic reaction; *Infrequent:* akinesia, alcohol misuse, antisocial reaction, ataxia, CNS stimulation, cogwheel rigidity, delirium, dementia, depersonalization, dysarthria, facial paralysis, hypesthesia, hypokinesia, hypotonia, incoordination, libido decreased, libido increased, obsessive compulsive symptoms, phobias, somatization, stimulant misuse, stupor, stuttering, tardive dyskinesia, vertigo, and withdrawal syndrome; *Rare:* circumoral paresthesia, coma, encephalopathy, neuralgia, neuropathy, nystagmus, paralysis, subarachnoid hemorrhage, and tobacco misuse.

Treatment–Emergent Extrapyramidal Symptoms Assessed by Rating Scales Incidence in a Fixed Dosage Range, Placebo–Controlled Clinical Trial of Oral Olanzapine in Schizophrenia — Acute Phase*

		Percentage of Patients Reporting Event		
	Placebo	Olanzapine 5 ± 2.5 mg/day	Olanzapine 10 ± 2.5 mg/day	Olanzapine 15 ± 2.5 mg/day
Parkinsonism[†]	15	14	12	14
Akathisia[‡]	23	16	19	27

* No statistically significant differences.
† Percentage of patients with a Simpson–Angus Scale total score >3.
‡ Percentage of patients with a Barnes Akathisia Scale global score ≥2.

Treatment–Emergent Extrapyramidal Symptoms Assessed by Adverse Events Incidence in a Fixed Dosage Range, Placebo–Controlled Clinical Trial of Oral Olanzapine in Schizophrenia — Acute Phase

		Percentage of Patients Reporting Event		
	Placebo (N=68)	Olanzapine 5 ± 2.5 mg/day (N=65)	Olanzapine 10 ± 2.5 mg/day (N=64)	Olanzapine 15 ± 2.5 mg/day (N=69)
Dystonic events*	1	3	2	3
Parkinsonism events[†]	10	8	14	20
Akathisia events[‡]	1	5	11[§]	10[§]
Dyskinetic events[¶]	4	0	2	1
Residual events[#]	1	2	5	1
Any extrapyramidal event	16	15	25	32[§]

* Patients with the following COSTART terms were counted in this category: dystonia, generalized spasm, neck rigidity, oculogyric crisis, opisthotonos, torticollis.
† Patients with the following COSTART terms were counted in this category: akinesia, cogwheel rigidity, extrapyramidal syndrome, hypertonia, hypokinesia, masked facies, tremor.
‡ Patients with the following COSTART terms were counted in this category: akathisia, hyperkinesia.
§ Statistically significantly different from placebo.
¶ Patients with the following COSTART terms were counted in this category: buccoglossal syndrome, choreoathetosis, dyskinesia, tardive dyskinesia.
# Patients with the following COSTART terms were counted in this category: movement disorder, myoclonus, twitching.

Treatment–Emergent Extrapyramidal Symptoms Assessed by Rating Scales Incidence in a Fixed Dose, Placebo–Controlled Clinical Trial of Intramuscular Olanzapine for Injection in Agitated Patients with Schizophrenia*

		Percentage of Patients Reporting Event		
	Placebo	Olanzapine IM 2.5 mg	Olanzapine IM 5 mg	Olanzapine IM 7.5 mg	Olanzapine IM 10 mg
Parkinsonism[†]	0	0	0	0	3
Akathisia[‡]	0	0	5	0	0

* No statistically significant differences.
† Percentage of patients with a Simpson–Angus total score >3.
‡ Percentage of patients with a Barnes Akathisia Scale global score ≥2.

Treatment–Emergent Extrapyramidal Symptoms Assessed by Adverse Events Incidence in a Fixed Dose, Placebo–Controlled Clinical Trial of Intramuscular Olanzapine for Injection in Agitated Patients with Schizophrenia*

		Percentage of Patients Reporting Event		
	Placebo (N=45)	Olanzapine IM 2.5 mg (N=48)	Olanzapine IM 5 mg (N=45)	Olanzapine IM 7.5 mg (N=46)	Olanzapine IM 10 mg (N=46)
Dystonic events[†]	0	0	0	0	0
Parkinsonism events[‡]	0	4	2	0	0
Akathisia events[§]	0	2	0	0	0
Dyskinetic events[¶]	0	0	0	0	0
Residual events[#]	0	0	0	0	0
Any extrapyramidal event	0	4	2	0	0

* No statistically significant differences.
† Patients with the following COSTART terms were counted in this category: dystonia, generalized spasm, neck rigidity, oculogyric crisis, opisthotonos, torticollis.
‡ Patients with the following COSTART terms were counted in this category: akinesia, cogwheel rigidity, extrapyramidal syndrome, hypertonia, hypokinesia, masked facies, tremor.
§ Patients with the following COSTART terms were counted in this category: akathisia, hyperkinesia.
¶ Patients with the following COSTART terms were counted in this category: buccoglossal syndrome, choreoathetosis, dyskinesia, tardive dyskinesia.
# Patients with the following COSTART terms were counted in this category: movement disorder, myoclonus, twitching.

Respiratory System—*Frequent:* dyspnea; *Infrequent:* apnea, asthma, epistaxis, hemoptysis, hyperventilation, hypoxia, laryngitis, and voice alteration; *Rare:* atelectasis, hiccup, hypoventilation, lung edema, and stridor.

Skin and Appendages—*Frequent:* sweating; *Infrequent:* alopecia, contact dermatitis, dry skin, eczema, maculopapular rash, pruritus, seborrhea, skin discoloration, skin ulcer, urticaria, and vesiculobullous rash; *Rare:* hirsutism and pustular rash.

Special Senses—*Frequent:* conjunctivitis; *Infrequent:* abnormality of accommodation, blepharitis, cataract, deafness, diplopia, dry eyes, ear pain, eye hemorrhage, eye inflammation, eye pain, ocular muscle abnormality, taste perversion, and tinnitus; *Rare:* corneal lesion, glaucoma, keratoconjunctivitis, macular hypopigmentation, miosis, mydriasis, and pigment deposits lens.

Urogenital System—*Frequent:* vaginitis[1]; *Infrequent:* abnormal ejaculation[1], amenorrhea[1], breast pain, cystitis, decreased menstruation[1], dysuria, female lactation[1], glycosuria, gynecomastia, hematuria, impotence[1], increased menstruation[1], menorrhagia[1], metrorrhagia[1], polyuria, premenstrual syndrome[1], pyuria, urinary frequency, urinary retention, urinary urgency, urination impaired, uterine fibroids enlarged[1], and vaginal hemorrhage[1]; *Rare:* albuminuria, breast enlargement, mastitis, and oliguria.

Following is a list of terms that reflect treatment–emergent adverse events reported by patients treated with intramuscular olanzapine for injection (at one or more doses ≥2.5 mg/injection) in clinical trials (722 patients). This listing may not include those events already listed in previous tables or elsewhere in labeling, those events for which a drug cause was remote, those event terms which were so general as to be uninformative, and those events reported only once which did not have a substantial probability of being acutely life–threatening.

Events are further categorized by body system and listed in order of decreasing frequency according to the following definitions: frequent adverse events are those occurring in at least 1/100 patients (only those not already listed in the tabulated results from placebo–controlled trials appear in this listing); infrequent adverse events are those occurring in 1/100 to 1/1000 patients.

Body as a Whole—*Frequent:* injection site pain; *Infrequent:* abdominal pain and fever.

Cardiovascular System—*Infrequent:* AV block, heart block, and syncope.

Digestive System—*Infrequent:* diarrhea and nausea.

Hemic and Lymphatic System—*Infrequent:* anemia.

Metabolic and Nutritional Disorders—*Infrequent:* creatine phosphokinase increased, dehydration, and hyperkalemia.

Musculoskeletal System—*Infrequent:* twitching.

Nervous System—*Infrequent:* abnormal gait, akathisia, articulation impairment, confusion, and emotional lability.

Skin and Appendages—*Infrequent:* sweating.

Postintroduction Reports

Adverse events reported since market introduction that were temporally (but not necessarily causally) related to ZYPREXA therapy include the following: allergic reaction (e.g., anaphylactoid reaction, angioedema, pruritus or urticaria), diabetic coma, jaundice, neutropenia, pancreatitis, priapism, rhabdomyolysis, and venous thromboembolic events (including pulmonary embolism and deep venous thrombosis). Random cholesterol levels of ≥240 mg/dL and random triglyceride levels of ≥1000 mg/dL have been reported.

[1]Adjusted for gender.

DRUG ABUSE AND DEPENDENCE

Controlled Substance Class

Olanzapine is not a controlled substance.

Physical and Psychological Dependence

In studies prospectively designed to assess abuse and dependence potential, olanzapine was shown to have acute depressive CNS effects but little or no potential of abuse or physical dependence in rats administered oral doses up to 15 times the maximum recommended human daily oral dose (20 mg) and rhesus monkeys administered oral doses up to 8 times the maximum recommended human daily oral dose on a mg/m^2 basis.

Olanzapine has not been systematically studied in humans for its potential for abuse, tolerance, or physical dependence. While the clinical trials did not reveal any tendency for any drug–seeking behavior, these observations were not systematic, and it is not possible to predict on the basis of this limited experience the extent to which a CNS–active drug will be misused, diverted, and/or abused once marketed. Consequently, patients should be evaluated carefully for a history of drug abuse, and such patients should be observed closely for signs of misuse or abuse of olanzapine (e.g., development of tolerance, increases in dose, drug–seeking behavior).

OVERDOSAGE

Human Experience

In premarketing trials involving more than 3100 patients and/or normal subjects, accidental or intentional acute overdosage of olanzapine was identified in 67 patients. In the patient taking the largest identified amount, 300 mg, the only symptoms reported were drowsiness and slurred speech. In the limited number of patients who were evaluated in hospitals, including the patient taking 300 mg, there were no observations indicating an adverse change in laboratory analytes or ECG. Vital signs were usually within normal limits following overdoses.

Adverse Event	Placebo (N=68)	Olanzapine 5 ± 2.5 mg/day (N=65)	Olanzapine 10 ± 2.5 mg/day (N=64)	Olanzapine 15 ± 2.5 mg/day (N=69)
		Percentage of Patients Reporting Event		
Asthenia	15	8	9	20
Dry mouth	4	3	5	13
Nausea	9	0	2	9
Somnolence	16	20	30	39
Tremor	3	0	5	7

In postmarketing reports of overdose with olanzapine alone, symptoms have been reported in the majority of cases. In symptomatic patients, symptoms with ≥10% incidence included agitation/aggressiveness, dysarthria, tachycardia, various extrapyramidal symptoms, and reduced level of consciousness ranging from sedation to coma. Among less commonly reported symptoms were the following potentially medically serious events: aspiration, cardiopulmonary arrest, cardiac arrhythmias (such as supraventricular tachycardia and one patient experiencing sinus pause with spontaneous resumption of normal rhythm), delirium, possible neuroleptic malignant syndrome, respiratory depression/arrest, convulsion, hypertension, and hypotension. Eli Lilly and Company has received reports of fatality in association with overdose of olanzapine alone. In one case of death, the amount of acutely ingested olanzapine was reported to be possibly as low as 450 mg of oral olanzapine; however, in another case, a patient was reported to survive an acute olanzapine ingestion of approximately 2 g of oral olanzapine.

Overdosage Management

The possibility of multiple drug involvement should be considered. In case of acute overdosage, establish and maintain an airway and ensure adequate oxygenation and ventilation, which may include intubation. Gastric lavage (after intubation, if patient is unconscious) and administration of activated charcoal together with a laxative should be considered. The possibility of obtundation, seizures, or dystonic reaction of the head and neck following overdose may create a risk of aspiration with induced emesis. Cardiovascular monitoring should commence immediately and should include continuous electrocardiographic monitoring to detect possible arrhythmias.

There is no specific antidote to olanzapine. Therefore, appropriate supportive measures should be initiated. Hypotension and circulatory collapse should be treated with appropriate measures such as intravenous fluids and/or sympathomimetic agents. (Do not use epinephrine, dopamine, or other sympathomimetics with beta–agonist activity, since beta stimulation may worsen hypotension in the setting of olanzapine–induced alpha blockade.) Close medical supervision and monitoring should continue until the patient recovers.

DOSAGE AND ADMINISTRATION

Schizophrenia

Usual Dose—Oral olanzapine should be administered on a once–a–day schedule without regard to meals, generally beginning with 5 to 10 mg initially, with a target dose of 10 mg/day within several days. Further dosage adjustments, if indicated, should generally occur at intervals of not less than 1 week, since steady state for olanzapine would not be achieved for approximately 1 week in the typical patient. When dosage adjustments are necessary, dose increments/decrements of 5 mg QD are recommended.

Efficacy in schizophrenia was demonstrated in a dose range of 10 to 15 mg/day in clinical trials. However, doses above 10 mg/day were not demonstrated to be more efficacious than the 10 mg/day dose. An increase to a dose greater than the target dose of 10 mg/day (i.e., to a dose of 15 mg/day or greater) is recommended only after clinical assessment. The safety of doses above 20 mg/day has not been evaluated in clinical trials.

Dosing in Special Populations—The recommended starting dose is 5 mg in patients who are debilitated, who have a predisposition to hypotensive reactions, who otherwise exhibit a combination of factors that may result in slower metabolism of olanzapine (e.g., nonsmoking female patients ≥65 years of age), or who may be more pharmacodynamically sensitive to olanzapine (*see* CLINICAL PHARMACOLOGY; also *see* Use in Patients with Concomitant Illness and Drug Interactions *under* PRECAUTIONS). When indicated, dose escalation should be performed with caution in these patients.

Maintenance Treatment—While there is no body of evidence available to answer the question of how long the patient treated with olanzapine should remain on it, the effectiveness of oral olanzapine, 10 mg/day to 20 mg/day, in maintaining treatment response in schizophrenic patients who had been stable on ZYPREXA for approximately 8 weeks and were then followed for a period of up to 8 months has been demonstrated in a placebo–controlled trial (*see* CLINICAL EFFICACY DATA). Patients should be periodically reassessed to determine the need for maintenance treatment with appropriate dose.

Bipolar Disorder

Usual Monotherapy Dose—Oral olanzapine should be administered on a once–a–day schedule without regard to meals, generally beginning with 10 or 15 mg. Dosage adjustments, if indicated, should generally occur at intervals of not less than 24 hours, reflecting the procedures in the placebo–controlled trials. When dosage adjustments are necessary, dose increments/decrements of 5 mg QD are recommended.

Short–term (3–4 weeks) antimanic efficacy was demonstrated in a dose range of 5 mg to 20 mg/day in clinical trials. The safety of doses above 20 mg/day has not been evaluated in clinical trials.

Maintenance Monotherapy—The benefit of maintaining bipolar patients on monotherapy with oral ZYPREXA at a dose of 5 to 20 mg/day, after achieving a responder status for an average duration of two weeks, was demonstrated in a controlled trial (*see* CLINICAL EFFICACY DATA). The physician who elects to use ZYPREXA for extended periods should periodically re–evaluate the long–term usefulness of the drug for the individual patient.

Bipolar Mania Usual Dose in Combination with Lithium or Valproate—When administered in combination with lithium or valproate, oral olanzapine dosing should generally begin with 10 mg once–a–day without regard to meals.

Short–term (6 weeks) antimanic efficacy was demonstrated in a dose range of 5 mg to 20 mg/day in clinical trials. The safety of doses above 20 mg/day has not been evaluated in clinical trials.

Dosing in Special Populations—*See* Dosing in Special Populations *under* DOSAGE AND ADMINISTRATION, Schizophrenia.

Administration of ZYPREXA ZYDIS (olanzapine orally disintegrating tablets)

After opening sachet, peel back foil on blister. Do not push tablet through foil. Immediately upon opening the blister, using dry hands, remove tablet and place entire ZYPREXA ZYDIS in the mouth. Tablet disintegration occurs rapidly in saliva so it can be easily swallowed with or without liquid.

Agitation Associated with Schizophrenia and Bipolar I Mania

Usual Dose for Agitated Patients with Schizophrenia or Bipolar Mania—The efficacy of intramuscular olanzapine for injection in controlling agitation in these disorders was demonstrated in a dose range of 2.5 mg to 10 mg. The recommended dose in these patients is 10 mg. A lower dose of 5 or 7.5 mg may be considered when clinical factors warrant (*see* CLINICAL EFFICACY DATA). If agitation warranting additional intramuscular doses persists following the initial dose, subsequent doses up to 10 mg may be given. However, the efficacy of repeated doses of intramuscular olanzapine for injection in agitated patients has not been systematically evaluated in controlled clinical trials. Also, the safety of total daily doses greater than 30 mg, or 10 mg injections given more frequently than 2 hours after the initial dose, and 4 hours after the second dose have not been evaluated in clinical trials. Maximal dosing of intramuscular olanzapine (e.g., three doses of 10 mg administered 2–4 hours apart) may be associated with a substantial occurrence of significant orthostatic hypotension (*see* PRECAUTIONS, Hemodynamic Effects). Thus, it is recommended that patients requiring subsequent intramuscular injections be assessed for orthostatic hypotension prior to the administration of any subsequent doses of intramuscular olanzapine for injection. The administration of an additional dose to a patient with a clinically significant postural change in systolic blood pressure is not recommended.

If ongoing olanzapine therapy is clinically indicated, oral olanzapine may be initiated in a range of 5–20 mg/day as soon as clinically appropriate (*see* Schizophrenia or Bipolar Disorder *under* DOSAGE AND ADMINISTRATION).

Intramuscular Dosing in Special Populations—A dose of 5 mg per injection should be considered for geriatric patients or when other clinical factors warrant. A lower dose of 2.5 mg per injection should be considered for patients who otherwise might be debilitated, be predisposed to hypotensive reactions, or be more pharmacodynamically sensitive to olanzapine (*see* CLINICAL PHARMACOLOGY; also *see* Use in Patients with Concomitant Illness and Drug Interactions *under* PRECAUTIONS).

Administration of ZYPREXA IntraMuscular

ZYPREXA IntraMuscular is intended for intramuscular use only. Do not administer intravenously or subcutaneously. Inject slowly, deep into the muscle mass.

Parenteral drug products should be inspected visually for particulate matter and discoloration prior to administration, whenever solution and container permit.

Directions for preparation of ZYPREXA IntraMuscular with Sterile Water for Injection

Dissolve the contents of the vial using 2.1 mL of Sterile Water for Injection to provide a solution containing approximately 5 mg/mL of olanzapine. The resulting solution should appear clear and yellow. ZYPREXA IntraMuscular

Continued on next page

This product information was prepared in March 2008. Current information on products of Eli Lilly and Company may be obtained by calling 1-800-545-5979.

			TABLET STRENGTH			
	2.5 mg	5 mg	7.5 mg	10 mg	15 mg	20 mg
Tablet No.	4112	4115	4116	4117	4415	4420
Identification	LILLY	LILLY	LILLY	LILLY	LILLY	LILLY
	4112	4115	4116	4117	4415	4420
NDC Codes:						
Bottles 30	NDC 0002-	NDC 0002-	NDC 0002-	NDC 0002-	NDC 0002-	NDC 0002-
	4112-30	4115-30	4116-30	4117-30	4415-30	4420-30
Blisters – ID* 100	NDC 0002-	NDC 0002-	NDC 0002-	NDC 0002-	NDC 0002-	NDC 0002-
	4112-33	4115-33	4116-33	4117-33	4415-33	4420-33
Bottles 1000	NDC 0002-	NDC 0002-	NDC 0002-	NDC 0002-	NDC 0002-	NDC 0002-
	4112-04	4115-04	4116-04	4117-04	4415-04	4420-04

* Identi-Dose® (unit dose medication, Lilly).

		TABLET STRENGTH		
ZYPREXA ZYDIS				
Tablets	5 mg	10 mg	15 mg	20 mg
Tablet No.	4453	4454	4455	4456
Debossed	5	10	15	20
NDC Codes:				
Dose Pack 30 (Child–Resistant)	NDC 0002-	NDC 0002-	NDC 0002-	NDC 0002-
	4453-85	4454-85	4455-85	4456-85

Zyprexa—Cont.

reconstituted with Sterile Water for Injection should be used immediately (within 1 hour) after reconstitution. **Discard any unused portion.**
The following table provides injection volumes for delivering various doses of intramuscular olanzapine for injection reconstituted with Sterile Water for Injection.

Dose, mg Olanzapine	Volume of Injection, mL
10	Withdraw total contents of vial
7.5	1.5
5	1
2.5	0.5

Physical Incompatibility Information
ZYPREXA IntraMuscular should be reconstituted only with Sterile Water for Injection. ZYPREXA IntraMuscular should not be combined in a syringe with diazepam injection because precipitation occurs when these products are mixed. Lorazepam injection should not be used to reconstitute ZYPREXA IntraMuscular as this combination results in a delayed reconstitution time. ZYPREXA IntraMuscular should not be combined in a syringe with haloperidol injection because the resulting low pH has been shown to degrade olanzapine over time.

HOW SUPPLIED

The ZYPREXA 2.5 mg, 5 mg, 7.5 mg, and 10 mg tablets are white, round, and imprinted in blue ink with LILLY and tablet number. The 15 mg tablets are elliptical, blue, and debossed with LILLY and tablet number. The 20 mg tablets are elliptical, pink, and debossed with LILLY and tablet number. The tablets are available as follows:
[See first table above]
ZYPREXA ZYDIS (olanzapine orally disintegrating tablets) are yellow, round, and debossed with the tablet strength. The tablets are available as follows:
[See second table above]
ZYPREXA is a registered trademark of Eli Lilly and Company.
ZYDIS is a registered trademark of Catalent Pharma Solutions.
ZYPREXA ZYDIS (olanzapine orally disintegrating tablets) is manufactured for Eli Lilly and Company by Catalent Pharma Solutions, United Kingdom, SN5 8RU.
ZYPREXA IntraMuscular is available in:
NDC 0002-7597-01 (No. VL7597) – 10 mg vial (1s)
Store ZYPREXA tablets, ZYPREXA ZYDIS, and ZYPREXA IntraMuscular vials (before reconstitution) at controlled room temperature, 20° to 25°C (68° to 77°F) [see USP]. Reconstituted ZYPREXA IntraMuscular may be stored at controlled room temperature, 20° to 25°C (68° to 77°F) [see USP] for up to 1 hour if necessary. **Discard any unused portion of reconstituted ZYPREXA IntraMuscular.** The USP defines controlled room temperature as a temperature maintained thermostatically that encompasses the usual and customary working environment of 20° to 25°C (68° to 77°F); that results in a mean kinetic temperature calculated to be not more than 25°C; and that allows for excursions between 15° and 30°C (59° and 86°F) that are experienced in pharmacies, hospitals, and warehouses.
Protect ZYPREXA tablets and ZYPREXA ZYDIS from light and moisture. Protect ZYPREXA IntraMuscular from light, do not freeze.

ANIMAL TOXICOLOGY

In animal studies with olanzapine, the principal hematologic findings were reversible peripheral cytopenias in individual dogs dosed at 10 mg/kg (17 times the maximum recommended human daily oral dose on a mg/m² basis), dose-related decreases in lymphocytes and neutrophils in mice, and lymphopenia in rats. A few dogs treated with 10 mg/kg developed reversible neutropenia and/or reversible hemolytic anemia between 1 and 10 months of treatment. Dose-related decreases in lymphocytes and neutrophils were seen in mice given doses of 10 mg/kg (equal to 2 times the maxi-

mum recommended human daily oral dose on a mg/m² basis) in studies of 3 months' duration. Nonspecific lymphopenia, consistent with decreased body weight gain, occurred in rats receiving 22.5 mg/kg (11 times the maximum recommended human daily oral dose on a mg/m² basis) for 3 months or 16 mg/kg (8 times the maximum recommended human daily oral dose on a mg/m² basis) for 6 or 12 months. No evidence of bone marrow cytotoxicity was found in any of the species examined. Bone marrows were normocellular or hypercellular, indicating that the reductions in circulating blood cells were probably due to peripheral (non–marrow) factors.
Literature revised March 10, 2008
Eli Lilly and Company
Indianapolis, IN 46285, USA
www.ZYPREXA.com
Copyright © 1997, 2008, Eli Lilly and Company. All rights reserved.
PV 6240 AMP

Merck & Co., Inc.
PO BOX 4 WP39-206
WEST POINT, PA 19486-0004

For Medical Information Contact:
Generally:
Product and service information:
Call the Merck National Service Center, 8:00 AM to 7:00 PM (ET), Monday through Friday:
(800) NSC-MERCK
(800) 672-6372
FAX: (800) MERCK-68
FAX: (800) 637-2568
Adverse Drug Experiences:
Call the Merck National Service Center, 8:00 AM to 7:00 PM (ET), Monday through Friday:
(800) NSC-MERCK
(800) 672-6372
Pregnancy Registries
(800) 986-8999
In Emergencies:
24-hour emergency information for healthcare professionals:
(800) NSC-MERCK
(800) 672-6372
Sales and Ordering:
For product orders and direct account inquiries only, call the Order Management Center,
8:00 AM to 7:00 PM (ET), Monday through Friday:
(800) MERCK RX
(800) 637-2579

CRIXIVAN®   ℞
(INDINAVIR SULFATE)
CAPSULES

Prescribing information for this product, which appears on pages 1951–1959 of the 2008 PDR, has been revised as follows. Please write "See Supplement A" next to product heading.
In the **WARNINGS** section under the *Drug Interactions* subhead, 5th line down, the contents of the parentheses have been changed to:
(e.g., atorvastatin or rosuvastatin)
In the **PRECAUTIONS** section, in Table 9, the row beginning "HMG-CoA Reductase" has been changed to:
1st column: HMG-CoA Reductase Inhibitors: atorvastatin, rosuvastatin
2nd column: ↑atorvastatin concentration ↑rosuvastatin concentration
3rd column: Use the lowest possible dose of atorvastatin or rosuvastatin with careful monitoring, or consider other

HMG-CoA reductase inhibitors that are not primarily metabolized by CYP3A4, such as pravastatin, or fluvastatin in combination with CRIXIVAN.
Revisions based on 9640606, Issued September 2007.
In the Patient Information, under the heading **MEDICINES YOU SHOULD NOT TAKE WITH CRIXIVAN**, in the paragraph beginning "It is not recommended," in the second sentence, after (atorvastatin), add:
or CRESTOR® (rosuvastatin);
Under the heading **MEDICINES YOU CAN TAKE WITH CRIXIVAN**, delete:
CRESTOR® (rosuvastatin)
Revisions based on 9640606, Issued September 2007.

CUPRIMINE® Capsules   ℞
(Penicillamine)

Physicians planning to use penicillamine should thoroughly familiarize themselves with its toxicity, special dosage considerations, and therapeutic benefits. Penicillamine should never be used casually. Each patient should remain constantly under the close supervision of the physician. Patients should be warned to report promptly any symptoms suggesting toxicity.

DESCRIPTION

Penicillamine is a chelating agent used in the treatment of Wilson's disease. It is also used to reduce cystine excretion in cystinuria and to treat patients with severe, active rheumatoid arthritis unresponsive to conventional therapy (see INDICATIONS). It is 3-mercapto-D-valine. It is a white or practically white, crystalline powder, freely soluble in water, slightly soluble in alcohol, and insoluble in ether, acetone, benzene, and carbon tetrachloride. Although its configuration is D, it is levorotatory as usually measured:
$[\alpha]25° = -62.5° \pm 2°$ (c = 1, 1N NaOH),
D
calculated on a dried basis.
The empirical formula is $C_5H_{11}NO_2S$, giving it a molecular weight of 149.21. The structural formula is:

$$\underset{(CH_3)_2C}{\overset{SH}{|}}\underset{—}{\quad}\underset{CHCOOH}{\overset{NH_2}{|}}$$

It reacts readily with formaldehyde or acetone to form a thiazolidine-carboxylic acid.
Capsules CUPRIMINE* (Penicillamine) for oral administration contain either 125 mg or 250 mg of penicillamine. Each capsule contains the following inactive ingredients: D & C Yellow 10, gelatin, lactose, magnesium stearate, and titanium dioxide. The 125 mg capsule also contains iron oxide.

*Registered trademark of MERCK & CO., Inc.

CLINICAL PHARMACOLOGY

Penicillamine is a chelating agent recommended for the removal of excess copper in patients with Wilson's disease. From *in vitro* studies which indicate that one atom of copper combines with two molecules of penicillamine, it would appear that one gram of penicillamine should be followed by the excretion of about 200 milligrams of copper; however, the actual amount excreted is about one percent of this.
Penicillamine also reduces excess cystine excretion in cystinuria. This is done, at least in part, by disulfide interchange between penicillamine and cystine, resulting in formation of penicillamine-cysteine disulfide, a substance that is much more soluble than cystine and is excreted readily.
Penicillamine interferes with the formation of cross-links between tropocollagen molecules and cleaves them when newly formed.
The mechanism of action of penicillamine in rheumatoid arthritis is unknown although it appears to suppress disease activity. Unlike cytotoxic immunosuppressants, penicillamine markedly lowers IgM rheumatoid factor but produces no significant depression in absolute levels of serum immunoglobulins. Also unlike cytotoxic immunosuppressants which act on both, penicillamine *in vitro* depresses T-cell activity but not B-cell activity.
In vitro, penicillamine dissociates macroglobulins (rheumatoid factor) although the relationship of the activity to its effect in rheumatoid arthritis is not known.
In rheumatoid arthritis, the onset of therapeutic response to CUPRIMINE may not be seen for two or three months. In those patients who respond, however, the first evidence of suppression of symptoms such as pain, tenderness, and swelling is generally apparent within three months. The optimum duration of therapy has not been determined. If remissions occur, they may last from months to years, but usually require continued treatment (see DOSAGE AND ADMINISTRATION).
In all patients receiving penicillamine, it is important that CUPRIMINE be given on an empty stomach, at least one hour before meals or two hours after meals, and at least one hour apart from any other drug, food, milk, antacid, zinc or iron-containing preparation. This permits maximum absorption and reduces the likelihood of inactivation by metal binding in the gastrointestinal tract.
Pharmacokinetics
Penicillamine is absorbed rapidly but incompletely (40–70%) from the gastrointestinal tract, with wide inter-

individual variations. Food, antacids, and iron reduce absorption of the drug. The peak plasma concentration of penicillamine occurs 1–3 hours after ingestion. It is approximately 1–2 mg/L after an oral dose of 250 mg. The drug appears in the plasma as free penicillamine, penicillamine disulfide, and cysteine-penicillamine disulfide. When prolonged treatment is stopped, there is a slow elimination phase lasting 4–6 days.

More than 80% of plasma penicillamine is bound to proteins, especially albumin and ceruloplasmin. The drug also binds to erythrocytes and macrophages. A small fraction of the dose is metabolized in the liver to S-methyl-D-penicillamine. Excretion is mainly renal, mainly as disulfides.

INDICATIONS

CUPRIMINE is indicated in the treatment of Wilson's disease, cystinuria, and in patients with severe, active rheumatoid arthritis who have failed to respond to an adequate trial of conventional therapy. Available evidence suggests that CUPRIMINE is not of value in ankylosing spondylitis.

Wilson's Disease—Wilson's disease (hepatolenticular degeneration) occurs in individuals who have inherited an autosomal recessive defect that leads to an accumulation of copper far in excess of metabolic requirements. The excess copper is deposited in several organs and tissues, and eventually produces pathological effects primarily in the liver, where damage progresses to postnecrotic cirrhosis, and in the brain, where degeneration is widespread. Copper is also deposited as characteristic, asymptomatic, golden-brown Kayser-Fleisher rings in the corneas of all patients with cerebral symptomatology and some patients who are either asymptomatic or manifest only hepatic symptomatology.

Two types of patients require treatment for Wilson's disease: (1) the symptomatic, and (2) the asymptomatic in whom it can be assumed the disease will develop in the future if the patient is not treated.

The diagnosis, if suspected on the basis of family or individual history or physical examination, can be confirmed if the plasma copper-protein ceruloplasmin** is <20 mg/dL and either a quantitative determination in a liver biopsy specimen shows an abnormally high concentration of copper (>250 mcg/g dry weight) or Kayser-Fleischer rings are present.

Treatment has two objectives:

(1) to minimize dietary intake of copper;

(2) to promote excretion and complex formation (i.e., detoxification) of excess tissue copper.

The first objective is attained by a daily diet that contains no more than one or two milligrams of copper. Such a diet should exclude, most importantly, chocolate, nuts, shellfish, mushrooms, liver, molasses, broccoli, and cereals and dietary supplements enriched with copper, and be composed to as great an extent as possible of foods with a low copper content. Distilled or demineralized water should be used if the patient's drinking water contains more than 0.1 mg of copper per liter.

For the second objective, a copper chelating agent is used. In symptomatic patients this treatment usually produces marked neurologic improvement, fading of Kayser-Fleischer rings, and gradual amelioration of hepatic dysfunction and psychic disturbances.

Clinical experience to date suggests that life is prolonged with the above regimen.

Noticeable improvement may not occur for one to three months. Occasionally, neurologic symptoms become worse during initiation of therapy with CUPRIMINE. Despite this, the drug should not be withdrawn. Temporary interruption carries an increased risk of developing a sensitivity reaction upon resumption of therapy, although it may result in clinical improvement of neurological symptoms (see WARNINGS). If the neurological symptoms and signs continue to worsen for a month after the initiation of CUPRIMINE therapy, several short courses of treatment with 2,3-dimercaprol (BAL) while continuing CUPRIMINE may be considered.

Treatment of asymptomatic patients has been carried out for over thirty years. Symptoms and signs of the disease appear to be prevented indefinitely if daily treatment with CUPRIMINE is continued.

Cystinuria—Cystinuria is characterized by excessive urinary excretion of the dibasic amino acids, arginine, lysine, ornithine, and cystine, and the mixed disulfide of cysteine and homocysteine. The metabolic defect that leads to cystinuria is inherited as an autosomal, recessive trait. Metabolism of the affected amino acids is influenced by at least two abnormal factors: (1) defective gastrointestinal absorption and (2) renal tubular dysfunction.

Arginine, lysine, ornithine, and cysteine are soluble substances, readily excreted. There is no apparent pathology connected with their excretion in excessive quantities.

Cystine, however, is so slightly soluble at the usual range of urinary pH that it is not excreted readily, and so crystallizes and forms stones in the urinary tract. Stone formation is the only known pathology in cystinuria.

Normal daily output of cystine is 40 to 80 mg. In cystinuria, output is greatly increased and may exceed 1 g/day. At 500 to 600 mg/day, stone formation is almost certain. When it is more than 300 mg/day, treatment is indicated.

Conventional treatment is directed at keeping urinary cystine diluted enough to prevent stone formation, keeping the urine alkaline enough to dissolve as much cystine as possible, and minimizing cystine production by a diet low in methionine (the major dietary precursor of cystine). Patients must drink enough fluid to keep urine specific gravity below 1.010, take enough alkali to keep urinary pH at 7.5 to 8, and maintain a diet low in methionine. This diet is not recommended in growing children and probably is contraindicated in pregnancy because of its low protein content (see PRECAUTIONS).

When these measures are inadequate to control recurrent stone formation, CUPRIMINE may be used as additional therapy, and when patients refuse to adhere to conventional treatment, CUPRIMINE may be a useful substitute. It is capable of keeping cystine excretion to near normal values, thereby hindering stone formation and the serious consequences of pyelonephritis and impaired renal function that develop in some patients.

Bartter and colleagues depict the process by which penicillamine interacts with cystine to form penicillamine-cysteine mixed disulfide as:

CSSC + PS′ ⇄ CS′ + CSSP
PSSP + CS′ ⇄ PS′ + CSSP
CSSC + PSSP ⇄ 2 CSSP

CSSC = cystine
CS′ = deprotonated cysteine
PSSP = penicillamine disulfide
PS′ = deprotonated penicillamine sulfhydryl
CSSP = penicillamine-cysteine mixed disulfide

In this process, it is assumed that the deprotonated form of penicillamine, PS′, is the active factor in bringing about the disulfide interchange.

Rheumatoid Arthritis—Because CUPRIMINE can cause severe adverse reactions, its use in rheumatoid arthritis should be restricted to patients who have severe, active disease and who have failed to respond to an adequate trial of conventional therapy. Even then, benefit-to-risk ratio should be carefully considered. Other measures, such as rest, physiotherapy, salicylates, and corticosteroids should be used, when indicated, in conjunction with CUPRIMINE (see PRECAUTIONS).

**For quantitative test for serum ceruloplasmin see: Morell, A.G.; Windsor, J.; Sternlieb, I.; Scheinberg, I.H.: Measurement of the concentration of ceruloplasmin in serum by determination of its oxidase activity, in "Laboratory Diagnosis of Liver Disease", F.W. Sunderman; F.W. Sunderman, Jr. (eds.), St. Louis, Warren H. Green, Inc., 1968, pp. 193-195.

CONTRAINDICATIONS

Except for the treatment of Wilson's disease or certain patients with cystinuria, use of penicillamine during pregnancy is contraindicated (see WARNINGS).

Although breast milk studies have not been reported in animals or humans, mothers on therapy with penicillamine should not nurse their infants.

Patients with a history of penicillamine-related aplastic anemia or agranulocytosis should not be restarted on penicillamine (see WARNINGS and ADVERSE REACTIONS). Because of its potential for causing renal damage, penicillamine should not be administered to rheumatoid arthritis patients with a history or other evidence of renal insufficiency.

WARNINGS

The use of penicillamine has been associated with fatalities due to certain diseases such as aplastic anemia, agranulocytosis, thrombocytopenia, Goodpasture's syndrome, and myasthenia gravis.

Because of the potential for serious hematological and renal adverse reactions to occur at any time, routine urinalysis, white and differential blood cell count, hemoglobin determination, and direct platelet count must be done twice weekly, together with monitoring of the patient's skin, lymph nodes and body temperature, during the first month of therapy, every two weeks for the next five months, and monthly thereafter. Patients should be instructed to report promptly the development of signs and symptoms of granulocytopenia and/or thrombocytopenia such as fever, sore throat, chills, bruising or bleeding. The above laboratory studies should then be promptly repeated.

Leukopenia and thrombocytopenia have been reported to occur in up to five percent of patients during penicillamine therapy. Leukopenia is of the granulocytic series and may or may not be associated with an increase in eosinophils. A confirmed reduction in WBC below 3500/mm^3 mandates discontinuance of penicillamine therapy. Thrombocytopenia may be on an idiosyncratic basis, with decreased or absent megakaryocytes in the marrow, when it is part of an aplastic anemia. In other cases the thrombocytopenia is presumably on an immune basis since the number of megakaryocytes in the marrow has been reported to be normal or sometimes increased. The development of a platelet count below 100,000/mm^3, even in the absence of clinical bleeding, requires at least temporary cessation of penicillamine therapy. A progressive fall in either platelet count or WBC in three successive determinations, even though values are still within the normal range, likewise requires at least temporary cessation.

Proteinuria and/or hematuria may develop during therapy and may be warning signs of membranous glomerulopathy which can progress to a nephrotic syndrome. Close observation of these patients is essential. In some patients the proteinuria disappears with continued therapy; in others, penicillamine must be discontinued. When a patient develops proteinuria or hematuria the physician must ascertain whether it is a sign of drug-induced glomerulopathy or is unrelated to penicillamine.

Rheumatoid arthritis patients who develop moderate degrees of proteinuria may be continued cautiously on penicillamine therapy, provided that quantitative 24-hour urinary protein determinations are obtained at intervals of one to two weeks. Penicillamine dosage should not be increased under these circumstances. Proteinuria which exceeds 1 g/24 hours, or proteinuria which is progressively increasing, requires either discontinuance of the drug or a reduction in the dosage. In some patients, proteinuria has been reported to clear following reduction in dosage.

In rheumatoid arthritis patients, penicillamine should be discontinued if unexplained gross hematuria or persistent microscopic hematuria develops.

In patients with Wilson's disease or cystinuria the risks of continued penicillamine therapy in patients manifesting potentially serious urinary abnormalities must be weighed against the expected therapeutic benefits.

When penicillamine is used in cystinuria, an annual x-ray for renal stones is advised. Cystine stones form rapidly, sometimes in six months.

Up to one year or more may be required for any urinary abnormalities to disappear after penicillamine has been discontinued.

Because of rare reports of intrahepatic cholestasis and toxic hepatitis, liver function tests are recommended every six months for the duration of therapy. In Wilson's disease, these are recommended every three months, at least during the first year of treatment.

Goodpasture's syndrome has occurred rarely. The development of abnormal urinary findings associated with hemoptysis and pulmonary infiltrates on x-ray requires immediate cessation of penicillamine.

Obliterative bronchiolitis has been reported rarely. The patient should be cautioned to report immediately pulmonary symptoms such as exertional dyspnea, unexplained cough or wheezing. Pulmonary function studies should be considered at that time.

Onset of new neurological symptoms has been reported with CUPRIMINE (see ADVERSE REACTIONS). Occasionally, neurological symptoms become worse during initiation of therapy with CUPRIMINE (see INDICATIONS). Myasthenic syndrome sometimes progressing to myasthenia gravis has been reported. Ptosis and diplopia, with weakness of the extraocular muscles, are often early signs of myasthenia. In the majority of cases, symptoms of myasthenia have receded after withdrawal of penicillamine.

Most of the various forms of pemphigus have occurred during treatment with penicillamine. Pemphigus vulgaris and pemphigus foliaceus are reported most frequently, usually as a late complication of therapy. The seborrhea-like characteristics of pemphigus foliaceus may obscure an early diagnosis. When pemphigus is suspected, CUPRIMINE should be discontinued. Treatment has consisted of high doses of corticosteroids alone or, in some cases, concomitantly with an immunosuppressant. Treatment may be required for only a few weeks or months, but may need to be continued for more than a year.

Once instituted for Wilson's disease or cystinuria, treatment with penicillamine should, as a rule, be continued on a daily basis. Interruptions for even a few days have been followed by sensitivity reactions after reinstitution of therapy.

Pregnancy Category D

Penicillamine can cause fetal harm when administered to a pregnant woman. Penicillamine has been shown to be teratogenic in rats when given in doses 6 times higher than the highest dose recommended for human use. Skeletal defects, cleft palates and fetal toxicity (resorptions) have been reported.

There are no controlled studies on the use of penicillamine in pregnant women. Although normal outcomes have been reported, characteristic congenital cutis laxa and associated birth defects have been reported in infants born of mothers who received therapy with penicillamine during pregnancy. Penicillamine should be used in women of childbearing potential only when the expected benefits outweigh the possible hazards. Women on therapy with penicillamine who are of childbearing potential should be apprised of this risk, advised to report promptly any missed menstrual periods or other indications of possible pregnancy, and followed closely for early recognition of pregnancy. If this drug is used during pregnancy, or if the patient becomes pregnant while taking this drug, the patient should be apprised of the potential hazard to the fetus.

Wilson's Disease—Reported experience*** shows that continued treatment with penicillamine throughout pregnancy protects the mother against relapse of the Wilson's disease, and that discontinuation of penicillamine has deleterious effects on the mother, which may be fatal.

If penicillamine is administered during pregnancy to patients with Wilson's disease, it is recommended that the daily dosage be limited to 750 mg. If cesarean section is planned the daily dose should be reduced to 250 mg, but not lower, for the last six weeks of pregnancy and postoperatively until wound healing is complete.

Cystinuria—If possible, penicillamine should not be given during pregnancy to women with cystinuria (see CONTRA-

Continued on next page

Information on the Merck & Co., Inc., products listed on these pages is from the full prescribing information in use March 1, 2008. For information, please call 1-800-NSC-MERCK [1-800-672-6372].

Cuprimine—Cont.

INDICATIONS). There are reports of women with cystinuria on therapy with penicillamine who gave birth to infants with generalized connective tissue defects who died following abdominal surgery. If stones continue to form in these patients, the benefits of therapy to the mother must be evaluated against the risk to the fetus.

Rheumatoid Arthritis—Penicillamine should not be administered to rheumatoid arthritis patients who are pregnant (see CONTRAINDICATIONS) and should be discontinued promptly in patients in whom pregnancy is suspected or diagnosed.

There is a report that a woman with rheumatoid arthritis treated with less than one gram a day of penicillamine during pregnancy gave birth (cesarean delivery) to an infant with growth retardation, flattened face with broad nasal bridge, low set ears, short neck with loose skin folds, and unusually lax body skin.

***Scheinberg, I.H., Sternlieb, I.: N. Engl. J. Med. *293:*1300-1302, Dec. 18, 1975.

PRECAUTIONS

Some patients may experience drug fever, a marked febrile response to penicillamine, usually in the second to third week following initiation of therapy. Drug fever may sometimes be accompanied by a macular cutaneous eruption.

In the case of drug fever in patients with Wilson's disease or cystinuria, penicillamine should be temporarily discontinued until the reaction subsides. Then penicillamine should be reinstituted with a small dose that is gradually increased until the desired dosage is attained. Systemic steroid therapy may be necessary, and is usually helpful, in such patients in whom drug fever and rash develop several times.

In the case of drug fever in rheumatoid arthritis patients, because other treatments are available, penicillamine should be discontinued and another therapeutic alternative tried since experience indicates that the febrile reaction will recur in a very high percentage of patients upon readministration of penicillamine.

The skin and mucous membranes should be observed for allergic reactions. Early and late rashes have occurred. Early rash occurs during the first few months of treatment and is more common. It is usually a generalized pruritic, erythematous, maculopapular or morbilliform rash and resembles the allergic rash seen with other drugs. Early rash usually disappears within days after stopping penicillamine and seldom recurs when the drug is restarted at a lower dosage.

Pruritus and early rash may often be controlled by the concomitant administration of antihistamines. Less commonly, a late rash may be seen, usually after six months or more of treatment, and requires discontinuation of penicillamine. It is usually on the trunk, is accompanied by intense pruritus, and is usually unresponsive to topical corticosteroid therapy. Late rash may take weeks to disappear after penicillamine is stopped and usually recurs if the drug is restarted.

The appearance of a drug eruption accompanied by fever, arthralgia, lymphadenopathy or other allergic manifestations usually requires discontinuation of penicillamine.

Certain patients will develop a positive antinuclear antibody (ANA) test and some of these may show a lupus erythematosus-like syndrome similar to drug-induced lupus associated with other drugs. The lupus erythematosus-like syndrome is not associated with hypocomplementemia and may be present without nephropathy. The development of a positive ANA test does not mandate discontinuance of the drug; however, the physician should be alerted to the possibility that a lupus erythematosus-like syndrome may develop in the future.

Some patients may develop oral ulcerations which in some cases have the appearance of aphthous stomatitis. The stomatitis usually recurs on rechallenge but often clears on a lower dosage. Although rare, cheilosis, glossitis and gingivostomatitis have also been reported. These oral lesions are frequently dose-related and may preclude further increase in penicillamine dosage or require discontinuation of the drug.

Hypogeusia (a blunting or diminution in taste perception) has occurred in some patients. This may last two to three months or more and may develop into a total loss of taste; however, it is usually self-limited despite continued penicillamine treatment. Such taste impairment is rare in patients with Wilson's disease.

Penicillamine should not be used in patients who are receiving concurrently gold therapy, antimalarial or cytotoxic drugs, oxyphenbutazone or phenylbutazone because these drugs are also associated with similar serious hematologic and renal adverse reactions. Patients who have had gold salt therapy discontinued due to a major toxic reaction may be at greater risk of serious adverse reactions with penicillamine but not necessarily of the same type.

Patients who are allergic to penicillin may theoretically have cross-sensitivity to penicillamine. The possibility of reactions from contamination of penicillamine by trace amounts of penicillin has been eliminated now that penicillamine is being produced synthetically rather than as a degradation product of penicillin.

Patients with Wilson's disease or cystinuria should be given 25 mg/day of pyridoxine during therapy, since penicillamine increases the requirement for this vitamin. Patients also may receive benefit from a multivitamin preparation, although there is no evidence that deficiency of any vitamin other than pyridoxine is associated with penicillamine. In Wilson's disease, multivitamin preparations must be copper-free.

Rheumatoid arthritis patients whose nutrition is impaired should also be given a daily supplement of pyridoxine. Mineral supplements should not be given, since they may block the response to penicillamine.

Iron deficiency may develop, especially in pediatric patients and in menstruating women. In Wilson's disease, this may be a result of adding the effects of the low copper diet, which is probably also low in iron, and the penicillamine to the effects of blood loss or growth. In cystinuria, a low methionine diet may contribute to iron deficiency, since it is necessarily low in protein. If necessary, iron may be given in short courses, but a period of two hours should elapse between administration of penicillamine and iron, since orally administered iron has been shown to reduce the effects of penicillamine.

Penicillamine causes an increase in the amount of soluble collagen. In the rat this results in inhibition of normal healing and also a decrease in tensile strength of intact skin. In man this may be the cause of increased skin friability at sites especially subject to pressure or trauma, such as shoulders, elbows, knees, toes, and buttocks. Extravasations of blood may occur and may appear as purpuric areas, with external bleeding if the skin is broken, or as vesicles containing dark blood. Neither type is progressive. There is no apparent association with bleeding elsewhere in the body and no associated coagulation defect has been found. Therapy with penicillamine may be continued in the presence of these lesions. They may not recur if dosage is reduced. Other reported effects probably due to the action of penicillamine on collagen are excessive wrinkling of the skin and development of small, white papules at venipuncture and surgical sites.

The effects of penicillamine on collagen and elastin make it advisable to consider a reduction in dosage to 250 mg/day, when surgery is contemplated. Reinstitution of full therapy should be delayed until wound healing is complete.

Carcinogenesis, Mutagenesis, Impariment of Fertility

Long-term animal carcinogenicity studies have not been done with penicillamine. There is a report that five of ten autoimmune disease-prone NZB hybrid mice developed lymphocytic leukemia after 6 months' intraperitoneal treatment with a dose of 400 mg/kg penicillamine 5 days per week.

Penicillamine is directly mutagenic to *S. typhimurium* strain TA92 in the Ames test; mutagenicity is enhanced by kidney postmitochondrial subcellular fraction 9. penicillamine does not induce gene mutations in Chinese hamster V79 cells.

Penicillamine induces sister-chromatid exchanges and chromosome aberrations in cultivated mammalian cells. No studies on the effect of penicillamine on fertility are available.

Pregnancy

Pregnancy Category D

(see WARNINGS, Pregnancy)

Nursing Mothers

See CONTRAINDICATIONS.

Pediatric Use

The efficacy of CUPRIMINE in juvenile rheumatoid arthritis has not been established.

Geriatric Use

Clinical studies of CUPRIMINE are limited in subjects aged 65 and over; they did not include sufficient numbers of elderly subjects aged 65 and over to adequately determine whether they respond differently from younger subjects. Review of reported clinical trials with penicillamine in the elderly suggest greater risk than in younger patients for overall skin rash and abnormality of taste. In general, dose selection for an elderly patient should be cautious, starting at the low end of the dosing range, reflecting the greater frequency of decreased hepatic, renal or cardiac function, and of concomitant disease or other drugs.

This drug is known to be substantially excreted by the kidney, and the risk of toxic reactions to this drug may be greater inpatients with impaired renal function. Because elderly patients are more likely to have decreased renal function, care should be taken in dose selection, and careful monitoring of renal function is recommended.

ADVERSE REACTIONS

Penicillamine is a drug with a high incidence of untoward reactions, some of which are potentially fatal. Therefore, it is mandatory that patients receiving penicillamine therapy remain under close medical supervision throughout the period of drug administration (see WARNINGS and PRECAUTIONS).

Reported incidences (%) for the most commonly occurring adverse reactions in rheumatoid arthritis patients are noted, based on 17 representative clinical trials reported in the literature (1270 patients).

Allergic—Generalized pruritus, early and late rashes (5%), pemphigus (see WARNINGS), and drug eruptions which may be accompanied by fever, arthralgia, or lymphadenopathy have occurred (see WARNINGS and PRECAUTIONS). Some patients may show a lupus erythematosus-like syndrome similar to drug-induced lupus produced by other pharmacological agents (see PRECAUTIONS).

Urticaria and exfoliative dermatitis have occurred.

Thyroiditis has been reported; hypoglycemia in association with anti-insulin antibodies has been reported. These reactions are extremely rare.

Some patients may develop a migratory polyarthralgia, often with objective synovitis (see DOSAGE AND ADMINISTRATION).

Gastrointestinal—Anorexia, epigastric pain, nausea, vomiting, or occasional diarrhea may occur (17%).

Isolated cases of reactivated peptic ulcer have occurred, as have hepatic dysfunction including hepatic failure, and pancreatitis. Intrahepatic cholestasis and toxic hepatitis have been reported rarely. There have been a few reports of increased serum alkaline phosphatase, lactic dehydrogenase, and positive cephalin flocculation and thymol turbidity tests.

Some patients may report a blunting, diminution, or total loss of taste perception (12%); or may develop oral ulcerations. Although rare, cheilosis, glossitis, and gingivostomatitis have been reported (see PRECAUTIONS).

Gastrointestinal side effects are usually reversible following cessation of therapy.

Hematological—Penicillamine can cause bone marrow depression (see WARNINGS). Leukopenia (2%) and thrombocytopenia (4%) have occurred. Fatalities have been reported as a result of thrombocytopenia, agranulocytosis, aplastic anemia, and sideroblastic anemia.

Thrombotic thrombocytopenic purpura, hemolytic anemia, red cell aplasia, monocytosis, leukocytosis, eosinophilia, and thrombocytosis have also been reported.

Renal—Patients on penicillamine therapy may develop proteinuria (6%) and/or hematuria which, in some, may progress to the development of the nephrotic syndrome as a result of an immune complex membranous glomerulopathy (see WARNINGS). Renal failure has been reported.

Central Nervous System—Tinnitus, optic neuritis and peripheral sensory and motor neuropathies (including polyradiculoneuropathy, i.e., Guillain-Barre syndrome) have been reported. Muscular weakness may or may not occur with the peripheral neuropathies. Visual and psychic disturbances; mental disorders; and agitation and anxiety have been reported.

Neuromuscular—Myasthenia gravis (see WARNINGS); dystonia.

Other—Adverse reactions that have been reported rarely include thrombophlebitis; hyperpyrexia (see PRECAUTIONS); falling hair or alopecia; lichen planus; polymyositis; dermatomyositis; mammary hyperplasia; elastosis perforans serpiginosa; toxic epidermal necrolysis; anetoderma (cutaneous macular atrophy); and Goodpasture's syndrome, a severe and ultimately fatal glomerulonephritis associated with intra-alveolar hemorrhage (see WARNINGS). Vasculitis, including fatal renal vasculitis, has also been reported. Allergic alveolitis, obliterative bronchiolitis, interstitial pneumonitis and pulmonary fibrosis have been reported in patients with severe rheumatoid arthritis, some of whom were receiving penicillamine. Bronchial asthma also has been reported.

Increased skin friability, excessive wrinkling of skin, and development of small white papules at venipuncture and surgical sites have been reported (see PRECAUTIONS); yellow nail syndrome.

The chelating action of the drug may cause increased excretion of other heavy metals such as zinc, mercury and lead.

There have been reports associating penicillamine with leukemia. However, circumstances involved in these reports are such that a cause and effect relationship to the drug has not been established.

DOSAGE AND ADMINISTRATION

In all patients receiving penicillamine, it is important that CUPRIMINE be given on an empty stomach, at least one hour before meals or two hours after meals, and at least one hour apart from any other drug, food, or milk. Because penicillamine increases the requirement for pyridoxine, patients may require a daily supplement of pyridoxine (see PRECAUTIONS).

Wilson's Disease—Optimal dosage can be determined by measurement of urinary copper excretion and the determination of free copper in the serum. The urine must be collected in copper-free glassware, and should be quantitatively analyzed for copper before and soon after initiation of therapy with CUPRIMINE.

Determination of 24-hour urinary copper excretion is of greatest value in the first week of therapy with penicillamine. In the absence of any drug reaction, a dose between 0.75 and 1.5 g that results in an initial 24-hour cupriuresis of over 2 mg should be continued for about three months, by which time the most reliable method of monitoring maintenance treatment is the determination of free copper in the serum. This equals the difference between quantitatively determined total copper and ceruloplasmin-copper. Adequately treated patients will usually have less than 10 mcg free copper/dL of serum. It is seldom necessary to exceed a dosage of 2 g/day. If the patient is intolerant to therapy with CUPRIMINE, alternative treatment is trientine hydrochloride.

In patients who cannot tolerate as much as 1 g/day initially, initiating dosage with 250 mg/day, and increasing gradually to the requisite amount, gives closer control of the effects of the drug and may help to reduce the incidence of adverse reactions.

Cystinuria—It is recommended that CUPRIMINE be used along with conventional therapy. By reducing urinary cystine, it decreases crystalluria and stone formation. In some instances, it has been reported to decrease the size of, and even to dissolve, stones already formed.

The usual dosage of CUPRIMINE in the treatment of cystinuria is 2 g/day for adults, with a range of 1 to 4 g/day. For pediatric patients, dosage can be based on 30 mg/kg/day. The total daily amount should be divided into four doses. If four equal doses are not feasible, give the larger portion at bedtime. If adverse reactions necessitate a reduction in dosage, it is important to retain the bedtime dose.

Initiating dosage with 250 mg/day, and increasing gradually to the requisite amount, gives closer control of the effects of the drug and may help to reduce the incidence of adverse reactions.

In addition to taking CUPRIMINE, patients should drink copiously. It is especially important to drink about a pint of fluid at bedtime and another pint once during the night when urine is more concentrated and more acid than during the day. The greater the fluid intake, the lower the required dosage of CUPRIMINE.

Dosage must be individualized to an amount that limits cystine excretion to 100-200 mg/day in those with no history of stones, and below 100 mg/day in those who have had stone formation and/or pain. Thus, in determining dosage, the inherent tubular defect, the patient's size, age, and rate of growth, and his diet and water intake all must be taken into consideration.

The standard nitroprusside cyanide test has been reported useful as a qualitative measure of the effective dose:† Add 2 mL of freshly prepared 5 percent sodium cyanide to 5 mL of a 24-hour aliquot of protein-free urine and let stand ten minutes. Add 5 drops of freshly prepared 5 percent sodium nitroprusside and mix. Cystine will turn the mixture magenta. If the result is negative, it can be assumed that cystine excretion is less than 100 mg/g creatinine.

Although penicillamine is rarely excreted unchanged, it also will turn the mixture magenta. If there is any question as to which substance is causing the reaction, a ferric chloride test can be done to eliminate doubt: Add 3 percent ferric chloride dropwise to the urine. Penicillamine will turn the urine an immediate and quickly fading blue. Cystine will not produce any change in appearance.

---

† Lotz, M., Potts, J.T. and Bartter, F.C.: Brit. Med. J. *2:* 521, Aug. 28, 1965 (in Medical Memoranda).

Rheumatoid Arthritis—The principal rule of treatment with CUPRIMINE in rheumatoid arthritis is patience. The onset of therapeutic response is typically delayed. Two or three months may be required before the first evidence of a clinical response is noted (see CLINICAL PHARMACOLOGY).

When treatment with CUPRIMINE has been interrupted because of adverse reactions or other reasons, the drug should be reintroduced cautiously by starting with a lower dosage and increasing slowly.

Initial Therapy—The currently recommended dosage regimen in rheumatoid arthritis begins with a single daily dose of 125 mg or 250 mg which is thereafter increased at one to three month intervals, by 125 mg or 250 mg/day, as patient response and tolerance indicate. If a satisfactory remission of symptoms is achieved, the dose associated with the remission should be continued (see *Maintenance Therapy*). If there is no improvement and there are no signs of potentially serious toxicity after two to three months of treatment with doses of 500-750 mg/day, increases of 250 mg/day at two to three month intervals may be continued until a satisfactory remission occurs (see *Maintenance Therapy*) or signs of toxicity develop (see WARNINGS and PRECAUTIONS). If there is no discernible improvement after three to four months of treatment with 1000 to 1500 mg of penicillamine/day, it may be assumed the patient will not respond and CUPRIMINE should be discontinued.

Maintenance Therapy—The maintenance dosage of CUPRIMINE must be individualized, and may require adjustment during the course of treatment. Many patients respond satisfactorily to a dosage within the 500-750 mg/day range. Some need less.

Changes in maintenance dosage levels may not be reflected clinically or in the erythrocyte sedimentation rate for two to three months after each dosage adjustment.

Some patients will subsequently require an increase in the maintenance dosage to achieve maximal disease suppression. In those patients who do respond, but who evidence incomplete suppression of their disease after the first six to nine months of treatment, the daily dosage of CUPRIMINE may be increased by 125 mg or 250 mg/day at three-month intervals. It is unusual in current practice to employ a dosage in excess of 1 g/day, but up to 1.5 g/day has sometimes been required.

Management of Exacerbations—During the course of treatment some patients may experience an exacerbation of disease activity following an initial good response. These may be self-limited and can subside within twelve weeks. They are usually controlled by the addition of non-steroidal anti-inflammatory drugs, and only if the patient has demonstrated a true "escape" phenomenon (as evidenced by failure of the flare to subside within this time period) should an increase in the maintenance dose ordinarily be considered.

In the rheumatoid patient, migratory polyarthralgia due to penicillamine is extremely difficult to differentiate from an exacerbation of the rheumatoid arthritis. Discontinuance or a substantial reduction in dosage of CUPRIMINE for up to several weeks will usually determine which of these processes is responsible for the arthralgia.

Duration of Therapy—The optimum duration of therapy with CUPRIMINE in rheumatoid arthritis has not been determined. If the patient has been in remission for six months or more, a gradual, stepwise dosage reduction in decrements of 125 mg or 250 mg/day at approximately three month intervals may be attempted.

Concomitant Drug Therapy—CUPRIMINE should not be used in patients who are receiving gold therapy, antimalarial or cytotoxic drugs, oxyphenbutazone, or phenylbutazone (see PRECAUTIONS). Other measures, such as salicylates, other non-steroidal anti-inflammatory drugs, or systemic corticosteroids, may be continued when penicillamine is initiated. After improvement commences, analgesic and anti-inflammatory drugs may be slowly discontinued as symptoms permit. Steroid withdrawal must be done gradually, and many months of treatment with CUPRIMINE may be required before steroids can be completely eliminated.

Dosage Frequency—Based on clinical experience dosages up to 500 mg/day can be given as a single daily dose. Dosages in excess of 500 mg/day should be administered in divided doses.

HOW SUPPLIED

No. 3299—Capsules CUPRIMINE, 250 mg, are ivory-colored capsules containing a white or nearly white powder, and are coded CUPRIMINE and MSD 602. They are supplied as follows:

NDC 0006-0602-68 in bottles of 100.

No. 3350—Capsules CUPRIMINE, 125 mg, are opaque ivory and gray capsules containing a white or nearly white powder, and are coded CUPRIMINE and MSD 672. They are supplied as follows:

NDC 0006-0672-68 in bottles of 100.

Storage

Keep container tightly closed.

7873244, Issued October 2004

COPYRIGHT © MERCK & CO., Inc., 1985, 1989, 1992
All rights reserved

DEMSER® Capsules ℞
(Metyrosine)

DESCRIPTION

DEMSER* (Metyrosine) is (−)-α-methyl-*L*-tyrosine or (α-MPT). It has the following structural formula:

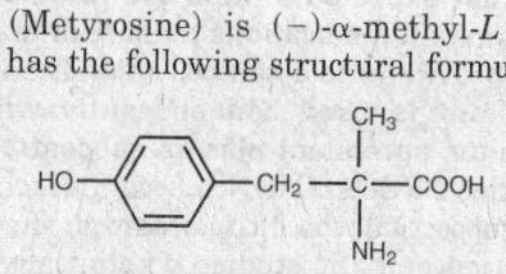

Metyrosine is a white, crystalline compound of molecular weight 195. It is very slightly soluble in water, acetone, and methanol, and insoluble in chloroform and benzene. It is soluble in acidic aqueous solutions. It is also soluble in alkaline aqueous solutions, but is subject to oxidative degradation under these conditions.

DEMSER is supplied as capsules, for oral administration. Each capsule contains 250 mg metyrosine. Inactive ingredients are colloidal silicon dioxide, gelatin, hydroxypropyl cellulose, magnesium stearate, titanium dioxide, and FD&C Blue 2.

---

*Registered trademark of MERCK & CO., Inc.

COPYRIGHT © MERCK & CO., Inc., 1985
All rights reserved

CLINICAL PHARMACOLOGY

DEMSER inhibits tyrosine hydroxylase, which catalyzes the first transformation in catecholamine biosynthesis, i.e., the conversion of tyrosine to dihydroxyphenylalanine (DOPA). Because the first step is also the rate-limiting step, blockade of tyrosine hydroxylase activity results in decreased endogenous levels of catecholamines, usually measured as decreased urinary excretion of catecholamines and their metabolites.

In patients with pheochromocytoma, who produce excessive amounts of norepinephrine and epinephrine, administration of one to four grams of DEMSER per day has reduced catecholamine biosynthesis from about 35 to 80 percent as measured by the total excretion of catecholamines and their metabolites (metanephrine and vanillylmandelic acid). The maximum biochemical effect usually occurs within two to three days, and the urinary concentration of catecholamines and their metabolites usually returns to pretreatment levels within three to four days after DEMSER is discontinued. In some patients the total excretion of catecholamines and catecholamine metabolites may be lowered to normal or near normal levels (less than 10 mg/24 hours). In most patients the duration of treatment has been two to eight weeks, but several patients have received DEMSER for periods of one to 10 years.

Most patients with pheochromocytoma treated with DEMSER experience decreased frequency and severity of hypertensive attacks with their associated headache, nausea, sweating, and tachycardia. In patients who respond, blood pressure decreases progressively during the first two days of therapy with DEMSER; after withdrawal, blood pressure usually increases gradually to pretreatment values within two to three days.

Metyrosine is well absorbed from the gastrointestinal tract. From 53 to 88 percent (mean 69 percent) was recovered in the urine as unchanged drug following maintenance oral doses of 600 to 4000 mg/24 hours in patients with pheochromocytoma or essential hypertension. Less than 1% of the dose was recovered as catechol metabolites. These metabolites are probably not present in sufficient amounts to contribute to the biochemical effects of metyrosine. The quantities excreted, however, are sufficient to interfere with accurate determination of urinary catecholamines determined by routine techniques.

Plasma half-life of metyrosine determined over an 8-hour period after single oral doses was 3.4–3.7 hours in three patients.

For further information, refer to: Sjoerdsma, A.; Engelman, K.; Waldman, T. A.; Cooperman, L. H.; Hammond, W. G.: Pheochromocytoma: Current concepts of diagnosis and treatment, Ann. Intern. Med. *65:* 1302–1326, Dec. 1966.

INDICATIONS AND USAGE

DEMSER is indicated in the treatment of patients with pheochromocytoma for:

1. Preoperative preparation of patients for surgery
2. Management of patients when surgery is contraindicated
3. Chronic treatment of patients with malignant pheochromocytoma.

DEMSER is not recommended for the control of essential hypertension.

CONTRAINDICATIONS

DEMSER is contraindicated in persons known to be hypersensitive to this compound.

WARNINGS

Maintain Fluid Volume During and After Surgery

When DEMSER is used preoperatively, alone or especially in combination with alpha-adrenergic blocking drugs, adequate intravascular volume must be maintained intraoperatively (especially after tumor removal) and postoperatively to avoid hypotension and decreased perfusion of vital organs resulting from vasodilatation and expanded volume capacity. Following tumor removal, large volumes of plasma may be needed to maintain blood pressure and central venous pressure within the normal range.

In addition, life-threatening arrhythmias may occur during anesthesia and surgery, and may require treatment with a beta blocker or lidocaine. During surgery, patients should have continuous monitoring of blood pressure and electrocardiogram.

Intraoperative Effects

While the preoperative use of DEMSER in patients with pheochromocytoma is thought to decrease intraoperative problems with blood pressure control, DEMSER does not eliminate the danger of hypertensive crises or arrhythmias during manipulation of the tumor, and the alpha-adrenergic blocking drug, phentolamine, may be needed.

Interaction with Alcohol

DEMSER may add to the sedative effects of alcohol and other CNS depressants, e.g., hypnotics, sedatives, and tranquilizers. (See PRECAUTIONS, *Information for Patients* and *Drug Interactions*.)

PRECAUTIONS

General

Metyrosine Crystalluria: **Crystalluria and urolithiasis have been found in dogs treated with DEMSER (Metyrosine) at doses similar to those used in humans, and crystalluria has also been observed in a few patients. To minimize the risk of crystalluria, patients should be urged to maintain water intake sufficient to achieve a daily urine volume of 2000 mL or more, particularly when doses greater than 2 g per day are given. Routine examination of the urine should be carried out. Metyrosine will crystallize as needles or rods. If metyrosine crystalluria occurs, fluid intake should be increased further. If crystalluria persists, the dosage should be reduced or the drug discontinued.**

Relatively Little Data Regarding Long-term Use: The total human experience with the drug is quite limited and few patients have been studied long-term. Chronic animal studies have not been carried out. Therefore, suitable laboratory tests should be carried out periodically in patients requiring prolonged use of DEMSER and caution should be observed in patients with impaired hepatic or renal function.

Information for Patients

When receiving DEMSER, patients should be warned about engaging in activities requiring mental alertness and motor coordination, such as driving a motor vehicle or operating machinery. DEMSER may have additive sedative effects with alcohol and other CNS depressants, e.g., hypnotics, sedatives, and tranquilizers.

Patients should be advised to maintain a liberal fluid intake. (See PRECAUTIONS, *General*.)

Drug Interactions

Caution should be observed in administering DEMSER to patients receiving phenothiazines or haloperidol because the extrapyramidal effects of these drugs can be expected to be potentiated by inhibition of catecholamine synthesis.

Concurrent use of DEMSER with alcohol or other CNS depressants can increase their sedative effects. (See WARNINGS and PRECAUTIONS, *Information for Patients*.)

Laboratory Test Interference

Spurious increases in urinary catecholamines may be observed in patients receiving DEMSER due to the presence of metabolites of the drug.

Carcinogenesis, Mutagenesis, Impairment of Fertility

Long-term carcinogenic studies in animals and studies on mutagenesis and impairment of fertility have not been performed with metyrosine.

Continued on next page

Information on the Merck & Co., Inc., products listed on these pages is from the full prescribing information in use March 1, 2008. For information, please call 1-800-NSC-MERCK [1-800-672-6372].

Demser—Cont.

Pregnancy

Pregnancy Category C. Animal reproduction studies have not been conducted with DEMSER. It is also not known whether DEMSER can cause fetal harm when administered to a pregnant woman or can affect reproduction capacity. DEMSER should be given to a pregnant woman only if clearly needed.

Nursing Mothers

It is not known whether DEMSER is excreted in human milk. Because many drugs are excreted in human milk, caution should be exercised when DEMSER is administered to a nursing woman.

Pediatric Use

Safety and effectiveness in pediatric patients below the age of 12 years have not been established.

Geriatric Use

Clinical studies of DEMSER did not include sufficient numbers of subjects aged 65 and over to determine whether they respond differently from younger subjects. Other reported clinical experience has not identified differences in responses between the elderly and younger patients. In general, dose selection for an elderly patient should be cautious, usually starting at the low end of the dosing range, reflecting the greater frequency of decreased hepatic, renal, or cardiac function, and of concomitant disease or other drug therapy.

ADVERSE REACTIONS

Central Nervous System

Sedation: The most common adverse reaction to DEMSER is moderate to severe sedation, which has been observed in almost all patients. It occurs at both low and high dosages. Sedative effects begin within the first 24 hours of therapy, are maximal after two to three days, and tend to wane during the next few days. Sedation usually is not obvious after one week unless the dosage is increased, but at dosages greater than 2000 mg/day some degree of sedation or fatigue may persist.

In most patients who experience sedation, temporary changes in sleep pattern occur following withdrawal of the drug. Changes consist of insomnia that may last for two or three days and feelings of increased alertness and ambition. Even patients who do not experience sedation while on DEMSER may report symptoms of psychic stimulation when the drug is discontinued.

Extrapyramidal Signs: Extrapyramidal signs such as drooling, speech difficulty, and tremor have been reported in approximately 10 percent of patients. These occasionally have been accompanied by trismus and frank parkinsonism.

Anxiety and Psychic Disturbances: Anxiety and psychic disturbances such as depression, hallucinations, disorientation, and confusion may occur. These effects seem to be dose-dependent and may disappear with reduction of dosage.

Diarrhea

Diarrhea occurs in about 10 percent of patients and may be severe. Anti-diarrheal agents may be required if continuation of DEMSER is necessary.

Miscellaneous

Infrequently, slight swelling of the breast, galactorrhea, nasal stuffiness, decreased salivation, dry mouth, headache, nausea, vomiting, abdominal pain, and impotence or failure of ejaculation may occur. Crystalluria (see PRECAUTIONS) and transient dysuria and hematuria have been observed in a few patients. Hematologic disorders (including eosinophilia, anemia, thrombocytopenia, and thrombocytosis), increased SGOT levels, peripheral edema, and hypersensitivity reactions such as urticaria and pharyngeal edema have been reported rarely.

OVERDOSAGE

Signs of metyrosine overdosage include those central nervous system effects observed in some patients even at low dosages.

At doses exceeding 2000 mg/day, some degree of sedation or feeling of fatigue may persist. Doses of 2000–4000 mg/day can result in anxiety or agitated depression, neuromuscular effects (including fine tremor of the hands, gross tremor of the trunk, tightening of the jaw with trismus), diarrhea, and decreased salivation with dry mouth.

Reduction of drug dose or cessation of treatment results in the disappearance of these symptoms.

The acute toxicity of metyrosine was 442 mg/kg and 752 mg/kg in the female mouse and rat respectively.

DOSAGE AND ADMINISTRATION

The recommended initial dosage of DEMSER for adults and children 12 years of age and older is 250 mg orally four times daily. This may be increased by 250 mg to 500 mg every day to a maximum of 4.0 g/day in divided doses. When used for preoperative preparation, the optimally effective dosage of DEMSER should be given for at least five to seven days.

Optimally effective dosages of DEMSER usually are between 2.0 and 3.0 g/day, and the dose should be titrated by monitoring clinical symptoms and catecholamine excretion. In patients who are hypertensive, dosage should be titrated to achieve normalization of blood pressure and control of clinical symptoms. In patients who are usually normotensive, dosage should be titrated to the amount that will reduce urinary metanephrines and/or vanillylmandelic acid by 50 percent or more.

If patients are not adequately controlled by the use of DEMSER, an alpha-adrenergic blocking agent (phenoxybenzamine) should be added.

Use of DEMSER in children under 12 years of age has been limited and a dosage schedule for this age group cannot be given.

HOW SUPPLIED

No. 3355—Capsules DEMSER, 250 mg, are opaque, two-toned blue capsules coded MSD 690 on one side and DEMSER on the other. They are supplied as follows:
NDC 0006-0690-68 bottles of 100.

7900809 Issued April 2002

EMEND® ℞
[ē' mĕnd]
(aprepitant)
CAPSULES

Prescribing information for this product, which appears on pages 1968–1975 of the 2008 PDR, has been revised as follows. Please write "See Supplement A" next to the product heading.

In the **CONTRAINDICATIONS** section, in the first paragraph, replace "CYP3A4" in the first sentence with "cytochrome P450 isoenzyme 3A4 (CYP3A)". In the third sentence, replace "cytochrome P450 isoenzyme 3A4 (CYP3A)" with "CYP3A4".

In the **PRECAUTIONS** section, the first 3 paragraphs in the *General* subsection should read: **EMEND, a dose-dependent inhibitor of CYP3A4, should be used with caution in patients receiving concomitant medications that are primarily metabolized through CYP3A4. Moderate inhibition of CYP3A4 by aprepitant, 125 mg/80 mg regimen, could result in elevated plasma concentrations of these concomitant medications.**

Weak inhibition of CYP3A4 by a single 40 mg dose of aprepitant is not expected to alter the plasma concentrations of concomitant medications that are primarily metabolized through CYP3A4 to a clinically significant degree.

When aprepitant is used concomitantly with another CYP3A4 inhibitor, aprepitant plasma concentrations could be elevated (See PRECAUTIONS, *Drug Interactions*).

In the same subsection, the fifth paragraph should read: In separate pharmacokinetic studies no clinically significant change in docetaxel or vinorelbine pharmacokinetics was observed when EMEND (125 mg/80 mg regimen) was co-administered.

In the subsection *Effect of aprepitant on the pharmacokinetics of other agents*, add the following new paragraph after the paragraph labeled *Docetaxel:*

Vinorelbine: In a pharmacokinetic study, EMEND (125mg/80 mg regimen) did not influence the pharmacokinetics of vinorelbine to a clinically significant degree.

In the **DOSAGE AND ADMINISTRATION** section, add the following sentence as a separate paragraph under the first bulleted subhead:

EMEND (aprepitant) is available as capsules for oral administration.

In the second paragraph, add "orally" between "80 mg" and "once daily". Then add the following new paragraph:

EMEND (fosaprepitant dimeglumine) for Injection is a lyophilized prodrug of aprepitant containing polysorbate 80 (PS80) and may be substituted for oral EMEND (125 mg), 30 minutes prior to chemotherapy, on Day 1 only of the CINV regimen as an intravenous infusion administered over 15 minutes.

In the **HOW SUPPLIED** section, replace the line directly under the first paragraph with:
NDC 0006-0461-02 unit-of-use bi-fold package of 2
In the same section, delete "**NDC** 0006-0461-30 bottles of 30 (with dessicant)".

Also, at the end of this section, add: U.S. Patent Nos.: 5,145,684; 5,719,147; 6,048,859; 6,096,742; 6,235,735 Revisions based on 9738707, issued November 2007, and 9852008, issued February 2008.
Patient Information
EMEND® (EE mend)
(aprepitant) Capsules
Patient information for this product, which appears on pages 1974 and 1975 of the 2008 PDR, has been revised as follows. Please write "See Supplement A" next to the product heading.
The section **How should I take EMEND?** should now read:
• Take EMEND exactly as prescribed.
• EMEND (aprepitant) is a capsule that you swallow with a drink.
If you are a cancer patient, the recommended 3-day regimen includes:
• **Day 1:** one 125-mg capsule of EMEND (white/pink) by mouth 1 hour before you start your chemotherapy treatment;
  AND
• **Day 2 and Day 3:** one 80-mg capsule (white) by mouth of EMEND each morning for the 2 days following your chemotherapy treatment.
Your doctor may substitute EMEND (fosaprepitant dimeglumine) for Injection (115 mg) for EMEND (aprepitant) capsules (125 mg) 30 minutes prior to your chemotherapy treatment on Day 1 only. You still need to take one 80-mg capsule (white) of EMEND by mouth each morning for the 2 days following your chemotherapy treatment.
In the same section, delete the bullets before the last 3 paragraphs.

At the end of the Patient Information, add: U.S. Patent Nos.: 5,145,684; 5,719,147; 6,048,859; 6,096,742; 6,235,735 Revisions based on 9738805, issued September 2006, and 9738806, issued February 2008.

GARDASIL® ℞
[GARD-ah-sill]
[Human Papillomavirus Quadrivalent (Types 6, 11, 16, and 18) Vaccine, Recombinant]

Prescribing information for this product, which appears on pages 1989–1994 of the 2008 PDR, has been revised as follows. Please write "See Supplement A" next to the product heading.

In the **ADVERSE REACTIONS** section, under *Post-marketing Reports*, after the line "Gastrointestinal disorders: Nausea, vomiting." insert the following 2 lines:
Musculoskeletal and connective tissue disorders: Arthralgia, myalgia.
General disorders and administrative site conditions: Asthenia, fatigue, malaise.

In the **DOSAGE AND ADMINISTRATION** section, under *Method of Administration*, replace the third paragraph with the following:
Syncope (fainting) may follow any vaccination, especially in adolescents and young adults. Syncope, sometimes associated with falling, has occurred after vaccination with GARDASIL. Therefore, vaccinees should be carefully observed for approximately 15 minutes after administration of GARDASIL (See ADVERSE REACTIONS, *Post-Marketing Reports*).

Replace the subheading *Prefilled Syringe Use* with *Prefilled Syringe Use With and Without Needle Guard (Safety) Device.*
Immediately after this subheading, insert the sub-subheading *Prefilled Syringe With Needle Guard (Safety) Device.*
After the *Prefilled Syringe With Needle Guard (Safety) Device* section, insert the following sub-subheading and text:
Prefilled Syringe Without Needle Guard (Safety) Device
This package does not contain a needle guard (safety device) or a needle. Shake well before use. Attach the needle by twisting in a clockwise direction until the needle fits securely on the syringe. Administer the entire dose as per standard protocol.

In the **HOW SUPPLIED** section, under *Syringes*, delete the first paragraph. After the second paragraph, insert the following paragraph:
No. 4109 — GARDASIL is supplied as a carton of six 0.5-mL single-dose prefilled Luer Lock syringes with tip caps. **NDC** 0006-4109-09.
Revisions based on 9682306, issued November 2007, and 9682307, issued December 2007.

In the **Patient Information**, in the **What are the possible side effects of GARDASIL?** section, replace the fifth paragraph with the following:
Additional side effects reported include swollen glands (neck, armpit, or groin), Guillain-Barré syndrome, headache, joint pain, aching muscles, unusual tiredness or weakness, and generally feeling unwell.
Revisions based on 9682306, issued November 2007, and 9682307, issued December 2007.

INVANZ® ℞
(ertapenem for injection)

Prescribing information for this product, which appears on pages 2005–2012 of the 2008 PDR, has been revised as follows. Please write "See Supplement A" next to the product heading.

In the **WARNINGS** section, after the first paragraph, add the subhead *Seizure Potential*, and after the next paragraph, add the following new paragraph:
Carbapenems, including ertapenem, may reduce serum valproic acid concentrations to subtherapeutic levels, resulting in loss of seizure control. Serum valproic acid concentrations should be monitored frequently after initiating carbapenem therapy. Alternative antibacterial or anticonvulsant therapy should be considered if serum valproic acid concentrations drop below the therapeutic range or a seizure occurs. (See PRECAUTIONS, *Drug Interactions*.)

In the **PRECAUTIONS** section, under *Drug Interactions*, delete the last paragraph and replace it with the following new paragraph:
A clinically significant reduction in serum valproic acid concentration has been reported in patients receiving carbapenem antibiotics and may result in loss of seizure control. Although the mechanism of this interaction is not fully understood, data from *in vitro* and animal studies suggest that carbapenem antibiotics may inhibit valproic acid glucuronide hydrolysis. Serum valproic acid concentrations should be monitored frequently after initiating carbapenem therapy. Alternative antibacterial or anticonvulsant therapy should be considered if serum valproic acid concentrations drop below the therapeutic range or a seizure occurs. (See WARNINGS, *Seizure Potential*.)

Revisions based on 9709705, issued December 2007, and 9709706, issued February 2008.

JANUMET™
(sitagliptin/metformin HCl) tablets

Rx

Prescribing information for this product, which appears on pages 2012–2017 of the 2008 PDR, has been completely revised as follows. Please write "See Supplement A" next to the product heading.

HIGHLIGHTS OF PRESCRIBING INFORMATION
These highlights do not include all the information needed to use JANUMET safely and effectively. See full prescribing information for JANUMET.
JANUMET™ (sitagliptin/metformin HCl) tablets
Initial U.S. Approval: 2007

WARNING: LACTIC ACIDOSIS

See full prescribing information for complete boxed warning.

- **Lactic acidosis can occur due to metformin accumulation. The risk increases with conditions such as sepsis, dehydration, excess alcohol intake, hepatic insufficiency, renal impairment, and acute congestive heart failure. (5.1)**
- **Symptoms include malaise, myalgias, respiratory distress, increasing somnolence, and nonspecific abdominal distress. Laboratory abnormalities include low pH, increased anion gap and elevated blood lactate. (5.1)**
- **If acidosis is suspected, discontinue JANUMET and hospitalize the patient immediately. (5.1)**

RECENT MAJOR CHANGES

Indications and Usage (1)	2/2008
Dosage and Administration	
Recommended Dosing (2.1)	2/2008
Contraindications (4)	1/2008
Warnings and Precautions	
Use with Medications Known to Cause Hypoglycemia (5.8)	2/2008
Hypersensitivity Reactions (5.13)	1/2008
Macrovascular Outcomes (5.14)	2/2008

INDICATIONS AND USAGE

JANUMET is a dipeptidyl peptidase-4 (DPP-4) inhibitor and biguanide combination product indicated as an adjunct to diet and exercise to improve glycemic control in adults with type 2 diabetes mellitus when treatment with both sitagliptin and metformin is appropriate. (1)
Important Limitations of Use:
- JANUMET should not be used in patients with type 1 diabetes or for the treatment of diabetic ketoacidosis. (1)
- JANUMET has not been studied in combination with insulin. (1)

DOSAGE AND ADMINISTRATION

- Individualize the starting dose of JANUMET based on the patient's current regimen. (2.1)
- May adjust the dosing based on effectiveness and tolerability while not exceeding the maximum recommended daily dose of 100 mg sitagliptin and 2000 mg metformin. (2.1)
- JANUMET should be given twice daily with meals, with gradual dose escalation, to reduce the gastrointestinal (GI) side effects due to metformin. (2.1)

DOSAGE FORMS AND STRENGTHS

Tablets: 50 mg sitagliptin/500 mg metformin HCl and 50 mg sitagliptin/1000 mg metformin HCl (3)

CONTRAINDICATIONS

- Renal dysfunction, e.g., serum creatinine ≥1.5 mg/dL [males], ≥1.4 mg/dL [females] or abnormal creatinine clearance. (4, 5.1, 5.3)
- Acute or chronic metabolic acidosis, including diabetic ketoacidosis, with or without coma. (4, 5.1)
- History of a serious hypersensitivity reaction to JANUMET or sitagliptin (one of the components of JANUMET), such as anaphylaxis or angioedema. (5.13, 6.2)
- Temporarily discontinue JANUMET in patients undergoing radiologic studies involving intravascular administration of iodinated contrast materials. (4, 5.1, 5.10)

WARNINGS AND PRECAUTIONS

- Do not use JANUMET in patients with hepatic disease. (5.1, 5.2)
- Before initiating JANUMET and at least annually thereafter, assess renal function and verify as normal. (4, 5.1, 5.3, 5.9)
- Measure hematologic parameters annually. (5.4, 6.1)
- Warn patients against excessive alcohol intake. (5.1, 5.5)
- May need to discontinue JANUMET and temporarily use insulin during periods of stress and decreased intake of fluids and food as may occur with fever, trauma, infection or surgery. (5.6, 5.7, 5.11, 5.12)
- Promptly evaluate patients previously controlled on JANUMET who develop laboratory abnormalities or clinical illness for evidence of ketoacidosis or lactic acidosis. (5.1, 5.7, 5.11, 5.12)
- When used with an insulin secretagogue (e.g., sulfonylurea, meglitinide), a lower dose of the insulin secretagogue may be required to reduce the risk of hypoglycemia. (2.1, 5.8)
- There have been postmarketing reports of serious allergic and hypersensitivity reactions in patients treated with sitagliptin (one of the components of JANUMET), such as anaphylaxis, angioedema, and exfoliative skin conditions including Stevens-Johnson syndrome. In such cases, promptly stop JANUMET, assess for other potential causes, institute appropriate monitoring and treatment, and initiate alternative treatment for diabetes. (5.13, 6.2)

- There have been no clinical studies establishing conclusive evidence of macrovascular risk reduction with JANUMET or any other oral anti-diabetic drug. (5.14)

ADVERSE REACTIONS

- The most common adverse reactions reported in ≥5% of patients simultaneously started on sitagliptin and metformin and more commonly than in patients treated with placebo were diarrhea, upper respiratory tract infection, and headache. (6.1)
- Adverse reactions reported in ≥5% of patients treated with sitagliptin in combination with sulfonylurea and metformin and more commonly than in patients treated with placebo in combination with sulfonylurea and metformin were hypoglycemia and headache. (6.1)
- Nasopharyngitis was the only adverse reaction reported in ≥5% of patients treated with sitagliptin monotherapy and more commonly than in patients given placebo. (6.1)
- The most common (>5%) adverse reactions due to initiation of metformin therapy are diarrhea, nausea/vomiting, flatulence, abdominal discomfort, indigestion, asthenia, and headache. (6.1)

To report SUSPECTED ADVERSE REACTIONS, contact Merck & Co., Inc. at 1-877-888-4231 or FDA at 1-800-FDA-1088 or www.fda.gov/medwatch.

DRUG INTERACTIONS

- Cationic drugs eliminated by renal tubular secretion: Use with caution. (5.9, 7.1)

USE IN SPECIFIC POPULATIONS

- Safety and effectiveness of JANUMET in children under 18 years have not been established. (8.4)
- There are no adequate and well-controlled studies in pregnant women. To report drug exposure during pregnancy call 1-800-986-8999. (8.1)

See 17 for PATIENT COUNSELING INFORMATION and FDA-approved patient labeling.

Revised: 2/2008

FULL PRESCRIBING INFORMATION: CONTENTS*

*Sections or subsections omitted from the full prescribing information are not listed.

FULL PRESCRIBING INFORMATION

WARNING: LACTIC ACIDOSIS

Lactic acidosis is a rare, but serious complication that can occur due to metformin accumulation. The risk increases with conditions such as sepsis, dehydration, excess alcohol intake, hepatic insufficiency, renal impairment, and acute congestive heart failure.

The onset is often subtle, accompanied only by nonspecific symptoms such as malaise, myalgias, respiratory distress, increasing somnolence, and nonspecific abdominal distress.

Laboratory abnormalities include low pH, increased anion gap and elevated blood lactate.

If acidosis is suspected, JANUMET[1] should be discontinued and the patient hospitalized immediately. [See Warnings and Precautions (5.1).]

---

1 INDICATIONS AND USAGE

JANUMET is indicated as an adjunct to diet and exercise to improve glycemic control in adults with type 2 diabetes mellitus when treatment with both sitagliptin and metformin is appropriate. [See Clinical Studies (14).]
Important Limitations of Use
JANUMET should not be used in patients with type 1 diabetes or for the treatment of diabetic ketoacidosis, as it would not be effective in these settings.
JANUMET has not been studied in combination with insulin.

2 DOSAGE AND ADMINISTRATION
2.1 Recommended Dosing
The dosage of antihyperglycemic therapy with JANUMET should be individualized on the basis of the patient's current regimen, effectiveness, and tolerability while not exceeding the maximum recommended daily dose of 100 mg sitagliptin and 2000 mg metformin. Initial combination therapy or maintenance of combination therapy should be individualized and left to the discretion of the health care provider.
JANUMET should generally be given twice daily with meals, with gradual dose escalation, to reduce the gastrointestinal (GI) side effects due to metformin.
The starting dose of JANUMET should be based on the patient's current regimen. JANUMET should be given twice daily with meals. The following doses are available:
  50 mg sitagliptin/500 mg metformin hydrochloride
  50 mg sitagliptin/1000 mg metformin hydrochloride.
Patients inadequately controlled with diet and exercise alone
If therapy with a combination tablet containing sitagliptin and metformin is considered appropriate for a patient with type 2 diabetes mellitus inadequately controlled with diet and exercise alone, the recommended starting dose is 50 mg sitagliptin/500 mg metformin hydrochloride twice daily. Patients with inadequate glycemic control on this dose can be titrated up to 50 mg sitagliptin/1000 mg metformin hydrochloride twice daily.
Patients inadequately controlled on metformin monotherapy
If therapy with a combination tablet containing sitagliptin and metformin is considered appropriate for a patient inadequately controlled on metformin alone, the recommended starting dose of JANUMET should provide sitagliptin dosed as 50 mg twice daily (100 mg total daily dose) and the dose of metformin already being taken. For patients taking metformin 850 mg twice daily, the recommended starting dose of JANUMET is 50 mg sitagliptin/1000 mg metformin hydrochloride twice daily.
Patients inadequately controlled on sitagliptin monotherapy
If therapy with a combination tablet containing sitagliptin and metformin is considered appropriate for a patient inadequately controlled on sitagliptin alone, the recommended starting dose of JANUMET is 50 mg sitagliptin/500 mg metformin hydrochloride twice daily. Patients with inadequate control on this dose can be titrated up to 50 mg sitagliptin/1000 mg metformin hydrochloride twice daily. Patients taking sitagliptin monotherapy dose-adjusted for renal insufficiency should not be switched to JANUMET [see Contraindications (4)].
Patients switching from co-administration of sitagliptin and metformin
For patients switching from sitagliptin co-administered with metformin, JANUMET may be initiated at the dose of sitagliptin and metformin already being taken.
Patients inadequately controlled on dual combination therapy with any two of the following antihyperglycemic agents: sitagliptin, metformin or a sulfonylurea
If therapy with a combination tablet containing sitagliptin and metformin is considered appropriate in this setting, the usual starting dose of JANUMET should provide sitagliptin dosed as 50 mg twice daily (100 mg total daily dose). In determining the starting dose of the metformin component, the patient's level of glycemic control and current dose (if any) of metformin should be considered. Gradual dose escalation to reduce the gastrointestinal (GI) side effects associated with metformin should be considered. Patients currently on or initiating a sulfonylurea may require lower sulfonylurea doses to reduce the risk of hypoglycemia [see Warnings and Precautions (5.9)].
No studies have been performed specifically examining the safety and efficacy of JANUMET in patients previously treated with other oral antihyperglycemic agents and switched to JANUMET. Any change in therapy of type 2 diabetes should be undertaken with care and appropriate monitoring as changes in glycemic control can occur.

Continued on next page

Information on the Merck & Co., Inc., products listed on these pages is from the full prescribing information in use March 1, 2008. For information, please call 1-800-NSC-MERCK [1-800-672-6372].

Janumet—Cont.

3 DOSAGE FORMS AND STRENGTHS

- 50 mg/500 mg tablets are light pink, capsule-shaped, film-coated tablets with "575" debossed on one side.
- 50 mg/1000 mg tablets are red, capsule-shaped, film-coated tablets with "577" debossed on one side.

4 CONTRAINDICATIONS

JANUMET (sitagliptin/metformin HCl) is contraindicated in patients with:

- Renal disease or renal dysfunction, e.g., as suggested by serum creatinine levels ≥1.5 mg/dL [males], ≥1.4 mg/dL [females] or abnormal creatinine clearance which may also result from conditions such as cardiovascular collapse (shock), acute myocardial infarction, and septicemia *[see Warnings and Precautions (5.1)].*
- Acute or chronic metabolic acidosis, including diabetic ketoacidosis, with or without coma.
- History of a serious hypersensitivity reaction to JANUMET or sitagliptin (one of the components of JANUMET), such as anaphylaxis or angioedema. *[See Warnings and Precautions (5.13) and Adverse Reactions (6.2).]*

JANUMET should be temporarily discontinued in patients undergoing radiologic studies involving intravascular administration of iodinated contrast materials, because use of such products may result in acute alteration of renal function *[see Warnings and Precautions (5.10)].*

5 WARNINGS AND PRECAUTIONS

5.1 Lactic Acidosis

Metformin hydrochloride

Lactic acidosis is a rare, but serious, metabolic complication that can occur due to metformin accumulation during treatment with JANUMET; when it occurs, it is fatal in approximately 50% of cases. Lactic acidosis may also occur in association with a number of pathophysiologic conditions, including diabetes mellitus, and whenever there is significant tissue hypoperfusion and hypoxemia. Lactic acidosis is characterized by elevated blood lactate levels (>5 mmol/L), decreased blood pH, electrolyte disturbances with an increased anion gap, and an increased lactate/pyruvate ratio. When metformin is implicated as the cause of lactic acidosis, metformin plasma levels >5 μg/mL are generally found. The reported incidence of lactic acidosis in patients receiving metformin hydrochloride is very low (approximately 0.03 cases/1000 patient-years, with approximately 0.015 fatal cases/1000 patient-years). In more than 20,000 patient-years exposure to metformin in clinical trials, there were no reports of lactic acidosis. Reported cases have occurred primarily in diabetic patients with significant renal insufficiency, including both intrinsic renal disease and renal hypoperfusion, often in the setting of multiple concomitant medical/surgical problems and multiple concomitant medications. Patients with congestive heart failure requiring pharmacologic management, in particular those with unstable or acute congestive heart failure who are at risk of hypoperfusion and hypoxemia, are at increased risk of lactic acidosis. The risk of lactic acidosis increases with the degree of renal dysfunction and the patient's age. The risk of lactic acidosis may, therefore, be significantly decreased by regular monitoring of renal function in patients taking metformin and by use of the minimum effective dose of metformin. In particular, treatment of the elderly should be accompanied by careful monitoring of renal function. Metformin treatment should not be initiated in patients ≥80 years of age unless measurement of creatinine clearance demonstrates that renal function is not reduced, as these patients are more susceptible to developing lactic acidosis. In addition, metformin should be promptly withheld in the presence of any condition associated with hypoxemia, dehydration, or sepsis. Because impaired hepatic function may significantly limit the ability to clear lactate, metformin should generally be avoided in patients with clinical or laboratory evidence of hepatic disease. Patients should be cautioned against excessive alcohol intake, either acute or chronic, when taking metformin, since alcohol potentiates the effects of metformin hydrochloride on lactate metabolism. In addition, metformin should be temporarily discontinued prior to any intravascular radiocontrast study and for any surgical procedure *[see Warnings and Precautions (5.3, 5.5, 5.6, 5.10)].*

The onset of lactic acidosis often is subtle, and accompanied only by nonspecific symptoms such as malaise, myalgias, respiratory distress, increasing somnolence, and nonspecific abdominal distress. There may be associated hypothermia, hypotension, and resistant bradyarrhythmias with more marked acidosis. The patient and the patient's physician must be aware of the possible importance of such symptoms and the patient should be instructed to notify the physician immediately if they occur *[see Warnings and Precautions (5.11)].* Metformin should be withdrawn until the situation is clarified. Serum electrolytes, ketones, blood glucose, and if indicated, blood pH, lactate levels, and even blood metformin levels may be useful. Once a patient is stabilized on any dose level of metformin, gastrointestinal symptoms, which are common during initiation of therapy, are unlikely to be drug related. Later occurrence of gastrointestinal symptoms could be due to lactic acidosis or other serious disease.

Levels of fasting venous plasma lactate above the upper limit of normal but less than 5 mmol/L in patients taking metformin do not necessarily indicate impending lactic acidosis and may be explainable by other mechanisms, such as poorly controlled diabetes or obesity, vigorous physical activity, or technical problems in sample handling *[see Warnings and Precautions (5.7, 5.12)].*

Lactic acidosis should be suspected in any diabetic patient with metabolic acidosis lacking evidence of ketoacidosis (ketonuria and ketonemia).

Lactic acidosis is a medical emergency that must be treated in a hospital setting. In a patient with lactic acidosis who is taking metformin, the drug should be discontinued immediately and general supportive measures promptly instituted. Because metformin hydrochloride is dialyzable (with a clearance of up to 170 mL/min under good hemodynamic conditions), prompt hemodialysis is recommended to correct the acidosis and remove the accumulated metformin. Such management often results in prompt reversal of symptoms and recovery *[see Contraindications (4); Warnings and Precautions (5.5, 5.6, 5.9, 5.10, 5.11)].*

5.2 Impaired Hepatic Function

Since impaired hepatic function has been associated with some cases of lactic acidosis, JANUMET should generally be avoided in patients with clinical or laboratory evidence of hepatic disease.

5.3 Assessment of Renal Function

Metformin and sitagliptin are known to be substantially excreted by the kidney. The risk of metformin accumulation and lactic acidosis increases with the degree of impairment of renal function. Thus, patients with serum creatinine levels above the upper limit of normal for their age should not receive JANUMET. In the elderly, JANUMET should be carefully titrated to establish the minimum dose for adequate glycemic effect, because aging can be associated with reduced renal function. *[See Warnings and Precautions (5.1) and Use in Specific Populations (8.5).]*

Before initiation of therapy with JANUMET and at least annually thereafter, renal function should be assessed and verified as normal. In patients in whom development of renal dysfunction is anticipated, particularly in elderly patients, renal function should be assessed more frequently and JANUMET discontinued if evidence of renal impairment is present.

5.4 Vitamin B₁₂ Levels

In controlled clinical trials of metformin of 29 weeks duration, a decrease to subnormal levels of previously normal serum Vitamin B_{12} levels, without clinical manifestations, was observed in approximately 7% of patients. Such decrease, possibly due to interference with B_{12} absorption from the B_{12}-intrinsic factor complex, is, however, very rarely associated with anemia and appears to be rapidly reversible with discontinuation of metformin or Vitamin B_{12} supplementation. Measurement of hematologic parameters on an annual basis is advised in patients on JANUMET and any apparent abnormalities should be appropriately investigated and managed. *[See Adverse Reactions (6.1).]*

Certain individuals (those with inadequate Vitamin B_{12} or calcium intake or absorption) appear to be predisposed to developing subnormal Vitamin B_{12} levels. In these patients, routine serum Vitamin B_{12} measurements at two- to three-year intervals may be useful.

5.5 Alcohol Intake

Alcohol is known to potentiate the effect of metformin on lactate metabolism. Patients, therefore, should be warned against excessive alcohol intake, acute or chronic, while receiving JANUMET.

5.6 Surgical Procedures

Use of JANUMET should be temporarily suspended for any surgical procedure (except minor procedures not associated with restricted intake of food and fluids) and should not be restarted until the patient's oral intake has resumed and renal function has been evaluated as normal.

5.7 Change in Clinical Status of Patients with Previously Controlled Type 2 Diabetes

A patient with type 2 diabetes previously well controlled on JANUMET who develops laboratory abnormalities or clinical illness (especially vague and poorly defined illness) should be evaluated promptly for evidence of ketoacidosis or lactic acidosis. Evaluation should include serum electrolytes and ketones, blood glucose and, if indicated, blood pH, lactate, pyruvate, and metformin levels. If acidosis of either form occurs, JANUMET must be stopped immediately and other appropriate corrective measures initiated.

5.8 Use with Medications Known to Cause Hypoglycemia

Sitagliptin

As is typical with other antihyperglycemic agents used in combination with a sulfonylurea, when sitagliptin was used in combination with metformin and a sulfonylurea, a medication known to cause hypoglycemia, the incidence of hypoglycemia was increased over that of placebo in combination with metformin and a sulfonylurea *[see Adverse Reactions (6)].* Therefore, patients also receiving an insulin secretagogue (e.g., sulfonylurea, meglitinide) may require a lower dose of the insulin secretagogue to reduce the risk of hypoglycemia *[see Dosage and Administration (2.1)].*

Metformin hydrochloride

Hypoglycemia does not occur in patients receiving metformin alone under usual circumstances of use, but could occur when caloric intake is deficient, when strenuous exercise is not compensated by caloric supplementation, or during concomitant use with other glucose-lowering agents (such as sulfonylureas and insulin) or ethanol. Elderly, debilitated, or malnourished patients, and those with adrenal or pituitary insufficiency or alcohol intoxication are particularly susceptible to hypoglycemic effects. Hypoglycemia may be difficult to recognize in the elderly, and in people who are taking β-adrenergic blocking drugs.

5.9 Concomitant Medications Affecting Renal Function or Metformin Disposition

Concomitant medication(s) that may affect renal function or result in significant hemodynamic change or may interfere with the disposition of metformin, such as cationic drugs that are eliminated by renal tubular secretion *[see Drug Interactions (7.1)],* should be used with caution.

5.10 Radiologic Studies with Intravascular Iodinated Contrast Materials

Intravascular contrast studies with iodinated materials (for example, intravenous urogram, intravenous cholangiography, angiography, and computed tomography (CT) scans with intravascular contrast materials) can lead to acute alteration of renal function and have been associated with lactic acidosis in patients receiving metformin *[see Contraindications (4)].* Therefore, in patients in whom any such study is planned, JANUMET should be temporarily discontinued at the time of or prior to the procedure, and withheld for 48 hours subsequent to the procedure and reinstituted only after renal function has been re-evaluated and found to be normal.

5.11 Hypoxic States

Cardiovascular collapse (shock) from whatever cause, acute congestive heart failure, acute myocardial infarction and other conditions characterized by hypoxemia have been associated with lactic acidosis and may also cause prerenal azotemia. When such events occur in patients on JANUMET therapy, the drug should be promptly discontinued.

5.12 Loss of Control of Blood Glucose

When a patient stabilized on any diabetic regimen is exposed to stress such as fever, trauma, infection, or surgery, a temporary loss of glycemic control may occur. At such times, it may be necessary to withhold JANUMET and temporarily administer insulin. JANUMET may be reinstituted after the acute episode is resolved.

5.13 Hypersensitivity Reactions

There have been postmarketing reports of serious hypersensitivity reactions in patients treated with sitagliptin, one of the components of JANUMET. These reactions include anaphylaxis, angioedema, and exfoliative skin conditions including Stevens-Johnson syndrome. Because these reactions are reported voluntarily from a population of uncertain size, it is generally not possible to reliably estimate their frequency or establish a causal relationship to drug exposure. Onset of these reactions occurred within the first 3 months after initiation of treatment with sitagliptin, with some reports occurring after the first dose. If a hypersensitivity reaction is suspected, discontinue JANUMET, assess for other potential causes for the event, and institute alternative treatment for diabetes. *[See Adverse Reactions (6.2).]*

5.14 Macrovascular Outcomes

There have been no clinical studies establishing conclusive evidence of macrovascular risk reduction with JANUMET or any other oral anti-diabetic drug.

6 ADVERSE REACTIONS

6.1 Clinical Trials Experience

Because clinical trials are conducted under widely varying conditions, adverse reaction rates observed in the clinical trials of a drug cannot be directly compared to rates in the clinical trials of another drug and may not reflect the rates observed in practice.

Sitagliptin and Metformin Co-administration in Patients with Type 2 Diabetes Inadequately Controlled on Diet and Exercise

Table 1 summarizes the most common (≥5% of patients) adverse reactions reported (regardless of investigator assessment of causality) in a 24-week placebo-controlled factorial study in which sitagliptin and metformin were co-administered to patients with type 2 diabetes inadequately controlled on diet and exercise.

[See table 1 at bottom of next page]

Sitagliptin Add-on Therapy in Patients with Type 2 Diabetes Inadequately Controlled on Metformin Alone

In a 24-week placebo-controlled trial of sitagliptin 100 mg administered once daily added to a twice daily metformin regimen, there were no adverse reactions reported regardless of investigator assessment of causality in ≥5% of patients and more commonly than in patients given placebo. Discontinuation of therapy due to clinical adverse reactions was similar to the placebo treatment group (sitagliptin and metformin, 1.9%; placebo and metformin, 2.5%).

Hypoglycemia

Adverse reactions of hypoglycemia were based on all reports of hypoglycemia; a concurrent glucose measurement was not required. The overall incidence of pre-specified adverse reactions of hypoglycemia in patients with type 2 diabetes inadequately controlled on diet and exercise was 0.6% in patients given placebo, 0.6% in patients given sitagliptin alone, 0.8% in patients given metformin alone, and 1.6% in patients given sitagliptin in combination with metformin. In patients with type 2 diabetes inadequately controlled on metformin alone, the overall incidence of adverse reactions of hypoglycemia was 1.3% in patients given add-on sitagliptin and 2.1% in patients given add-on placebo.

Gastrointestinal Adverse Reactions

The incidences of pre-selected gastrointestinal adverse experiences in patients treated with sitagliptin and metformin were similar to those reported for patients treated with metformin alone. See Table 2.

[See table 2 at bottom of next page]

Sitagliptin in Combination with Metformin and Glimepiride
In a 24-week placebo-controlled study of sitagliptin 100 mg as add-on therapy in patients with type 2 diabetes inadequately controlled on metformin and glimepiride (sitagliptin, N=116; placebo, N=113), the adverse reactions reported regardless of investigator assessment of causality in ≥5% of patients treated with sitagliptin and more commonly than in patients treated with placebo were: hypoglycemia (sitagliptin, 16.4%; placebo, 0.9%) and headache (6.9%, 2.7%).

No clinically meaningful changes in vital signs or in ECG (including in QTc interval) were observed with the combination of sitagliptin and metformin.

The most common adverse experience in sitagliptin monotherapy reported regardless of investigator assessment of causality in ≥5% of patients and more commonly than in patients given placebo was nasopharyngitis.

The most common (>5%) established adverse reactions due to initiation of metformin therapy are diarrhea, nausea/vomiting, flatulence, abdominal discomfort, indigestion, asthenia, and headache.

Laboratory Tests
Sitagliptin
The incidence of laboratory adverse reactions was similar in patients treated with sitagliptin and metformin (7.6%) compared to patients treated with placebo and metformin (8.7%). In most but not all studies, a small increase in white blood cell count (approximately 200 cells/microL difference in WBC vs placebo; mean baseline WBC approximately 6600 cells/microL) was observed due to a small increase in neutrophils. This change in laboratory parameters is not considered to be clinically relevant.

Metformin hydrochloride
In controlled clinical trials of metformin of 29 weeks duration, a decrease to subnormal levels of previously normal serum Vitamin B_{12} levels, without clinical manifestations, was observed in approximately 7% of patients. Such decrease, possibly due to interference with B_{12} absorption from the B_{12}-intrinsic factor complex, is, however, very rarely associated with anemia and appears to be rapidly reversible with discontinuation of metformin or Vitamin B_{12} supplementation. *[See Warnings and Precautions (5.4).]*

6.2 Postmarketing Experience
The following additional adverse reactions have been identified during postapproval use of JANUMET or sitagliptin, one of the components of JANUMET. Because these reactions are reported voluntarily from a population of uncer-

tain size, it is generally not possible to reliably estimate their frequency or establish a causal relationship to drug exposure.

Hypersensitivity reactions include anaphylaxis, angioedema, rash, urticaria and exfoliative skin conditions including Stevens-Johnson syndrome *[see Warnings and Precautions (5.13)]*; upper respiratory tract infection.

7 DRUG INTERACTIONS
7.1 Cationic Drugs
Cationic drugs (e.g., amiloride, digoxin, morphine, procainamide, quinidine, quinine, ranitidine, triamterene, trimethoprim, or vancomycin) that are eliminated by renal tubular secretion theoretically have the potential for interaction with metformin by competing for common renal tubular transport systems. Such interaction between metformin and oral cimetidine has been observed in normal healthy volunteers in both single- and multiple-dose metformin-cimetidine drug interaction studies, with a 60% increase in peak metformin plasma and whole blood concentrations and a 40% increase in plasma and whole blood metformin AUC. There was no change in elimination half-life in the single-dose study. Metformin had no effect on cimetidine pharmacokinetics. Although such interactions remain theoretical (except for cimetidine), careful patient monitoring and dose adjustment of JANUMET and/or the interfering drug is recommended in patients who are taking cationic medications that are excreted via the proximal renal tubular secretory system.

7.2 Digoxin
There was a slight increase in the area under the curve (AUC, 11%) and mean peak drug concentration (C_{max}, 18%) of digoxin with the co-administration of 100 mg sitagliptin for 10 days. These increases are not considered likely to be clinically meaningful. Digoxin, as a cationic drug, has the potential to compete with metformin for common renal tubular transport systems, thus affecting the serum concentrations of either digoxin, metformin or both. Patients receiving digoxin should be monitored appropriately. No dosage adjustment of digoxin or JANUMET is recommended.

7.3 Glyburide
In a single-dose interaction study in type 2 diabetes patients, co-administration of metformin and glyburide did not result in any changes in either metformin pharmacokinetics or pharmacodynamics. Decreases in glyburide AUC and C_{max} were observed, but were highly variable. The single-dose nature of this study and the lack of correlation

between glyburide blood levels and pharmacodynamic effects make the clinical significance of this interaction uncertain.

7.4 Furosemide
A single-dose, metformin-furosemide drug interaction study in healthy subjects demonstrated that pharmacokinetic parameters of both compounds were affected by co-administration. Furosemide increased the metformin plasma and blood C_{max} by 22% and blood AUC by 15%, without any significant change in metformin renal clearance. When administered with metformin, the C_{max} and AUC of furosemide were 31% and 12% smaller, respectively, than when administered alone, and the terminal half-life was decreased by 32%, without any significant change in furosemide renal clearance. No information is available about the interaction of metformin and furosemide when co-administered chronically.

7.5 Nifedipine
A single-dose, metformin-nifedipine drug interaction study in normal healthy volunteers demonstrated that co-administration of nifedipine increased plasma metformin C_{max} and AUC by 20% and 9%, respectively, and increased the amount excreted in the urine. T_{max} and half-life were unaffected. Nifedipine appears to enhance the absorption of metformin. Metformin had minimal effects on nifedipine.

7.6 The Use of Metformin with Other Drugs
Certain drugs tend to produce hyperglycemia and may lead to loss of glycemic control. These drugs include the thiazides and other diuretics, corticosteroids, phenothiazines, thyroid products, estrogens, oral contraceptives, phenytoin, nicotinic acid, sympathomimetics, calcium channel blocking drugs, and isoniazid. When such drugs are administered to a patient receiving JANUMET the patient should be closely observed to maintain adequate glycemic control.

In healthy volunteers, the pharmacokinetics of metformin and propranolol, and metformin and ibuprofen were not affected when co-administered in single-dose interaction studies.

Metformin is negligibly bound to plasma proteins and is, therefore, less likely to interact with highly protein-bound drugs such as salicylates, sulfonamides, chloramphenicol, and probenecid, as compared to the sulfonylureas, which are extensively bound to serum proteins.

8 USE IN SPECIFIC POPULATIONS
8.1 Pregnancy
Pregnancy Category B:
JANUMET
There are no adequate and well-controlled studies in pregnant women with JANUMET or its individual components; therefore, the safety of JANUMET in pregnant women is not known. JANUMET should be used during pregnancy only if clearly needed.

Merck & Co., Inc. maintains a registry to monitor the pregnancy outcomes of women exposed to JANUMET while pregnant. Health care providers are encouraged to report any prenatal exposure to JANUMET by calling the Pregnancy Registry at (800) 986-8999.

No animal studies have been conducted with the combined products in JANUMET to evaluate effects on reproduction. The following data are based on findings in studies performed with sitagliptin or metformin individually.

Sitagliptin
Reproduction studies have been performed in rats and rabbits. Doses of sitagliptin up to 125 mg/kg (approximately 12 times the human exposure at the maximum recommended human dose) did not impair fertility or harm the fetus. There are, however, no adequate and well-controlled studies with sitagliptin in pregnant women.

Sitagliptin administered to pregnant female rats and rabbits from gestation day 6 to 20 (organogenesis) was not teratogenic at oral doses up to 250 mg/kg (rats) and 125 mg/kg (rabbits), or approximately 30 and 20 times human exposure at the maximum recommended human dose (MRHD) of 100 mg/day based on AUC comparisons. Higher doses increased the incidence of rib malformations in offspring at 1000 mg/kg, or approximately 100 times human exposure at the MRHD.

Sitagliptin administered to female rats from gestation day 6 to lactation day 21 decreased body weight in male and female offspring at 1000 mg/kg. No functional or behavioral toxicity was observed in offspring of rats.

Placental transfer of sitagliptin administered to pregnant rats was approximately 45% at 2 hours and 80% at 24 hours postdose. Placental transfer of sitagliptin administered to pregnant rabbits was approximately 66% at 2 hours and 30% at 24 hours.

Metformin hydrochloride
Metformin was not teratogenic in rats and rabbits at doses up to 600 mg/kg/day. This represents an exposure of about 2 and 6 times the maximum recommended human daily dose of 2,000 mg based on body surface area comparisons for rats and rabbits, respectively. Determination of fetal concentrations demonstrated a partial placental barrier to metformin.

Continued on next page

Table 1: Sitagliptin and Metformin Co-administered to Patients with Type 2 Diabetes Inadequately Controlled on Diet and Exercise:
Adverse Reactions Reported (Regardless of Investigator Assessment of Causality) in ≥5% of Patients Receiving Combination Therapy (and Greater than in Patients Receiving Placebo)[†]

	Number of Patients (%)			
	Placebo	Sitagliptin 100 mg QD	Metformin 500 mg/ Metformin 1000 mg bid[††]	Sitagliptin 50 mg bid + Metformin 500 mg/ Metformin 1000 mg bid[††]
	N = 176	N = 179	N = 364[††]	N = 372[††]
Diarrhea	7 (4.0)	5 (2.8)	28 (7.7)	28 (7.5)
Upper Respiratory Tract Infection	9 (5.1)	8 (4.5)	19 (5.2)	23 (6.2)
Headache	5 (2.8)	2 (1.1)	14 (3.8)	22 (5.9)

[†] Intent-to-treat population.
[††] Data pooled for the patients given the lower and higher doses of metformin.

Table 2: Pre-selected Gastrointestinal Adverse Reactions (Regardless of Investigator Assessment of Causality) Reported in Patients with Type 2 Diabetes Receiving Sitagliptin and Metformin

	Number of Patients (%)					
	Study of Sitagliptin and Metformin in Patients Inadequately Controlled on Diet and Exercise				Study of Sitagliptin Add-on in Patients Inadequately Controlled on Metformin Alone	
	Placebo	Sitagliptin 100 mg QD	Metformin 500 mg/ Metformin 1000 mg bid[†]	Sitagliptin 50 mg bid + Metformin 500 mg/ Metformin 1000 mg bid[†]	Placebo and Metformin ≥1500 mg daily	Sitagliptin 100 mg QD and Metformin ≥1500 mg daily
	N = 176	N = 179	N = 364	N = 372	N = 237	N = 464
Diarrhea	7 (4.0)	5 (2.8)	28 (7.7)	28 (7.5)	6 (2.5)	11 (2.4)
Nausea	2 (1.1)	2 (1.1)	20 (5.5)	18 (4.8)	2 (0.8)	6 (1.3)
Vomiting	1 (0.6)	0 (0.0)	2 (0.5)	8 (2.2)	2 (0.8)	5 (1.1)
Abdominal Pain[††]	4 (2.3)	6 (3.4)	14 (3.8)	11 (3.0)	9 (3.8)	10 (2.2)

[†] Data pooled for the patients given the lower and higher doses of metformin.
[††] Abdominal discomfort was included in the analysis of abdominal pain in the study of initial therapy.

Information on the Merck & Co., Inc., products listed on these pages is from the full prescribing information in use March 1, 2008. For information, please call 1-800-NSC-MERCK [1-800-672-6372].

Janumet—Cont.

8.3 Nursing Mothers
No studies in lactating animals have been conducted with the combined components of JANUMET. In studies performed with the individual components, both sitagliptin and metformin are secreted in the milk of lactating rats. It is not known whether sitagliptin is excreted in human milk. Because many drugs are excreted in human milk, caution should be exercised when JANUMET is administered to a nursing woman.

8.4 Pediatric Use
Safety and effectiveness of JANUMET in pediatric patients under 18 years have not been established.

8.5 Geriatric Use
JANUMET
Because sitagliptin and metformin are substantially excreted by the kidney, and because aging can be associated with reduced renal function, JANUMET should be used with caution as age increases. Care should be taken in dose selection and should be based on careful and regular monitoring of renal function. *[See Warnings and Precautions (5.1, 5.3); Clinical Pharmacology (12.3).]*
Sitagliptin
Of the total number of subjects (N=3884) in Phase II and III clinical studies of sitagliptin, 725 patients were 65 years and over, while 61 patients were 75 years and over. No overall differences in safety or effectiveness were observed between subjects 65 years and over and younger subjects. While this and other reported clinical experience have not identified differences in responses between the elderly and younger patients, greater sensitivity of some older individuals cannot be ruled out.
Metformin hydrochloride
Controlled clinical studies of metformin did not include sufficient numbers of elderly patients to determine whether they respond differently from younger patients, although other reported clinical experience has not identified differences in responses between the elderly and young patients. Metformin should only be used in patients with normal renal function. The initial and maintenance dosing of metformin should be conservative in patients with advanced age, due to the potential for decreased renal function in this population. Any dose adjustment should be based on a careful assessment of renal function. *[See Contraindications (4); Warnings and Precautions (5.3); and Clinical Pharmacology (12.3).]*

10 OVERDOSAGE
Sitagliptin
During controlled clinical trials in healthy subjects, single doses of up to 800 mg sitagliptin were administered. Maximal mean increases in QTc of 8.0 msec were observed in one study at a dose of 800 mg sitagliptin, a mean effect that is not considered clinically important *[see Clinical Pharmacology (12.2)]*. There is no experience with doses above 800 mg in humans. In Phase I multiple-dose studies, there were no dose-related clinical adverse reactions observed with sitagliptin with doses of up to 400 mg per day for periods of up to 28 days.
In the event of an overdose, it is reasonable to employ the usual supportive measures, e.g., remove unabsorbed material from the gastrointestinal tract, employ clinical monitoring (including obtaining an electrocardiogram), and institute supportive therapy as indicated by the patient's clinical status.
Sitagliptin is modestly dialyzable. In clinical studies, approximately 13.5% of the dose was removed over a 3- to 4-hour hemodialysis session. Prolonged hemodialysis may be considered if clinically appropriate. It is not known if sitagliptin is dialyzable by peritoneal dialysis.
Metformin hydrochloride
Overdose of metformin hydrochloride has occurred, including ingestion of amounts greater than 50 grams. Hypoglycemia was reported in approximately 10% of cases, but no causal association with metformin hydrochloride has been established. Lactic acidosis has been reported in approximately 32% of metformin overdose cases *[see Warnings and Precautions (5.1)]*. Metformin is dialyzable with a clearance of up to 170 mL/min under good hemodynamic conditions. Therefore, hemodialysis may be useful for removal of accumulated drug from patients in whom metformin overdosage is suspected.

11 DESCRIPTION
JANUMET (sitagliptin/metformin HCl) tablets contain two oral antihyperglycemic drugs used in the management of type 2 diabetes: sitagliptin and metformin hydrochloride.
Sitagliptin
Sitagliptin is an orally-active inhibitor of the dipeptidyl peptidase-4 (DPP-4) enzyme. Sitagliptin is present in JANUMET tablets in the form of sitagliptin phosphate monohydrate. Sitagliptin phosphate monohydrate is described chemically as 7-[(3*R*)-3-amino-1-oxo-4-(2,4,5-trifluorophenyl)butyl]-5,6,7,8-tetrahydro-3-(trifluoromethyl)-1,2,4-triazolo[4,3-*a*]pyrazine phosphate (1:1) monohydrate with an empirical formula of $C_{16}H_{15}F_6N_5O \bullet H_3PO_4 \bullet H_2O$ and a molecular weight of 523.32. The structural formula is:
[See chemical structure at top of next column]
Sitagliptin phosphate monohydrate is a white to off-white, crystalline, non-hygroscopic powder. It is soluble in water and N,N-dimethyl formamide; slightly soluble in methanol; very slightly soluble in ethanol, acetone, and acetonitrile; and insoluble in isopropanol and isopropyl acetate.

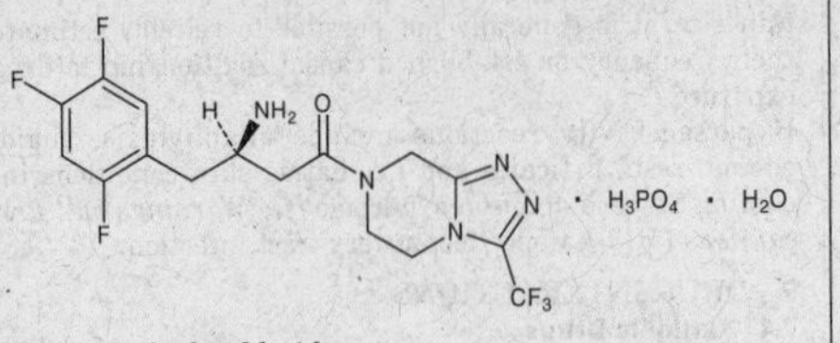

Metformin hydrochloride
Metformin hydrochloride (*N,N*-dimethylimidodicarbonimidic diamide hydrochloride) is not chemically or pharmacologically related to any other classes of oral antihyperglycemic agents. Metformin hydrochloride is a white to off-white crystalline compound with a molecular formula of $C_4H_{11}N_5 \bullet HCl$ and a molecular weight of 165.63. Metformin hydrochloride is freely soluble in water and is practically insoluble in acetone, ether, and chloroform. The pK_a of metformin is 12.4. The pH of a 1% aqueous solution of metformin hydrochloride is 6.68. The structural formula is as shown:

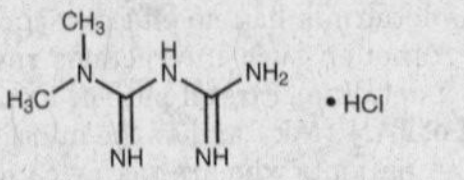

JANUMET
JANUMET is available for oral administration as tablets containing 64.25 mg sitagliptin phosphate monohydrate and metformin hydrochloride equivalent to: 50 mg sitagliptin as free base and 500 mg metformin hydrochloride (JANUMET 50 mg/500 mg) or 1000 mg metformin hydrochloride (JANUMET 50 mg/1000 mg). Each film-coated tablet of JANUMET contains the following inactive ingredients: microcrystalline cellulose, polyvinylpyrrolidone, sodium lauryl sulfate, and sodium stearyl fumarate. In addition, the film coating contains the following inactive ingredients: polyvinyl alcohol, polyethylene glycol, talc, titanium dioxide, red iron oxide, and black iron oxide.

12 CLINICAL PHARMACOLOGY
12.1 Mechanism of Action
JANUMET
JANUMET combines two antihyperglycemic agents with complementary mechanisms of action to improve glycemic control in patients with type 2 diabetes: sitagliptin, a dipeptidyl peptidase-4 (DPP-4) inhibitor, and metformin hydrochloride, a member of the biguanide class.
Sitagliptin
Sitagliptin is a DPP-4 inhibitor, which is believed to exert its actions in patients with type 2 diabetes by slowing the inactivation of incretin hormones. Concentrations of the active intact hormones are increased by sitagliptin, thereby increasing and prolonging the action of these hormones. Incretin hormones, including glucagon-like peptide-1 (GLP-1) and glucose-dependent insulinotropic polypeptide (GIP), are released by the intestine throughout the day, and levels are increased in response to a meal. These hormones are rapidly inactivated by the enzyme DPP-4. The incretins are part of an endogenous system involved in the physiologic regulation of glucose homeostasis. When blood glucose concentrations are normal or elevated, GLP-1 and GIP increase insulin synthesis and release from pancreatic beta cells by intracellular signaling pathways involving cyclic AMP. GLP-1 also lowers glucagon secretion from pancreatic alpha cells, leading to reduced hepatic glucose production. By increasing and prolonging active incretin levels, sitagliptin increases insulin release and decreases glucagon levels in the circulation in a glucose-dependent manner. Sitagliptin demonstrates selectivity for DPP-4 and does not inhibit DPP-8 or DPP-9 activity *in vitro* at concentrations approximating those from therapeutic doses.
Metformin hydrochloride
Metformin is an antihyperglycemic agent which improves glucose tolerance in patients with type 2 diabetes, lowering both basal and postprandial plasma glucose. Its pharmacologic mechanisms of action are different from other classes of oral antihyperglycemic agents. Metformin decreases hepatic glucose production, decreases intestinal absorption of glucose, and improves insulin sensitivity by increasing peripheral glucose uptake and utilization. Unlike sulfonylureas, metformin does not produce hypoglycemia in either patients with type 2 diabetes or normal subjects (except in special circumstances *[see Warnings and Precautions (5.8)]*) and does not cause hyperinsulinemia. With metformin therapy, insulin secretion remains unchanged while fasting insulin levels and day-long plasma insulin response may actually decrease.

12.2 Pharmacodynamics
Sitagliptin
General
In patients with type 2 diabetes, administration of sitagliptin led to inhibition of DPP-4 enzyme activity for a 24-hour period. After an oral glucose load or a meal, this DPP-4 inhibition resulted in a 2- to 3-fold increase in circulating levels of active GLP-1 and GIP, decreased glucagon concentrations, and increased responsiveness of insulin release to glucose, resulting in higher C-peptide and insulin concentrations. The rise in insulin with the decrease in glucagon was associated with lower fasting glucose concentrations and reduced glucose excursion following an oral glucose load or a meal.
Sitagliptin and Metformin hydrochloride Co-administration
In a two-day study in healthy subjects, sitagliptin alone increased active GLP-1 concentrations, whereas metformin alone increased active and total GLP-1 concentrations to similar extents. Co-administration of sitagliptin and metformin had an additive effect on active GLP-1 concentrations. Sitagliptin, but not metformin, increased active GIP concentrations. It is unclear what these findings mean for changes in glycemic control in patients with type 2 diabetes.
In studies with healthy subjects, sitagliptin did not lower blood glucose or cause hypoglycemia.
Cardiac Electrophysiology
In a randomized, placebo-controlled crossover study, 79 healthy subjects were administered a single oral dose of sitagliptin 100 mg, sitagliptin 800 mg (8 times the recommended dose), and placebo. At the recommended dose of 100 mg, there was no effect on the QTc interval obtained at the peak plasma concentration, or at any other time during the study. Following the 800-mg dose, the maximum increase in the placebo-corrected mean change in QTc from baseline at 3 hours postdose was 8.0 msec. This increase is not considered to be clinically significant. At the 800-mg dose, peak sitagliptin plasma concentrations were approximately 11 times higher than the peak concentrations following a 100-mg dose.
In patients with type 2 diabetes administered sitagliptin 100 mg (N=81) or sitagliptin 200 mg (N=63) daily, there were no meaningful changes in QTc interval based on ECG data obtained at the time of expected peak plasma concentration.

12.3 Pharmacokinetics
JANUMET
The results of a bioequivalence study in healthy subjects demonstrated that the JANUMET (sitagliptin/metformin HCl) 50 mg/500 mg and 50 mg/1000 mg combination tablets are bioequivalent to co-administration of corresponding doses of sitagliptin (JANUVIA™[2]) and metformin hydrochloride as individual tablets.
Absorption
Sitagliptin
The absolute bioavailability of sitagliptin is approximately 87%. Co-administration of a high-fat meal with sitagliptin had no effect on the pharmacokinetics of sitagliptin.
Metformin hydrochloride
The absolute bioavailability of a metformin hydrochloride 500-mg tablet given under fasting conditions is approximately 50-60%. Studies using single oral doses of metformin hydrochloride tablets 500 mg to 1500 mg, and 850 mg to 2550 mg, indicate that there is a lack of dose proportionality with increasing doses, which is due to decreased absorption rather than an alteration in elimination. Food decreases the extent of and slightly delays the absorption of metformin, as shown by approximately a 40% lower mean peak plasma concentration (C_{max}), a 25% lower area under the plasma concentration versus time curve (AUC), and a 35-minute prolongation of time to peak plasma concentration (T_{max}) following administration of a single 850-mg tablet of metformin with food, compared to the same tablet strength administered fasting. The clinical relevance of these decreases is unknown.
Distribution
Sitagliptin
The mean volume of distribution at steady state following a single 100-mg intravenous dose of sitagliptin to healthy subjects is approximately 198 liters. The fraction of sitagliptin reversibly bound to plasma proteins is low (38%).
Metformin hydrochloride
The apparent volume of distribution (V/F) of metformin following single oral doses of metformin hydrochloride tablets 850 mg averaged 654 ± 358 L. Metformin is negligibly bound to plasma proteins, in contrast to sulfonylureas, which are more than 90% protein bound. Metformin partitions into erythrocytes, most likely as a function of time. At usual clinical doses and dosing schedules of metformin hydrochloride tablets, steady-state plasma concentrations of metformin are reached within 24-48 hours and are generally <1 mcg/mL. During controlled clinical trials of metformin, maximum metformin plasma levels did not exceed 5 mcg/mL, even at maximum doses.
Metabolism
Sitagliptin
Approximately 79% of sitagliptin is excreted unchanged in the urine with metabolism being a minor pathway of elimination.
Following a [^{14}C]sitagliptin oral dose, approximately 16% of the radioactivity was excreted as metabolites of sitagliptin. Six metabolites were detected at trace levels and are not expected to contribute to the plasma DPP-4 inhibitory activity of sitagliptin. *In vitro* studies indicated that the primary enzyme responsible for the limited metabolism of sitagliptin was CYP3A4, with contribution from CYP2C8.
Metformin hydrochloride
Intravenous single-dose studies in normal subjects demonstrate that metformin is excreted unchanged in the urine and does not undergo hepatic metabolism (no metabolites have been identified in humans) nor biliary excretion.
Excretion
Sitagliptin
Following administration of an oral [^{14}C]sitagliptin dose to healthy subjects, approximately 100% of the administered radioactivity was eliminated in feces (13%) or urine (87%) within one week of dosing. The apparent terminal $t_{½}$ following a 100-mg oral dose of sitagliptin was approximately 12.4 hours and renal clearance was approximately 350 mL/min.
Elimination of sitagliptin occurs primarily via renal excretion and involves active tubular secretion. Sitagliptin is a substrate for human organic anion transporter-3 (hOAT-3),

which may be involved in the renal elimination of sitagliptin. The clinical relevance of hOAT-3 in sitagliptin transport has not been established. Sitagliptin is also a substrate of p-glycoprotein, which may also be involved in mediating the renal elimination of sitagliptin. However, cyclosporine, a p-glycoprotein inhibitor, did not reduce the renal clearance of sitagliptin.

Metformin hydrochloride

Renal clearance is approximately 3.5 times greater than creatinine clearance, which indicates that tubular secretion is the major route of metformin elimination. Following oral administration, approximately 90% of the absorbed drug is eliminated via the renal route within the first 24 hours, with a plasma elimination half-life of approximately 6.2 hours. In blood, the elimination half-life is approximately 17.6 hours, suggesting that the erythrocyte mass may be a compartment of distribution.

Special Populations

Renal Insufficiency

JANUMET

JANUMET should not be used in patients with renal insufficiency *[see Contraindications (4); Warnings and Precautions (5.3)]*.

Sitagliptin

An approximately 2-fold increase in the plasma AUC of sitagliptin was observed in patients with moderate renal insufficiency, and an approximately 4-fold increase was observed in patients with severe renal insufficiency including patients with ESRD on hemodialysis, as compared to normal healthy control subjects.

Metformin hydrochloride

In patients with decreased renal function (based on measured creatinine clearance), the plasma and blood half-life of metformin is prolonged and the renal clearance is decreased in proportion to the decrease in creatinine clearance.

Hepatic Insufficiency

Sitagliptin

In patients with moderate hepatic insufficiency (Child-Pugh score 7 to 9), mean AUC and C_{max} of sitagliptin increased approximately 21% and 13%, respectively, compared to healthy matched controls following administration of a single 100-mg dose of sitagliptin. These differences are not considered to be clinically meaningful.

There is no clinical experience in patients with severe hepatic insufficiency (Child-Pugh score >9).

Metformin hydrochloride

No pharmacokinetic studies of metformin have been conducted in patients with hepatic insufficiency.

Gender

Sitagliptin

Gender had no clinically meaningful effect on the pharmacokinetics of sitagliptin based on a composite analysis of Phase I pharmacokinetic data and on a population pharmacokinetic analysis of Phase I and Phase II data.

Metformin hydrochloride

Metformin pharmacokinetic parameters did not differ significantly between normal subjects and patients with type 2 diabetes when analyzed according to gender. Similarly, in controlled clinical studies in patients with type 2 diabetes, the antihyperglycemic effect of metformin was comparable in males and females.

Geriatric

Sitagliptin

When the effects of age on renal function are taken into account, age alone did not have a clinically meaningful impact on the pharmacokinetics of sitagliptin based on a population pharmacokinetic analysis. Elderly subjects (65 to 80 years) had approximately 19% higher plasma concentrations of sitagliptin compared to younger subjects.

Metformin hydrochloride

Limited data from controlled pharmacokinetic studies of metformin in healthy elderly subjects suggest that total plasma clearance of metformin is decreased, the half life is prolonged, and C_{max} is increased, compared to healthy young subjects. From these data, it appears that the change in metformin pharmacokinetics with aging is primarily accounted for by a change in renal function (see **GLUCOPHAGE**[3] prescribing information: **CLINICAL PHARMACOLOGY**, Special Populations, Geriatrics).

JANUMET treatment should not be initiated in patients ≥80 years of age unless measurement of creatinine clearance demonstrates that renal function is not reduced *[see Warnings and Precautions (5.1, 5.3)]*.

Pediatric

No studies with JANUMET have been performed in pediatric patients.

Race

Sitagliptin

Race had no clinically meaningful effect on the pharmacokinetics of sitagliptin based on a composite analysis of available pharmacokinetic data, including subjects of white, Hispanic, black, Asian, and other racial groups.

Metformin hydrochloride

No studies of metformin pharmacokinetic parameters according to race have been performed. In controlled clinical studies of metformin in patients with type 2 diabetes, the antihyperglycemic effect was comparable in whites (n=249), blacks (n=51), and Hispanics (n=24).

Body Mass Index (BMI)

Sitagliptin

Body mass index had no clinically meaningful effect on the pharmacokinetics of sitagliptin based on a composite analysis of Phase I pharmacokinetic data and on a population pharmacokinetic analysis of Phase I and Phase II data.

Table 3:
Glycemic Parameters at Final Visit (24-Week Study) for Sitagliptin and Metformin, Alone and in Combination in Patients with Type 2 Diabetes Inadequately Controlled on Diet and Exercise†

	Placebo	Sitagliptin 100 mg QD	Metformin 500 mg bid	Metformin 1000 mg bid	Sitagliptin 50 mg bid + Metformin 500 mg bid	Sitagliptin 50 mg bid + Metformin 1000 mg bid
A1C (%)	**N = 165**	**N = 175**	**N = 178**	**N = 177**	**N = 183**	**N = 178**
Baseline (mean)	8.7	8.9	8.9	8.7	8.8	8.8
Change from baseline (adjusted mean‡)	0.2	-0.7	-0.8	-1.1	-1.4	-1.9
Difference from placebo (adjusted mean‡) (95% CI)		-0.8§ (-1.1, -0.6)	-1.0§ (-1.2, -0.8)	-1.3§ (-1.5, -1.1)	-1.6§ (-1.8, -1.3)	-2.1§ (-2.3, -1.8)
Patients (%) achieving A1C <7%	15 (9%)	35 (20%)	41 (23%)	68 (38%)	79 (43%)	118 (66%)
% Patients receiving rescue medication	32	21	17	12	8	2
FPG (mg/dL)	**N = 169**	**N = 178**	**N = 179**	**N = 179**	**N = 183**	**N = 180**
Baseline (mean)	196	201	205	197	204	197
Change from baseline (adjusted mean‡)	6	-17	-27	-29	-47	-64
Difference from placebo (adjusted mean‡) (95% CI)		-23§ (-33, -14)	-33§ (-43, -24)	-35§ (-45, -26)	-53§ (-62, -43)	-70§ (-79, -60)
2-hour PPG (mg/dL)	**N = 129**	**N = 136**	**N = 141**	**N = 138**	**N = 147**	**N = 152**
Baseline (mean)	277	285	293	283	292	287
Change from baseline (adjusted mean‡)	0	-52	-53	-78	-93	-117
Difference from placebo (adjusted mean‡) (95% CI)		-52§ (-67, -37)	-54§ (-69, -39)	-78§ (-93, -63)	-93§ (-107, -78)	-117§ (-131, -102)

† Intent to Treat Population using last observation on study prior to glyburide (glibenclamide) rescue therapy.
‡ Least squares means adjusted for prior antihyperglycemic therapy status and baseline value.
§ p<0.001 compared to placebo.

Drug Interactions

Sitagliptin and Metformin hydrochloride

Co-administration of multiple doses of sitagliptin (50 mg) and metformin (1000 mg) given twice daily did not meaningfully alter the pharmacokinetics of either sitagliptin or metformin in patients with type 2 diabetes.

Pharmacokinetic drug interaction studies with JANUMET have not been performed; however, such studies have been conducted with the individual components of JANUMET (sitagliptin and metformin hydrochloride).

Sitagliptin

In Vitro Assessment of Drug Interactions

Sitagliptin is not an inhibitor of CYP isozymes CYP3A4, 2C8, 2C9, 2D6, 1A2, 2C19 or 2B6, and is not an inducer of CYP3A4. Sitagliptin is a p-glycoprotein substrate, but does not inhibit p-glycoprotein mediated transport of digoxin. Based on these results, sitagliptin is considered unlikely to cause interactions with other drugs that utilize these pathways.

Sitagliptin is not extensively bound to plasma proteins. Therefore, the propensity of sitagliptin to be involved in clinically meaningful drug-drug interactions mediated by plasma protein binding displacement is very low.

In Vivo Assessment of Drug Interactions

Effect of Sitagliptin on Other Drugs

In clinical studies, as described below, sitagliptin did not meaningfully alter the pharmacokinetics of metformin, glyburide, simvastatin, rosiglitazone, warfarin, or oral contraceptives, providing *in vivo* evidence of a low propensity for causing drug interactions with substrates of CYP3A4, CYP2C8, CYP2C9, and organic cationic transporter (OCT).

Digoxin: Sitagliptin had a minimal effect on the pharmacokinetics of digoxin. Following administration of 0.25 mg digoxin concomitantly with 100 mg of sitagliptin daily for 10 days, the plasma AUC of digoxin was increased by 11%, and the plasma C_{max} by 18%.

Sulfonylureas: Single-dose pharmacokinetics of glyburide, a CYP2C9 substrate, was not meaningfully altered in subjects receiving multiple doses of sitagliptin. Clinically meaningful interactions would not be expected with other sulfonylureas (e.g., glipizide, tolbutamide, and glimepiride) which, like glyburide, are primarily eliminated by CYP2C9 *[see Warnings and Precautions (5.8)]*.

Simvastatin: Single-dose pharmacokinetics of simvastatin, a CYP3A4 substrate, was not meaningfully altered in subjects receiving multiple daily doses of sitagliptin. Therefore, sitagliptin is not an inhibitor of CYP3A4-mediated metabolism.

Thiazolidinediones: Single-dose pharmacokinetics of rosiglitazone was not meaningfully altered in subjects receiving multiple daily doses of sitagliptin, indicating that sitagliptin is not an inhibitor of CYP2C8-mediated metabolism.

Warfarin: Multiple daily doses of sitagliptin did not meaningfully alter the pharmacokinetics, as assessed by measurement of S(-) or R(+) warfarin enantiomers, or pharmacodynamics (as assessed by measurement of prothrombin INR) of a single dose of warfarin. Because S(-) warfarin is primarily metabolized by CYP2C9, these data also support the conclusion that sitagliptin is not a CYP2C9 inhibitor.

Oral Contraceptives: Co-administration with sitagliptin did not meaningfully alter the steady-state pharmacokinetics of norethindrone or ethinyl estradiol.

Effect of Other Drugs on Sitagliptin

Clinical data described below suggest that sitagliptin is not susceptible to clinically meaningful interactions by co-administered medications.

Cyclosporine: A study was conducted to assess the effect of cyclosporine, a potent inhibitor of p-glycoprotein, on the pharmacokinetics of sitagliptin. Co-administration of a single 100-mg oral dose of sitagliptin and a single 600-mg oral dose of cyclosporine increased the AUC and C_{max} of sitagliptin by approximately 29% and 68%, respectively. These modest changes in sitagliptin pharmacokinetics were not considered to be clinically meaningful. The renal clearance of sitagliptin was also not meaningfully altered. Therefore, meaningful interactions would not be expected with other p-glycoprotein inhibitors.

Metformin hydrochloride

[See Drug Interactions (7.1, 7.3, 7.4, 7.5, 7.6).]

13 NONCLINICAL TOXICOLOGY

13.1 Carcinogenesis, Mutagenesis, Impairment of Fertility

JANUMET

No animal studies have been conducted with the combined products in JANUMET to evaluate carcinogenesis, mutagenesis or impairment of fertility. The following data are based on the findings in studies with sitagliptin and metformin individually.

Sitagliptin

A two-year carcinogenicity study was conducted in male and female rats given oral doses of sitagliptin of 50, 150, and 500 mg/kg/day. There was an increased incidence of combined liver adenoma/carcinoma in males and females and of liver carcinoma in females at 500 mg/kg. This dose results in exposures approximately 60 times the human exposure at the maximum recommended daily adult human dose (MRHD) of 100 mg/day based on AUC comparisons. Liver tumors were not observed at 150 mg/kg, approximately 20 times the human exposure at the MRHD. A two-year carcinogenicity study was conducted in male and female mice given oral doses of sitagliptin of 50, 125, 250, and 500 mg/kg/day. There was no increase in the incidence of tumors in any organ up to 500 mg/kg, approximately 70 times human

Continued on next page

Information on the Merck & Co., Inc., products listed on these pages is from the full prescribing information in use March 1, 2008. For information, please call 1-800-NSC-MERCK [1-800-672-6372].

Janumet—Cont.

exposure at the MRHD. Sitagliptin was not mutagenic or clastogenic with or without metabolic activation in the Ames bacterial mutagenicity assay, a Chinese hamster ovary (CHO) chromosome aberration assay, an *in vitro* cytogenetics assay in CHO, an *in vitro* rat hepatocyte DNA alkaline elution assay, and an *in vivo* micronucleus assay.

In rat fertility studies with oral gavage doses of 125, 250, and 1000 mg/kg, males were treated for 4 weeks prior to mating, during mating, up to scheduled termination (approximately 8 weeks total), and females were treated 2 weeks prior to mating through gestation day 7. No adverse effect on fertility was observed at 125 mg/kg (approximately 12 times human exposure at the MRHD of 100 mg/day based on AUC comparisons). At higher doses, nondose-related increased resorptions in females were observed (approximately 25 and 100 times human exposure at the MRHD based on AUC comparison).

Metformin hydrochloride

Long-term carcinogenicity studies have been performed in rats (dosing duration of 104 weeks) and mice (dosing duration of 91 weeks) at doses up to and including 900 mg/kg/day and 1500 mg/kg/day, respectively. These doses are both approximately four times the maximum recommended human daily dose of 2000 mg based on body surface area comparisons. No evidence of carcinogenicity with metformin was found in either male or female mice. Similarly, there was no tumorigenic potential observed with metformin in male rats. There was, however, an increased incidence of benign stromal uterine polyps in female rats treated with 900 mg/kg/day.

There was no evidence of a mutagenic potential of metformin in the following *in vitro* tests: Ames test (*S. typhimurium*), gene mutation test (mouse lymphoma cells), or chromosomal aberrations test (human lymphocytes). Results in the *in vivo* mouse micronucleus test were also negative. Fertility of male or female rats was unaffected by metformin when administered at doses as high as 600 mg/kg/day, which is approximately three times the maximum recommended human daily dose based on body surface area comparisons.

14 CLINICAL STUDIES

The co-administration of sitagliptin and metformin has been studied in patients with type 2 diabetes inadequately controlled on diet and exercise and in combination with glimepiride.

There have been no clinical efficacy studies conducted with JANUMET; however, bioequivalence of JANUMET with co-administered sitagliptin and metformin hydrochloride tablets was demonstrated.

Sitagliptin and Metformin Co-administration in Patients with Type 2 Diabetes Inadequately Controlled on Diet and Exercise

A total of 1091 patients with type 2 diabetes and inadequate glycemic control on diet and exercise participated in a 24-week, randomized, double-blind, placebo-controlled factorial study designed to assess the efficacy of sitagliptin and metformin co-administration. Patients on an antihyperglycemic agent (N=541) underwent a diet, exercise, and drug washout period of up to 12 weeks duration. After the washout period, patients with inadequate glycemic control (A1C 7.5% to 11%) were randomized after completing a 2-week single-blind placebo run-in period. Patients not on antihyperglycemic agents at study entry (N=550) with inadequate glycemic control (A1C 7.5% to 11%) immediately entered the 2-week single-blind placebo run-in period and then were randomized. Approximately equal numbers of patients were randomized to receive placebo, 100 mg of sitagliptin once daily, 500 mg or 1000 mg of metformin twice daily, or 50 mg of sitagliptin twice daily in combination with 500 mg or 1000 mg of metformin twice daily. Patients who failed to meet specific glycemic goals during the study were treated with glyburide (glibenclamide) rescue.

Sitagliptin and metformin co-administration provided significant improvements in A1C, FPG, and 2-hour PPG compared to placebo, to metformin alone, and to sitagliptin alone (Table 3, Figure 1). Mean reductions from baseline in A1C were generally greater for patients with higher baseline A1C values. For patients not on an antihyperglycemic agent at study entry, mean reductions from baseline in A1C were: sitagliptin 100 mg once daily, -1.1%; metformin 500 mg bid, -1.1%; metformin 1000 mg bid, -1.2%; sitagliptin 50 mg bid with metformin 500 mg bid, -1.6%; sitagliptin 50 mg bid with metformin 1000 mg bid, -1.9%; and for patients receiving placebo, -0.2%. The decrease in body weight in the groups given sitagliptin in combination with metformin was similar to that in the groups given metformin alone or placebo.

[See table 3 at top of previous page]
[See figure 1 at top of next column]

In addition, this study included patients (N=117) with more severe hyperglycemia (A1C >11% or blood glucose >280 mg/dL) who were treated with twice daily open-label sitagliptin 50 mg and metformin 1000 mg. In this group of patients, the mean baseline A1C value was 11.2%, mean FPG was 314 mg/dL, and mean 2-hour PPG was 441 mg/dL. After 24 weeks, mean decreases from baseline of -2.9% for A1C, -127 mg/dL for FPG, and -208 mg/dL for 2-hour PPG were observed.

Initial combination therapy or maintenance of combination therapy should be individualized and are left to the discretion of the health care provider.

Table 4: Glycemic Parameters at Final Visit (24-Week Study) of Sitagliptin in Add-on Combination Therapy with Metformin[†]

	Sitagliptin 100 mg QD + Metformin	Placebo + Metformin
A1C (%)	N = 453	N = 224
Baseline (mean)	8.0	8.0
Change from baseline (adjusted mean[‡])	-0.7	-0.0
Difference from placebo + metformin (adjusted mean[‡]) (95% CI)	-0.7[§] (-0.8, -0.5)	
Patients (%) achieving A1C <7%	213 (47%)	41 (18%)
FPG (mg/dL)	N = 454	N = 226
Baseline (mean)	170	174
Change from baseline (adjusted mean[‡])	-17	9
Difference from placebo + metformin (adjusted mean[‡]) (95% CI)	-25[§] (-31, -20)	
2-hour PPG (mg/dL)	N = 387	N = 182
Baseline (mean)	275	272
Change from baseline (adjusted mean[‡])	-62	-11
Difference from placebo + metformin (adjusted mean[‡]) (95% CI)	-51[§] (-61, -41)	

[†] Intent to Treated Population using last observation on study prior to pioglitazone rescue therapy.
[‡] Least squares means adjusted for prior antihyperglycemic therapy and baseline value.
[§] p<0.001 compared to placebo + metformin

Table 5: Glycemic Parameters at Final Visit (24-Week Study) for Sitagliptin in Combination with Metformin and Glimepiride[†]

	Sitagliptin 100 mg + Metformin and Glimepiride	Placebo + Metformin and Glimepiride
A1C (%)	N = 115	N = 105
Baseline (mean)	8.3	8.3
Change from baseline (adjusted mean[‡])	-0.6	0.3
Difference from placebo (adjusted mean[‡]) (95% CI)	-0.9[§] (-1.1, -0.7)	
Patients (%) achieving A1C <7%	26 (23%)	1 (1%)
FPG (mg/dL)	N = 115	N = 109
Baseline (mean)	179	179
Change from baseline (adjusted mean[‡])	-8	13
Difference from placebo (adjusted mean[‡]) (95% CI)	-21[§] (-32, -10)	

[†] Intent to Treat Population using last observation on study prior to pioglitazone rescue therapy.
[‡] Least squares means adjusted for prior antihyperglycemic therapy status and baseline value.
[§] p<0.001 compared to placebo.

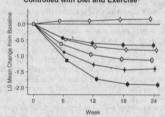

Figure 1: Mean Change from Baseline for A1C (%) over 24 Weeks with Sitagliptin and Metformin, Alone and in Combination in Patients with Type 2 Diabetes Inadequately Controlled with Diet and Exercise[†]

○ Placebo   □ Metformin 1000 mg b.i.d.
● Sitagliptin 100 mg q.d.   ◆ Sitagliptin 50 mg b.i.d. + Metformin 500 mg b.i.d.
◇ Metformin 500 mg b.i.d.   ■ Sitagliptin 50 mg b.i.d. + Metformin 1000 mg b.i.d.

[†]Intention to Treat Population; Least squares means adjusted for prior antihyperglycemic therapy and baseline value.

Sitagliptin Add-on Therapy in Patients with Type 2 Diabetes Inadequately Controlled on Metformin Alone

A total of 701 patients with type 2 diabetes participated in a 24-week, randomized, double-blind, placebo-controlled study designed to assess the efficacy of sitagliptin in combination with metformin. Patients already on metformin (N=431) at a dose of at least 1500 mg per day were randomized after completing a 2-week, single-blind placebo run-in period. Patients on metformin and another antihyperglycemic agent (N=229) and patients not on any antihyperglycemic agent (N=41) were randomized after a run-in period of approximately 10 weeks on metformin (at a dose of at least 1500 mg per day) in mono-

therapy. Patients were randomized to the addition of either 100 mg of sitagliptin or placebo, administered once daily. Patients who failed to meet specific glycemic goals during the studies were treated with pioglitazone rescue.

In combination with metformin, sitagliptin provided significant improvements in A1C, FPG, and 2-hour PPG compared to placebo with metformin (Table 4). Rescue glycemic therapy was used in 5% of patients treated with sitagliptin 100 mg and 14% of patients treated with placebo. A similar decrease in body weight was observed for both treatment groups.

[See table 4 above]

Sitagliptin Add-on Therapy in Patients with Type 2 Diabetes Inadequately Controlled on the Combination of Metformin and Glimepiride

A total of 441 patients with type 2 diabetes participated in a 24-week, randomized, double-blind, placebo-controlled study designed to assess the efficacy of sitagliptin in combination with glimepiride, with or without metformin. Patients entered a run-in treatment period on glimepiride (≥4 mg per day) alone or glimepiride in combination with metformin (≥1500 mg per day). After a dose-titration and dose-stable run-in period of up to 16 weeks and a 2-week placebo run-in period, patients with inadequate glycemic control (A1C 7.5% to 10.5%) were randomized to the addition of either 100 mg of sitagliptin or placebo, administered once daily. Patients who failed to meet specific glycemic goals during the studies were treated with pioglitazone rescue.

Patients receiving sitagliptin with metformin and glimepiride had significant improvements in A1C and FPG compared to patients receiving placebo with metformin and glimepiride (Table 5), with mean reductions from baseline relative to placebo in A1C of -0.9% and in FPG of -21 mg/dL.

Rescue therapy was used in 8% of patients treated with add-on sitagliptin 100 mg and 29% of patients treated with add-on placebo. The patients treated with add-on sitagliptin had a mean increase in body weight of 1.1 kg vs. add-on placebo (+0.4 kg vs. -0.7 kg). In addition, add-on sitagliptin resulted in an increased rate of hypoglycemia compared to add-on placebo. *[See Warnings and Precautions (5.2); Adverse Reactions (6.1).]*

[See table 5 at top of previous page]

Sitagliptin Add-on Therapy vs. Glipizide Add-on Therapy in Patients with Type 2 Diabetes Inadequately Controlled on Metformin

The efficacy of sitagliptin was evaluated in a 52-week, double-blind, glipizide-controlled noninferiority trial in patients with type 2 diabetes. Patients not on treatment or on other antihyperglycemic agents entered a run-in treatment period of up to 12 weeks duration with metformin monotherapy (dose of ≥1500 mg per day) which included washout of medications other than metformin, if applicable. After the run-in period, those with inadequate glycemic control (A1C 6.5% to 10%) were randomized 1:1 to the addition of sitagliptin 100 mg once daily or glipizide for 52 weeks. Patients receiving glipizide were given an initial dosage of 5 mg/day and then electively titrated over the next 18 weeks to a maximum dosage of 20 mg/day as needed to optimize glycemic control. Thereafter, the glipizide dose was to be kept constant, except for down-titration to prevent hypoglycemia. The mean dose of glipizide after the titration period was 10 mg.

After 52 weeks, sitagliptin and glipizide had similar mean reductions from baseline in A1C in the intent-to-treat analysis (Table 6). These results were consistent with the per protocol analysis (Figure 2). A conclusion in favor of the non-inferiority of sitagliptin to glipizide may be limited to patients with baseline A1C comparable to those included in the study (over 70% of patients had baseline A1C <8% and over 90% had A1C <9%).

Table 6: Glycemic Parameters in a 52-Week Study Comparing Sitagliptin to Glipizide as Add-On Therapy in Patients Inadequately Controlled on Metformin (Intent-to-Treat Population)†

	Sitagliptin 100 mg + Metformin	Glipizide + Metformin
A1C (%)	N = 576	N = 559
Baseline (mean)	7.7	7.6
Change from baseline (adjusted mean‡)	-0.5	-0.6
FPG (mg/dL)	N = 583	N = 568
Baseline (mean)	166	164
Change from baseline (adjusted mean‡)	-8	-8

† The Intent to Treat Analysis used the patients' last observation in the study prior to discontinuation.
‡ Least squares means adjusted for prior anti-hyperglycemic therapy status and baseline A1C value.

Figure 2: Mean Change from Baseline for A1C (%) Over 52 Weeks in a Study Comparing Sitagliptin to Glipizide as Add-On Therapy in Patients Inadequately Controlled on Metformin (Per Protocol Population)†

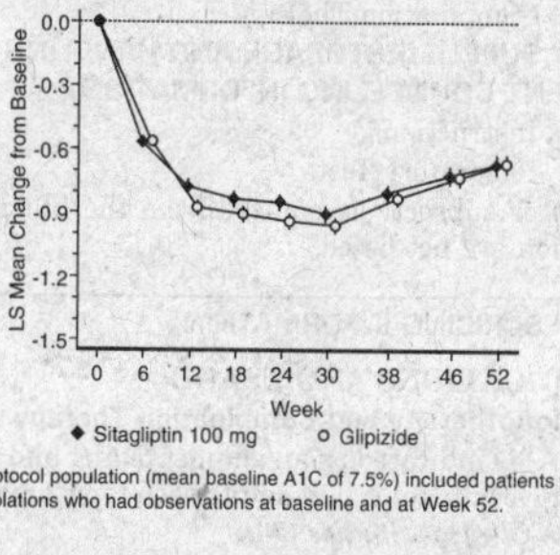

† The per protocol population (mean baseline A1C of 7.5%) included patients without major protocol violations who had observations at baseline and at Week 52.

The incidence of hypoglycemia in the sitagliptin group (4.9%) was significantly (p<0.001) lower than that in the glipizide group (32.0%). Patients treated with sitagliptin exhibited a significant mean decrease from baseline in body weight compared to a significant weight gain in patients administered glipizide (-1.5 kg vs. +1.1 kg).

16 HOW SUPPLIED/STORAGE AND HANDLING

No. 6747 — Tablets JANUMET, 50 mg/500 mg, are light pink, capsule-shaped, film-coated tablets with "575" debossed on one side. They are supplied as follows:
NDC 0006-0575-61 unit-of-use bottles of 60
NDC 0006-0575-62 unit-of-use bottles of 180
NDC 0006-0575-52 unit dose blister packages of 50
NDC 0006-0575-82 bulk bottles of 1000.

No. 6749 — Tablets JANUMET, 50 mg/1000 mg, are red, capsule-shaped, film-coated tablets with "577" debossed on one side. They are supplied as follows:
NDC 0006-0577-61 unit-of-use bottles of 60
NDC 0006-0577-62 unit-of-use bottles of 180
NDC 0006-0577-52 unit dose blister packages of 50
NDC 0006-0577-82 bulk bottles of 1000.
Store at 20-25°C (68-77°F), excursions permitted to 15-30°C (59-86°F), [See USP Controlled Room Temperature].

17 PATIENT COUNSELING INFORMATION

See FDA-Approved Patient Labeling.

17.1 Instructions

Patients should be informed of the potential risks and benefits of JANUMET and of alternative modes of therapy. They should also be informed about the importance of adherence to dietary instructions, regular physical activity, periodic blood glucose monitoring and A1C testing, recognition and management of hypoglycemia and hyperglycemia, and assessment for diabetes complications. During periods of stress such as fever, trauma, infection, or surgery, medication requirements may change and patients should be advised to seek medical advice promptly.

The risks of lactic acidosis due to the metformin component, its symptoms, and conditions that predispose to its development, as noted in Warnings and Precautions (5.1), should be explained to patients. Patients should be advised to discontinue JANUMET immediately and to promptly notify their health practitioner if unexplained hyperventilation, myalgia, malaise, unusual somnolence, dizziness, slow or irregular heart beat, sensation of feeling cold (especially in the extremities) or other nonspecific symptoms occur. Gastrointestinal symptoms are common during initiation of metformin treatment and may occur during initiation of JANUMET therapy; however, patients should consult their physician if they develop unexplained symptoms. Although gastrointestinal symptoms that occur after stabilization are unlikely to be drug related, such an occurrence of symptoms should be evaluated to determine if it may be due to lactic acidosis or other serious disease.

Patients should be counseled against excessive alcohol intake, either acute or chronic, while receiving JANUMET.

Patients should be informed about the importance of regular testing of renal function and hematological parameters when receiving treatment with JANUMET.

Patients should be informed that allergic reactions have been reported during postmarketing use of sitagliptin, one of the components of JANUMET. If symptoms of allergic reactions (including rash, hives, and swelling of the face, lips, tongue, and throat that may cause difficulty in breathing or swallowing) occur, patients must stop taking JANUMET and seek medical advice promptly.

Physicians should instruct their patients to read the Patient Package Insert before starting JANUMET therapy and to reread each time the prescription is renewed. Patients should be instructed to inform their doctor if they develop any bothersome or unusual symptom, or if any symptom persists or worsens.

17.2 Laboratory Tests

Response to all diabetic therapies should be monitored by periodic measurements of blood glucose and A1C levels, with a goal of decreasing these levels towards the normal range. A1C is especially useful for evaluating long-term glycemic control.

Initial and periodic monitoring of hematologic parameters (e.g., hemoglobin/hematocrit and red blood cell indices) and renal function (serum creatinine) should be performed, at least on an annual basis. While megaloblastic anemia has rarely been seen with metformin therapy, if this is suspected, Vitamin B_{12} deficiency should be excluded.

Distributed by:
MERCK & CO., INC., Whitehouse Station, NJ 08889, USA
9794106
US Patent No.: 6,699,871
[1]Trademark of MERCK & CO., Inc., Whitehouse Station, New Jersey 08889 USA
[2]Trademark of MERCK & CO., Inc., Whitehouse Station, New Jersey 08889 USA
[3]**GLUCOPHAGE®** is a registered trademark of Merck Sante S.A.S, an associate of Merck KGaA of Darmstadt, Germany. Licensed to Bristol-Myers Squibb Company.

COPYRIGHT © 2007, 2008 MERCK & CO., Inc.
All rights reserved

Patient Information

JANUMET™ (JAN-you-met)
(sitagliptin/metformin HCl)
Tablets

Read the Patient Information that comes with JANUMET[1] before you start taking it and each time you get a refill. There may be new information. This leaflet does not take the place of talking with your doctor about your medical condition or treatment.

What is the most important information I should know about JANUMET?

Metformin hydrochloride, one of the ingredients in JANUMET, can cause a rare but serious side effect called lactic acidosis (a build-up of lactic acid in the blood) that can cause death. Lactic acidosis is a medical emergency and must be treated in a hospital.

Stop taking JANUMET and call your doctor right away if you get any of the following symptoms of lactic acidosis:

- You feel very weak and tired.
- You have unusual (not normal) muscle pain.
- You have trouble breathing.
- You have unexplained stomach or intestinal problems with nausea and vomiting, or diarrhea.
- You feel cold, especially in your arms and legs.
- You feel dizzy or lightheaded.
- You have a slow or irregular heart beat.

You have a higher chance of getting lactic acidosis if you:

- have kidney problems.
- have liver problems.
- have congestive heart failure that requires treatment with medicines.
- drink a lot of alcohol (very often or short-term "binge" drinking).
- get dehydrated (lose a large amount of body fluids). This can happen if you are sick with a fever, vomiting, or diarrhea. Dehydration can also happen when you sweat a lot with activity or exercise and don't drink enough fluids.
- have certain x-ray tests with injectable dyes or contrast agents.
- have surgery.
- have a heart attack, severe infection, or stroke.
- are 80 years of age or older and have not had your kidney function tested.

What is JANUMET?

JANUMET tablets contain two prescription medicines, sitagliptin (JANUVIA™[2]) and metformin. JANUMET can be used along with diet and exercise to lower blood sugar in adult patients with type 2 diabetes. Your doctor will determine if JANUMET is right for you and will determine the best way to start and continue to treat your diabetes.

JANUMET:

- helps to improve the levels of insulin after a meal.
- helps the body respond better to the insulin it makes naturally.
- decreases the amount of sugar made by the body.
- is unlikely to cause low blood sugar (hypoglycemia) when it is taken by itself to treat high blood sugar.

JANUMET has not been studied in children under 18 years of age.

JANUMET has not been studied with insulin, a medicine known to cause low blood sugar.

Who should not take JANUMET?

Do not take JANUMET if you:

- **have type 1 diabetes.**
- **have certain kidney problems.**
- **have conditions called metabolic acidosis or diabetic ketoacidosis** (increased ketones in the blood or urine).
- **have had an allergic reaction to JANUMET or sitagliptin (JANUVIA), one of the components of JANUMET.**
- **are going to receive an injection of dye or contrast agents for an x-ray procedure,** JANUMET will need to be stopped for a short time. Talk to your doctor about when to stop JANUMET and when to start again. See *"What is the most important information I should know about JANUMET?"*

What should I tell my doctor before and during treatment with JANUMET?

JANUMET may not be right for you. Tell your doctor about all of your medical conditions, including if you:

- have kidney problems.
- have liver problems.
- have had an allergic reaction to JANUMET or sitagliptin (JANUVIA), one of the components of JANUMET.
- have heart problems, including congestive heart failure.
- are older than 80 years. Patients over 80 years should not take JANUMET unless their kidney function is checked and it is normal.
- drink alcohol a lot (all the time or short-term "binge" drinking).
- are pregnant or plan to become pregnant. It is not known if JANUMET will harm your unborn baby. If you are pregnant, talk with your doctor about the best way to control your blood sugar while you are pregnant. If you use JANUMET during pregnancy, talk with your doctor about how you can be on the JANUMET registry. The toll-free telephone number for the pregnancy registry is 1-800-986-8999.
- are breast-feeding or plan to breast-feed. It is not known if JANUMET will pass into your breast milk. Talk with your doctor about the best way to feed your baby if you are taking JANUMET.

Tell your doctor about all the medicines you take, including prescription and non-prescription medicines, vitamins, and herbal supplements. JANUMET may affect how well other drugs work and some drugs can affect how well JANUMET works.

Know the medicines you take. Keep a list of your medicines and show it to your doctor and pharmacist when you get a new medicine. Talk to your doctor before you start any new medicine.

Continued on next page

Information on the Merck & Co., Inc., products listed on these pages is from the full prescribing information in use March 1, 2008. For information, please call 1-800-NSC-MERCK [1-800-672-6372].

Janumet—Cont.

How should I take JANUMET?

- Your doctor will tell you how many JANUMET tablets to take and how often you should take them. Take JANUMET exactly as your doctor tells you.
- Your doctor may need to increase your dose to control your blood sugar.
- Your doctor may prescribe JANUMET along with a sulfonylurea (another medicine to lower blood sugar). See *"What are the possible side effects of JANUMET?"* for information about increased risk of low blood sugar.
- Take JANUMET with meals to lower your chance of an upset stomach.
- Continue to take JANUMET as long as your doctor tells you.
- If you take too much JANUMET, call your doctor or poison control center right away.
- If you miss a dose, take it with food as soon as you remember. If you do not remember until it is time for your next dose, skip the missed dose and go back to your regular schedule. Do not take two doses of JANUMET at the same time.
- **You may need to stop taking JANUMET for a short time. Call your doctor for instructions if you:**
  - are dehydrated (have lost too much body fluid). Dehydration can occur if you are sick with severe vomiting, diarrhea or fever, or if you drink a lot less fluid than normal.
  - plan to have surgery.
  - are going to receive an injection of dye or contrast agent for an x-ray procedure.
  See *"What is the most important information I should know about JANUMET?"* and *"Who should not take JANUMET?"*
- **When your body is under some types of stress, such as fever, trauma (such as a car accident), infection or surgery, the amount of diabetes medicine that you need may change. Tell your doctor right away if you have any of these conditions and follow your doctor's instructions.**
- Monitor your blood sugar as your doctor tells you to.
- Stay on your prescribed diet and exercise program while taking JANUMET.
- Talk to your doctor about how to prevent, recognize and manage low blood sugar (hypoglycemia), high blood sugar (hyperglycemia), and complications of diabetes.
- Your doctor will monitor your diabetes with regular blood tests, including your blood sugar levels and your hemoglobin A1C.
- Your doctor will do blood tests to check your kidney function before and during treatment with JANUMET.

What are the possible side effects of JANUMET?

JANUMET can cause serious side effects. See "What is the most important information I should know about JANUMET?"

Common side effects when taking JANUMET include:
- stuffy or runny nose and sore throat
- upper respiratory infection
- diarrhea
- nausea and vomiting
- gas, stomach discomfort, indigestion
- weakness
- headache

Taking JANUMET with meals can help reduce the common stomach side effects of metformin that usually occur at the beginning of treatment. If you have unusual or unexpected stomach problems, talk with your doctor. Stomach problems that start up later during treatment may be a sign of something more serious.

Certain diabetes medicines, such as sulfonylureas and meglitinides, can cause low blood sugar (hypoglycemia). When JANUMET is used with these medicines, you may have blood sugars that are too low. Your doctor may prescribe lower doses of the sulfonylurea or meglitinide medicine. Tell your doctor if you are having problems with low blood sugar.

Serious allergic reactions can happen with JANUMET or sitagliptin, one of the medicines in JANUMET. Symptoms of a serious allergic reaction may include rash, hives, and swelling of the face, lips, tongue, and throat, difficulty breathing or swallowing. If you have an allergic reaction, stop taking JANUMET and call your doctor right away. Your doctor may prescribe a medication to treat your allergic reaction and a different medication for your diabetes.

These are not all the possible side effects of JANUMET. For more information, ask your doctor.

Tell your doctor if you have any side effect that bothers you, is unusual, or does not go away.

How should I store JANUMET?

Store JANUMET at room temperature, 68-77°F (20-25°C).

Keep JANUMET and all medicines out of the reach of children.

General information about the use of JANUMET

Medicines are sometimes prescribed for conditions that are not mentioned in patient information leaflets. Do not use JANUMET for a condition for which it was not prescribed. Do not give JANUMET to other people, even if they have the same symptoms you have. It may harm them.

This leaflet summarizes the most important information about JANUMET. If you would like to know more informa-

tion, talk with your doctor. You can ask your doctor or pharmacist for information about JANUMET that is written for health professionals. For more information call 1-800-622-4477.

What are the ingredients in JANUMET?

Active ingredients: sitagliptin and metformin hydrochloride.

Inactive ingredients: microcrystalline cellulose, polyvinylpyrrolidone, sodium lauryl sulfate, and sodium stearyl fumarate. The tablet film coating contains the following inactive ingredients: polyvinyl alcohol, polyethylene glycol, talc, titanium dioxide, red iron oxide, and black iron oxide.

What is type 2 diabetes?

Type 2 diabetes is a condition in which your body does not make enough insulin, and the insulin that your body produces does not work as well as it should. Your body can also make too much sugar. When this happens, sugar (glucose) builds up in the blood. This can lead to serious medical problems.

The main goal of treating diabetes is to lower your blood sugar to a normal level. Lowering and controlling blood sugar may help prevent or delay complications of diabetes, such as heart problems, kidney problems, blindness, and amputation.

High blood sugar can be lowered by diet and exercise, and by certain medicines when necessary.

Issued February 2008

Distributed by:

MERCK & CO., INC., Whitehouse Station, NJ 08889, USA
9794106

JANUVIA™ ℞

[ja-new'-vee-a]

(sitagliptin)
Tablets

Prescribing information for this product, which appears on pages 2017-2021 of the 2008 PDR, has been completely revised as follows. Please write "See Supplement A" next to the product heading.

HIGHLIGHTS OF PRESCRIBING INFORMATION

These highlights do not include all the information needed to use JANUVIA safely and effectively. See full prescribing information for JANUVIA.

JANUVIA™ (sitagliptin) Tablets
Initial U.S. Approval: 2006

RECENT MAJOR CHANGES

Indications and Usage	
Monotherapy and Combination Therapy (1.1)	10/2007
Important Limitations of Use (1.2)	10/2007
Dosage and Administration	
Recommended Dosing (2.1)	10/2007
Concomitant Use with a Sulfonylurea (2.3)	10/2007
Contraindications (4)	10/2007
Warnings and Precautions	
Use with Medications Known to Cause	
Hypoglycemia (5.2)	10/2007
Hypersensitivity Reactions (5.3)	10/2007

INDICATIONS AND USAGE

JANUVIA is a dipeptidyl peptidase-4 (DPP-4) inhibitor indicated as an adjunct to diet and exercise to improve glycemic control in adults with type 2 diabetes mellitus. (1.1)

Important Limitations of Use:
- JANUVIA should not be used in patients with type 1 diabetes or for the treatment of diabetic ketoacidosis. (1.2)
- JANUVIA has not been studied in combination with insulin. (1.2)

DOSAGE AND ADMINISTRATION

The recommended dose of JANUVIA is 100 mg once daily. JANUVIA can be taken with or without food. (2.1)
Dosage adjustment is recommended for patients with moderate or severe renal insufficiency or end-stage renal disease. (2.2)

Dosage Adjustment in Patients With Moderate, Severe and End Stage Renal Disease (ESRD) (2.2)	
50 mg once daily	25 mg once daily
Moderate	Severe and ESRD
CrCl ≥30 to <50 mL/min	CrCl <30 mL/min
~Serum Cr levels [mg/dL]	~Serum Cr levels [mg/dL]
Men: >1.7-≤3.0;	Men: >3.0;
Women: >1.5-≤2.5	Women: >2.5; or on dialysis

DOSAGE FORMS AND STRENGTHS

Tablets: 100 mg, 50 mg, and 25 mg (3)

CONTRAINDICATIONS

History of a serious hypersensitivity reaction to sitagliptin, such as anaphylaxis or angioedema (5.3, 6.2)

WARNINGS AND PRECAUTIONS

- Dosage adjustment is recommended in patients with moderate or severe renal insufficiency and in patients with

ESRD. Assessment of renal function is recommended prior to initiating JANUVIA and periodically thereafter. (2.2, 5.1)
- When used with a sulfonylurea, a lower dose of sulfonylurea may be required to reduce the risk of hypoglycemia. (2.3, 5.2)
- There have been postmarketing reports of serious allergic and hypersensitivity reactions in patients treated with JANUVIA such as anaphylaxis, angioedema, and exfoliative skin conditions including Stevens-Johnson syndrome. In such cases, promptly stop JANUVIA, assess for other potential causes, institute appropriate monitoring and treatment, and initiate alternative treatment for diabetes. (5.3, 6.2)

ADVERSE REACTIONS

Adverse reactions reported in ≥5% of patients treated with JANUVIA and more commonly than in patients treated with placebo are: upper respiratory tract infection, nasopharyngitis and headache. Hypoglycemia was also reported more commonly in patients treated with the combination of JANUVIA and sulfonylurea, with or without metformin, than in patients given the combination of placebo and sulfonylurea, with or without metformin. (6.1)

To report SUSPECTED ADVERSE REACTIONS, contact Merck & Co., Inc. at 1-877-888-4231 or FDA at 1-800-FDA-1088 or www.fda.gov/medwatch.

USE IN SPECIFIC POPULATIONS

- Safety and effectiveness of JANUVIA in children under 18 years have not been established. (8.4)
- There are no adequate and well-controlled studies in pregnant women. To report drug exposure during pregnancy call 1-800-986-8999. (8.1)

See 17 for PATIENT COUNSELING INFORMATION and FDA-approved patient labeling.

Revised: 10/2007

FULL PRESCRIBING INFORMATION: CONTENTS*

FULL PRESCRIBING INFORMATION

1 INDICATIONS AND USAGE

1.1 Monotherapy and Combination Therapy

JANUVIA[1] is indicated as an adjunct to diet and exercise to improve glycemic control in adults with type 2 diabetes mellitus. *[See Clinical Studies (14).]*

1.2 Important Limitations of Use

JANUVIA should not be used in patients with type 1 diabetes or for the treatment of diabetic ketoacidosis, as it would not be effective in these settings.

JANUVIA has not been studied in combination with insulin.

2 DOSAGE AND ADMINISTRATION

2.1 Recommended Dosing

The recommended dose of JANUVIA is 100 mg once daily. JANUVIA can be taken with or without food.

2.2 Patients with Renal Insufficiency

For patients with mild renal insufficiency (creatinine clearance [CrCl] ≥50 mL/min, approximately corresponding to serum creatinine levels of ≤1.7 mg/dL in men and ≤1.5 mg/dL in women), no dosage adjustment for JANUVIA is required.

For patients with moderate renal insufficiency (CrCl ≥30 to <50 mL/min, approximately corresponding to serum creatinine levels of >1.7 to ≤3.0 mg/dL in men and >1.5 to ≤2.5 mg/dL in women), the dose of JANUVIA is 50 mg once daily.

For patients with severe renal insufficiency (CrCl <30 mL/min, approximately corresponding to serum creatinine levels of >3.0 mg/dL in men and >2.5 mg/dL in women) or with end-stage renal disease (ESRD) requiring hemodialysis or peritoneal dialysis, the dose of JANUVIA is 25 mg once daily. JANUVIA may be administered without regard to the timing of hemodialysis.

Because there is a need for dosage adjustment based upon renal function, assessment of renal function is recommended prior to initiation of JANUVIA and periodically thereafter. Creatinine clearance can be estimated from serum creatinine using the Cockcroft-Gault formula. *[See Clinical Pharmacology (12.3).]*

2.3 Concomitant Use with a Sulfonylurea

When JANUVIA is used in combination with a sulfonylurea, a lower dose of sulfonylurea may be required to reduce the risk of hypoglycemia. *[See Warnings and Precautions (5.2).]*

3 DOSAGE FORMS AND STRENGTHS

- 100 mg tablets are beige, round, film-coated tablets with "277" on one side.
- 50 mg tablets are light beige, round, film-coated tablets with "112" on one side.
- 25 mg tablets are pink, round, film-coated tablets with "221" on one side.

4 CONTRAINDICATIONS

History of a serious hypersensitivity reaction to sitagliptin, such as anaphylaxis or angioedema. *[See Warnings and Precautions (5.3) and Adverse Reactions (6.2).]*

5 WARNINGS AND PRECAUTIONS

5.1 Use in Patients with Renal Insufficiency

A dosage adjustment is recommended in patients with moderate or severe renal insufficiency and in patients with ESRD requiring hemodialysis or peritoneal dialysis. *[See Dosage and Administration (2.2); Clinical Pharmacology (12.3).]*

5.2 Use with Medications Known to Cause Hypoglycemia

As is typical with other antihyperglycemic agents used in combination with a sulfonylurea, when JANUVIA was used in combination with a sulfonylurea, a class of medications known to cause hypoglycemia, the incidence of hypoglycemia was increased over that of placebo. *[See Adverse Reactions (6.1).]* Therefore, a lower dose of sulfonylurea may be required to reduce the risk of hypoglycemia. *[See Dosage and Administration (2.3).]*

5.3 Hypersensitivity Reactions

There have been postmarketing reports of serious hypersensitivity reactions in patients treated with JANUVIA. These reactions include anaphylaxis, angioedema, and exfoliative skin conditions including Stevens-Johnson syndrome. Because these reactions are reported voluntarily from a population of uncertain size, it is generally not possible to reliably estimate their frequency or establish a causal relationship to drug exposure. Onset of these reactions occurred within the first 3 months after initiation of treatment with JANUVIA, with some reports occurring after the first dose. If a hypersensitivity reaction is suspected, discontinue JANUVIA, assess for other potential causes for the event, and institute alternative treatment for diabetes. *[See Adverse Reactions (6.2).]*

6 ADVERSE REACTIONS

6.1 Clinical Trials Experience

Because clinical trials are conducted under widely varying conditions, adverse reaction rates observed in the clinical trials of a drug cannot be directly compared to rates in the clinical trials of another drug and may not reflect the rates observed in practice.

In controlled clinical studies as both monotherapy and combination therapy with metformin or pioglitazone, the overall incidence of adverse reactions, hypoglycemia, and discontinuation of therapy due to clinical adverse reactions with JANUVIA were similar to placebo. In combination with glimepiride, with or without metformin, the overall incidence of clinical adverse reactions with JANUVIA was higher than with placebo, in part related to a higher incidence of hypoglycemia (see Table 1); the incidence of discontinuation due to clinical adverse reactions was similar to placebo.

Two placebo-controlled monotherapy studies, one of 18- and one of 24-week duration, included patients treated with JANUVIA 100 mg daily, JANUVIA 200 mg daily, and placebo. Three 24-week, placebo-controlled add-on combination therapy studies, one with metformin, one with pioglitazone, and one with glimepiride with or without metformin, were also conducted. In addition to a stable dose of metformin, pioglitazone, glimepiride, or glimepiride and metformin, patients whose diabetes was not adequately controlled were given either JANUVIA 100 mg daily or placebo. The adverse reactions, reported regardless of investigator assessment of causality in ≥5% of patients treated with JANUVIA 100 mg daily as monotherapy, JANUVIA in combination with pioglitazone, or JANUVIA in combination with glimepiride, with or without metformin, and more commonly than in patients treated with placebo, are shown in Table 1.

Table 2
Initial Therapy with Combination of Sitagliptin and Metformin: Adverse Reactions Reported (Regardless of Investigator Assessment of Causality) in ≥5% of Patients Receiving Combination Therapy (and Greater than in Patients Receiving Metformin alone, Sitagliptin alone, and Placebo)†

	Number of Patients (%)			
	Placebo	**Sitagliptin (JANUVIA) 100 mg QD**	**Metformin 500 or 1000 mg bid††**	**Sitagliptin 50 mg bid + Metformin 500 or 1000 mg bid††**
	N = 176	N = 179	N = 364††	N = 372††
Upper Respiratory Infection	9 (5.1)	8 (4.5)	19 (5.2)	23 (6.2)
Headache	5 (2.8)	2 (1.1)	14 (3.8)	22 (5.9)

† Intent-to-treat population.
†† Data pooled for the patients given the lower and higher doses of metformin.

Table 1
Placebo-Controlled Clinical Studies of JANUVIA Monotherapy or Add-on Combination Therapy with Pioglitazone or Glimepiride +/− Metformin: Adverse Reactions Reported in ≥5% of Patients and More Commonly than in Patients Given Placebo, Regardless of Investigator Assessment of Causality†

	Number of Patients (%)	
Monotherapy	**JANUVIA 100 mg**	**Placebo**
	N = 443	N = 363
Nasopharyngitis	23 (5.2)	12 (3.3)
Combination with Pioglitazone	**JANUVIA 100 mg + Pioglitazone**	**Placebo + Pioglitazone**
	N = 175	N = 178
Upper Respiratory Tract Infection	11 (6.3)	6 (3.4)
Headache	9 (5.1)	7 (3.9)
Combination with Glimepiride (+/− Metformin)	**JANUVIA 100 mg + Glimepiride (+/− Metformin)**	**Placebo + Glimepiride (+/− Metformin)**
	N = 222	N = 219
Hypoglycemia	27 (12.2)	4 (1.8)
Nasopharyngitis	14 (6.3)	10 (4.6)
Headache	13 (5.9)	5 (2.3)

† Intent to treat population

In the study of patients receiving JANUVIA as add-on combination therapy with metformin, there were no adverse reactions reported regardless of investigator assessment of causality in ≥5% of patients and more commonly than in patients given placebo.

In the prespecified pooled analysis of the two monotherapy studies, the add-on to metformin study, and the add-on to pioglitazone study, the overall incidence of adverse reactions of hypoglycemia in patients treated with JANUVIA 100 mg was similar to placebo (1.2% vs 0.9%). Adverse reactions of hypoglycemia were based on all reports of hypoglycemia; a concurrent glucose measurement was not required. The incidence of selected gastrointestinal adverse reactions in patients treated with JANUVIA was as follows: abdominal pain (JANUVIA 100 mg, 2.3%; placebo, 2.1%), nausea (1.4%, 0.6%), and diarrhea (3.0%, 2.3%).

In an additional, 24-week, placebo-controlled factorial study of initial therapy with sitagliptin in combination with metformin, the adverse reactions reported (regardless of investigator assessment of causality) in ≥5% of patients are shown in Table 2. The incidence of hypoglycemia was 0.6% in patients given placebo, 0.6% in patients given sitagliptin alone, 0.8% in patients given metformin alone, and 1.6% in patients given sitagliptin in combination with metformin. [See table 2 above]

No clinically meaningful changes in vital signs or in ECG (including in QTc interval) were observed in patients treated with JANUVIA.

Laboratory Tests

Across clinical studies, the incidence of laboratory adverse reactions was similar in patients treated with JANUVIA 100 mg compared to patients treated with placebo. A small increase in white blood cell count (WBC) was observed due to an increase in neutrophils. This increase in WBC (of approximately 200 cells/microL vs placebo, in four pooled placebo-controlled clinical studies, with a mean baseline WBC count of approximately 6600 cells/microL) is not considered to be clinically relevant. In a 12-week study of 91 patients with chronic renal insufficiency, 37 patients with moderate renal insufficiency were randomized to JANUVIA 50 mg daily, while 14 patients with the same magnitude of renal impairment were randomized to placebo. Mean (SE) increases in serum creatinine were observed in patients treated with JANUVIA [0.12 mg/dL (0.04)] and in patients treated with placebo [0.07 mg/dL (0.07)]. The clinical significance of this added increase in serum creatinine relative to placebo is not known.

6.2 Postmarketing Experience

The following additional adverse reactions have been identified during postapproval use of JANUVIA. Because these reactions are reported voluntarily from a population of uncertain size, it is generally not possible to reliably estimate their frequency or establish a causal relationship to drug exposure.

Hypersensitivity reactions include anaphylaxis, angioedema, rash, urticaria, and exfoliative skin conditions including Stevens-Johnson syndrome. *[See Warnings and Precautions (5.3).]*

7 DRUG INTERACTIONS

7.1 Digoxin

There was a slight increase in the area under the curve (AUC, 11%) and mean peak drug concentration (C_{max}, 18%) of digoxin with the co-administration of 100 mg sitagliptin for 10 days. Patients receiving digoxin should be monitored appropriately. No dosage adjustment of digoxin or JANUVIA is recommended.

8 USE IN SPECIFIC POPULATIONS

8.1 Pregnancy

Pregnancy Category B:

Reproduction studies have been performed in rats and rabbits. Doses of sitagliptin up to 125 mg/kg (approximately 12 times the human exposure at the maximum recommended human dose) did not impair fertility or harm the fetus. There are, however, no adequate and well-controlled studies in pregnant women. Because animal reproduction studies are not always predictive of human response, this drug should be used during pregnancy only if clearly needed.

Merck & Co., Inc. maintains a registry to monitor the pregnancy outcomes of women exposed to JANUVIA while pregnant. Health care providers are encouraged to report any prenatal exposure to JANUVIA by calling the Pregnancy Registry at (800) 986-8999.

Sitagliptin administered to pregnant female rats and rabbits from gestation day 6 to 20 (organogenesis) was not teratogenic at oral doses up to 250 mg/kg (rats) and 125 mg/kg (rabbits), or approximately 30- and 20-times human exposure at the maximum recommended human dose (MRHD) of 100 mg/day based on AUC comparisons. Higher doses increased the incidence of rib malformations in offspring at 1000 mg/kg, or approximately 100 times human exposure at the MRHD.

Sitagliptin administered to female rats from gestation day 6 to lactation day 21 decreased body weight in male and female offspring at 1000 mg/kg. No functional or behavioral toxicity was observed in offspring of rats.

Placental transfer of sitagliptin administered to pregnant rats was approximately 45% at 2 hours and 80% at 24 hours postdose. Placental transfer of sitagliptin administered to pregnant rabbits was approximately 66% at 2 hours and 30% at 24 hours.

8.3 Nursing Mothers

Sitagliptin is secreted in the milk of lactating rats at a milk to plasma ratio of 4:1. It is not known whether sitagliptin is excreted in human milk. Because many drugs are excreted in human milk, caution should be exercised when JANUVIA is administered to a nursing woman.

8.4 Pediatric Use

Safety and effectiveness of JANUVIA in pediatric patients under 18 years of age have not been established.

8.5 Geriatric Use

Of the total number of subjects (N=3884) in pre-approval clinical safety and efficacy studies of JANUVIA, 725 patients were 65 years and over, while 61 patients were 75 years and over. No overall differences in safety or effectiveness were observed between subjects 65 years and over and

Continued on next page

Information on the Merck & Co., Inc., products listed on these pages is from the full prescribing information in use March 1, 2008. For information, please call 1-800-NSC-MERCK [1-800-672-6372].

Januvia—Cont.

younger subjects. While this and other reported clinical experience have not identified differences in responses between the elderly and younger patients, greater sensitivity of some older individuals cannot be ruled out.

This drug is known to be substantially excreted by the kidney. Because elderly patients are more likely to have decreased renal function, care should be taken in dose selection in the elderly, and it may be useful to assess renal function in these patients prior to initiating dosing and periodically thereafter *[see Dosage and Administration (2.2); Clinical Pharmacology (12.3)]*.

10 OVERDOSAGE

During controlled clinical trials in healthy subjects, single doses of up to 800 mg JANUVIA were administered. Maximal mean increases in QTc of 8.0 msec were observed in one study at a dose of 800 mg JANUVIA, a mean effect that is not considered clinically important *[see Clinical Pharmacology (12.2)]*. There is no experience with doses above 800 mg in humans. In Phase I multiple-dose studies, there were no dose-related clinical adverse reactions observed with JANUVIA with doses of up to 600 mg per day for periods of up to 10 days and 400 mg per day for up to 28 days.

In the event of an overdose, it is reasonable to employ the usual supportive measures, e.g., remove unabsorbed material from the gastrointestinal tract, employ clinical monitoring (including obtaining an electrocardiogram), and institute supportive therapy as dictated by the patient's clinical status.

Sitagliptin is modestly dialyzable. In clinical studies, approximately 13.5% of the dose was removed over a 3- to 4-hour hemodialysis session. Prolonged hemodialysis may be considered if clinically appropriate. It is not known if sitagliptin is dialyzable by peritoneal dialysis.

11 DESCRIPTION

JANUVIA Tablets contain sitagliptin phosphate, an orally-active inhibitor of the dipeptidyl peptidase-4 (DPP-4) enzyme.

Sitagliptin phosphate monohydrate is described chemically as 7-[(3*R*)-3-amino-1-oxo-4-(2,4,5-trifluorophenyl) butyl]-5,6,7,8-tetrahydro-3-(trifluoromethyl)-1,2,4-triazolo[4,3-*a*]pyrazine phosphate (1:1) monohydrate.

The empirical formula is $C_{16}H_{15}F_6N_5O{\bullet}H_3PO_4{\bullet}H_2O$ and the molecular weight is 523.32. The structural formula is:

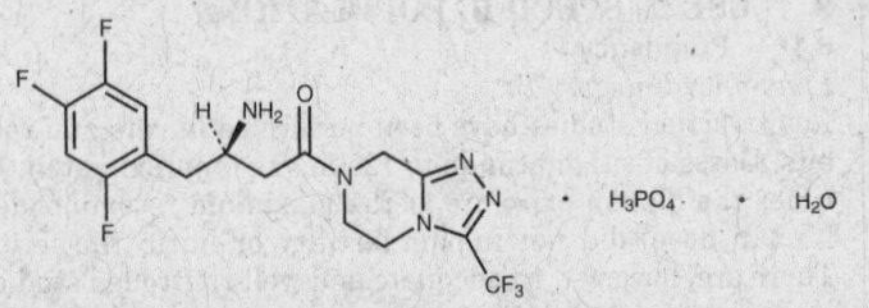

Sitagliptin phosphate monohydrate is a white to off-white, crystalline, non-hygroscopic powder. It is soluble in water and N,N-dimethyl formamide; slightly soluble in methanol; very slightly soluble in ethanol, acetone, and acetonitrile; and insoluble in isopropanol and isopropyl acetate.

Each film-coated tablet of JANUVIA contains 32.13, 64.25, or 128.5 mg of sitagliptin phosphate monohydrate, which is equivalent to 25, 50, or 100 mg, respectively, of free base and the following inactive ingredients: microcrystalline cellulose, anhydrous dibasic calcium phosphate, croscarmellose sodium, magnesium stearate, and sodium stearyl fumarate. In addition, the film coating contains the following inactive ingredients: polyvinyl alcohol, polyethylene glycol, talc, titanium dioxide, red iron oxide, and yellow iron oxide.

12 CLINICAL PHARMACOLOGY

12.1 Mechanism of Action

Sitagliptin is a DPP-4 inhibitor, which is believed to exert its actions in patients with type 2 diabetes by slowing the inactivation of incretin hormones. Concentrations of the active intact hormones are increased by JANUVIA, thereby increasing and prolonging the action of these hormones. Incretin hormones, including glucagon-like peptide-1 (GLP-1) and glucose-dependent insulinotropic polypeptide (GIP), are released by the intestine throughout the day, and levels are increased in response to a meal. These hormones are rapidly inactivated by the enzyme, DPP-4. The incretins are part of an endogenous system involved in the physiologic regulation of glucose homeostasis. When blood glucose concentrations are normal or elevated, GLP-1 and GIP increase insulin synthesis and release from pancreatic beta cells by intracellular signaling pathways involving cyclic AMP. GLP-1 also lowers glucagon secretion from pancreatic alpha cells, leading to reduced hepatic glucose production. By increasing and prolonging active incretin levels, JANUVIA increases insulin release and decreases glucagon levels in the circulation in a glucose-dependent manner. Sitagliptin demonstrates selectivity for DPP-4 and does not inhibit DPP-8 or DPP-9 activity *in vitro* at concentrations approximating those from therapeutic doses.

12.2 Pharmacodynamics

General

In patients with type 2 diabetes, administration of JANUVIA led to inhibition of DPP-4 enzyme activity for a 24-hour period. After an oral glucose load or a meal, this DPP-4 inhibition resulted in a 2- to 3-fold increase in circulating levels of active GLP-1 and GIP, decreased glucagon concentrations, and increased responsiveness of insulin release to glucose, resulting in higher C-peptide and insulin concentrations. The rise in insulin with the decrease in glucagon was associated with lower fasting glucose concentrations and reduced glucose excursion following an oral glucose load or a meal.

In a two-day study in healthy subjects, sitagliptin alone increased active GLP-1 concentrations, whereas metformin alone increased active and total GLP-1 concentrations to similar extents. Co-administration of sitagliptin and metformin had an additive effect on active GLP-1 concentrations. Sitagliptin, but not metformin, increased active GIP concentrations. It is unclear how these findings relate to changes in glycemic control in patients with type 2 diabetes.

In studies with healthy subjects, JANUVIA did not lower blood glucose or cause hypoglycemia.

Cardiac Electrophysiology

In a randomized, placebo-controlled crossover study, 79 healthy subjects were administered a single oral dose of JANUVIA 100 mg, JANUVIA 800 mg (8 times the recommended dose), and placebo. At the recommended dose of 100 mg, there was no effect on the QTc interval obtained at the peak plasma concentration, or at any other time during the study. Following the 800 mg dose, the maximum increase in the placebo-corrected mean change in QTc from baseline was observed at 3 hours postdose and was 8.0 msec. This increase is not considered to be clinically significant. At the 800 mg dose, peak sitagliptin plasma concentrations were approximately 11 times higher than the peak concentrations following a 100 mg dose.

In patients with type 2 diabetes administered JANUVIA 100 mg (N=81) or JANUVIA 200 mg (N=63) daily, there were no meaningful changes in QTc interval based on ECG data obtained at the time of expected peak plasma concentration.

12.3 Pharmacokinetics

The pharmacokinetics of sitagliptin has been extensively characterized in healthy subjects and patients with type 2 diabetes. After oral administration of a 100 mg dose to healthy subjects, sitagliptin was rapidly absorbed, with peak plasma concentrations (median T_{max}) occurring 1 to 4 hours postdose. Plasma AUC of sitagliptin increased in a dose-proportional manner. Following a single oral 100 mg dose to healthy volunteers, mean plasma AUC of sitagliptin was 8.52 μM•hr, C_{max} was 950 nM, and apparent terminal half-life ($t_{1/2}$) was 12.4 hours. Plasma AUC of sitagliptin increased approximately 14% following 100 mg doses at steady-state compared to the first dose. The intra-subject and inter-subject coefficients of variation for sitagliptin AUC were small (5.8% and 15.1%). The pharmacokinetics of sitagliptin was generally similar in healthy subjects and in patients with type 2 diabetes.

Absorption

The absolute bioavailability of sitagliptin is approximately 87%. Because coadministration of a high-fat meal with JANUVIA had no effect on the pharmacokinetics, JANUVIA may be administered with or without food.

Distribution

The mean volume of distribution at steady state following a single 100 mg intravenous dose of sitagliptin to healthy subjects is approximately 198 liters. The fraction of sitagliptin reversibly bound to plasma proteins is low (38%).

Metabolism

Approximately 79% of sitagliptin is excreted unchanged in the urine with metabolism being a minor pathway of elimination.

Following a [^{14}C]sitagliptin oral dose, approximately 16% of the radioactivity was excreted as metabolites of sitagliptin. Six metabolites were detected at trace levels and are not expected to contribute to the plasma DPP-4 inhibitory activity of sitagliptin. *In vitro* studies indicated that the primary enzyme responsible for the limited metabolism of sitagliptin was CYP3A4, with contribution from CYP2C8.

Excretion

Following administration of an oral [^{14}C]sitagliptin dose to healthy subjects, approximately 100% of the administered radioactivity was eliminated in feces (13%) or urine (87%) within one week of dosing. The apparent terminal $t_{1/2}$ following a 100 mg oral dose of sitagliptin was approximately 12.4 hours and renal clearance was approximately 350 mL/min.

Elimination of sitagliptin occurs primarily via renal excretion and involves active tubular secretion. Sitagliptin is a substrate for human organic anion transporter-3 (hOAT-3), which may be involved in the renal elimination of sitagliptin. The clinical relevance of hOAT-3 in sitagliptin transport has not been established. Sitagliptin is also a substrate of p-glycoprotein, which may also be involved in mediating the renal elimination of sitagliptin. However, cyclosporine, a p-glycoprotein inhibitor, did not reduce the renal clearance of sitagliptin.

Special Populations

Renal Insufficiency

A single-dose, open-label study was conducted to evaluate the pharmacokinetics of JANUVIA (50 mg dose) in patients with varying degrees of chronic renal insufficiency compared to normal healthy control subjects. The study included patients with renal insufficiency classified on the basis of creatinine clearance as mild (50 to <80 mL/min), moderate (30 to <50 mL/min), and severe (<30 mL/min), as well as patients with ESRD on hemodialysis. In addition, the effects of renal insufficiency on sitagliptin pharmacokinetics in patients with type 2 diabetes and mild or moderate renal insufficiency were assessed using population pharmacokinetic analyses. Creatinine clearance was measured by 24-hour urinary creatinine clearance measurements or estimated from serum creatinine based on the Cockcroft-Gault formula:

$$CrCl = \frac{[140 - \text{age (years)}] \times \text{weight (kg)}}{[72 \times \text{serum creatinine (mg/dL)}]} \quad \{\times 0.85 \text{ for female patients}\}$$

Compared to normal healthy control subjects, an approximate 1.1- to 1.6-fold increase in plasma AUC of sitagliptin was observed in patients with mild renal insufficiency. Because increases of this magnitude are not clinically relevant, dosage adjustment in patients with mild renal insufficiency is not necessary. Plasma AUC levels of sitagliptin were increased approximately 2-fold and 4-fold in patients with moderate renal insufficiency and in patients with severe renal insufficiency, including patients with ESRD on hemodialysis, respectively. Sitagliptin was modestly removed by hemodialysis (13.5% over a 3- to 4-hour hemodialysis session starting 4 hours postdose). To achieve plasma concentrations of sitagliptin similar to those in patients with normal renal function, lower dosages are recommended in patients with moderate and severe renal insufficiency, as well as in ESRD patients requiring hemodialysis. *[See Dosage and Administration (2.2).]*

Hepatic Insufficiency

In patients with moderate hepatic insufficiency (Child-Pugh score 7 to 9), mean AUC and C_{max} of sitagliptin increased approximately 21% and 13%, respectively, compared to healthy matched controls following administration of a single 100 mg dose of JANUVIA. These differences are not considered to be clinically meaningful. No dosage adjustment for JANUVIA is necessary for patients with mild or moderate hepatic insufficiency.

There is no clinical experience in patients with severe hepatic insufficiency (Child-Pugh score >9).

Body Mass Index (BMI)

No dosage adjustment is necessary based on BMI. Body mass index had no clinically meaningful effect on the pharmacokinetics of sitagliptin based on a composite analysis of Phase I pharmacokinetic data and on a population pharmacokinetic analysis of Phase I and Phase II data.

Gender

No dosage adjustment is necessary based on gender. Gender had no clinically meaningful effect on the pharmacokinetics of sitagliptin based on a composite analysis of Phase I pharmacokinetic data and on a population pharmacokinetic analysis of Phase I and Phase II data.

Geriatric

No dosage adjustment is required based solely on age. When the effects of age on renal function are taken into account, age alone did not have a clinically meaningful impact on the pharmacokinetics of sitagliptin based on a population pharmacokinetic analysis. Elderly subjects (65 to 80 years) had approximately 19% higher plasma concentrations of sitagliptin compared to younger subjects.

Pediatric

Studies characterizing the pharmacokinetics of sitagliptin in pediatric patients have not been performed.

Race

No dosage adjustment is necessary based on race. Race had no clinically meaningful effect on the pharmacokinetics of sitagliptin based on a composite analysis of available pharmacokinetic data, including subjects of white, Hispanic, black, Asian, and other racial groups.

Drug Interactions

In Vitro Assessment of Drug Interactions

Sitagliptin is not an inhibitor of CYP isozymes CYP3A4, 2C8, 2C9, 2D6, 1A2, 2C19 or 2B6, and is not an inducer of CYP3A4. Sitagliptin is a p-glycoprotein substrate, but does not inhibit p-glycoprotein mediated transport of digoxin. Based on these results, sitagliptin is considered unlikely to cause interactions with other drugs that utilize these pathways.

Sitagliptin is not extensively bound to plasma proteins. Therefore, the propensity of sitagliptin to be involved in clinically meaningful drug-drug interactions mediated by plasma protein binding displacement is very low.

In Vivo Assessment of Drug Interactions

Effects of Sitagliptin on Other Drugs

In clinical studies, as described below, sitagliptin did not meaningfully alter the pharmacokinetics of metformin, glyburide, simvastatin, rosiglitazone, warfarin, or oral contraceptives, providing *in vivo* evidence of a low propensity for causing drug interactions with substrates of CYP3A4, CYP2C8, CYP2C9, and organic cationic transporter (OCT).

Digoxin: Sitagliptin had a minimal effect on the pharmacokinetics of digoxin. Following administration of 0.25 mg digoxin concomitantly with 100 mg of JANUVIA daily for 10 days, the plasma AUC of digoxin was increased by 11%, and the plasma C_{max} by 18%.

Metformin: Co-administration of multiple twice-daily doses of sitagliptin with metformin, an OCT substrate, did not meaningfully alter the pharmacokinetics of metformin in patients with type 2 diabetes. Therefore, sitagliptin is not an inhibitor of OCT-mediated transport.

Sulfonylureas: Single-dose pharmacokinetics of glyburide, a CYP2C9 substrate, was not meaningfully altered in subjects receiving multiple doses of sitagliptin. Clinically meaningful interactions would not be expected with other sulfonylureas (e.g., glipizide, tolbutamide, and glimepiride) which, like glyburide, are primarily eliminated by CYP2C9.

Simvastatin: Single-dose pharmacokinetics of simvastatin, a CYP3A4 substrate, was not meaningfully altered in subjects receiving multiple daily doses of sitagliptin.

Therefore, sitagliptin is not an inhibitor of CYP3A4-mediated metabolism.

Thiazolidinediones: Single-dose pharmacokinetics of rosiglitazone was not meaningfully altered in subjects receiving multiple daily doses of sitagliptin, indicating that JANUVIA is not an inhibitor of CYP2C8-mediated metabolism.

Warfarin: Multiple daily doses of sitagliptin did not meaningfully alter the pharmacokinetics, as assessed by measurement of $S(-)$ or $R(+)$ warfarin enantiomers, or pharmacodynamics (as assessed by measurement of prothrombin INR) of a single dose of warfarin. Because $S(-)$ warfarin is primarily metabolized by CYP2C9, these data also support the conclusion that sitagliptin is not a CYP2C9 inhibitor.

Oral Contraceptives: Co-administration with sitagliptin did not meaningfully alter the steady-state pharmacokinetics of norethindrone or ethinyl estradiol.

Effects of Other Drugs on Sitagliptin

Clinical data described below suggest that sitagliptin is not susceptible to clinically meaningful interactions by co-administered medications.

Metformin: Co-administration of multiple twice-daily doses of metformin with sitagliptin did not meaningfully alter the pharmacokinetics of sitagliptin in patients with type 2 diabetes.

Cyclosporine: A study was conducted to assess the effect of cyclosporine, a potent inhibitor of p-glycoprotein, on the pharmacokinetics of sitagliptin. Co-administration of a single 100 mg oral dose of JANUVIA and a single 600 mg oral dose of cyclosporine increased the AUC and C_{max} of sitagliptin by approximately 29% and 68%, respectively. These modest changes in sitagliptin pharmacokinetics were not considered to be clinically meaningful. The renal clearance of sitagliptin was also not meaningfully altered. Therefore, meaningful interactions would not be expected with other p-glycoprotein inhibitors.

13 NONCLINICAL TOXICOLOGY

13.1 Carcinogenesis, Mutagenesis, Impairment of Fertility

A two-year carcinogenicity study was conducted in male and female rats given oral doses of sitagliptin of 50, 150, and 500 mg/kg/day. There was an increased incidence of combined liver adenoma/carcinoma in males and females and of liver carcinoma in females at 500 mg/kg. This dose results in exposures approximately 60 times the human exposure at the maximum recommended daily adult human dose (MRHD) of 100 mg/day based on AUC comparisons. Liver tumors were not observed at 150 mg/kg, approximately 20 times the human exposure at the MRHD. A two-year carcinogenicity study was conducted in male and female mice given oral doses of sitagliptin of 50, 125, 250, and 500 mg/kg/day. There was no increase in the incidence of tumors in any organ up to 500 mg/kg, approximately 70 times human exposure at the MRHD. Sitagliptin was not mutagenic or clastogenic with or without metabolic activation in the Ames bacterial mutagenicity assay, a Chinese hamster ovary (CHO) chromosome aberration assay, an *in vitro* cytogenetics assay in CHO, an *in vitro* rat hepatocyte DNA alkaline elution assay, and an *in vivo* micronucleus assay.

In rat fertility studies with oral gavage doses of 125, 250, and 1000 mg/kg, males were treated for 4 weeks prior to mating, during mating, up to scheduled termination (approximately 8 weeks total) and females were treated 2 weeks prior to mating through gestation day 7. No adverse effect on fertility was observed at 125 mg/kg (approximately 12 times human exposure at the MRHD of 100 mg/day based on AUC comparisons). At higher doses, nondose-related increased resorptions in females were observed (approximately 25 and 100 times human exposure at the MRHD based on AUC comparison).

14 CLINICAL STUDIES

JANUVIA has been studied as monotherapy and in combination with metformin, pioglitazone, glimepiride, and glimepiride+metformin.

There were approximately 3800 patients with type 2 diabetes randomized in six double-blind, placebo-controlled clinical safety and efficacy studies conducted to evaluate the effects of sitagliptin on glycemic control. The ethnic/racial distribution in these studies was approximately 60% white, 20% Hispanic, 8% Asian, 6% black, and 6% other groups. Patients had an overall mean age of approximately 55 years (range 18 to 87 years). In addition, an active (glipizide)-controlled study of 52-weeks duration was conducted in 1172 patients with type 2 diabetes who had inadequate glycemic control on metformin.

In patients with type 2 diabetes, treatment with JANUVIA produced clinically significant improvements in hemoglobin A1C, fasting plasma glucose (FPG) and 2-hour postprandial glucose (PPG) compared to placebo.

14.1 Monotherapy

A total of 1262 patients with type 2 diabetes participated in two double-blind, placebo-controlled studies, one of 18-week and another of 24-week duration, to evaluate the efficacy and safety of JANUVIA monotherapy. In both monotherapy studies, patients currently on an antihyperglycemic agent discontinued the agent, and underwent a diet, exercise, and drug washout period of about 7 weeks. Patients with inadequate glycemic control (A1C 7% to 10%) after the washout period were randomized after completing a 2-week single-blind placebo run-in period; patients not currently on antihyperglycemic agents (off therapy for at least 8 weeks) with inadequate glycemic control (A1C 7% to 10%) were randomized after completing the 2-week single-blind placebo run-in period. In the 18-week study, 521 patients were randomized

to placebo, JANUVIA 100 mg, or JANUVIA 200 mg, and in the 24-week study 741 patients were randomized to placebo, JANUVIA 100 mg, or JANUVIA 200 mg. Patients who failed to meet specific glycemic goals during the studies were treated with metformin rescue, added on to placebo or JANUVIA.

Treatment with JANUVIA at 100 mg daily provided significant improvements in A1C, FPG, and 2-hour PPG compared to placebo (Table 3). In the 18-week study, 9% of patients receiving JANUVIA 100 mg and 17% who received placebo required rescue therapy. In the 24-week study, 9% of patients receiving JANUVIA 100 mg and 21% of patients receiving placebo required rescue therapy. The improvement in A1C compared to placebo was not affected by gender, age, race, prior antihyperglycemic therapy, or baseline BMI. As is typical for trials of agents to treat type 2 diabetes, the mean reduction in A1C with JANUVIA appears to be related to the degree of A1C elevation at baseline. In these 18- and 24-week studies, among patients who were not on an antihyperglycemic agent at study entry, the reductions from baseline in A1C were -0.7% and -0.8%, respectively, for those given JANUVIA, and -0.1% and -0.2%, respectively, for those given placebo. Overall, the 200 mg daily dose did not provide greater glycemic efficacy than the 100 mg daily dose. The effect of JANUVIA on lipid endpoints was similar to placebo. Body weight did not increase from baseline with JANUVIA therapy in either study, compared to a small reduction in patients given placebo.

[See table 3 above]

Additional Monotherapy Study

A multinational, randomized, double-blind, placebo-controlled study was also conducted to assess the safety and tolerability of JANUVIA in 91 patients with type 2 diabetes and chronic renal insufficiency (creatinine clearance <50 mL/min). Patients with moderate renal insufficiency received 50 mg daily of JANUVIA and those with severe renal insufficiency or with ESRD on hemodialysis or peritoneal dialysis received 25 mg daily. In this study, the safety and tolerability of JANUVIA were generally similar to placebo. A small increase in serum creatinine was reported in patients with moderate renal insufficiency treated with JANUVIA relative to those on placebo. In addition, the reductions in A1C and FPG with JANUVIA compared to placebo were generally similar to those observed in other monotherapy studies. [See Clinical Pharmacology (12.3).]

14.2 Combination Therapy

Add-on Combination Therapy with Metformin

A total of 701 patients with type 2 diabetes participated in a 24-week, randomized, double-blind, placebo-controlled study designed to assess the efficacy of JANUVIA in combination with metformin. Patients already on metformin (N=431) at a dose of at least 1500 mg per day were randomized after completing a 2-week single-blind placebo run-in period. Patients on metformin and another antihyperglycemic agent (N=229) and patients not on any antihyperglycemic agents (off therapy for at least 8 weeks, N=41) were randomized after a run-in period of approximately 10 weeks on metformin (at a dose of at least 1500 mg per day) in monotherapy. Patients with inadequate glycemic control (A1C 7% to 10%) were randomized to the addition of either 100 mg of JANUVIA or placebo, administered once daily. Patients who failed to meet specific glycemic goals during the studies were treated with pioglitazone rescue.

In combination with metformin, JANUVIA provided significant improvements in A1C, FPG, and 2-hour PPG compared to placebo with metformin (Table 4). Rescue glycemic therapy was used in 5% of patients treated with JANUVIA 100 mg and 14% of patients treated with placebo. A similar decrease in body weight was observed for both treatment groups.

Table 3
Glycemic Parameters in 18- and 24-Week Placebo-Controlled Studies of JANUVIA in Patients with Type 2 Diabetes[†]

	18-Week Study		24-Week Study	
	JANUVIA 100 mg	Placebo	JANUVIA 100 mg	Placebo
A1C (%)	N = 193	N = 103	N = 229	N = 244
Baseline (mean)	8.0	8.1	8.0	8.0
Change from baseline (adjusted mean[‡])	-0.5	0.1	-0.6	0.2
Difference from placebo (adjusted mean[‡]) (95% CI)	-0.6[§] (-0.8, -0.4)		-0.8[§] (-1.0, -0.6)	
Patients (%) achieving A1C <7%	69 (36%)	16 (16%)	93 (41%)	41 (17%)
FPG (mg/dL)	N = 201	N = 107	N = 234	N = 247
Baseline (mean)	180	184	170	176
Change from baseline (adjusted mean[‡])	-13	7	-12	5
Difference from placebo (adjusted mean[‡]) (95% CI)	-20[§] (-31, -9)		-17[§] (-24, -10)	
2-hour PPG (mg/dL)	‖	‖	N = 201	N = 204
Baseline (mean)			257	271
Change from baseline (adjusted mean[‡])			-49	-2
Difference from placebo (adjusted mean[‡]) (95% CI)			-47[§] (-59, -34)	

[†] Intent to Treat Population using last observation on study prior to metformin rescue therapy.
[‡] Least squares means adjusted for prior antihyperglycemic therapy status and baseline value.
[§] p<0.001 compared to placebo.
‖ Data not available.

Table 4
Glycemic Parameters at Final Visit (24-Week Study) for JANUVIA in Add-on Combination Therapy with Metformin[†]

	JANUVIA 100 mg + Metformin	Placebo + Metformin
A1C (%)	N = 453	N = 224
Baseline (mean)	8.0	8.0
Change from baseline (adjusted mean[‡])	-0.7	-0.0
Difference from placebo + metformin (adjusted mean[‡]) (95% CI)	-0.7[§] (-0.8, -0.5)	
Patients (%) achieving A1C <7%	213 (47%)	41 (18%)
FPG (mg/dL)	N = 454	N = 226
Baseline (mean)	170	174
Change from baseline (adjusted mean[‡])	-17	9
Difference from placebo + metformin (adjusted mean[‡]) (95% CI)	-25[§] (-31, -20)	
2-hour PPG (mg/dL)	N = 387	N = 182
Baseline (mean)	275	272
Change from baseline (adjusted mean[‡])	-62	-11
Difference from placebo + metformin (adjusted mean[‡]) (95% CI)	-51[§] (-61, -41)	

[†] Intent to Treat Population using last observation on study prior to pioglitazone rescue therapy.

Continued on next page

Januvia—Cont.

‡ Least squares means adjusted for prior antihyperglycemic therapy and baseline value.
§ p<0.001 compared to placebo + metformin.

Initial Combination Therapy with Metformin
A total of 1091 patients with type 2 diabetes and inadequate glycemic control on diet and exercise participated in a 24-week, randomized, double-blind, placebo-controlled factorial study designed to assess the efficacy of sitagliptin as initial therapy in combination with metformin. Patients on an antihyperglycemic agent (N=541) discontinued the agent, and underwent a diet, exercise, and drug washout period of up to 12 weeks duration. After the washout period, patients with inadequate glycemic control (A1C 7.5% to 11%) were randomized after completing a 2-week single-blind placebo run-in period. Patients not on antihyperglycemic agents at study entry (N=550) with inadequate glycemic control (A1C 7.5% to 11%) immediately entered the 2-week single-blind placebo run-in period and then were randomized. Approximately equal numbers of patients were randomized to receive initial therapy with placebo, 100 mg of JANUVIA once daily, 500 mg or 1000 mg of metformin twice daily, or 50 mg of sitagliptin twice daily in combination with 500 mg or 1000 mg of metformin twice daily. Patients who failed to meet specific glycemic goals during the study were treated with glyburide (glibenclamide) rescue.
Initial therapy with the combination of JANUVIA and metformin provided significant improvements in A1C, FPG, and 2-hour PPG compared to placebo, to metformin alone, and to JANUVIA alone (Table 5, Figure 1). Mean reductions from baseline in A1C were generally greater for patients with higher baseline A1C values. For patients not on an antihyperglycemic agent at study entry, mean reductions from baseline in A1C were: JANUVIA 100 mg once daily, -1.1%; metformin 500 mg bid, -1.1%; metformin 1000 mg bid, -1.2%; sitagliptin 50 mg bid with metformin 500 mg bid, -1.6%; sitagliptin 50 mg bid with metformin 1000 mg bid, -1.9%; and for patients receiving placebo, -0.2%. Lipid effects were generally neutral. The decrease in body weight in the groups given sitagliptin in combination with metformin was similar to that in the groups given metformin alone or placebo.
[See table 5 above]

Table 5
Glycemic Parameters at Final Visit (24-Week Study)
for Sitagliptin and Metformin, Alone and in Combination as Initial Therapy[†]

	Placebo	Sitagliptin (JANUVIA) 100 mg QD	Metformin 500 mg bid	Metformin 1000 mg bid	Sitagliptin 50 mg bid + Metformin 500 mg bid	Sitagliptin 50 mg bid + Metformin 1000 mg bid
A1C (%)	N = 165	N = 175	N = 178	N = 177	N = 183	N = 178
Baseline (mean)	8.7	8.9	8.9	8.7	8.8	8.8
Change from baseline (adjusted mean[‡])	0.2	-0.7	-0.8	-1.1	-1.4	-1.9
Difference from placebo (adjusted mean[‡]) (95% CI)		-0.8[§] (-1.1, -0.6)	-1.0[§] (-1.2, -0.8)	-1.3[§] (-1.5, -1.1)	-1.6[§] (-1.8, -1.3)	-2.1[§] (-2.3, -1.8)
Patients (%) achieving A1C <7%	15 (9%)	35 (20%)	41 (23%)	68 (38%)	79 (43%)	118 (66%)
% Patients receiving rescue medication	32	21	17	12	8	2
FPG (mg/dL)	N = 169	N = 178	N = 179	N = 179	N = 183	N = 180
Baseline (mean)	196	201	205	197	204	197
Change from baseline (adjusted mean[‡])	6	-17	-27	-29	-47	-64
Difference from placebo (adjusted mean[‡]) (95% CI)		-23[§] (-33, -14)	-33[§] (-43, -24)	-35[§] (-45, -26)	-53[§] (-62, -43)	-70[§] (-79, -60)
2-hour PPG (mg/dL)	N = 129	N = 136	N = 141	N = 138	N = 147	N = 152
Baseline (mean)	277	285	293	283	292	287
Change from baseline (adjusted mean[‡])	0	-52	-53	-78	-93	-117
Difference from placebo (adjusted mean[‡]) (95% CI)		-52[§] (-67, -37)	-54[§] (-69, -39)	-78[§] (-93, -63)	-93[§] (-107, -78)	-117[§] (-131, -102)

† Intent to Treat Population using last observation on study prior to glyburide (glibenclamide) rescue therapy.
‡ Least squares means adjusted for prior antihyperglycemic therapy status and baseline value.
§ p<0.001 compared to placebo.

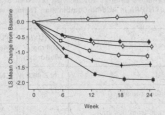

Figure 1: Mean Change from Baseline for A1C (%) over 24 Weeks with Sitagliptin and Metformin, Alone and in Combination as Initial Therapy in Patients with Type 2 Diabetes[†]

○ Placebo   ☐ Metformin 1000 mg b.i.d.
● Sitagliptin 100 mg q.d.   ◆ Sitagliptin 50 mg b.i.d. + Metformin 500 mg b.i.d.
◇ Metformin 500 mg b.i.d.   ✦ Sitagliptin 50 mg b.i.d. + Metformin 1000 mg b.i.d.

[†]All Patients Treated Population Least squares means adjusted for prior antihyperglycemic therapy and baseline value.

In addition, this study included patients (N=117) with more severe hyperglycemia (A1C >11% or blood glucose >280 mg/dL) who were treated with twice daily open-label JANUVIA 50 mg and metformin 1000 mg. In this group of patients, the mean baseline A1C value was 11.2%, mean FPG was 314 mg/dL, and mean 2-hour PPG was 441 mg/dL. After 24 weeks, mean decreases from baseline of -2.9% for A1C, -127 mg/dL for FPG, and -208 mg/dL for 2-hour PPG were observed.
Initial combination therapy or maintenance of combination therapy may not be appropriate for all patients. These management options are left to the discretion of the health care provider.
Active-Controlled Study vs Glipizide in Combination with Metformin
The efficacy of JANUVIA was evaluated in a 52-week, double-blind, glipizide-controlled noninferiority trial in patients with type 2 diabetes. Patients not on treatment or on other antihyperglycemic agents entered a run-in treatment period of up to 12 weeks duration with metformin monotherapy (dose of ≥1500 mg per day) which included washout of medications other than metformin, if applicable. After the run-in period, those with inadequate glycemic control (A1C 6.5% to 10%) were randomized 1:1 to the addition of JANUVIA 100 mg once daily or glipizide for 52 weeks. Patients receiving glipizide were given an initial dosage of 5 mg/day and then electively titrated over the next 18 weeks to a maximum dosage of 20 mg/day as needed to optimize glycemic control. Thereafter, the glipizide dose was to be kept constant, except for down-titration to prevent hypoglycemia. The mean dose of glipizide after the titration period was 10 mg.
After 52 weeks, JANUVIA and glipizide had similar mean reductions from baseline in A1C in the intent-to-treat analysis (Table 6). These results were consistent with the per protocol analysis (Figure 2). A conclusion in favor of the non-

inferiority of JANUVIA to glipizide may be limited to patients with baseline A1C comparable to those included in the study (over 70% of patients had baseline A1C <8% and over 90% had A1C <9%).

Table 6
Glycemic Parameters in a 52-Week Study Comparing JANUVIA to Glipizide as Add-On Therapy in Patients Inadequately Controlled on Metformin (Intent-to-Treat Population)[†]

	JANUVIA 100 mg	Glipizide
A1C (%)	N = 576	N = 559
Baseline (mean)	7.7	7.6
Change from baseline (adjusted mean[‡])	-0.5	-0.6
FPG (mg/dL)	N = 583	N = 568
Baseline (mean)	166	164
Change from baseline (adjusted mean[‡])	-8	-8

† The Intent to Treat Analysis used the patients' last observation in the study prior to discontinuation.
‡ Least squares means adjusted for prior antihyperglycemic therapy status and baseline A1C value.

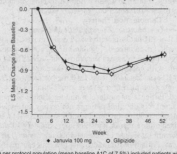

Figure 2: Mean Change from Baseline for A1C (%) Over 52 Weeks in a Study Comparing JANUVIA to Glipizide as Add-On Therapy in Patients Inadequately Controlled on Metformin (Per Protocol Population)[†]

◆ Januvia 100 mg   ◇ Glipizide

† The per protocol population (mean baseline A1C of 7.5%) included patients without major protocol violations who had observations at baseline and at Week 52.

The incidence of hypoglycemia in the JANUVIA group (4.9%) was significantly (p<0.001) lower than that in the

glipizide group (32.0%). Patients treated with JANUVIA exhibited a significant mean decrease from baseline in body weight compared to a significant weight gain in patients administered glipizide (-1.5 kg vs +1.1 kg).
Add-on Combination Therapy with Pioglitazone
A total of 353 patients with type 2 diabetes participated in a 24-week, randomized, double-blind, placebo-controlled study designed to assess the efficacy of JANUVIA in combination with pioglitazone. Patients on any oral antihyperglycemic agent in monotherapy (N=212) or on a PPARγ agent in combination therapy (N=106) or not on an antihyperglycemic agent (off therapy for at least 8 weeks, N=34) were switched to monotherapy with pioglitazone (at a dose of 30-45 mg per day), and completed a run-in period of approximately 12 weeks in duration. After the run-in period on pioglitazone monotherapy, patients with inadequate glycemic control (A1C 7% to 10%) were randomized to the addition of either 100 mg of JANUVIA or placebo, administered once daily. Patients who failed to meet specific glycemic goals during the studies were treated with metformin rescue. Glycemic endpoints measured were A1C and fasting glucose.
In combination with pioglitazone, JANUVIA provided significant improvements in A1C and FPG compared to placebo with pioglitazone (Table 7). Rescue therapy was used in 7% of patients treated with JANUVIA 100 mg and 14% of patients treated with placebo. There was no significant difference between JANUVIA and placebo in body weight change.

Table 7
Glycemic Parameters at Final Visit (24-Week Study) for JANUVIA in Add-on Combination Therapy with Pioglitazone[†]

	JANUVIA 100 mg + Pioglitazone	Placebo + Pioglitazone
A1C (%)	N = 163	N = 174
Baseline (mean)	8.1	8.0
Change from baseline (adjusted mean[‡])	-0.9	-0.2
Difference from placebo + pioglitazone (adjusted mean[‡]) (95% CI)	-0.7[§] (-0.9, -0.5)	
Patients (%) achieving A1C <7%	74 (45%)	40 (23%)
FPG (mg/dL)	N = 163	N = 174
Baseline (mean)	168	166

Change from baseline (adjusted mean‡)	-17	1
Difference from placebo + pioglitazone (adjusted mean‡) (95% CI)	-18§ (-24, -11)	

† Intent to Treat Population using last observation on study prior to metformin rescue therapy.
‡ Least squares means adjusted for prior antihyperglycemic therapy status and baseline value.
§ p<0.001 compared to placebo + pioglitazone.

Add-on Combination Therapy with Glimepiride, with or without Metformin

A total of 441 patients with type 2 diabetes participated in a 24-week, randomized, double-blind, placebo-controlled study designed to assess the efficacy of JANUVIA in combination with glimepiride, with or without metformin. Patients entered a run-in treatment period on glimepiride (≥4 mg per day) alone or glimepiride in combination with metformin (≥1500 mg per day). After a dose-titration and dose-stable run-in period of up to 16 weeks and a 2-week placebo run-in period, patients with inadequate glycemic control (A1C 7.5% to 10.5%) were randomized to the addition of either 100 mg of JANUVIA or placebo, administered once daily. Patients who failed to meet specific glycemic goals during the studies were treated with pioglitazone rescue.

In combination with glimepiride, with or without metformin, JANUVIA provided significant improvements in A1C and FPG compared to placebo (Table 8). In the entire study population (patients on JANUVIA in combination with glimepiride and patients on JANUVIA in combination with glimepiride and metformin), a mean reduction from baseline relative to placebo in A1C of -0.7% and in FPG of -20 mg/dL was seen. Rescue therapy was used in 12% of patients treated with JANUVIA 100 mg and 27% of patients treated with placebo. In this study, patients treated with JANUVIA had a mean increase in body weight of 1.1 kg vs. placebo (+0.8 kg vs. -0.4 kg). In addition, there was an increased rate of hypoglycemia. *[See Warnings and Precautions (5.2); Adverse Reactions (6.1).]*
[See table 8 above]

16 HOW SUPPLIED/STORAGE AND HANDLING

No. 6737 — Tablets JANUVIA, 25 mg, are pink, round, film-coated tablets with "221" on one side.
They are supplied as follows:
  NDC 0006-0221-31 unit-of-use bottles of 30
  NDC 0006-0221-54 unit-of-use bottles of 90
  NDC 0006-0221-28 unit dose blister packages of 100.
No. 6738 — Tablets JANUVIA, 50 mg, are light beige, round, film-coated tablets with "112" on one side.
They are supplied as follows:
  NDC 0006-0112-31 unit-of-use bottles of 30
  NDC 0006-0112-54 unit-of-use bottles of 90
  NDC 0006-0112-28 unit dose blister packages of 100.
No. 6739 — Tablets JANUVIA, 100 mg, are beige, round, film-coated tablets with "277" on one side.
They are supplied as follows:
  NDC 0006-0277-31 unit-of-use bottles of 30
  NDC 0006-0277-54 unit-of-use bottles of 90
  NDC 0006-0277-28 unit dose blister packages of 100
  NDC 0006-0277-74 bottles of 500
  NDC 0006-0277-82 bottles of 1000.

Storage
Store at 20-25°C (68-77°F), excursions permitted to 15-30°C (59-86°F), [see USP Controlled Room Temperature].

17 PATIENT COUNSELING INFORMATION

See FDA-Approved Patient Labeling.

17.1 Instructions
Patients should be informed of the potential risks and benefits of JANUVIA and of alternative modes of therapy. Patients should also be informed about the importance of adherence to dietary instructions, regular physical activity, periodic blood glucose monitoring and A1C testing, recognition and management of hypoglycemia and hyperglycemia, and assessment for diabetes complications. During periods of stress such as fever, trauma, infection, or surgery, medication requirements may change and patients should be advised to seek medical advice promptly.
Patients should be informed that allergic reactions have been reported during postmarketing use of JANUVIA. If symptoms of allergic reactions (including rash, hives, and swelling of the face, lips, tongue, and throat that may cause difficulty in breathing or swallowing) occur, patients must stop taking JANUVIA and seek medical advice promptly.
Physicians should instruct their patients to read the Patient Package Insert before starting JANUVIA therapy and to re-read each time the prescription is renewed. Patients should be instructed to inform their doctor or pharmacist if they develop any unusual symptom, or if any known symptom persists or worsens.

17.2 Laboratory Tests
Patients should be informed that response to all diabetic therapies should be monitored by periodic measurements of blood glucose and A1C levels, with a goal of decreasing these levels towards the normal range. A1C is especially useful for evaluating long-term glycemic control. Patients should be informed of the potential need to adjust dose based on changes in renal function tests over time.

Table 8
Glycemic Parameters at Final Visit (24-Week Study) for JANUVIA in Combination with Glimepiride, with or without Metformin†

	JANUVIA 100 mg + Glimepiride	Placebo + Glimepiride	JANUVIA 100 mg + Glimepiride + Metformin	Placebo + Glimepiride + Metformin
A1C (%)	N = 102	N = 103	N = 115	N = 105
Baseline (mean)	8.4	8.5	8.3	8.3
Change from baseline (adjusted mean‡)	-0.3	0.3	-0.6	0.3
Difference from placebo (adjusted mean‡) (95% CI)	-0.6§ (-0.8, -0.3)		-0.9§ (-1.1, -0.7)	
Patients (%) achieving A1C <7%	11 (11%)	9 (9%)	26 (23%)	1 (1%)
FPG (mg/dL)	N = 104	N = 104	N = 115	N = 109
Baseline (mean)	183	185	179	179
Change from baseline (adjusted mean‡)	-1	18	-8	13
Difference from placebo (adjusted mean‡) (95% CI)	-19‖ (-32, -7)		-21§ (-32, -10)	

† Intent to Treat Population using last observation on study prior to pioglitazone rescue therapy.
‡ Least squares means adjusted for prior antihyperglycemic therapy status and baseline value.
§ p<0.001 compared to placebo.
‖ p<0.01 compared to placebo.

Manufactured for:
MERCK & CO., INC., Whitehouse Station, NJ 08889, USA
Manufactured by:
Merck Sharp & Dohme (Italia) S.p.A.
Via Emilia, 21
27100 – Pavia, Italy
9762704
US Patent No.: 6,699,871

Patient Information
JANUVIA™ (jah-NEW-vee-ah)
(sitagliptin)
Tablets

Read the Patient Information that comes with JANUVIA* before you start taking it and each time you get a refill. There may be new information. This leaflet does not take the place of talking with your doctor about your medical condition or treatment.

What is JANUVIA?
JANUVIA is a prescription medicine used along with diet and exercise to lower blood sugar in adult patients with type 2 diabetes. JANUVIA may be taken alone or along with certain other medicines to control blood sugar.
• JANUVIA lowers blood sugar when blood sugar is high, especially after a meal. JANUVIA also lowers blood sugar between meals.
• JANUVIA helps to improve the levels of insulin produced by your own body after a meal.
• JANUVIA decreases the amount of sugar made by the body. JANUVIA is unlikely to cause your blood sugar to be lowered to a dangerous level (hypoglycemia) because it does not work when your blood sugar is low.
JANUVIA has not been studied in children under 18 years of age.
JANUVIA has not been studied with insulin, a medicine known to cause low blood sugar.

Who should not take JANUVIA?
Do not take JANUVIA if you:
• have had an allergic reaction to JANUVIA.
JANUVIA should not be used to treat patients with:
• Type 1 diabetes.
• Diabetic ketoacidosis (increased ketones in the blood or urine).

What should I tell my doctor before and during treatment with JANUVIA?
Tell your doctor about all of your medical conditions, including if you:
• have had an allergic reaction to JANUVIA.
• have kidney problems.
• are pregnant or plan to become pregnant. It is not known if JANUVIA will harm your unborn baby. If you are pregnant, talk with your doctor about the best way to control your blood sugar while you are pregnant. If you use JANUVIA during pregnancy, talk with your doctor about how you can be on the JANUVIA registry. The toll-free telephone number for the pregnancy registry is: 1-800-986-8999.
• are breast-feeding or plan to breast-feed. It is not known if JANUVIA will pass into your breast milk. Talk with your doctor about the best way to feed your baby if you are taking JANUVIA.
Tell your doctor about all the medicines you take, including prescription and non-prescription medicines, vitamins, and herbal supplements.

Know the medicines you take. Keep a list of your medicines and show it to your doctor and pharmacist when you get a new medicine.
How should I take JANUVIA?
• Take JANUVIA exactly as your doctor tells you to take it.
• Take JANUVIA by mouth once a day.
• Take JANUVIA with or without food.
• If you have kidney problems, your doctor may prescribe lower doses of JANUVIA. Your doctor may perform blood tests on you from time to time to measure how well your kidneys are working.
• Your doctor may prescribe JANUVIA along with certain other medicines that lower blood sugar.
• If you miss a dose, take it as soon as you remember. If you do not remember until it is time for your next dose, skip the missed dose and go back to your regular schedule. Do not take two doses of JANUVIA at the same time.
• If you take too much JANUVIA, call your doctor or local Poison Control Center right away.
• **When your body is under some types of stress, such as fever, trauma (such as a car accident), infection or surgery, the amount of diabetes medicine that you need may change. Tell your doctor right away if you have any of these conditions and follow your doctor's instructions.**
• Monitor your blood sugar as your doctor tells you to.
• Stay on your prescribed diet and exercise program while taking JANUVIA.
• Talk to your doctor about how to prevent, recognize and manage low blood sugar (hypoglycemia), high blood sugar (hyperglycemia), and complications of diabetes.
• Your doctor will monitor your diabetes with regular blood tests, including your blood sugar levels and your hemoglobin A1C.
What are the possible side effects of JANUVIA?
The most common side effects of JANUVIA include:
• Upper respiratory infection
• Stuffy or runny nose and sore throat
• Headache
JANUVIA may occasionally cause stomach discomfort and diarrhea.
When JANUVIA is used in combination with another type of diabetes medicine known as a sulfonylurea, low blood sugar (hypoglycemia) due to the sulfonylurea can occur. Your doctor may prescribe lower doses of the sulfonylurea medicine.
The following additional side effects have been reported in general use with JANUVIA:
• Allergic reactions, which may be serious, including rash, hives, and swelling of the face, lips, tongue, and throat that may cause difficulty in breathing or swallowing. If you have an allergic reaction, stop taking JANUVIA and call your doctor right away. Your doctor may prescribe a medication to treat your allergic reaction and a different medication for your diabetes.
Tell your doctor if you have any side effect that bothers you or that does not go away.
Other side effects may occur when using JANUVIA. For more information, ask your doctor.
How should I store JANUVIA?
• Store JANUVIA at room temperature, 68 to 77°F (20 to 25°C).

Continued on next page

Information on the Merck & Co., Inc., products listed on these pages is from the full prescribing information in use March 1, 2008. For information, please call 1-800-NSC-MERCK [1-800-672-6372].

Januvia—Cont.

Keep JANUVIA and all medicines out of the reach of children.
General information about the use of JANUVIA
Medicines are sometimes prescribed for conditions that are not mentioned in patient information leaflets. Do not use JANUVIA for a condition for which it was not prescribed. Do not give JANUVIA to other people, even if they have the same symptoms you have. It may harm them.
This leaflet summarizes the most important information about JANUVIA. If you would like to know more information, talk with your doctor. You can ask your doctor or pharmacist for additional information about JANUVIA that is written for health professionals. For more information call 1-800-622-4477.
What are the ingredients in JANUVIA?
Active ingredient: sitagliptin
Inactive ingredients: microcrystalline cellulose, anhydrous dibasic calcium phosphate, croscarmellose sodium, magnesium stearate, and sodium stearyl fumarate. The tablet film coating contains the following inactive ingredients: polyvinyl alcohol, polyethylene glycol, talc, titanium dioxide, red iron oxide, and yellow iron oxide.
What is type 2 diabetes?
Type 2 diabetes is a condition in which your body does not make enough insulin, and the insulin that your body produces does not work as well as it should. Your body can also make too much sugar. When this happens, sugar (glucose) builds up in the blood. This can lead to serious medical problems.
The main goal of treating diabetes is to lower your blood sugar to a normal level. Lowering and controlling blood sugar may help prevent or delay complications of diabetes, such as heart disease, kidney disease, blindness, and amputation.
High blood sugar can be lowered by diet and exercise, and by certain medicines when necessary.
Revised October 2007
Manufactured for:
MERCK & CO., INC., Whitehouse Station, NJ 08889, USA
Manufactured by:
Merck Sharp & Dohme (Italia) S.p.A.
Via Emilia, 21
27100 – Pavia, Italy
9762704

M-M-R® II ℞
(MEASLES, MUMPS, AND RUBELLA VIRUS VACCINE LIVE)

Prescribing Information for this product, which appears on pages 2022–2024 of the 2008 PDR, has been revised as follows. Please write "see Supplement A" next to the product heading.
In the **ADVERSE REACTIONS** section, under *Urogenital System*, add "Epididymitis" so it reads:
Urogenital System
Epididymitis, orchitis.
Revisions based on 9739304, issued December 2007.

MAXALT® ℞
(rizatriptan benzoate)
Tablets
and
MAXALT-MLT®
(rizatriptan benzoate)
Orally Disintegrating Tablets

Prescribing information for this product, which appears on pages 2024–2028 of the 2008 PDR, has been revised as follows. Please write "See Supplement A" next to the product heading.
In the **Adverse Reactions** section, under *Postmarketing Experience*, **General:**, the text that follows "**General:**" should read as follows: Hypersensitivity reaction, anaphylaxis/anaphylactoid reaction, angioedema (e.g., facial edema, tongue swelling, pharyngeal edema), wheezing, toxic epidermal necrolysis.
Revisions based on 9652505, issued August 2007.

MEVACOR® TABLETS ℞
(Lovastatin)

Prescribing information for this product, which appears on pages 2033–2038 of the 2008 PDR, has been revised as follows. Please write "See Supplement A" next to the product heading.
Under **HOW SUPPLIED**, 1st sentence, replace "3561" with "8123"; replace "MEVACOR" with "plain". Add a period at the end of the 2nd sentence after "60". Delete the 3rd and 4th sentences, beginning with "**NDC** 0006-0731-94" and ending with "1,000." In the 5th sentence, replace "3562" with "8124"; replace "MEVACOR" with "plain". Add a period at the end of the 6th sentence after "60". Delete the last 2 sentences, beginning with "**NDC** 0006-0732-94" and ending with "1,000."
Revisions based on 9844657, issued December 2007.

PEPCID® TABLETS ℞
[*pep' sid*]
(famotidine)
PEPCID®
(famotidine) for Oral Suspension

Prescribing information for this product, which appears on pages 2050–2053 of the 2008 PDR, has been revised as follows. Please write "See Supplement A" next to the product heading.
In the Header, delete "**PEPCID® (famotidine) for Oral Suspension**". In the **DESCRIPTION** section, delete the entire fourth paragraph. In the **CLINICAL PHARMACOLOGY IN ADULTS** section, under *Pharmacokinetics*, delete the third sentence "PEPCID Tablets and PEPCID for Oral Suspension are bioequivalent.". In the **PRECAUTIONS** section, delete the entire *Information for Patients* header and the paragraph that follows. In the **DOSAGE AND ADMINISTRATION** section, delete the *Oral Suspension* header and the 3 paragraphs that follow. In the **HOW SUPPLIED** section, delete "No. 3538" through the end of that subsection "400 mg famotidine". Under *Storage*, delete the second paragraph. In the signoff, delete "PEPCID (famotidine) for Oral Suspension is manufactured by: Merck logo, Merck & Co., Inc., Whitehouse Station, NJ 08889, USA"
Revisions based on 7825039, issued January 2007.

PNEUMOVAX® 23 ℞
(Pneumoccal Vaccine Polyvalent)

Prescribing information for this product, which appears on pages 2056–2057 of the 2008 PDR, has been revised as follows. Please write "See Supplement A" next to the product heading.
In the **PRECAUTIONS** section, under *Geriatric Use*, second sentence after "...65 years of age and older" delete "(n=629)". After "...64 years of age" delete "(n=379).". Replace the text "The data did not suggest an increased rate of adverse reactions among subjects ≥ 65 years of age compared to those 50 to 64 years of age." with "Of 1007 subjects enrolled in this study, 433 subjects were 65 to 74 years of age, and 195 subjects were 75 years of age or older. No overall difference in safety was observed between these subjects and younger subjects."
In the **ADVERSE REACTIONS** section, delete first and second paragraphs, "The following adverse experiences have been reported with PNEUMOVAX 23 in clinical trials and/or post-marketing experience:
Local reactions at injection site including pain, soreness, warmth, erythema, swelling, induration, decreased limb mobility and peripheral edema in the injected extremity. Also reported was an increase in the laboratory value for serum C-reactive protein."
Third and forth paragraphs, change from "The most common adverse experiences reported in clinical trials and post-marketing experience were:
fever ≤ 102°F, injection site reactions including soreness, erythema, warmth, swelling and local induration." with "The most common adverse experiences reported with PNEUMOVAX 23 in clinical trials were:
Local reaction at injection site including soreness, erythema, warmth, swelling and induration Fever ≤102°F"
In the **ADVERSE REACTIONS** section, delete the fifth and sixth paragraphs: "In a clinical trial, an increased rate of local reactions has been observed with revaccination at 3-5 years following primary vaccination. It was reported that the overall injection-site adverse experiences rate for subjects ≥65 years of age was higher following revaccination (79.3%) than following primary vaccination (52.9%). The reported overall injection-site adverse experiences rate for re-vaccinees and primary vaccinees who were 50 to 64 years of age were similar (79.6% and 72.8% respectively). In both age groups, re-vaccinees reported a higher rate of a composite endpoint (any of the following: moderate pain, severe pain, and/or large induration at the injection site) than primary vaccinees. Among subjects ≥ 65 years of age, the composite endpoint was reported by 30.6% and 10.4% of revaccination and primary vaccination subjects, respectively, while among subjects 50-64 years of age, the endpoint was reported by 35.5% and 18.9% respectively. The injection site reactions occurred within the 3 day monitoring period and typically resolved by day 5. The rate of overall systemic adverse experiences was similar among both primary vaccinees and re-vaccinees within each age group. The rate of vaccine-related systemic adverse experiences was higher following revaccination (33.1%) than following primary vaccination (21.7%) in subjects ≥65 years of age, and was similar following revaccination (37.5%) and primary vaccination (35.5%) in subjects 50-64 years of age. The most common systemic adverse experiences were as follows: asthenia/fatigue, myalgia and headache. Regardless of age, the observed increase in post vaccination use of analgesics (≤13% in the re-vaccinees and ≤4% in the primary vaccinees) returned to baseline by day 5.
In post-marketing experience, injection site cellulitis-like reactions were reported rarely; between 1989 and 2002, when approximately 43 million doses were distributed, the annual reporting rate was <2/100,000 doses. These cellulitis-like reactions occurred with initial and repeat vaccination at a median onset time of 2 days after vaccine administration and were transient in nature."
In the **ADVERSE REACTIONS** section, seventh paragraph, after "...in post-marketing experience" add "with PNEUMOVAX 23"
In the **ADVERSE REACTIONS** section, *Body as a Whole*, Change "*Body as a Whole*" to "*General disorders and administration site conditions*"
After "Chills" add
"Pain
Decreased limb mobility
Peripheral edema in the injected extremity"
In the **ADVERSE REACTIONS** section, *Skin*, add new section (following style) under *Skin*,
"*Investigations*
Increased serum C-reactive protein"
Add new paragraph "In post-marketing experience, injection site cellulitis-like reactions were reported rarely; between 1989 and 2002, when approximately 43 million doses were distributed, the annual reporting rate was <2/100,000 doses. These cellulitis-like reactions occurred with initial and repeat vaccination at a median onset time of 2 days after vaccine administration."
In the **ADVERSE REACTIONS** section, second paragraph after the New Paragraph, first sentence, change "It was reported that the overall injection-site adverse experiences rate for subjects ≥65 years of age was higher following revaccination..." to "For subjects aged >65 years, it was reported that the overall injection-site adverse experiences rate was higher following revaccination (79.3%) than following primary vaccination (52.9%). For subjects aged 50-64 years, the reported overall...".
In the **ADVERSE REACTIONS** section, second paragraph after the New Paragraph, second sentence, change "The reported overall injection-site adverse experiences rate for revaccinees and primary vaccinees who were 50 to 64 years of age were similar..." to "For subjects aged 50-64 years, the reported overall injection-site adverse experiences rate for re-vaccinees and primary vaccinees were similar..."
In the **ADVERSE REACTIONS** section, forth paragraph after the New Paragraph, third sentence, after "The most common systemic adverse experiences" add "reported after PNEUMOVAX 23"
Revisions based on 7999828, issued September 2007.

PROQUAD® ℞
[*prō-kwăd*]
(Measles, Mumps, Rubella and Varicella Virus Vaccine Live)

Prescribing information for this product, which appears on pages 2076–2079 of the 2008 PDR, has been revised as follows. Please write "See Supplement A" next to the product heading.
"(Oka/Merck)" has been removed from the generic name.
In the **CONTRAINDICATIONS** section, in the fifth bullet, clarification regarding disseminated varicella vaccine virus infection in children with underlying immunodeficiency disorders has been added by inclusion of the sentence "In addition, disseminated varicella vaccine virus infection has been reported in children with underlying immunodeficiency disorders who were inadvertently vaccinated with a varicella-containing vaccine." to the end of the paragraph of the fifth bullet.
In the **ADVERSE REACTIONS** section, the adverse event "encephalitis" was relocated to the ProQuad *Post-marketing reports* subsection because it has now been reported following use of ProQuad, and "febrile seizure (see below)" has also been added. "Abnormal coordination" was revised to "ataxia". Thus, the *Post-marketing reports* section now reads:
Post-marketing reports
The following additional adverse events have been reported with ProQuad in post-marketing experience.
Infections and infestations: herpes zoster, varicella.
Immune system disorders: anaphylactic reaction.
Nervous system disorders: ataxia, convulsion, encephalitis (see below), febrile seizure (see below).
Skin and subcutaneous tissue disorders: pruritus.
In the *Post-marketing surveillance* section, add "either" and "or ProQuad" as follows:
Post-marketing surveillance
The discussion that follows describes adverse reactions which have been identified postapproval for either the monovalent components of ProQuad or ProQuad.
In the *Post-marketing surveillance* section, add the following text as the last paragraph before the Dosage and Administration section:
Febrile seizures have been reported in children receiving ProQuad. Consistent with clinical study data on the timing of fever and measles-like rash, an interim analysis of a post marketing observational study in children (N=14,263) receiving their first dose of vaccine has shown that febrile seizures occurred more frequently 5-12 days following vaccination with ProQuad (0.5 per 1000) when compared with data from children in a historical, age- and gender-matched, control group vaccinated with M-M-R II and VARIVAX (N=14,263) concomitantly (0.2 per 1000). In the 0-30 day time period following vaccination, the incidence of febrile seizures with ProQuad (1.0 per 1000) was not greater than that observed in children receiving M-M-R II and VARIVAX concomitantly (1.3 per 1000).
In *Adverse Experiences after vaccination with M-M-R II or VARIVAX*, "epididymitis" has been added based on post-marketing reports for M-M-R II. Add the following text after the *Musculoskeletal, connective tissue and bone disorders* section:
Reproductive system and breast disorders
Epididymitis.
Revisions based on 9633807, issued February 2008.

ROTATEQ® ℞

[roō-tă-těk]

(Rotavirus Vaccine, Live, Oral, Pentavalent)
Oral Solution
Initial U.S. Approval: 2006

Prescribing information for this product, which appears on pages 2087–2091 of the 2008 PDR, has been completely revised as follows. Please write "See Supplement A" next to the product heading.

HIGHLIGHTS OF PRESCRIBING INFORMATION
These highlights do not include all the information needed to use RotaTeq safely and effectively. See full prescribing information for RotaTeq.

INDICATIONS AND USAGE
RotaTeq® is indicated for the prevention of rotavirus gastroenteritis in infants and children caused by the G1, G2, G3 and G4 serotypes contained in the vaccine. (1)

DOSAGE AND ADMINISTRATION
- FOR ORAL USE ONLY. NOT FOR INJECTION. (2)
- The vaccination series consists of three ready-to-use liquid doses of RotaTeq administered orally starting at 6 to 12 weeks of age, with the subsequent doses administered at 4- to 10-week intervals. The third dose should not be given after 32 weeks of age. (2)

DOSAGE FORMS AND STRENGTHS
2 mL, oral solution of 5 live human-bovine reassortant rotaviruses which contains a minimum of $2.0 - 2.8 \times 10^6$ infectious units (IU) per reassortant dose, depending on the serotype, and not greater than 116×10^6 IU per aggregate dose. (3)

CONTRAINDICATIONS
- A demonstrated history of hypersensitivity to the vaccine or any component of the vaccine. (4)

WARNINGS AND PRECAUTIONS
- No safety or efficacy data are available for the administration of RotaTeq to infants who are potentially immunocompromised (e.g., HIV/AIDS). (5.1)
- No safety or efficacy data are available for the administration of RotaTeq to infants with a history of gastrointestinal disorders (e.g., active acute gastrointestinal illness, chronic diarrhea, failure to thrive, history of congenital abdominal disorders, abdominal surgery and intussusception). (5.2)
- Caution is advised when considering whether to administer RotaTeq to individuals with immunodeficient contacts. (5.4)

ADVERSE REACTIONS
Most common adverse events included diarrhea, vomiting, irritability, otitis media, nasopharyngitis, and bronchospasm. (6.1)

To report SUSPECTED ADVERSE REACTIONS, contact Merck & Co., Inc. at 1-877-888-4231 or FDA at 1-800-822-7967 or www.vaers.hhs.gov[2].

USE IN SPECIFIC POPULATIONS
Pediatric Use: Safety and efficacy have not been established in infants less than 6 weeks of age or greater than 32 weeks of age. Data are available from clinical studies to support the use of RotaTeq in:
- Pre-term infants according to their age in weeks since birth
- Infants with controlled gastroesophageal reflux disease. (8.4)

See 17 for PATIENT COUNSELING INFORMATION and FDA-approved patient labeling.

Revised: 09/2007

FULL PRESCRIBING INFORMATION: CONTENTS*

FULL PRESCRIBING INFORMATION

1   INDICATIONS AND USAGE

RotaTeq[1] is indicated for the prevention of rotavirus gastroenteritis in infants and children caused by the serotypes G1, G2, G3, and G4 when administered as a 3-dose series to infants between the ages of 6 to 32 weeks. The first dose of RotaTeq should be administered between 6 and 12 weeks of age *[see Dosage and Administration (2)]*.

[1] Registered trademark of MERCK & CO., Inc., Whitehouse Station, New Jersey 08889 USA
COPYRIGHT © 2006, 2007 MERCK & CO., Inc.
All rights reserved

2   DOSAGE AND ADMINISTRATION

FOR ORAL USE ONLY. NOT FOR INJECTION.
The vaccination series consists of three ready-to-use liquid doses of RotaTeq administered orally starting at 6 to 12 weeks of age, with the subsequent doses administered at 4- to 10-week intervals. The third dose should not be given after 32 weeks of age *[see Clinical Studies (14)]*.

There are no restrictions on the infant's consumption of food or liquid, including breast milk, either before or after vaccination with RotaTeq.

Do not mix the RotaTeq vaccine with any other vaccines or solutions. Do not reconstitute or dilute *[see Dosage and Administration (2.2)]*.

For storage instructions *[see How Supplied/Storage and Handling (16.1)]*.

Each dose is supplied in a container consisting of a squeezable plastic, latex-free dosing tube with a twist-off cap, allowing for direct oral administration. The dosing tube is contained in a pouch *[see Dosage and Administration (2.2)]*.

2.1   Use with Other Vaccines
In clinical trials, RotaTeq was administered concomitantly with other licensed pediatric vaccines *[see Adverse Reactions (6.1), Drug Interactions (7.1), and Clinical Studies (14)]*.

2.2   Instructions for Use

To administer the vaccine:

Tear open the pouch and remove the dosing tube.

Clear the fluid from the dispensing tip by holding tube vertically and tapping cap.
Open the dosing tube in 2 easy motions:

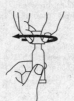

1. Puncture the dispensing tip by screwing cap *clockwise* until it becomes tight.

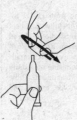

2. Remove cap by turning it *counterclockwise*.

Administer dose by gently squeezing liquid into infant's mouth toward the inner cheek until dosing tube is empty. (A residual drop may remain in the tip of the tube.)
If for any reason an incomplete dose is administered (e.g., infant spits or regurgitates the vaccine), a replacement dose is not recommended, since such dosing was not studied in the clinical trials. The infant should continue to receive any remaining doses in the recommended series.
Discard the empty tube and cap in approved biological waste containers according to local regulations.

3   DOSAGE FORMS AND STRENGTHS
RotaTeq, 2 mL for oral use, is a ready-to-use solution of live reassortant rotaviruses, containing G1, G2, G3, G4 and P1A[8] which contains a minimum of $2.0 - 2.8 \times 10^6$ infectious units (IU) per individual reassortant dose, depending on the serotype, and not greater than 116×10^6 IU per aggregate dose.
Each dose is supplied in a container consisting of a squeezable plastic, latex-free dosing tube with a twist-off cap, allowing for direct oral administration. The dosing tube is contained in a pouch.

4   CONTRAINDICATIONS
A demonstrated history of hypersensitivity to any component of the vaccine.
Infants who develop symptoms suggestive of hypersensitivity after receiving a dose of RotaTeq should not receive further doses of RotaTeq.

5   WARNINGS AND PRECAUTIONS
5.1   Immunocompromised Populations
No safety or efficacy data are available for the administration of RotaTeq to infants who are potentially immunocompromised including:
- Infants with blood dyscrasias, leukemia, lymphomas of any type, or other malignant neoplasms affecting the bone marrow or lymphatic system.
- Infants on immunosuppressive therapy (including high-dose systemic corticosteroids). RotaTeq may be administered to infants who are being treated with topical corticosteroids or inhaled steroids.
- Infants with primary and acquired immunodeficiency states, including HIV/AIDS or other clinical manifestations of infection with human immunodeficiency viruses; cellular immune deficiencies; and hypogammaglobulinemic and dysgammaglobulinemic states. There are insufficient data from the clinical trials to support administration of RotaTeq to infants with indeterminate HIV status who are born to mothers with HIV/AIDS.
- Infants who have received a blood transfusion or blood products, including immunoglobulins within 42 days.

No data are available regarding potential vaccine virus transmission from vaccine recipient to non-vaccinated household or other contacts *[see Warnings and Precautions (5.4)]*.

5.2   Gastrointestinal Illness
No safety or efficacy data are available for administration of RotaTeq to infants with a history of gastrointestinal disorders including infants with active acute gastrointestinal illness, infants with chronic diarrhea and failure to thrive, and infants with a history of congenital abdominal disorders, abdominal surgery, and intussusception. Caution is advised when considering administration of RotaTeq to these infants.

5.3   Intussusception
Following administration of a previously licensed live rhesus rotavirus-based vaccine, an increased risk of intussusception was observed.[1] In the Rotavirus Efficacy and Safety Trial [REST] (n=69,625), the data did not show an increased risk of intussusception for RotaTeq when compared to placebo. In post-marketing experience, cases of intussusception have been reported in temporal association with RotaTeq. *[See Adverse Reactions (6.1 and 6.2).]*

5.4   Shedding and Transmission
Shedding was evaluated among a subset of subjects in REST 4 to 6 days after each dose and among all subjects who submitted a stool antigen rotavirus positive sample at any time. RotaTeq was shed in the stools of 32 of 360 [8.9%, 95% CI (6.2%, 12.3%)] vaccine recipients tested after dose 1; 0 of 249 [0.0%, 95% CI (0.0%, 1.5%)] vaccine recipients tested after dose 2; and in 1 of 385 [0.3%, 95% CI (<0.1%, 1.4%)] vaccine recipients after dose 3. In phase 3 studies, shedding was observed as early as 1 day and as late as 15 days after a dose. Transmission was not evaluated.
Caution is advised when considering whether to administer RotaTeq to individuals with immunodeficient close contacts such as:
- Individuals with malignancies or who are otherwise immunocompromised; or
- Individuals receiving immunosuppressive therapy.

RotaTeq is a solution of live reassortant rotaviruses and can potentially be transmitted to persons who have contact with the vaccine. The potential risk of transmission of vaccine virus should be weighed against the risk of acquiring and transmitting natural rotavirus.

5.5   Febrile Illness
Febrile illness may be reason for delaying use of RotaTeq except when, in the opinion of the physician, withholding the vaccine entails a greater risk. Low-grade fever

Continued on next page

RotaTeq—Cont.

(<100.5°F [38.1°C]) itself and mild upper respiratory infection do not preclude vaccination with RotaTeq.

5.6   Incomplete Regimen

The clinical studies were not designed to assess the level of protection provided by only one or two doses of RotaTeq.

5.7   Limitations of Vaccine Effectiveness

RotaTeq may not protect all vaccine recipients against rotavirus.

5.8   Post-Exposure Prophylaxis

No clinical data are available for RotaTeq when administered after exposure to rotavirus.

6   ADVERSE REACTIONS

6.1   Clinical Studies Experience

71,725 infants were evaluated in 3 placebo-controlled clinical trials including 36,165 infants in the group that received RotaTeq and 35,560 infants in the group that received placebo. Parents/guardians were contacted on days 7, 14, and 42 after each dose regarding intussusception and any other serious adverse events. The racial distribution was as follows: White (69% in both groups); Hispanic-American (14% in both groups); Black (8% in both groups); Multiracial (5% in both groups); Asian (2% in both groups); Native American (RotaTeq 2%, placebo 1%); and Other (<1% in both groups). The gender distribution was 51% male and 49% female in both vaccination groups.

Because clinical trials are conducted under conditions that may not be typical of those observed in clinical practice, the adverse reaction rates presented below may not be reflective of those observed in clinical practice.

Serious Adverse Events

Serious adverse events occurred in 2.4% of recipients of RotaTeq when compared to 2.6% of placebo recipients within the 42-day period of a dose in the phase 3 clinical studies of RotaTeq. The most frequently reported serious adverse events for RotaTeq compared to placebo were:

bronchiolitis   (0.6% RotaTeq vs. 0.7% Placebo),
gastroenteritis   (0.2% RotaTeq vs. 0.3% Placebo),
pneumonia   (0.2% RotaTeq vs. 0.2% Placebo),
fever   (0.1% RotaTeq vs. 0.1% Placebo),
                     and
urinary tract infection (0.1% RotaTeq vs. 0.1% Placebo).

Deaths

Across the clinical studies, 52 deaths were reported. There were 25 deaths in the RotaTeq recipients compared to 27 deaths in the placebo recipients. The most commonly reported cause of death was sudden infant death syndrome, which was observed in 8 recipients of RotaTeq and 9 placebo recipients.

Intussusception

In REST, 34,837 vaccine recipients and 34,788 placebo recipients were monitored by active surveillance to identify potential cases of intussusception at 7, 14, and 42 days after each dose, and every 6 weeks thereafter for 1 year after the first dose.

For the primary safety outcome, cases of intussusception occurring within 42 days of any dose, there were 6 cases among RotaTeq recipients and 5 cases among placebo recipients (see Table 1). The data did not suggest an increased risk of intussusception relative to placebo.

Table 1
Confirmed cases of intussusception in recipients of RotaTeq as compared with placebo recipients during REST

	RotaTeq (n=34,837)	Placebo (n=34,788)
Confirmed intussusception cases within 42 days of any dose	6	5
Relative risk (95% CI) *	1.6 (0.4, 6.4)	
Confirmed intussusception cases within 365 days of dose 1	13	15
Relative risk (95% CI)	0.9 (0.4, 1.9)	

*Relative risk and 95% confidence interval based upon group sequential design stopping criteria employed in REST.

Among vaccine recipients, there were no confirmed cases of intussusception within the 42-day period after the first dose, which was the period of highest risk for the rhesus rotavirus-based product (see Table 2).

[See table 2 above]

All of the children who developed intussusception recovered without sequelae with the exception of a 9-month-old male who developed intussusception 98 days after dose 3 and died of post-operative sepsis. There was a single case of intussusception among 2,470 recipients of RotaTeq in a 7-month-old male in the phase 1 and 2 studies (716 placebo recipients).

Hematochezia

Hematochezia reported as an adverse experience occurred in 0.6% (39/6,130) of vaccine and 0.6% (34/5,560) of placebo recipients within 42 days of any dose. Hematochezia reported as a serious adverse experience occurred in <0.1% (4/36,150) of vaccine and <0.1% (7/35,536) of placebo recipients within 42 days of any dose.

Table 2
Intussusception cases by day range in relation to dose in REST

Day Range	Dose 1 RotaTeq	Dose 1 Placebo	Dose 2 RotaTeq	Dose 2 Placebo	Dose 3 RotaTeq	Dose 3 Placebo	Any Dose RotaTeq	Any Dose Placebo
1-7	0	0	1	0	0	0	1	0
1-14	0	0	1	0	0	1	1	1
1-21	0	0	3	0	0	1	3	1
1-42	0	1	4	1	2	3	6	5

Table 4
Solicited adverse experiences within the first week after doses 1, 2, and 3 (Detailed Safety Cohort)

Adverse experience	Dose 1 RotaTeq	Dose 1 Placebo	Dose 2 RotaTeq	Dose 2 Placebo	Dose 3 RotaTeq	Dose 3 Placebo
Elevated temperature*	n=5,616 17.1%	n=5,077 16.2%	n=5,215 20.0%	n=4,725 19.4%	n=4,865 18.2%	n=4,382 17.6%
	n=6,130	n=5,560	n=5,703	n=5,173	n=5,496	n=4,989
Vomiting	6.7%	5.4%	5.0%	4.4%	3.6%	3.2%
Diarrhea	10.4%	9.1%	8.6%	6.4%	6.1%	5.4%
Irritability	7.1%	7.1%	6.0%	6.5%	4.3%	4.5%

*Temperature ≥100.5°F [38.1°C] rectal equivalent obtained by adding 1 degree F to otic and oral temperatures and 2 degrees F to axillary temperatures

Table 6
Solicited adverse experiences within the first week of doses 1, 2, and 3 among pre-term infants

Adverse event	Dose 1 RotaTeq	Dose 1 Placebo	Dose 2 RotaTeq	Dose 2 Placebo	Dose 3 RotaTeq	Dose 3 Placebo
Elevated temperature*	N=127 18.1%	N=133 17.3%	N=124 25.0%	N=121 28.1%	N=115 14.8%	N=108 20.4%
	N=154	N=154	N=137	N=137	N=135	N=129
Vomiting	5.8%	7.8%	2.9%	2.2%	4.4%	4.7%
Diarrhea	6.5%	5.8%	7.3%	7.3%	3.7%	3.9%
Irritability	3.9%	5.2%	2.9%	4.4%	8.1%	5.4%

*Temperature ≥100.5°F [38.1°C] rectal equivalent obtained by adding 1 degree F to otic and oral temperatures and 2 degrees F to axillary temperatures

Seizures

All seizures reported in the phase 3 trials of RotaTeq (by vaccination group and interval after dose) are shown in Table 3.

Table 3
Seizures reported by day range in relation to any dose in the phase 3 trials of RotaTeq

Day range	1-7	1-14	1-42
RotaTeq	10	15	33
Placebo	5	8	24

Seizures reported as serious adverse experiences occurred in <0.1% (27/36,150) of vaccine and <0.1% (18/35,536) of placebo recipients (not significant). Ten febrile seizures were reported as serious adverse experiences, 5 were observed in vaccine recipients and 5 in placebo recipients.

Kawasaki Disease

In the phase 3 clinical trials, infants were followed for up to 42 days of vaccine dose. Kawasaki disease was reported in 5 of 36,150 vaccine recipients and in 1 of 35,536 placebo recipients with unadjusted relative risk 4.9 (95% CI 0.6, 239.1).

Most Common Adverse Events

Solicited Adverse Events

Detailed safety information was collected from 11,711 infants (6,138 recipients of RotaTeq) which included a subset of subjects in REST and all subjects from Studies 007 and 009 (Detailed Safety Cohort). A Vaccination Report Card was used by parents/guardians to record the child's temperature and any episodes of diarrhea and vomiting on a daily basis during the first week following each vaccination. Table 4 summarizes the frequencies of these adverse events and irritability.

[See table 4 above]

Other Adverse Events

Parents/guardians of the 11,711 infants were also asked to report the presence of other events on the Vaccination Report Card for 42 days after each dose.

Fever was observed at similar rates in vaccine (N=6,138) and placebo (N=5,573) recipients (42.6% vs. 42.8%). Adverse events that occurred at a statistically higher incidence (i.e., 2-sided p-value <0.05) within the 42 days of any dose among recipients of RotaTeq as compared with placebo recipients are shown in Table 5.

Table 5
Adverse events that occurred at a statistically higher incidence within 42 days of any dose among recipients of RotaTeq as compared with placebo recipients

Adverse event	RotaTeq N=6,138 n (%)	Placebo N=5,573 n (%)
Diarrhea	1,479 (24.1%)	1,186 (21.3%)
Vomiting	929 (15.2%)	758 (13.6%)
Otitis media	887 (14.5%)	724 (13.0%)
Nasopharyngitis	422 (6.9%)	325 (5.8%)
Bronchospasm	66 (1.1%)	40 (0.7%)

Safety in Pre-Term Infants

RotaTeq or placebo was administered to 2,070 pre-term infants (25 to 36 weeks gestational age, median 34 weeks) according to their age in weeks since birth in REST. All pre-term infants were followed for serious adverse experiences; a subset of 308 infants was monitored for all adverse experiences. There were 4 deaths throughout the study, 2 among vaccine recipients (1 SIDS and 1 motor vehicle accident) and 2 among placebo recipients (1 SIDS and 1 unknown cause). No cases of intussusception were reported. Serious adverse experiences occurred in 5.5% of vaccine and 5.8% of placebo recipients. The most common serious adverse experience was bronchiolitis, which occurred in 1.4% of vaccine and 2.0% of placebo recipients. Parents/guardians were asked to record the child's temperature and any episodes of vomiting and diarrhea daily for the first week following vaccination. The frequencies of these adverse experiences and irritability within the week after dose 1 are summarized in Table 6.

[See table 6 above]

6.2   Post-Marketing Experience

The following adverse events have been identified during post-approval use of RotaTeq from reports to the Vaccine Adverse Event Reporting System (VAERS).

Reporting of adverse events following immunization to VAERS is voluntary, and the number of doses of vaccine administered is not known; therefore, it is not always possible to reliably estimate the adverse event frequency or establish a causal relationship to vaccine exposure using VAERS data.

In post-marketing experience, the following adverse events have been reported in infants who have received RotaTeq:

Gastrointestinal disorders:
Intussusception
Hematochezia
Skin and subcutaneous tissue disorders:
Urticaria
Infections and infestations:
Kawasaki disease
Reporting Adverse Events
Parents or guardians should be instructed to report any adverse reactions to their health care provider.
Health care providers should report all adverse events to the U.S. Department of Health and Human Services' Vaccine Adverse Events Reporting System (VAERS). VAERS accepts all reports of suspected adverse events after the administration of any vaccine, including but not limited to the reporting of events required by the National Childhood Vaccine Injury Act of 1986. For information or a copy of the vaccine reporting form, call the VAERS toll-free number at 1-800-822-7967 or report on line to **www.vaers.hhs.gov**.[2]

7   DRUG INTERACTIONS

Immunosuppressive therapies including irradiation, antimetabolites, alkylating agents, cytotoxic drugs and corticosteroids (used in greater than physiologic doses), may reduce the immune response to vaccines.

7.1   Concomitant Vaccine Administration
In clinical trials, RotaTeq was administered concomitantly with diphtheria and tetanus toxoids and acellular pertussis (DTaP), inactivated poliovirus vaccine (IPV), H. influenzae type b conjugate (Hib), hepatitis B vaccine, and pneumococcal conjugate vaccine *[see Clinical Studies (14)]*. The safety data available are in the ADVERSE REACTIONS section *[see Adverse Reactions (6.1)]*.
There was no evidence for reduced antibody responses to the diphtheria or tetanus toxoid components of DTaP or to the other vaccines that were concomitantly administered with RotaTeq. However, insufficient immunogenicity data are available to confirm lack of interference of immune responses when RotaTeq is concomitantly administered with childhood vaccines to prevent pertussis.

8   USE IN SPECIFIC POPULATIONS

8.1   Pregnancy
Pregnancy Category C: Animal reproduction studies have not been conducted with RotaTeq. It is also not known whether RotaTeq can cause fetal harm when administered to a pregnant woman or can affect reproduction capacity. RotaTeq is not indicated in women of child-bearing age and should not be administered to pregnant females.

8.4   Pediatric Use
Safety and efficacy have not been established in infants less than 6 weeks of age or greater than 32 weeks of age.
Data are available from clinical studies to support the use of RotaTeq in pre-term infants according to their age in weeks since birth *[see Adverse Reactions (6.1)]*.
Data are available from clinical studies to support the use of RotaTeq in infants with controlled gastroesophageal reflux disease.

11   DESCRIPTION

RotaTeq is a live, oral pentavalent vaccine that contains 5 live reassortant rotaviruses. The rotavirus parent strains of the reassortants were isolated from human and bovine hosts. Four reassortant rotaviruses express one of the outer capsid proteins (G1, G2, G3, or G4) from the human rotavirus parent strain and the attachment protein (serotype P7) from the bovine rotavirus parent strain. The fifth reassortant virus expresses the attachment protein, P1A (genotype P[8]), herein referred to as serotype P1A[8], from the human rotavirus parent strain and the outer capsid protein of serotype G6 from the bovine rotavirus parent strain (see Table 7).
[See table 7 above]
The reassortants are propagated in Vero cells using standard cell culture techniques in the absence of antifungal agents.
The reassortants are suspended in a buffered stabilizer solution. Each vaccine dose contains sucrose, sodium citrate, sodium phosphate monobasic monohydrate, sodium hydroxide, polysorbate 80, cell culture media, and trace amounts of fetal bovine serum. RotaTeq contains no preservatives.
RotaTeq is a pale yellow clear liquid that may have a pink tint.

12   CLINICAL PHARMACOLOGY

Rotavirus is a leading cause of severe acute gastroenteritis in infants and young children, with over 95% of these children infected by the time they are 5 years old.[3] The most severe cases occur among infants and young children between 6 months and 24 months of age.[4]

12.1   Mechanism of Action
The exact immunologic mechanism by which RotaTeq protects against rotavirus gastroenteritis is unknown *[see Clinical Studies (14.6)]*. RotaTeq is a live viral vaccine that replicates in the small intestine and induces immunity.

13   NONCLINICAL TOXICOLOGY

13.1   Carcinogenesis, Mutagenesis, Impairment of Fertility
RotaTeq has not been evaluated for its carcinogenic or mutagenic potential or its potential to impair fertility.

14   CLINICAL STUDIES

Overall, 72,324 infants were randomized in 3 placebo-controlled, phase 3 studies conducted in 11 countries on 3 continents. The data demonstrating the efficacy of RotaTeq in preventing rotavirus gastroenteritis come from 6,983 of

Table 7

Name of Reassortant	Human Rotavirus Parent Strains and Outer Surface Protein Compositions	Bovine Rotavirus Parent Strain and Outer Surface Protein Composition	Reassortant Outer Surface Protein Composition (Human Rotavirus Component in Bold)	Minimum Dose Levels (10^6 infectious units)
G1	WI79 – G1P1A[8]		**G1**P7[5]	2.2
G2	SC2 – G2P2[6]		**G2**P7[5]	2.8
G3	WI78 – G3P1A[8]	WC3 - G6, P7[5]	**G3**P7[5]	2.2
G4	BrB – G4P2[6]		**G4**P7[5]	2.0
P1A[8]	WI79 – G1P1A[8]		G6**P1A[8]**	2.3

Table 8
Efficacy of RotaTeq against any grade of severity of and severe* G1-4 rotavirus gastroenteritis through the first rotavirus season postvaccination in REST

	Per Protocol		Intent-to-Treat[†]	
	RotaTeq	Placebo	RotaTeq	Placebo
Subjects vaccinated	2,834	2,839	2,834	2,839
		Gastroenteritis cases		
Any grade of severity	82	315	150	371
Severe*	1	51	2	55
	Efficacy estimate % and (95% confidence interval)			
Any grade of severity	74.0 (66.8, 79.9)		60.0 (51.5, 67.1)	
Severe*	98.0 (88.3, 100.0)		96.4 (86.2, 99.6)	

*Severe gastroenteritis defined by a clinical scoring system based on the intensity and duration of symptoms of fever, vomiting, diarrhea, and behavioral changes
[†]ITT analysis includes all subjects in the efficacy cohort who received at least one dose of vaccine.

Table 9
Efficacy of RotaTeq in reducing G1-4 rotavirus-related hospitalizations in REST

	Per Protocol		Intent-to-Treat*	
	RotaTeq	Placebo	RotaTeq	Placebo
Subjects vaccinated	34,035	34,003	34,035	34,003
Number of hospitalizations	6	144	10	187
Efficacy estimate % and (95% confidence interval)	95.8 (90.5, 98.2)		94.7 (89.3, 97.3)	

* ITT analysis includes all subjects who received at least one dose of vaccine.

these infants from the US (including Navajo and White Mountain Apache Nations) and Finland who were enrolled in 2 of these studies: REST and Study 007. The third trial, Study 009, provided clinical evidence supporting the consistency of manufacture and contributed data to the overall safety evaluation.
The racial distribution of the efficacy subset was as follows: White (RotaTeq 68%, placebo 69%); Hispanic-American (RotaTeq 10%, placebo 9%); Black (2% in both groups); Multiracial (RotaTeq 4%, placebo 5%); Asian (<1% in both groups); Native American (RotaTeq 15%, placebo 14%); and Other (<1% in both groups). The gender distribution was 52% male and 48% female in both vaccination groups.
The efficacy evaluations in these studies included: 1) Prevention of any grade of severity of rotavirus gastroenteritis; 2) Prevention of severe rotavirus gastroenteritis, as defined by a clinical scoring system; and 3) Reduction in hospitalizations due to rotavirus gastroenteritis.
The vaccine was given as a three-dose series to healthy infants with the first dose administered between 6 and 12 weeks of age and followed by two additional doses administered at 4- to 10-week intervals. The age of infants receiving the third dose was 32 weeks of age or less. Oral polio vaccine administration was not permitted; however, other childhood vaccines could be concomitantly administered. Breastfeeding was permitted in all studies.
The case definition for rotavirus gastroenteritis used to determine vaccine efficacy required that a subject meet both of the following clinical and laboratory criteria: (1) greater than or equal to 3 watery or looser-than-normal stools within a 24-hour period and/or forceful vomiting; and (2) rotavirus antigen detection by enzyme immunoassay (EIA) in a stool specimen taken within 14 days of onset of symptoms. The severity of rotavirus acute gastroenteritis was determined by a clinical scoring system that took into account the intensity and duration of symptoms of fever, vomiting, diarrhea, and behavioral changes.
The primary efficacy analyses included cases of rotavirus gastroenteritis caused by serotypes G1, G2, G3, and G4 that occurred at least 14 days after the third dose through the first rotavirus season post vaccination.
Analyses were also done to evaluate the efficacy of RotaTeq against rotavirus gastroenteritis caused by serotypes G1, G2, G3, and G4 at any time following the first dose through the first rotavirus season postvaccination among infants who received at least one vaccination (Intent-to-treat, ITT).

14.1   Rotavirus Efficacy and Safety Trial
Primary efficacy against any grade of severity of rotavirus gastroenteritis caused by naturally occurring serotypes G1, G2, G3, or G4 through the first rotavirus season after vaccination was 74.0% (95% CI: 66.8, 79.9) and the ITT efficacy was 60.0% (95% CI: 51.5, 67.1). Primary efficacy against severe rotavirus gastroenteritis caused by naturally occurring serotypes G1, G2, G3, or G4 through the first rotavirus season after vaccination was 98.0% (95% CI: 88.3, 100.0), and ITT efficacy was 96.4% (95% CI: 86.2, 99.6). See Table 8.
[See table 8 above]
The efficacy of RotaTeq against severe disease was also demonstrated by a reduction in hospitalizations for rotavirus gastroenteritis among all subjects enrolled in REST. RotaTeq reduced hospitalizations for rotavirus gastroenteritis caused by serotypes G1, G2, G3, and G4 through the first two years after the third dose by 95.8% (95% CI: 90.5, 98.2). The ITT efficacy in reducing hospitalizations was 94.7% (95% CI: 89.3, 97.3) as shown in Table 9.
[See table 9 above]

14.2   Study 007
Primary efficacy against any grade of severity of rotavirus gastroenteritis caused by naturally occurring serotypes G1, G2, G3, or G4 through the first rotavirus season after vaccination was 72.5% (95% CI: 50.6, 85.6) and the ITT efficacy was 58.4% (95% CI: 33.8, 74.5). Primary efficacy against severe rotavirus gastroenteritis caused by naturally occurring serotypes G1, G2, G3, or G4 through the first rotavirus season after vaccination was 100% (95% CI: 13.0, 100.0) and ITT efficacy against severe rotavirus disease was 100%, (95% CI: 30.2, 100.0) as shown in Table 10.
[See table 10 at top of next page]

14.3   Multiple Rotavirus Seasons
The efficacy of RotaTeq through a second rotavirus season was evaluated in a single study (REST). Efficacy against any grade of severity of rotavirus gastroenteritis caused by rotavirus serotypes G1, G2, G3, and G4 through the two ro-

Continued on next page

Information on the Merck & Co., Inc., products listed on these pages is from the full prescribing information in use March 1, 2008. For information, please call 1-800-NSC-MERCK [1-800-672-6372].

RotaTeq—Cont.

tavirus seasons after vaccination was 71.3% (95% CI: 64.7, 76.9). The efficacy of RotaTeq in preventing cases occurring only during the second rotavirus season postvaccination was 62.6% (95% CI: 44.3, 75.4). The efficacy of RotaTeq beyond the second season postvaccination was not evaluated.

14.4 Rotavirus Gastroenteritis Regardless of Serotype

The rotavirus serotypes identified in the efficacy subset of REST and Study 007 were G1P1A[8]; G2P1[4]; G3P1A[8]; G4P1A[8]; and G9P1A[8].

In REST, the efficacy of RotaTeq against any grade of severity of naturally occurring rotavirus gastroenteritis regardless of serotype was 71.8% (95% CI: 64.5, 77.8) and efficacy against severe rotavirus disease was 98.0% (95% CI: 88.3, 99.9). The ITT efficacy starting at dose 1 was 50.9% (95% CI: 41.6, 58.9) for any grade of severity of rotavirus disease and was 96.4% (95% CI: 86.3, 99.6) for severe rotavirus disease. In Study 007, the primary efficacy of RotaTeq against any grade of severity of rotavirus gastroenteritis regardless of serotype was 72.7% (95% CI: 51.9, 85.4) and efficacy against severe rotavirus disease was 100% (95% CI: 12.7, 100). The ITT efficacy starting at dose 1 was 48.0% (95% CI: 21.6, 66.1) for any grade of severity of rotavirus disease and was 100% (95% CI: 30.4, 100.0) for severe rotavirus disease.

14.5 Rotavirus Gastroenteritis by Serotype

The efficacy against any grade of severity of rotavirus gastroenteritis by serotype in the REST efficacy cohort is shown in Table 11.

[See table 11 above]

In a separate post hoc analysis of health care utilization data from 68,038 infants (RotaTeq 34,035 and placebo 34,003) in REST, using a case definition that included culture confirmation, hospitalization and emergency departments visits due to G9P1A[8] rotavirus gastroenteritis were reduced (RotaTeq 0 cases: placebo 14 cases) by 100% (95% CI: 69.6%, 100.0%).

14.6 Immunogenicity

A relationship between antibody responses to RotaTeq and protection against rotavirus gastroenteritis has not been established. In phase 3 studies, 92.9% to 100% of 439 recipients of RotaTeq achieved a 3-fold or more rise in serum antirotavirus IgA after a three-dose regimen when compared to 12.3%-20.0% of 397 placebo recipients.

15 REFERENCES

1. Murphy TV, Gargiullo PM, Massoudi MS et al. Intussusception among infants given an oral rotavirus vaccine. N Engl J Med 2001;344:564-572.
2. Centers for Disease Control and Prevention. General recommendations on immunization: recommendations of the Advisory Committee on Immunization Practices (ACIP) and the American Academy of Family Physicians (AAFP). MMWR 2002;51(RR-2):1-35.
3. Parashar UD et al. Global illness and deaths caused by rotavirus disease in children. Emerg Infect Dis 2003;9(5):565-572.
4. Parashar UD, Holman RC, Clarke MJ, Bresee JS, Glass RI. Hospitalizations associated with rotavirus diarrhea in the United States, 1993 through 1995: surveillance based on the new ICD-9-CM rotavirus-specific diagnostic code. J Infect Dis 1998;177:13-7.

16 HOW SUPPLIED/STORAGE AND HANDLING

No. 4047—RotaTeq, 2 mL, a solution for oral use, is a pale yellow clear liquid that may have a pink tint. It is supplied as follows:

NDC 0006-4047-31 package of 1 individually pouched single-dose tube

NDC 0006-4047-41 package of 10 individually pouched single-dose tubes.

16.1 Storage and Handling

Store and transport refrigerated at 2-8°C (36-46°F). RotaTeq should be administered as soon as possible after being removed from refrigeration. For information regarding stability under conditions other than those recommended, call 1-800-MERCK-90.

Protect from light.

RotaTeq should be discarded in approved biological waste containers according to local regulations.

The product must be used before the expiration date.

17 PATIENT COUNSELING INFORMATION

[See FDA-Approved Patient Labeling (17.2).]

17.1 Information for Parents/Guardians

Parents or guardians should be given a copy of the required vaccine information and be given the "Patient Information" appended to this insert. Parents and/or guardians should be encouraged to read the patient information that describes the benefits and risks associated with the vaccine and ask any questions they may have during the visit. See PRECAUTIONS and Patient Information.

Manuf. and Dist. by:

MERCK & CO., INC., Whitehouse Station, NJ 08889, USA

Issued September 2007

Printed in USA

9714305

17.2 FDA-Approved Patient Labeling

Revisions based on Label 9714305, Issued September 2007.

PATIENT INFORMATION

RotaTeq®* (pronounced "RŌ-tuh-tek")

rotavirus vaccine, live, oral, pentavalent

You should read this information before your child receives the RotaTeq vaccine and ask your child's doctor any questions you may have. Your child will need 3 doses of the vac-

---

Table 10
Efficacy of RotaTeq against any grade of severity of and severe* G1-4 rotavirus gastroenteritis through the first rotavirus season postvaccination in Study 007

	Per Protocol		Intent-to-Treat[†]	
	RotaTeq	Placebo	RotaTeq	Placebo
Subjects vaccinated	650	660	650	660
Gastroenteritis cases				
Any grade of severity	15	54	27	64
Severe*	0	6	0	7
Efficacy estimate % and (95% confidence interval)				
Any grade of severity	72.5 (50.6, 85.6)		58.4 (33.8, 74.5)	
Severe*	100.0 (13.0, 100.0)		100.0 (30.2, 100.0)	

*Severe gastroenteritis defined by a clinical scoring system based on the intensity and duration of symptoms of fever, vomiting, diarrhea, and behavioral change
[†]ITT analysis includes all subjects in the efficacy cohort who received at least one dose of vaccine.

Table 11
Serotype-specific efficacy of RotaTeq against any grade of severity of rotavirus gastroenteritis among infants in the REST efficacy cohort through the first rotavirus season postvaccination (Per Protocol)

	Number of cases		
Serotype identified by PCR	RotaTeq (N=2,834)	Placebo (N=2,839)	% Efficacy (95% Confidence Interval)
Serotypes present in RotaTeq			
G1P1A[8]	72	286	74.9 (67.3, 80.9)
G2P1[4]	6	17	63.4 (2.6, 88.2)
G3P1A[8]	1	6	NS
G4P1A[8]	3	6	NS
Serotypes not present in RotaTeq			
G9P1A[8]	1	3	NS
Unidentified*	11	15	NS

N = number vaccinated
NS = not significant

* Includes rotavirus antigen-positive samples in which the specific serotype could not be identified by PCR

---

cine over the course of a few months. So read the leaflet before your child receives each dose of the vaccine in case any of the information about the vaccine changes. This leaflet is a summary of certain information about the vaccine. If you would like additional information, your health care provider can give you more complete information about this vaccine that is written for health care professionals. This leaflet does not take the place of talking with your child's doctor.

What is RotaTeq and How Does it Work?

RotaTeq is a vaccine that can help protect your child from getting a virus infection that can cause fever, vomiting, and diarrhea. The vaccine is given by mouth at 3 different times, each about one to two months apart. Nearly all children become infected with the rotavirus by the time they are 5 years old.

RotaTeq helps protect against diarrhea and vomiting only if they are caused by the rotavirus. It does not protect against diarrhea and vomiting that are caused by anything else.

RotaTeq may not fully protect all children that get the vaccine, and if your child already has the virus it will not help them.

What are the Symptoms of a Rotavirus Infection?

Infection with the Rotavirus is the most common cause of severe diarrhea in infants. Sometimes the diarrhea and vomiting can be severe and lead to the loss of body fluids (dehydration) and even to death.

Signs that your infant is dehydrated include:
- Sleepiness
- Dry mouth and tongue
- Fussiness
- Dry diaper for several hours

If your infant shows signs that they are dehydrated, you should call the doctor immediately.

What should I tell the doctor before my child gets RotaTeq?

There are some things your doctor should know before your child gets the vaccine. You should tell your doctor if your child:
- Has any illness with fever. A mild fever or cold by itself is not a reason to delay taking the vaccination.
- Has diarrhea or has been vomiting.
- Has not been gaining weight.
- Is not growing as expected.
- Has a blood disorder.
- Has any type of cancer.
- Has a weak immune system because of a disease (this includes HIV/AIDS).

- Gets treatment or takes medicines that may weaken the immune system (such as high doses of steroids) or has received a blood transfusion or blood products within the past 42 days.
- Was born with gastrointestinal problems, or has had a blockage or abdominal surgery.
- Has regular close contact with a member of the family or household who has a weakened immune system. For example, a person in the house with cancer or one who is taking medicines that may weaken their immune system.

Who should not receive RotaTeq?

Your child should not get the vaccine if:
- He or she had an allergic reaction after getting a dose of this vaccine.
- He or she is allergic to any of the ingredients of the vaccine. A list of ingredients can be found at the end of this leaflet.

What important information should I know about RotaTeq?

Intussusception is a serious and life-threatening event that occurs when a part of the intestine (the tube that goes from the stomach to the anus) gets blocked or twisted. Cases of intussusception can occur when no vaccine has been given and the cause is usually unknown. However, a different rotavirus vaccine was associated with intussusception and is no longer available.

In clinical trials, RotaTeq was studied in 70,000 infants (35,000 infants received RotaTeq and 35,000 received placebo), and no increased risk of intussusception was found. However, since RotaTeq has been on the market, cases of intussusception in infants who received RotaTeq have been reported to the Vaccine Adverse Event Reporting System (VAERS). Intussusception occurred at various times after vaccination with RotaTeq. Some of these infants required hospitalization and surgery on their intestine or a special enema to treat this problem.

Call your child's doctor right away if your child has vomiting, diarrhea, severe stomach pain, blood in their stool or change in their bowel movements as these may be signs of intussusception. It is important to contact your doctor if you have questions or if your child has any of these symptoms, at any time after vaccination, even if it has been several weeks since the last vaccine dose.

What are the possible side effects of RotaTeq?

The most common side effects reported after taking RotaTeq were diarrhea, vomiting, fever, runny nose and sore throat, wheezing or coughing, and ear infection.

Other reported side effects include hives.

These are NOT all the possible side effects of RotaTeq. You can ask your doctor or health care provider for a more complete list.

If your child seems to be having any side effects that are not mentioned in this leaflet, please call your doctor or other health care provider. If the condition continues or worsens, you should seek medical attention.

You, as a parent or guardian, may also report any adverse reactions to your child's health care provider or directly to the Vaccine Adverse Event Reporting System (VAERS). The VAERS toll-free number is 1-800-822-7967 or report online to www.vaers.hhs.gov.

Can RotaTeq be given with other vaccines?

Your child may get RotaTeq at the same time as other childhood vaccines.

How is RotaTeq given?

The vaccine is given by mouth. Your child will receive 3 doses of the vaccine. The first dose is given when your child is 6 to 12 weeks of age, the second dose is given 4 to 10 weeks later and the third dose is given 4 to 10 weeks after the second dose. The last (third) dose should be given to your child by 32 weeks of age.

Your health care provider will gently squeeze the vaccine into your child's mouth (see Figure 1). Your infant may spit out some or all of it. If this happens, the dose does not need to be given again during that visit.

Figure 1:

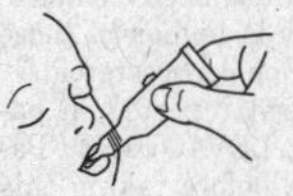

What do I do if my child misses a dose of RotaTeq?

All 3 doses of the vaccine should be given to your child by 32 weeks of age. Your health care provider will tell you when your child should come for the follow-up doses. It is important to keep those appointments. If you forget or are not able to go back at the planned time, ask your health care provider for advice.

What else should I know about RotaTeq?

This leaflet gives a summary of certain information about the vaccine. If you have any questions or concerns about RotaTeq, talk to your health care provider. You can also visit www.rotateq.com.

What are the ingredients in RotaTeq?

Active Ingredient: 5 live rotavirus strains (G1, G2, G3, G4, and P1).

Inactive Ingredients: sucrose, sodium citrate, sodium phosphate monobasic monohydrate, sodium hydroxide, polysorbate 80 and also fetal bovine serum.

Rx only

Issued September 2007

Manuf. and Dist. by:

MERCK & CO., INC., Whitehouse Station, NJ 08889, USA

Revisions based on 9714305, issued September 2007.

SINGULAIR® ℞

[*sing u lair*]

(montelukast sodium)

TABLETS, CHEWABLE TABLETS, AND ORAL GRANULES

Prescribing information for this product, which appears on pages 2091–2097 of the 2008 PDR, has been revised as follows. Please write "See Supplement A" next to the product heading.

In the **CLINICAL PHARMACOLOGY** section, add the following new subsection:

Clinical Studies – Exercise-Induced Bronchoconstriction

SINGLE-DOSE ADMINISTRATION (ADULTS AND ADOLESCENTS)

The efficacy of SINGULAIR, 10 mg, when given as a single dose 2 hours before exercise for the prevention of exercise-induced bronchoconstriction (EIB) was investigated in three (U.S. and Multinational), randomized, double-blind, placebo-controlled crossover studies that included a total of 160 adult and adolescent patients 15 years of age and older with exercise-induced bronchoconstriction. Exercise challenge testing was conducted at 2 hours, 8.5 or 12 hours, and 24 hours following administration of a single dose of study drug (SINGULAIR 10 mg or placebo). The primary endpoint was the mean maximum percent fall in FEV_1 following the 2 hours post-dose exercise challenge in all three studies (Study A, Study B, and Study C). In Study A, a single dose of SINGULAIR 10 mg demonstrated a statistically significant protective benefit against EIB when taken 2 hours prior to exercise. Some patients were protected from exercise-induced bronchoconstriction at 8.5 and 24 hours after administration; however, some patients were not. The results for the mean maximum percent fall at each timepoint in Study A are shown in the TABLE 3 below and are representative of the results from the other two studies.

TABLE 3
Mean Maximum Percent Fall in FEV_1 Following Exercise Challenge in Study A (N=47)

Time of exercise challenge following medication administration	Mean Maximum percent fall in FEV_1*		Treatment difference % for SINGULAIR versus Placebo (95%CI)*
	SINGULAIR	Placebo	
2 hours	13	22	-9 (-12, -5)
8.5 hours	12	17	-5 (-9, -2)
24 hours	10	14	-4 (-7, -1)

*Least squares-mean

CHRONIC ADMINISTRATION (ADULTS AND PEDIATRIC PATIENTS)

In a 12-week, randomized, double-blind, parallel group study of 110 adult and adolescent asthmatics 15 years of age and older, with a mean baseline FEV_1 percent of predicted of 83% and with documented exercise-induced exacerbation of asthma, treatment with SINGULAIR, 10 mg, once daily in the evening, resulted in a statistically significant reduction in mean maximal percent fall in FEV_1 and mean time to recovery to within 5% of the pre-exercise FEV_1. Exercise challenge was conducted at the end of the dosing interval (i.e., 20 to 24 hours after the preceding dose). This effect was maintained throughout the 12-week treatment period indicating that tolerance did not occur. SINGULAIR did not, however, prevent clinically significant deterioration in maximal percent fall in FEV_1 after exercise (i.e., ≥20% decrease from pre-exercise baseline) in 52% of patients studied. In a separate crossover study in adults, a similar effect was observed after two once-daily 10-mg doses of SINGULAIR.

In pediatric patients 6 to 14 years of age, using the 5-mg chewable tablet, a 2-day crossover study demonstrated effects similar to those observed in adults when exercise challenge was conducted at the end of the dosing interval (i.e., 20 to 24 hours after the preceding dose).

Daily administration of SINGULAIR for the chronic treatment of asthma has not been established to prevent acute episodes of exercise-induced bronchoconstriction.

In the **INDICATIONS AND USAGE** section, after the first paragraph add the following paragraph: SINGULAIR is indicated for prevention of exercised-induced bronchoconstriction in patients 15 years of age and older.

In the **PRECAUTIONS** section, in the *General* subsection, at the end of the second paragraph, add: Patients who have exacerbations of asthma after exercise should have available for rescue a short-acting inhaled β-agonist.

In the same subsection, delete the fourth paragraph.

In the *Information for Patients* subsection, at the end of the second bulleted paragraph, add: Patients who have exacerbations of asthma after exercise should be instructed to have available for rescue a short-acting inhaled β-agonist. Daily administration of SINGULAIR for the chronic treatment of asthma has not been established to prevent acute episodes of exercise-induced bronchoconstriction.

In the same subsection, delete the fifth bulleted paragraph.

In the **ADVERSE REACTIONS** section, in the first sentence in the *Adults and Adolescents 15 Years of Age and Older with Asthma* subsection, change 2600 to 2950.

In the same subsection, after the second paragraph, add the following new paragraph: The safety profile of SINGULAIR when administered as a single dose for prevention of EIB in adult and adolescent patients 15 years of age and older was consistent with the safety profile previously described for SINGULAIR.

The *Post-Marketing Experience* subsection has been completely reorganized in the following format:

The following additional adverse reactions have been reported in post-marketing use:

Blood and lymphatic system disorders: increased bleeding tendency

Immune system disorders: hypersensitivity reactions including anaphylaxis, very rarely hepatic eosinophilic infiltration

Psychiatric disorders: agitation including aggressive behavior, anxiousness, dream abnormalities and hallucinations, depression, insomnia, irritability, restlessness, suicidal thinking and behavior (suicidality), tremor

Nervous system disorders: drowsiness, paraesthesia/hypoesthesia, very rarely seizures

Cardiac disorders: palpitations

Gastrointestinal disorders: diarrhea, dyspepsia, nausea, very rarely pancreatitis, vomiting

Hepatobiliary disorders: Rare cases of cholestatic hepatitis, hepatocellular liver-injury, and mixed-pattern liver injury have been reported in patients treated with SINGULAIR. Most of these occurred in combination with other confounding factors, such as use of other medications, or when SINGULAIR was administered to patients who had underlying potential for liver disease, such as alcohol use or other forms of hepatitis.

Skin and subcutaneous tissue disorders: angioedema, bruising, erythema nodosum, pruritus, urticaria

Musculoskeletal and connective tissue disorders: arthralgia, myalgia including muscle cramps

General disorders and administration site conditions: edema

The second paragraph in this subsection has not been changed.

The **DOSAGE AND ADMINISTRATION** section has completely changed to the following:

Dosage Information

The dosage for adults and adolescents 15 years of age and older is one 10-mg tablet.

The dosage for pediatric patients 6 to 14 years of age is one 5-mg chewable tablet.

The dosage for pediatric patients 2 to 5 years of age is one 4-mg chewable tablet or one packet of 4-mg oral granules.

The dosage for pediatric patients 6 to 23 months of age is one packet of 4-mg oral granules.

Asthma in Patients 12 Months of Age and Older

SINGULAIR should be taken once daily in the evening. Safety and effectiveness in pediatric patients less than 12 months of age have not been established.

Exercise-Induced Bronchoconstriction (EIB) in Patients 15 Years of Age and Older:

For prevention of EIB, a single dose of SINGULAIR should be taken at least 2 hours before exercise. An additional dose of SINGULAIR should not be taken within 24 hours of a previous dose. Patients already taking one tablet daily for another indication (including chronic asthma) should not take an additional dose to prevent EIB. All patients should have available for rescue a short-acting β-agonist. Safety and effectiveness in patients younger than 15 years of age have not been established. Daily administration of SINGULAIR for the chronic treatment of asthma has not been established to prevent acute episodes of exercise-induced bronchoconstriction.

Allergic Rhinitis

Seasonal Allergic Rhinitis in Patients 2 Years and Older

Perennial Allergic Rhinitis in Patients 6 Months and Older

For allergic rhinitis SINGULAIR should be taken once daily. The time of administration may be individualized to suit patient needs.

Safety and effectiveness in pediatric patients younger than 2 years of age with seasonal allergic rhinitis and less than 6 months of age with perennial allergic rhinitis have not been established.

Asthma and Allergic Rhinitis in Patients 12 Months of Age and Older:

Patients with both asthma and allergic rhinitis should take only one tablet daily in the evening.

Administration of SINGULAIR Oral Granules

SINGULAIR 4-mg oral granules can be administered either directly in the mouth, dissolved in 1 teaspoonful (5 mL) of cold or room temperature baby formula or breast milk, or mixed with a spoonful of cold or room temperature soft foods; based on stability studies, only applesauce, carrots, rice, or ice cream should be used. The packet should not be opened until ready to use. After opening the packet, the full dose (with or without mixing with baby formula, breast milk, or food) must be administered within 15 minutes. If mixed with baby formula, breast milk, or food, SINGULAIR oral granules must not be stored for future use. Discard any unused portion. SINGULAIR oral granules are not intended to be dissolved in any liquid other than baby formula or breast milk for administration. However, liquids may be taken subsequent to administration. SINGULAIR oral granules can be administered without regard to the time of meals.

Revisions based on 9628409, issued April 2007, 9628410, issued September 2007, and 9628412, issued February 2008.

Patient Information

SINGULAIR® (SING-u-lair) Tablets, Chewable Tablets, and Oral Granules

Generic name: montelukast (mon-te-LOO-kast) sodium

Patient information for this product, which appears on pages 2096 and 2097 of the 2008 PDR, has been revised as follows. Please write "See Supplement A" next to the product heading.

In the section **What is SINGULAIR?**, the second paragraph should now read:

SINGULAIR is prescribed for the treatment of asthma, the prevention of exercise-induced asthma, and allergic rhinitis.

In the same section, replace the fifth paragraph, with:

2. Prevention of exercise-induced asthma.

SINGULAIR is used for the prevention of exercise-induced asthma in patients 15 years of age and older.

Change the sixth paragraph from Number **2.** to Number **3.**

In the section **How should I take SINGULAIR?**, in the subsection **For adults and children 12 months of age and older with asthma:**, delete the last bulleted statement. Then add the following subsection:

For patients 15 years of age and older for the prevention of exercise-induced asthma:,

- Take SINGULAIR at least 2 hours before exercise.
- Always have your inhaled rescue medicine for asthma attacks with you.
- If you are taking SINGULAIR daily for chronic asthma or

Continued on next page

Information on the Merck & Co., Inc., products listed on these pages is from the full prescribing information in use March 1, 2008. For information, please call 1-800-NSC-MERCK [1-800-672-6372].

Singulair—Cont.

allergic rhinitis, do not take an additional dose to prevent exercise-induced asthma. Speak to your doctor about your treatment of exercise-induced asthma.
- Do not take an additional dose of SINGULAIR within 24 hours of a previous dose.

In the section **What is the daily dose of SINGULAIR for asthma or allergic rhinitis?**, delete "**daily**" and "**for asthma or allergic rhinitis**". Change the bold subhead under that to:
For asthma – Take once daily in the evening:
In the same section, add the following subheads and bullet after the fourth bulleted paragraph:
For exercise-induced asthma – Take at least 2 hours before exercise, but not more than once daily:
- One 10-mg tablet for adults and adolescents 15 years of age and older.

For allergic rhinitis – Take once daily at about the same time each day:
The section **What are the possible side effects of SINGULAIR?**, has a completely reorganized third paragraph in the following format:
Less common side effects that have happened with SINGULAIR include:
- increased bleeding tendency
- allergic reactions [including swelling of the face, lips, tongue, and/or throat (which may cause trouble breathing or swallowing), hives and itching]
- behavior and mood related changes [agitation including aggressive behavior, bad/vivid dreams, depression, feeling anxious, hallucinations (seeing things that are not there), irritability, restlessness, suicidal thoughts and actions, tremor, trouble sleeping]
- palpitations
- drowsiness, pins and needles/numbness, seizures (convulsions or fits)
- diarrhea, indigestion, inflammation of the pancreas, nausea, vomiting
- hepatitis
- bruising
- joint pain, muscle aches and muscle cramps
- swelling

After the section **What is asthma?**, add the following new section:
What is exercise-induced asthma?
Exercise-induced asthma, more accurately called exercise-induced bronchoconstriction occurs when exercise triggers symptoms of asthma.
Revisions based on 9628409, issued April 2007, 9628410, issued September 2007, and 9628412, issued February 2008.

Merck/Schering-Plough Pharmaceuticals

PO BOX 1000
UG4B–75
351 N. SUMNEYTOWN PIKE
NORTH WALES, PA 19454

For Product and Service Information, Medical Information, and Adverse Drug Experience Reporting:
Call: Merck/Schering-Plough National Service Center
Monday through Friday, 8:00 AM to 7:00 PM (ET)
866-637-2501
Fax: 800-637-2568
For 24-hour emergency information, healthcare professionals should call:
Merck/Schering-Plough National Service Center at
866-637-2501
For Product Ordering,
Call: Order Management Center
Monday through Friday, 8:00 AM to 7:00 PM (ET)
800-637-2579

VYTORIN® ℞
[vī-tōr-in]
(ezetimibe/simvastatin)
Tablets

Prescribing information for this product, which appears on pages 2127–2134 of the 2008 PDR, has been revised as follows. Please write "See Supplement A" next to the product heading.
In the **ADVERSE REACTIONS** section, under *Post-marketing Experience, Ezetimibe*, after "dizziness;", add "depression;".
Revisions based on 9619508, issued September 2007.
In the **Patient Information about VYTORIN**, under **What are the possible side effects of VYTORIN?**, in the bulleted copy of the third paragraph, after "dizziness;", add "depression;".
Revisions based on 9619508, issued September 2007.

ZETIA® ℞
[zĕt' ē ă]
(ezetimibe)
TABLETS

Prescribing information for this product, which appears on pages 2134–2139 of the 2008 PDR, has been revised as follows. Please write "See Supplement A" next to the product heading.
In the **ADVERSE REACTIONS** section, under *"Post-marketing Experience,"* in the second paragraph, after "dizziness;" add "depression;".
Revisions based on 29480958T, REV 14, issued September 2007.
In the **Patient Information about ZETIA**, under **What are the possible side effects of ZETIA?**, in the third paragraph, after "dizziness;" add "depression;".
Revisions based on 29480826T, Rev 14, issued September 2007.

Ortho-McNeil, Inc.

RARITAN, NJ 08869-0602

www.ortho-mcneil.com
For Medical Information Contact:
(800) 682-6532
In Emergencies:
(908) 218-7325
For Patient Education Materials Contact:
877-323-2200
For Customer Service (Sales and Ordering):
800-631-5273

LEVAQUIN® ℞
(levofloxacin)
TABLETS
LEVAQUIN®
(levofloxacin)
ORAL SOLUTION
LEVAQUIN®
(levofloxacin)
INJECTION
LEVAQUIN®
(levofloxacin in 5% dextrose)
INJECTION

Prescribing information for this product, which appears on pages 2358–2365 of the 2008 PDR, has been revised as follows. Please write "See Supplement A" next to the product heading.
In the WARNINGS & PRECAUTIONS section, a new subsection has been added:
Hepatotoxicity
Post-marketing reports of severe hepatotoxicity (including acute hepatitis and fatal events) have been received for patients treated with LEVAQUIN®. No evidence of serious drug-associated hepatotoxicity was detected in clinical trials of over 7,000 patients. Severe hepatotoxicity generally occurred within 14 days of initiation of therapy and most cases occurred within 6 days. Most cases of severe hepatotoxicity were not associated with hypersensitivity *[see Warnings and Precautions (5.2)]*. The majority of fatal hepatotoxicity reports occurred in patients 65 years of age or older and most were not associated with hypersensitivity. LEVAQUIN® should be discontinued immediately if the patient develops signs and symptoms of hepatitis *[see Adverse Reactions (6); Patient Counseling Information (17.3)]*.
In the WARNINGS & PRECAUTIONS section, a new subsection has been added:
Photosensitivity/Phototoxicity
Moderate to severe photosensitivity/phototoxicity reactions, the latter of which may manifest as exaggerated sunburn reactions (e.g., burning, erythema, exudation, vesicles, blistering, edema) involving areas exposed to light (typically the face, "V" area of the neck, extensor surfaces of the forearms, dorsa of the hands), can be associated with the use of quinolones after sun or UV light exposure. Therefore, excessive exposure to these sources of light should be avoided. Drug therapy should be discontinued if photosensitivity/phototoxicity occurs *[see Adverse Reactions (6.3); Patient Counseling Information (17.3)]*.
The PATIENT COUNSELING INFORMATION section has been added:
PATIENT COUNSELING INFORMATION
Antibacterial Resistance
Antibacterial drugs including LEVAQUIN® should only be used to treat bacterial infections. They do not treat viral infections (e.g., the common cold). When LEVAQUIN® is prescribed to treat a bacterial infection, patients should be told that although it is common to feel better early in the course of therapy, the medication should be taken exactly as directed. Skipping doses or not completing the full course of therapy may (1) decrease the effectiveness of the immediate treatment and (2) increase the likelihood that bacteria will develop resistance and will not be treatable by LEVAQUIN® or other antibacterial drugs in the future.
Administration with Food, Fluids, and Concomitant Medications
Patients should be informed that LEVAQUIN® Tablets may be taken with or without food. LEVAQUIN® Oral Solution should be taken 1 hour before or 2 hours after eating. The tablet and oral solution should be taken at the same time each day.
Patients should drink fluids liberally while taking LEVAQUIN® to avoid formation of a highly concentrated urine and crystal formation in the urine.
Antacids containing magnesium, or aluminum, as well as sucralfate, metal cations such as iron, and multivitamin preparations with zinc or didanosine should be taken at least two hours before or two hours after oral LEVAQUIN® administration.
Serious and Potentially Serious Adverse Reactions
Patients should be informed of the following serious adverse reactions that have been associated with LEVAQUIN® or other quinolone use:
- **Hypersensitivity Reactions:** Patients should be informed that LEVAQUIN® can cause hypersensitivity reactions, even following the first dose. Patients should discontinue the drug at the first sign of a skin rash, hives or other skin reactions, a rapid heartbeat, difficulty in swallowing or breathing, any swelling suggesting angioedema (e.g., swelling of the lips, tongue, face, tightness of the throat, hoarseness), or other symptoms of an allergic reaction.
- **Hepatotoxicity:** Severe hepatotoxicity (including acute hepatitis and fatal events) has been reported in patients taking LEVAQUIN®. Patients should inform their physician and be instructed to discontinue LEVAQUIN® treatment immediately if they experience any signs or symptoms of liver injury including: loss of appetite, nausea, vomiting, fever, weakness, tiredness, right upper quadrant tenderness, itching, yellowing of the skin and eyes, light colored bowel movements or dark colored urine.
- **Tendon Disorders:** Patients should discontinue LEVAQUIN® treatment and inform their physician if they experience pain, inflammation, or rupture of a tendon, and to rest and refrain from exercise until the diagnosis of tendonitis or tendon rupture has been excluded. The risk of serious tendon disorders is higher in those over 65 years of age, especially those on corticosteroids.
- **Convulsions:** Convulsions have been reported in patients taking quinolones, including LEVAQUIN®. Patients should notify their physician before taking this drug if they have a history of convulsions.
- **Neurologic Adverse Effects (e.g., dizziness, lightheadedness):** Patients should know how they react to LEVAQUIN® before they operate an automobile or machinery or engage in other activities requiring mental alertness and coordination.
- **Diarrhea:** Diarrhea is a common problem caused by antibiotics which usually ends when the antibiotic is discontinued. Sometimes after starting treatment with antibiotics, patients can develop watery and bloody stools (with or without stomach cramps and fever) even as late as two or more months after having taken the last dose of the antibiotic. If this occurs, patients should contact their physician as soon as possible.
- **Peripheral Neuropathies:** If symptoms of peripheral neuropathy including pain, burning, tingling, numbness, and/or weakness develop, patients should discontinue treatment and contact their physician.
- **Prolongation of the QT Interval:** Patients should inform their physician of any personal or family history of QT prolongation or proarrhythmic conditions such as hypokalemia, bradycardia, or recent myocardial ischemia; if they are taking any class IA (quinidine, procainamide), or class III (amiodarone, sotalol) antiarrhythmic agents. Patients should notify their physicians if they have any symptoms of prolongation of the QT interval, including prolonged heart palpitations or a loss of consciousness.
- **Photosensitivity/Phototoxicity:** Patients should be advised that photosensitivity/phototoxicity has been reported in patients receiving quinolone antibiotics. Patients should minimize or avoid exposure to natural or artificial sunlight (tanning beds or UVA/B treatment) while taking quinolones. If patients need to be outdoors when taking quinolones, they should wear loose-fitting clothes that protect skin from sun exposure and discuss other sun protection measures with their physician. If a sunburn like reaction or skin eruption occurs, patients should contact their physician.

Drug Interactions with Insulin, Oral Hypoglycemic Agents, and Warfarin
Patients should be informed that if they are diabetic and are being treated with insulin or an oral hypoglycemic agent and a hypoglycemic reaction occurs, they should discontinue LEVAQUIN® and consult a physician.
Patients should be informed that concurrent administration of warfarin and LEVAQUIN® has been associated with increases of the International Normalized Ratio (INR) or prothrombin time and clinical episodes of bleeding. Patients should notify their physician if they are taking warfarin, be monitored for evidence of bleeding, and also have their anticoagulation tests closely monitored while taking warfarin concomitantly.
In the PATIENT INFORMATION section, "What are possible side effects of LEVAQUIN®?" subsection, a new paragraph on hepatotoxicity has been added after the 3rd paragraph:
Hepatotoxicity (liver damage) has been reported in patients receiving LEVAQUIN®. Call your doctor right away if you have unexplained symptoms such as: nausea or vomiting, stomach pain, fever, weakness, abdominal pain or tenderness, itching, unusual or unexplained tiredness, loss of appetite, light colored bowel movements, dark colored urine or yellowing of your skin or the whites of your eyes.
In the PATIENT INFORMATION section, "What are possible side effects of LEVAQUIN®?" subsection, the 5th paragraph on phototoxicity has been updated as follows:
Sun sensitivity (photosensitivity), which can appear as skin eruption or severe sunburn, can occur in some patients taking quinolone antibiotics after exposure to sunlight or artificial ultraviolet (UV) light (e.g., tanning beds). LEVAQUIN® has been infrequently associated with photosensitivity. Avoid excessive exposure to sunlight or artificial

UV light while taking LEVAQUIN®. Use a sunscreen and wear protective clothing if out in the sun. If photosensitivity develops, contact your physician.
7518221 Revised 2/2008

TYLENOL® WITH CODEINE Ⓒ℞

[*ti 'len-awl-co' dēn*]
(acetaminophen and codeine phosphate)
tablets, USP

Prescribing information for this product, which appears on pages 2365–2366 of the 2008 PDR, has been completely revised as follows. Please write "See Supplement A" next to the product heading.

DESCRIPTION

TYLENOL® with Codeine is supplied in tablet form for oral administration.
Acetaminophen, 4'-hydroxyacetanilide, a slightly bitter, white, odorless, crystalline powder, is a non-opiate, non-salicylate analgesic and antipyretic. It has the following structural formula:

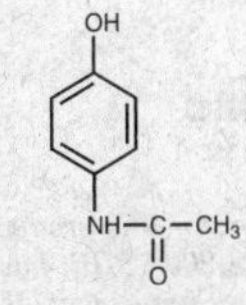

$C_8H_9NO_2$ M.W. 151.16

Codeine phosphate, 7,8-didehydro-4, 5α-epoxy-3-methoxy-17-methylmorphinan-6α-ol phosphate (1:1) (salt) hemihydrate, a white crystalline powder, is a narcotic analgesic and antitussive. It has the following structural formula:

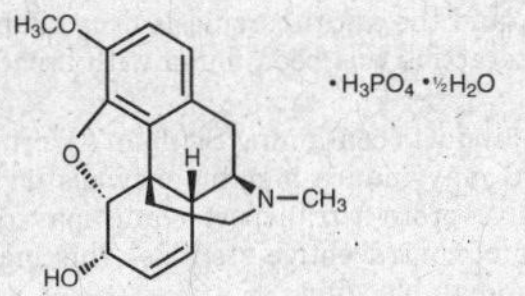

$C_{18}H_{21}NO_3 \cdot H_3PO_4 \cdot 1/2\, H_2O$ M.W. 406.37

Each tablet contains:

Acetaminophen	300 mg
No. 3 Codeine Phosphate	30 mg
(Warning: May be habit forming)	
Acetaminophen	300 mg
No. 4 Codeine Phosphate	60 mg
(Warning: May be habit forming)	

In addition, each tablet contains the following inactive ingredients:
TYLENOL® with Codeine No. 3 contains powdered cellulose, magnesium stearate, sodium metabisulfite†, pregelatinized starch (corn), and modified starch (corn).
TYLENOL® with Codeine No. 4 contains powdered cellulose, magnesium stearate, sodium metabisulfite†, pregelatinized starch (corn), and corn starch.
†See WARNINGS

CLINICAL PHARMACOLOGY

This product combines the analgesic effects of a centrally acting analgesic, codeine, with a peripherally acting analgesic, acetaminophen.

Pharmacokinetics
The behavior of the individual components is described below.
Codeine
Codeine is rapidly absorbed from the gastrointestinal tract. It is rapidly distributed from the intravascular spaces to the various body tissues, with preferential uptake by parenchymatous organs such as the liver, spleen, and kidney. Codeine crosses the blood-brain barrier and is found in fetal tissue and breast milk. The plasma concentration does not correlate with brain concentration or relief of pain; however, codeine is not bound to plasma proteins and does not accumulate in body tissues.
The plasma half-life is about 2.9 hours. The elimination of codeine is primarily via the kidneys, and about 90% of an oral dose is excreted by the kidneys within 24 hours of dosing. The urinary secretion products consist of free and glucuronide conjugated codeine (about 70%), free and conjugated norcodeine (about 10%), free and conjugated morphine (about 10%) normorphine (4%), and hydrocodone (1%). The remainder of the dose is excreted in the feces.
At therapeutic doses, the analgesic effect reaches a peak within 2 hours and persists between 4 and 6 hours.
See OVERDOSAGE for toxicity information.
Acetaminophen
Acetaminophen is rapidly absorbed from the gastrointestinal tract and is distributed throughout most body tissues. The plasma half-life is 1.25 to 3 hours, but may be increased by liver damage and following overdosage. Elimination of acetaminophen is principally by liver metabolism (conjugation) and subsequent renal excretion of metabolites. Approximately 85% of an oral dose appears in the urine within 24 hours of administration, most as the glucuronide conjugate, with small amounts of other conjugates and unchanged drug.
See OVERDOSAGE for toxicity information.

INDICATIONS AND USAGE

TYLENOL® with Codeine (acetaminophen and codeine phosphate) tablets are indicated for the relief of mild to moderately severe pain.

CONTRAINDICATIONS

This product should not be administered to patients who have previously exhibited hypersensitivity to codeine or acetaminophen.

WARNINGS

In the presence of head injury or other intracranial lesions, the respiratory depressant effects of codeine and other narcotics may be markedly enhanced, as well as their capacity for elevating cerebrospinal fluid pressure. Narcotics also produce other CNS depressant effects, such as drowsiness, that may further obscure the clinical course of the patients with head injuries.
Codeine or other narcotics may obscure signs on which to judge the diagnosis or clinical course of patients with acute abdominal conditions.
Codeine is habit forming and potentially abusable. Consequently, the extended use of this product is not recommended.
TYLENOL® with Codeine (acetaminophen and codeine phosphate) tablets contain sodium metabisulfite, a sulfite that may cause allergic-type reactions including anaphylactic symptoms and life-threatening or less severe asthmatic episodes in certain susceptible people. The overall prevalence of sulfite sensitivity in the general population is unknown and probably low. Sulfite sensitivity is seen more frequently in asthmatic than in nonasthmatic people.

PRECAUTIONS

General
TYLENOL® with Codeine (acetaminophen and codeine phosphate) tablets should be prescribed with caution in certain special-risk patients, such as the elderly or debilitated, and those with severe impairment of renal or hepatic function, head injuries, elevated intracranial pressure, acute abdominal conditions, hypothyroidism, urethral stricture, Addison's disease, or prostatic hypertrophy.
Ultra-Rapid Metabolizers of Codeine
Some individuals may be ultra-rapid metabolizers due to a specific CYP2D6*2×2 genotype. These individuals convert codeine into its active metabolite, morphine, more rapidly and completely than other people. This rapid conversion results in higher than expected serum morphine levels. Even at labeled dosage regimens, individuals who are ultra-rapid metabolizers may experience overdose symptoms such as extreme sleepiness, confusion, or shallow breathing.
The prevalence of this CYP2D6 phenotype varies widely and has been estimated at 0.5 to 1% in Chinese and Japanese, 0.5 to 1% in Hispanics, 1 to 10% in Caucasians, 3% in African Americans, and 16 to 28% in North Africans, Ethiopians, and Arabs. Data are not available for other ethnic groups.
When physicians prescribe codeine-containing drugs, they should choose the lowest effective dose for the shortest period of time and inform their patients about these risks and the signs of morphine overdose (see **PRECAUTIONS – Nursing Mothers**).

Information for Patients
Codeine may impair the mental and/or physical abilities required for the performance of potentially hazardous tasks such as driving a car or operating machinery. Such tasks should be avoided while taking this product.
Alcohol and other CNS depressants may produce an additive CNS depression, when taken with this combination product, and should be avoided.
Codeine may be habit forming. Patients should take the drug only for as long as it is prescribed, in the amounts prescribed, and no more frequently than prescribed.
Caution patients that some people have a variation in a liver enzyme and change codeine into morphine more rapidly and completely than other people. These people are ultra-rapid metabolizers and are more likely to have higher-than-normal levels of morphine in their blood after taking codeine, which can result in overdose symptoms such as extreme sleepiness, confusion, or shallow breathing. In most cases, it is unknown if someone is an ultra-rapid codeine metabolizer.
Nursing mothers taking codeine can also have higher morphine levels in their breast milk if they are ultra-rapid metabolizers. These higher levels of morphine in breast milk may lead to life-threatening or fatal side effects in nursing babies. Instruct nursing mothers to watch for signs of morphine toxicity in their infants including increased sleepiness (more than usual), difficulty breastfeeding, breathing difficulties, or limpness. Instruct nursing mothers to talk to the baby's doctor immediately if they notice these signs and, if they cannot reach the doctor right away, to take the baby to an emergency room or call 911 (or local emergency services).

Laboratory Tests
In patients with severe hepatic or renal disease, effects of therapy should be monitored with serial liver and/or renal function tests.

Drug Interactions
This drug may enhance the effects of other narcotic analgesics, alcohol, general anesthetics, tranquilizers such as chlordiazepoxide, sedative-hypnotics, or other CNS depressants, causing increased CNS depression.

Drug/Laboratory Test Interactions
Codeine may increase serum amylase levels.
Acetaminophen may produce false-positive test results for urinary 5-hydroxyindoleacetic acid.

Carcinogenesis, Mutagenesis, Impairment of Fertility
No adequate studies have been conducted in animals to determine whether acetaminophen and codeine have a potential for carcinogenesis or mutagenesis. No adequate studies have been conducted in animals to determine whether acetaminophen has a potential for impairment of fertility.
Acetaminophen and codeine have been found to have no mutagenic potential using the Ames Salmonella-Microsomal Activation test, the Basc test on Drosophila germ cells, and the Micronucleus test on mouse bone marrow.

Pregnancy
Teratogenic Effects: Pregnancy Category C.
Codeine:
A study in rats and rabbits reported no teratogenic effect of codeine administered during the period of organogenesis in doses ranging from 5 to 120 mg/kg. In the rat, doses at the 120 mg/kg level, in the toxic range for the adult animal, were associated with an increase in embryo resorption at the time of implantation. In another study a single 100 mg/kg dose of codeine administered to pregnant mice reportedly resulted in delayed ossification in the offspring. There are no adequate and well-controlled studies in pregnant women. TYLENOL® with Codeine (acetaminophen and codeine phosphate) tablets should be used during pregnancy only if the potential benefit justifies the potential risk to the fetus.
Nonteratogenic Effects:
Dependence has been reported in newborns whose mothers took opiates regularly during pregnancy. Withdrawal signs include irritability, excessive crying, tremors, hyperreflexia, fever, vomiting, and diarrhea. These signs usually appear during the first few days of life.

Labor and Delivery
Narcotic analgesics cross the placental barrier. The closer to delivery and the larger the dose used, the greater the possibility of respiratory depression in the newborn. Narcotic analgesics should be avoided during labor if delivery of a premature infant is anticipated. If the mother has received narcotic analgesics during labor, newborn infants should be observed closely for signs of respiratory depression. Resuscitation may be required (see OVERDOSAGE). The effect of codeine, if any, on the later growth, development, and functional maturation of the child is unknown.

Nursing Mothers
Acetaminophen is excreted in breast milk in small amounts, but the significance of its effect on nursing infants is not known. Because of the potential for serious adverse reactions in nursing infants from acetaminophen, a decision should be made whether to discontinue the drug, taking into account the importance of the drug to the mother.
Codeine is secreted into human milk. In women with normal codeine metabolism (normal CYP2D6 activity), the amount of codeine secreted into human milk is low and dose-dependent. Despite the common use of codeine products to manage postpartum pain, reports of adverse events in infants are rare. However, some women are ultra-rapid metabolizers of codeine. These women achieve higher-than-expected serum levels of codeine's active metabolite, morphine, leading to higher-than-expected levels of morphine in breast milk and potentially dangerously high serum morphine levels in their breastfed infants. Therefore, maternal use of codeine can potentially lead to serious adverse reactions, including death, in nursing infants.
The prevalence of this CYP2D6 phenotype varies widely and has been estimated at 0.5 to 1% in Chinese and Japanese, 0.5 to 1% in Hispanics, 1 to 10% in Caucasians, 3% in African Americans, and 16 to 28% in North Africans, Ethiopians, and Arabs. Data are not available for other ethnic groups.
The risk of infant exposure to codeine and morphine through breast milk should be weighed against the benefits of breastfeeding for both the mother and baby. Caution should be exercised when codeine is administered to a nursing woman. If a codeine containing product is selected, the lowest dose should be prescribed for the shortest period of time to achieve the desired clinical effect. Mothers using codeine should be informed about when to seek immediate medical care and how to identify the signs and symptoms of neonatal toxicity, such as drowsiness or sedation, difficulty breastfeeding, breathing difficulties, and decreased tone, in their baby. Nursing mothers who are ultra-rapid metabolizers may also experience overdose symptoms such as extreme sleepiness, confusion, or shallow breathing. Prescribers should closely monitor mother-infant pairs and notify treating pediatricians about the use of codeine during breastfeeding (see **PRECAUTIONS – General, Ultra-Rapid Metabolizers of Codeine**).

ADVERSE REACTIONS

The most frequently observed adverse reactions include drowsiness, lightheadedness, dizziness, sedation, shortness of breath, nausea, and vomiting. These effects seem to be more prominent in ambulatory than in non-ambulatory patients, and some of these adverse reactions may be alleviated if the patient lies down.
Other adverse reactions include allergic reactions, euphoria, dysphoria, constipation, abdominal pain, pruritus, rash, thrombocytopenia, and agranulocytosis.
At higher doses, codeine has most of the disadvantages of morphine including respiratory depression.

Continued on next page

Tylenol with Codeine—Cont.

DRUG ABUSE AND DEPENDENCE
Controlled Substance
TYLENOL® with Codeine (acetaminophen and codeine phosphate) tablets are classified as a Schedule III controlled substance.
Abuse and Dependence
Codeine can produce drug dependence of the morphine type and, therefore, has the potential for being abused. Psychological dependence, physical dependence, and tolerance may develop upon repeated administration and it should be prescribed and administered with the same degree of caution appropriate to the use of other oral narcotic medications.

OVERDOSAGE
Following an acute overdosage, toxicity may result from codeine or acetaminophen.
Signs and Symptoms:
Codeine
Toxicity from codeine poisoning includes the opioid triad of pinpoint pupils, depression of respiration, and loss of consciousness. Convulsions may occur.
Acetaminophen
In acetaminophen overdosage, dose-dependent, potentially fatal hepatic necrosis is the most serious adverse effect. Renal tubular necrosis, hypoglycemic coma and thrombocytopenia may also occur.
Early symptoms following a potentially hepatotoxic overdose may include: nausea, vomiting, diaphoresis and general malaise. Clinical and laboratory evidence of hepatic toxicity may not be apparent until 48 to 72 hours postingestion.
In adults, hepatic toxicity has rarely been reported with acute overdoses of less than 10 grams or fatalities with less than 15 grams.
Treatment:
A single or multiple overdose with acetaminophen and codeine is a potentially lethal polydrug overdose and consultation with a regional poison control center is recommended.
Immediate treatment includes support of cardiorespiratory function and measures to reduce drug absorption. Vomiting should be induced mechanically, or with syrup of ipecac, if the patient is alert (adequate pharyngeal and laryngeal reflexes). Oral activated charcoal (1g/kg) should follow gastric emptying. The first dose should be accompanied by an appropriate cathartic. If repeated doses are used, the cathartic might be included with alternate doses as required. Hypotension is usually hypovolemic and should respond to fluids. Vasopressors and other supportive measures should be employed as indicated. A cuffed endo-tracheal tube should be inserted before gastric lavage of the unconscious patient and, when necessary, to provide assisted respiration.
Meticulous attention should be given to maintaining adequate pulmonary ventilation. In severe cases of intoxication, peritoneal dialysis, or preferably hemodialysis, may be considered. If hypoprothrombinemia occurs due to acetaminophen overdose, vitamin K should be administered intravenously.
Naloxone, a narcotic antagonist, can reverse respiratory depression and coma associated with opioid overdose. Naloxone hydrochloride 0.4 mg to 2 mg is given parenterally. Since the duration of action of codeine may exceed that of the naloxone, the patient should be kept under continuous surveillance and repeated doses of the antagonist should be administered as needed to maintain adequate respiration. A narcotic antagonist should not be administered in the absence of clinically significant respiratory or cardiovascular depression.
If the dose of acetaminophen may have exceeded 140 mg/kg, acetylcysteine should be administered as early as possible. Serum acetaminophen levels should be obtained, since levels four or more hours following ingestion help predict acetaminophen toxicity. Do not await acetaminophen assay results before initiating treatment. Hepatic enzymes should be obtained initially and repeated at 24-hour intervals. Methemoglobinemia over 30% should be treated with methylene blue by slow intravenous administration.
Toxic Doses (for adults):
Acetaminophen: toxic dose 10 g
Codeine: toxic dose 240 mg

DOSAGE AND ADMINISTRATION
Dosage should be adjusted according to severity of pain and response of the patient.
The usual adult dosage is:

	Single Doses (Range)	Maximum 24-Hour Dose
Codeine phosphate	15 mg to 60 mg	360 mg
Acetaminophen	300 mg to 1000 mg	4000 mg

Doses may be repeated up to every 4 hours.
The prescriber must determine the number of tablets per dose, and the maximum number of tablets per 24 hours, based upon the above dosage guidance. This information should be conveyed in the prescription.
It should be kept in mind, however, that tolerance to codeine can develop with continued use and that the incidence of

untoward effects is dose related. Adult doses of codeine higher than 60 mg fail to give commensurate relief of pain but merely prolong analgesia and are associated with an appreciably increased incidence of undesirable side effects. Equivalently high doses in children would have similar effects.

HOW SUPPLIED
TYLENOL® with Codeine (acetaminophen and codeine phosphate) tablets are white, round, flat-faced, beveled edged tablet imprinted "McNEIL" on one side and "TYLENOL CODEINE" and either "3" or "4" on the other side and are supplied as follows: No. 3 - NDC 0045-0513-60 bottles of 100, NDC 0045-0513-80 bottles of 1000, No. 4 - NDC 0045-0515-60 bottles of 100, NDC 0045-0515-70 bottles of 500.
Store TYLENOL® with Codeine tablets at 20° to 25°C (68° to 77°F). (See USP Controlled Room Temperature).
Dispense in tight, light-resistant container as defined in the official compendium.
Manufactured by:
JOLLC
Gurabo, Puerto Rico 00778
Distributed by:
ORTHO-McNEIL
OMP DIVISION
ORTHO-McNEIL PHARMACEUTICAL, INC.
Raritan, New Jersey 08869

Revised January 2008
© OMP 2000   7518407

Ortho Women's Health & Urology
A Division of Ortho-McNeil Pharmaceutical, Inc.
RARITAN, NJ 08869-0602

For Medical Information Contact:
(800) 682-6532
In Emergencies:
(908) 218-7325
For Patient Education Materials Contact:
(877) 323-2200
For Customer Service (Sales and Ordering):
(800) 631-5273

ORTHO EVRA®   ℞
(norelgestromin/ethinyl estradiol transdermal system)

Prescribing information for this product, which appears on pages 2390–2399 of the 2008 PDR, has been revised as follows. Please write "See Supplement A" next to the product heading.
The WARNINGS section, 3rd paragraph has been revised as follows (and Table 5 added):
Epidemiologic, case-control studies[107–110] were conducted in the U.S. using electronic healthcare claims data to evaluate the risk of venous thromboembolism (VTE) among women aged 15–44 who used ORTHO EVRA® compared to women who used oral contraceptives containing 30–35 mcg of ethinyl estradiol (EE) and either norgestimate (NGM) or levonorgestrel (LNG). NGM is the prodrug for norelgestromin, the progestin in ORTHO EVRA®. These studies (see Table 5) used slightly different designs and reported odds ratios ranging from 0.9 (indicating no increase in risk) to 2.4 (indicating an approximate doubling of risk). One study (i3 Ingenix) included patient chart review to confirm the VTE occurrence.
[See table 5 below]
In the DETAILED PATIENT LABELING section, OTHER CONSIDERATIONS BEFORE USING ORTHO EVRA® subsection, the 1st & 2nd paragraphs have been revised as follows:
OTHER CONSIDERATIONS BEFORE USING ORTHO EVRA®
Hormones from ORTHO EVRA® get into the blood stream

and are processed by the body differently than hormones from birth control pills. **You will be exposed to about 60% more estrogen if you use ORTHO EVRA® than if you use a typical birth control pill containing 35 micrograms of estrogen.** In general, increased estrogen may increase the risk of side effects.
The risk of venous thromboembolic events (blood clots in the legs and/or the lungs) may be increased with ORTHO EVRA® use compared with use of birth control pills. Studies examined the risk of these serious blood clots in women who used either ORTHO EVRA® or birth control pills containing one of two progestins (levonorgestrel or norgestimate) and 30–35 micrograms of estrogen. Results of these studies ranged from an approximate doubling of risk of serious blood clots to no increase in risk in women using ORTHO EVRA® compared to women using birth control pills.
You should discuss this possible increased risk with your healthcare professional before using ORTHO EVRA®. Call your healthcare professional immediately if any of the adverse side effects listed under "WARNING SIGNALS" occur while you are using ORTHO EVRA®. (See below.)

10154401   Revised January 2008

ORTHO MICRONOR®   ℞
(norethindrone) Tablets

Prescribing information for this product, which appears on pages 2399–2402 of the 2008 PDR, has been revised as follows. Please write "See Supplement A" next to the product heading.
The PRECAUTIONS section, item 4 has been revised as follows:
4. Drug Interactions—The effectiveness of progestin-only pills is reduced by hepatic enzyme-inducing drugs such as the anticonvulsants phenytoin, carbamazepine, and barbiturates, and the antituberculosis drug rifampin. No significant interaction has been found with broad-spectrum antibiotics.
Herbal products containing St. John's Wort (hypericum perforatum) may induce hepatic enzymes (cytochrome P450) and p-glycoprotein transporter and may reduce the effectiveness of contraceptive steroids. This may also result in breakthrough bleeding.
Concurrent use of bosentan and norethindrone containing products may result in decreased concentrations of these contraceptive hormones thereby increasing the risk of unintended pregnancy and unscheduled bleeding.

In the DETAILED PATIENT LABELING section, YOU SHOULD NOT TAKE POPs subsection, 4th bullet has been revised as follows:
• If you are taking certain drugs for epilepsy (seizures) or for TB, or medicine for pulmonary hypertension or certain herbal products. (See "Using POPs with Other Medicines" below.)
In the DETAILED PATIENT LABELING section, the USING POPS WITH OTHER MEDICINES subsection has been revised as follows:
USING POPs WITH OTHER MEDICINES
Before taking a POP, inform your healthcare professional of any other medication, including over-the-counter medicine, that you may be taking.
These medicines can make POPs less effective:
Medicines for seizures such as:
  • Phenytoin (Dilantin®)
  • Carbamazepine (Tegretol)
  • Phenobarbital
Medicine for TB:
  • Rifampin (Rifampicin)
Medicine for pulmonary hypertension such as:
  • Bosentan (Tracleer®)
Herbal products such as:
  • St. John's Wort
Before you begin taking any new medicines be sure your healthcare professional knows you are taking a progestin-only birth control pill.
635-50-894-4   Revised August 2007

Table 5: Estimates (Odds Ratios) of Venous Thromboembolism Risk in Current Users of ORTHO EVRA® Compared to Oral Contraceptive Users

Epidemiologic Study	Comparator Product	Odds Ratio (95% C.I.)
i3 Ingenix[107]	NGM/35 mcg EE[A]	2.4 (1.1–5.5)[B]
BCDSP NGM[108,109,C]	NGM/35 mcg EE	0.9 (0.5–1.6)[108]
		1.1 (0.6–2.1)[109,D]
BCDSP LNG[110]	LNG[E]/30 mcg EE	2.0 (0.9–4.1)

[A] NGM = norgestimate; EE = ethinyl estradiol
[B] Increase in risk of VTE is statistically significant.
[C] BCDSP = Boston Collaborative Drug Surveillance Program
[D] Reference 109: Separate estimate from 17 months of data on new cases not included in the previous estimate (reference 108).
[E] LNG = levonorgestrel

ORTHO TRI-CYCLEN® TABLETS
ORTHO-CYCLEN® TABLETS
(norgestimate/ethinyl estradiol)   ℞

Prescribing information for this product, which appears on pages 2402–2411 of the 2008 PDR, has been revised as follows. Please write "See Supplement A" next to the product heading.

The ADVERSE REACTIONS section, 3rd paragraph, 17th bullet has been revised as follows:
• Allergic reaction, including rash, urticaria, angioedema

In the DETAILED PATIENT LABELING section, SIDE EFFECTS OF ORAL CONTRACEPTIVES subsection, item 5 has been revised as follows:
5. Other Side Effects - Other side effects may include nausea and vomiting, change in appetite, headache, nervousness, depression, dizziness, loss of scalp hair, rash, vaginal infections, and allergic reactions.

635-50-900-9   Revised July 2007

Otsuka America Pharmaceutical, Inc.

**2440 RESEARCH BOULEVARD
ROCKVILLE, MD 20850**

For Medical Information about products marketed by Otsuka America Pharmaceutical, Inc., or to report an adverse event, please contact: 1-800-562-3974

ABILIFY®   ℞
[ă-bĭl-ifĭ]
(aripiprazole)

Prescribing information for this product, which appears on pages 2424–2431 of the 2008 PDR, has been completely revised as follows. Please write "See Supplement A" next to the product heading.

HIGHLIGHTS OF PRESCRIBING INFORMATION
These highlights do not include all the information needed to use ABILIFY safely and effectively. See full prescribing information for ABILIFY.

ABILIFY® (aripiprazole) Tablets
ABILIFY® DISCMELT™ (aripiprazole) Orally Disintegrating Tablets
ABILIFY® (aripiprazole) Oral Solution
ABILIFY® (aripiprazole) Injection FOR INTRAMUSCULAR USE ONLY
Initial U.S. Approval: 2002

WARNINGS: INCREASED MORTALITY IN ELDERLY PATIENTS WITH DEMENTIA-RELATED PSYCHOSIS and SUICIDALITY AND ANTIDEPRESSANT DRUGS
See full prescribing information for complete boxed warning.

• Elderly patients with dementia-related psychosis treated with atypical antipsychotic drugs are at an increased risk of death compared to placebo. ABILIFY is not approved for the treatment of patients with dementia-related psychosis. (5.1)
• Children, adolescents, and young adults taking antidepressants for Major Depressive Disorder (MDD) and other psychiatric disorders are at increased risk of suicidal thinking and behavior. (5.2)

RECENT MAJOR CHANGES
Boxed Warning, Suicidality and Antidepressant
  Drugs   11/2007
Indications and Usage,
  Pediatric (13 to 17 years) Schizophrenia (1.1)   10/2007
  Pediatric (10 to 17 years) Bipolar Mania (1.2)   02/2008
  Adjunctive Treatment in Adults with MDD (1.3)   11/2007
Dosage and Administration,
  Pediatric Schizophrenia (2.1)   10/2007
  Pediatric Bipolar Mania (2.2)   02/2008
  Adjunctive Treatment in Adults with MDD (2.3)   11/2007
Warnings and Precautions, Clinical Worsening
  of Depression and Suicide Risk (5.2)   11/2007

INDICATIONS AND USAGE
ABILIFY is an atypical antipsychotic indicated as oral formulations for:
• Treatment of Schizophrenia in adults and adolescents aged 13 to 17 years (1.1)
• Treatment of acute manic or mixed episodes associated with Bipolar I Disorder in adults and pediatric patients aged 10 to 17 years (1.2)
• Adjunctive treatment of Major Depressive Disorder in adults (1.3)
as an injection for:
• Treatment of adults with agitation associated with Schizophrenia or Bipolar I Disorder, manic or mixed (1.4)

DOSAGE AND ADMINISTRATION

	Initial Dose	Recommended Dose	Maximum Dose
Schizophrenia – adults (2.1)	10-15 mg/day	10-15 mg/day	30 mg/day
Schizophrenia – adolescents (2.1)	2 mg/day	10 mg/day	30 mg/day
Bipolar Mania – adults (2.2)	15-30 mg/day	15-30 mg/day	30 mg/day
Bipolar Mania – pediatric patients (2.2)	2 mg/day	10 mg/day	30 mg/day
As an adjunct to antidepressants for the treatment of Major Depressive Disorder (2.3)	2-5 mg/day	5-10 mg/day	15 mg/day
Agitation associated with Schizophrenia or Bipolar Mania – adults (2.4)	9.75 mg/1.3 mL injected IM		30 mg/day injected IM

• Oral formulations: Administer once daily without regard to meals (2)
• IM injection: Wait at least 2 hours between doses. Maximum daily dose 30 mg (2.4)

DOSAGE FORMS AND STRENGTHS
• Tablets: 2 mg, 5 mg, 10 mg, 15 mg, 20 mg, and 30 mg (3)
• Orally Disintegrating Tablets: 10 mg and 15 mg (3)
• Oral Solution: 1 mg/mL (3)
• Injection: 9.75 mg/1.3 mL single-dose vial (3)

CONTRAINDICATIONS
Known hypersensitivity to ABILIFY (4)

WARNINGS AND PRECAUTIONS
• *Elderly Patients with Dementia-Related Psychosis:* Increased incidence of cerebrovascular adverse events (eg, stroke, transient ischemic attack, including fatalities) (5.1)
• *Suicidality and Antidepressants:* Increased risk of suicidality in children, adolescents, and young adults with Major Depressive Disorder (5.2)
• *Neuroleptic Malignant Syndrome:* Manage with immediate discontinuation and close monitoring (5.3)
• *Tardive Dyskinesia:* Discontinue if clinically appropriate (5.4)
• *Hyperglycemia and Diabetes Mellitus:* Monitor glucose regularly in patients with and at risk for diabetes (5.5)
• *Orthostatic Hypotension:* Use with caution in patients with known cardiovascular or cerebrovascular disease (5.6)
• *Seizures/Convulsions:* Use cautiously in patients with a history of seizures or with conditions that lower the seizure threshold (5.7)
• *Potential for Cognitive and Motor Impairment:* Use caution when operating machinery (5.8)
• *Suicide:* Closely supervise high-risk patients (5.10)

ADVERSE REACTIONS
Commonly observed adverse reactions (incidence ≥5% and at least twice that for placebo) were (6.2):
• Adult patients with Schizophrenia: akathisia
• Pediatric patients (13 to 17 years) with Schizophrenia: extrapyramidal disorder, somnolence, and tremor
• Adult patients with Bipolar Mania: constipation, akathisia, sedation, tremor, restlessness, and extrapyramidal disorder
• Pediatric patients (10 to 17 years) with Bipolar Mania: somnolence, extrapyramidal disorder, fatigue, nausea, akathisia, blurred vision, salivary hypersecretion, and dizziness
• Adult patients with Major Depressive Disorder (adjunctive treatment to antidepressant therapy): akathisia, restlessness, insomnia, constipation, fatigue, and blurred vision
• Adult patients with agitation associated with Schizophrenia or Bipolar Mania: nausea.

To report SUSPECTED ADVERSE REACTIONS, contact Bristol-Myers Squibb at 1-800-721-5072 or FDA at 1-800-FDA-1088 or www.fda.gov/medwatch

DRUG INTERACTIONS
• *Strong CYP3A4 (eg, ketoconazole) or CYP2D6 (eg, fluoxetine) inhibitors* will increase ABILIFY drug concentrations; reduce ABILIFY dose by one-half when used concomitantly (2.5, 7.1), except when used as adjunctive treatment with antidepressants (2.5)
• *CYP3A4 inducers (eg, carbamazepine)* will decrease ABILIFY drug concentrations; double ABILIFY dose when used concomitantly (2.5, 7.1)

See 17 for PATIENT COUNSELING INFORMATION and Medication Guide

                                        Revised: 02/2008

FULL PRESCRIBING INFORMATION: CONTENTS*
WARNINGS: INCREASED MORTALITY IN ELDERLY PATIENTS WITH DEMENTIA-RELATED PSYCHOSIS and SUICIDALITY AND ANTIDEPRESSANT DRUGS

FULL PRESCRIBING INFORMATION

WARNINGS: INCREASED MORTALITY IN ELDERLY PATIENTS WITH DEMENTIA-RELATED PSYCHOSIS and SUICIDALITY AND ANTIDEPRESSANT DRUGS
Elderly patients with dementia-related psychosis treated with atypical antipsychotic drugs are at an increased risk of death compared to placebo. Analyses of seventeen placebo-controlled trials (modal duration of 10 weeks) in these patients revealed a risk of death in the drug-treated patients of between 1.6 to 1.7 times that seen in placebo-treated patients. Over the course of a typical 10-week controlled trial, the rate of death in drug-treated patients was about 4.5%, compared to a rate of about 2.6% in the placebo group. Although the causes of death were varied, most of the deaths appeared to be either cardiovascular (eg, heart failure, sudden death) or infectious (eg, pneumonia) in nature. ABILIFY (aripiprazole) is not approved for the treatment

Continued on next page

Abilify—Cont.

of patients with dementia-related psychosis *[see WARNINGS AND PRECAUTIONS (5.1)]*.
Antidepressants increased the risk compared to placebo of suicidal thinking and behavior (suicidality) in children, adolescents, and young adults in short-term studies of Major Depressive Disorder (MDD) and other psychiatric disorders. Anyone considering the use of adjunctive ABILIFY or any other antidepressant in a child, adolescent, or young adult must balance this risk with the clinical need. Short-term studies did not show an increase in the risk of suicidality with antidepressants compared to placebo in adults beyond age 24; there was a reduction in risk with antidepressants compared to placebo in adults aged 65 and older. Depression and certain other psychiatric disorders are themselves associated with increases in the risk of suicide. Patients of all ages who are started on antidepressant therapy should be monitored appropriately and observed closely for clinical worsening, suicidality, or unusual changes in behavior. Families and caregivers should be advised of the need for close observation and communication with the prescriber. ABILIFY is not approved for use in pediatric patients with depression *[see WARNINGS AND PRECAUTIONS (5.2)]*.

1 INDICATIONS AND USAGE

1.1 Schizophrenia

Adults

ABILIFY is indicated for acute and maintenance treatment of Schizophrenia *[see CLINICAL STUDIES (14.1)]*.

Adolescents

ABILIFY is indicated for the treatment of Schizophrenia in adolescents 13 to 17 years of age *[see CLINICAL STUDIES (14.1)]*.

1.2 Bipolar Disorder

Adults

ABILIFY is indicated for acute and maintenance treatment of manic and mixed episodes associated with Bipolar I Disorder with or without psychotic features *[see CLINICAL STUDIES (14.2)]*.

Pediatric Patients

ABILIFY is indicated for the acute treatment of manic and mixed episodes associated with Bipolar Disorder with or without psychotic features in pediatric patients 10 to 17 years of age *[see CLINICAL STUDIES (14.2)]*.

1.3 Adjunctive Treatment of Major Depressive Disorder

Adults

ABILIFY is indicated for use as an adjunctive treatment to antidepressants for Major Depressive Disorder *[see CLINICAL STUDIES (14.3)]*.

1.4 Agitation Associated with Schizophrenia or Bipolar Mania

Adults

ABILIFY Injection is indicated for the treatment of agitation associated with Schizophrenia or Bipolar Disorder, manic or mixed. "Psychomotor agitation" is defined in DSM-IV as "excessive motor activity associated with a feeling of inner tension." Patients experiencing agitation often manifest behaviors that interfere with their diagnosis and care (eg, threatening behaviors, escalating or urgently distressing behavior, or self-exhausting behavior), leading clinicians to the use of intramuscular antipsychotic medications to achieve immediate control of the agitation *[see CLINICAL STUDIES (14.4)]*.

2 DOSAGE AND ADMINISTRATION

2.1 Schizophrenia

Usual Dose

Adults

The recommended starting and target dose for ABILIFY is 10 mg/day or 15 mg/day administered on a once-a-day schedule without regard to meals. ABILIFY has been systematically evaluated and shown to be effective in a dose range of 10 mg/day to 30 mg/day, when administered as the tablet formulation; however, doses higher than 10 mg/day or 15 mg/day were not more effective than 10 mg/day or 15 mg/day. Dosage increases should not be made before 2 weeks, the time needed to achieve steady-state *[see CLINICAL STUDIES (14.1)]*.

Adolescents

The recommended target dose of ABILIFY is 10 mg/day. Aripiprazole was studied in pediatric patients 13 to 17 years of age with Schizophrenia at daily doses of 10 mg and 30 mg. The starting daily dose of the tablet formulation in these patients was 2 mg, which was titrated to 5 mg after 2 days and to the target dose of 10 mg after 2 additional days. Subsequent dose increases should be administered in 5 mg increments. The 30 mg/day dose was not shown to be more efficacious than the 10 mg/day dose. ABILIFY can be administered without regard to meals *[see CLINICAL STUDIES (14.1)]*.

Maintenance Therapy

Adults

While there is no body of evidence available to answer the question of how long a patient treated with aripiprazole should remain on it, systematic evaluation of patients with Schizophrenia who had been symptomatically stable on other antipsychotic medications for periods of 3 months or longer, were discontinued from those medications, and were then administered ABILIFY 15 mg/day and observed for relapse during a period of up to 26 weeks, has demonstrated a benefit of such maintenance treatment *[see CLINICAL STUDIES (14.1)]*. Patients should be periodically reassessed to determine the need for maintenance treatment.

Pediatric Patients

The efficacy of ABILIFY for the maintenance treatment of Schizophrenia in the pediatric population has not been evaluated.

Switching from Other Antipsychotics

There are no systematically collected data to specifically address switching patients with Schizophrenia from other antipsychotics to ABILIFY or concerning concomitant administration with other antipsychotics. While immediate discontinuation of the previous antipsychotic treatment may be acceptable for some patients with Schizophrenia, more gradual discontinuation may be most appropriate for others. In all cases, the period of overlapping antipsychotic administration should be minimized.

2.2 Bipolar Disorder

Usual Dose

Adults

In clinical trials, the starting dose was 30 mg given once a day, without regard to meals. A dose of 30 mg/day was found to be effective when administered as the tablet formulation. Approximately 15% of patients had their dose decreased to 15 mg based on assessment of tolerability. The safety of doses above 30 mg/day has not been evaluated in clinical trials *[see CLINICAL STUDIES (14.2)]*.

Pediatric Patients

The efficacy of aripiprazole has been established in the treatment of pediatric patients 10 to 17 years of age with Bipolar I Disorder at doses of 10 mg/day or 30 mg/day. The recommended target dose of ABILIFY is 10 mg/day. The starting daily dose of the tablet formulation in these patients was 2 mg/day, which was titrated to 5 mg/day after 2 days and to the target dose of 10 mg/day after 2 additional days. Subsequent dose increases should be administered in 5 mg/day increments. ABILIFY can be administered without regard to meals. *[See CLINICAL STUDIES (14.2).]*

Maintenance Therapy

Adults

While there is no body of evidence available to answer the question of how long a patient treated with aripiprazole should remain on it, adult patients with Bipolar I Disorder who had been symptomatically stable on ABILIFY Tablets (15 mg/day or 30 mg/day with a starting dose of 30 mg/day) for at least 6 consecutive weeks and then randomized to ABILIFY Tablets (15 mg/day or 30 mg/day) or placebo and monitored for relapse, demonstrated a benefit of such maintenance treatment *[see CLINICAL STUDIES (14.2)]*. While it is generally agreed that pharmacological treatment beyond an acute response in Mania is desirable, both for maintenance of the initial response and for prevention of new manic episodes, there are no systematically obtained data to support the use of aripiprazole in such longer-term treatment (beyond 6 weeks). Physicians who elect to use ABILIFY for extended periods, that is, longer than 6 weeks, should periodically re-evaluate the long-term usefulness of the drug for the individual.

Pediatric Patients

The efficacy of ABILIFY for the maintenance treatment of Bipolar I Disorder in the pediatric population has not been evaluated.

2.3 Adjunctive Treatment of Major Depressive Disorder

Usual Dose

Adults

The recommended starting dose for ABILIFY as adjunctive treatment for patients already taking an antidepressant is 2 mg/day to 5 mg/day. The efficacy of ABILIFY as an adjunctive therapy for Major Depressive Disorder was established within a dose range of 2 mg/day to 15 mg/day. Dose adjustments of up to 5 mg/day should occur gradually, at intervals of no less than 1 week. The long-term efficacy of ABILIFY for the adjunctive treatment of Major Depressive Disorder has not been established *[see CLINICAL STUDIES (14.3)]*.

Pediatric Patients

The efficacy of ABILIFY for the adjunctive treatment of Major Depressive Disorder in the pediatric population has not been evaluated.

2.4 Agitation Associated with Schizophrenia or Bipolar Mania (Intramuscular Injection)

Usual Dose

Adults

The recommended dose in these patients is 9.75 mg. The effectiveness of aripiprazole injection in controlling agitation in Schizophrenia and Bipolar Mania was demonstrated over a dose range of 5.25 mg to 15 mg. No additional benefit was demonstrated for 15 mg compared to 9.75 mg. A lower dose of 5.25 mg may be considered when clinical factors warrant. If agitation warranting a second dose persists following the initial dose, cumulative doses up to a total of 30 mg/day may be given. However, the efficacy of repeated doses of aripiprazole injection in agitated patients has not been systematically evaluated in controlled clinical trials. The safety of total daily doses greater than 30 mg or injections given more frequently than every 2 hours have not been adequately evaluated in clinical trials *[see CLINICAL STUDIES (14.4)]*.

If ongoing aripiprazole therapy is clinically indicated, oral aripiprazole in a range of 10 mg/day to 30 mg/day should replace aripiprazole injection as soon as possible *[see DOSAGE AND ADMINISTRATION (2.1 and 2.2)]*.

Administration of ABILIFY Injection

To administer ABILIFY Injection, draw up the required volume of solution into the syringe as shown in Table 1. Discard any unused portion.

Table 1: ABILIFY Injection Dosing Recommendations

Single-Dose	Required Volume of Solution
5.25 mg	0.7 mL
9.75 mg	1.3 mL
15 mg	2 mL

ABILIFY Injection is intended for intramuscular use only. Do not administer intravenously or subcutaneously. Inject slowly, deep into the muscle mass.

Parenteral drug products should be inspected visually for particulate matter and discoloration prior to administration, whenever solution and container permit.

Pediatric Patients

ABILIFY Intramuscular Injection has not been evaluated in pediatric patients.

2.5 Dosage Adjustment

Dosage adjustments in adults are not routinely indicated on the basis of age, gender, race, or renal or hepatic impairment status *[see USE IN SPECIFIC POPULATIONS (8.4-8.10)]*.

Dosage adjustment for patients taking aripiprazole concomitantly with strong CYP3A4 inhibitors: When concomitant administration of aripiprazole with strong CYP3A4 inhibitors such as ketoconazole or clarithromycin is indicated, the aripiprazole dose should be reduced to one-half the usual dose. When the CYP3A4 inhibitor is withdrawn from the combination therapy, the aripiprazole dose should then be increased *[see DRUG INTERACTIONS (7.1)]*.

Dosage adjustment for patients taking aripiprazole concomitantly with potential CYP2D6 inhibitors: When concomitant administration of potential CYP2D6 inhibitors such as quinidine, fluoxetine, or paroxetine with aripiprazole occurs, aripiprazole dose should be reduced at least to one-half of its normal dose. When the CYP2D6 inhibitor is withdrawn from the combination therapy, the aripiprazole dose should then be increased *[see DRUG INTERACTIONS (7.1)]*. When adjunctive ABILIFY is administered to patients with Major Depressive Disorder, ABILIFY should be administered without dosage adjustment as specified in *DOSAGE AND ADMINISTRATION (2.3)*.

Dosage adjustment for patients taking potential CYP3A4 inducers: When a potential CYP3A4 inducer such as carbamazepine is added to aripiprazole therapy, the aripiprazole dose should be doubled. Additional dose increases should be based on clinical evaluation. When the CYP3A4 inducer is withdrawn from the combination therapy, the aripiprazole dose should be reduced to 10 mg to 15 mg *[see DRUG INTERACTIONS (7.1)]*.

2.6 Dosing of Oral Solution

The oral solution can be substituted for tablets on a mg-per-mg basis up to the 25 mg dose level. Patients receiving 30 mg tablets should receive 25 mg of the solution *[see CLINICAL PHARMACOLOGY (12.3)]*.

2.7 Dosing of Orally Disintegrating Tablets

The dosing for ABILIFY Orally Disintegrating Tablets is the same as for the oral tablets *[see DOSAGE AND ADMINISTRATION (2.1, 2.2 and 2.3)]*.

3 DOSAGE FORMS AND STRENGTHS

ABILIFY® (aripiprazole) Tablets are available as described in Table 2.

Table 2: ABILIFY Tablet Presentations

Tablet Strength	Tablet Color/Shape	Tablet Markings
2 mg	green modified rectangle	"A-006" and "2"
5 mg	blue modified rectangle	"A-007" and "5"
10 mg	pink modified rectangle	"A-008" and "10"
15 mg	yellow round	"A-009" and "15"
20 mg	white round	"A-010" and "20"
30 mg	pink round	"A-011" and "30"

ABILIFY® DISCMELT™ (aripiprazole) Orally Disintegrating Tablets are available as described in Table 3.

Table 3: ABILIFY DISCMELT Orally Disintegrating Tablet Presentations

Tablet Strength	Tablet Color/Shape	Tablet Markings
10 mg	pink (with scattered specks) round	"A" and "640" "10"
15 mg	yellow (with scattered specks) round	"A" and "641" "15"

ABILIFY® (aripiprazole) Oral Solution (1 mg/mL) is a clear, colorless to light yellow solution, supplied in child-resistant bottles along with a calibrated oral dosing cup.

ABILIFY® (aripiprazole) Injection for Intramuscular Use is a clear, colorless solution available as a ready-to-use, 9.75 mg/1.3 mL (7.5 mg/mL) solution in clear, Type 1 glass vials.

4 CONTRAINDICATIONS

Known hypersensitivity reaction to ABILIFY. Reactions have ranged from pruritus/urticaria to anaphylaxis [see ADVERSE REACTIONS (6.3)].

5 WARNINGS AND PRECAUTIONS

5.1 Use in Elderly Patients with Dementia-Related Psychosis

Increased Mortality

Elderly patients with dementia-related psychosis treated with atypical antipsychotic drugs are at an increased risk of death compared to placebo. ABILIFY (aripiprazole) is not approved for the treatment of patients with dementia-related psychosis [see BOXED WARNING].

Cerebrovascular Adverse Events, Including Stroke

In placebo-controlled clinical studies (two flexible dose and one fixed dose study) of dementia-related psychosis, there was an increased incidence of cerebrovascular adverse events (eg, stroke, transient ischemic attack), including fatalities, in aripiprazole-treated patients (mean age: 84 years; range: 78-88 years). In the fixed-dose study, there was a statistically significant dose response relationship for cerebrovascular adverse events in patients treated with aripiprazole. Aripiprazole is not approved for the treatment of patients with dementia-related psychosis [see also BOXED WARNING].

Safety Experience in Elderly Patients with Psychosis Associated with Alzheimer's Disease

In three, 10-week, placebo-controlled studies of aripiprazole in elderly patients with psychosis associated with Alzheimer's disease (n=938; mean age: 82.4 years; range: 56-99 years), the treatment-emergent adverse events that were reported at an incidence of ≥3% and aripiprazole incidence at least twice that for placebo were lethargy [placebo 2%, aripiprazole 5%], somnolence (including sedation) [placebo 3%, aripiprazole 8%], and incontinence (primarily, urinary incontinence) [placebo 1%, aripiprazole 5%], excessive salivation (placebo 0%, aripiprazole 4%), and lightheadedness (placebo 1%, aripiprazole 4%).

The safety and efficacy of ABILIFY in the treatment of patients with psychosis associated with dementia have not been established. If the prescriber elects to treat such patients with ABILIFY, vigilance should be exercised, particularly for the emergence of difficulty swallowing or excessive somnolence, which could predispose to accidental injury or aspiration [see also BOXED WARNING].

5.2 Clinical Worsening of Depression and Suicide Risk

Patients with Major Depressive Disorder (MDD), both adult and pediatric, may experience worsening of their depression and/or the emergence of suicidal ideation and behavior (suicidality) or unusual changes in behavior, whether or not they are taking antidepressant medications, and this risk may persist until significant remission occurs. Suicide is a known risk of depression and certain other psychiatric disorders, and these disorders themselves are the strongest predictors of suicide. There has been a long-standing concern, however, that antidepressants may have a role in inducing worsening of depression and the emergence of suicidality in certain patients during the early phases of treatment. Pooled analyses of short-term placebo-controlled trials of antidepressant drugs (SSRIs and others) showed that these drugs increase the risk of suicidal thinking and behavior (suicidality) in children, adolescents, and young adults (ages 18-24) with Major Depressive Disorder (MDD) and other psychiatric disorders. Short-term studies did not show an increase in the risk of suicidality with antidepressants compared to placebo in adults beyond age 24; there was a reduction with antidepressants compared to placebo in adults aged 65 and older.

The pooled analyses of placebo-controlled trials in children and adolescents with MDD, Obsessive Compulsive Disorder (OCD), or other psychiatric disorders included a total of 24 short-term trials of 9 antidepressant drugs in over 4400 patients. The pooled analyses of placebo-controlled trials in adults with MDD or other psychiatric disorders included a total of 295 short-term trials (median duration of 2 months) of 11 antidepressant drugs in over 77,000 patients. There was considerable variation in risk of suicidality among drugs, but a tendency toward an increase in the younger patients for almost all drugs studied. There were differences in absolute risk of suicidality across the different indications, with the highest incidence in MDD. The risk differences (drug vs. placebo), however, were relatively stable within age strata and across indications. These risk differences (drug-placebo difference in the number of cases of suicidality per 1000 patients treated) are provided in Table 4.

Table 4

Age Range	Drug-Placebo Difference in Number of Cases of Suicidality per 1000 Patients Treated
	Increases Compared to Placebo
<18	14 additional cases
18-24	5 additional cases
	Decreases Compared to Placebo
25-64	1 fewer case
≥65	6 fewer cases

No suicides occurred in any of the pediatric trials. There were suicides in the adult trials, but the number was not sufficient to reach any conclusion about drug effect on suicide.

It is unknown whether the suicidality risk extends to longer-term use, ie, beyond several months. However, there is substantial evidence from placebo-controlled maintenance trials in adults with depression that the use of antidepressants can delay the recurrence of depression.

All patients being treated with antidepressants for any indication should be monitored appropriately and observed closely for clinical worsening, suicidality, and unusual changes in behavior, especially during the initial few months of a course of drug therapy, or at times of dose changes, either increases or decreases.

The following symptoms, anxiety, agitation, panic attacks, insomnia, irritability, hostility, aggressiveness, impulsivity, akathisia (psychomotor restlessness), hypomania, and mania, have been reported in adult and pediatric patients being treated with antidepressants for Major Depressive Disorder as well as for other indications, both psychiatric and nonpsychiatric. Although a causal link between the emergence of such symptoms and either the worsening of depression and/or the emergence of suicidal impulses has not been established, there is concern that such symptoms may represent precursors to emerging suicidality.

Consideration should be given to changing the therapeutic regimen, including possibly discontinuing the medication, in patients whose depression is persistently worse, or who are experiencing emergent suicidality or symptoms that might be precursors to worsening depression or suicidality, especially if these symptoms are severe, abrupt in onset, or were not part of the patient's presenting symptoms.

Families and caregivers of patients being treated with antidepressants for Major Depressive Disorder or other indications, both psychiatric and nonpsychiatric, should be alerted about the need to monitor patients for the emergence of agitation, irritability, unusual changes in behavior, and the other symptoms described above, as well as the emergence of suicidality, and to report such symptoms immediately to healthcare providers. Such monitoring should include daily observation by families and caregivers. Prescriptions for ABILIFY should be written for the smallest quantity of tablets consistent with good patient management, in order to reduce the risk of overdose.

Screening Patients for Bipolar Disorder: A major depressive episode may be the initial presentation of Bipolar Disorder. It is generally believed (though not established in controlled trials) that treating such an episode with an antidepressant alone may increase the likelihood of precipitation of a mixed/manic episode in patients at risk for Bipolar Disorder. Whether any of the symptoms described above represent such a conversion is unknown. However, prior to initiating treatment with an antidepressant, patients with depressive symptoms should be adequately screened to determine if they are at risk for Bipolar Disorder; such screening should include a detailed psychiatric history, including a family history of suicide, Bipolar Disorder, and depression. It should be noted that ABILIFY is not approved for use in treating depression in the pediatric population.

5.3 Neuroleptic Malignant Syndrome (NMS)

A potentially fatal symptom complex sometimes referred to as Neuroleptic Malignant Syndrome (NMS) may occur with administration of antipsychotic drugs, including aripiprazole. Rare cases of NMS occurred during aripiprazole treatment in the worldwide clinical database. Clinical manifestations of NMS are hyperpyrexia, muscle rigidity, altered mental status, and evidence of autonomic instability (irregular pulse or blood pressure, tachycardia, diaphoresis, and cardiac dysrhythmia). Additional signs may include elevated creatine phosphokinase, myoglobinuria (rhabdomyolysis), and acute renal failure.

The diagnostic evaluation of patients with this syndrome is complicated. In arriving at a diagnosis, it is important to exclude cases where the clinical presentation includes both serious medical illness (eg, pneumonia, systemic infection) and untreated or inadequately treated extrapyramidal signs and symptoms (EPS). Other important considerations in the differential diagnosis include central anticholinergic toxicity, heat stroke, drug fever, and primary central nervous system pathology.

The management of NMS should include: 1) immediate discontinuation of antipsychotic drugs and other drugs not essential to concurrent therapy; 2) intensive symptomatic treatment and medical monitoring; and 3) treatment of any concomitant serious medical problems for which specific treatments are available. There is no general agreement about specific pharmacological treatment regimens for uncomplicated NMS.

If a patient requires antipsychotic drug treatment after recovery from NMS, the potential reintroduction of drug therapy should be carefully considered. The patient should be carefully monitored, since recurrences of NMS have been reported.

5.4 Tardive Dyskinesia

A syndrome of potentially irreversible, involuntary, dyskinetic movements may develop in patients treated with antipsychotic drugs. Although the prevalence of the syndrome appears to be highest among the elderly, especially elderly women, it is impossible to rely upon prevalence estimates to predict, at the inception of antipsychotic treatment, which patients are likely to develop the syndrome. Whether antipsychotic drug products differ in their potential to cause tardive dyskinesia is unknown.

The risk of developing tardive dyskinesia and the likelihood that it will become irreversible are believed to increase as the duration of treatment and the total cumulative dose of antipsychotic drugs administered to the patient increase. However, the syndrome can develop, although much less commonly, after relatively brief treatment periods at low doses.

There is no known treatment for established cases of tardive dyskinesia, although the syndrome may remit, partially or completely, if antipsychotic treatment is withdrawn. Antipsychotic treatment, itself, however, may suppress (or partially suppress) the signs and symptoms of the syndrome and, thereby, may possibly mask the underlying process. The effect that symptomatic suppression has upon the long-term course of the syndrome is unknown.

Given these considerations, ABILIFY should be prescribed in a manner that is most likely to minimize the occurrence of tardive dyskinesia. Chronic antipsychotic treatment should generally be reserved for patients who suffer from a chronic illness that (1) is known to respond to antipsychotic drugs and (2) for whom alternative, equally effective, but potentially less harmful treatments are not available or appropriate. In patients who do require chronic treatment, the smallest dose and the shortest duration of treatment producing a satisfactory clinical response should be sought. The need for continued treatment should be reassessed periodically.

If signs and symptoms of tardive dyskinesia appear in a patient on ABILIFY, drug discontinuation should be considered. However, some patients may require treatment with ABILIFY despite the presence of the syndrome.

5.5 Hyperglycemia and Diabetes Mellitus

Hyperglycemia, in some cases extreme and associated with ketoacidosis or hyperosmolar coma or death, has been reported in patients treated with atypical antipsychotics. There have been few reports of hyperglycemia in patients treated with ABILIFY [see ADVERSE REACTIONS (6.2, 6.3)]. Although fewer patients have been treated with ABILIFY, it is not known if this more limited experience is the sole reason for the paucity of such reports. Assessment of the relationship between atypical antipsychotic use and glucose abnormalities is complicated by the possibility of an increased background risk of diabetes mellitus in patients with Schizophrenia and the increasing incidence of diabetes mellitus in the general population. Given these confounders, the relationship between atypical antipsychotic use and hyperglycemia-related adverse events is not completely understood. However, epidemiological studies which did not include ABILIFY suggest an increased risk of treatment-emergent hyperglycemia-related adverse events in patients treated with the atypical antipsychotics included in these studies. Because ABILIFY was not marketed at the time these studies were performed, it is not known if ABILIFY is associated with this increased risk. Precise risk estimates for hyperglycemia-related adverse events in patients treated with atypical antipsychotics are not available.

Patients with an established diagnosis of diabetes mellitus who are started on atypical antipsychotics should be monitored regularly for worsening of glucose control. Patients with risk factors for diabetes mellitus (eg, obesity, family history of diabetes) who are starting treatment with atypical antipsychotics should undergo fasting blood glucose testing at the beginning of treatment and periodically during treatment. Any patient treated with atypical antipsychotics should be monitored for symptoms of hyperglycemia including polydipsia, polyuria, polyphagia, and weakness. Patients who develop symptoms of hyperglycemia during treatment with atypical antipsychotics should undergo fasting blood glucose testing. In some cases, hyperglycemia has resolved when the atypical antipsychotic was discontinued; however, some patients required continuation of antidiabetic treatment despite discontinuation of the suspect drug.

5.6 Orthostatic Hypotension

Aripiprazole may cause orthostatic hypotension, perhaps due to its α_1-adrenergic receptor antagonism. The incidence of orthostatic hypotension-associated events from short-term, placebo-controlled trials of adult patients on oral ABILIFY (n=1894) included (aripiprazole incidence, placebo incidence) orthostatic hypotension (1.2%, 0.3%), postural dizziness (0.6%, 0.4%), and syncope (0.6%, 0.5%); of pediatric patients 10 to 17 years of age (n=399) on oral ABILIFY included orthostatic hypotension (1.0%, 0%), postural dizziness (0.5%, 0%), and syncope (0.3%, 0%); and of patients on ABILIFY Injection (n=501) included orthostatic hypotension (0.6%, 0%), postural dizziness (0.2%, 0.5%), and syncope (0.4%, 0%).

The incidence of a significant orthostatic change in blood pressure (defined as a decrease in systolic blood pressure ≥20 mmHg accompanied by an increase in heart rate ≥25 when comparing standing to supine values) for aripiprazole was not meaningfully different from placebo (aripiprazole incidence, placebo incidence): in adult oral aripiprazole-treated patients (5%, 3%), in pediatric oral aripiprazole-treated patients aged 10 to 17 years (0%, 0.5%), or in aripiprazole injection-treated patients (3%, 2%).

Aripiprazole should be used with caution in patients with known cardiovascular disease (history of myocardial infarction or ischemic heart disease, heart failure or conduction abnormalities), cerebrovascular disease, or conditions which would predispose patients to hypotension (dehydration, hypovolemia, and treatment with antihypertensive medications).

Continued on next page

Abilify—Cont.

If parenteral benzodiazepine therapy is deemed necessary in addition to aripiprazole injection treatment, patients should be monitored for excessive sedation and for orthostatic hypotension [see DRUG INTERACTIONS (7.3)].

5.7   Seizures/Convulsions
In short-term, placebo-controlled trials, seizures/convulsions occurred in 0.2% (3/1894) of adult patients treated with oral aripiprazole, in 0.3% (1/399) of pediatric patients (10 to 17 years), and in 0.2% (1/501) of adult aripiprazole injection-treated patients.

As with other antipsychotic drugs, aripiprazole should be used cautiously in patients with a history of seizures or with conditions that lower the seizure threshold, eg, Alzheimer's dementia. Conditions that lower the seizure threshold may be more prevalent in a population of 65 years or older.

5.8   Potential for Cognitive and Motor Impairment
ABILIFY (aripiprazole), like other antipsychotics, may have the potential to impair judgment, thinking, or motor skills. For example, in short-term, placebo-controlled trials, somnolence (including sedation) was reported as follows (aripiprazole incidence, placebo incidence): in adult patients (n=1894) treated with oral ABILIFY (11%, 7%), in pediatric patients ages 10 to 17 (21%, 5%), and in adult patients on ABILIFY Injection (9%, 6%). Somnolence (including sedation) led to discontinuation in 0.2% (4/1894) of adult patients, and 1% (4/399) of pediatric patients (10 to 17 years) on oral ABILIFY in short-term, placebo-controlled trials, but did not lead to discontinuation of any adult patients on ABILIFY Injection.

Despite the relatively modest increased incidence of these events compared to placebo, patients should be cautioned about operating hazardous machinery, including automobiles, until they are reasonably certain that therapy with ABILIFY does not affect them adversely.

5.9   Body Temperature Regulation
Disruption of the body's ability to reduce core body temperature has been attributed to antipsychotic agents. Appropriate care is advised when prescribing aripiprazole for patients who will be experiencing conditions which may contribute to an elevation in core body temperature, (eg, exercising strenuously, exposure to extreme heat, receiving concomitant medication with anticholinergic activity, or being subject to dehydration) [see ADVERSE REACTIONS (6.3)].

5.10   Suicide
The possibility of a suicide attempt is inherent in psychotic illnesses, Bipolar Disorder, and Major Depressive Disorder, and close supervision of high-risk patients should accompany drug therapy. Prescriptions for ABILIFY should be written for the smallest quantity consistent with good patient management in order to reduce the risk of overdose [see ADVERSE REACTIONS (6.2, 6.3)].

In two 6-week placebo-controlled studies of aripiprazole as adjunctive treatment of Major Depressive Disorder, the incidences of suicidal ideation and suicide attempts were 0% (0/371) for aripiprazole and 0.5% (2/366) for placebo.

5.11   Dysphagia
Esophageal dysmotility and aspiration have been associated with antipsychotic drug use, including ABILIFY. Aspiration pneumonia is a common cause of morbidity and mortality in elderly patients, in particular those with advanced Alzheimer's dementia. Aripiprazole and other antipsychotic drugs should be used cautiously in patients at risk for aspiration pneumonia [see WARNINGS AND PRECAUTIONS (5.1) and ADVERSE REACTIONS (6.3)].

5.12   Use in Patients with Concomitant Illness
Clinical experience with ABILIFY in patients with certain concomitant systemic illnesses is limited [see USE IN SPECIFIC POPULATIONS (8.6, 8.7)].

ABILIFY has not been evaluated or used to any appreciable extent in patients with a recent history of myocardial infarction or unstable heart disease. Patients with these diagnoses were excluded from premarketing clinical studies [see WARNINGS AND PRECAUTIONS (5.1, 5.6)].

6   ADVERSE REACTIONS
6.1   Overall Adverse Reactions Profile
The following are discussed in more detail in other sections of the labeling:
- Use in Elderly Patients with Dementia-Related Psychosis [see BOXED WARNING and WARNINGS AND PRECAUTIONS (5.1)]
- Clinical Worsening of Depression and Suicide Risk [see BOXED WARNING and WARNINGS AND PRECAUTIONS (5.2)]
- Neuroleptic Malignant Syndrome (NMS) [see WARNINGS AND PRECAUTIONS (5.3)]
- Tardive Dyskinesia [see WARNINGS AND PRECAUTIONS (5.4)]
- Hyperglycemia and Diabetes Mellitus [see WARNINGS AND PRECAUTIONS (5.5)]
- Orthostatic Hypotension [see WARNINGS AND PRECAUTIONS (5.6)]
- Seizures/Convulsions [see WARNINGS AND PRECAUTIONS (5.7)]
- Potential for Cognitive and Motor Impairment [see WARNINGS AND PRECAUTIONS (5.8)]
- Body Temperature Regulation [see WARNINGS AND PRECAUTIONS (5.9)]
- Suicide [see WARNINGS AND PRECAUTIONS (5.10)]
- Dysphagia [see WARNINGS AND PRECAUTIONS (5.11)]
- Use in Patients with Concomitant Illness [see WARNINGS AND PRECAUTIONS (5.12)]

The most common adverse reactions in adult patients in clinical trials (≥10%) were nausea, vomiting, constipation, headache, dizziness, akathisia, anxiety, insomnia, and restlessness.

The most common adverse reactions in the pediatric clinical trials (≥10%) were somnolence, extrapyramidal disorder, headache, and nausea.

Aripiprazole has been evaluated for safety in 12,925 adult patients who participated in multiple-dose, clinical trials in Schizophrenia, Bipolar Disorder, Major Depressive Disorder, and Dementia of the Alzheimer's type, and who had approximately 7482 patient-years of exposure to oral aripiprazole and 749 patients with exposure to aripiprazole injection. A total of 3338 patients were treated with oral aripiprazole for at least 180 days and 1898 patients treated with oral aripiprazole had at least 1 year of exposure.

Aripiprazole has been evaluated for safety in 514 patients (10 to 17 years) who participated in multiple-dose, clinical trials in Schizophrenia or Bipolar Mania and who had approximately 205 patient-years of exposure to oral aripiprazole. A total of 278 pediatric patients were treated with oral aripiprazole for at least 180 days.

The conditions and duration of treatment with aripiprazole included (in overlapping categories) double-blind, comparative and noncomparative open-label studies, inpatient and outpatient studies, fixed- and flexible-dose studies, and short- and longer-term exposure.

Adverse events during exposure were obtained by collecting volunteered adverse events, as well as results of physical examinations, vital signs, weights, laboratory analyses, and ECG. Adverse experiences were recorded by clinical investigators using terminology of their own choosing. In the tables and tabulations that follow, MedDRA dictionary terminology has been used to classify reported adverse events into a smaller number of standardized event categories, in order to provide a meaningful estimate of the proportion of individuals experiencing adverse events.

The stated frequencies of adverse reactions represent the proportion of individuals who experienced at least once, a treatment-emergent adverse event of the type listed. An event was considered treatment emergent if it occurred for the first time or worsened while receiving therapy following baseline evaluation. There was no attempt to use investigator causality assessments; ie, all events meeting the defined criteria, regardless of investigator causality are included.

Throughout this section, adverse reactions are reported. These are adverse events that were considered to be reasonably associated with the use of ABILIFY (adverse drug reactions) based on the comprehensive assessment of the available adverse event information. A causal association for ABILIFY often cannot be reliably established in individual cases.

The figures in the tables and tabulations cannot be used to predict the incidence of side effects in the course of usual medical practice where patient characteristics and other factors differ from those that prevailed in the clinical trials. Similarly, the cited frequencies cannot be compared with figures obtained from other clinical investigations involving different treatment, uses, and investigators. The cited figures, however, do provide the prescriber with some basis for estimating the relative contribution of drug and nondrug factors to the adverse reaction incidence in the population studied.

6.2   Clinical Studies Experience
Adult Patients with Schizophrenia
The following findings are based on a pool of five placebo-controlled trials (four 4-week and one 6-week) in which oral aripiprazole was administered in doses ranging from 2 mg/day to 30 mg/day.

Adverse Reactions Associated with Discontinuation of Treatment

Overall, there was little difference in the incidence of discontinuation due to adverse reactions between aripiprazole-treated (7%) and placebo-treated (9%) patients. The types of adverse reactions that led to discontinuation were similar for the aripiprazole- and placebo-treated patients.

Commonly Observed Adverse Reactions

The only commonly observed adverse reaction associated with the use of aripiprazole in patients with Schizophrenia (incidence of 5% or greater and aripiprazole incidence at least twice that for placebo) was akathisia (aripiprazole 8%; placebo 4%).

Adult Patients with Bipolar Mania
The following findings are based on a pool of 3-week, placebo-controlled, Bipolar Mania trials in which oral aripiprazole was administered at doses of 15 mg/day or 30 mg/day.

Adverse Reactions Associated with Discontinuation of Treatment

Overall, in patients with Bipolar Mania, there was little difference in the incidence of discontinuation due to adverse reactions between aripiprazole-treated (11%) and placebo-treated (9%) patients. The types of adverse reactions that led to discontinuation were similar between the aripiprazole- and placebo-treated patients.

Commonly Observed Adverse Reactions

Commonly observed adverse reactions associated with the use of aripiprazole in patients with Bipolar Mania (incidence of 5% or greater and aripiprazole incidence at least twice that for placebo) are shown in Table 5.

Table 5:   Commonly Observed Adverse Reactions in Short-Term, Placebo-Controlled Trials of Adult Patients with Bipolar Mania Treated with Oral ABILIFY

Preferred Term	Percentage of Patients Reporting Reaction	
	Aripiprazole (n=597)	Placebo (n=436)
Constipation	13	6
Akathisia	15	3
Sedation	8	3
Tremor	7	3
Restlessness	6	3
Extrapyramidal Disorder	5	2

Less Common Adverse Reactions in Adults
Table 6 enumerates the pooled incidence, rounded to the nearest percent, of adverse reactions that occurred during acute therapy (up to 6 weeks in Schizophrenia and up to 3 weeks in Bipolar Mania), including only those reactions that occurred in 2% or more of patients treated with aripiprazole (doses ≥2 mg/day) and for which the incidence in patients treated with aripiprazole was greater than the incidence in patients treated with placebo in the combined dataset.

Table 6:   Adverse Reactions in Short-Term, Placebo-Controlled Trials in Adult Patients Treated with Oral ABILIFY (aripiprazole)

System Organ Class Preferred Term	Percentage of Patients Reporting Reaction[a]	
	Aripiprazole (n=1523)	Placebo (n=849)
Eye Disorders		
Blurred Vision	3	1
Gastrointestinal Disorders		
Nausea	16	12
Vomiting	12	6
Constipation	11	7
Dyspepsia	10	8
Dry Mouth	5	4
Abdominal Discomfort	3	2
Stomach Discomfort	3	2
Salivary Hypersecretion	2	1
General Disorders and Administration Site Conditions		
Fatigue	6	5
Pain	3	2
Peripheral Edema	2	1
Musculoskeletal and Connective Tissue Disorders		
Arthralgia	5	4
Pain in Extremity	4	2
Nervous System Disorders		
Headache	30	25
Dizziness	11	8
Akathisia	10	4
Sedation	7	4
Extrapyramidal Disorder	6	4
Tremor	5	3
Somnolence	5	4
Psychiatric Disorders		
Anxiety	20	17
Insomnia	19	14
Restlessness	5	3
Respiratory, Thoracic, and Mediastinal Disorders		
Pharyngolaryngeal Pain	4	3
Cough	3	2
Nasal Congestion	3	2
Vascular Disorders		
Hypertension[b]	2	1

[a] Adverse reactions reported by at least 2% of patients treated with oral aripiprazole, except adverse reactions which had an incidence equal to or less than placebo.
[b] Including blood pressure increased.

An examination of population subgroups did not reveal any clear evidence of differential adverse reaction incidence on the basis of age, gender, or race.

Pediatric Patients (13 to 17 years) with Schizophrenia
The following findings are based on one 6-week placebo-controlled trial in which oral aripiprazole was administered in doses ranging from 2 mg/day to 30 mg/day.

Adverse Reactions Associated with Discontinuation of Treatment

The incidence of discontinuation due to adverse reactions between aripiprazole-treated and placebo-treated pediatric patients (13 to 17 years) was 5% and 2%, respectively.

Commonly Observed Adverse Reactions

Commonly observed adverse reactions associated with the use of aripiprazole in adolescent patients with Schizophrenia (incidence of 5% or greater and aripiprazole incidence at least twice that for placebo) were extrapyramidal disorder, somnolence, and tremor.

Pediatric Patients (10 to 17 years) with Bipolar Mania
The following findings are based on one 4-week placebo-controlled trial in which oral aripiprazole was administered in doses of 10 mg/day or 30 mg/day.

Adverse Reactions Associated with Discontinuation of Treatment

The incidence of discontinuation due to adverse reactions between aripiprazole- and placebo-treated pediatric patients (10 to 17 years) was 7% and 2%, respectively.

Commonly Observed Adverse Reactions

Commonly observed adverse reactions associated with the use of aripiprazole in pediatric patients with Bipolar Mania (incidence of 5% or greater and aripiprazole incidence at least twice that for placebo) are shown in Table 7.

Table 7:　Commonly Observed Adverse Reactions in Short-Term, Placebo-Controlled Trials of Pediatric Patients (10 to 17 years) with Bipolar Mania Treated with Oral ABILIFY

	Percentage of Patients Reporting Reaction[a]	
Preferred Term	Aripiprazole (n=197)	Placebo (n=97)
Somnolence	23	3
Extrapyramidal Disorder	20	3
Fatigue	11	4
Nausea	11	4
Akathisia	10	2
Blurred Vision	8	0
Salivary Hypersecretion	6	0
Dizziness	5	1

Less Common Adverse Reactions in Pediatric Patients (10 to 17 years) with Schizophrenia or Bipolar Mania

Table 8 enumerates the pooled incidence, rounded to the nearest percent, of adverse reactions that occurred during acute therapy (up to 6 weeks in Schizophrenia and up to 4 weeks in Bipolar Mania), including only those reactions that occurred in 1% or more of pediatric patients treated with aripiprazole (doses ≥2 mg/day) and for which the incidence in patients treated with aripiprazole was greater than the incidence in patients treated with placebo.

Table 8:　Adverse Reactions in Short-Term, Placebo-Controlled Trials of Pediatric Patients (10 to 17 years) Treated with Oral ABILIFY

	Percentage of Patients Reporting Reaction[a]	
System Organ Class Preferred Term	Aripiprazole (n=399)	Placebo (n=197)
Eye Disorders		
Blurred Vision	5	0
Gastrointestinal Disorders		
Nausea	10	5
Salivary Hypersecretion	4	1
Diarrhea	3	0
Stomach Discomfort	2	1
Dry Mouth	2	1
General Disorders and Administration Site Conditions		
Fatigue	7	3
Pyrexia	3	1
Infections and Infestations		
Nasopharyngitis	4	3
Investigations		
Weight Increased	3	1
Metabolism and Nutrition Disorders		
Increased Appetite	4	2
Musculoskeletal and Connective Tissue Disorders		
Arthralgia	2	0
Nervous System Disorders		
Somnolence	20	5
Extrapyramidal Disorder	19	4
Headache	16	13
Akathisia	9	4
Dizziness	5	2
Tremor	5	2
Dystonia	2	0
Dyskinesia	1	0
Sedation	1	0
Skin and Subcutaneous Disorders		
Rash	2	1
Vascular Disorders		
Orthostatic Hypotension	1	0

[a] Adverse reactions reported by at least 1% of pediatric patients treated with oral aripiprazole, except adverse reactions which had an incidence equal to or less than placebo.

Adult Patients Receiving ABILIFY as Adjunctive Treatment of Major Depressive Disorder

The following findings are based on a pool of two placebo-controlled trials of patients with Major Depressive Disorder in which aripiprazole was administered at doses of 2 mg to 20 mg as adjunctive treatment to continued antidepressant therapy.

Adverse Reactions Associated with Discontinuation of Treatment

The incidence of discontinuation due to adverse reactions was 6% for adjunctive aripiprazole-treated patients and 2% for adjunctive placebo-treated patients.

Commonly Observed Adverse Reactions

The commonly observed adverse reactions associated with the use of adjunctive aripiprazole in patients with Major Depressive Disorder (incidence of 5% or greater and aripiprazole incidence at least twice that for placebo) were: akathisia, restlessness, insomnia, constipation, fatigue, and blurred vision.

Less Common Adverse Reactions in Adult Patients with Major Depressive Disorder

Table 9 enumerates the pooled incidence, rounded to the nearest percent, of adverse reactions that occurred during acute therapy (up to 6 weeks), including only those adverse reactions that occurred in 2% or more of patients treated with adjunctive aripiprazole (doses ≥2 mg/day) and for which the incidence in patients treated with adjunctive aripiprazole was greater than the incidence in patients treated with adjunctive placebo in the combined dataset.

Table 9:　Adverse Reactions in Short-Term, Placebo-Controlled Adjunctive Trials in Patients with Major Depressive Disorder

	Percentage of Patients Reporting Reaction[a]	
System Organ Class Preferred Term	Aripiprazole +ADT* (n=371)	Placebo +ADT* (n=366)
Eye Disorders		
Blurred Vision	6	1
Gastrointestinal Disorders		
Constipation	5	2
General Disorders and Administration Site Conditions		
Fatigue	8	4
Feeling Jittery	3	1
Infections and Infestations		
Upper Respiratory Tract Infection	6	4
Investigations		
Weight Increased	3	2
Metabolism and Nutrition Disorders		
Increased Appetite	3	2
Musculoskeletal and Connective Tissue Disorders		
Arthralgia	4	3
Myalgia	3	1
Nervous System Disorders		
Akathisia	25	4
Somnolence	6	4
Tremor	5	4
Sedation	4	2
Dizziness	4	2
Disturbance in Attention	3	1
Extrapyramidal Disorder	2	0
Psychiatric Disorders		
Restlessness	12	2
Insomnia	8	2

[a] Adverse reactions reported by at least 2% of patients treated with adjunctive aripiprazole, except adverse reactions which had an incidence equal to or less than placebo.

* Antidepressant Therapy

Patients with Agitation Associated with Schizophrenia or Bipolar Mania (Intramuscular Injection)

The following findings are based on a pool of three placebo-controlled trials of patients with agitation associated with Schizophrenia or Bipolar Mania in which aripiprazole injection was administered at doses of 5.25 mg to 15 mg.

Adverse Reactions Associated with Discontinuation of Treatment

Overall, in patients with agitation associated with Schizophrenia or Bipolar Mania, there was little difference in the incidence of discontinuation due to adverse reactions between aripiprazole-treated (0.8%) and placebo-treated (0.5%) patients.

Commonly Observed Adverse Reactions

There was one commonly observed adverse reaction (nausea) associated with the use of aripiprazole injection in patients with agitation associated with Schizophrenia and Bipolar Mania (incidence of 5% or greater and aripiprazole incidence at least twice that for placebo).

Less Common Adverse Reactions in Patients with Agitation Associated with Schizophrenia or Bipolar Mania

Table 10 enumerates the pooled incidence, rounded to the nearest percent, of adverse reactions that occurred during acute therapy (24-hour) including only those adverse reactions that occurred in 2% or more of patients treated with aripiprazole injection (doses ≥5.25 mg/day) and for which the incidence in patients treated with aripiprazole injection was greater than the incidence in patients treated with placebo in the combined dataset.

Table 10:　Adverse Reactions in Short-Term, Placebo-Controlled Trials in Patients Treated with ABILIFY Injection

	Percentage of Patients Reporting Reaction[a]	
System Organ Class Preferred Term	Aripiprazole (n=501)	Placebo (n=220)
Cardiac Disorders		
Tachycardia	2	<1
Gastrointestinal Disorders		
Nausea	9	3
Vomiting	3	1
General Disorders and Administration Site Conditions		
Fatigue	2	1
Nervous System Disorders		
Headache	12	7
Dizziness	8	5
Somnolence	7	4
Sedation	3	2
Akathisia	2	0

[a] Adverse reactions reported by at least 2% of patients treated with aripiprazole injection, except adverse reactions which had an incidence equal to or less than placebo.

Dose-Related Adverse Reactions

Schizophrenia

Dose response relationships for the incidence of treatment-emergent adverse events were evaluated from four trials in adult patients with Schizophrenia comparing various fixed doses (2 mg/day, 5 mg/day, 10 mg/day, 15 mg/day, 20 mg/day, and 30 mg/day) of oral aripiprazole to placebo. This analysis, stratified by study, indicated that the only adverse reaction to have a possible dose response relationship, and then most prominent only with 30 mg, was somnolence [including sedation]; (incidences were placebo, 7.1%; 10 mg, 8.5%; 15 mg, 8.7%; 20 mg, 7.5%; 30 mg, 12.6%).

In the study of pediatric patients (13 to 17 years of age) with Schizophrenia, three common adverse reactions appeared to have a possible dose response relationship: extrapyramidal disorder (incidences were placebo, 5.0%; 10 mg, 13.0%; 30 mg, 21.6%); somnolence (incidences were placebo, 6.0%; 10 mg, 11.0%; 30 mg, 21.6%); and tremor (incidences were placebo, 2.0%; 10 mg, 2.0%; 30 mg, 11.8%).

Bipolar Mania

In the study of pediatric patients (10 to 17 years of age) with Bipolar Mania, four common adverse reactions had a possible dose response relationship at 4 weeks; extrapyramidal disorder (incidences were placebo, 3.1%; 10 mg, 12.2%; 30 mg, 27.3%); somnolence (incidences were placebo, 3.1%; 10 mg, 19.4%; 30 mg, 26.3%); akathisia (incidences were placebo, 2.1%, 10 mg, 8.2%; 30 mg, 11.1%); and salivary hypersecretion (incidences were placebo, 0%; 10 mg, 3.1%; 30 mg, 8.1%).

Extrapyramidal Symptoms

In short-term, placebo-controlled trials in Schizophrenia in adults, the incidence of reported EPS-related events, excluding events related to akathisia, for aripiprazole-treated patients was 13% vs. 12% for placebo; and the incidence of akathisia-related events for aripiprazole-treated patients was 8% vs. 4% for placebo. In the short-term, placebo-controlled trial of Schizophrenia in pediatric (13 to 17 years) patients, the incidence of reported EPS-related events, excluding events related to akathisia, for aripiprazole-treated patients was 25% vs. 7% for placebo; and the incidence of akathisia-related events for aripiprazole-treated patients was 9% vs. 6% for placebo. In the short-term, placebo-controlled trials in Bipolar Mania in adults, the incidence of reported EPS-related events, excluding events related to akathisia, for aripiprazole-treated patients was 15% vs. 8% for placebo and the incidence of akathisia-related events for aripiprazole-treated patients was 15% vs. 4% for placebo. In the short-term, placebo-controlled trial in Bipolar Mania in pediatric (10 to 17 years) patients, the incidence of reported EPS-related events, excluding events related to akathisia, for aripiprazole-treated patients was 26% vs. 5% for placebo and the incidence of akathisia-related events for aripiprazole-treated patients was 10% vs. 2% for placebo. In the short-term, placebo-controlled trials in Major Depressive Disorder, the incidence of reported EPS-related events, excluding events related to akathisia, for adjunctive aripiprazole-treated patients was 8% vs. 5% for adjunctive placebo-treated patients; and the incidence of akathisia-related events for adjunctive aripiprazole-treated patients was 25% vs. 4% for adjunctive placebo-treated patients.

Objectively collected data from those trials was collected on the Simpson Angus Rating Scale (for EPS), the Barnes Akathisia Scale (for akathisia), and the Assessments of Involuntary Movement Scales (for dyskinesias). In the adult Schizophrenia trials, the objectively collected data did not show a difference between aripiprazole and placebo, with the exception of the Barnes Akathisia Scale (aripiprazole, 0.08; placebo, -0.05). In the pediatric (13 to 17 years) Schizophrenia trial, the objectively collected data did not show a difference between aripiprazole and placebo, with the exception of the Simpson Angus Rating Scale (aripiprazole, 0.24; placebo, -0.29). In the adult Bipolar Mania trials, the Simpson Angus Rating Scale and the Barnes Akathisia Scale showed a significant difference between aripiprazole and placebo (aripiprazole, 0.61; placebo, 0.03 and aripiprazole, 0.25; placebo, -0.06). Changes in the Assessments of Involuntary Movement Scales were similar for the aripiprazole and placebo groups. In the pediatric (10 to 17 years) short-term Bipolar Mania trial, the Simpson Angus Rating Scale showed a significant difference between aripiprazole and placebo (aripiprazole, 0.90; placebo, -0.05). Changes in the Barnes Akathisia Scale and the Assessments of Involuntary Movement Scales were similar for the aripiprazole and placebo groups. In the Major Depressive Disorder trials, the Simpson Angus Rating Scale and the Barnes Akathisia Scale showed a significant difference between adjunctive aripiprazole and adjunctive placebo (aripiprazole, 0.31; placebo, 0.03 and aripiprazole, 0.22; placebo, 0.02). Changes in the Assessments of Involuntary Movement Scales were similar for the adjunctive aripiprazole and adjunctive placebo groups.

Similarly, in a long-term (26-week), placebo-controlled trial of Schizophrenia in adults, objectively collected data on the

Continued on next page

Abilify—Cont.

Simpson Angus Rating Scale (for EPS), the Barnes Akathisia Scale (for akathisia), and the Assessments of Involuntary Movement Scales (for dyskinesias) did not show a difference between aripiprazole and placebo.
In the placebo-controlled trials in patients with agitation associated with Schizophrenia or Bipolar Mania, the incidence of reported EPS-related events excluding events related to akathisia for aripiprazole-treated patients was 2% vs. 2% for placebo and the incidence of akathisia-related events for aripiprazole-treated patients was 2% vs. 0% for placebo. Objectively collected data on the Simpson Angus Rating Scale (for EPS) and the Barnes Akathisia Scale (for akathisia) for all treatment groups did not show a difference between aripiprazole and placebo.

Dystonia

Class Effect: Symptoms of dystonia, prolonged abnormal contractions of muscle groups, may occur in susceptible individuals during the first few days of treatment. Dystonic symptoms include: spasm of the neck muscles, sometimes progressing to tightness of the throat, swallowing difficulty, difficulty breathing, and/or protrusion of the tongue. While these symptoms can occur at low doses, they occur more frequently and with greater severity with high potency and at higher doses of first generation antipsychotic drugs. An elevated risk of acute dystonia is observed in males and younger age groups.

Laboratory Test Abnormalities

A between group comparison for 3-week to 6-week, placebo-controlled trials in adults or 4-week to 6-week, placebo-controlled trials in pediatric patients (10 to 17 years) revealed no medically important differences between the aripiprazole and placebo groups in the proportions of patients experiencing potentially clinically significant changes in routine serum chemistry, hematology, or urinalysis parameters. Similarly, there were no aripiprazole/placebo differences in the incidence of discontinuations for changes in serum chemistry, hematology, or urinalysis in adult or pediatric patients.
In the 6-week trials of aripiprazole as adjunctive therapy for Major Depressive Disorder, there were no clinically important differences between the adjunctive aripiprazole-treated and adjunctive placebo-treated patients in the median change from baseline in prolactin, fasting glucose, HDL, LDL, or total cholesterol measurements. The median % change from baseline in triglycerides was 5% for adjunctive aripiprazole-treated patients vs. 0% for adjunctive placebo-treated patients.
In a long-term (26-week), placebo-controlled trial there were no medically important differences between the aripiprazole and placebo patients in the mean change from baseline in prolactin, fasting glucose, triglyceride, HDL, LDL, or total cholesterol measurements.

Weight Gain

In 4-week to 6-week trials in adults with Schizophrenia, there was a slight difference in mean weight gain between aripiprazole and placebo patients (+0.7 kg vs. -0.05 kg, respectively) and also a difference in the proportion of patients meeting a weight gain criterion of ≥7% of body weight [aripiprazole (8%) compared to placebo (3%)]. In a 6-week trial in pediatric patients (13 to 17 years) with Schizophrenia, there was a slight difference in mean weight gain between aripiprazole and placebo patients (+0.13 kg vs. -0.83 kg, respectively) and also a difference in the proportion of patients meeting a weight gain criterion of ≥7% of body weight [aripiprazole (5%) compared to placebo (1%)]. In 3-week trials in adults with Mania, the mean weight gain for aripiprazole and placebo patients was 0.0 kg vs. -0.2 kg, respectively. The proportion of patients meeting a weight gain criterion of ≥7% of body weight was aripiprazole (3%) compared to placebo (2%).
In the trials adding aripiprazole to antidepressants, patients first received 8 weeks of antidepressant treatment followed by 6 weeks of adjunctive aripiprazole or placebo in addition to their ongoing antidepressant treatment. The mean weight gain with adjunctive aripiprazole was 1.7 kg vs. 0.4 kg with adjunctive placebo. The proportion of patients meeting a weight gain criterion of ≥7% of body weight was 5% with adjunctive aripiprazole compared to 1% with adjunctive placebo.
Table 11 provides the weight change results from a long-term (26-week), placebo-controlled study of aripiprazole, both mean change from baseline and proportions of patients meeting a weight gain criterion of ≥7% of body weight relative to baseline, categorized by BMI at baseline. Although there was no mean weight increase, the aripiprazole group tended to show more patients with a ≥7% weight gain.
[See table 11 below]
Table 12 provides the weight change results from a long-term (52-week) study of aripiprazole, both mean change from baseline and proportions of patients meeting a weight gain criterion of ≥7% of body weight relative to baseline, categorized by BMI at baseline:

Table 12: Weight Change Results Categorized by BMI at Baseline: Active-Controlled Study in Schizophrenia, Safety Sample

	BMI <23 (n=314)	BMI 23-27 (n=265)	BMI >27 (n=260)
Mean change from baseline (kg)	2.6	1.4	-1.2
% with ≥7% increase BW	30%	19%	8%

ECG Changes

Between group comparisons for a pooled analysis of placebo-controlled trials in patients with Schizophrenia, Bipolar Mania, or Major Depressive Disorder revealed no significant differences between oral aripiprazole and placebo in the proportion of patients experiencing potentially important changes in ECG parameters. Aripiprazole was associated with a median increase in heart rate of 3 beats per minute compared to no increase among placebo patients.
In the pooled, placebo-controlled trials in patients with agitation associated with Schizophrenia or Bipolar Mania, there were no significant differences between aripiprazole injection and placebo in the proportion of patients experiencing potentially important changes in ECG parameters, as measured by standard 12-lead ECGs.

Additional Findings Observed in Clinical Trials

Adverse Reactions in Long-Term, Double-Blind, Placebo-Controlled Trials

The adverse reactions reported in a 26-week, double-blind trial comparing oral ABILIFY and placebo in patients with Schizophrenia were generally consistent with those reported in the short-term, placebo-controlled trials, except for a higher incidence of tremor [8% (12/153) for ABILIFY vs. 2% (3/153) for placebo]. In this study, the majority of the cases of tremor were of mild intensity (8/12 mild and 4/12 moderate), occurred early in therapy (9/12 ≤49 days), and were of limited duration (7/12 ≤10 days). Tremor infrequently led to discontinuation (<1%) of ABILIFY. In addition, in a long-term (52-week), active-controlled study, the incidence of tremor was 5% (40/859) for ABILIFY. A similar profile was observed in a long-term study in Bipolar Disorder.

Other Adverse Reactions Observed During the Premarketing Evaluation of Aripiprazole

Following is a list of MedDRA terms that reflect adverse reactions as defined in *ADVERSE REACTIONS (6.1)* reported by patients treated with oral aripiprazole at multiple doses ≥2 mg/day during any phase of a trial within the database of 12,925 adult patients. All events assessed as possible adverse drug reactions have been included with the exception of more commonly occurring events. In addition, medically/clinically meaningful adverse reactions, particularly those that are likely to be useful to the prescriber or that have pharmacologic plausibility, have been included. Events already listed in other parts of *ADVERSE REACTIONS (6)*, or those considered in *WARNINGS AND PRECAUTIONS (5)* or *OVERDOSAGE (10)* have been excluded. Although the reactions reported occurred during treatment with aripiprazole, they were not necessarily caused by it.
Events are further categorized by MedDRA system organ class and listed in order of decreasing frequency according to the following definitions: those occurring in at least 1/100 patients (only those not already listed in the tabulated results from placebo-controlled trials appear in this listing); those occurring in 1/100 to 1/1000 patients; and those occurring in fewer than 1/1000 patients.

Adults - Oral Administration

Blood and Lymphatic System Disorders:
≥1/1000 patients and <1/100 patients - leukopenia, neutropenia; *<1/1000 patients* - thrombocytopenia, agranulocytosis, idiopathic thrombocytopenic purpura
Cardiac Disorders:
≥1/1000 patients and <1/100 patients - cardiopulmonary failure, bradycardia, cardio-respiratory arrest, atrioventricular block, atrial fibrillation, angina pectoris, bundle branch block; *<1/1000 patients* - atrial flutter, ventricular tachycardia, complete atrioventricular block, supraventricular tachycardia
Eye Disorders:
≥1/1000 patients and <1/100 patients - eyelid edema, photophobia, diplopia, photopsia; *<1/1000 patients* - excessive blinking
Gastrointestinal Disorders:
≥1/1000 patients and <1/100 patients - dysphagia, gastroesophageal reflux disease, gastrointestinal hemorrhage, swollen tongue, ulcer, esophagitis, angioedema; *<1/1000 patients* - pancreatitis
General Disorders and Administration Site Conditions:
≥1/100 patients - asthenia; *≥1/1000 patients and <1/100 patients* - mobility decreased, face edema; *<1/1000 patients* - hypothermia
Hepatobiliary Disorders:
≥1/1000 patients and <1/100 patients - cholecystitis, cholelithiasis; *<1/1000 patients* - hepatitis, jaundice
Injury, Poisoning, and Procedural Complications:
≥1/100 patients - fall; *≥1/1000 patients and <1/100 patients* - self mutilation; *<1/1000 patients* - heat stroke
Investigations:
≥1/100 patients - creatine phosphokinase increased; *≥1/1000 patients and <1/100 patients* - hepatic enzyme increased, blood urea increased, blood bilirubin increased, blood creatinine increased, electrocardiogram QT corrected interval prolonged, blood prolactin increased; *<1/1000 patients* - blood lactate dehydrogenase increased, glycosylated hemoglobin increased, GGT increased
Metabolism and Nutrition Disorders:
≥1/1000 patients and <1/100 patients - anorexia, hyperlipidemia
Musculoskeletal and Connective Tissue Disorders:
≥1/100 patients - muscle spasms; *≥1/1000 patients and <1/100 patients* - muscle rigidity; *<1/1000 patients* - rhabdomyolysis
Nervous System Disorders:
≥1/100 patients - coordination abnormal; *≥1/1000 patients and <1/100 patients* - speech disorder, parkinsonism, cogwheel rigidity, memory impairment, cerebrovascular accident, hypokinesia, tardive dyskinesia, hypotonia, hypertonia, akinesia, myoclonus, bradykinesia; *<1/1000 patients* - Grand Mal convulsion, choreoathetosis
Psychiatric Disorders:
≥1/100 patients - agitation, irritability, suicidal ideation; *≥1/1000 patients and <1/100 patients* - aggression, loss of libido, libido decreased, hostility, suicide attempt, libido increased, anger, anorgasmia, delirium, intentional self injury, completed suicide, tic, homicidal ideation; *<1/1000 patients* - psychomotor agitation, premature ejaculation, catatonia, sleep walking
Renal and Urinary Disorders:
≥1/1000 patients and <1/100 patients - urinary retention, polyuria, nocturia
Reproductive System and Breast Disorders:
≥1/1000 patients and <1/100 patients - erectile dysfunction, amenorrhea, menstruation irregular, breast pain; *<1/1000 patients* - gynaecomastia, priapism, galactorrhea
Respiratory, Thoracic, and Mediastinal Disorders:
≥1/100 patients - dyspnea; *≥1/1000 patients and <1/100 patients* - pneumonia aspiration, respiratory distress; *<1/1000 patients* - pulmonary embolism, asphyxia
Skin and Subcutaneous Tissue Disorders:
≥1/100 patients - hyperhydrosis; *≥1/1000 patients and <1/100 patients* - erythema, pruritus, ecchymosis, face edema, photosensitivity reaction, alopecia, urticaria
Vascular Disorders:
≥1/1000 patients and <1/100 patients - hypotension, deep vein thrombosis, phlebitis; *<1/1000 patients* - shock, thrombophlebitis

Pediatric Patients - Oral Administration

Most adverse events observed in the pooled database of 514 pediatric patients aged 10 to 17 years were also observed in the adult population. Additional adverse reactions observed in the pediatric population are listed below.
Gastrointestinal Disorders:
≥1/1000 patients and <1/100 patients - tongue dry, tongue spasm
Investigations:
≥1/100 patients - blood insulin increased
Nervous System Disorders:
≥1/1000 patients and <1/100 patients - sleep talking
Skin and Subcutaneous Tissue Disorders:
≥1/1000 patients and <1/100 patients - hirsutism

Adults - Intramuscular Injection

All adverse reactions observed in the pooled database of 749 adult patients treated with aripiprazole injection, were also observed in the adult population treated with oral aripiprazole. Additional adverse reactions observed in the aripiprazole injection population are listed below.
General Disorders and Administration Site Conditions:
≥1/100 patients - injection site reaction; *≥1/1000 patients and <1/100 patients* - venipuncture site bruise

6.3 Postmarketing Experience

The following adverse reactions have been identified during postapproval use of ABILIFY. Because these reactions are reported voluntarily from a population of uncertain size, it is not always possible to establish a causal relationship to drug exposure: rare occurrences of allergic reaction (anaphylactic reaction, angioedema, laryngospasm, pruritus/urticaria, or oropharyngeal spasm), and blood glucose fluctuation.

7 DRUG INTERACTIONS

Given the primary CNS effects of aripiprazole, caution should be used when ABILIFY is taken in combination with other centrally-acting drugs or alcohol.
Due to its alpha adrenergic antagonism, aripiprazole has the potential to enhance the effect of certain antihypertensive agents.

7.1 Potential for Other Drugs to Affect ABILIFY

Aripiprazole is not a substrate of CYP1A1, CYP1A2, CYP2A6, CYP2B6, CYP2C8, CYP2C9, CYP2C19, or

Table 11: Weight Change Results Categorized by BMI at Baseline: Placebo-Controlled Study in Schizophrenia, Safety Sample

	BMI <23		BMI 23-27		BMI >27	
	Placebo (n=54)	Aripiprazole (n=59)	Placebo (n=48)	Aripiprazole (n=39)	Placebo (n=49)	Aripiprazole (n=53)
Mean change from baseline (kg)	-0.5	-0.5	-0.6	-1.3	-1.5	-2.1
% with ≥7% increase BW	3.7%	6.8%	4.2%	5.1%	4.1%	5.7%

CYP2E1 enzymes. Aripiprazole also does not undergo direct glucuronidation. This suggests that an interaction of aripiprazole with inhibitors or inducers of these enzymes, or other factors, like smoking, is unlikely.

Both CYP3A4 and CYP2D6 are responsible for aripiprazole metabolism. Agents that induce CYP3A4 (eg, carbamazepine) could cause an increase in aripiprazole clearance and lower blood levels. Inhibitors of CYP3A4 (eg, ketoconazole) or CYP2D6 (eg, quinidine, fluoxetine, or paroxetine) can inhibit aripiprazole elimination and cause increased blood levels.

Ketoconazole and Other CYP3A4 Inhibitors

Coadministration of ketoconazole (200 mg/day for 14 days) with a 15 mg single dose of aripiprazole increased the AUC of aripiprazole and its active metabolite by 63% and 77%, respectively. The effect of a higher ketoconazole dose (400 mg/day) has not been studied. When ketoconazole is given concomitantly with aripiprazole, the aripiprazole dose should be reduced to one-half of its normal dose. Other strong inhibitors of CYP3A4 (itraconazole) would be expected to have similar effects and need similar dose reductions; moderate inhibitors (erythromycin, grapefruit juice) have not been studied. When the CYP3A4 inhibitor is withdrawn from the combination therapy, the aripiprazole dose should be increased.

Quinidine and Other CYP2D6 Inhibitors

Coadministration of a 10 mg single dose of aripiprazole with quinidine (166 mg/day for 13 days), a potent inhibitor of CYP2D6, increased the AUC of aripiprazole by 112% but decreased the AUC of its active metabolite, dehydro-aripiprazole, by 35%. Aripiprazole dose should be reduced to one-half of its normal dose when quinidine is given concomitantly with aripiprazole. Other significant inhibitors of CYP2D6, such as fluoxetine or paroxetine, would be expected to have similar effects and should lead to similar dose reductions. When the CYP2D6 inhibitor is withdrawn from the combination therapy, the aripiprazole dose should be increased. When adjunctive ABILIFY is administered to patients with Major Depressive Disorder, ABILIFY should be administered without dosage adjustment as specified in *DOSAGE AND ADMINISTRATION (2.3)*.

Carbamazepine and Other CYP3A4 Inducers

Coadministration of carbamazepine (200 mg twice daily), a potent CYP3A4 inducer, with aripiprazole (30 mg/day) resulted in an approximate 70% decrease in Cmax and AUC values of both aripiprazole and its active metabolite, dehydro-aripiprazole. When carbamazepine is added to aripiprazole therapy, aripiprazole dose should be doubled. Additional dose increases should be based on clinical evaluation. When carbamazepine is withdrawn from the combination therapy, the aripiprazole dose should be reduced.

7.2 Potential for ABILIFY to Affect Other Drugs

Aripiprazole is unlikely to cause clinically important pharmacokinetic interactions with drugs metabolized by cytochrome P450 enzymes. In *in vivo* studies, 10 mg/day to 30 mg/day doses of aripiprazole had no significant effect on metabolism by CYP2D6 (dextromethorphan), CYP2C9 (warfarin), CYP2C19 (omeprazole, warfarin), and CYP3A4 (dextromethorphan) substrates. Additionally, aripiprazole and dehydro-aripiprazole did not show potential for altering CYP1A2-mediated metabolism *in vitro*.

Alcohol

There was no significant difference between aripiprazole coadministered with ethanol and placebo coadministered with ethanol on performance of gross motor skills or stimulus response in healthy subjects. As with most psychoactive medications, patients should be advised to avoid alcohol while taking ABILIFY (aripiprazole).

7.3 Drugs Having No Clinically Important Interactions with ABILIFY

Famotidine

Coadministration of aripiprazole (given in a single dose of 15 mg) with a 40 mg single dose of the H_2 antagonist famotidine, a potent gastric acid blocker, decreased the solubility of aripiprazole and, hence, its rate of absorption, reducing by 37% and 21% the Cmax of aripiprazole and dehydro-aripiprazole, respectively, and by 13% and 15%, respectively, the extent of absorption (AUC). No dosage adjustment of aripiprazole is required when administered concomitantly with famotidine.

Valproate

When valproate (500 mg/day-1500 mg/day) and aripiprazole (30 mg/day) were coadministered, at steady-state the Cmax and AUC of aripiprazole were decreased by 25%. No dosage adjustment of aripiprazole is required when administered concomitantly with valproate.

When aripiprazole (30 mg/day) and valproate (1000 mg/day) were coadministered, at steady-state there were no clinically significant changes in the Cmax or AUC of valproate. No dosage adjustment of valproate is required when administered concomitantly with aripiprazole.

Lithium

A pharmacokinetic interaction of aripiprazole with lithium is unlikely because lithium is not bound to plasma proteins, is not metabolized, and is almost entirely excreted unchanged in urine. Coadministration of therapeutic doses of lithium (1200 mg/day-1800 mg/day) for 21 days with aripiprazole (30 mg/day) did not result in clinically significant changes in the pharmacokinetics of aripiprazole or its active metabolite, dehydro-aripiprazole (Cmax and AUC increased by less than 20%). No dosage adjustment of aripiprazole is required when administered concomitantly with lithium.

Coadministration of aripiprazole (30 mg/day) with lithium (900 mg/day) did not result in clinically significant changes in the pharmacokinetics of lithium. No dosage adjustment of lithium is required when administered concomitantly with aripiprazole.

Dextromethorphan

Aripiprazole at doses of 10 mg/day to 30 mg/day for 14 days had no effect on dextromethorphan's O-dealkylation to its major metabolite, dextrorphan, a pathway dependent on CYP2D6 activity. Aripiprazole also had no effect on dextromethorphan's N-demethylation to its metabolite 3-methyoxymorphinan, a pathway dependent on CYP3A4 activity. No dosage adjustment of dextromethorphan is required when administered concomitantly with aripiprazole.

Warfarin

Aripiprazole 10 mg/day for 14 days had no effect on the pharmacokinetics of R-warfarin and S-warfarin or on the pharmacodynamic end point of International Normalized Ratio, indicating the lack of a clinically relevant effect of aripiprazole on CYP2C9 and CYP2C19 metabolism or the binding of highly protein-bound warfarin. No dosage adjustment of warfarin is required when administered concomitantly with aripiprazole.

Omeprazole

Aripiprazole 10 mg/day for 15 days had no effect on the pharmacokinetics of a single 20 mg dose of omeprazole, a CYP2C19 substrate, in healthy subjects. No dosage adjustment of omeprazole is required when administered concomitantly with aripiprazole.

Lorazepam

Coadministration of lorazepam injection (2 mg) and aripiprazole injection (15 mg) to healthy subjects (n=40: 35 males and 5 females; ages 19-45 years old) did not result in clinically important changes in the pharmacokinetics of either drug. No dosage adjustment of aripiprazole is required when administered concomitantly with lorazepam. However, the intensity of sedation was greater with the combination as compared to that observed with aripiprazole alone and the orthostatic hypotension observed was greater with the combination as compared to that observed with lorazepam alone *[see WARNINGS AND PRECAUTIONS (5.6)]*.

Escitalopram

Coadministration of 10 mg/day oral doses of aripiprazole for 14 days to healthy subjects had no effect on the steady-state pharmacokinetics of 10 mg/day escitalopram, a substrate of CYP2C19 and CYP3A4. No dosage adjustment of escitalopram is required when aripiprazole is added to escitalopram.

Venlafaxine

Coadministration of 10 mg/day to 20 mg/day oral doses of aripiprazole for 14 days to healthy subjects had no effect on the steady-state pharmacokinetics of venlafaxine and O-desmethylvenlafaxine following 75 mg/day venlafaxine XR, a CYP2D6 substrate. No dosage adjustment of venlafaxine is required when aripiprazole is added to venlafaxine.

Fluoxetine, Paroxetine, and Sertraline

A population pharmacokinetic analysis in patients with Major Depressive Disorder showed no substantial change in plasma concentrations of fluoxetine (20 mg/day or 40 mg/day), paroxetine CR (37.5 mg/day or 50 mg/day), or sertraline (100 mg/day or 150 mg/day) dosed to steady-state. The steady-state plasma concentrations of fluoxetine and norfluoxetine increased by about 18% and 36%, respectively and concentrations of paroxetine decreased by about 27%. The steady-state plasma concentrations of sertraline and desmethylsertraline were not substantially changed when these antidepressant therapies were coadministered with aripiprazole. Aripiprazole dosing was 2 mg/day to 15 mg/day (when given with fluoxetine or paroxetine) or 2 mg/day to 20 mg/day (when given with sertraline).

8 USE IN SPECIFIC POPULATIONS

In general, no dosage adjustment for ABILIFY (aripiprazole) is required on the basis of a patient's age, gender, race, smoking status, hepatic function, or renal function *[see DOSAGE AND ADMINISTRATION (2.5)]*.

8.1 Pregnancy

Pregnancy Category C: In animal studies, aripiprazole demonstrated developmental toxicity, including possible teratogenic effects in rats and rabbits.

Pregnant rats were treated with oral doses of 3 mg/kg/day, 10 mg/kg/day, and 30 mg/kg/day (1 times, 3 times, and 10 times the maximum recommended human dose [MRHD] on a mg/m^2 basis) of aripiprazole during the period of organogenesis. Gestation was slightly prolonged at 30 mg/kg. Treatment caused a slight delay in fetal development, as evidenced by decreased fetal weight (30 mg/kg), undescended testes (30 mg/kg), and delayed skeletal ossification (10 mg/kg and 30 mg/kg). There were no adverse effects on embryofetal or pup survival. Delivered offspring had decreased bodyweights (10 mg/kg and 30 mg/kg), and increased incidences of hepatodiaphragmatic nodules and diaphragmatic hernia at 30 mg/kg (the other dose groups were not examined for these findings). A low incidence of diaphragmatic hernia was also seen in the fetuses exposed to 30 mg/kg. Postnatally, delayed vaginal opening was seen at 10 mg/kg and 30 mg/kg and impaired reproductive performance (decreased fertility rate, corpora lutea, implants, live fetuses, and increased post-implantation loss, likely mediated through effects on female offspring) was seen at 30 mg/kg. Some maternal toxicity was seen at 30 mg/kg; however, there was no evidence to suggest that these developmental effects were secondary to maternal toxicity.

In pregnant rats receiving aripiprazole injection intravenously (3 mg/kg/day, 9 mg/kg/day, and 27 mg/kg/day) during the period of organogenesis, decreased fetal weight and delayed skeletal ossification were seen at the highest dose, which also caused some maternal toxicity.

Pregnant rabbits were treated with oral doses of 10 mg/kg/day, 30 mg/kg/day, and 100 mg/kg/day (2 times, 3 times, and 11 times human exposure at MRHD based on AUC and 6 times, 19 times, and 65 times the MRHD based on mg/m^2) of aripiprazole during the period of organogenesis. Decreased maternal food consumption and increased abortions were seen at 100 mg/kg. Treatment caused increased fetal mortality (100 mg/kg), decreased fetal weight (30 mg/kg and 100 mg/kg), increased incidence of a skeletal abnormality (fused sternebrae at 30 mg/kg and 100 mg/kg), and minor skeletal variations (100 mg/kg).

In pregnant rabbits receiving aripiprazole injection intravenously (3 mg/kg/day, 10 mg/kg/day, and 30 mg/kg/day) during the period of organogenesis, the highest dose, which caused pronounced maternal toxicity, resulted in decreased fetal weight, increased fetal abnormalities (primarily skeletal), and decreased fetal skeletal ossification. The fetal no-effect dose was 10 mg/kg, which produced 15 times the human exposure at the MRHD based on AUC and is 6 times the MRHD based on mg/m^2.

In a study in which rats were treated with oral doses of 3 mg/kg/day, 10 mg/kg/day, and 30 mg/kg/day (1 times, 3 times, and 10 times the MRHD on a mg/m^2 basis) of aripiprazole perinatally and postnatally (from day 17 of gestation through day 21 postpartum), slight maternal toxicity and slightly prolonged gestation were seen at 30 mg/kg. An increase in stillbirths and decreases in pup weight (persisting into adulthood) and survival were seen at this dose.

In rats receiving aripiprazole injection intravenously (3 mg/kg/day, 8 mg/kg/day, and 20 mg/kg/day) from day 6 of gestation through day 20 postpartum, an increase in stillbirths was seen at 8 mg/kg and 20 mg/kg, and decreases in early postnatal pup weights and survival were seen at 20 mg/kg. These doses produced some maternal toxicity. There were no effects on postnatal behavioral and reproductive development.

There are no adequate and well-controlled studies in pregnant women. It is not known whether aripiprazole can cause fetal harm when administered to a pregnant woman or can affect reproductive capacity. Aripiprazole should be used during pregnancy only if the potential benefit outweighs the potential risk to the fetus.

8.2 Labor and Delivery

The effect of aripiprazole on labor and delivery in humans is unknown.

8.3 Nursing Mothers

Aripiprazole was excreted in milk of rats during lactation. It is not known whether aripiprazole or its metabolites are excreted in human milk. It is recommended that women receiving aripiprazole should not breast-feed.

8.4 Pediatric Use

Safety and effectiveness in pediatric patients with Major Depressive Disorder or agitation associated with Schizophrenia or Bipolar Mania have not been established.

Safety and effectiveness in pediatric patients with Schizophrenia were established in a 6-week, placebo-controlled clinical trial in 202 pediatric patients aged 13 to 17 years *[see INDICATIONS AND USAGE (1.1), DOSAGE AND ADMINISTRATION (2.1), ADVERSE REACTIONS (6.2), and CLINICAL STUDIES (14.1)]*.

Safety and effectiveness in pediatric patients with Bipolar Mania were established in a 4-week, placebo-controlled clinical trial in 197 pediatric patients aged 10 to 17 years. *[See INDICATIONS AND USAGE (1.2), DOSAGE AND ADMINISTRATION (2.2), ADVERSE REACTIONS (6.2), and CLINICAL STUDIES (14.2)]*.

The pharmacokinetics of aripiprazole and dehydro-aripiprazole in pediatric patients 10 to 17 years of age were similar to those in adults after correcting for the differences in body weights.

8.5 Geriatric Use

In formal single-dose pharmacokinetic studies (with aripiprazole given in a single dose of 15 mg), aripiprazole clearance was 20% lower in elderly (≥65 years) subjects compared to younger adult subjects (18 to 64 years). There was no detectable age effect, however, in the population pharmacokinetic analysis in Schizophrenia patients. Also, the pharmacokinetics of aripiprazole after multiple doses in elderly patients appeared similar to that observed in young, healthy subjects. No dosage adjustment is recommended for elderly patients *[see also BOXED WARNING and WARNINGS AND PRECAUTIONS (5.1)]*.

Of the 12,925 patients treated with oral aripiprazole in clinical trials, 1061 (8%) were ≥65 years old and 799 (6%) were ≥75 years old. The majority (97%) of the 799 patients were diagnosed with Dementia of the Alzheimer's type.

Placebo-controlled studies of oral aripiprazole in Schizophrenia, Bipolar Mania, or Major Depressive Disorder did not include sufficient numbers of subjects aged 65 and over to determine whether they respond differently from younger subjects.

Of the 749 patients treated with aripiprazole injection in clinical trials, 99 (13%) were ≥65 years old and 78 (10%) were ≥75 years old. Placebo-controlled studies of aripiprazole injection in patients with agitation associated with Schizophrenia or Bipolar Mania did not include sufficient numbers of subjects aged 65 and over to determine whether they respond differently from younger subjects.

Continued on next page

Abilify—Cont.

Studies of elderly patients with psychosis associated with Alzheimer's disease have suggested that there may be a different tolerability profile in this population compared to younger patients with Schizophrenia *[see also BOXED WARNING and WARNINGS AND PRECAUTIONS (5.1)]*. The safety and efficacy of ABILIFY in the treatment of patients with psychosis associated with Alzheimer's disease has not been established. If the prescriber elects to treat such patients with ABILIFY, vigilance should be exercised.

8.6 Renal Impairment

In patients with severe renal impairment (creatinine clearance <30 mL/min), Cmax of aripiprazole (given in a single dose of 15 mg) and dehydro-aripiprazole increased by 36% and 53%, respectively, but AUC was 15% lower for aripiprazole and 7% higher for dehydro-aripiprazole. Renal excretion of both unchanged aripiprazole and dehydro-aripiprazole is less than 1% of the dose. No dosage adjustment is required in subjects with renal impairment.

8.7 Hepatic Impairment

In a single-dose study (15 mg of aripiprazole) in subjects with varying degrees of liver cirrhosis (Child-Pugh Classes A, B, and C), the AUC of aripiprazole, compared to healthy subjects, increased 31% in mild HI, increased 8% in moderate HI, and decreased 20% in severe HI. None of these differences would require dose adjustment.

8.8 Gender

Cmax and AUC of aripiprazole and its active metabolite, dehydro-aripiprazole, are 30% to 40% higher in women than in men, and correspondingly, the apparent oral clearance of aripiprazole is lower in women. These differences, however, are largely explained by differences in body weight (25%) between men and women. No dosage adjustment is recommended based on gender.

8.9 Race

Although no specific pharmacokinetic study was conducted to investigate the effects of race on the disposition of aripiprazole, population pharmacokinetic evaluation revealed no evidence of clinically significant race-related differences in the pharmacokinetics of aripiprazole. No dosage adjustment is recommended based on race.

8.10 Smoking

Based on studies utilizing human liver enzymes *in vitro*, aripiprazole is not a substrate for CYP1A2 and also does not undergo direct glucuronidation. Smoking should, therefore, not have an effect on the pharmacokinetics of aripiprazole. Consistent with these *in vitro* results, population pharmacokinetic evaluation did not reveal any significant pharmacokinetic differences between smokers and nonsmokers. No dosage adjustment is recommended based on smoking status.

9 DRUG ABUSE AND DEPENDENCE

9.1 Controlled Substance

ABILIFY is not a controlled substance.

9.2 Abuse and Dependence

Aripiprazole has not been systematically studied in humans for its potential for abuse, tolerance, or physical dependence. In physical dependence studies in monkeys, withdrawal symptoms were observed upon abrupt cessation of dosing. While the clinical trials did not reveal any tendency for any drug-seeking behavior, these observations were not systematic and it is not possible to predict on the basis of this limited experience the extent to which a CNS-active drug will be misused, diverted, and/or abused once marketed. Consequently, patients should be evaluated carefully for a history of drug abuse, and such patients should be observed closely for signs of ABILIFY misuse or abuse (eg, development of tolerance, increases in dose, drug-seeking behavior).

10 OVERDOSAGE

MedDRA terminology has been used to classify the adverse reactions.

10.1 Human Experience

A total of 76 cases of deliberate or accidental overdosage with oral aripiprazole have been reported worldwide. These include overdoses with oral aripiprazole alone and in combination with other substances. No fatality was reported from these cases. Of the 44 cases with known outcome, 33 cases recovered without sequelae and one case recovered with sequelae (mydriasis and feeling abnormal). The largest known case of acute ingestion with a known outcome involved 1080 mg of oral aripiprazole (36 times the maximum recommended daily dose) in a patient who fully recovered. Included in the 76 cases are 10 cases of deliberate or accidental overdosage in children (age 12 and younger) involving oral aripiprazole ingestions up to 195 mg with no fatalities.

Common adverse reactions (reported in at least 5% of all overdose cases) reported with oral aripiprazole overdosage (alone or in combination with other substances) include vomiting, somnolence, and tremor. Other clinically important signs and symptoms observed in one or more patients with aripiprazole overdoses (alone or with other substances) include acidosis, aggression, aspartate aminotransferase increased, atrial fibrillation, bradycardia, coma, confusional state, convulsion, blood creatine phosphokinase increased, depressed level of consciousness, hypertension, hypokalemia, hypotension, lethargy, loss of consciousness, QRS complex prolonged, QT prolonged, pneumonia aspiration, respiratory arrest, status epilepticus, and tachycardia.

10.2 Management of Overdosage

No specific information is available on the treatment of overdose with aripiprazole. An electrocardiogram should be obtained in case of overdosage and if QT interval prolongation is present, cardiac monitoring should be instituted. Otherwise, management of overdose should concentrate on supportive therapy, maintaining an adequate airway, oxygenation and ventilation, and management of symptoms. Close medical supervision and monitoring should continue until the patient recovers.

Charcoal: In the event of an overdose of ABILIFY, an early charcoal administration may be useful in partially preventing the absorption of aripiprazole. Administration of 50 g of activated charcoal, one hour after a single 15 mg oral dose of aripiprazole, decreased the mean AUC and Cmax of aripiprazole by 50%.

Hemodialysis: Although there is no information on the effect of hemodialysis in treating an overdose with aripiprazole, hemodialysis is unlikely to be useful in overdose management since aripiprazole is highly bound to plasma proteins.

11 DESCRIPTION

Aripiprazole is a psychotropic drug that is available as ABILIFY® (aripiprazole) tablets, ABILIFY® DISCMELT™ (aripiprazole) orally disintegrating tablets, ABILIFY® (aripiprazole) oral solution, and ABILIFY® (aripiprazole) injection, a solution for intramuscular injection. Aripiprazole is 7-[4-[4-(2,3-dichlorophenyl)-1-piperazinyl] butoxy]-3,4-dihydrocarbostyril. The empirical formula is $C_{23}H_{27}Cl_2N_3O_2$ and its molecular weight is 448.38. The chemical structure is:

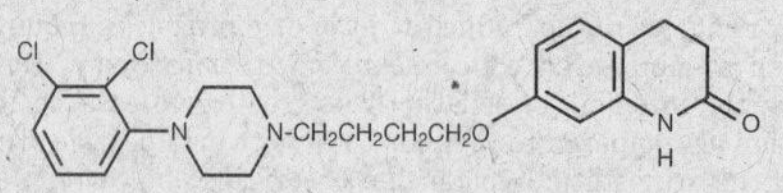

ABILIFY Tablets are available in 2 mg, 5 mg, 10 mg, 15 mg, 20 mg, and 30 mg strengths. Inactive ingredients include cornstarch, hydroxypropyl cellulose, lactose monohydrate, magnesium stearate, and microcrystalline cellulose. Colorants include ferric oxide (yellow or red) and FD&C Blue No. 2 Aluminum Lake.

ABILIFY DISCMELT Orally Disintegrating Tablets are available in 10 mg and 15 mg strengths. Inactive ingredients include acesulfame potassium, aspartame, calcium silicate, croscarmellose sodium, crospovidone, crème de vanilla (natural and artificial flavors), magnesium stearate, microcrystalline cellulose, silicon dioxide, tartaric acid, and xylitol. Colorants include ferric oxide (yellow or red) and FD&C Blue No. 2 Aluminum Lake.

ABILIFY Oral Solution is a clear, colorless to light yellow solution available in a concentration of 1 mg/mL. The inactive ingredients for this solution include disodium edetate, fructose, glycerin, dl-lactic acid, methylparaben, propylene glycol, propylparaben, sodium hydroxide, sucrose, and purified water. The oral solution is flavored with natural orange cream and other natural flavors.

ABILIFY Injection is available in single-dose vials as a ready-to-use, 9.75 mg/1.3 mL (7.5 mg/mL) clear, colorless, sterile, aqueous solution for intramuscular use only. Inactive ingredients for this solution include 150 mg/mL of sulfobutylether β-cyclodextrin (SBECD), tartaric acid, sodium hydroxide, and water for injection.

12 CLINICAL PHARMACOLOGY

12.1 Mechanism of Action

The mechanism of action of aripiprazole, as with other drugs having efficacy in Schizophrenia, Bipolar Disorder, Major Depressive Disorder, and agitation associated with Schizophrenia or Bipolar Disorder, is unknown. However, it has been proposed that the efficacy of aripiprazole is mediated through a combination of partial agonist activity at D_2 and 5-HT_{1A} receptors and antagonist activity at 5-HT_{2A} receptors. Actions at receptors other than D_2, 5-HT_{1A}, and 5-HT_{2A} may explain some of the other clinical effects of aripiprazole (eg, the orthostatic hypotension observed with aripiprazole may be explained by its antagonist activity at adrenergic $alpha_1$ receptors).

12.2 Pharmacodynamics

Aripiprazole exhibits high affinity for dopamine D_2 and D_3, serotonin 5-HT_{1A} and 5-HT_{2A} receptors (K_i values of 0.34 nM, 0.8 nM, 1.7 nM, and 3.4 nM, respectively), moderate affinity for dopamine D_4, serotonin 5-HT_{2C} and 5-HT_7, $alpha_1$-adrenergic and histamine H_1 receptors (K_i values of 44 nM, 15 nM, 39 nM, 57 nM, and 61 nM, respectively), and moderate affinity for the serotonin reuptake site (K_i=98 nM). Aripiprazole has no appreciable affinity for cholinergic muscarinic receptors (IC_{50}>1000 nM). Aripiprazole functions as a partial agonist at the dopamine D_2 and the serotonin 5-HT_{1A} receptors, and as an antagonist at serotonin 5-HT_{2A} receptor.

12.3 Pharmacokinetics

ABILIFY activity is presumably primarily due to the parent drug, aripiprazole, and to a lesser extent, to its major metabolite, dehydro-aripiprazole, which has been shown to have affinities for D_2 receptors similar to the parent drug and represents 40% of the parent drug exposure in plasma. The mean elimination half-lives are about 75 hours and 94 hours for aripiprazole and dehydro-aripiprazole, respectively. Steady-state concentrations are attained within 14 days of dosing for both active moieties. Aripiprazole accumulation is predictable from single-dose pharmacokinetics. At steady-state, the pharmacokinetics of aripiprazole are dose-proportional. Elimination of aripiprazole is mainly through hepatic metabolism involving two P450 isozymes, CYP2D6 and CYP3A4.

Pharmacokinetic studies showed that ABILIFY DISCMELT Orally Disintegrating Tablets are bioequivalent to ABILIFY Tablets.

ORAL ADMINISTRATION

Absorption

Tablet: Aripiprazole is well absorbed after administration of the tablet, with peak plasma concentrations occurring within 3 hours to 5 hours; the absolute oral bioavailability of the tablet formulation is 87%. ABILIFY can be administered with or without food. Administration of a 15 mg ABILIFY Tablet with a standard high-fat meal did not significantly affect the Cmax or AUC of aripiprazole or its active metabolite, dehydro-aripiprazole, but delayed Tmax by 3 hours for aripiprazole and 12 hours for dehydro-aripiprazole.

Oral Solution: Aripiprazole is well absorbed when administered orally as the solution. At equivalent doses, the plasma concentrations of aripiprazole from the solution were higher than that from the tablet formulation. In a relative bioavailability study comparing the pharmacokinetics of 30 mg aripiprazole as the oral solution to 30 mg aripiprazole tablets in healthy subjects, the solution to tablet ratios of geometric mean Cmax and AUC values were 122% and 114%, respectively *[see DOSAGE AND ADMINISTRATION (2.6)]*. The single-dose pharmacokinetics of aripiprazole were linear and dose-proportional between the doses of 5 mg to 30 mg.

Distribution

The steady-state volume of distribution of aripiprazole following intravenous administration is high (404 L or 4.9 L/kg), indicating extensive extravascular distribution. At therapeutic concentrations, aripiprazole and its major metabolite are greater than 99% bound to serum proteins, primarily to albumin. In healthy human volunteers administered 0.5 mg/day to 30 mg/day aripiprazole for 14 days, there was dose-dependent D_2 receptor occupancy indicating brain penetration of aripiprazole in humans.

Metabolism and Elimination

Aripiprazole is metabolized primarily by three biotransformation pathways: dehydrogenation, hydroxylation, and N-dealkylation. Based on *in vitro* studies, CYP3A4 and CYP2D6 enzymes are responsible for dehydrogenation and hydroxylation of aripiprazole, and N-dealkylation is catalyzed by CYP3A4. Aripiprazole is the predominant drug moiety in the systemic circulation. At steady-state, dehydro-aripiprazole, the active metabolite, represents about 40% of aripiprazole AUC in plasma.

Approximately 8% of Caucasians lack the capacity to metabolize CYP2D6 substrates and are classified as poor metabolizers (PM), whereas the rest are extensive metabolizers (EM). PMs have about an 80% increase in aripiprazole exposure and about a 30% decrease in exposure to the active metabolite compared to EMs, resulting in about a 60% higher exposure to the total active moieties from a given dose of aripiprazole compared to EMs. Coadministration of ABILIFY with known inhibitors of CYP2D6, such as quinidine or fluoxetine in EMs, approximately doubles aripiprazole plasma exposure, and dose adjustment is needed *[see DRUG INTERACTIONS (7.1)]*. The mean elimination half-lives are about 75 hours and 146 hours for aripiprazole in EMs and PMs, respectively. Aripiprazole does not inhibit or induce the CYP2D6 pathway.

Following a single oral dose of [^{14}C]-labeled aripiprazole, approximately 25% and 55% of the administered radioactivity was recovered in the urine and feces, respectively. Less than 1% of unchanged aripiprazole was excreted in the urine and approximately 18% of the oral dose was recovered unchanged in the feces.

INTRAMUSCULAR ADMINISTRATION

In two pharmacokinetic studies of aripiprazole injection administered intramuscularly to healthy subjects, the median times to the peak plasma concentrations were at 1 hour and 3 hours. A 5 mg intramuscular injection of aripiprazole had an absolute bioavailability of 100%. The geometric mean maximum concentration achieved after an intramuscular dose was on average 19% higher than the Cmax of the oral tablet. While the systemic exposure over 24 hours was generally similar between aripiprazole injection given intramuscularly and after oral tablet administration, the aripiprazole AUC in the first 2 hours after an intramuscular injection was 90% greater than the AUC after the same dose as a tablet. In stable patients with Schizophrenia or Schizoaffective Disorder, the pharmacokinetics of aripiprazole after intramuscular administration were linear over a dose range of 1 mg to 45 mg. Although the metabolism of aripiprazole injection was not systematically evaluated, the intramuscular route of administration would not be expected to alter the metabolic pathways.

13 NONCLINICAL TOXICOLOGY

13.1 Carcinogenesis, Mutagenesis, Impairment of Fertility

Carcinogenesis

Lifetime carcinogenicity studies were conducted in ICR mice and in Sprague-Dawley (SD) and F344 rats. Aripiprazole was administered for 2 years in the diet at doses of 1 mg/kg/day, 3 mg/kg/day, 10 mg/kg/day, and 30 mg/kg/day to ICR mice and 1 mg/kg/day, 3 mg/kg/day, and 10 mg/kg/day to F344 rats (0.2 times to 5 times and 0.3 times to 3 times the maximum recommended human dose [MRHD] based on mg/m^2, respectively). In addition, SD rats were dosed orally for 2 years at 10 mg/kg/day, 20 mg/kg/day,

40 mg/kg/day, and 60 mg/kg/day (3 times to 19 times the MRHD based on mg/m^2). Aripiprazole did not induce tumors in male mice or rats. In female mice, the incidences of pituitary gland adenomas and mammary gland adenocarcinomas and adenoacanthomas were increased at dietary doses of 3 mg/kg/day to 30 mg/kg/day (0.1 times to 0.9 times human exposure at MRHD based on AUC and 0.5 times to 5 times the MRHD based on mg/m^2). In female rats, the incidence of mammary gland fibroadenomas was increased at a dietary dose of 10 mg/kg/day (0.1 times human exposure at MRHD based on AUC and 3 times the MRHD based on mg/m^2); and the incidences of adrenocortical carcinomas and combined adrenocortical adenomas/carcinomas were increased at an oral dose of 60 mg/kg/day (14 times human exposure at MRHD based on AUC and 19 times the MRHD based on mg/m^2).

Proliferative changes in the pituitary and mammary gland of rodents have been observed following chronic administration of other antipsychotic agents and are considered prolactin-mediated. Serum prolactin was not measured in the aripiprazole carcinogenicity studies. However, increases in serum prolactin levels were observed in female mice in a 13-week dietary study at the doses associated with mammary gland and pituitary tumors. Serum prolactin was not increased in female rats in 4-week and 13-week dietary studies at the dose associated with mammary gland tumors. The relevance for human risk of the findings of prolactin-mediated endocrine tumors in rodents is unknown.

Mutagenesis

The mutagenic potential of aripiprazole was tested in the *in vitro* bacterial reverse-mutation assay, the *in vitro* bacterial DNA repair assay, the *in vitro* forward gene mutation assay in mouse lymphoma cells, the *in vitro* chromosomal aberration assay in Chinese hamster lung (CHL) cells, the *in vivo* micronucleus assay in mice, and the unscheduled DNA synthesis assay in rats. Aripiprazole and a metabolite (2,3-DCPP) were clastogenic in the *in vitro* chromosomal aberration assay in CHL cells with and without metabolic activation. The metabolite, 2,3-DCPP, produced increases in numerical aberrations in the *in vitro* assay in CHL cells in the absence of metabolic activation. A positive response was obtained in the *in vivo* micronucleus assay in mice; however, the response was due to a mechanism not considered relevant to humans.

Impairment of Fertility

Female rats were treated with oral doses of 2 mg/kg/day, 6 mg/kg/day, and 20 mg/kg/day (0.6 times, 2 times, and 6 times the maximum recommended human dose [MRHD] on a mg/m^2 basis) of aripiprazole from 2 weeks prior to mating through day 7 of gestation. Estrus cycle irregularities and increased corpora lutea were seen at all doses, but no impairment of fertility was seen. Increased pre-implantation loss was seen at 6 mg/kg and 20 mg/kg and decreased fetal weight was seen at 20 mg/kg.

Male rats were treated with oral doses of 20 mg/kg/day, 40 mg/kg/day, and 60 mg/kg/day (6 times, 13 times, and 19 times the MRHD on a mg/m^2 basis) of aripiprazole from 9 weeks prior to mating through mating. Disturbances in spermatogenesis were seen at 60 mg/kg and prostate atrophy was seen at 40 mg/kg and 60 mg/kg, but no impairment of fertility was seen.

13.2 Animal Toxicology and/or Pharmacology

Aripiprazole produced retinal degeneration in albino rats in a 26-week chronic toxicity study at a dose of 60 mg/kg and in a 2-year carcinogenicity study at doses of 40 mg/kg and 60 mg/kg. The 40 mg/kg and 60 mg/kg doses are 13 times and 19 times the maximum recommended human dose (MRHD) based on mg/m^2 and 7 times to 14 times human exposure at MRHD based on AUC. Evaluation of the retinas of albino mice and of monkeys did not reveal evidence of retinal degeneration. Additional studies to further evaluate the mechanism have not been performed. The relevance of this finding to human risk is unknown.

14 CLINICAL STUDIES

14.1 Schizophrenia

Adult

The efficacy of ABILIFY in the treatment of Schizophrenia was evaluated in five short-term (4-week and 6-week), placebo-controlled trials of acutely relapsed inpatients who predominantly met DSM-III/IV criteria for Schizophrenia. Four of the five trials were able to distinguish aripiprazole from placebo, but one study, the smallest, did not. Three of these studies also included an active control group consisting of either risperidone (one trial) or haloperidol (two trials), but they were not designed to allow for a comparison of ABILIFY and the active comparators.

In the four positive trials for ABILIFY, four primary measures were used for assessing psychiatric signs and symptoms. The Positive and Negative Syndrome Scale (PANSS) is a multi-item inventory of general psychopathology used to evaluate the effects of drug treatment in Schizophrenia. The PANSS positive subscale is a subset of items in the PANSS that rates seven positive symptoms of Schizophrenia (delusions, conceptual disorganization, hallucinatory behavior, excitement, grandiosity, suspiciousness/persecution, and hostility). The PANSS negative subscale is a subset of items in the PANSS that rates seven negative symptoms of Schizophrenia (blunted affect, emotional withdrawal, poor rapport, passive apathetic withdrawal, difficulty in abstract thinking, lack of spontaneity/flow of conversation, stereotyped thinking). The Clinical Global Impression (CGI) assessment reflects the impression of a skilled observer, fully familiar with the manifestations of Schizophrenia, about the overall clinical state of the patient.

In a 4-week trial (n=414) comparing two fixed doses of ABILIFY (15 mg/day or 30 mg/day) and haloperidol (10 mg/day) to placebo, both doses of ABILIFY were superior to placebo in the PANSS total score, PANSS positive subscale, and CGI-severity score. In addition, the 15 mg dose was superior to placebo in the PANSS negative subscale.

In a 4-week trial (n=404) comparing two fixed doses of ABILIFY (20 mg/day or 30 mg/day) and risperidone (6 mg/day) to placebo, both doses of ABILIFY were superior to placebo in the PANSS total score, PANSS positive subscale, PANSS negative subscale, and CGI-severity score.

In a 6-week trial (n=420) comparing three fixed doses of ABILIFY (10 mg/day, 15 mg/day, or 20 mg/day) to placebo, all three doses of ABILIFY were superior to placebo in the PANSS total score, PANSS positive subscale, and the PANSS negative subscale.

In a 6-week trial (n=367) comparing three fixed doses of ABILIFY (2 mg/day, 5 mg/day, or 10 mg/day) to placebo, the 10 mg dose of ABILIFY was superior to placebo in the PANSS total score, the primary outcome measure of the study. The 2 mg and 5 mg doses did not demonstrate superiority to placebo on the primary outcome measure.

In a fifth study, a 4-week trial (n=103) comparing ABILIFY in a range of 5 mg/day to 30 mg/day or haloperidol 5 mg/day to 20 mg/day to placebo, haloperidol was superior to placebo, in the Brief Psychiatric Rating Scale (BPRS), a multi-item inventory of general psychopathology traditionally used to evaluate the effects of drug treatment in psychosis, and in a responder analysis based on the CGI-severity score, the primary outcomes for that trial. ABILIFY was only significantly different compared to placebo in a responder analysis based on the CGI-severity score.

Thus, the efficacy of 10 mg, 15 mg, 20 mg, and 30 mg daily doses was established in two studies for each dose. Among these doses, there was no evidence that the higher dose groups offered any advantage over the lowest dose group of these studies.

An examination of population subgroups did not reveal any clear evidence of differential responsiveness on the basis of age, gender, or race.

A longer-term trial enrolled 310 inpatients or outpatients meeting DSM-IV criteria for Schizophrenia who were, by history, symptomatically stable on other antipsychotic medications for periods of 3 months or longer. These patients were discontinued from their antipsychotic medications and randomized to ABILIFY 15 mg/day or placebo for up to 26 weeks of observation for relapse. Relapse during the double-blind phase was defined as CGI-Improvement score of ≥5 (minimally worse), scores ≥5 (moderately severe) on the hostility or uncooperativeness items of the PANSS, or ≥20% increase in the PANSS total score. Patients receiving ABILIFY 15 mg/day experienced a significantly longer time to relapse over the subsequent 26 weeks compared to those receiving placebo.

Pediatric

The efficacy of ABILIFY (aripiprazole) in the treatment of Schizophrenia in pediatric patients (13 to 17 years of age) was evaluated in one 6-week, placebo-controlled trial of outpatients who met DSM-IV criteria for Schizophrenia and had a PANSS score ≥70 at baseline. In this trial (n=302) comparing two fixed doses of ABILIFY (10 mg/day or 30 mg/day) to placebo, ABILIFY was titrated starting from 2 mg/day to the target dose in 5 days in the 10 mg/day treatment arm and in 11 days in the 30 mg/day treatment arm. Both doses of ABILIFY were superior to placebo in the PANSS total score, the primary outcome measure of the study. The 30 mg/day dosage was not shown to be more efficacious than the 10 mg/day dose.

14.2 Bipolar Disorder

Adults

The efficacy of ABILIFY in the treatment of acute manic episodes was established in two 3-week, placebo-controlled trials in hospitalized patients who met the DSM-IV criteria for Bipolar I Disorder with manic or mixed episodes (in one trial, 21% of placebo and 42% of ABILIFY-treated patients had data beyond two weeks). These trials included patients with or without psychotic features and with or without a rapid-cycling course.

The primary instrument used for assessing manic symptoms was the Young Mania Rating Scale (Y-MRS), an 11-item clinician-rated scale traditionally used to assess the degree of manic symptomatology (irritability, disruptive/aggressive behavior, sleep, elevated mood, speech, increased activity, sexual interest, language/thought disorder, thought content, appearance, and insight) in a range from 0 (no manic features) to 60 (maximum score). A key secondary instrument included the Clinical Global Impression - Bipolar (CGI-BP) Scale.

In the two positive, 3-week, placebo-controlled trials (n=268; n=248) which evaluated ABILIFY 30 mg, once daily (with a starting dose of 30 mg/day and an allowed reduction to 15 mg/day), ABILIFY was superior to placebo in the reduction of Y-MRS total score and CGI-BP Severity of Illness score (mania).

A trial was conducted in patients meeting DSM-IV criteria for Bipolar I Disorder with a recent manic or mixed episode who had been stabilized on open-label ABILIFY and who had maintained a clinical response for at least 6 weeks. The first phase of this trial was an open-label stabilization period in which inpatients and outpatients were clinically stabilized and then maintained on open-label ABILIFY (15 mg/day or 30 mg/day, with a starting dose of 30 mg/day) for at least 6 consecutive weeks. One hundred sixty-one outpatients were then randomized in a double-blind fashion, to either the same dose of ABILIFY they were on at the end of the stabilization and maintenance period or placebo and were then monitored for manic or depressive relapse. During the randomization phase, ABILIFY was superior to placebo on time to the number of combined affective relapses (manic plus depressive), the primary outcome measure for this study. The majority of these relapses were due to manic rather than depressive symptoms. There is insufficient data to know whether ABILIFY is effective in delaying the time to occurrence of depression in patients with Bipolar I Disorder.

An examination of population subgroups did not reveal any clear evidence of differential responsiveness on the basis of age and gender; however, there were insufficient numbers of patients in each of the ethnic groups to adequately assess inter-group differences.

Pediatric Patients

The efficacy of ABILIFY in the treatment of Bipolar I Disorder in pediatric patients (10 to 17 years of age) was evaluated in one four-week placebo-controlled trial (n=296) of outpatients who met DSM-IV criteria for Bipolar I Disorder manic or mixed episodes with or without psychotic features and had a Y-MRS score ≥20 at baseline. This double-blind, placebo-controlled trial compared two fixed doses of ABILIFY (10 mg/day or 30 mg/day) to placebo. The ABILIFY dose was started at 2 mg/day, which was titrated to 5 mg/day after 2 days, and to the target dose in 5 days in the 10 mg/day treatment arm and in 13 days in the 30 mg/day treatment arm. Both doses of ABILIFY were superior to placebo in change from baseline to week 4 on the Y-MRS total score.

14.3 Adjunctive Treatment of Major Depressive Disorder

The efficacy of ABILIFY in the adjunctive treatment of Major Depressive Disorder was demonstrated in two short-term (6-week), placebo-controlled trials of adult patients meeting DSM-IV criteria for Major Depressive Disorder who had had an inadequate response to prior antidepressant therapy (1 to 3 courses) in the current episode and who had also demonstrated an inadequate response to 8 weeks of prospective antidepressant therapy (paroxetine controlled-release, venlafaxine extended-release, fluoxetine, escitalopram, or sertraline). Inadequate response for prospective treatment was defined as less than 50% improvement on the 17-item version of the Hamilton Depression Rating Scale (HAMD17), minimal HAMD17 score of 14, and a Clinical Global Impressions Improvement rating of no better than minimal improvement. Inadequate response to prior treatment was defined as less than 50% improvement as perceived by the patient after a minimum of 6 weeks of antidepressant therapy at or above the minimal effective dose.

The primary instrument used for assessing depressive symptoms was the Montgomery-Asberg Depression Rating Scale (MADRS), a 10-item clinician-rated scale used to assess the degree of depressive symptomatology (apparent sadness, reported sadness, inner tension, reduced sleep, reduced appetite, concentration difficulties, lassitude, inability to feel, pessimistic thoughts, and suicidal thoughts). The key secondary instrument was the Sheehan Disability Scale (SDS), a 3-item self-rated instrument used to assess the impact of depression on three domains of functioning (work/school, social life, and family life) with each item scored from 0 (not at all) to 10 (extreme).

In the two trials (n=381, n=362), ABILIFY was superior to placebo in reducing mean MADRS total scores. In one study, ABILIFY was also superior to placebo in reducing the mean SDS score.

In both trials, patients received ABILIFY adjunctive to antidepressants at a dose of 5 mg/day. Based on tolerability and efficacy, doses could be adjusted by 5 mg increments, one week apart. Allowable doses were: 2 mg/day, 5 mg/day, 10 mg/day, 15 mg/day, and for patients who were not on potent CYP2D6 inhibitors fluoxetine and paroxetine, 20 mg/day. The mean final dose at the end point for the two trials was 10.7 mg/day and 11.4 mg/day.

An examination of population subgroups did not reveal evidence of differential response based on age, choice of prospective antidepressant, or race. With regard to gender, a smaller mean reduction on the MADRS total score was seen in males than in females.

14.4 Agitation Associated with Schizophrenia or Bipolar Mania

The efficacy of intramuscular aripiprazole for injection for the treatment of agitation was established in three short-term (24-hour), placebo-controlled trials in agitated inpatients from two diagnostic groups: Schizophrenia and Bipolar I Disorder (manic or mixed episodes, with or without psychotic features). Each of the trials included a single active comparator treatment arm of either haloperidol injection (Schizophrenia studies) or lorazepam injection (Bipolar Mania study). Patients could receive up to three injections during the 24-hour treatment periods; however, patients could not receive the second injection until after the initial 2-hour period when the primary efficacy measure was assessed. Patients enrolled in the trials needed to be: (1) judged by the clinical investigators as clinically agitated and clinically appropriate candidates for treatment with intramuscular medication, and (2) exhibiting a level of agitation that met or exceeded a threshold score of ≥15 on the

Continued on next page

Abilify—Cont.

five items comprising the Positive and Negative Syndrome Scale (PANSS) Excited Component (ie, poor impulse control, tension, hostility, uncooperativeness, and excitement items) with at least two individual item scores ≥4 using a 1-7 scoring system (1 = absent, 4 = moderate, 7 = extreme). In the studies, the mean baseline PANSS Excited Component score was 19, with scores ranging from 15 to 34 (out of a maximum score of 35), thus suggesting predominantly moderate levels of agitation with some patients experiencing mild or severe levels of agitation. The primary efficacy measure used for assessing agitation signs and symptoms in these trials was the change from baseline in the PANSS Excited Component at 2 hours post-injection. A key secondary measure was the Clinical Global Impression of Improvement (CGI-I) Scale. The results of the trials follow:

In a placebo-controlled trial in agitated inpatients predominantly meeting DSM-IV criteria for Schizophrenia (n=350), four fixed aripiprazole injection doses of 1 mg, 5.25 mg, 9.75 mg, and 15 mg were evaluated. At 2 hours post-injection, the 5.25 mg, 9.75 mg, and 15 mg doses were statistically superior to placebo in the PANSS Excited Component and on the CGI-I Scale.

In a second placebo-controlled trial in agitated inpatients predominantly meeting DSM-IV criteria for Schizophrenia (n=445), one fixed aripiprazole injection dose of 9.75 mg was evaluated. At 2 hours post-injection, aripiprazole for injection was statistically superior to placebo in the PANSS Excited Component and on the CGI-I Scale.

In a placebo-controlled trial in agitated inpatients meeting DSM-IV criteria for Bipolar I Disorder (manic or mixed) (n=291), two fixed aripiprazole injection doses of 9.75 mg and 15 mg were evaluated. At 2 hours post-injection, both doses were statistically superior to placebo in the PANSS Excited Component.

Examination of population subsets (age, race, and gender) did not reveal any differential responsiveness on the basis of these subgroupings.

16 HOW SUPPLIED/STORAGE AND HANDLING

16.1 How Supplied

ABILIFY® (aripiprazole) Tablets have markings on one side and are available in the strengths and packages listed in Table 13.

[See table 13 above]

ABILIFY® DISCMELT™ (aripiprazole) Orally Disintegrating Tablets are round tablets with markings on either side. ABILIFY DISCMELT is available in the strengths and packages listed in Table 14.

[See table 14 above]

ABILIFY® (aripiprazole) Oral Solution (1 mg/mL) is supplied in child-resistant bottles along with a calibrated oral dosing cup. ABILIFY Oral Solution is available as follows:

150 mL bottle   NDC 59148-013-15

ABILIFY® (aripiprazole) Injection for intramuscular use is available as a ready-to-use, 9.75 mg/1.3 mL (7.5 mg/mL) solution in clear, Type 1 glass vials as follows:

9.75 mg/1.3 mL single-dose vial   NDC 59148-016-65

16.2 Storage

Tablets

Store at 25° C (77° F); excursions permitted between 15° C to 30° C (59° F to 86° F) [see USP Controlled Room Temperature].

Oral Solution

Store at 25° C (77° F); excursions permitted between 15° C to 30° C (59° F to 86° F) [see USP Controlled Room Temperature]. Opened bottles of ABILIFY Oral Solution can be used for up to 6 months after opening, but not beyond the expiration date on the bottle. The bottle and its contents should be discarded after the expiration date.

Injection

Store at 25° C (77° F); excursions permitted between 15° C to 30° C (59° F to 86° F) [see USP Controlled Room Temperature]. Protect from light by storing in the original container. Retain in carton until time of use.

17 PATIENT COUNSELING INFORMATION

See Medication Guide (17.2)

17.1 Information for Patients

Physicians are advised to discuss the following issues with patients for whom they prescribe ABILIFY:

Increased Mortality in Elderly Patients with Dementia-Related Psychosis

Patients and caregivers should be advised that elderly patients with dementia-related psychoses treated with atypical antipsychotic drugs are at increased risk of death compared with placebo. ABILIFY is not approved for elderly patients with dementia-related psychosis [see WARNINGS AND PRECAUTIONS (5.1)].

Clinical Worsening of Depression and Suicide Risk

Patients, their families, and their caregivers should be encouraged to be alert to the emergence of anxiety, agitation, panic attacks, insomnia, irritability, hostility, aggressiveness, impulsivity, akathisia (psychomotor restlessness), hypomania, mania, other unusual changes in behavior, worsening of depression, and suicidal ideation, especially early during antidepressant treatment and when the dose is adjusted up or down. Families and caregivers of patients should be advised to look for the emergence of such symptoms on a day-to-day basis, since changes may be abrupt. Such symptoms should be reported to the patient's prescriber or health professional, especially if they are severe, abrupt in onset, or were not part of the patient's presenting

Table 13: ABILIFY Tablet Presentations

Tablet Strength	Tablet Color/Shape	Tablet Markings	Pack Size	NDC Code
2 mg	green modified rectangle	"A-006" and "2"	Bottle of 30	59148-006-13
5 mg	blue modified rectangle	"A-007" and "5"	Bottle of 30 Blister of 100	59148-007-13 59148-007-35
10 mg	pink modified rectangle	"A-008" and "10"	Bottle of 30 Blister of 100	59148-008-13 59148-008-35
15 mg	yellow round	"A-009" and "15"	Bottle of 30 Blister of 100	59148-009-13 59148-009-35
20 mg	white round	"A-010" and "20"	Bottle of 30 Blister of 100	59148-010-13 59148-010-35
30 mg	pink round	"A-011" and "30"	Bottle of 30 Blister of 100	59148-011-13 59148-011-35

Table 14: ABILIFY DISCMELT Orally Disintegrating Tablet Presentations

Tablet Strength	Tablet Color	Tablet Markings	Pack Size	NDC Code
10 mg	pink (with scattered specks)	"A" and "640" "10"	Blister of 30	59148-640-23
15 mg	yellow (with scattered specks)	"A" and "641" "15"	Blister of 30	59148-641-23

symptoms. Symptoms such as these may be associated with an increased risk for suicidal thinking and behavior and indicate a need for very close monitoring and possibly changes in the medication [see WARNINGS AND PRECAUTIONS (5.2)].

Prescribers or other health professionals should inform patients, their families, and their caregivers about the benefits and risks associated with treatment with ABILIFY and should counsel them in its appropriate use. A patient Medication Guide about "Antidepressant Medicines, Depression and other Serious Mental Illness, and Suicidal Thoughts or Actions" is available for ABILIFY. The prescriber or health professional should instruct patients, their families, and their caregivers to read the Medication Guide and should assist them in understanding its contents. Patients should be given the opportunity to discuss the contents of the Medication Guide and to obtain answers to any questions they may have. It should be noted that ABILIFY is not approved as a single agent for treatment of depression and has not been evaluated in pediatric Major Depressive Disorder.

Use of Orally Disintegrating Tablet

Do not open the blister until ready to administer. For single tablet removal, open the package and peel back the foil on the blister to expose the tablet. Do not push the tablet through the foil because this could damage the tablet. Immediately upon opening the blister, using dry hands, remove the tablet and place the entire ABILIFY DISCMELT Orally Disintegrating Tablet on the tongue. Tablet disintegration occurs rapidly in saliva. It is recommended that ABILIFY DISCMELT be taken without liquid. However, if needed, it can be taken with liquid. Do not attempt to split the tablet.

Interference with Cognitive and Motor Performance

Because aripiprazole may have the potential to impair judgment, thinking, or motor skills, patients should be cautioned about operating hazardous machinery, including automobiles, until they are reasonably certain that aripiprazole therapy does not affect them adversely [see WARNINGS AND PRECAUTIONS (5.8)].

Pregnancy

Patients should be advised to notify their physician if they become pregnant or intend to become pregnant during therapy with ABILIFY [see USE IN SPECIFIC POPULATIONS (8.1)].

Nursing

Patients should be advised not to breast-feed an infant if they are taking ABILIFY [see USE IN SPECIFIC POPULATIONS (8.3)].

Concomitant Medication

Patients should be advised to inform their physicians if they are taking, or plan to take, any prescription or over-the-counter drugs, since there is a potential for interactions [see DRUG INTERACTIONS (7)].

Alcohol

Patients should be advised to avoid alcohol while taking ABILIFY [see DRUG INTERACTIONS (7.2)].

Heat Exposure and Dehydration

Patients should be advised regarding appropriate care in avoiding overheating and dehydration [see WARNINGS AND PRECAUTIONS (5.9)].

Sugar Content

Patients should be advised that each mL of ABILIFY Oral Solution contains 400 mg of sucrose and 200 mg of fructose.

Phenylketonurics

Phenylalanine is a component of aspartame. Each ABILIFY DISCMELT Orally Disintegrating Tablet contains the following amounts: 10 mg - 1.12 mg phenylalanine and 15 mg - 1.68 mg phenylalanine.

Tablets manufactured by Otsuka Pharmaceutical Co, Ltd, Tokyo, 101-8535 Japan or Bristol-Myers Squibb Company, Princeton, NJ 08543 USA

Orally Disintegrating Tablets, Oral Solution, and Injection manufactured by Bristol-Myers Squibb Company, Princeton, NJ 08543 USA

Distributed and marketed by Otsuka America Pharmaceutical, Inc, Rockville, MD 20850 USA

Marketed by Bristol-Myers Squibb Company, Princeton, NJ 08543 USA

Bristol-Myers Squibb Company

Otsuka

Otsuka America Pharmaceutical, Inc.

US Patent Nos: 5,006,528; 6,977,257; and 7,115,587

1239550A2   0308L-0818   Rev February 2008

© 2008, Otsuka Pharmaceutical Co, Ltd, Tokyo, 101-8535 Japan

17.2 Medication Guide

MEDICATION GUIDE

ABILIFY® (a BIL ĭ fī)

Generic name: aripiprazole

Antidepressant Medicines, Depression and other Serious Mental Illnesses, and Suicidal Thoughts or Actions

Read the Medication Guide that comes with your or your family member's antidepressant medicine. This Medication Guide is only about the risk of suicidal thoughts and actions with antidepressant medicines. **Talk to your, or your family member's, healthcare provider** about:

• all risks and benefits of treatment with antidepressant medicines

• all treatment choices for depression or other serious mental illness

What is the most important information I should know about antidepressant medicines, depression and other serious mental illnesses, and suicidal thoughts or actions?

1. Antidepressant medicines may increase suicidal thoughts or actions in some children, teenagers, and young adults within the first few months of treatment.

2. Depression and other serious mental illnesses are the most important causes of suicidal thoughts and actions. Some people may have a particularly high risk of having suicidal thoughts or actions. These include people who have (or have a family history of) bipolar illness (also called manic-depressive illness) or suicidal thoughts or actions.

3. How can I watch for and try to prevent suicidal thoughts and actions in myself or a family member?

• Pay close attention to any changes, especially sudden changes, in mood, behaviors, thoughts, or feelings. This is very important when an antidepressant medicine is started or when the dose is changed.

• Call the healthcare provider right away to report new or sudden changes in mood, behavior, thoughts, or feelings.

• Keep all follow-up visits with the healthcare provider as scheduled. Call the healthcare provider between visits as needed, especially if you have concerns about symptoms.

Call a healthcare provider right away if you or your family member has any of the following symptoms, especially if they are new, worse, or worry you:

• thoughts about suicide or dying

• attempts to commit suicide

• new or worse depression

• new or worse anxiety

• feeling very agitated or restless

• panic attacks

• trouble sleeping (insomnia)

• new or worse irritability

• acting aggressive, being angry, or violent

• acting on dangerous impulses

• an extreme increase in activity and talking (mania)
• other unusual changes in behavior or mood

What else do I need to know about antidepressant medicines?

• **Never stop an antidepressant medicine without first talking to a healthcare provider.** Stopping an antidepressant medicine suddenly can cause other symptoms.
• **Antidepressants are medicines used to treat depression and other illnesses.** It is important to discuss all the risks of treating depression and also the risks of not treating it. Patients and their families or other caregivers should discuss all treatment choices with the healthcare provider, not just the use of antidepressants.
• **Antidepressant medicines have other side effects.** Talk to the healthcare provider about the side effects of the medicine prescribed for you or your family member.
• **Antidepressant medicines can interact with other medicines.** Know all of the medicines that you or your family member takes. Keep a list of all medicines to show the healthcare provider. Do not start new medicines without first checking with your healthcare provider.
• **Not all antidepressant medicines prescribed for children are FDA approved for use in children.** Talk to your child's healthcare provider for more information.

This Medication Guide has been approved by the U.S. Food and Drug Administration for all antidepressants.

It should be noted that ABILIFY is approved to be added to an antidepressant when the response from the antidepressant alone is not adequate. ABILIFY is not approved for pediatric patients with depression.

Call your doctor for medical advice about side effects. You may report side effects to FDA at 1-800-FDA-1088.

ABILIFY is a trademark of Otsuka Pharmaceutical Company.

1239550A2 0308L-0818 Rev February 2008

© 2008, Otsuka Pharmaceutical Co, Ltd, Tokyo, 101-8535 Japan

Parke-Davis

A Division of Warner-Lambert Company LLC
A Pfizer Company
235 EAST 42ND STREET
NEW YORK, NY 10017-5755

For updates to the product information listed below, please check the Pfizer Web site, http://www.pfizerpro.com, or call (800) 438-1985. For complete product listing, please see the Manufacturer's' Index.

For Medical Information, Contact:
(800) 438-1985
24 hours a day, seven days a week

Distribution:
1855 Shelby Oaks Drive North
Memphis, TN 38134
(901) 387-5200

Customer Service:
(800) 533-4535

LIPITOR® ℞

[lĭ′pĭ-tōr]
(Atorvastatin Calcium)
Tablets

Prescribing information for this product, which appears on pages 2457–2462 of the 2008 PDR, has been completely revised as follows. Please write "See Supplement A" next to the product heading.

DESCRIPTION

LIPITOR® (atorvastatin calcium) is a synthetic lipid-lowering agent. Atorvastatin is an inhibitor of 3-hydroxy-3-methylglutaryl-coenzyme A (HMG-CoA) reductase. This enzyme catalyzes the conversion of HMG-CoA to mevalonate, an early and rate-limiting step in cholesterol biosynthesis.

Atorvastatin calcium is [R-(R*,R*)]-2-(4-fluorophenyl)-ß, δ-dihydroxy-5-(1-methylethyl)-3-phenyl-4-[(phenylamino) carbonyl]-1H-pyrrole-1-heptanoic acid, calcium salt (2:1) trihydrate. The empirical formula of atorvastatin calcium is $(C_{33}H_{34}FN_2O_5)_2Ca \cdot 3H_2O$ and its molecular weight is 1209.42. Its structural formula is:

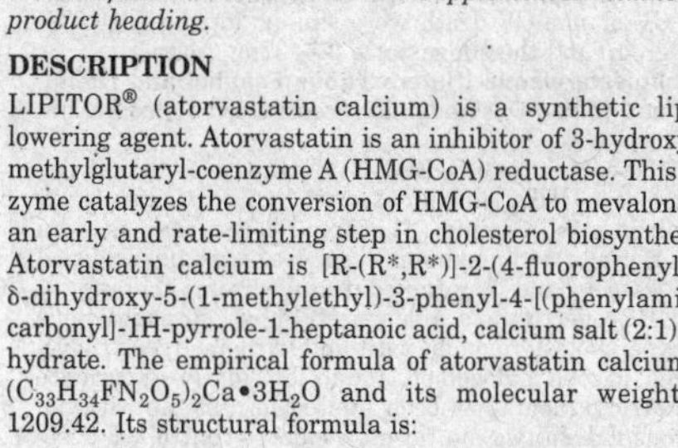

Atorvastatin calcium is a white to off-white crystalline powder that is insoluble in aqueous solutions of pH 4 and below. Atorvastatin calcium is very slightly soluble in distilled water, pH 7.4 phosphate buffer, and acetonitrile, slightly soluble in ethanol, and freely soluble in methanol.

LIPITOR tablets for oral administration contain 10, 20, 40 or 80 mg atorvastatin and the following inactive ingredients: calcium carbonate, USP; candelilla wax, FCC; croscarmellose sodium, NF; hydroxypropyl cellulose, NF; lactose monohydrate, NF; magnesium stearate, NF; microcrystalline cellulose, NF; Opadry White YS-1-7040 (hypromellose, polyethylene glycol, talc, titanium dioxide); polysorbate 80, NF; simethicone emulsion.

CLINICAL PHARMACOLOGY

Mechanism of Action

Atorvastatin is a selective, competitive inhibitor of HMG-CoA reductase, the rate-limiting enzyme that converts 3-hydroxy-3-methylglutaryl-coenzyme A to mevalonate, a precursor of sterols, including cholesterol. Cholesterol and triglycerides circulate in the bloodstream as part of lipoprotein complexes. With ultracentrifugation, these complexes separate into HDL (high-density lipoprotein), IDL (intermediate-density lipoprotein), LDL (low-density lipoprotein), and VLDL (very-low-density lipoprotein) fractions. Triglycerides (TG) and cholesterol in the liver are incorporated into VLDL and released into the plasma for delivery to peripheral tissues. LDL is formed from VLDL and is catabolized primarily through the high-affinity LDL receptor. Clinical and pathologic studies show that elevated plasma levels of total cholesterol (total-C), LDL-cholesterol (LDL-C), and apolipoprotein B (apo B) promote human atherosclerosis and are risk factors for developing cardiovascular disease, while increased levels of HDL-C are associated with a decreased cardiovascular risk.

In animal models, LIPITOR lowers plasma cholesterol and lipoprotein levels by inhibiting HMG-CoA reductase and cholesterol synthesis in the liver and by increasing the number of hepatic LDL receptors on the cell-surface to enhance uptake and catabolism of LDL; LIPITOR also reduces LDL production and the number of LDL particles. LIPITOR reduces LDL-C in some patients with homozygous familial hypercholesterolemia (FH), a population that rarely responds to other lipid-lowering medication(s).

A variety of clinical studies have demonstrated that elevated levels of total-C, LDL-C, and apo B (a membrane complex for LDL-C) promote human atherosclerosis. Similarly, decreased levels of HDL-C (and its transport complex, apo A) are associated with the development of atherosclerosis. Epidemiologic investigations have established that cardiovascular morbidity and mortality vary directly with the level of total-C and LDL-C, and inversely with the level of HDL-C.

LIPITOR reduces total-C, LDL-C, and apo B in patients with homozygous and heterozygous FH, nonfamilial forms of hypercholesterolemia, and mixed dyslipidemia. LIPITOR also reduces VLDL-C and TG and produces variable increases in HDL-C and apolipoprotein A-1. LIPITOR reduces total-C, LDL-C, VLDL-C, apo B, TG, and non-HDL-C, and increases HDL-C in patients with isolated hypertriglyceridemia. LIPITOR reduces intermediate density lipoprotein cholesterol (IDL-C) in patients with dysbetalipoproteinemia.

Like LDL, cholesterol-enriched triglyceride-rich lipoproteins, including VLDL, intermediate density lipoprotein (IDL), and remnants, can also promote atherosclerosis. Elevated plasma triglycerides are frequently found in a triad with low HDL-C levels and small LDL particles, as well as in association with non-lipid metabolic risk factors for coronary heart disease. As such, total plasma TG has not consistently been shown to be an independent risk factor for CHD. Furthermore, the independent effect of raising HDL or lowering TG on the risk of coronary and cardiovascular morbidity and mortality has not been determined.

Pharmacodynamics

Atorvastatin as well as some of its metabolites are pharmacologically active in humans. The liver is the primary site of action and the principal site of cholesterol synthesis and LDL clearance. Drug dosage rather than systemic drug concentration correlates better with LDL-C reduction. Individualization of drug dosage should be based on therapeutic response (see DOSAGE AND ADMINISTRATION).

Pharmacokinetics and Drug Metabolism

Absorption: Atorvastatin is rapidly absorbed after oral administration; maximum plasma concentrations occur within 1 to 2 hours. Extent of absorption increases in proportion to atorvastatin dose. The absolute bioavailability of atorvastatin (parent drug) is approximately 14% and the systemic availability of HMG-CoA reductase inhibitory activity is approximately 30%. The low systemic availability is attributed to presystemic clearance in gastrointestinal mucosa and/or hepatic first-pass metabolism. Although food decreases the rate and extent of drug absorption by approximately 25% and 9%, respectively, as assessed by Cmax and AUC, LDL-C reduction is similar whether atorvastatin is given with or without food. Plasma atorvastatin concentrations are lower (approximately 30% for Cmax and AUC) following evening drug administration compared with morning. However, LDL-C reduction is the same regardless of the time of day of drug administration (see DOSAGE AND ADMINISTRATION).

Distribution: Mean volume of distribution of atorvastatin is approximately 381 liters. Atorvastatin is ≥98% bound to plasma proteins. A blood/plasma ratio of approximately 0.25 indicates poor drug penetration into red blood cells. Based on observations in rats, atorvastatin is likely to be secreted in human milk (see CONTRAINDICATIONS, Pregnancy and Lactation, and PRECAUTIONS, Nursing Mothers).

Metabolism: Atorvastatin is extensively metabolized to ortho- and parahydroxylated derivatives and various beta-oxidation products. *In vitro* inhibition of HMG-CoA reductase by ortho- and parahydroxylated metabolites is equivalent to that of atorvastatin. Approximately 70% of circulating inhibitory activity for HMG-CoA reductase is attributed to active metabolites. *In vitro* studies suggest the importance of atorvastatin metabolism by cytochrome P450 3A4, consistent with increased plasma concentrations of atorvastatin in humans following coadministration with erythromycin, a known inhibitor of this isozyme (see PRECAUTIONS, Drug Interactions). In animals, the ortho-hydroxy metabolite undergoes further glucuronidation.

Excretion: Atorvastatin and its metabolites are eliminated primarily in bile following hepatic and/or extra-hepatic metabolism; however, the drug does not appear to undergo enterohepatic recirculation. Mean plasma elimination half-life of atorvastatin in humans is approximately 14 hours, but the half-life of inhibitory activity for HMG-CoA reductase is 20 to 30 hours due to the contribution of active metabolites. Less than 2% of a dose of atorvastatin is recovered in urine following oral administration.

Special Populations

Geriatric: Plasma concentrations of atorvastatin are higher (approximately 40% for Cmax and 30% for AUC) in healthy elderly subjects (age ≥65 years) than in young adults. Clinical data suggest a greater degree of LDL-lowering at any dose of drug in the elderly patient population compared to younger adults (see PRECAUTIONS section; Geriatric Use subsection).

Pediatric: Pharmacokinetic data in the pediatric population are not available.

Gender: Plasma concentrations of atorvastatin in women differ from those in men (approximately 20% higher for Cmax and 10% lower for AUC); however, there is no clinically significant difference in LDL-C reduction with LIPITOR between men and women.

Renal Insufficiency: Renal disease has no influence on the plasma concentrations or LDL-C reduction of atorvastatin; thus, dose adjustment in patients with renal dysfunction is not necessary (see DOSAGE AND ADMINISTRATION).

Hemodialysis: While studies have not been conducted in patients with end-stage renal disease, hemodialysis is not expected to significantly enhance clearance of atorvastatin since the drug is extensively bound to plasma proteins.

Hepatic Insufficiency: In patients with chronic alcoholic liver disease, plasma concentrations of atorvastatin are markedly increased. Cmax and AUC are each 4-fold greater in patients with Childs-Pugh A disease. Cmax and AUC are approximately 16-fold and 11-fold increased, respectively, in patients with Childs-Pugh B disease (see CONTRAINDICATIONS).

Clinical Studies

Prevention of Cardiovascular Disease

In the Anglo-Scandinavian Cardiac Outcomes Trial (ASCOT), the effect of LIPITOR (atorvastatin calcium) on fatal and non-fatal coronary heart disease was assessed in 10,305 hypertensive patients 40-80 years of age (mean of 63 years), without a previous myocardial infarction and with TC levels ≤251 mg/dl (6.5 mmol/l). Additionally all patients had at least 3 of the following cardiovascular risk factors: male gender (81.1%), age >55 years (84.5%), smoking (33.2%), diabetes (24.3%), history of CHD in a first-degree relative (26%), TC:HDL >6 (14.3%), peripheral vascular disease (5.1%), left ventricular hypertrophy (14.4%), prior cerebrovascular event (9.8%), specific ECG abnormality (14.3%), proteinuria/albuminuria (62.4%). In this double-blind, placebo-controlled study patients were treated with anti-hypertensive therapy (Goal BP <140/90 mm Hg for non-diabetic patients, <130/80 mm Hg for diabetic patients) and allocated to either LIPITOR 10 mg daily (n=5168) or placebo (n=5137), using a covariate adaptive method which took into account the distribution of nine baseline characteristics of patients already enrolled and minimized the imbalance of those characteristics across the groups. Patients were followed for a median duration of 3.3 years.

The effect of 10 mg/day of LIPITOR on lipid levels was similar to that seen in previous clinical trials.

LIPITOR significantly reduced the rate of coronary events [either fatal coronary heart disease (46 events in the placebo group vs. 40 events in the LIPITOR group) or nonfatal MI (108 events in the placebo group vs. 60 events in the LIPITOR group)] with a relative risk reduction of 36% [(based on incidences of 1.9% for LIPITOR vs. 3.0% for placebo), p=0.0005 (see Figure 1)]. The risk reduction was consistent regardless of age, smoking status, obesity or presence of renal dysfunction. The effect of LIPITOR was seen regardless of baseline LDL levels. Due to the small number of events, results for women were inconclusive.

Figure 1: Effect of LIPITOR 10 mg/day on Cumulative Incidence of Nonfatal Myocardial Infarction or Coronary Heart Disease Death (in ASCOT-LLA)

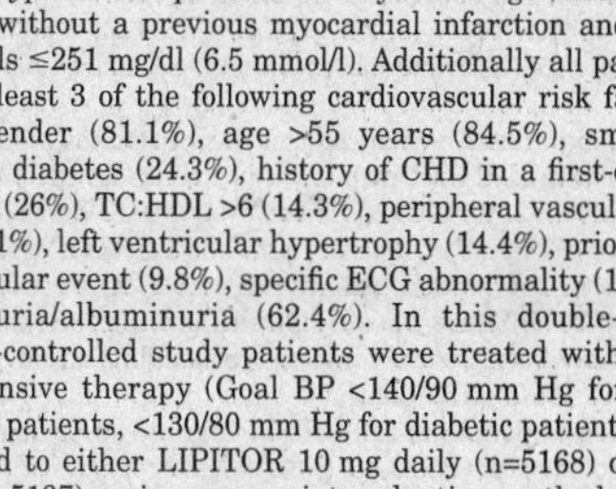

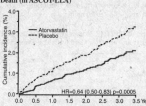

LIPITOR also significantly decreased the relative risk for revascularization procedures by 42%. Although the reduction of fatal and non-fatal strokes did not reach a pre-defined significance level (p=0.01), a favorable trend was observed with a 26% relative risk reduction (incidences of 1.7% for LIPITOR and 2.3% for placebo). There was no significant difference between the treatment groups for death

Continued on next page

Lipitor—Cont.

due to cardiovascular causes (p=0.51) or noncardiovascular causes (p=0.17).

In the Collaborative Atorvastatin Diabetes Study (CARDS), the effect of LIPITOR (atorvastatin calcium) on cardiovascular disease (CVD) endpoints was assessed in 2838 subjects (94% White, 68% male), ages 40-75 with type 2 diabetes based on WHO criteria, without prior history of cardiovascular disease and with LDL≤160 mg/dL and TG ≤600 mg/dL. In addition to diabetes, subjects had 1 or more of the following risk factors: current smoking (23%), hypertension (80%), retinopathy (30%), or microalbuminuria (9%) or macroalbuminuria (3%). No subjects on hemodialysis were enrolled in the study. In this multicenter, placebo-controlled, double-blind clinical trial, subjects were randomly allocated to either LIPITOR 10 mg daily (1429) or placebo (1411) in a 1:1 ratio and were followed for a median duration of 3.9 years. The primary endpoint was the occurrence of any of the major cardiovascular events: myocardial infarction, acute CHD death, unstable angina, coronary revascularization, or stroke. The primary analysis was the time to first occurrence of the primary endpoint.

Baseline characteristics of subjects were: mean age of 62 years, mean HbA$_{1c}$ 7.7%; median LDL-C 120 mg/dL; median TC 207 mg/dL; median TG 151 mg/dL; median HDL-C 52mg/dL.

The effect of LIPITOR 10 mg/day on lipid levels was similar to that seen in previous clinical trials.

LIPITOR significantly reduced the rate of major cardiovascular events (primary endpoint events) (83 events in the LIPITOR group vs. 127 events in the placebo group) with a relative risk reduction of 37%, HR 0.63, 95% CI (0.48,0.83) (p=0.001) (see Figure 2). An effect of LIPITOR was seen regardless of age, sex, or baseline lipid levels.

Figure 2. Effect of LIPITOR 10 mg/day on Time to Occurrence of Major Cardiovascular Event (myocardial infarction, acute CHD death, unstable angina, coronary revascularization, or stroke) in CARDS.

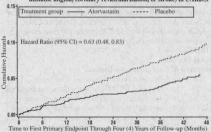

LIPITOR significantly reduced the risk of stroke by 48% (21 events in the LIPITOR group vs 39 events in the placebo group), HR 0.52, 95% CI (0.31,0.89) (p=0.016) and reduced the risk of MI by 42% (38 events in the LIPITOR group vs 64 events in the placebo group), HR 0.58, 95.1% CI (0.39, 0.86) (p=0.007). There was no significant difference between the treatment groups for angina, revascularization procedures, and acute CHD death.

There were 61 deaths in the LIPITOR group vs 82 deaths in the placebo group, (HR 0.73, p=0.059).

In the Treating to New Targets Study (TNT), the effect of LIPITOR 80 mg/day vs. LIPITOR 10 mg/day on the reduction in cardiovascular events was assessed in 10,001 subjects (94% white, 81% male, 38% ≥65 years) with clinically evident coronary heart disease who had achieved a target LDL-C level <130 mg/dL after completing an 8-week, open-label, run-in period with LIPITOR 10 mg/day. Subjects were randomly assigned to either 10 mg/day or 80 mg/day of LIPITOR and followed for a median duration of 4.9 years. The primary endpoint was the time-to-first occurrence of any of the following major cardiovascular events (MCVE): death due to CHD, non-fatal myocardial infarction, resuscitated cardiac arrest, and fatal and non-fatal stroke. The mean LDL-C, TC, TG, non-HDL and HDL cholesterol levels at 12 weeks were 73, 145, 128, 98 and 47 mg/dL during treatment with 80 mg of LIPITOR and 99, 177, 152, 129 and 48 mg/dL during treatment with 10 mg of LIPITOR.

Treatment with LIPITOR 80 mg/day significantly reduced the rate of MCVE (434 events in the 80mg/day group vs 548 events in the 10 mg/day group) with a relative risk reduction of 22%, HR 0.78, 95% CI (0.69,0.89), p=0.0002 (see Figure 3 and Table 1). The overall risk reduction was consistent regardless of age (<65, ≥65) or gender.

Figure 3. Effect of LIPITOR 80 mg/day vs. 10 mg/day on Time to Occurrence of Major Cardiovascular Events (TNT)

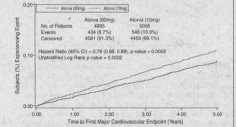

[See table 1 above]

Of the events that comprised the primary efficacy endpoint, treatment with LIPITOR 80 mg/day significantly reduced the rate of nonfatal, non-procedure related MI and fatal and non-fatal stroke, but not CHD death or resuscitated cardiac arrest (Table 1). Of the predefined secondary endpoints, treatment with LIPITOR 80 mg/day significantly reduced the rate of coronary revascularization, angina and hospitalization for heart failure, but not peripheral vascular disease. The reduction in the rate of CHF with hospitalization was only observed in the 8% of patients with a prior history of CHF.

There was no significant difference between the treatment groups for all-cause mortality (Table 1). The proportions of subjects who experienced cardiovascular death, including the components of CHD death and fatal stroke were numerically smaller in the LIPITOR 80 mg group than in the LIPITOR 10 mg treatment group. The proportions of subjects who experienced noncardiovascular death were numerically larger in the LIPITOR 80 mg group than in the LIPITOR 10 mg treatment group.

In the Incremental Decrease in Endpoints Through Aggressive Lipid Lowering Study (IDEAL), treatment with LIPITOR 80 mg/day was compared to treatment with simvastatin 20-40 mg/day in 8,888 subjects up to 80 years of age with a history of CHD to assess whether reduction in CV risk could be achieved. Patients were mainly male (81%), white (99%) with an average age of 61.7 years, and an average LDL-C of 121.5 mg/dL at randomization; 76% were on statin therapy. In this prospective, randomized, open-label, blinded endpoint (PROBE) trial with no run-in period, subjects were followed for a median duration of 4.8 years. The mean LDL-C, TC, TG, HDL and non-HDL cholesterol levels at Week 12 were 78, 145, 115, 45 and 100 mg/dL during treatment with 80 mg of LIPITOR and 105, 179, 142, 47 and 132 mg/dL during treatment with 20-40 mg of simvastatin.

There was no significant difference between the treatment groups for the primary endpoint, the rate of first major coronary event (fatal CHD, nonfatal MI and resuscitated car-

diac arrest): 411 (9.3%) in the LIPITOR 80 mg/day group vs. 463 (10.4%) in the simvastatin 20-40 mg/day group, HR 0.89, 95% CI (0.78,1.01), p=0.07.

There were no significant differences between the treatment groups for all-cause mortality: 366 (8.2%) in the LIPITOR 80 mg/day group vs. 374 (8.4%) in the simvastatin 20-40 mg/day group. The proportions of subjects who experienced CV or non-CV death were similar for the LIPITOR 80 mg group and the simvastatin 20-40 mg group.

Hypercholesterolemia (Heterozygous Familial and Nonfamilial) and Mixed Dyslipidemia (*Fredrickson* Types IIa and IIb)

LIPITOR reduces total-C, LDL-C, VLDL-C, apo B, and TG, and increases HDL-C in patients with hypercholesterolemia and mixed dyslipidemia. Therapeutic response is seen within 2 weeks, and maximum response is usually achieved within 4 weeks and maintained during chronic therapy.

LIPITOR is effective in a wide variety of patient populations with hypercholesterolemia, with and without hypertriglyceridemia, in men and women, and in the elderly. Experience in pediatric patients has been limited to patients with homozygous FH. In two multicenter, placebo-controlled, dose-response studies in patients with hypercholesterolemia, LIPITOR given as a single dose over 6 weeks significantly reduced total-C, LDL-C, apo B, and TG (Pooled results are provided in Table 2).

[See table 2 above]

In patients with *Fredrickson* Types IIa and IIb hyperlipoproteinemia pooled from 24 controlled trials, the median (25th and 75th percentile) percent changes from baseline in HDL-C for atorvastatin 10, 20, 40, and 80 mg were 6.4 (-1.4, 14), 8.7(0, 17), 7.8(0, 16), and 5.1 (-2.7, 15), respectively. Additionally, analysis of the pooled data demonstrated consistent and significant decreases in total-C, LDL-C, TG, total-C/HDL-C, and LDL-C/HDL-C.

In three multicenter, double-blind studies in patients with hypercholesterolemia, LIPITOR was compared to other HMG-CoA reductase inhibitors. After randomization, patients were treated for 16 weeks with either LIPITOR 10 mg per day or a fixed dose of the comparative agent (Table 3).

TABLE 1. Overview of Efficacy Results in TNT

Endpoint	Atorvastatin 10 mg (N=5006)		Atorvastatin 80 mg (N=4995)		HR[a] (95%CI)
PRIMARY ENDPOINT	n	(%)	n	(%)	
First major cardiovascular endpoint	548	(10.9)	434	(8.7)	0.78 (0.69, 0.89)
Components of the Primary Endpoint					
CHD death	127	(2.5)	101	(2.0)	0.80 (0.61, 1.03)
Nonfatal, non-procedure related MI	308	(6.2)	243	(4.9)	0.78 (0.66, 0.93)
Resuscitated cardiac arrest	26	(0.5)	25	(0.5)	0.96 (0.56, 1.67)
Stroke (fatal and non-fatal)	155	(3.1)	117	(2.3)	0.75 (0.59, 0.96)
SECONDARY ENDPOINTS*					
First CHF with hospitalization	164	(3.3)	122	(2.4)	0.74 (0.59, 0.94)
First PVD endpoint	282	(5.6)	275	(5.5)	0.97 (0.83, 1.15)
First CABG or other coronary revascularization procedure[b]	904	(18.1)	667	(13.4)	0.72 (0.65, 0.80)
First documented angina endpoint[b]	615	(12.3)	545	(10.9)	0.88 (0.79, 0.99)
All cause mortality	282	(5.6)	284	(5.7)	1.01 (0.85, 1.19)
Components of all cause mortality					
Cardiovascular death	155	(3.1)	126	(2.5)	0.81 (0.64, 1.03)
Noncardiovascular death	127	(2.5)	158	(3.2)	1.25 (0.99, 1.57)
Cancer death	75	(1.5)	85	(1.7)	1.13 (0.83, 1.55)
Other non-CV death	43	(0.9)	58	(1.2)	1.35 (0.91, 2.00)
Suicide, homicide and other traumatic non-CV death	9	(0.2)	15	(0.3)	1.67 (0.73, 3.82)

[a] Atorvastatin 80 mg: atorvastatin 10 mg
[b] component of other secondary endpoints
* secondary endpoints not included in primary endpoint
HR=hazard ratio; CHD=coronary heart disease; CI=confidence interval; MI=myocardial infarction; CHF=congestive heart failure; CV=cardiovascular; PVD=peripheral vascular disease; CABG=coronary artery bypass graft
Confidence intervals for the Secondary Endpoints were not adjusted for multiple comparisons

TABLE 2. Dose-Response in Patients With Primary Hypercholesterolemia (Adjusted Mean % Change From Baseline)[a]

Dose	N	TC	LDL-C	Apo B	TG	HDL-C	Non-HDL-C/HDL-C
Placebo	21	4	4	3	10	-3	7
10	22	-29	-39	-32	-19	6	-34
20	20	-33	-43	-35	-26	9	-41
40	21	-37	-50	-42	-29	6	-45
80	23	-45	-60	-50	-37	5	-53

[a] Results are pooled from 2 dose-response studies.

[See table 3 above]

The impact on clinical outcomes of the differences in lipid-altering effects between treatments shown in Table 3 is not known. Table 3 does not contain data comparing the effects of atorvastatin 10 mg and higher doses of lovastatin, pravastatin, and simvastatin. The drugs compared in the studies summarized in the table are not necessarily interchangeable.

Hypertriglyceridemia (*Fredrickson* Type IV)

The response to LIPITOR in 64 patients with isolated hypertriglyceridemia treated across several clinical trials is shown in the table below. For the atorvastatin-treated patients, median (min, max) baseline TG level was 565 (267-1502).

[See table 4 above]

Dysbetalipoproteinemia (*Fredrickson* Type III)

The results of an open-label crossover study of 16 patients (genotypes: 14 apo E2/E2 and 2 apo E3/E2) with dysbetalipoproteinemia (*Fredrickson* Type III) are shown in the table below.

[See table 5 above]

Homozygous Familial Hypercholesterolemia

In a study without a concurrent control group, 29 patients ages 6 to 37 years with homozygous FH received maximum daily doses of 20 to 80 mg of LIPITOR. The mean LDL-C reduction in this study was 18%. Twenty-five patients with a reduction in LDL-C had a mean response of 20% (range of 7% to 53%, median of 24%); the remaining 4 patients had 7% to 24% increases in LDL-C. Five of the 29 patients had absent LDL-receptor function. Of these, 2 patients also had a portacaval shunt and had no significant reduction in LDL-C. The remaining 3 receptor-negative patients had a mean LDL-C reduction of 22%.

Heterozygous Familial Hypercholesterolemia in Pediatric Patients

In a double-blind, placebo-controlled study followed by an open-label phase, 187 boys and postmenarchal girls 10-17 years of age (mean age 14.1 years) with heterozygous familial hypercholesterolemia (FH) or severe hypercholesterolemia were randomized to LIPITOR (n=140) or placebo (n=47) for 26 weeks and then all received LIPITOR for 26 weeks. Inclusion in the study required 1) a baseline LDL-C level ≥ 190 mg/dL or 2) a baseline LDL-C ≥ 160 mg/dL and a positive family history of FH or documented premature cardiovascular disease in a first- or second-degree relative. The mean baseline LDL-C value was 218.6 mg/dL (range: 138.5-385.0 mg/dL) in the LIPITOR group compared to 230.0 mg/dL (range: 160.0-324.5 mg/dL) in the placebo group. The dosage of LIPITOR (once daily) was 10 mg for the first 4 weeks and up-titrated to 20 mg if the LDL-C level was > 130 mg/dL. The number of LIPITOR-treated patients who required up-titration to 20 mg after Week 4 during the double-blind phase was 80 (57.1%).

LIPITOR significantly decreased plasma levels of total-C, LDL-C, triglycerides, and apolipoprotein B during the 26 week double-blind phase (see Table 6).

[See table 6 above]

The mean achieved LDL-C value was 130.7 mg/dL (range: 70.0-242.0 mg/dL) in the LIPITOR group compared to 228.5 mg/dL (range: 152.0-385.0 mg/dL) in the placebo group during the 26 week double-blind phase.

The safety and efficacy of doses above 20 mg have not been studied in controlled trials in children. The long-term efficacy of LIPITOR therapy in childhood to reduce morbidity and mortality in adulthood has not been established.

INDICATIONS AND USAGE

Prevention of Cardiovascular Disease

In adult patients without clinically evident coronary heart disease, but with multiple risk factors for coronary heart disease such as age, smoking, hypertension, low HDL-C, or a family history of early coronary heart disease, LIPITOR is indicated to:

• Reduce the risk of myocardial infarction

• Reduce the risk of stroke

• Reduce the risk for revascularization procedures and angina

In patients with type 2 diabetes, and without clinically evident coronary heart disease, but with multiple risk factors for coronary heart disease such as retinopathy, albuminuria, smoking, or hypertension, LIPITOR is indicated to:

• Reduce the risk of myocardial infarction

• Reduce the risk of stroke

In patients with clinically evident coronary heart disease, LIPITOR is indicated to:

• Reduce the risk of non-fatal myocardial infarction

• Reduce the risk of fatal and non-fatal stroke

• Reduce the risk for revascularization procedures

• Reduce the risk of hospitalization for CHF

• Reduce the risk of angina

Hypercholesterolemia

LIPITOR is indicated:

1. as an adjunct to diet to reduce elevated total-C, LDL-C, apo B, and TG levels and to increase HDL-C in patients with primary hypercholesterolemia (heterozygous familial and nonfamilial) and mixed dyslipidemia (*Fredrickson* Types IIa and IIb);

2. as an adjunct to diet for the treatment of patients with elevated serum TG levels (*Fredrickson* Type IV);

3. for the treatment of patients with primary dysbetalipoproteinemia (*Fredrickson* Type III) who do not respond

TABLE 3. Mean Percent Change From Baseline at Endpoint (Double-Blind, Randomized, Active-Controlled Trials)

Treatment (Daily Dose)	N	Total-C	LDL-C	Apo B	TG	HDL-C	Non-HDL-C/ HDL-C
Study 1							
Atorvastatin 10 mg	707	-27[a]	-36[a]	-28[a]	-17[a]	+7	-37[a]
Lovastatin 20 mg	191	-19	-27	-20	-6	+7	-28
95% CI for Diff [1]		-9.2, -6.5	-10.7, -7.1	-10.0, -6.5	-15.2, -7.1	-1.7, 2.0	-11.1, -7.1
Study 2							
Atorvastatin 10 mg	222	-25[b]	-35[b]	-27[b]	-17[b]	+6	-36[b]
Pravastatin 20 mg	77	-17	-23	-17	-9	+8	-28
95% CI for Diff [1]		-10.8, -6.1	-14.5, -8.2	-13.4, -7.4	-14.1, -0.7	-4.9, 1.6	-11.5, -4.1
Study 3							
Atorvastatin 10 mg	132	-29[c]	-37[c]	-34[c]	-23[c]	+7	-39[c]
Simvastatin 10 mg	45	-24	-30	-30	-15	+7	-33
95% CI for Diff [1]		-8.7, -2.7	-10.1, -2.6	-8.0, -1.1	-15.1, -0.7	-4.3, 3.9	-9.6, -1.9

[1] A negative value for the 95% CI for the difference between treatments favors atorvastatin for all except HDL-C, for which a positive value favors atorvastatin. If the range does not include 0, this indicates a statistically significant difference.
[a] Significantly different from lovastatin, ANCOVA, p ≤0.05
[b] Significantly different from pravastatin, ANCOVA, p ≤0.05
[c] Significantly different from simvastatin, ANCOVA, p ≤0.05

TABLE 4. Combined Patients With Isolated Elevated TG: Median (min, max) Percent Changes From Baseline

	Placebo (N=12)	Atorvastatin 10 mg (N=37)	Atorvastatin 20 mg (N=13)	Atorvastatin 80 mg (N=14)
Triglycerides	-12.4 (-36.6, 82.7)	-41.0 (-76.2, 49.4)	-38.7 (-62.7, 29.5)	-51.8 (-82.8, 41.3)
Total-C	-2.3 (-15.5, 24.4)	-28.2 (-44.9, 6.8)	-34.9 (-49.6, -15.2)	-44.4 (-63.5, -3.8)
LDL-C	3.6 (-31.3, 31.6)	-26.5 (-57.7, 9.8)	-30.4 (-53.9, 0.3)	-40.5 (-60.6, -13.8)
HDL-C	3.8 (-18.6, 13.4)	13.8 (-9.7, 61.5)	11.0 (-3.2, 25.2)	7.5 (-10.8, 37.2)
VLDL-C	-1.0 (-31.9, 53.2)	-48.8 (-85.8, 57.3)	-44.6 (-62.2, -10.8)	-62.0 (-88.2, 37.6)
non-HDL-C	-2.8 (-17.6, 30.0)	-33.0 (-52.1, -13.3)	-42.7 (-53.7, -17.4)	-51.5 (-72.9, -4.3)

TABLE 5. Open-Label Crossover Study of 16 Patients With Dysbetalipoproteinemia (*Fredrickson* Type III)

	Median (min, max) at Baseline (mg/dL)	Median % Change (min, max)	
		Atorvastatin 10 mg	Atorvastatin 80 mg
Total-C	442 (225, 1320)	-37 (-85, 17)	-58 (-90, -31)
Triglycerides	678 (273, 5990)	-39 (-92, -8)	-53 (-95, -30)
IDL-C + VLDL-C	215 (111, 613)	-32 (-76, 9)	-63 (-90, -8)
non-HDL-C	411 (218, 1272)	-43 (-87, -19)	-64 (-92, -36)

TABLE 6
Lipid-altering Effects of LIPITOR in Adolescent Boys and Girls with Heterozygous Familial Hypercholesterolemia or Severe Hypercholesterolemia
(Mean Percent Change from Baseline at Endpoint in Intention-to-Treat Population)

DOSAGE	N	Total-C	LDL-C	HDL-C	TG	Apolipoprotein B
Placebo	47	-1.5	-0.4	-1.9	1.0	0.7
LIPITOR	140	-31.4	-39.6	2.8	-12.0	-34.0

4. to reduce total-C and LDL-C in patients with homozygous familial hypercholesterolemia as an adjunct to other lipid-lowering treatments (eg, LDL apheresis) or if such treatments are unavailable;

5. as an adjunct to diet to reduce total-C, LDL-C, and apo B levels in boys and postmenarchal girls, 10 to 17 years of age, with heterozygous familial hypercholesterolemia if after an adequate trial of diet therapy the following findings are present:

a. LDL-C remains ≥ 190 mg/dL or

b. LDL-C remains ≥ 160 mg/dL and:

• there is a positive family history of premature cardiovascular disease or

• two or more other CVD risk factors are present in the pediatric patient

Therapy with lipid-altering agents should be a component of multiple-risk-factor intervention in individuals at increased risk for atherosclerotic vascular disease due to hypercholesterolemia. Lipid-altering agents should be used in addition to a diet restricted in saturated fat and cholesterol only when the response to diet and other nonpharmacological measures has been inadequate (see *National Cholesterol Education Program (NCEP) Guidelines*, summarized in Table 7).

[See table 7 at top of next page]

After the LDL-C goal has been achieved, if the TG is still ≥200 mg/dL, non-HDL-C (total-C minus HDL-C) becomes a secondary target of therapy. Non-HDL-C goals are set 30 mg/dL higher than LDL-C goals for each risk category.

Prior to initiating therapy with LIPITOR, secondary causes

mellitus, hypothyroidism, nephrotic syndrome, dysproteinemias, obstructive liver disease, other drug therapy, and alcoholism) should be excluded, and a lipid profile performed to measure total-C, LDL-C, HDL-C, and TG. For patients with TG <400 mg/dL (<4.5 mmol/L), LDL-C can be estimated using the following equation: LDL-C = total-C - (0.20 × [TG] + HDL-C). For TG levels >400 mg/dL (>4.5 mmol/L), this equation is less accurate and LDL-C concentrations should be determined by ultracentrifugation.

LIPITOR has not been studied in conditions where the major lipoprotein abnormality is elevation of chylomicrons (*Fredrickson* Types I and V).

The NCEP classification of cholesterol levels in pediatric patients with a familial history of hypercholesterolemia or premature cardiovascular disease is summarized below:

Category	Total-C (mg/dL)	LDL-C (mg/dL)
Acceptable	<170	<110
Borderline	170-199	110-129
High	≥200	≥130

CONTRAINDICATIONS

Active liver disease or unexplained persistent elevations of serum transaminases.

Hypersensitivity to any component of this medication.

Lipitor—Cont.

Pregnancy and Lactation

Atherosclerosis is a chronic process and discontinuation of lipid-lowering drugs during pregnancy should have little impact on the outcome of long-term therapy of primary hypercholesterolemia. Cholesterol and other products of cholesterol biosynthesis are essential components for fetal development (including synthesis of steroids and cell membranes). Since HMG-CoA reductase inhibitors decrease cholesterol synthesis and possibly the synthesis of other biologically active substances derived from cholesterol, they may cause fetal harm when administered to pregnant women. Therefore, HMG-CoA reductase inhibitors are contraindicated during pregnancy and in nursing mothers. ATORVASTATIN SHOULD BE ADMINISTERED TO WOMEN OF CHILDBEARING AGE ONLY WHEN SUCH PATIENTS ARE HIGHLY UNLIKELY TO CONCEIVE AND HAVE BEEN INFORMED OF THE POTENTIAL HAZARDS. If the patient becomes pregnant while taking this drug, therapy should be discontinued and the patient apprised of the potential hazard to the fetus.

WARNINGS

Liver Dysfunction

HMG-CoA reductase inhibitors, like some other lipid-lowering therapies, have been associated with biochemical abnormalities of liver function. **Persistent elevations (>3 times the upper limit of normal [ULN] occurring on 2 or more occasions) in serum transaminases occurred in 0.7% of patients who received atorvastatin in clinical trials. The incidence of these abnormalities was 0.2%, 0.2%, 0.6%, and 2.3% for 10, 20, 40, and 80 mg, respectively.**

One patient in clinical trials developed jaundice. Increases in liver function tests (LFT) in other patients were not associated with jaundice or other clinical signs or symptoms. Upon dose reduction, drug interruption, or discontinuation, transaminase levels returned to or near pretreatment levels without sequelae. Eighteen of 30 patients with persistent LFT elevations continued treatment with a reduced dose of atorvastatin.

It is recommended that liver function tests be performed prior to and at 12 weeks following both the initiation of therapy and any elevation of dose, and periodically (e.g., semiannually) thereafter. Liver enzyme changes generally occur in the first 3 months of treatment with atorvastatin. Patients who develop increased transaminase levels should be monitored until the abnormalities resolve. Should an increase in ALT or AST of >3 times ULN persist, reduction of dose or withdrawal of atorvastatin is recommended.

Atorvastatin should be used with caution in patients who consume substantial quantities of alcohol and/or have a history of liver disease. Active liver disease or unexplained persistent transaminase elevations are contraindications to the use of atorvastatin (see CONTRAINDICATIONS).

Skeletal Muscle

Rare cases of rhabdomyolysis with acute renal failure secondary to myoglobinuria have been reported with atorvastatin and with other drugs in this class.

Uncomplicated myalgia has been reported in atorvastatin-treated patients (see ADVERSE REACTIONS). Myopathy, defined as muscle aches or muscle weakness in conjunction with increases in creatine phosphokinase (CPK) values >10 times ULN, should be considered in any patient with diffuse myalgias, muscle tenderness or weakness, and/or marked elevation of CPK. Patients should be advised to report promptly unexplained muscle pain, tenderness or weakness, particularly if accompanied by malaise or fever. Atorvastatin therapy should be discontinued if markedly elevated CPK levels occur or myopathy is diagnosed or suspected.

The risk of myopathy during treatment with drugs in this class is increased with concurrent administration of cyclosporine, fibric acid derivatives, erythromycin, clarithromycin, combination of ritonavir plus saquinavir or lopinavir plus ritonavir, niacin, or azole antifungals. Physicians considering combined therapy with atorvastatin and fibric acid derivatives, erythromycin, clarithromycin, a combination of ritonavir plus saquinavir or lopinavir plus ritonavir, immunosuppressive drugs, azole antifungals, or lipid-modifying doses of niacin should carefully weigh the potential benefits and risks and should carefully monitor patients for any signs or symptoms of muscle pain, tenderness, or weakness, particularly during the initial months of therapy and during any periods of upward dosage titration of either drug. Lower starting and maintenance doses of atorvastatin should be considered when taken concomitantly with the aforementioned drugs (See DRUG INTERACTIONS). Periodic creatine phosphokinase (CPK) determinations may be considered in such situations, but there is no assurance that such monitoring will prevent the occurrence of severe myopathy. **Atorvastatin therapy should be temporarily withheld or discontinued in any patient with an acute, serious condition suggestive of a myopathy or having a risk factor predisposing to the development of renal failure secondary to rhabdomyolysis (e.g., severe acute infection, hypotension, major surgery, trauma, severe metabolic, endocrine and electrolyte disorders, and uncontrolled seizures).**

PRECAUTIONS

General

Before instituting therapy with atorvastatin, an attempt should be made to control hypercholesterolemia with appropriate diet, exercise, and weight reduction in obese patients, and to treat other underlying medical problems (see INDICATIONS AND USAGE).

TABLE 7. NCEP Treatment Guidelines: LDL-C Goals and Cutpoints for Therapeutic Lifestyle Changes and Drug Therapy in Different Risk Categories

Risk Category	LDL-C Goal (mg/dL)	LDL Level at Which to Initiate Therapeutic Lifestyle Changes (mg/dL)	LDL Level at Which to Consider Drug Therapy (mg/dL)
CHD[a] or CHD risk equivalents (10-year risk >20%)	<100	≥100	≥130 (100-129: drug optional)[b]
2+ Risk Factors (10-year risk ≤20%)	<130	≥130	10-year risk 10%-20%: ≥130 10-year risk <10%: ≥ 160
0-1 Risk factor[c]	<160	≥160	≥190 (160-189: LDL-lowering drug optional)

[a] CHD, coronary heart disease

[b] Some authorities recommend use of LDL-lowering drugs in this category if an LDL-C level of < 100 mg/dL cannot be achieved by therapeutic lifestyle changes. Others prefer use of drugs that primarily modify triglycerides and HDL-C, e.g., nicotinic acid or fibrate. Clinical judgement also may call for deferring drug therapy in this subcategory.

[c] Almost all people with 0-1 risk factor have 10-year risk <10%; thus, 10-year risk assessment in people with 0-1 risk factor is not necessary.

Information for Patients

Patients should be advised to report promptly unexplained muscle pain, tenderness, or weakness, particularly if accompanied by malaise or fever.

Drug Interactions

The risk of myopathy during treatment with HMG-CoA reductase inhibitors is increased with concurrent administration of fibric acid derivatives, lipid-modifying doses of niacin or cytochrome P450 3A4 inhibitors (e.g. cyclosporine, erythromycin, clarithromycin, and azole antifungals) (see WARNINGS, Skeletal Muscle).

Inhibitors of cytochrome P450 3A4: Atorvastatin is metabolized by cytochrome P450 3A4. Concomitant administration of atorvastatin with inhibitors of cytochrome P450 3A4 can lead to increases in plasma concentrations of atorvastatin. The extent of interaction and potentiation of effects depends on the variability of effect on cytochrome P450 3A4.

Clarithromycin: Concomitant administration of atorvastatin 80 mg with clarithromycin (500 mg twice daily) resulted in a 4.4-fold increase in atorvastatin AUC (see WARNINGS, Skeletal Muscle, and DOSAGE AND ADMINISTRATION).

Erythromycin: In healthy individuals, plasma concentrations of atorvastatin increased approximately 40% with co-administration of atorvastatin and erythromycin, a known inhibitor of cytochrome P450 3A4 (see WARNINGS, Skeletal Muscle).

Combination of Protease Inhibitors: Concomitant administration of atorvastatin 40 mg with ritonavir plus saquinavir (400 mg twice daily) resulted in a 3-fold increase in atorvastatin AUC. Concomitant administration of atorvastatin 20 mg with lopinavir plus ritonavir (400 mg+100 mg twice daily) resulted in a 5.9-fold increase in atorvastatin AUC (see WARNINGS, Skeletal Muscle, and DOSAGE AND ADMINISTRATION).

Itraconazole: Concomitant administration of atorvastatin (20 to 40 mg) and itraconazole (200 mg) was associated with a 2.5-3.3-fold increase in atorvastatin AUC.

Diltiazem hydrochloride: Co-administration of atorvastatin (40 mg) with diltiazem (240 mg) was associated with higher plasma concentrations of atorvastatin.

Cimetidine: Atorvastatin plasma concentrations and LDL-C reduction were not altered by co-administration of cimetidine.

Grapefruit juice: Contains one or more components that inhibit CYP 3A4 and can increase plasma concentrations of atorvastatin, especially with excessive grapefruit juice consumption (>1.2 liters per day).

Cyclosporine: Atorvastatin and atorvastatin-metabolites are substrates of the OATP1B1 transporter. Inhibitors of the OATP1B1 (e.g. cyclosporine) can increase the bioavailability of atorvastatin. Concomitant administration of atorvastatin 10 mg and cyclosporine 5.2 mg/kg/day resulted in an 8.7-fold increase in atorvastatin AUC. In cases where co-administration of atorvastatin with cyclosporine is necessary, the dose of atorvastatin should not exceed 10 mg (see WARNINGS, Skeletal Muscle).

Inducers of cytochrome P450 3A4: Concomitant administration of atorvastatin with inducers of cytochrome P450 3A4 (eg efavirenz, rifampin) can lead to variable reductions in plasma concentrations of atorvastatin. Due to the dual interaction mechanism of rifampin, simultaneous co-administration of atorvastatin with rifampin is recommended, as delayed administration of atorvastatin after administration of rifampin has been associated with a significant reduction in atorvastatin plasma concentrations.

Antacid: When atorvastatin and Maalox® TC suspension were coadministered, plasma concentrations of atorvastatin decreased approximately 35%. However, LDL-C reduction was not altered.

Antipyrine: Because atorvastatin does not affect the pharmacokinetics of antipyrine, interactions with other drugs metabolized via the same cytochrome isozymes are not expected.

Colestipol: Plasma concentrations of atorvastatin decreased approximately 25% when colestipol and atorvastatin were coadministered. However, LDL-C reduction was greater when atorvastatin and colestipol were coadministered than when either drug was given alone.

Digoxin: When multiple doses of atorvastatin and digoxin were coadministered, steady-state plasma digoxin concentrations increased by approximately 20%. Patients taking digoxin should be monitored appropriately.

Oral Contraceptives: Coadministration of atorvastatin and an oral contraceptive increased AUC values for norethindrone and ethinyl estradiol by approximately 30% and 20%. These increases should be considered when selecting an oral contraceptive for a woman taking atorvastatin.

Warfarin: Atorvastatin had no clinically significant effect on prothrombin time when administered to patients receiving chronic warfarin treatment.

Amlodipine: In a drug-drug interaction study in healthy subjects, co-administration of atorvastatin 80 mg and amlodipine 10 mg resulted in an 18% increase in exposure to atorvastatin which was not clinically meaningful.

Endocrine Function

HMG-CoA reductase inhibitors interfere with cholesterol synthesis and theoretically might blunt adrenal and/or gonadal steroid production. Clinical studies have shown that atorvastatin does not reduce basal plasma cortisol concentration or impair adrenal reserve. The effects of HMG-CoA reductase inhibitors on male fertility have not been studied in adequate numbers of patients. The effects, if any, on the pituitary-gonadal axis in premenopausal women are unknown. Caution should be exercised if an HMG-CoA reductase inhibitor is administered concomitantly with drugs that may decrease the levels or activity of endogenous steroid hormones, such as ketoconazole, spironolactone, and cimetidine.

CNS Toxicity

Brain hemorrhage was seen in a female dog treated for 3 months at 120 mg/kg/day. Brain hemorrhage and optic nerve vacuolation were seen in another female dog that was sacrificed in moribund condition after 11 weeks of escalating doses up to 280 mg/kg/day. The 120 mg/kg dose resulted in a systemic exposure approximately 16 times the human plasma area-under-the-curve (AUC, 0-24 hours) based on the maximum human dose of 80 mg/day. A single tonic convulsion was seen in each of 2 male dogs (one treated at 10 mg/kg/day and one at 120 mg/kg/day) in a 2-year study. No CNS lesions have been observed in mice after chronic treatment for up to 2 years at doses up to 400 mg/kg/day or in rats at doses up to 100 mg/kg/day. These doses were 6 to 11 times (mouse) and 8 to 16 times (rat) the human AUC (0-24) based on the maximum recommended human dose of 80 mg/day.

CNS vascular lesions, characterized by perivascular hemorrhages, edema, and mononuclear cell infiltration of perivascular spaces, have been observed in dogs treated with other members of this class. A chemically similar drug in this class produced optic nerve degeneration (Wallerian degeneration of retinogeniculate fibers) in clinically normal dogs in a dose-dependent fashion at a dose that produced plasma drug levels about 30 times higher than the mean drug level in humans taking the highest recommended dose.

Carcinogenesis, Mutagenesis, Impairment of Fertility

In a 2-year carcinogenicity study in rats at dose levels of 10, 30, and 100 mg/kg/day, 2 rare tumors were found in muscle in high-dose females: in one, there was a rhabdomyosarcoma and, in another, there was a fibrosarcoma. This dose represents a plasma AUC (0-24) value of approximately 16 times the mean human plasma drug exposure after an 80 mg oral dose.

A 2-year carcinogenicity study in mice given 100, 200, or 400 mg/kg/day resulted in a significant increase in liver adenomas in high-dose males and liver carcinomas in high-dose females. These findings occurred at plasma AUC (0-24) values of approximately 6 times the mean human plasma drug exposure after an 80 mg oral dose.

In vitro, atorvastatin was not mutagenic or clastogenic in the following tests with and without metabolic activation: the Ames test with *Salmonella typhimurium* and *Escherichia coli*, the HGPRT forward mutation assay in Chinese hamster lung cells, and the chromosomal aberration assay in Chinese hamster lung cells. Atorvastatin was negative in the *in vivo* mouse micronucleus test.

Studies in rats performed at doses up to 175 mg/kg (15 times the human exposure) produced no changes in fertility. There was aplasia and aspermia in the epididymis of 2 of 10 rats treated with 100 mg/kg/day of atorvastatin for 3 months (16 times the human AUC at the 80 mg dose); testis weights were significantly lower at 30 and 100 mg/kg and epididymal weight was lower at 100 mg/kg. Male rats given 100 mg/kg/day for 11 weeks prior to mating had decreased sperm motility, spermatid head concentration, and increased abnormal sperm. Atorvastatin caused no adverse effects on semen parameters, or reproductive organ histopathology in dogs given doses of 10, 40, or 120 mg/kg for two years.

Pregnancy

Pregnancy Category X

See CONTRAINDICATIONS

Safety in pregnant women has not been established. Atorvastatin crosses the rat placenta and reaches a level in fetal liver equivalent to that of maternal plasma. Atorvastatin was not teratogenic in rats at doses up to 300 mg/kg/day or in rabbits at doses up to 100 mg/kg/day. These doses resulted in multiples of about 30 times (rat) or 20 times (rabbit) the human exposure based on surface area (mg/m^2).

In a study in rats given 20, 100, or 225 mg/kg/day, from gestation day 7 through to lactation day 21 (weaning), there was decreased pup survival at birth, neonate, weaning, and maturity in pups of mothers dosed with 225 mg/kg/day. Body weight was decreased on days 4 and 21 in pups of mothers dosed at 100 mg/kg/day; pup body weight was decreased at birth and at days 4, 21, and 91 at 225 mg/kg/day. Pup development was delayed (rotorod performance at 100 mg/kg/day and acoustic startle at 225 mg/kg/day; pinnae detachment and eye opening at 225 mg/kg/day). These doses correspond to 6 times (100 mg/kg) and 22 times (225 mg/kg) the human AUC at 80 mg/day. Rare reports of congenital anomalies have been received following intrauterine exposure to HMG-CoA reductase inhibitors. There has been one report of severe congenital bony deformity, tracheo-esophageal fistula, and anal atresia (VATER association) in a baby born to a woman who took lovastatin with dextroamphetamine sulfate during the first trimester of pregnancy. LIPITOR should be administered to women of child-bearing potential only when such patients are highly unlikely to conceive and have been informed of the potential hazards. If the woman becomes pregnant while taking LIPITOR, it should be discontinued and the patient advised again as to the potential hazards to the fetus.

Nursing Mothers

Nursing rat pups had plasma and liver drug levels of 50% and 40%, respectively, of that in their mother's milk. Because of the potential for adverse reactions in nursing infants, women taking LIPITOR should not breast-feed (see CONTRAINDICATIONS).

Pediatric Use

Safety and effectiveness in patients 10-17 years of age with heterozygous familial hypercholesterolemia have been evaluated in a controlled clinical trial of 6 months duration in adolescent boys and postmenarchal girls. Patients treated with LIPITOR had an adverse experience profile generally similar to that of patients treated with placebo, the most common adverse experiences observed in both groups, regardless of causality assessment, were infections. **Doses greater than 20 mg have not been studied in this patient population.** In this limited controlled study, there was no detectable effect on growth or sexual maturation in boys or on menstrual cycle length in girls (see CLINICAL PHARMACOLOGY, Clinical Studies section; ADVERSE REACTIONS, Pediatric Patients (ages 10-17 years); and DOSAGE AND ADMINISTRATION, Heterozygous Familial Hypercholesterolemia in Pediatric Patients (10-17 years of age). Adolescent females should be counseled on appropriate contraceptive methods while on LIPITOR therapy (see CONTRAINDICATIONS and PRECAUTIONS, Pregnancy). **LIPITOR has not been studied in controlled clinical trials involving pre-pubertal patients or patients younger than 10 years of age.**

Clinical efficacy with doses up to 80 mg/day for 1 year have been evaluated in an uncontrolled study of patients with homozygous FH including 8 pediatric patients (see CLINICAL PHARMACOLOGY, Clinical Studies: Homozygous Familial Hypercholesterolemia).

Geriatric Use

The safety and efficacy of atorvastatin (10-80 mg) in the geriatric population (≥65 years of age) was evaluated in the ACCESS study. In this 54-week open-label trial 1,958 patients initiated therapy with atorvastatin 10 mg. Of these, 835 were elderly (≥65 years) and 1,123 were non-elderly. The mean change in LDL-C from baseline after 6 weeks of treatment with atorvastatin 10 mg was −38.2% in the elderly patients versus −34.6% in the non-elderly group.

The rates of discontinuation due to adverse events were similar between the two age groups. There were no differences in clinically relevant laboratory abnormalities between the age groups.

Use in Patients with Recent Stroke or TIA

In a post-hoc analysis of the Stroke Prevention by Aggressive Reduction in Cholesterol Levels (SPARCL) study where LIPITOR 80 mg vs placebo was administered in 4,731 subjects without CHD who had a stroke or TIA within the preceding 6 months, a higher incidence of hemorrhagic stroke was seen in the LIPITOR 80 mg group compared to placebo. Subjects with hemorrhagic stroke on study entry appeared to be at increased risk for hemorrhagic stroke.

TABLE 8. Adverse Events in Placebo-Controlled Studies (% of Patients)

BODY SYSTEM/ Adverse Event	Placebo N = 270	Atorvastatin 10 mg N = 863	Atorvastatin 20 mg N = 36	Atorvastatin 40 mg N = 79	Atorvastatin 80 mg N = 94
BODY AS A WHOLE					
Infection	10.0	10.3	2.8	10.1	7.4
Headache	7.0	5.4	16.7	2.5	6.4
Accidental Injury	3.7	4.2	0.0	1.3	3.2
Flu Syndrome	1.9	2.2	0.0	2.5	3.2
Abdominal Pain	0.7	2.8	0.0	3.8	2.1
Back Pain	3.0	2.8	0.0	3.8	1.1
Allergic Reaction	2.6	0.9	2.8	1.3	0.0
Asthenia	1.9	2.2	0.0	3.8	0.0
DIGESTIVE SYSTEM					
Constipation	1.8	2.1	0.0	2.5	1.1
Diarrhea	1.5	2.7	0.0	3.8	5.3
Dyspepsia	4.1	2.3	2.8	1.3	2.1
Flatulence	3.3	2.1	2.8	1.3	1.1
RESPIRATORY SYSTEM					
Sinusitis	2.6	2.8	0.0	2.5	6.4
Pharyngitis	1.5	2.5	0.0	1.3	2.1
SKIN AND APPENDAGES					
Rash	0.7	3.9	2.8	3.8	1.1
MUSCULOSKELETAL SYSTEM					
Arthralgia	1.5	2.0	0.0	5.1	0.0
Myalgia	1.1	3.2	5.6	1.3	0.0

ADVERSE REACTIONS

LIPITOR is generally well-tolerated. Adverse reactions have usually been mild and transient. In controlled clinical studies of 2502 patients, <2% of patients were discontinued due to adverse experiences attributable to atorvastatin. The most frequent adverse events thought to be related to atorvastatin were constipation, flatulence, dyspepsia, and abdominal pain.

Clinical Adverse Experiences

Adverse experiences reported in ≥2% of patients in placebo-controlled clinical studies of atorvastatin, regardless of causality assessment, are shown in Table 8.

[See table 8 above]

Anglo-Scandinavian Cardiac Outcomes Trial (ASCOT)

In ASCOT (see CLINICAL PHARMACOLOGY, *Clinical Studies*) involving 10,305 participants treated with LIPITOR 10 mg daily (n=5,168) or placebo (n=5,137), the safety and tolerability profile of the group treated with LIPITOR was comparable to that of the group treated with placebo during a median of 3.3 years of follow-up.

Collaborative Atorvastatin Diabetes Study (CARDS)

In CARDS (see CLINICAL PHARMACOLOGY, *Clinical Studies*) involving 2838 subjects with type 2 diabetes treated with LIPITOR 10 mg daily (n=1428) or placebo (n=1410), there was no difference in the overall frequency of adverse events or serious adverse events between the treatment groups during a median follow-up of 3.9 years. No cases of rhabdomyolysis were reported.

Treating to New Targets Study (TNT)

In TNT (see CLINICAL PHARMACOLOGY, *Clinical Studies*) involving 10,001 subjects with clinically evident CHD treated with LIPITOR 10 mg daily (n=5006) or LIPITOR 80 mg daily (n=4995), there were more serious adverse events and discontinuations due to adverse events in the high-dose atorvastatin group (92, 1.8%; 497, 9.9%, respectively) as compared to the low-dose group (69, 1.4%; 404, 8.1%, respectively) during a median follow-up of 4.9 years. Persistent transaminase elevations (≥3 × ULN twice within 4-10 days) occurred in 62 (1.3%) individuals with atorvastatin 80 mg and in nine (0.2%) individuals with atorvastatin 10 mg. Elevations of CK (≥ 10 × ULN) were low overall, but were higher in the high-dose atorvastatin treatment group (13, 0.3%) compared to the low-dose atorvastatin group (6, 0.1%).

Incremental Decrease in Endpoints Through Aggressive Lipid Lowering Study (IDEAL)

In IDEAL (see CLINICAL PHARMACOLOGY, *Clinical Studies*) involving 8,888 subjects treated with LIPITOR 80 mg/day (n=4439) or simvastatin 20-40 mg daily (n=4449), there was no difference in the overall frequency of adverse events or serious adverse events between the treatment groups during a median follow-up of 4.8 years.

The following adverse events were reported, regardless of causality assessment in patients treated with atorvastatin in clinical trials. The events in italics occurred in ≥2% of patients and the events in plain type occurred in <2% of patients.

Body as a Whole: *Chest pain*, face edema, fever, neck rigidity, malaise, photosensitivity reaction, generalized edema.

Digestive System: *Nausea*, gastroenteritis, liver function tests abnormal, colitis, vomiting, gastritis, dry mouth, rectal hemorrhage, esophagitis, eructation, glossitis, mouth ulceration, anorexia, increased appetite, stomatitis, biliary pain, cheilitis, duodenal ulcer, dysphagia, enteritis, melena, gum hemorrhage, stomach ulcer, tenesmus, ulcerative stomatitis, hepatitis, pancreatitis, cholestatic jaundice.

Respiratory System: *Bronchitis, rhinitis*, pneumonia, dyspnea, asthma, epistaxis.

Nervous System: *Insomnia, dizziness*, paresthesia, somnolence, amnesia, abnormal dreams, libido decreased, emotional lability, incoordination, peripheral neuropathy, torticollis, facial paralysis, hyperkinesia, depression, hypesthesia, hypertonia.

Musculoskeletal System: *Arthritis*, leg cramps, bursitis, tenosynovitis, myasthenia, tendinous contracture, myositis.

Skin and Appendages: Pruritus, contact dermatitis, alopecia, dry skin, sweating, acne, urticaria, eczema, seborrhea, skin ulcer.

Urogenital System: *Urinary tract infection, hematuria, albuminuria*, urinary frequency, cystitis, impotence, dysuria, kidney calculus, nocturia, epididymitis, fibrocystic breast, vaginal hemorrhage, breast enlargement, metrorrhagia, nephritis, urinary incontinence, urinary retention, urinary urgency, abnormal ejaculation, uterine hemorrhage.

Special Senses: Amblyopia, tinnitus, dry eyes, refraction disorder, eye hemorrhage, deafness, glaucoma, parosmia, taste loss, taste perversion.

Cardiovascular System: Palpitation, vasodilatation, syncope, migraine, postural hypotension, phlebitis, arrhythmia, angina pectoris, hypertension.

Metabolic and Nutritional Disorders: *Peripheral edema*, hyperglycemia, creatine phosphokinase increased, gout, weight gain, hypoglycemia.

Hemic and Lymphatic System: Ecchymosis, anemia, lymphadenopathy, thrombocytopenia, petechia.

Postintroduction Reports

Adverse events associated with LIPITOR therapy reported since market introduction, that are not listed above, regardless of causality assessment, include the following: anaphylaxis, angioneurotic edema, bullous rashes (including erythema multiforme, Stevens-Johnson syndrome, and toxic epidermal necrolysis), rhabdomyolysis, fatigue, and tendon rupture.

Pediatric Patients (ages 10-17 years)

In a 26-week controlled study in boys and postmenarchal girls (n=140), the safety and tolerability profile of LIPITOR 10 to 20 mg daily was generally similar to that of placebo (see CLINICAL PHARMACOLOGY, Clinical Studies section and PRECAUTIONS, Pediatric Use).

OVERDOSAGE

There is no specific treatment for atorvastatin overdosage. In the event of an overdose, the patient should be treated symptomatically, and supportive measures instituted as required. Due to extensive drug binding to plasma proteins, hemodialysis is not expected to significantly enhance atorvastatin clearance.

DOSAGE AND ADMINISTRATION

The patient should be placed on a standard cholesterol-lowering diet before receiving LIPITOR and should continue on this diet during treatment with LIPITOR.

Hypercholesterolemia (Heterozygous Familial and Nonfamilial) and Mixed Dyslipidemia (*Fredrickson* Types IIa and IIb)

The recommended starting dose of LIPITOR is 10 or 20 mg once daily. Patients who require a large reduction in LDL-C (more than 45%) may be started at 40 mg once daily. The dosage range of LIPITOR is 10 to 80 mg once daily. LIPITOR can be administered as a single dose at any time of the day, with or without food. The starting dose and maintenance doses of LIPITOR should be individualized according to patient characteristics such as goal of therapy and response (see *NCEP Guidelines*, summarized in Table 7). After initiation and/or upon titration of LIPITOR, lipid levels should be analyzed within 2 to 4 weeks and dosage adjusted accordingly.

Since the goal of treatment is to lower LDL-C, the NCEP recommends that LDL-C levels be used to initiate and assess treatment response. Only if LDL-C levels are not available, should total-C be used to monitor therapy.

Heterozygous Familial Hypercholesterolemia in Pediatric Patients (10-17 years of age)

The recommended starting dose of LIPITOR is 10 mg/day; the maximum recommended dose is 20 mg/day (doses

Continued on next page

Lipitor—Cont.

greater than 20 mg have not been studied in this patient population). Doses should be individualized according to the recommended goal of therapy (see NCEP Pediatric Panel Guidelines[1], CLINICAL PHARMACOLOGY, and INDICATIONS AND USAGE). Adjustments should be made at intervals of 4 weeks or more.

[1] National Cholesterol Education Program (NCEP): Highlights of the Report of the Expert Panel on Blood Cholesterol Levels in Children Adolescents, *Pediatrics*. 89(3):495-501. 1992.

Homozygous Familial Hypercholesterolemia
The dosage of LIPITOR in patients with homozygous FH is 10 to 80 mg daily. LIPITOR should be used as an adjunct to other lipid-lowering treatments (e.g., LDL apheresis) in these patients or if such treatments are unavailable.

Concomitant Lipid Lowering Therapy
LIPITOR may be used in combination with a bile acid binding resin for additive effect. The combination of HMG-CoA reductase inhibitors and fibrates should generally be avoided (see WARNINGS, Skeletal Muscle, and PRECAUTIONS, Drug Interactions for other drug-drug interactions).

Dosage in Patients With Renal Insufficiency
Renal disease does not affect the plasma concentrations nor LDL-C reduction of atorvastatin; thus, dosage adjustment in patients with renal dysfunction is not necessary (see CLINICAL PHARMACOLOGY, Pharmacokinetics).

Dosage in Patients Taking Cyclosporine, Clarithromycin or A Combination of Ritonavir plus Saquinavir or Lopinavir plus Ritonavir
In patients taking cyclosporine, therapy should be limited to LIPITOR 10 mg once daily.

In patients taking clarithromycin or in patients with HIV taking a combination of ritonavir plus saquinavir or lopinavir plus ritonavir, for doses of atorvastatin exceeding 20 mg appropriate clinical assessment is recommended to ensure that the lowest dose necessary of atorvastatin is employed (see WARNINGS, Skeletal Muscle, and PRECAUTIONS, Drug Interactions).

HOW SUPPLIED
LIPITOR® (atorvastatin calcium) is supplied as white, elliptical, film-coated tablets of atorvastatin calcium containing 10, 20, 40 and 80 mg atorvastatin.

10 mg tablets: coded "PD 155" on one side and "10" on the other.
NDC 0071-0155-23 bottles of 90
NDC 0071-0155-34 bottles of 5000
NDC 0071-0155-40 10 × 10 unit dose blisters
20 mg tablets: coded "PD 156" on one side and "20" on the other.
NDC 0071-0156-23 bottles of 90
NDC 0071-0156-40 10 × 10 unit dose blisters
NDC 0071-0156-94 bottles of 5000
40 mg tablets: coded "PD 157" on one side and "40" on the other.
NDC 0071-0157-23 bottles of 90
NDC 0071-0157-73 bottles of 500
NDC 0071-0157-88 bottles of 2500
NDC 0071-0157-40 10 × 10 unit dose blisters
80 mg tablets: coded "PD 158" on one side and "80" on the other.
NDC 0071-0158-23 bottles of 90
NDC 0071-0158-73 bottles of 500
NDC 0071-0158-88 bottles of 2500
NDC 0071-0158-92 8 × 8 unit dose blisters
Storage
Store at controlled room temperature 20-25°C (68-77°F) [see USP].
Rx Only
Manufactured by:
Pfizer Ireland Pharmaceuticals
Dublin, Ireland
Distributed by:
Parke-Davis
Division of Pfizer Inc, NY, NY 10017
LAB-0021-20.0   Revised November 2007

Pfizer Inc.
235 EAST 42ND STREET
NEW YORK, NY 10017–5755

For updates to the product information listed below, please check the Pfizer Web site, http://www.pfizerpro.com, or call (800) 438-1985. For complete product listing, please see the Manufacturers' Index.

For Medical Information, Contact:
(800) 438-1985
24 hours a day, seven days a week

Distribution:
1855 Shelby Oaks Drive North
Memphis, TN 38134
(901) 387-5200

Customer Service:
(800) 533-4535

Pfizer Companies Include:
Agouron Pharmaceuticals
Parke-Davis – see Parke-Davis
Pharmacia & Upjohn – see Pharmacia & Upjohn
G.D. Searle & Co. – see G.D. Searle & Co.

CADUET®   ℞
[kă-dew-ĕt]
(amlodipine besylate/atorvastatin calcium) Tablets

Prescribing information for this product, which appears on pages 2484–2492 of the 2008 PDR, has been completely revised as follows. Please write "See Supplement A" next to the product heading.

DESCRIPTION
CADUET® (amlodipine besylate and atorvastatin calcium) tablets combine the long-acting calcium channel blocker amlodipine besylate with the synthetic lipid-lowering agent atorvastatin calcium.

The amlodipine besylate component of CADUET is chemically described as 3-Ethyl-5-methyl (±)-2-[(2-aminoethoxy)methyl]-4-(o-chlorophenyl)-1,4-dihydro-6-methyl-3,5-pyridinedicarboxylate, monobenzenesulphonate. Its empirical formula is $C_{20}H_{25}ClN_2O_5 \cdot C_6H_6O_3S$.

The atorvastatin calcium component of CADUET is chemically described as [R-(R*, R*)]-2-(4-fluorophenyl)-β,δ-dihydroxy-5-(1-methylethyl)-3-phenyl-4-[(phenylamino)carbonyl]-1H-pyrrole-1-heptanoic acid, calcium salt (2:1) trihydrate. Its empirical formula is $(C_{33}H_{34}FN_2O_5)_2Ca \cdot 3H_2O$. The structural formulae for amlodipine besylate and atorvastatin calcium are shown below.

Amlodipine besylate

Atorvastatin calcium

CADUET contains amlodipine besylate, a white to off-white crystalline powder, and atorvastatin calcium, also a white to off-white crystalline powder. Amlodipine besylate has a molecular weight of 567.1 and atorvastatin calcium has a molecular weight of 1209.42. Amlodipine besylate is slightly soluble in water and sparingly soluble in ethanol. Atorvastatin calcium is insoluble in aqueous solutions of pH 4 and below. Atorvastatin calcium is very slightly soluble in distilled water, pH 7.4 phosphate buffer, and acetoni-

trile; slightly soluble in ethanol, and freely soluble in methanol.

CADUET tablets are formulated for oral administration in the following strength combinations:
[See table 1 below]

Each tablet also contains calcium carbonate, croscarmellose sodium, microcrystalline cellulose, pregelatinized starch, polysorbate 80, hydroxypropyl cellulose, purified water, colloidal silicon dioxide (anhydrous), magnesium stearate, Opadry® II White 85F28751 (polyvinyl alcohol, titanium dioxide, PEG 3000 and talc) or Opadry® II Blue 85F10919 (polyvinyl alcohol, titanium dioxide, PEG 3000, talc and FD&C blue #2). Combinations of atorvastatin with 2.5 mg and 5 mg amlodipine are film coated white, and combinations of atorvastatin with 10 mg amlodipine are film coated blue.

CLINICAL PHARMACOLOGY
Mechanism of Action
CADUET
CADUET is a combination of two drugs, a dihydropyridine calcium antagonist (calcium ion antagonist or slow-channel blocker) amlodipine (antihypertensive/antianginal agent) and an HMG-CoA reductase inhibitor atorvastatin (cholesterol lowering agent). The amlodipine component of CADUET inhibits the transmembrane influx of calcium ions into vascular smooth muscle and cardiac muscle. The atorvastatin component of CADUET is a selective, competitive inhibitor of HMG-CoA reductase, the rate-limiting enzyme that converts 3-hydroxy-3-methylglutaryl-coenzyme A to mevalonate, a precursor of sterols, including cholesterol.

The Amlodipine Component of CADUET
Experimental data suggest that amlodipine binds to both dihydropyridine and nondihydropyridine binding sites. The contractile processes of cardiac muscle and vascular smooth muscle are dependent upon the movement of extracellular calcium ions into these cells through specific ion channels. Amlodipine inhibits calcium ion influx across cell membranes selectively, with a greater effect on vascular smooth muscle cells than on cardiac muscle cells. Negative inotropic effects can be detected *in vitro* but such effects have not been seen in intact animals at therapeutic doses. Serum calcium concentration is not affected by amlodipine. Within the physiologic pH range, amlodipine is an ionized compound (pKa=8.6), and its kinetic interaction with the calcium channel receptor is characterized by a gradual rate of association and dissociation with the receptor binding site, resulting in a gradual onset of effect.

Amlodipine is a peripheral arterial vasodilator that acts directly on vascular smooth muscle to cause a reduction in peripheral vascular resistance and reduction in blood pressure.

The precise mechanisms by which amlodipine relieves angina have not been fully delineated, but are thought to include the following:

Exertional Angina: In patients with exertional angina, amlodipine reduces the total peripheral resistance (afterload) against which the heart works and reduces the rate pressure product, and thus myocardial oxygen demand, at any given level of exercise.

Vasospastic Angina: Amlodipine has been demonstrated to block constriction and restore blood flow in coronary arteries and arterioles in response to calcium, potassium epinephrine, serotonin, and thromboxane A_2 analog in experimental animal models and in human coronary vessels in vitro. This inhibition of coronary spasm is responsible for the effectiveness of amlodipine in vasospastic (Prinzmetal's or variant) angina.

The Atorvastatin Component of CADUET
Cholesterol and triglycerides circulate in the bloodstream as part of lipoprotein complexes. With ultracentrifugation, these complexes separate into HDL (high-density lipoprotein), IDL (intermediate-density lipoprotein), LDL (low-density lipoprotein), and VLDL (very-low-density lipoprotein) fractions. Triglycerides (TG) and cholesterol in the liver are incorporated into VLDL and released into the plasma for delivery to peripheral tissues. LDL is formed from VLDL and is catabolized primarily through the high-affinity LDL receptor.

Clinical and pathologic studies show that elevated plasma levels of total cholesterol (total-C), LDL-cholesterol (LDL-C), and apolipoprotein B (apo B) promote human atherosclerosis and are risk factors for developing cardiovascular disease, while increased levels of HDL-C are associated with a decreased cardiovascular risk.

Epidemiologic investigations have established that cardiovascular morbidity and mortality vary directly with the level of total-C and LDL-C, and inversely with the level of HDL-C.

In animal models, atorvastatin lowers plasma cholesterol and lipoprotein levels by inhibiting HMG-CoA reductase and cholesterol synthesis in the liver and by increasing the number of hepatic LDL receptors on the cell-surface to en-

Table 1. CADUET Tablet Strengths

	2.5 mg/ 10 mg	2.5 mg/ 20 mg	2.5 mg/ 40 mg	5 mg/ 10 mg	5 mg/ 20 mg	5 mg/ 40 mg	5 mg/ 80 mg	10 mg/ 10 mg	10 mg/ 20 mg	10 mg/ 40 mg	10 mg/ 80 mg
amlodipine equivalent (mg)	2.5	2.5	2.5	5	5	5	5	10	10	10	10
atorvastatin equivalent (mg)	10	20	40	10	20	40	80	10	20	40	80

hance uptake and catabolism of LDL; atorvastatin also reduces LDL production and the number of LDL particles.

Atorvastatin reduces total-C, LDL-C, and apo B in patients with homozygous and heterozygous familial hypercholesterolemia (FH), nonfamilial forms of hypercholesterolemia, and mixed dyslipidemia. Atorvastatin also reduces VLDL-C and TG and produces variable increases in HDL-C and apolipoprotein A-1. Atorvastatin reduces total-C, LDL-C, VLDL-C, apo B, TG, and non-HDL-C, and increases HDL-C in patients with isolated hypertriglyceridemia. Atorvastatin reduces intermediate density lipoprotein cholesterol (IDL-C) in patients with dysbetalipoproteinemia.

Like LDL, cholesterol-enriched triglyceride-rich lipoproteins, including VLDL, intermediate density lipoprotein (IDL), and remnants, can also promote atherosclerosis. Elevated plasma triglycerides are frequently found in a triad with low HDL-C levels and small LDL particles, as well as in association with non-lipid metabolic risk factors for coronary heart disease. As such, total plasma TG has not consistently been shown to be an independent risk factor for CHD. Furthermore, the independent effect of raising HDL or lowering TG on the risk of coronary and cardiovascular morbidity and mortality has not been determined.

Pharmacokinetics and Metabolism

Absorption

Studies with amlodipine: After oral administration of therapeutic doses of amlodipine alone, absorption produces peak plasma concentrations between 6 and 12 hours. Absolute bioavailability has been estimated to be between 64% and 90%. The bioavailability of amlodipine when administered alone is not altered by the presence of food.

Studies with atorvastatin: After oral administration alone, atorvastatin is rapidly absorbed; maximum plasma concentrations occur within 1 to 2 hours. Extent of absorption increases in proportion to atorvastatin dose. The absolute bioavailability of atorvastatin (parent drug) is approximately 14% and the systemic availability of HMG-CoA reductase inhibitory activity is approximately 30%. The low systemic availability is attributed to presystemic clearance in gastrointestinal mucosa and/or hepatic first-pass metabolism. Although food decreases the rate and extent of drug absorption by approximately 25% and 9%, respectively, as assessed by Cmax and AUC, LDL-C reduction is similar whether atorvastatin is given with or without food. Plasma atorvastatin concentrations are lower (approximately 30% for Cmax and AUC) following evening drug administration compared with morning. However, LDL-C reduction is the same regardless of the time of day of drug administration (see **DOSAGE AND ADMINISTRATION**).

Studies with CADUET: Following oral administration of CADUET peak plasma concentrations of amlodipine and atorvastatin are seen at 6 to 12 hours and 1 to 2 hours post dosing, respectively. The rate and extent of absorption (bioavailability) of amlodipine and atorvastatin from CADUET are not significantly different from the bioavailability of amlodipine and atorvastatin administered separately (see above).

The bioavailability of amlodipine from CADUET was not affected by food. Although food decreases the rate and extent of absorption of atorvastatin from CADUET by approximately 32% and 11%, respectively, as it does with atorvastatin when given alone. LDL-C reduction is similar whether atorvastatin is given with or without food.

Distribution

Studies with amlodipine: Ex vivo studies have shown that approximately 93% of the circulating amlodipine drug is bound to plasma proteins in hypertensive patients. Steady-state plasma levels of amlodipine are reached after 7 to 8 days of consecutive daily dosing.

Studies with atorvastatin: Mean volume of distribution of atorvastatin is approximately 381 liters. Atorvastatin is ≥98% bound to plasma proteins. A blood/plasma ratio of approximately 0.25 indicates poor drug penetration into red blood cells. Based on observations in rats, atorvastatin calcium is likely to be secreted in human milk (see **CONTRAINDICATIONS, Pregnancy and Lactation,** and **PRECAUTIONS, Nursing Mothers**).

Metabolism

Studies with amlodipine: Amlodipine is extensively (about 90%) converted to inactive metabolites via hepatic metabolism.

Studies with atorvastatin: Atorvastatin is extensively metabolized to ortho- and parahydroxylated derivatives and various beta-oxidation products. *In vitro* inhibition of HMG-CoA reductase by ortho- and parahydroxylated metabolites is equivalent to that of atorvastatin. Approximately 70% of circulating inhibitory activity for HMG-CoA reductase is attributed to active metabolites. *In vitro* studies suggest the importance of atorvastatin metabolism by cytochrome P450 3A4, consistent with increased plasma concentrations of atorvastatin in humans following coadministration with erythromycin, a known inhibitor of this isozyme (see **PRECAUTIONS, Drug Interactions**). In animals, the ortho-hydroxy metabolite undergoes further glucuronidation.

Excretion

Studies with amlodipine: Elimination from the plasma is biphasic with a terminal elimination half-life of about 30-50 hours. Ten percent of the parent amlodipine compound and 60% of the metabolites of amlodipine are excreted in the urine.

Studies with atorvastatin: Atorvastatin and its metabolites are eliminated primarily in bile following hepatic and/or extra-hepatic metabolism; however, the drug does not appear to undergo enterohepatic recirculation. Mean plasma elimination half-life of atorvastatin in humans is approximately 14 hours, but the half-life of inhibitory activity for HMG-CoA reductase is 20 to 30 hours due to the contribution of active metabolites. Less than 2% of a dose of atorvastatin is recovered in urine following oral administration.

Special Populations

Geriatric

Studies with amlodipine: Elderly patients have decreased clearance of amlodipine with a resulting increase in AUC of approximately 40-60%, and a lower initial dose of amlodipine may be required.

Studies with atorvastatin: Plasma concentrations of atorvastatin are higher (approximately 40% for Cmax and 30% for AUC) in healthy elderly subjects (age ≥65 years) than in young adults. Clinical data suggest a greater degree of LDL-lowering at any dose of atorvastatin in the elderly population compared to younger adults (see **PRECAUTIONS** section, **Geriatric Use**).

Pediatric

Studies with amlodipine: Sixty-two hypertensive patients aged 6 to 17 years received doses of amlodipine between 1.25 mg and 20 mg. Weight-adjusted clearance and volume of distribution were similar to values in adults.

Studies with atorvastatin: Pharmacokinetic data in the pediatric population are not available.

Gender

Studies with atorvastatin: Plasma concentrations of atorvastatin in women differ from those in men (approximately 20% higher for Cmax and 10% lower for AUC); however, there is no clinically significant difference in LDL-C reduction with atorvastatin between men and women.

Renal Insufficiency

Studies with amlodipine: The pharmacokinetics of amlodipine are not significantly influenced by renal impairment. Patients with renal failure may therefore receive the usual initial amlodipine dose.

Studies with atorvastatin: Renal disease has no influence on the plasma concentrations or LDL-C reduction of atorvastatin; thus, dose adjustment of atorvastatin in patients with renal dysfunction is not necessary (see **DOSAGE AND ADMINISTRATION**).

Hemodialysis

While studies have not been conducted in patients with end-stage renal disease, hemodialysis is not expected to significantly enhance clearance of atorvastatin and/or amlodipine since both drugs are extensively bound to plasma proteins.

Hepatic Insufficiency

Studies with amlodipine: Elderly patients and patients with hepatic insufficiency have decreased clearance of amlodipine with a resulting increase in AUC of approximately 40-60%, and a lower initial dose may be required.

Studies with atorvastatin: In patients with chronic alcoholic liver disease, plasma concentrations of atorvastatin are markedly increased. Cmax and AUC are each 4-fold greater in patients with Childs-Pugh A disease. Cmax and AUC of atorvastatin are approximately 16-fold and 11-fold increased, respectively, in patients with Childs-Pugh B disease (see **CONTRAINDICATIONS**).

Heart Failure

Studies with amlodipine: In patients with moderate to severe heart failure, the increase in AUC for amlodipine was similar to that seen in the elderly and in patients with hepatic insufficiency.

Pharmacodynamics

Hemodynamic Effects of Amlodipine: Following administration of therapeutic doses to patients with hypertension, amlodipine produces vasodilation resulting in a reduction of supine and standing blood pressures. These decreases in blood pressure are not accompanied by a significant change in heart rate or plasma catecholamine levels with chronic dosing. Although the acute intravenous administration of amlodipine decreases arterial blood pressure and increases heart rate in hemodynamic studies of patients with chronic stable angina, chronic administration of oral amlodipine in clinical trials did not lead to clinically significant changes in heart rate or blood pressures in normotensive patients with angina.

With chronic once daily oral administration of amlodipine, antihypertensive effectiveness is maintained for at least 24 hours. Plasma concentrations correlate with effect in both young and elderly patients. The magnitude of reduction in blood pressure with amlodipine is also correlated with the height of pretreatment elevation; thus, individuals with moderate hypertension (diastolic pressure 105-114 mmHg) had about a 50% greater response than patients with mild hypertension (diastolic pressure 90-104 mmHg). Normotensive subjects experienced no clinically significant change in blood pressures (+1/–2 mmHg).

In hypertensive patients with normal renal function, therapeutic doses of amlodipine resulted in a decrease in renal vascular resistance and an increase in glomerular filtration rate and effective renal plasma flow without change in filtration fraction or proteinuria.

As with other calcium channel blockers, hemodynamic measurements of cardiac function at rest and during exercise (or pacing) in patients with normal ventricular function treated with amlodipine have generally demonstrated a small increase in cardiac index without significant influence on dP/dt or on left ventricular end diastolic pressure or volume. In hemodynamic studies, amlodipine has not been associated with a negative inotropic effect when administered in the therapeutic dose range to intact animals and man, even when co-administered with beta-blockers to man. Similar findings, however, have been observed in normals or well-compensated patients with heart failure with agents possessing significant negative inotropic effects.

Electrophysiologic Effects of Amlodipine: Amlodipine does not change sinoatrial nodal function or atrioventricular conduction in intact animals or man. In patients with chronic stable angina, intravenous administration of 10 mg did not significantly alter A-H and H-V conduction and sinus node recovery time after pacing. Similar results were obtained in patients receiving amlodipine and concomitant beta blockers. In clinical studies in which amlodipine was administered in combination with beta-blockers to patients with either hypertension or angina, no adverse effects on electrocardiographic parameters were observed. In clinical trials with angina patients alone, amlodipine therapy did not alter electrocardiographic intervals or produce higher degrees of AV blocks.

LDL-C Reduction with Atorvastatin: Atorvastatin as well as some of its metabolites are pharmacologically active in humans. The liver is the primary site of action and the principal site of cholesterol synthesis and LDL clearance. Drug dosage rather than systemic drug concentration correlates better with LDL-C reduction. Individualization of drug dosage should be based on therapeutic response (see **DOSAGE AND ADMINISTRATION**).

Clinical Studies

Clinical Studies with Amlodipine

Amlodipine Effects in Hypertension

Adult Patients: The antihypertensive efficacy of amlodipine has been demonstrated in a total of 15 double-blind, placebo-controlled, randomized studies involving 800 patients on amlodipine and 538 on placebo. Once daily administration produced statistically significant placebo-corrected reductions in supine and standing blood pressures at 24 hours postdose, averaging about 12/6 mmHg in the standing position and 13/7 mmHg in the supine position in patients with mild to moderate hypertension. Maintenance of the blood pressure effect over the 24-hour dosing interval was observed, with little difference in peak and trough effect. Tolerance was not demonstrated in patients studied for up to 1 year. The 3 parallel, fixed doses, dose response studies showed that the reduction in supine and standing blood pressures was dose-related within the recommended dosing range. Effects on diastolic pressure were similar in young and older patients. The effect on systolic pressure was greater in older patients, perhaps because of greater baseline systolic pressure. Effects were similar in black patients and in white patients.

Pediatric Patients: Two-hundred sixty-eight hypertensive patients aged 6 to 17 years were randomized first to amlodipine 2.5 or 5 mg once daily for 4 weeks and then randomized again to the same dose or to placebo for another 4 weeks. Patients receiving 5 mg amlodipine at the end of 8 weeks had lower blood pressure than those secondarily randomized to placebo. The magnitude of the treatment effect is difficult to interpret, but it is probably less than 5 mmHg systolic on the 5 mg dose. Adverse events were similar to those seen in adults.

Amlodipine Effects in Chronic Stable Angina: The effectiveness of 5-10 mg/day of amlodipine in exercise-induced angina has been evaluated in 8 placebo-controlled, double-blind clinical trials of up to 6 weeks duration involving 1038 patients (684 amlodipine, 354 placebo) with chronic stable angina. In 5 of the 8 studies, significant increases in exercise time (bicycle or treadmill) were seen with the 10 mg dose. Increases in symptom-limited exercise time averaged 12.8% (63 sec) for amlodipine 10 mg, and averaged 7.9% (38 sec) for amlodipine 5 mg. Amlodipine 10 mg also increased time to 1 mm ST segment deviation in several studies and decreased angina attack rate. The sustained efficacy of amlodipine in angina patients has been demonstrated over long-term dosing. In patients with angina, there were no clinically significant reductions in blood pressures (4/1 mmHg) or changes in heart rate (+0.3 bpm).

Amlodipine Effects in Vasospastic Angina: In a double-blind, placebo-controlled clinical trial of 4 weeks duration in 50 patients, amlodipine therapy decreased attacks by approximately 4/week compared with a placebo decrease of approximately 1/week ($p<0.01$). Two of 23 amlodipine and 7 of 27 placebo patients discontinued from the study due to lack of clinical improvement.

Amlodipine Effects in Documented Coronary Artery Disease: In PREVENT, 825 patients with angiographically documented coronary artery disease were randomized to amlodipine (5-10 mg once daily) or placebo and followed for 3 years. Although the study did not show significance on the primary objective of change in coronary luminal diameter as assessed by quantitative coronary angiography, the data suggested a favorable outcome with respect to fewer hospitalizations for angina and revascularization procedures in patients with CAD.

CAMELOT enrolled 1318 patients with CAD recently documented by angiography, without left main coronary disease and without heart failure or an ejection fraction <40%. Patients (76% males, 89% Caucasian, 93% enrolled at US sites, 89% with a history of angina, 52% without PCI, 4% with PCI and no stent, and 44% with a stent) were randomized to double-blind treatment with either amlodipine (5-10 mg once daily) or placebo in addition to standard care that included aspirin (89%), statins (83%), beta-blockers (74%), nitroglycerin (50%), anti-coagulants (40%), and diuretics (32%), but excluded other calcium channel blockers. The mean duration of follow-up was 19 months. The primary endpoint was the time to first occurrence of one of the following events: hospitalization for angina pectoris, coro-

Continued on next page

Caduet—Cont.

nary revascularization, myocardial infarction, cardiovascular death, resuscitated cardiac arrest, hospitalization for heart failure, stroke/TIA, or peripheral vascular disease. A total of 110 (16.6%) and 151 (23.1%) first events occurred in the amlodipine and placebo groups respectively for a hazard ratio of 0.691 (95% CI: 0.540-0.884, p= 0.003). The primary endpoint is summarized in Figure 1 below. The outcome of this study was largely derived from the prevention of hospitalizations for angina and the prevention of revascularization procedures (see Table 2). Effects in various subgroups are shown in Figure 2.

In a angiographic substudy (n=274) conducted within CAMELOT, there was no significant difference between amlodipine and placebo on the change of atheroma volume in the coronary artery as assessed by intravascular ultrasound.

Figure 1: Kaplan-Meier analysis of composite clinical outcomes for amlodipine versus placebo

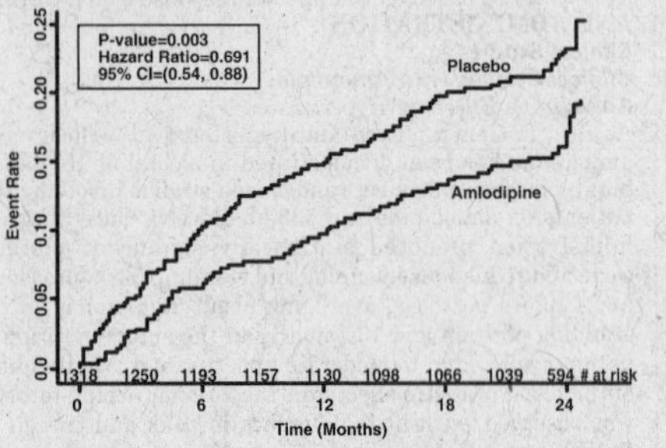

Figure 2 – Effects on primary endpoint of amlodipine versus placebo across subgroups

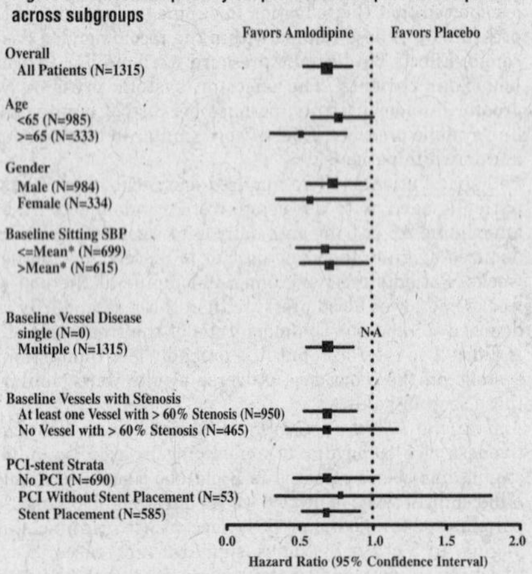

*The mean sitting baseline SBP is 129 mmHg

Table 2 below summarizes the significant clinical outcomes from the composites of the primary endpoint. The other components of the primary endpoint including cardiovascular death, resuscitated cardiac arrest, myocardial infarction, hospitalization for heart failure, stroke/TIA, or peripheral vascular disease did not demonstrate a significant difference between amlodipine and placebo.

Table 2. Incidence of Significant Clinical Outcomes for CAMELOT

Clinical Outcomes N (%)	Amlodipine (N=663)	Placebo (N=655)	Risk Reduction (p-value)
Composite CV Endpoint	**110 (16.6)**	**151 (23.1)**	**31% (0.003)**
Hospitalization for Angina*	51 (7.7)	84 (12.8)	42% (0.002)
Coronary Revascularization*	78 (11.8)	103 (15.7)	27% (0.033)

*Total patients with these events

Amlodipine Effects in Patients with Congestive Heart Failure: Amlodipine has been compared to placebo in four 8-12 week studies of patients with NYHA class II/III heart failure, involving a total of 697 patients. In these studies, there was no evidence of worsened heart failure based on measures of exercise tolerance, NYHA classification, symptoms, or LVEF. In a long-term (follow-up at least 6 months, mean 13.8 months) placebo-controlled mortality/morbidity study of amlodipine 5-10 mg in 1153 patients with NYHA classes III (n=931) or IV (n=222) heart failure on stable doses of diuretics, digoxin, and ACE inhibitors, amlodipine had no effect on the primary endpoint of the study which was the combined endpoint of all-cause mortality and cardiac morbidity (as defined by life-threatening arrhythmia, acute myocardial infarction, or hospitalization for worsened heart failure), or on NYHA classification, or symptoms of heart failure. Total combined all-cause mortality and cardiac morbidity events were 222/571 (39%) for patients on amlodipine and 246/583 (42%) for patients on placebo; the cardiac morbid events represented about 25% of the endpoints in the study.

Another study (PRAISE-2) randomized patients with NYHA class III (80%) or IV (20%) heart failure without clinical symptoms or objective evidence of underlying ischemic disease, on stable doses of ACE inhibitor (99%), digitalis (99%) and diuretics (99%), to placebo (n=827) or amlodipine (n=827) and followed them for a mean of 33 months. There was no statistically significant difference between amlodipine and placebo in the primary endpoint of all cause mortality (95% confidence limits from 8% reduction to 29% increase on amlodipine). With amlodipine there were more reports of pulmonary edema.

Clinical Studies with Atorvastatin

Prevention of Cardiovascular Disease: In the Anglo-Scandinavian Cardiac Outcomes Trial (ASCOT), the effect of atorvastatin on fatal and non-fatal coronary heart disease was assessed in 10,305 hypertensive patients 40-80 years of age (mean of 63 years), without a previous myocardial infarction and with TC levels ≤251 mg/dl (6.5 mmol/l). Additionally all patients had at least 3 of the following cardiovascular risk factors: male gender (81.1%), age >55 years (84.5%), smoking (33.2%), diabetes (24.3%), history of CHD in a first-degree relative (26%), TC:HDL >6 (14.3%), peripheral vascular disease (5.1%), left ventricular hypertrophy (14.4%), prior cerebrovascular event (9.8%), specific ECG abnormality (14.3%), proteinuria/albuminuria (62.4%)]. In this double-blind, placebo-controlled study patients were treated with anti-hypertensive therapy (Goal BP <140/90 mm Hg for non-diabetic patients, <130/80 mm Hg for diabetic patients) and allocated to either atorvastatin 10 mg daily (n=5168) or placebo (n=5137), using a covariate adaptive method which took into account the distribution of nine baseline characteristics of patients already enrolled and minimized the imbalance of those characteristics across the groups. Patients were followed for a median duration of 3.3 years.

The effect of 10 mg/day of atorvastatin on lipid levels was similar to that seen in previous clinical trials.

Atorvastatin significantly reduced the rate of coronary events [either fatal coronary heart disease (46 events in the placebo group vs 40 events in the atorvastatin group) or nonfatal MI (108 events in the placebo group vs 60 events in the atorvastatin group)] with a relative risk reduction of 36% [(based on incidences of 1.9% for atorvastatin vs 3.0% for placebo), p=0.0005 (see Figure 3)]. The risk reduction was consistent regardless of age, smoking status, obesity or presence of renal dysfunction. The effect of atorvastatin was seen regardless of baseline LDL levels. Due to the small number of events, results for women were inconclusive.

Figure 3: Effects of Atorvastatin 10 mg/day on Cumulative Incidence of Nonfatal Myocardial Infarction or Coronary Heart Disease Death (in ASCOT-LLA)

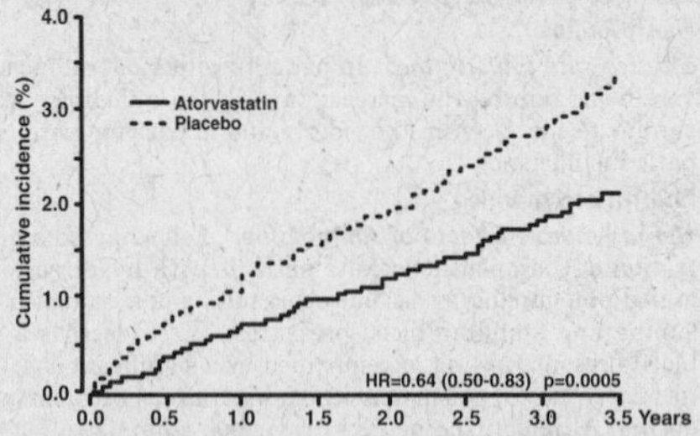

Atorvastatin also significantly decreased the relative risk for revascularization procedures by 42%. Although the reduction of fatal and non-fatal strokes did not reach a predefined significance level (p 0.01), a favorable trend was observed with a 26% relative risk reduction (incidences of 1.7% for atorvastatin and 2.3% for placebo). There was no significant difference between the treatment groups for death due to cardiovascular causes (p=0.51) or noncardiovascular causes (p=0.17).

In the Collaborative Atorvastatin Diabetes Study (CARDS), the effect of atorvastatin on cardiovascular disease (CVD) endpoints was assessed in 2838 subjects (94% White, 68% male), ages 40-75 with type 2 diabetes based on WHO criteria, without prior history of cardiovascular disease and with LDL≤ 160 mg/dL and TG ≤600 mg/dL. In addition to diabetes, subjects had 1 or more of the following risk factors: current smoking (23%), hypertension (80%), retinopathy (30%), or microalbuminuria (9%) or macroalbuminuria (3%). No subjects on hemodialysis were enrolled in the study. In this multicenter, placebo-controlled, double-blind clinical trial, subjects were randomly allocated to either atorvastatin 10 mg daily (1429) or placebo (1411) in a 1:1 ratio and were followed for a median duration of 3.9 years. The primary endpoint was the occurrence of any of the major cardiovascular events: myocardial infarction, acute CHD death, unstable angina, coronary revascularization, or stroke. The primary analysis was the time to first occurrence of the primary endpoint.

Baseline characteristics of subjects were: mean age of 62 years, mean HbA_{1c} 7.7%; median LDL-C 120 mg/dL; median TC 207 mg/dL; median TG 151 mg/dL; median HDL-C 52mg/dL.

The effect of atorvastatin 10 mg/day on lipid levels was similar to that seen in previous clinical trials.

Atorvastatin significantly reduced the rate of major cardiovascular events (primary endpoint events) (83 events in the atorvastatin group vs 127 events in the placebo group) with a relative risk reduction of 37%, HR 0.63, 95% CI (0.48,0.83) (p=0.001) (see Figure 4). An effect of atorvastatin was seen regardless of age, sex, or baseline lipid levels.

Figure 4: Effect of Atorvastatin 10 mg/day on Time Occurrence of Major Cardivascular Events (myocardial infarction, acute CHD death, unstable angina, coronary revascularization, or stroke) in CARDS.

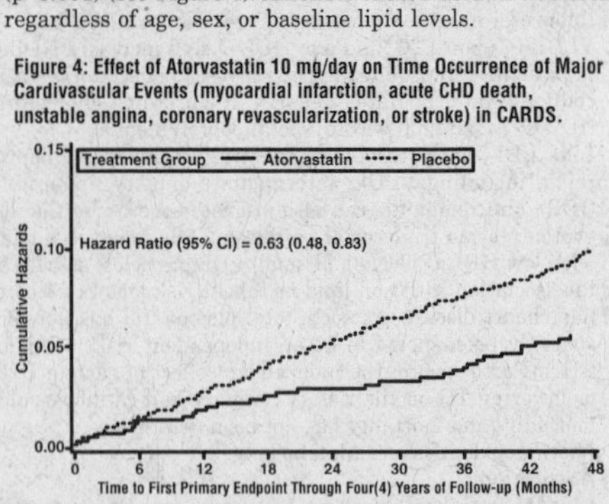

Atorvastatin significantly reduced the risk of stroke by 48% (21 events in the atorvastatin group vs 39 events in the placebo group), HR 0.52, 95% CI (0.31,0.89) (p=0.016) and reduced the risk of MI by 42% (38 events in the atorvastatin group vs 64 events in the placebo group), HR 0.58, 95.1% CI (0.39, 0.86) (p=0.007). There was no significant difference between the treatment groups for angina, revascularization procedures, and acute CHD death.

There were 61 deaths in the atorvastatin group vs. 82 deaths in the placebo group, (HR 0.73, p=0.059).

In the Treating to New Targets Study (TNT), the effect of LIPITOR 80 mg/day vs. LIPITOR 10 mg/day on the reduction in cardiovascular events was assessed in 10,001 subjects (94% white, 81% male, 38% ≥65 years) with clinically evident coronary heart disease who had achieved a target LDL-C level <130 mg/dL after completing an 8-week, open-label, run-in period with LIPITOR 10 mg/day. Subjects were randomly assigned to either 10 mg/day or 80 mg/day of LIPITOR and followed for a median duration of 4.9 years. The primary endpoint was the time-to-first occurrence of any of the following major cardiovascular events (MCVE): death due to CHD, non-fatal myocardial infarction, resuscitated cardiac arrest, and fatal and non-fatal stroke. The mean LDL-C, TC, TG, non-HDL and HDL cholesterol levels at 12 weeks were 73, 145, 128, 98 and 47 mg/dL during treatment with 80 mg of LIPITOR and 99, 177, 152, 129 and 48 mg/dL during treatment with 10 mg of LIPITOR.

Treatment with LIPITOR 80 mg/day significantly reduced the rate of MCVE (434 events in the 80mg/day group vs 548 events in the 10 mg/day group) with a relative risk reduction of 22%, HR 0.78, 95% CI (0.69,0.89), p=0.0002 (see Figure 5 and Table 3). The overall risk reduction was consistent regardless of age (<65, ≥65) or gender.

Figure 5. Effect of LIPITOR 80 mg/day vs. 10 mg/day on Time to Occurrence of Major Cardiovascular Events (TNT)

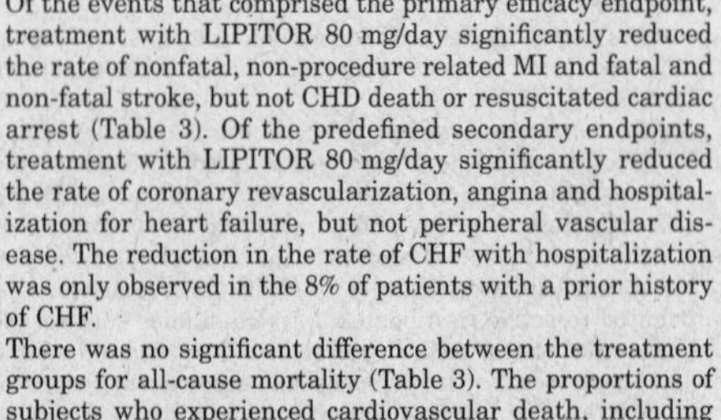

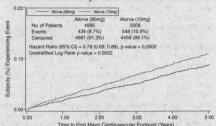

[See table 3 at top of next page]

Of the events that comprised the primary efficacy endpoint, treatment with LIPITOR 80 mg/day significantly reduced the rate of nonfatal, non-procedure related MI and fatal and non-fatal stroke, but not CHD death or resuscitated cardiac arrest (Table 3). Of the predefined secondary endpoints, treatment with LIPITOR 80 mg/day significantly reduced the rate of coronary revascularization, angina and hospitalization for heart failure, but not peripheral vascular disease. The reduction in the rate of CHF with hospitalization was only observed in the 8% of patients with a prior history of CHF.

There was no significant difference between the treatment groups for all-cause mortality (Table 3). The proportions of subjects who experienced cardiovascular death, including the components of CHD death and fatal stroke were numerically smaller in the LIPITOR 80 mg group than in the LIPITOR 10 mg treatment group. The proportions of subjects who experienced noncardiovascular death were numerically larger in the LIPITOR 80 mg group than in the LIPITOR 10 mg treatment group.

In the Incremental Decrease in Endpoints Through Aggressive Lipid Lowering Study (IDEAL), treatment with LIPITOR 80 mg/day was compared to treatment with simvastatin 20-40 mg/day in 8,888 subjects up to 80 years of age with a history of CHD to assess whether reduction in CV risk could be achieved. Patients were mainly male (81%), white (99%) with an average age of 61.7 years, and an average LDL-C of 121.5 mg/dL at randomization; 76%

were on statin therapy. In this prospective, randomized, open-label, blinded endpoint (PROBE) trial with no run-in period, subjects were followed for a median duration of 4.8 years. The mean LDL-C, TC, TG, HDL and non-HDL cholesterol levels at Week 12 were 78, 145, 115, 45 and 100 mg/dL during treatment with 80 mg of LIPITOR and 105, 179, 142, 47 and 132 mg/dL during treatment with 20-40 mg of simvastatin.

There was no significant difference between the treatment groups for the primary endpoint, the rate of first major coronary event (fatal CHD, nonfatal MI and resuscitated cardiac arrest): 411 (9.3%) in the LIPITOR 80 mg/day group vs. 463 (10.4%) in the simvastatin 20-40 mg/day group, HR 0.89, 95% CI (0.78,1.01), p=0.07.

There were no significant differences between the treatment groups for all-cause mortality: 366 (8.2%) in the LIPITOR 80 mg/day group vs. 374 (8.4%) in the simvastatin 20-40 mg/day group. The proportions of subjects who experienced CV or non-CV death were similar for the LIPITOR 80 mg group and the simvastatin 20-40 mg group.

Atorvastatin Studies in Hypercholesterolemia (Heterozygous Familial and Nonfamilial) and Mixed Dyslipidemia (Fredrickson Types IIa and IIb): Atorvastatin reduces total-C, LDL-C, VLDL-C, apo B, and TG, and increases HDL-C in patients with hypercholesterolemia and mixed dyslipidemia. Therapeutic response is seen within 2 weeks, and maximum response is usually achieved within 4 weeks and maintained during chronic therapy.

Atorvastatin is effective in a wide variety of patient populations with hypercholesterolemia, with and without hypertriglyceridemia, in men and women, and in the elderly.

In two multicenter, placebo-controlled, dose-response studies in patients with hypercholesterolemia, atorvastatin given as a single dose over 6 weeks significantly reduced total-C, LDL-C, apo B, and TG (pooled results are provided in Table 4).

[See table 4 above]

In patients with *Fredrickson* Types IIa and IIb hyperlipoproteinemia pooled from 24 controlled trials, the median (25th and 75th percentile) percent changes from baseline in HDL-C for atorvastatin 10, 20, 40, and 80 mg were 6.4 (-1.4, 14), 8.7 (0, 17), 7.8 (0, 16), and 5.1 (-2.7, 15), respectively. Additionally, analysis of the pooled data demonstrated consistent and significant decreases in total-C, LDL-C, TG, total-C/HDL-C, and LDL-C/HDL-C.

In three multicenter, double-blind studies in patients with hypercholesterolemia, atorvastatin was compared to other HMG-CoA reductase inhibitors. After randomization, patients were treated for 16 weeks with either atorvastatin 10 mg per day or a fixed dose of the comparative agent (Table 5).

[See table 5 above]

The impact on clinical outcomes of the differences in lipid-altering effects between treatments shown in Table 5 is not known. Table 5 does not contain data comparing the effects of atorvastatin 10 mg and higher doses of lovastatin, pravastatin, and simvastatin. The drugs compared in the studies summarized in the table are not necessarily interchangeable.

Atorvastatin Effects in Hypertriglyceridemia (Fredrickson Type IV): The response to atorvastatin in 64 patients with isolated hypertriglyceridemia treated across several clinical trials is shown in the table below. For the atorvastatin-treated patients, median (min, max) baseline TG level was 565 (267-1502).

[See table 6 at top of next page]

Atorvastatin Effects in Dysbetalipoproteinemia (Fredrickson Type III): The results of an open-label crossover study of atorvastatin in 16 patients (genotypes: 14 apo E2/E2 and 2 apo E3/E2) with dysbetalipoproteinemia (*Fredrickson* Type III) are shown in the table below.

[See table 7 at top of next page]

Atorvastatin Effects in Homozygous Familial Hypercholesterolemia: In a study without a concurrent control group, 29 patients ages 6 to 37 years with homozygous FH received maximum daily doses of 20 to 80 mg of atorvastatin. The mean LDL-C reduction in this study was 18%. Twenty-five patients with a reduction in LDL-C had a mean response of 20% (range of 7% to 53%, median of 24%); the remaining 4 patients had 7% to 24% increases in LDL-C. Five of the 29 patients had absent LDL-receptor function. Of these, 2 patients also had a portacaval shunt and had no significant reduction in LDL-C. The remaining 3 receptor-negative patients had a mean LDL-C reduction of 22%.

Atorvastatin Effects in Heterozygous Familial Hypercholesterolemic Pediatric Patients: In a double-blind, placebo-controlled study followed by an open-label phase, 187 boys and postmenarchal girls 10-17 years of age (mean age 14.1 years) with heterozygous FH or severe hypercholesterolemia were randomized to atorvastatin (n=140) or placebo (n=47) for 26 weeks and then all received atorvastatin for 26 weeks. Inclusion in the study required 1) a baseline LDL-C level ≥ 190 mg/dL or 2) a baseline LDL-C ≥ 160 mg/dL and positive family history of FH or documented premature cardiovascular disease in a first- or second-degree relative. The mean baseline LDL-C value was 218.6 mg/dL (range: 138.5–385.0 mg/dL) in the atorvastatin group compared to 230.0 mg/dL (range: 160.0–324.5 mg/dL) in placebo group. The dosage of atorvastatin (once daily) was 10 mg for the first 4 weeks and up-titrated to 20 mg if the LDL-C level was >130 mg/dL. The number of atorvastatin-treated patients who required up-titration to 20 mg after Week 4 during the double-blind phase was 80 (57.1%).

Atorvastatin significantly decreased plasma levels of total-C, LDL-C, triglycerides, and apolipoprotein B during the 26 week double-blind phase (see Table 8).

[See table 8 at top of next page]

The mean achieved LDL-C value was 130.7 mg/dL (range: 70.0-242.0 mg/dL) in the atorvastatin group compared to 228.5 mg/dL (range: 152.0–385.0 mg/dL) in the placebo group during the 26 week double-blind phase.

The safety and efficacy of atorvastatin doses above 20 mg have not been studied in controlled trials in children. The long-term efficacy of atorvastatin therapy in childhood to reduce morbidity and mortality in adulthood has not been established.

Clinical Study of Combined Amlodipine and Atorvastatin in Patients with Hypertension and Dyslipidemia

In a double-blind, placebo-controlled study, a total of 1660 patients with co-morbid hypertension and dyslipidemia received once daily treatment with eight dose combinations of amlodipine and atorvastatin (5/10, 10/10, 5/20, 10/20, 5/40, 10/40, 5/80, or 10/80 mg), amlodipine alone (5 mg or 10 mg), atorvastatin alone (10 mg, 20 mg, 40 mg, or 80 mg) or placebo. In addition to concomitant hypertension and dyslipidemia, 15% of the patients had diabetes mellitus, 22% were smokers and 14% had a positive family history of cardiovascular disease. At eight weeks, all eight combination-treatment groups of amlodipine and atorvastatin demonstrated statistically significant dose-related reductions in systolic blood pressure (SBP), diastolic blood pressure (DBP) and LDL-C compared to placebo, with no overall modification of effect of either component on SBP, DBP and LDL-C (Table 9).

[See table 9 at top of next page]

TABLE 3. Overview of Efficacy Results in TNT

Endpoint	Atorvastatin 10 mg (N=5006)		Atorvastatin 80 mg (N=4995)		HR[a] (95%CI)
PRIMARY ENDPOINT	n	(%)	n	(%)	
First major cardiovascular endpoint	548	(10.9)	434	(8.7)	0.78 (0.69, 0.89)
Components of the Primary Endpoint					
CHD death	127	(2.5)	101	(2.0)	0.80 (0.61, 1.03)
Nonfatal, non-procedure related MI	308	(6.2)	243	(4.9)	0.78 (0.66, 0.93)
Resuscitated cardiac arrest	26	(0.5)	25	(0.5)	0.96 (0.56, 1.67)
Stroke (fatal and non-fatal)	155	(3.1)	117	(2.3)	0.75 (0.59, 0.96)
SECONDARY ENDPOINTS*					
First CHF with hospitalization	164	(3.3)	122	(2.4)	0.74 (0.59, 0.94)
First PVD endpoint	282	(5.6)	275	(5.5)	0.97 (0.83, 1.15)
First CABG or other coronary revascularization procedure[b]	904	(18.1)	667	(13.4)	0.72 (0.65, 0.80)
First documented angina endpoint[b]	615	(12.3)	545	(10.9)	0.88 (0.79, 0.99)
All cause mortality	282	(5.6)	284	(5.7)	1.01 (0.85, 1.19)
Components of all cause mortality					
Cardiovascular death	155	(3.1)	126	(2.5)	0.81 (0.64, 1.03)
Noncardiovascular death	127	(2.5)	158	(3.2)	1.25 (0.99, 1.57)
Cancer death	75	(1.5)	85	(1.7)	1.13 (0.83, 1.55)
Other non-CV death	43	(0.9)	58	(1.2)	1.35 (0.91, 2.00)
Suicide, homicide and other traumatic non-CV death	9	(0.2)	15	(0.3)	1.67 (0.73, 3.82)

a Atorvastatin 80 mg: atorvastatin 10 mg
b component of other secondary endpoints
* secondary endpoints not included in primary endpoint
HR=hazard ratio; CHD=coronary heart disease; CI=confidence interval; MI=myocardial infarction; CHF=congestive heart failure; CV=cardiovascular; PVD=peripheral vascular disease; CABG=coronary artery bypass graft
Confidence intervals for the Secondary Endpoints were not adjusted for multiple comparisons

Table 4. Dose-Response in Patients With Primary Hypercholesterolemia (Adjusted Mean Percent Change From Baseline)[a]

DOSE	N	TC	LDL-C	ApoB	TG	HDL-C	Non-HDL-C/ HDL-C
Placebo	21	4	4	3	10	-3	7
10 mg	22	-29	-39	-32	-19	6	-34
20 mg	20	-33	-43	-35	-26	9	-41
40 mg	21	-37	-50	-42	-29	6	-45
80 mg	23	-45	-60	-50	-37	5	-53

a Results are pooled from 2 dose-response studies.

Table 5. Mean Percent Change From Baseline at Endpoint (Double-Blind, Randomized, Active-Controlled Trials)

Treatment (Daily Dose)	N	Total-C	LDL-C	Apo B	TG	HDL-C	Non-HDL-C/ HDL-C
Study 1							
Atorvastatin 10 mg	707	-27[a]	-36[a]	-28[a]	-17[a]	+7	-37[a]
Lovastatin 20 mg	191	-19	-27	-20	-6	+7	-28
95% CI for Diff[1]		-9.2, -6.5	-10.7, -7.1	-10.0, -6.5	-15.2, -7.1	-1.7, 2.0	-11.1, -7.1
Study 2							
Atorvastatin 10 mg	222	-25[b]	-35[b]	-27[b]	-17[b]	+6	-36[b]
Pravastatin 20 mg	77	-17	-23	-17	-9	+8	-28
95% CI for Diff[1]		-10.8, -6.1	-14.5, -8.2	-13.4, -7.4	-14.1, -0.7	-4.9, 1.6	-11.5, -4.1
Study 3							
Atorvastatin 10 mg	132	-29[c]	-37[c]	-34[c]	-23[c]	+7	-39[c]
Simvastatin 10 mg	45	-24	-30	-30	-15	+7	-33
95% CI for Diff[1]		-8.7, -2.7	-10.1, -2.6	-8.0, -1.1	-15.1, -0.7	-4.3, 3.9	-9.6, -1.9

[1] A negative value for the 95% CI for the difference between treatments favors atorvastatin for all except HDL-C, for which a positive value favors atorvastatin. If the range does not include 0, this indicates a statistically significant difference.
a Significantly different from lovastatin, ANCOVA, p ≤0.05
b Significantly different from pravastatin, ANCOVA, p ≤0.05
c Significantly different from simvastatin, ANCOVA, p ≤0.05

Caduet—Cont.

INDICATIONS AND USAGE

CADUET (amlodipine and atorvastatin) is indicated in patients for whom treatment with both amlodipine and atorvastatin is appropriate.

Amlodipine

1. *Hypertension:* Amlodipine is indicated for the treatment of hypertension. It may be used alone or in combination with other antihypertensive agents;

2. *Coronary Artery Disease (CAD)*
   Chronic Stable Angina: Amlodipine is indicated for the treatment of chronic stable angina. Amlodipine may be used alone or in combination with other antianginal or antihypertensive agents;
   Vasospastic Angina (Prinzmetal's or Variant Angina): Amlodipine is indicated for the treatment of confirmed or suspected vasospastic angina. Amlodipine may be used as monotherapy or in combination with other antianginal drugs.
   Angiographically Documented CAD: In patients with recently documented CAD by angiography and without heart failure or an ejection fraction <40%, amlodipine is indicated to reduce the risk of hospitalization due to angina and to reduce the risk of a coronary revascularization procedure.

AND

Atorvastatin

1. *Prevention of Cardiovascular Disease:* In adult patients without clinically evident coronary heart disease, but with multiple risk factors for coronary heart disease such as age, smoking, hypertension, low HDL-C, or a family history of early coronary heart disease, atorvastatin is indicated to:
   - Reduce the risk of myocardial infarction
   - Reduce the risk of stroke
   - Reduce the risk for revascularization procedures and angina
   In patients with type 2 diabetes, and without clinically evident coronary heart disease, but with multiple risk factors for coronary heart disease such as retinopathy, albuminuria, smoking, or hypertension, LIPITOR is indicated to:
   - Reduce the risk of myocardial infarction
   - Reduce the risk of stroke;
   In patients with clinically evident coronary heart disease, LIPITOR is indicated to:
   • Reduce the risk of non-fatal myocardial infarction
   • Reduce the risk of fatal and non-fatal stroke
   • Reduce the risk for revascularization procedures
   • Reduce the risk of hospitalization for CHF
   • Reduce the risk of angina

2. *Heterozygous Familial and Nonfamilial Hypercholesterolemia:* Atorvastatin is indicated as an adjunct to diet to reduce elevated total-C, LDL-C, apo B, and TG levels and to increase HDL-C in patients with primary hypercholesterolemia (heterozygous familial and nonfamilial) and mixed dyslipidemia (*Fredrickson* Types IIa and IIb);

3. *Elevated Serum TG Levels:* Atorvastatin is indicated as an adjunct to diet for the treatment of patients with elevated serum TG levels (*Fredrickson* Type IV);

4. *Primary Dysbetalipoproteinemia:* Atorvastatin is indicated for the treatment of patients with primary dysbetalipoproteinemia (*Fredrickson* Type III) who do not respond adequately to diet;

5. *Homozygous Familial Hypercholesterolemia:* Atorvastatin is indicated to reduce total-C and LDL-C in patients with homozygous familial hypercholesterolemia as an adjunct to other lipid-lowering treatments (e.g., LDL apheresis) or if such treatments are unavailable;

6. *Pediatric Patients:* Atorvastatin is indicated as an adjunct to diet to reduce total-C, LDL-C, and apo B levels in boys and postmenarchal girls, 10 to 17 years of age, with heterozygous familial hypercholesterolemia if after an adequate trial of diet therapy the following findings are present:
   a. LDL-C remains ≥ 190 mg/dL or
   b. LDL-C remains ≥ 160 mg/dL and:
      • there is a positive family history of premature cardiovascular disease or
      • two or more other CVD risk factors are present in the pediatric patients.

Therapy with lipid-altering agents should be a component of multiple-risk-factor intervention in individuals at increased risk for atherosclerotic vascular disease due to hypercholesterolemia. Lipid-altering agents should be used, in addition to a diet restricted in saturated fat and cholesterol, only when the response to diet and other nonpharmacological measures has been inadequate (see *National Cholesterol Education Program (NCEP) Guidelines,* summarized in Table 10).

[See table 10 at top of next page]

After the LDL-C goal has been achieved, if the TG is still ≥200 mg/dL, non-HDL-C (total-C minus HDL-C) becomes a secondary target of therapy. Non-HDL-C goals are set 30 mg/dL higher than LDL-C goals for each risk category.

Prior to initiating therapy with atorvastatin, secondary causes for hypercholesterolemia (e.g., poorly controlled diabetes mellitus, hypothyroidism, nephrotic syndrome, dysproteinemias, obstructive liver disease, other drug therapy, and alcoholism) should be excluded, and a lipid profile performed to measure total-C, LDL-C, HDL-C, and TG. For pa-

Table 6. Combined Patients With Isolated Elevated TG: Median (min, max) Percent Changes From Baseline

	Placebo (N=12)	Atorvastatin 10 mg (N=37)	Atorvastatin 20 mg (N=13)	Atorvastatin 80 mg (N=14)
Triglycerides	-12.4 (-36.6, 82.7)	-41.0 (-76.2, 49.4)	-38.7 (-62.7, 29.5)	-51.8 (-82.8, 41.3)
Total-C	-2.3 (-15.5, 24.4)	-28.2 (-44.9, -6.8)	-34.9 (-49.6, -15.2)	-44.4 (-63.5, -3.8)
LDL-C	3.6 (-31.3, 31.6)	-26.5 (-57.7, 9.8)	-30.4 (-53.9, 0.3)	-40.5 (-60.6, -13.8)
HDL-C	3.8 (-18.6, 13.4)	13.8 (-9.7, 61.5)	11.0 (-3.2, 25.2)	7.5 (-10.8, 37.2)
VLDL-C	-1.0 (-31.9, 53.2)	-48.8 (-85.8, 57.3)	-44.6 (-62.2, -10.8)	-62.0 (-88.2, 37.6)
non-HDL-C	-2.8 (-17.6, 30.0)	-33.0 (-52.1, -13.3)	-42.7 (-53.7, -17.4)	-51.5 (-72.9, -4.3)

Table 7. Open-Label Crossover Study of 16 Patients With Dysbetalipoproteinemia (*Fredrickson* Type III)

	Median (min, max) at Baseline (mg/dL)	Median % Change (min, max) Atorvastatin 10 mg	Atorvastatin 80 mg
Total-C	442 (225, 1320)	-37 (-85, 17)	-58 (-90, -31)
Triglycerides	678 (273, 5990)	-39 (-92, -8)	-53 (-95, -30)
IDL-C + VLDL-C	215 (111, 613)	-32 (-76, 9)	-63 (-90, -8)
non-HDL-C	411 (218, 1272)	-43 (-87, -19)	-64 (-92, -36)

Table 8. Lipid-altering Effects of Atorvastatin in Adolescent Boys and Girls with Heterozygous Familial Hypercholesterolemia or Severe Hypercholesterolemia (Mean Percent Change from Baseline at Endpoint in Intention-to-Treat Population)

DOSAGE	N	Total-C	LDL-C	HDL-C	TG	Apolipoprotein B
Placebo	47	-1.5	-0.4	-1.9	1.0	0.7
Atorvastatin	140	-31.4	-39.6	2.8	-12.0	-34.0

Table 9. Efficacy in Terms of Reduction in Blood Pressure and LDL-C
Efficacy of the Combined Treatments in Reducing Systolic BP

Parameter / Analysis		ATO 0 mg	ATO 10 mg	ATO 20 mg	ATO 40 mg	ATO 80 mg
AML 0 mg	Mean change (mmHg)	-3.0	-4.5	-6.2	-6.2	-6.4
	Difference versus placebo (mmHg)	–	-1.5	-3.2	-3.2	-3.4
AML 5 mg	Mean change (mmHg)	-12.8	-13.7	-15.3	-12.7	-12.2
	Difference versus placebo (mmHg)	-9.8	-10.7	-12.3	-9.7	-9.2
AML 10 mg	Mean change (mmHg)	-16.2	-15.9	-16.1	-16.3	-17.6
	Difference versus placebo (mmHg)	-13.2	-12.9	-13.1	-13.3	-14.6

Efficacy of the Combined Treatments in Reducing Diastolic BP

Parameter / Analysis		ATO 0 mg	ATO 10 mg	ATO 20 mg	ATO 40 mg	ATO 80 mg
AML 0 mg	Mean change (mmHg)	-3.3	-4.1	-3.9	-5.1	-4.1
	Difference versus placebo (mmHg)	–	-0.8	-0.6	-1.8	-0.8
AML 5 mg	Mean change (mmHg)	-7.6	-8.2	-9.4	-7.3	-8.4
	Difference versus placebo (mmHg)	-4.3	-4.9	-6.1	-4.0	-5.1
AML 10 mg	Mean change (mmHg)	-10.4	-9.1	-10.6	-9.8	-11.1
	Difference versus placebo (mmHg)	-7.1	-5.8	-7.3	-6.5	-7.8

Efficacy of the Combined Treatments in Reducing LDL-C (% change)

Parameter / Analysis		ATO 0 mg	ATO 10 mg	ATO 20 mg	ATO 40 mg	ATO 80 mg
AML 0 mg	Mean % change	-1.1	-33.4	-39.5	-43.1	-47.2
AML 5 mg	Mean % change	-0.1	-38.7	-42.3	-44.9	-48.4
AML 10 mg	Mean % change	-2.5	-36.6	-38.6	-43.2	-49.1

tients with TG <400 mg/dL (<4.5 mmol/L), LDL-C can be estimated using the following equation: LDL-C = total-C - (0.20 × [TG] + HDL-C). For TG levels >400 mg/dL (>4.5 mmol/L), this equation is less accurate and LDL-C concentrations should be determined by ultracentrifugation.

The antidyslipidemic component of CADUET has not been studied in conditions where the major lipoprotein abnormality is elevation of chylomicrons (*Fredrickson* Types I and V). The NCEP classification of cholesterol levels in pediatric patients with a familial history of hypercholesterolemia or premature cardiovascular disease is summarized below:

Table 11. NCEP Classification of Cholesterol Levels in Pediatric Patients

Category	Total-C (mg/dL)	LDL-C (mg/dL)
Acceptable	<170	<110
Borderline	170-199	110-129
High	≥200	≥130

Table 10. NCEP Treatment Guidelines: LDL-C Goals and Cutpoints for Therapeutic Lifestyle Changes and Drug Therapy in Different Risk Categories

Risk Category	LDL-C Goal (mg/dL)	LDL-C Level at Which to Initiate Therapeutic Lifestyle Changes (mg/dL)	LDL-C Level at Which to Consider Drug Therapy (mg/dL)
CHD[a] or CHD risk equivalents (10-year risk >20%)	<100	≥100	≥130 (100-129: drug optional)[b]
2+ Risk Factors (10-year risk ≤20%)	<130	≥130	10-year risk 10%-20%: ≥ 130 10-year risk <10%: ≥ 160
0-1 Risk Factor[c]	<160	≥160	≥190 (160-189: LDL-lowering drug optional)

[a] CHD, coronary heart disease
[b] Some authorities recommend use of LDL-lowering drugs in this category if an LDL-C level of < 100 mg/dL cannot be achieved by therapeutic lifestyle changes. Others prefer use of drugs that primarily modify triglycerides and HDL-C, e.g., nicotinic acid or fibrate. Clinical judgment also may call for deferring drug therapy in this subcategory.
[c] Almost all people with 0-1 risk factor have 10-year risk <10%; thus, 10-year risk assessment in people with 0-1 risk factor is not necessary.

CONTRAINDICATIONS

CADUET contains atorvastatin and is therefore contraindicated in patients with active liver disease or unexplained persistent elevations of serum transaminases.
CADUET is contraindicated in patients with known hypersensitivity to any component of this medication.

Pregnancy and Lactation

Atherosclerosis is a chronic process and discontinuation of lipid-lowering drugs during pregnancy should have little impact on the outcome of long-term therapy of primary hypercholesterolemia. Cholesterol and other products of cholesterol biosynthesis are essential components for fetal development (including synthesis of steroids and cell membranes). Since HMG-CoA reductase inhibitors decrease cholesterol synthesis and possibly the synthesis of other biologically active substances derived from cholesterol, they may cause fetal harm when administered to pregnant women. Therefore, HMG-CoA reductase inhibitors are contraindicated during pregnancy and in nursing mothers. CADUET, WHICH INCLUDES ATORVASTATIN, SHOULD BE ADMINISTERED TO WOMEN OF CHILDBEARING AGE ONLY WHEN SUCH PATIENTS ARE HIGHLY UNLIKELY TO CONCEIVE AND HAVE BEEN INFORMED OF THE POTENTIAL HAZARDS. If the patient becomes pregnant while taking this drug, therapy should be discontinued and the patient apprised of the potential hazard to the fetus.

WARNINGS

Increased Angina and/or Myocardial Infarction

Rarely, patients, particularly those with severe obstructive coronary artery disease, have developed documented increased frequency, duration and/or severity of angina or acute myocardial infarction on starting calcium channel blocker therapy or at the time of dosage increase. The mechanism of this effect has not been elucidated.

Liver Dysfunction

HMG-CoA reductase inhibitors, like some other lipid-lowering therapies, have been associated with biochemical abnormalities of liver function. **Persistent elevations (>3 times the upper limit of normal [ULN] occurring on 2 or more occasions) in serum transaminases occurred in 0.7% of patients who received atorvastatin in clinical trials. The incidence of these abnormalities was 0.2%, 0.2%, 0.6%, and 2.3% for 10, 20, 40, and 80 mg, respectively.**

In clinical trials in patients taking atorvastatin the following has been observed. One patient in clinical trials developed jaundice. Increases in liver function tests (LFT) in other patients were not associated with jaundice or other clinical signs or symptoms. Upon dose reduction, drug interruption, or discontinuation, transaminase levels returned to or near pretreatment levels without sequelae. Eighteen of 30 patients, with persistent LFT elevations continued treatment with a reduced dose of atorvastatin.

It is recommended that liver function tests be performed prior to and at 12 weeks following both the initiation of therapy and any elevation of dose, and periodically (e.g., semiannually) thereafter. Liver enzyme changes generally occur in the first 3 months of treatment with atorvastatin. Patients who develop increased transaminase levels should be monitored until the abnormalities resolve. Should an increase in ALT or AST of >3 times ULN persist, reduction of dose or withdrawal of CADUET is recommended.

CADUET should be used with caution in patients who consume substantial quantities of alcohol and/or have a history of liver disease. Active liver disease or unexplained persistent transaminase elevations are contraindications to the use of CADUET (see **CONTRAINDICATIONS**).

Skeletal Muscle

Rare cases of rhabdomyolysis with acute renal failure secondary to myoglobinuria have been reported with the atorvastatin component of CADUET and with other drugs in the HMG-CoA reductase inhibitor class.

Uncomplicated myalgia has been reported in atorvastatin-treated patients (see **ADVERSE REACTIONS**). Myopathy, defined as muscle aches or muscle weakness in conjunction with increases in creatine phosphokinase (CPK) values >10 times ULN, should be considered in any patient with diffuse myalgias, muscle tenderness or weakness, and/or marked elevation of CPK. Patients should be advised to report promptly unexplained muscle pain, tenderness or weakness, particularly if accompanied by malaise or fever. CADUET therapy should be discontinued if markedly elevated CPK levels occur or myopathy is diagnosed or suspected.

The risk of myopathy during treatment with drugs in the HMG-CoA reductase inhibitor class is increased with concurrent administration of cyclosporine, fibric acid derivatives, erythromycin, clarithromycin, combination of ritonavir plus saquinavir or lopinavir plus ritonavir, niacin, or azole antifungals. Physicians considering combined therapy with CADUET and fibric acid derivatives, erythromycin, clarithromycin, a combination of ritonavir plus saquinavir or lopinavir plus ritonavir, immunosuppressive drugs, azole antifungals, or lipid-modifying doses of niacin should carefully weigh the potential benefits and risks and should carefully monitor patients for any signs or symptoms of muscle pain, tenderness, or weakness, particularly during the initial months of therapy and during any periods of upward dosage titration of either drug. Lower starting and maintenance doses of atorvastatin should be considered when taken concomitantly with the aforementioned drugs (See **DRUG INTERACTIONS**). Periodic creatine phosphokinase (CPK) determinations may be considered in such situations, but there is no assurance that such monitoring will prevent the occurrence of severe myopathy.

In patients taking CADUET, therapy should be temporarily withheld or discontinued in any patient with an acute, serious condition suggestive of a myopathy or having a risk factor predisposing to the development of renal failure secondary to rhabdomyolysis (e.g., severe acute infection, hypotension, major surgery, trauma, severe metabolic, endocrine and electrolyte disorders, and uncontrolled seizures).

PRECAUTIONS

General

Since the vasodilation induced by the amlodipine component of CADUET is gradual in onset, acute hypotension has rarely been reported after oral administration of amlodipine. Nonetheless, caution should be exercised when administering CADUET as with any other peripheral vasodilator particularly in patients with severe aortic stenosis. Before instituting therapy with CADUET, an attempt should be made to control hypercholesterolemia with appropriate diet, exercise, and weight reduction in obese patients, and to treat other underlying medical problems (see **INDICATIONS AND USAGE**).

Use in Patients with Congestive Heart Failure

In general, calcium channel blockers should be used with caution in patients with heart failure. The amlodipine component of CADUET (5-10 mg per day) has been studied in a placebo-controlled trial of 1153 patients with NYHA Class III or IV heart failure (see **CLINICAL PHARMACOLOGY**) on stable doses of ACE inhibitor, digoxin, and diuretics. Follow-up was at least 6 months, with a mean of about 14 months. There was no overall adverse effect on survival or cardiac morbidity (as defined by life-threatening arrhythmia, acute myocardial infarction, or hospitalization for worsened heart failure). Amlodipine has been compared to placebo in four 8-12 week studies of patients with NYHA class II/III heart failure, involving a total of 697 patients. In these studies, there was no evidence of worsened heart failure based on measures of exercise tolerance, NYHA classification, symptoms, or LVEF.

Beta-Blocker Withdrawal

The amlodipine component of CADUET is not a beta-blocker and therefore gives no protection against the dangers of abrupt beta-blocker withdrawal; any such withdrawal should be by gradual reduction of the dose of beta-blocker.

Endocrine Function

HMG-CoA reductase inhibitors, such as the atorvastatin component of CADUET interfere with cholesterol synthesis and theoretically might blunt adrenal and/or gonadal steroid production. Clinical studies have shown that atorvastatin does not reduce basal plasma cortisol concentration or impair adrenal reserve. The effects of HMG-CoA reductase inhibitors on male fertility have not been studied in adequate numbers of patients. The effects, if any, on the pituitary-gonadal axis in premenopausal women are unknown. Caution should be exercised if an HMG-CoA reductase inhibitor is administered concomitantly with drugs that may decrease the levels or activity of endogenous steroid hormones, such as ketoconazole, spironolactone, and cimetidine.

CNS Toxicity

Studies with atorvastatin: Brain hemorrhage was seen in a female dog treated with atorvastatin calcium for 3 months at a dose equivalent to 120 mg atorvastatin/kg/day. Brain hemorrhage and optic nerve vacuolation were seen in another female dog that was sacrificed in moribund condition after 11 weeks of escalating doses of atorvastatin calcium equivalent to up to 280 mg atorvastatin/kg/day. The 120 mg/kg dose of atorvastatin resulted in a systemic exposure approximately 16 times the human plasma area-under-the-curve (AUC, 0-24 hours) based on the maximum human dose of 80 mg/day. A single tonic convulsion was seen in each of 2 male dogs (one treated with atorvastatin calcium at a dose equivalent to 10 mg atorvastatin/kg/day and one at a dose equivalent to 120 mg atorvastatin/kg/day) in a 2-year study. No CNS lesions have been observed in mice after chronic treatment for up to 2 years at doses of atorvastatin calcium equivalent to up to 400 mg atorvastatin/kg/day or in rats at doses equivalent to up to 100 mg atorvastatin/kg/day. These doses were 6 to 11 times (mouse) and 8 to 16 times (rat) the human AUC (0-24) based on the maximum recommended human dose of 80 mg atorvastatin/day.

CNS vascular lesions, characterized by perivascular hemorrhages, edema, and mononuclear cell infiltration of perivascular spaces, have been observed in dogs treated with other members of the HMG-CoA reductase class. A chemically similar drug in this class produced optic nerve degeneration (Wallerian degeneration of retinogeniculate fibers) in clinically normal dogs in a dose-dependent fashion at a dose that produced plasma drug levels about 30 times higher than the mean drug level in humans taking the highest recommended dose.

Information for Patients

Due to the risk of myopathy with drugs of the HMG-CoA reductase class, to which the atorvastatin component of CADUET belongs, patients should be advised to report promptly unexplained muscle pain, tenderness, or weakness, particularly if accompanied by malaise or fever.

Drug Interactions

Data from a drug-drug interaction study involving 10 mg of amlodipine and 80 mg of atorvastatin in healthy subjects indicate that the pharmacokinetics of amlodipine are not altered when the drugs are coadministered. The effect of amlodipine on the pharmacokinetics of atorvastatin showed no effect on the Cmax: 91% (90% confidence interval: 80 to 103%), but the AUC of atorvastatin increased by 18% (90% confidence interval: 109 to 127%) in the presence of amlodipine.

No drug interaction studies have been conducted with CADUET and other drugs, although studies have been conducted in the individual amlodipine and atorvastatin components, as described below:

Studies with Amlodipine:

In vitro data in human plasma indicate that amlodipine has no effect on the protein binding of drugs tested (digoxin, phenytoin, warfarin, and indomethacin).

Cimetidine: Co-administration of amlodipine with cimetidine did not alter the pharmacokinetics of amlodipine.

Maalox® (antacid): Co-administration of the antacid Maalox with a single dose of amlodipine had no significant effect on the pharmacokinetics of amlodipine.

Sildenafil: A single 100 mg dose of sildenafil (Viagra®) in subjects with essential hypertension had no effect on the pharmacokinetic parameters of amlodipine. When amlodipine and sildenafil were used in combination, each agent independently exerted its own blood pressure lowering effect.

Digoxin: Co-administration of amlodipine with digoxin did not change serum digoxin levels or digoxin renal clearance in normal volunteers.

Ethanol (alcohol): Single and multiple 10 mg doses of amlodipine had no significant effect on the pharmacokinetics of ethanol.

Warfarin: Co-administration of amlodipine with warfarin did not change the warfarin prothrombin response time.

In clinical trials, amlodipine has been safely administered with thiazide diuretics, beta-blockers, angiotensin-converting enzyme inhibitors, long-acting nitrates, sublingual nitroglycerin, digoxin, warfarin, non-steroidal anti-inflammatory drugs, antibiotics, and oral hypoglycemic drugs.

Continued on next page

Caduet—Cont.

Studies with Atorvastatin:
The risk of myopathy during treatment with HMG-CoA reductase inhibitors is increased with concurrent administration of fibric acid derivatives, lipid-modifying doses of niacin or cytochrome P450 3A4 inhibitors (e.g. cyclosporine, erythromycin, clarithromycin, and azole antifungals) (see **WARNINGS, Skeletal Muscle**).

Inhibitors of cytochrome P450 3A4: Atorvastatin is metabolized by cytochrome P450 3A4. Concomitant administration of atorvastatin with inhibitors of cytochrome P450 3A4 can lead to increases in plasma concentrations of atorvastatin. The extent of interaction and potentiation of effects depends on the variability of effect on cytochrome P450 3A4.

  Clarithromycin: Concomitant administration of atorvastatin 80 mg with clarithromycin (500 mg twice daily) resulted in a 4.4-fold increase in atorvastatin AUC (see **WARNINGS, Skeletal Muscle,** and **DOSAGE AND ADMINISTRATION**).

  Erythromycin: In healthy individuals, plasma concentrations of atorvastatin increased approximately 40% with co-administration of atorvastatin and erythromycin, a known inhibitor of cytochrome P450 3A4 (see **WARNINGS, Skeletal Muscle**).

  Combination of Protease Inhibitors: Concomitant administration of atorvastatin 40 mg with ritonavir plus saquinavir (400 mg twice daily) resulted in a 3-fold increase in atorvastatin AUC. Concomitant administration of atorvastatin 20 mg with lopinavir plus ritonavir (400 mg+100 mg twice daily) resulted in a 5.9-fold increase in atorvastatin AUC (see **WARNINGS, Skeletal Muscle,** and **DOSAGE AND ADMINISTRATION**).

  Itraconazole: Concomitant administration of atorvastatin (20 to 40 mg) and itraconazole (200 mg) was associated with a 2.5–3.3-fold increase in atorvastatin AUC.

  Diltiazem hydrochloride: Co-administration of atorvastatin (40 mg) with diltiazem (240 mg) was associated with higher plasma concentrations of atorvastatin.

  Cimetidine: Atorvastatin plasma concentrations and LDL-C reduction were not altered by co-administration of cimetidine.

  Grapefruit juice: Contains one or more components that inhibit CYP 3A4 and can increase plasma concentrations of atorvastatin, especially with excessive grapefruit juice consumption (>1.2 liters per day).

Cyclosporine: Atorvastatin and atorvastatin-metabolites are substrates of the OATP1B1 transporter. Inhibitors of the OATP1B1 (e.g. cyclosporine) can increase the bioavailability of atorvastatin. Concomitant administration of atorvastatin 10 mg and cyclosporine 5.2 mg/kg/day resulted in an 8.7-fold increase in atorvastatin AUC. In cases where co-administration of atorvastatin with cyclosporine is necessary, the dose of atorvastatin should not exceed 10 mg (see **WARNINGS, Skeletal Muscle**).

Inducers of cytochrome P450 3A4: Concomitant administration of atorvastatin with inducers of cytochrome P450 3A4 (eg efavirenz, rifampin) can lead to variable reductions in plasma concentrations of atorvastatin. Due to the dual interaction mechanism of rifampin, simultaneous co-administration of atorvastatin with rifampin is recommended, as delayed administration of atorvastatin after administration of rifampin has been associated with a significant reduction in atorvastatin plasma concentrations.

Antacid: When atorvastatin and Maalox TC suspension were coadministered, plasma concentrations of atorvastatin decreased approximately 35%. However, LDL-C reduction was not altered.

Antipyrine: Because atorvastatin does not affect the pharmacokinetics of antipyrine, interactions with other drugs metabolized via the same cytochrome isozymes are not expected.

Colestipol: Plasma concentrations of atorvastatin decreased approximately 25% when colestipol and atorvastatin were coadministered. However, LDL-C reduction was greater when atorvastatin and colestipol were co-administered than when either drug was given alone.

Digoxin: When multiple doses of atorvastatin and digoxin were coadministered, steady-state plasma digoxin concentrations increased by approximately 20%. Patients taking digoxin should be monitored appropriately.

Oral Contraceptives: Coadministration of atorvastatin and an oral contraceptive increased AUC values for norethindrone and ethinyl estradiol by approximately 30% and 20%. These increases should be considered when selecting an oral contraceptive for a woman taking CADUET.

Warfarin: Atorvastatin had no clinically significant effect on prothrombin time when administered to patients receiving chronic warfarin treatment.

Amlodipine: In a drug-drug interaction study in healthy subjects, co-administration of atorvastatin 80 mg and amlodipine 10 mg resulted in an 18% increase in exposure to atorvastatin which was not clinically meaningful.

Drug/Laboratory Test Interactions
None known.

Carcinogenesis, Mutagenesis, Impairment of Fertility
Studies with amlodipine: Rats and mice treated with amlodipine maleate in the diet for up to two years, at concentrations calculated to provide daily dosage levels of 0.5, 1.25, and 2.5 mg amlodipine/kg/day, showed no evidence of a carcinogenic effect of the drug. For the mouse, the highest dose was, on a mg/m² basis, similar to the maximum recommended human dose of 10 mg amlodipine/day*. For the rat, the highest dose level was, on a mg/m² basis, about twice the maximum recommended human dose*.

Mutagenicity studies conducted with amlodipine maleate revealed no drug related effects at either the gene or chromosome levels.

There was no effect on the fertility of rats treated orally with amlodipine maleate (males for 64 days and females for 14 days prior to mating) at doses up to 10 mg amlodipine/kg/day (8 times* the maximum recommended human dose of 10 mg/day on a mg/m² basis).

Studies with atorvastatin: In a 2-year carcinogenicity study with atorvastatin calcium in rats at dose levels equivalent to 10, 30, and 100 mg atorvastatin/kg/day, 2 rare tumors were found in muscle in high-dose females: in one, there was a rhabdomyosarcoma and, in another, there was a fibrosarcoma. This dose represents a plasma AUC (0-24) value of approximately 16 times the mean human plasma drug exposure after an 80 mg oral dose.

A 2-year carcinogenicity study in mice given atorvastatin calcium at dose levels equivalent to 100, 200, and 400 mg atorvastatin/kg/day resulted in a significant increase in liver adenomas in high-dose males and liver carcinomas in high-dose females. These findings occurred at plasma AUC (0-24) values of approximately 6 times the mean human plasma drug exposure after an 80 mg oral dose.

In vitro, atorvastatin was not mutagenic or clastogenic in the following tests with and without metabolic activation: the Ames test with *Salmonella typhimurium* and *Escherichia coli,* the HGPRT forward mutation assay in Chinese hamster lung cells, and the chromosomal aberration assay in Chinese hamster lung cells. Atorvastatin was negative in the *in vivo* mouse micronucleus test.

*Based on patient weight of 50 kg.

There were no effects on fertility when rats were given atorvastatin calcium at doses equivalent to up to 175 mg atorvastatin/kg/day (15 times the human exposure). There was aplasia and aspermia in the epididymides of 2 of 10 rats treated with atorvastatin calcium at a dose equivalent to 100 mg atorvastatin/kg/day for 3 months (16 times the human AUC at the 80 mg dose); testis weights were significantly lower at 30 and 100 mg/kg/day and epididymal weight was lower at 100 mg/kg/day. Male rats given the equivalent of 100 mg atorvastatin/kg/day for 11 weeks prior to mating had decreased sperm motility, spermatid head concentration, and increased abnormal sperm. Atorvastatin caused no adverse effects on semen parameters, or reproductive organ histopathology in dogs given doses of atorvastatin calcium equivalent to 10, 40, or 120 mg atorvastatin/kg/day for two years.

Pregnancy

Pregnancy Category X (see CONTRAINDICATIONS)
Safety in pregnant women has not been established with CADUET. CADUET should be administered to women of child-bearing potential only when such patients are highly unlikely to conceive and have been informed of the potential hazards. If the woman becomes pregnant while taking CADUET, it should be discontinued and the patient advised again as to the potential hazards to the fetus.

Studies with amlodipine: No evidence of teratogenicity or other embryo/fetal toxicity was found when pregnant rats and rabbits were treated orally with amlodipine maleate at doses up to 10 mg amlodipine/kg/day (respectively 8 times* and 23 times* the maximum recommended human dose of 10 mg/day on a mg/m² basis) during their respective periods of major organogenesis. However, litter size was significantly decreased (by about 50%) and the number of intrauterine deaths was significantly increased (about 5-fold) in rats receiving amlodipine maleate at 10 mg amlodipine/kg/day for 14 days before mating and throughout mating and gestation. Amlodipine maleate has been shown to prolong both the gestation period and the duration of labor in rats at this dose. There are no adequate and well-controlled studies in pregnant women.

*Based on patient weight of 50 kg.

Studies with atorvastatin: Atorvastatin crosses the rat placenta and reaches a level in fetal liver equivalent to that of maternal plasma. Atorvastatin was not teratogenic in rats at doses of atorvastatin calcium equivalent to up to 300 mg atorvastatin/kg/day or in rabbits at doses of atorvastatin calcium equivalent to up to 100 mg atorvastatin/kg/day. These doses resulted in multiples of about 30 times (rat) or 20 times (rabbit) the human exposure based on surface area (mg/m²).

In a study in rats given atorvastatin calcium at doses equivalent to 20, 100, or 225 mg atorvastatin/kg/day, from gestation day 7 through to lactation day 21 (weaning), there was decreased pup survival at birth, neonate, weaning, and maturity for pups of mothers dosed with 225 mg/kg/day. Body weight was decreased on days 4 and 21 for pups of mothers dosed at 100 mg/kg/day; pup body weight was decreased at birth and at days 4, 21, and 91 at 225 mg/kg/day. Pup development was delayed (rotorod performance at 100 mg/kg/day and acoustic startle at 225 mg/kg/day; pinnae detachment and eye opening at 225 mg/kg/day). These doses of atorvastatin correspond to 6 times (100 mg/kg) and 22 times (225 mg/kg) the human AUC at 80 mg/day.

Rare reports of congenital anomalies have been received following intrauterine exposure to HMG-CoA reductase inhibitors. There has been one report of severe congenital bony deformity, tracheo-esophageal fistula, and anal atresia (VATER association) in a baby born to a woman who took lovastatin with dextroamphetamine sulfate during the first trimester of pregnancy.

Labor and Delivery
No studies have been conducted in pregnant women on the effect of CADUET, amlodipine or atorvastatin on the mother or the fetus during labor or delivery, or on the duration of labor or delivery. Amlodipine has been shown to prolong the duration of labor in rats.

Nursing Mothers
It is not known whether the amlodipine component of CADUET is excreted in human milk. Nursing rat pups taking atorvastatin had plasma and liver drug levels of 50% and 40%, respectively, of that in their mother's milk. Because of the potential for adverse reactions in nursing infants, women taking CADUET should not breast-feed (see **CONTRAINDICATIONS**).

Pediatric Use
There have been no studies conducted to determine the safety or effectiveness of CADUET in pediatric populations. *Studies with amlodipine:* The effect of amlodipine on blood pressure in patients less than 6 years of age is not known. *Studies with atorvastatin:* Safety and effectiveness in patients 10-17 years of age with heterozygous familial hypercholesterolemia have been evaluated in controlled clinical trials of 6 months duration in adolescent boys and postmenarchal girls. Patients treated with atorvastatin had an adverse experience profile generally similar to that of patients treated with placebo, the most common adverse experiences observed in both groups, regardless of causality assessment, were infections. **Doses greater than 20 mg have not been studied in this patient population.** In this limited controlled study, there was no detectable effect on growth or sexual maturation in boys or on menstrual cycle length in girls. See **CLINICAL PHARMACOLOGY**, Clinical Studies section; **ADVERSE REACTIONS**, *Pediatric Patients;* and **DOSAGE AND ADMINISTRATION**, *Pediatric Patients (10-17 years of age) with Heterozygous Familial Hypercholesterolemia.* Adolescent females should be counseled on appropriate contraceptive methods while on atorvastatin therapy (see **CONTRAINDICATIONS** and **PRECAUTIONS**, *Pregnancy*). **Atorvastatin has not been studied in controlled clinical trials involving pre-pubertal patients or patients younger than 10 years of age.**

Clinical efficacy with doses of atorvastatin up to 80 mg/day for 1 year have been evaluated in an uncontrolled study of patients with homozygous FH including 8 pediatric patients. See **CLINICAL PHARMACOLOGY**, Clinical Studies, *Atorvastatin Effects in Homozygous Familial Hypercholesterolemia.*

Geriatric Use
There have been no studies conducted to determine the safety or effectiveness of CADUET in geriatric populations. *In studies with amlodipine:* Clinical studies of amlodipine did not include sufficient numbers of subjects aged 65 and over to determine whether they respond differently from younger subjects. Other reported clinical experience has not identified differences in responses between the elderly and younger patients. In general, dose selection of the amlodipine component of CADUET for an elderly patient should be cautious, usually starting at the low end of the dosing range, reflecting the greater frequency of decreased hepatic, renal, or cardiac function, and of concomitant disease or other drug therapy. Elderly patients have decreased clearance of amlodipine with a resulting increase of AUC of approximately 40-60%, and a lower initial dose may be required (see **DOSAGE AND ADMINISTRATION**).

In studies with atorvastatin: The safety and efficacy of atorvastatin (10-80 mg) in the geriatric population (≥65 years of age) was evaluated in the ACCESS study. In this 54-week open-label trial 1,958 patients initiated therapy with atorvastatin calcium 10 mg. Of these, 835 were elderly (≥65 years) and 1,123 were non-elderly. The mean change in LDL-C from baseline after 6 weeks of treatment with atorvastatin calcium 10 mg was –38.2% in the elderly patients versus –34.6% in the non-elderly group.

The rates of discontinuation in patients on atorvastatin due to adverse events were similar between the two age groups. There were no differences in clinically relevant laboratory abnormalities between the age groups.

In studies with Atorvastatin

Use in Patients with Recent Stroke or TIA
In a post-hoc analysis of the Stroke Prevention by Aggressive Reduction in Cholesterol Levels (SPARCL) study where LIPITOR 80 mg vs placebo was administered in 4,731 subjects without CHD who had a stroke or TIA within the preceding 6 months, a higher incidence of hemorrhagic stroke was seen in the LIPITOR 80 mg group compared to placebo. Subjects with hemorrhagic stroke on study entry appeared to be at increased risk for hemorrhagic stroke.

ADVERSE REACTIONS
CADUET
CADUET (amlodipine besylate/atorvastatin calcium) has been evaluated for safety in 1092 patients in double-blind placebo controlled studies treated for co-morbid hypertension and dyslipidemia. In general, treatment with CADUET was well tolerated. For the most part, adverse experiences have been mild or moderate in severity. In clinical trials with CADUET, no adverse experiences peculiar to this combination have been observed. Adverse experiences are similar in terms of nature, severity, and frequency to those reported previously with amlodipine and atorvastatin.

The following information is based on the clinical experience with amlodipine and atorvastatin.

The Amlodipine Component of CADUET
Amlodipine has been evaluated for safety in more than 11,000 patients in U.S. and foreign clinical trials. In gen-

eral, treatment with amlodipine was well tolerated at doses up to 10 mg daily. Most adverse reactions reported during therapy with amlodipine were of mild or moderate severity. In controlled clinical trials directly comparing amlodipine (N=1730) in doses up to 10 mg to placebo (N=1250), discontinuation of amlodipine due to adverse reactions was required in only about 1.5% of patients and was not significantly different from placebo (about 1%). The most common side effects are headache and edema. The incidence (%) of side effects which occurred in a dose related manner are as follows:

Adverse Event	amlodipine			
	2.5 mg N=275	5.0 mg N=296	10.0 mg N=268	Placebo N=520
Edema	1.8	3.0	10.8	0.6
Dizziness	1.1	3.4	3.4	1.5
Flushing	0.7	1.4	2.6	0.0
Palpitations	0.7	1.4	4.5	0.6

Other adverse experiences which were not clearly dose related but which were reported with an incidence greater than 1.0% in placebo-controlled clinical trials include the following:

Placebo-Controlled Studies

Adverse Event	amlodipine (%) (N=1730)	Placebo (%) (N=1250)
Headache	7.3	7.8
Fatigue	4.5	2.8
Nausea	2.9	1.9
Abdominal Pain	1.6	0.3
Somnolence	1.4	0.6

For several adverse experiences that appear to be drug and dose related, there was a greater incidence in women than men associated with amlodipine treatment as shown in the following table:

Adverse Event	amlodipine		Placebo	
	M=% (N=1218)	F=% (N=512)	M=% (N=914)	F=% (N=336)
Edema	5.6	14.6	1.4	5.1
Flushing	1.5	4.5	0.3	0.9
Palpitations	1.4	3.3	0.9	0.9
Somnolence	1.3	1.6	0.8	0.3

The following events occurred in ≤1% but >0.1% of patients treated with amlodipine in controlled clinical trials or under conditions of open trials or marketing experience where a causal relationship is uncertain; they are listed to alert the physician to a possible relationship:

Cardiovascular: arrhythmia (including ventricular tachycardia and atrial fibrillation), bradycardia, chest pain, hypotension, peripheral ischemia, syncope, tachycardia, postural dizziness, postural hypotension, vasculitis.

Central and Peripheral Nervous System: hypoesthesia, neuropathy peripheral, paresthesia, tremor, vertigo.

Gastrointestinal: anorexia, constipation, dyspepsia,** dysphagia, diarrhea, flatulence, pancreatitis, vomiting, gingival hyperplasia.

General: allergic reaction, asthenia,** back pain, hot flushes, malaise, pain, rigors, weight gain, weight decrease.

Musculoskeletal System: arthralgia, arthrosis, muscle cramps,** myalgia.

Psychiatric: sexual dysfunction (male** and female), insomnia, nervousness, depression, abnormal dreams, anxiety, depersonalization.

Respiratory System: dyspnea,** epistaxis.

Skin and Appendages: angioedema, erythema multiforme, pruritus,** rash,** rash erythematous, rash maculopapular.

**These events occurred in less than 1% in placebo-controlled trials, but the incidence of these side effects was between 1% and 2% in all multiple dose studies.

Special Senses: abnormal vision, conjunctivitis, diplopia, eye pain, tinnitus.

Urinary System: micturition frequency, micturition disorder, nocturia.

Autonomic Nervous System: dry mouth, sweating increased.

Metabolic and Nutritional: hyperglycemia, thirst.

Hemopoietic: leukopenia, purpura, thrombocytopenia.

The following events occurred in ≤0.1% of patients treated with amlodipine in controlled clinical trials or under conditions of open trials or marketing experience: cardiac failure, pulse irregularity, extrasystoles, skin discoloration, urticaria, skin dryness, alopecia, dermatitis, muscle weakness, twitching, ataxia, hypertonia, migraine, cold and clammy skin, apathy, agitation, amnesia, gastritis, increased appetite, loose stools, coughing, rhinitis, dysuria, polyuria, parosmia, taste perversion, abnormal visual accommodation, and xerophthalmia.

Other reactions occurred sporadically and cannot be distinguished from medications or concurrent disease states such as myocardial infarction and angina.

Amlodipine therapy has not been associated with clinically significant changes in routine laboratory tests. No clinically relevant changes were noted in serum potassium, serum glucose, total triglycerides, total cholesterol, HDL cholesterol, uric acid, blood urea nitrogen, or creatinine.

In the CAMELOT and PREVENT studies (see **CLINICAL PHARMACOLOGY Clinical Studies, Clinical Studies with Amlodipine**) the adverse event profile was similar to that reported previously (see above), with the most common adverse event being peripheral edema.

Table 12. Adverse Events in Placebo-Controlled Studies (% of Patients)

Body System/ Adverse Event	Placebo N=270	atorvastatin 10 mg N=863	20 mg N=36	40 mg N=79	80 mg N=94
BODY AS A WHOLE					
Infection	10.0	10.3	2.8	10.1	7.4
Headache	7.0	5.4	16.7	2.5	6.4
Accidental Injury	3.7	4.2	0.0	1.3	3.2
Flu Syndrome	1.9	2.2	0.0	2.5	3.2
Abdominal Pain	0.7	2.8	0.0	3.8	2.1
Back Pain	3.0	2.8	0.0	3.8	1.1
Allergic Reaction	2.6	0.9	2.8	1.3	0.0
Asthenia	1.9	2.2	0.0	3.8	0.0
DIGESTIVE SYSTEM					
Constipation	1.8	2.1	0.0	2.5	1.1
Diarrhea	1.5	2.7	0.0	3.8	5.3
Dyspepsia	4.1	2.3	2.8	1.3	2.1
Flatulence	3.3	2.1	2.8	1.3	1.1
RESPIRATORY SYSTEM					
Sinusitis	2.6	2.8	0.0	2.5	6.4
Pharyngitis	1.5	2.5	0.0	1.3	2.1
SKIN AND APPENDAGES					
Rash	0.7	3.9	2.8	3.8	1.1
MUSCULOSKELETAL SYSTEM					
Arthralgia	1.5	2.0	0.0	5.1	0.0
Myalgia	1.1	3.2	5.6	1.3	0.0

The following postmarketing event has been reported infrequently with amlodipine treatment where a causal relationship is uncertain: gynecomastia. In postmarketing experience, jaundice and hepatic enzyme elevations (mostly consistent with cholestasis or hepatitis) in some cases severe enough to require hospitalization have been reported in association with use of amlodipine.

Amlodipine has been used safely in patients with chronic obstructive pulmonary disease, well-compensated congestive heart failure, peripheral vascular disease, diabetes mellitus, and abnormal lipid profiles.

The Atorvastatin Component of CADUET

Atorvastatin is generally well-tolerated. Adverse reactions have usually been mild and transient. In controlled clinical studies of 2502 patients, <2% of patients were discontinued due to adverse experiences attributable to atorvastatin calcium. The most frequent adverse events thought to be related to atorvastatin calcium were constipation, flatulence, dyspepsia, and abdominal pain.

Clinical Adverse Experiences

Adverse experiences reported in ≥2% of patients in placebo-controlled clinical studies of atorvastatin, regardless of causality assessment, are shown in Table 12.

[See table 12 above]

Anglo-Scandinavian Cardiac Outcomes Trial (ASCOT)

In ASCOT (see **CLINICAL PHARMACOLOGY, Clinical Studies, Clinical Studies with Atorvastatin**) involving 10,305 participants treated with atorvastatin 10 mg daily (n=5,168) or placebo (n=5,137), the safety and tolerability profile of the group treated with atorvastatin was comparable to that of the group treated with placebo during a median of 3.3 years of follow-up.

Collaborative Atorvastatin Diabetes Study (CARDS)

In CARDS (see **CLINICAL PHARMACOLOGY, Clinical Studies, Clinical Studies with Atorvastatin**) involving 2838 subjects with type 2 diabetes treated with LIPITOR 10 mg daily (n=1428) or placebo (n=1410), there was no difference in the overall frequency of adverse events or serious adverse events between the treatment groups during a median follow-up of 3.9 years. No cases of rhabdomyolysis were reported.

Treating to New Targets Study (TNT)

In TNT (see CLINICAL PHARMACOLOGY, *Clinical Studies*) involving 10,001 subjects with clinically evident CHD treated with LIPITOR 10 mg daily (n=5006) or LIPITOR 80 mg daily (n=4995), there were more serious adverse events and discontinuations due to adverse events in the high-dose atorvastatin group (92, 1.8%; 497, 9.9%, respectively) as compared to the low-dose group (69, 1.4%; 404, 8.1%, respectively) during a median follow-up of 4.9 years. Persistent transaminase elevations (≥3 × ULN twice within 4-10 days) occurred in 62 (1.3%) individuals with atorvastatin 80 mg and in nine (0.2%) individuals with atorvastatin 10 mg. Elevations of CK (≥ 10 × ULN) were low overall, but were higher in the high-dose atorvastatin treatment group (13, 0.3%) compared to the low-dose atorvastatin group (6, 0.1%).

Incremental Decrease in Endpoints Through Aggressive Lipid Lowering Study (IDEAL)

In IDEAL (see CLINICAL PHARMACOLOGY, *Clinical Studies*) involving 8,888 subjects treated with LIPITOR 80 mg/day (n=4439) or simvastatin 20-40 mg daily (n=4449), there was no difference in the overall frequency of adverse events or serious adverse events between the treatment groups during a median follow-up of 4.8 years.

The following adverse events were reported, regardless of causality assessment, in patients treated with atorvastatin in clinical trials. The events in italics occurred in ≥2% of patients and the events in plain type occurred in <2% of patients.

Body as a Whole: *Chest pain*, face edema, fever, neck rigidity, malaise, photosensitivity reaction, generalized edema.

Digestive System: *Nausea*, gastroenteritis, liver function tests abnormal, colitis, vomiting, gastritis, dry mouth, rectal hemorrhage, esophagitis, eructation, glossitis, mouth ulceration, anorexia, increased appetite, stomatitis, biliary pain, cheilitis, duodenal ulcer, dysphagia, enteritis, melena, gum hemorrhage, stomach ulcer, tenesmus, ulcerative stomatitis, hepatitis, pancreatitis, cholestatic jaundice.

Respiratory System: *Bronchitis, rhinitis*, pneumonia, dyspnea, asthma, epistaxis.

Nervous System: *Insomnia, dizziness*, paresthesia, somnolence, amnesia, abnormal dreams, libido decreased, emotional lability, incoordination, peripheral neuropathy, torticollis, facial paralysis, hyperkinesia, depression, hypesthesia, hypertonia.

Musculoskeletal System: *Arthritis*, leg cramps, bursitis, tenosynovitis, myasthenia, tendinous contracture, myositis.

Skin and Appendages: Pruritus, contact dermatitis, alopecia, dry skin, sweating, acne, urticaria, eczema, seborrhea, skin ulcer.

Urogenital System: *Urinary tract infection, hematuria, albuminuria*, urinary frequency, cystitis, impotence, dysuria, kidney calculus, nocturia, epididymitis, fibrocystic breast, vaginal hemorrhage, breast enlargement, metrorrhagia, nephritis, urinary incontinence, urinary retention, urinary urgency, abnormal ejaculation, uterine hemorrhage.

Special Senses: Amblyopia, tinnitus, dry eyes, refraction disorder, eye hemorrhage, deafness, glaucoma, parosmia, taste loss, taste perversion.

Cardiovascular System: Palpitation, vasodilatation, syncope, migraine, postural hypotension, phlebitis, arrhythmia, angina pectoris, hypertension.

Metabolic and Nutritional Disorders: *Peripheral edema*, hyperglycemia, creatine phosphokinase increased, gout, weight gain, hypoglycemia.

Hemic and Lymphatic System: Ecchymosis, anemia, lymphadenopathy, thrombocytopenia, petechia.

Postintroduction Reports with Atorvastatin

Adverse events associated with atorvastatin therapy reported since market introduction, that are not listed above, regardless of causality assessment, include the following: anaphylaxis, angioneurotic edema, bullous rashes (including erythema multiforme, Stevens-Johnson syndrome, and toxic epidermal necrolysis), rhabdomyolysis, fatigue and tendon rupture

Pediatric Patients (ages 10-17 years)

In a 26-week controlled study in boys and postmenarchal girls (n=140), the safety and tolerability profile of atorvastatin 10 to 20 mg daily was generally similar to that of placebo (see **CLINICAL PHARMACOLOGY, Clinical Studies** section and **PRECAUTIONS, Pediatric Use**).

OVERDOSAGE

There is no information on overdosage with CADUET in humans.

Information on Amlodipine

Single oral doses of amlodipine maleate equivalent to 40 mg amlodipine/kg and 100 mg amlodipine/kg in mice and rats, respectively, caused deaths. Single oral amlodipine maleate doses equivalent to 4 or more mg amlodipine/kg in dogs (11 or more times the maximum recommended clinical dose on a mg/m^2 basis) caused a marked peripheral vasodilation and hypotension.

Overdosage might be expected to cause excessive peripheral vasodilation with marked hypotension and possibly a reflex tachycardia. In humans, experience with intentional overdosage of amlodipine is limited. Reports of intentional overdosage include a patient who ingested 250 mg and was asymptomatic and was not hospitalized; another (120 mg) was hospitalized, underwent gastric lavage and remained normotensive; the third (105 mg) was hospitalized and had hypotension (90/50 mmHg) which normalized following plasma expansion. A patient who took 70 mg amlodipine and an unknown quantity of benzodiazepine in a suicide attempt developed shock which was refractory to treatment

Continued on next page

Caduet—Cont.

and died the following day with abnormally high benzodiazepine plasma concentration. A case of accidental drug overdose has been documented in a 19-month-old male who ingested 30 mg amlodipine (about 2 mg/kg). During the emergency room presentation, vital signs were stable with no evidence of hypotension, but a heart rate of 180 bpm. Ipecac was administered 3.5 hours after ingestion and on subsequent observation (overnight) no sequelae were noted. If massive overdose should occur, active cardiac and respiratory monitoring should be instituted. Frequent blood pressure measurements are essential. Should hypotension occur, cardiovascular support including elevation of the extremities and the judicious administration of fluids should be initiated. If hypotension remains unresponsive to these conservative measures, administration of vasopressors (such as phenylephrine) should be considered with attention to circulating volume and urine output. Intravenous calcium gluconate may help to reverse the effects of calcium entry blockade. As amlodipine is highly protein bound, hemodialysis is not likely to be of benefit.

Information on Atorvastatin

There is no specific treatment for atorvastatin overdosage. In the event of an overdose, the patient should be treated symptomatically, and supportive measures instituted as required. Due to extensive drug binding to plasma proteins, hemodialysis is not expected to significantly enhance atorvastatin clearance.

DOSAGE AND ADMINISTRATION

Dosage of CADUET must be individualized on the basis of both effectiveness and tolerance for each individual component in the treatment of hypertension/angina and hyperlipidemia.

Amlodipine (Hypertension or angina)

Adults: The usual initial antihypertensive oral dose of amlodipine is 5 mg once daily with a maximum dose of 10 mg once daily. Small, fragile, or elderly individuals, or patients with hepatic insufficiency may be started on 2.5 mg once daily and this dose may be used when adding amlodipine to other antihypertensive therapy.

Dosage should be adjusted according to each patient's need. In general, titration should proceed over 7 to 14 days so that the physician can fully assess the patient's response to each dose level. Titration may proceed more rapidly, however, if clinically warranted, provided the patient is assessed frequently.

The recommended dose of amlodipine for chronic stable or vasospastic angina is 5-10 mg, with the lower dose suggested in the elderly and in patients with hepatic insufficiency. Most patients will require 10 mg for adequate effect. See **ADVERSE REACTIONS** section for information related to dosage and side effects.

The recommended dose range of amlodipine for patients with coronary artery disease is 5-10 mg once daily. In clinical studies the majority of patients required 10 mg (see **CLINICAL PHARMACOLOGY, Clinical studies**).

Children: The effective antihypertensive oral dose of amlodipine in pediatric patients ages 6-17 years is 2.5 mg to 5 mg once daily. Doses in excess of 5 mg daily have not been studied in pediatric patients. See **CLINICAL PHARMACOLOGY.**

Atorvastatin (Hyperlipidemia)

The patient should be placed on a standard cholesterol-lowering diet before receiving atorvastatin and should continue on this diet during treatment with atorvastatin.

Hypercholesterolemia (Heterozygous Familial and Nonfamilial) and Mixed Dyslipidemia (Fredrickson Types IIa and IIb)

The recommended starting dose of atorvastatin is 10 or 20 mg once daily. Patients who require a large reduction in LDL-C (more than 45%) may be started at 40 mg once daily. The dosage range of atorvastatin is 10 to 80 mg once daily. Atorvastatin can be administered as a single dose at any time of the day, with or without food. The starting dose and maintenance doses of atorvastatin should be individualized according to patient characteristics such as goal of therapy and response (see *NCEP Guidelines*, summarized in Table 9). After initiation and/or upon titration of atorvastatin, lipid levels should be analyzed within 2 to 4 weeks and dosage adjusted accordingly.

Since the goal of treatment is to lower LDL-C, the NCEP recommends that LDL-C levels be used to initiate and assess treatment response. Only if LDL-C levels are not available, should total-C be used to monitor therapy.

Heterozygous Familial Hypercholesterolemia in Pediatric Patients (10-17 years of age)

The recommended starting dose of atorvastatin is 10 mg/day; the maximum recommended dose is 20 mg/day (doses greater than 20 mg have not been studied in this patient population). Doses should be individualized according to the recommended goal of therapy (see NCEP Pediatric Panel Guidelines[1], **CLINICAL PHARMACOLOGY,** and **INDICATIONS AND USAGE**). Adjustments should be made at intervals of 4 weeks or more.

Homozygous Familial Hypercholesterolemia

The dosage of atorvastatin in patients with homozygous FH is 10 to 80 mg daily. Atorvastatin should be used as an adjunct to other lipid-lowering treatments (e.g., LDL apheresis) in these patients or if such treatments are unavailable. Note: a 2.5/80 mg CADUET tablet is not available. Management of patients needing a 2.5/80 mg combination requires individual assessments of dyslipidemia and therapy with the individual components as a 2.5/80 mg CADUET tablet is not available.

Concomitant Lipid Lowering Therapy

Atorvastatin may be used in combination with a bile acid binding resin for additive effect. The combination of HMG-CoA reductase inhibitors and fibrates should generally be avoided (see **WARNINGS, Skeletal Muscle,** and **PRECAUTIONS, Drug Interactions** for other drug-drug interactions).

Dosage in Patients With Renal Insufficiency

Renal disease does not affect the plasma concentrations nor LDL-C reduction of atorvastatin; thus, dosage adjustment in patients with renal dysfunction is not necessary (see **CLINICAL PHARMACOLOGY, Pharmacokinetics**).

Dosage in Patients Taking Cyclosporine, Clarithromycin or A Combination of Ritonavir plus Saquinavir or Lopinavir plus Ritonavir

In patients taking cyclosporine, therapy should be limited to LIPITOR 10 mg once daily. In patients taking clarithromycin or in patients with HIV taking a combination of ritonavir plus saquinavir or lopinavir plus ritonavir, for doses of atorvastatin exceeding 20 mg appropriate clinical assessment is recommended to ensure that the lowest dose necessary of atorvastatin is employed (see **WARNINGS, Skeletal Muscle,** and **PRECAUTIONS, *Drug Interactions***).

CADUET

CADUET may be substituted for its individually titrated components. Patients may be given the equivalent dose of CADUET or a dose of CADUET with increased amounts of amlodipine, atorvastatin or both for additional antianginal effects, blood pressure lowering, or lipid lowering effect.

[1]National Cholesterol Education Program (NCEP): Highlights of the Report of the Expert Panel on Blood Cholesterol Levels in Children Adolescents. *Pediatrics*. 89(3): 495-501. 1992.

CADUET may be used to provide additional therapy for patients already on one of its components. As initial therapy for one indication and continuation of treatment of the other, the recommended starting dose of CADUET should be selected based on the continuation of the component being used and the recommended starting dose for the added monotherapy.

CADUET may be used to initiate treatment in patients with hyperlipidemia and either hypertension or angina. The recommended starting dose of CADUET should be based on the appropriate combination of recommendations for the monotherapies. The maximum dose of the amlodipine component of CADUET is 10 mg once daily. The maximum dose of the atorvastatin component of CADUET is 80 mg once daily.

See above for detailed information related to the dosing and administration of amlodipine and atorvastatin.

HOW SUPPLIED

CADUET® tablets contain amlodipine besylate and atorvastatin calcium equivalent to amlodipine and atorvastatin in the dose strengths described below.

CADUET tablets are differentiated by tablet color/size and are engraved with "Pfizer" on one side and a unique number on the other side. CADUET tablets are supplied for oral administration in the following strengths and package configurations:

[See table 13 below]

Store at 25°C (77°F); excursions permitted to 15-30°C (59-86°F) [see USP Controlled Room Temperature].

Rx only

Manufactured by:

Pfizer Ireland Pharmaceuticals

Dublin, Ireland

Distributed by

Pfizer Labs

Division of Pfizer Inc, NY, NY 10017

LAB-0276-12.0

Revised December 2007

Table 13. CADUET Packaging Configurations

	CADUET			
Package Configuration	Tablet Strength (amlodipine besylate/ atorvastatin calcium) mg	NDC #	Engraving	Tablet Color
Bottle of 30	2.5/10	0069-2960-30	CDT 251	White
Bottle of 30	2.5/20	0069-2970-30	CDT 252	White
Bottle of 30	2.5/40	0069-2980-30	CDT 254	White
Bottle of 30	5/10	0069-2150-30	CDT 051	White
Bottle of 30	5/20	0069-2170-30	CDT 052	White
Bottle of 30	5/40	0069-2190-30	CDT 054	White
Bottle of 30	5/80	0069-2260-30	CDT 058	White
Bottle of 30	10/10	0069-2160-30	CDT 101	Blue
Bottle of 30	10/20	0069-2180-30	CDT 102	Blue
Bottle of 30	10/40	0069-2250-30	CDT 104	Blue
Bottle of 30	10/80	0069-2270-30	CDT 108	Blue

CHANTIX™ ℞

[*chan-tiks*]

(varenicline) Tablets

Prescribing information for this product, which appears on pages 2494–2498 of the 2008 PDR, has been completely revised as follows. Please write "See Supplement A" next to the product heading.

DESCRIPTION

CHANTIX™ tablets contain the active ingredient, varenicline (as the tartrate salt), which is a partial agonist selective for $\alpha_4\beta_2$ nicotinic acetylcholine receptor subtypes. *Varenicline,* as the tartrate salt, is a powder which is a white to off-white to slightly yellow solid with the following chemical name: 7,8,9,10-tetrahydro-6,10-methano-6*H*-pyrazino[2,3-h][3]benzazepine, (2*R*,3*R*)-2,3-dihydroxybutanedioate (1:1). It is highly soluble in water. Varenicline tartrate has a molecular weight of 361.35 Daltons, and a molecular formula of $C_{13}H_{13}N_3 \bullet C_4H_6O_6$. The chemical structure is:

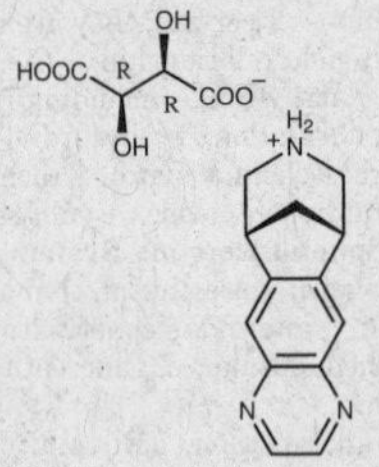

CHANTIX is supplied for oral administration in two strengths: a 0.5 mg capsular biconvex, white to off-white, film-coated tablet debossed with "*Pfizer*" on one side and "CHX 0.5" on the other side and a 1 mg capsular biconvex, light blue film-coated tablet debossed with "*Pfizer*" on one side and "CHX 1.0" on the other side. Each 0.5 mg CHANTIX tablet contains 0.85 mg of varenicline tartrate equivalent to 0.5 mg of varenicline free base; each 1mg CHANTIX tablet contains 1.71 mg of varenicline tartrate equivalent to 1 mg of varenicline free base. The following inactive ingredients are included in the tablets: microcrystalline cellulose, anhydrous dibasic calcium phosphate, croscarmellose sodium, colloidal silicon dioxide, magnesium stearate, Opadry® White (for 0.5 mg), Opadry® Blue (for 1 mg), and Opadry® Clear.

CLINICAL PHARMACOLOGY

Mechanism Of Action

Varenicline binds with high affinity and selectivity at $\alpha_4\beta_2$ neuronal nicotinic acetylcholine receptors. The efficacy of CHANTIX in smoking cessation is believed to be the result of varenicline's activity at a sub-type of the nicotinic receptor where its binding produces agonist activity, while simultaneously preventing nicotine binding to $\alpha_4\beta_2$ receptors.

Electrophysiology studies *in vitro* and neurochemical studies *in vivo* have shown that varenicline binds to $\alpha_4\beta_2$ neuronal nicotinic acetylcholine receptors and stimulates receptor-mediated activity, but at a significantly lower level than nicotine. Varenicline blocks the ability of nicotine to activate $\alpha_4\beta_2$ receptors and thus to stimulate the central nervous mesolimbic dopamine system, believed to be the neuronal mechanism underlying reinforcement and reward experienced upon smoking. Varenicline is highly selective and binds more potently to $\alpha_4\beta_2$ receptors than to other common nicotinic receptors (>500-fold $\alpha_3\beta_4$, >3500-fold α_7, >20,000-fold $\alpha_1\beta\gamma\delta$), or to non-nicotinic receptors and transporters (>2000-fold). Varenicline also binds with moderate affinity (Ki = 350 nM) to the 5-HT3 receptor.

Pharmacokinetics

Absorption/Distribution

Maximum plasma concentrations of varenicline occur typically within 3-4 hours after oral administration. Following administration of multiple oral doses of varenicline, steady-state conditions were reached within 4 days. Over the recommended dosing range, varenicline exhibits linear pharmacokinetics after single or repeated doses. In a mass balance study, absorption of varenicline was virtually complete after oral administration and systemic availability was high. Oral bioavailability of varenicline is unaffected by food or time-of-day dosing. Plasma protein binding of varenicline is low (≤20%) and independent of both age and renal function.

Metabolism/Elimination

The elimination half-life of varenicline is approximately 24 hours. Varenicline undergoes minimal metabolism with 92% excreted unchanged in the urine. Renal elimination of varenicline is primarily through glomerular filtration along with active tubular secretion possibly via the organic cation transporter, OCT2.

Pharmacokinetics In Special Patient Populations

There are no clinically meaningful differences in varenicline pharmacokinetics due to age, race, gender, smoking status, or use of concomitant medications, as demonstrated in specific pharmacokinetic studies and in population pharmacokinetic analyses.

Renal impairment

Varenicline pharmacokinetics were unchanged in subjects with mild renal impairment (estimated creatinine clearance >50 mL/min and ≤80 mL/min). In patients with moderate renal impairment (estimated creatinine clearance ≥30 mL/min and ≤50 mL/min), varenicline exposure increased 1.5-fold compared with subjects with normal renal function (estimated creatinine clearance >80 mL/min). In subjects with severe renal impairment (estimated creatinine clearance <30 mL/min), varenicline exposure was increased 2.1-fold. In subjects with end-stage-renal disease (ESRD) undergoing a three hour session of hemodialysis for three days a week, varenicline exposure was increased 2.7-fold following 0.5 mg once daily administration for 12 days. The plasma C_{max} and AUC of varenicline noted in this setting were similar to healthy subjects receiving about 1 mg twice daily. Caution is warranted with the use of CHANTIX in subjects with renal impairment (See **DOSAGE AND ADMINISTRATION**). Additionally, in subjects with ESRD, varenicline was efficiently removed by hemodialysis (See **OVERDOSAGE**).

Geriatric

A combined single and multiple-dose pharmacokinetic study demonstrated that the pharmacokinetics of 1 mg varenicline given QD or BID to 16 healthy elderly male and female smokers (aged 65-75 yrs) for 7 consecutive days was similar to that of younger subjects.

Pediatric

Because the safety and effectiveness of CHANTIX in pediatric patients have not been established, CHANTIX is not recommended for use in patients under 18 years of age.

When 22 pediatric patients aged 12 to 17 years (inclusive) received a single 0.5 mg and 1 mg-dose of varenicline, the pharmacokinetics of varenicline was approximately dose proportional between the 0.5 mg and 1 mg doses. Systemic exposure, as assessed by AUC(0-∞), and renal clearance of varenicline were comparable to those of an adult population.

Hepatic impairment

Due to the absence of significant hepatic metabolism, varenicline pharmacokinetics should be unaffected in patients with hepatic insufficiency.

Drug-Drug Interactions

Drug interaction studies were performed with varenicline and digoxin, warfarin, transdermal nicotine, bupropion, cimetidine and metformin. No clinically meaningful pharmacokinetic drug-drug interactions have been identified.

In vitro studies demonstrated that varenicline does not inhibit the following cytochrome P450 enzymes (IC50 >6400 ng/mL): 1A2, 2A6, 2B6, 2C8, 2C9, 2C19, 2D6, 2E1, and 3A4/5. Also, in human hepatocytes *in vitro*, varenicline does not induce the cytochrome P450 enzymes 1A2 and 3A4.

In vitro studies demonstrated that varenicline does not inhibit human renal transport proteins at therapeutic concentrations. Therefore, drugs that are cleared by renal secretion (e.g. metformin - see below) are unlikely to be affected by varenicline.

In vitro studies demonstrated the active renal secretion of varenicline is mediated by the human organic cation transporter, OCT2. Co-administration with inhibitors of OCT2 may not require a dose adjustment of CHANTIX as the increase in systemic exposure to CHANTIX is not expected to be clinically meaningful (see Cimetidine interaction below). Furthermore, since metabolism of varenicline represents less than 10% of its clearance, drugs known to affect the cytochrome P450 system are unlikely to alter the pharmacokinetics of CHANTIX (see **Pharmacokinetics**) and therefore a dose adjustment of CHANTIX would not be required.

Metformin: When co-administered to 30 smokers varenicline (1 mg BID) did not alter the steady-state pharmacokinetics of metformin (500 mg BID), which is a substrate of OCT2. Metformin had no effect on varenicline steady-state pharmacokinetics.

Cimetidine: Co-administration of an OCT2 inhibitor, cimetidine (300 mg QID), with varenicline (2 mg single dose) to 12 smokers increased the systemic exposure of varenicline by 29% (90% CI: 21.5%, 36.9%) due to a reduction in varenicline renal clearance.

Digoxin: Varenicline (1 mg BID) did not alter the steady-state pharmacokinetics of digoxin administered as a 0.25 mg daily dose in 18 smokers.

Warfarin: Varenicline (1 mg BID) did not alter the pharmacokinetics of a single 25 mg dose of (R, S)-warfarin in 24 smokers. Prothrombin time (INR) was not affected by varenicline. Smoking cessation itself may result in changes to warfarin pharmacokinetics (see **PRECAUTIONS**).

Use with other therapies for smoking cessation:

Bupropion: Varenicline (1 mg BID) did not alter the steady-state pharmacokinetics of bupropion (150 mg BID) in 46 smokers. The safety of the combination of bupropion and varenicline has not been established.

Nicotine replacement therapy (NRT): Although co-administration of varenicline (1 mg BID) and transdermal nicotine (21 mg/day) for up to 12 days did not affect nicotine pharmacokinetics, the incidence of nausea, headache, vomiting, dizziness, dyspepsia and fatigue was greater for the combination than for NRT alone. In this study, eight of twenty-two (36%) subjects treated with the combination of varenicline and NRT prematurely discontinued treatment due to adverse events, compared to 1 of 17 (6%) of subjects treated with NRT and placebo.

Safety and efficacy of CHANTIX in combination with other smoking cessation therapies have not been studied.

CLINICAL STUDIES

The efficacy of CHANTIX in smoking cessation was demonstrated in six clinical trials in which a total of 3659 chronic cigarette smokers (≥10 cigarettes per day) were treated with CHANTIX. In all clinical studies, abstinence from smoking was determined by patient self-report and verified by measurement of exhaled carbon monoxide (CO≤10 ppm) at weekly visits. Among the CHANTIX treated patients enrolled in these studies, the completion rate was 65%. Except for the initial Phase 2 study (Study 1) and the maintenance of abstinence study (Study 6), patients were treated for 12 weeks and then were followed for 40 weeks post-treatment. Most subjects enrolled in these trials were white (79%-96%). All studies enrolled almost equal numbers of men and women. The average age of subjects in these studies was 43 years. Subjects on average had smoked about 21 cigarettes per day for an average of approximately 25 years.

In all studies, patients were provided with an educational booklet on smoking cessation and received up to 10 minutes of smoking cessation counseling at each weekly treatment visit according to Agency for Healthcare Research and Quality guidelines. Patients set a date to stop smoking (target quit date, TQD) with dosing starting 1 week before this date.

Initiation of Abstinence

Study 1: This was a six-week dose-ranging study comparing CHANTIX to placebo. This study provided initial evidence that CHANTIX at a total dose of 1 mg per day or 2 mg per day was effective as an aid to smoking cessation.

Study 2: This study of 627 subjects compared CHANTIX 1 mg per day and 2 mg per day with placebo. Patients were treated for 12 weeks (including one week titration) and then were followed for 40 weeks post-treatment. CHANTIX was given in two divided doses. Each dose of CHANTIX was given in two different regimens, with and without initial dose titration, to explore the effect of different dosing regimens on tolerability. For the titrated groups, dosage was titrated up over the course of one week, with full dosage achieved starting with the second week of dosing. The titrated and nontitrated groups were pooled for efficacy analysis.

Forty five percent of subjects receiving CHANTIX 1 mg per day (0.5 mg BID) and 51% of subjects receiving 2 mg per day (1 mg BID) had CO-confirmed continuous abstinence during weeks 9 through 12 compared to 12% of subjects in the placebo group (Figure 1). In addition, 31% of the 1 mg per day group and 31% of the 2 mg per day group were continuously abstinent from one week after TQD through the end of treatment as compared to 8% of the placebo group.

Study 3: This flexible-dosing study of 312 subjects examined the effect of a patient-directed dosing strategy of CHANTIX or placebo. After an initial one-week titration to a dose of 0.5 mg BID, subjects could adjust their dosage as often as they wished between 0.5 mg QD to 1 mg BID per day. Sixty nine percent of patients titrated to the maximum allowable dose at any time during the study. For 44% of patients, the modal dose selected was 1 mg BID; for slightly over half of the study participants, the modal dose selected was 1 mg/day or less.

Of the subjects treated with CHANTIX, 40% had CO-confirmed continuous abstinence during weeks 9 through 12 compared to 12% in the placebo group. In addition, 29% of the CHANTIX group were continuously abstinent from one week after TQD through the end of treatment as compared to 9% of the placebo group.

Study 4 and Study 5: These identical double-blind studies compared CHANTIX 2 mg per day, bupropion sustained release (SR) 150 mg BID, and placebo. Patients were treated for 12 weeks and then were followed for 40 weeks post-treatment. The CHANTIX dosage of 1 mg BID was achieved using a titration of 0.5 mg QD for the initial 3 days followed by 0.5 mg BID for the next 4 days. The bupropion SR dosage of 150 mg BID was achieved using a 3-day titration of 150 mg QD. Study 4 enrolled 1022 subjects and Study 5 enrolled 1023 subjects. Patients inappropriate for bupropion treatment or patients who had previously used bupropion were excluded.

Table 1: Continuous Abstinence, Week 9 through 12 (95% confidence interval) across different studies

	CHANTIX 0.5 mg BID	CHANTIX 1 mg BID	CHANTIX Flexible	Bupropion SR	Placebo
Study 2	45% (39%, 51%)	51% (44%, 57%)			12% (6%, 18%)
Study 3			40% (32%, 48%)		12% (7%, 17%)
Study 4		44% (38%, 49%)		30% (25%, 35%)	17% (13%, 22%)
Study 5		44% (38%, 49%)		30% (25%, 35%)	18% (14%, 22%)

In Study 4, subjects treated with CHANTIX had a superior rate of CO-confirmed abstinence during weeks 9 through 12 (44%) compared to patients treated with bupropion SR (30%) or placebo (17%). The bupropion SR quit rate was also superior to placebo. In addition, 29% of the CHANTIX group were continuously abstinent from one week after TQD through the end of treatment as compared to 12% of the placebo group and 23% of the bupropion SR group.

Similarly in Study 5, subjects treated with CHANTIX had a superior rate of CO-confirmed abstinence during weeks 9 through 12 (44%) compared to patients treated with bupropion SR (30%) or placebo (18%). The bupropion SR quit rate was also superior to placebo. In addition, 29% of the CHANTIX group were continuously abstinent from one week after TQD through the end of treatment as compared to 11% of the placebo group and 21% of the bupropion SR group.

Figure 1: Continuous Abstinence, Weeks 9 through 12

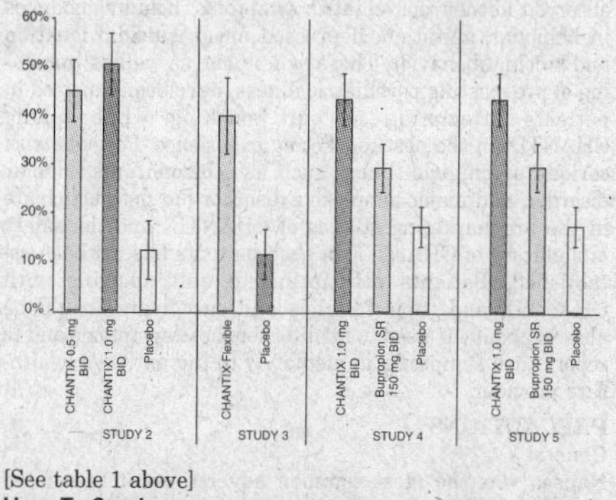

[See table 1 above]

Urge To Smoke

Based on responses to the Brief Questionnaire of Smoking Urges and the Minnesota Nicotine Withdrawal scale "Urge to Smoke" item, CHANTIX reduced urge to smoke compared to placebo in all studies.

Long-Term Abstinence

Studies 1 through 5 included 40 weeks of post-treatment follow-up. In each study, CHANTIX treated patients were more likely to maintain abstinence throughout the follow-up period than were patients treated with placebo (Figure 2, Table 2).

Figure 2: Continuous Abstinence, Weeks 9 through 52

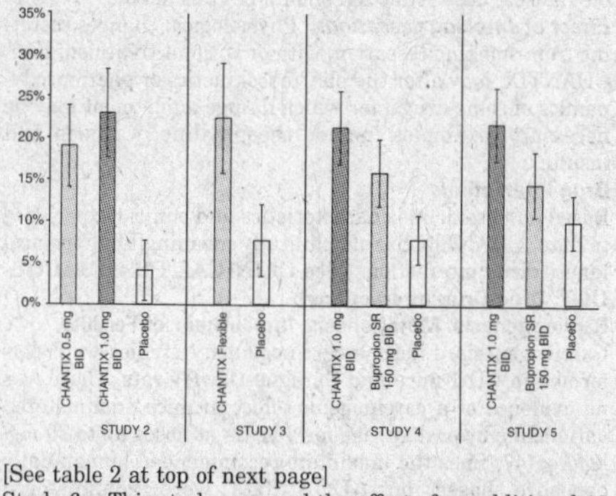

[See table 2 at top of next page]

Study 6: This study assessed the effect of an additional 12 weeks of CHANTIX therapy on the likelihood of long-term abstinence. Patients in this study (n=1927) were treated with open-label CHANTIX 1 mg BID for 12 weeks. Patients who had stopped smoking by Week 12 were then randomized to double-blind treatment with CHANTIX (1 mg BID) or placebo for an additional 12 weeks and then followed for 28 weeks post-treatment.

The continuous abstinence rate from Week 13 through Week 24 was higher for subjects continuing treatment with CHANTIX (70%) than for subjects switching to placebo (50%). Superiority to placebo was also maintained during 28 weeks post-treatment follow-up (CHANTIX 54% versus placebo 39%).

Continued on next page

Chantix—Cont.

In Figure 3 below, the x-axis represents the study week for each observation allowing a comparison of groups at similar times after discontinuation of CHANTIX. Post-CHANTIX follow-up begins at Week 13 for the placebo group and Week 25 for the CHANTIX group. The y-axis represents the percent of subjects who had been abstinent for the last week of CHANTIX treatment and remained abstinent at the given timepoint.

Figure 3: Continuous Abstinence Rate during nontreatment follow-up

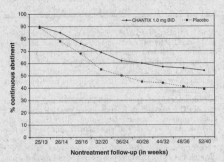

INDICATIONS AND USAGE
CHANTIX is indicated as an aid to smoking cessation treatment.

WARNINGS
Neuropsychiatric Symptoms
Serious neuropsychiatric symptoms have occurred in patients being treated with CHANTIX. Some cases may have been complicated by the symptoms of nicotine withdrawal in patients who stopped smoking; however, some of these symptoms have occurred in patients who continued to smoke. All patients being treated with CHANTIX should be observed for neuropsychiatric symptoms including changes in behavior, agitation, depressed mood, suicidal ideation and suicidal behavior. These symptoms, as well as worsening of pre-existing psychiatric illness, have been reported in patients attempting to quit smoking while taking CHANTIX in the post-marketing experience. Patients with serious psychiatric illness such as schizophrenia, bipolar disorder, and major depressive disorder did not participate in the pre-marketing studies of CHANTIX and the safety and efficacy of CHANTIX in such patients has not been established. Patients attempting to quit smoking with CHANTIX and their families and caregivers should be alerted about the need to monitor for these symptoms and to report such symptoms immediately to the patient's health-care provider.

PRECAUTIONS
General
Nausea was the most common adverse event associated with CHANTIX treatment. Nausea was generally described as mild or moderate and often transient; however, for some subjects, it was persistent over several months. The incidence of nausea was dose-dependent. Initial dose-titration was beneficial in reducing the occurrence of nausea. Nausea was reported by approximately 30% of patients treated with CHANTIX 1 mg BID after an initial week of dose titration. In patients taking CHANTIX 0.5 mg BID, the incidence of nausea was 16% following initial titration. Approximately 3% of subjects treated with CHANTIX 1 mg BID in studies involving 12 weeks of treatment discontinued treatment prematurely because of nausea. For patients with intolerable nausea, dose reduction should be considered.

Effect of smoking cessation: Physiological changes resulting from smoking cessation, with or without treatment with CHANTIX, may alter the pharmacokinetics or pharmacodynamics of some drugs, for which dosage adjustment may be necessary (examples include theophylline, warfarin and insulin).

Drug Interactions
Based on varenicline characteristics and clinical experience to date, CHANTIX has no clinically meaningful pharmacokinetic drug interactions (See **CLINICAL PHARMACOLOGY, Drug-Drug Interactions**).

Carcinogenesis, Mutagenesis, Impairment of Fertility
Carcinogenesis. Lifetime carcinogenicity studies were performed in CD-1 mice and Sprague-Dawley rats. There was no evidence of a carcinogenic effect in mice administered varenicline by oral gavage for 2 years at doses up to 20 mg/kg/day (47 times the maximum recommended human daily exposure based on AUC). Rats were administered varenicline (1, 5, and 15 mg/kg/day) by oral gavage for 2 years. In male rats (n = 65 per sex per dose group), incidences of hibernoma (tumor of the brown fat) were increased at the mid dose (1 tumor, 5 mg/kg/day, 23 times the maximum recommended human daily exposure based on AUC) and maximum dose (2 tumors, 15 mg/kg/day, 67 times the maximum recommended human daily exposure based on AUC). The clinical relevance of this finding to humans has not been established. There was no evidence of carcinogenicity in female rats.
Mutagenesis. Varenicline was not genotoxic, with or without metabolic activation, in the following assays: Ames bacterial mutation assay; mammalian CHO/HGPRT assay; and tests for cytogenetic aberrations *in vivo* in rat bone marrow and *in vitro* in human lymphocytes.

Table 2: Continuous Abstinence, Weeks 9 through 52 (95% confidence interval) across different studies

	CHANTIX 0.5 mg BID	CHANTIX 1 mg BID	CHANTIX Flexible	Bupropion SR	Placebo
Study 2	19% (14%, 24%)	23% (18%, 28%)			4% (1%, 8%)
Study 3			22% (16%, 29%)		8% (3%, 12%)
Study 4		21% (17%, 26%)		16% (12%, 20%)	8% (5%, 11%)
Study 5		22% (17%, 26%)		14% (11%, 18%)	10% (7%, 13%)

Impairment of fertility. There was no evidence of impairment of fertility in either male or female Sprague-Dawley rats administered varenicline succinate up to 15 mg/kg/day (67 and 36 times, respectively, the maximum recommended human daily exposure based on AUC at 1 mg BID). However, a decrease in fertility was noted in the offspring of pregnant rats who were administered varenicline succinate at an oral dose of 15 mg/kg/day (36 times the maximum recommended human daily exposure based on AUC at 1 mg BID). This decrease in fertility in the offspring of treated female rats was not evident at an oral dose of 3 mg/kg/day (9 times the maximum recommended human daily exposure based on AUC at 1 mg BID).

Pregnancy
Pregnancy Category C.
Varenicline succinate was not teratogenic in rats and rabbits at oral doses up to 15 and 30 mg/kg/day, respectively (36 and 50-times the maximum recommended human daily exposure based on AUC at 1 mg BID, respectively).

Nonteratogenic effects
Varenicline succinate has been shown to have an adverse effect on the fetus in animal reproduction studies. Administration of varenicline succinate to pregnant rabbits resulted in reduced fetal weights at an oral dose of 30 mg/kg/day (50 times the human AUC at 1 mg BID); this reduction was not evident following treatment with 10 mg/kg/day (23 times the maximum recommended daily human exposure based on AUC). In addition, in the offspring of pregnant rats treated with varenicline succinate there were decreases in fertility and increases in auditory startle response at an oral dose of 15 mg/kg/day (36 times the maximum recommended human daily exposure based on AUC at 1 mg BID). There are no adequate and well-controlled studies in pregnant women. CHANTIX should be used during pregnancy only if the potential benefit justifies the potential risk to the fetus.

Nursing mothers
Although it is not known whether this drug is excreted in human milk, animal studies have demonstrated that varenicline can be transferred to nursing pups. Because many drugs are excreted in human milk and because of the potential for serious adverse reactions in nursing infants from CHANTIX, a decision should be made whether to discontinue nursing or to discontinue the drug, taking into account the importance of the drug to the mother.

Labor and delivery
The potential effects of CHANTIX on labor and delivery are not known.

Pediatric Use
Safety and effectiveness of CHANTIX in pediatric patients have not been established; therefore, CHANTIX is not recommended for use in patients under 18 years of age.

Geriatric Use
A combined single and multiple-dose pharmacokinetic study demonstrated that the pharmacokinetics of 1 mg varenicline given QD or BID to 16 healthy elderly male and female smokers (aged 65-75 yrs) for 7 consecutive days was similar to that of younger subjects. No overall differences in safety or effectiveness were observed between these subjects and younger subjects, and other reported clinical experience has not identified differences in responses between the elderly and younger patients, but greater sensitivity of some older individuals cannot be ruled out.
Varenicline is known to be substantially excreted by the kidney, and the risk of toxic reactions to this drug may be greater in patients with impaired renal function. Because elderly patients are more likely to have decreased renal function, care should be taken in dose selection, and it may be useful to monitor renal function (see **DOSAGE AND ADMINISTRATION, Special Populations, Patients with impaired renal function**).
No dosage adjustment is recommended for elderly patients (see **DOSAGE AND ADMINISTRATION, Special Populations**).

Information for Patients:
- Patients should be instructed to set a date to quit smoking and to initiate CHANTIX treatment one week before the quit date.
- Patients should be advised that CHANTIX should be taken after eating, and with a full glass of water.
- Patients should be instructed how to titrate CHANTIX, beginning at a dose of 0.5 mg/day. Prescribers should explain that one 0.5 mg tablet should be taken daily for the first three days, and that for the next four days, one 0.5 mg tablet should be taken in the morning and one 0.5 mg tablet should be taken in the evening.
- Patients should be advised that, after the first seven days, the dose should be increased to one 1 mg tablet in the morning and one 1 mg tablet in the evening.

- Patients should be encouraged to continue to attempt to quit if they have early lapses after quit day.
- Patients should also be provided with educational materials and necessary counseling to support an attempt at quitting smoking.
- Patients should be informed that nausea and insomnia are side effects of CHANTIX and are usually transient; however, patients should be advised that if they are persistently troubled by these symptoms, they should notify the prescribing physician so that a dose reduction can be considered.
- Patients should be informed that they may experience vivid, unusual or strange dreams during treatment with CHANTIX.
- Patients should be informed that quitting smoking, with or without CHANTIX, may be associated with nicotine withdrawal symptoms (depression, agitation) or exacerbation of pre-existing psychiatric illness. Some patients have experienced depressed mood, agitation, changes in behavior, suicidal ideation and suicide when attempting to quit smoking while taking CHANTIX. They should be urged to report any such symptoms to their health care providers, and to reveal any history of psychiatric illness prior to initiating treatment.
- Patients should be informed that some medications may require dose adjustment after quitting smoking.
- Patients intending to become pregnant or planning to breast-feed an infant should be advised of the risks of smoking and risks and benefits of smoking cessation with CHANTIX.
- Patients should be advised to use caution driving or operating machinery until they know how quitting smoking with varenicline may affect them.

ADVERSE REACTIONS
During the premarketing development of CHANTIX, over 4500 individuals were exposed to CHANTIX, with over 450 treated for at least 24 weeks and approximately 100 for a year. Most study participants were treated for 12 weeks or less.
In Phase 2 and 3 placebo-controlled studies, the treatment discontinuation rate due to adverse events in patients dosed with 1 mg BID was 12% for CHANTIX compared to 10% for placebo in studies of three months' treatment. In this group, the discontinuation rates for the most common adverse events in CHANTIX treated patients were as follows: nausea (3% vs. 0.5% for placebo), headache (0.6% vs. 0.9% for placebo), insomnia (1.2% vs. 1.1% for placebo), and abnormal dreams (0.3% vs. 0.2% for placebo).
Adverse Events were categorized using the Medical Dictionary for Regulatory Activities (MedDRA, Version 7.1).
The most common adverse events associated with CHANTIX (>5% and twice the rate seen in placebo-treated patients) were nausea, sleep disturbance, constipation, flatulence, and vomiting.
Smoking cessation, with or without treatment, is associated with nicotine withdrawal symptoms.
The most common adverse event associated with CHANTIX treatment is nausea. For patients treated to the maximum recommended dose of 1 mg BID following initial dosage titration, the incidence of nausea was 30% compared with 10% in patients taking a comparable placebo regimen. In patients taking CHANTIX 0.5 mg BID following initial titration, the incidence was 16% compared with 11% for placebo. Nausea was generally described as mild or moderate and often transient; however, for some subjects, it was persistent throughout the treatment period.
Table 3 shows the adverse events for CHANTIX and placebo in the 12 week fixed dose studies with titration in the first week (Studies 2 (titrated arm only), 4, and 5). MedDRA High Level Group Terms (HLGT) reported in ≥ 5% of patients in the CHANTIX 1 mg BID dose group, and more commonly than in the placebo group, are listed, along with subordinate Preferred Terms (PT) reported in ≥ 1% of CHANTIX patients (and at least 0.5% more frequent than placebo). Closely related Preferred Terms such as 'Insomnia', 'Initial insomnia', 'Middle insomnia', 'Early morning awakening' were grouped, but individual patients reporting two or more grouped events are only counted once.
[See table 3 at top of next page]
The overall pattern, and the frequency of adverse events during the longer-term trials was very similar to that described in Table 3, though several of the most common events were reported by a greater proportion of patients. Nausea, for instance, was reported in 40% of patients treated with CHANTIX 1 mg BID in a one-year study, compared to 8% of placebo-treated patients.
Following is a list of treatment-emergent adverse events reported by patients treated with CHANTIX during all clini-

cal trials. The listing does not include those events already listed in the previous tables or elsewhere in labeling, those events for which a drug cause was remote, those events which were so general as to be uninformative, and those events reported only once which did not have a substantial probability of being acutely life-threatening.

BLOOD AND LYMPHATIC SYSTEM DISORDERS. *Infrequent:* Anemia, Lymphadenopathy. *Rare:* Leukocytosis, Thrombocytopenia, Splenomegaly.

CARDIAC DISORDERS. *Infrequent:* Angina pectoris, Arrhythmia, Bradycardia, Ventricular extrasystoles, Myocardial infarction, Palpitations, Tachycardia. *Rare:* Atrial fibrillation, Cardiac flutter, Coronary artery disease, Cor pulmonale, Acute coronary syndrome.

EAR AND LABYRINTH DISORDERS. *Infrequent:* Tinnitus, Vertigo. *Rare:* Deafness, Meniere's disease.

ENDOCRINE DISORDERS. *Infrequent:* Thyroid gland disorders.

EYE DISORDERS. *Infrequent:* Conjunctivitis, Dry eye, Eye irritation, Vision blurred, Visual disturbance, Eye pain. *Rare:* Acquired night blindness, Blindness transient, Cataract subcapsular, Ocular vascular disorder, Photophobia, Vitreous floaters.

GASTROINTESTINAL DISORDERS. *Frequent:* Diarrhea, Gingivitis. *Infrequent:* Dysphagia, Enterocolitis, Eructation, Gastritis, Gastrointestinal hemorrhage, Mouth ulceration, Esophagitis. *Rare:* Gastric ulcer, Intestinal obstruction, Pancreatitis acute.

GENERAL DISORDERS AND ADMINISTRATION SITE CONDITIONS. *Frequent:* Chest pain, Influenza like illness, Edema, Thirst. *Infrequent:* Chest discomfort, Chills, Pyrexia.

HEPATOBILIARY DISORDERS. *Infrequent:* Gall bladder disorder.

IMMUNE SYSTEM DISORDERS. *Infrequent:* Hypersensitivity. *Rare:* Drug hypersensitivity.

INVESTIGATIONS. *Frequent:* Liver function test abnormal, Weight increased. *Infrequent:* Electrocardiogram abnormal, Muscle enzyme increased, Urine analysis abnormal.

METABOLISM AND NUTRITION DISORDERS. *Infrequent:* Diabetes mellitus, Hyperlipidemia, Hypokalemia. *Rare:* Hyperkalemia, Hypoglycemia.

MUSCULOSKELETAL AND CONNECTIVE TISSUE DISORDERS. *Frequent:* Arthralgia, Back pain, Muscle cramp, Musculoskeletal pain, Myalgia. *Infrequent:* Arthritis, Osteoporosis. *Rare:* Myositis.

NERVOUS SYSTEM DISORDERS. *Frequent:* Disturbance in attention, Dizziness, Sensory disturbance. *Infrequent:* Amnesia, Migraine, Parosmia, Psychomotor hyperactivity, Restless legs syndrome, Syncope, Tremor. *Rare:* Balance disorder, Cerebrovascular accident, Convulsion, Dysarthria, Facial palsy, Mental impairment, Multiple sclerosis, Nystagmus, Psychomotor skills impaired, Transient ischemic attack, Visual field defect.

PSYCHIATRIC DISORDERS. *Frequent:* Anxiety, Depression, Emotional disorder, Irritability, Restlessness. *Infrequent:* Aggression, Agitation, Disorientation, Dissociation, Libido decreased, Mood swings, Thinking abnormal. *Rare:* Bradyphrenia, Euphoric mood, Hallucination, Psychotic disorder, Suicidal ideation.

RENAL AND URINARY DISORDERS. *Frequent:* Polyuria. *Infrequent:* Nephrolithiasis, Nocturia, Urine abnormality, Urethral syndrome. *Rare:* Renal failure acute, Urinary retention.

REPRODUCTIVE SYSTEM AND BREAST DISORDERS. *Frequent:* Menstrual disorder. *Infrequent:* Erectile dysfunction. *Rare:* Sexual dysfunction.

RESPIRATORY, THORACIC AND MEDIASTINAL DISORDERS. *Frequent:* Epistaxis, Respiratory disorders. *Infrequent:* Asthma. *Rare:* Pleurisy, Pulmonary embolism.

SKIN AND SUBCUTANEOUS TISSUE DISORDERS. *Frequent:* Hyperhidrosis. *Infrequent:* Acne, Dermatitis, Dry skin, Eczema, Erythema, Psoriasis, Urticaria. *Rare:* Photosensitivity reaction.

VASCULAR DISORDERS. *Frequent:* Hot flush, Hypertension. *Infrequent:* Hypotension, Peripheral ischemia, Thrombosis.

Post-Marketing Experience:
The following adverse events have been reported during post-approval use of Chantix. Because these events are reported voluntarily from a population of uncertain size, it is not always possible to reliably estimate their frequency or establish a causal relationship to drug exposure.

There have been reports of depressed mood, agitation, changes in behavior, suicidal ideation and suicide in patients attempting to quit smoking while taking Chantix. Smoking cessation with or without treatment is associated with nicotine withdrawal symptoms and the exacerbation of underlying psychiatric illness. Not all patients had known pre-existing psychiatric illness and not all had discontinued smoking. The role of Chantix in these reports is not known (see **WARNINGS**).

DRUG ABUSE AND DEPENDENCE

Controlled Substance Class
Varenicline is not a controlled substance.

Humans: Fewer than 1 out of 1000 patients reported euphoria in clinical trials with CHANTIX. At higher doses (greater than 2 mg), CHANTIX produced more frequent reports of gastrointestinal disturbances such as nausea and vomiting. There is no evidence of dose-escalation to maintain therapeutic effects in clinical studies, which suggests that tolerance does not develop. Abrupt discontinuation of

Table 3: Common Treatment Emergent AEs (%) in the Fixed-Dose, Placebo-Controlled Studies (≥ 1% in the 1 mg BID CHANTIX Group, and 1 mg BID CHANTIX at least 0.5% more than Placebo)

SYSTEM ORGAN CLASS High Level Group Term Preferred Term	CHANTIX 0.5 mg BID N=129	CHANTIX 1 mg BID N=821	Placebo N=805
GASTROINTESTINAL			
GI Signs and Symptoms			
Nausea	16	30	10
Abdominal Pain *	5	7	5
Flatulence	9	6	3
Dyspepsia	5	5	3
Vomiting	1	5	2
GI Motility/Defecation Conditions			
Constipation	5	8	3
Gastroesophageal reflux disease	1	1	0
Salivary Gland Conditions			
Dry mouth	4	6	4
PSYCHIATRIC DISORDERS			
Sleep Disorder/Disturbances			
Insomnia **	19	18	13
Abnormal dreams	9	13	5
Sleep disorder	2	5	3
Nightmare	2	1	0
NERVOUS SYSTEM			
Headaches			
Headache	19	15	13
Neurological Disorders NEC			
Dysgeusia	8	5	4
Somnolence	3	3	2
Lethargy	2	1	0
GENERAL DISORDERS			
General Disorders NEC			
Fatigue/Malaise/Asthenia	4	7	6
RESPIR/THORACIC/MEDIAST			
Respiratory Disorders NEC			
Rhinorrhea	0	1	0
Dyspnoea	2	1	1
Upper Respiratory Tract Disorder	7	5	4
SKIN/SUBCUTANEOUS TISSUE			
Epidermal and Dermal Conditions			
Rash	1	3	2
Pruritus	0	1	1
METABOLISM & NUTRITION			
Appetite/General Nutrit. Disorders			
Increased appetite	4	3	2
Decreased appetite/Anorexia	1	2	1

* Includes PTs Abdominal (pain, pain upper, pain lower, discomfort, tenderness, distension) and Stomach discomfort
** Includes PTs Insomnia/Initial insomnia/Middle insomnia/Early morning awakening

CHANTIX was associated with an increase in irritability and sleep disturbances in up to 3% of patients. This suggests that, in some patients, varenicline may produce mild physical dependence which is not associated with addiction. In a human laboratory abuse liability study, a single oral dose of 1 mg varenicline did not produce any significant positive or negative subjective responses in smokers. In nonsmokers, 1 mg varenicline produced an increase in some positive subjective effects, but this was accompanied by an increase in negative adverse effects, especially nausea. A single oral dose of 3 mg varenicline uniformly produced unpleasant subjective responses in both smokers and nonsmokers.

Animals: Studies in rodents have shown that varenicline produces behavioral responses similar to those produced by nicotine. In rats trained to discriminate nicotine from saline, varenicline produced full generalization to the nicotine cue. In self-administration studies, the degree to which varenicline substitutes for nicotine is dependent upon the requirement of the task. Rats trained to self-administer nicotine under easy conditions continued to self-administer varenicline to a degree comparable to that of nicotine, however in a more demanding task, rats self-administered varenicline to a lesser extent than nicotine. Varenicline pretreatment also reduced nicotine self-administration.

OVERDOSAGE
In case of overdose, standard supportive measures should be instituted as required.

Varenicline has been shown to be dialyzed in patients with end stage renal disease (see **CLINICAL PHARMACOLOGY, Pharmacokinetics, Pharmacokinetics in Special Patient Populations**), however, there is no experience in dialysis following overdose.

DOSAGE AND ADMINISTRATION
Usual Dosage for Adults
Smoking cessation therapies are more likely to succeed for patients who are motivated to stop smoking and who are provided additional advice and support. Patients should be provided with appropriate educational materials and counseling to support the quit attempt.

The patient should set a date to stop smoking. CHANTIX dosing should start one week before this date.

CHANTIX should be taken after eating and with a full glass of water.

The recommended dose of CHANTIX is 1 mg twice daily following a 1-week titration as follows:

Days 1 – 3:	0.5 mg once daily
Days 4 – 7:	0.5 mg twice daily
Day 8 – End of treatment:	1 mg twice daily

Patients who cannot tolerate adverse effects of CHANTIX may have the dose lowered temporarily or permanently.

Patients should be treated with CHANTIX for 12 weeks. For patients who have successfully stopped smoking at the end of 12 weeks, an additional course of 12 weeks treatment with CHANTIX is recommended to further increase the likelihood of long-term abstinence.

Patients who do not succeed in stopping smoking during 12 weeks of initial therapy, or who relapse after treatment, should be encouraged to make another attempt once factors contributing to the failed attempt have been identified and addressed.

Special Populations
Patients with impaired renal function
No dosage adjustment is necessary for patients with mild to moderate renal impairment. For patients with severe renal impairment, the recommended starting dose of CHANTIX is 0.5 mg once daily. Patients may then titrate as needed to a maximum dose of 0.5 mg twice a day. For patients with end-stage renal disease undergoing hemodialysis, a maximum dose of 0.5 mg once daily may be administered if tolerated well (See **CLINICAL PHARMACOLOGY, Pharmacokinetics, Pharmacokinetics in Special Populations, Renal impairment**).

Dosing in elderly patients and patients with impaired hepatic function
No dosage adjustment is necessary for patients with hepatic impairment. Because elderly patients are more likely to have decreased renal function, care should be taken in dose selection, and it may be useful to monitor renal function (See **PRECAUTIONS, Geriatric Use**).

Continued on next page

Chantix—Cont.

Use in children
Safety and effectiveness of CHANTIX in pediatric patients have not been established; therefore, CHANTIX is not recommended for use in patients under 18 years of age.

HOW SUPPLIED

CHANTIX is supplied for oral administration in two strengths: a 0.5 mg capsular biconvex, white to off-white, film-coated tablet debossed with *"Pfizer"* on one side and "CHX 0.5" on the other side and a 1 mg capsular biconvex, light blue film-coated tablet debossed with *"Pfizer"* on one side and "CHX 1.0" on the other side. CHANTIX is supplied in the following package configurations:

	Description	NDC
Packs		
	First month of therapy: Pack (Includes 1 card - 0.5 mg × 11 tablets and 3 cards - 1 mg × 14 tablets)	NDC 0069-0471-97
	Continuing months of therapy: Pack (Includes 4 cards - 1 mg × 14 tablets)	NDC 0069-0469-97
Bottles		
	0.5 mg - bottle of 56	NDC 0069-0468-56
	1 mg - bottle of 56	NDC 0069-0469-56

STORAGE AND HANDLING
Store at 25°C (77°F); excursions permitted to 15–30°C (59–86°F) (see USP Controlled Room Temperature).
Rx only
Distributed by
Pfizer Labs
Division of Pfizer Inc, NY, NY 10017
LAB-0327-7.0
January 2008

REVATIO® ℞

[*rĕ-vă-tē-ō*]
(sildenafil citrate)
Tablets

Prescribing information for this product, which appears on pages 2537–2540 of the 2008 PDR, has been completely revised as follows. Please write "See Supplement A" next to the product heading.

DESCRIPTION

REVATIO®, an oral therapy for pulmonary arterial hypertension, is the citrate salt of sildenafil, a selective inhibitor of cyclic guanosine monophosphate (cGMP)-specific phosphodiesterase type-5 (PDE5). Sildenafil is also marketed as VIAGRA® for male erectile dysfunction.

Sildenafil citrate is designated chemically as 1-[[3-(6,7-dihydro-1-methyl-7-oxo-3-propyl-1*H*-pyrazolo [4,3-*d*] pyrimidin-5-yl)-4-ethoxyphenyl] sulfonyl]-4-methylpiperazine citrate and has the following structural formula:

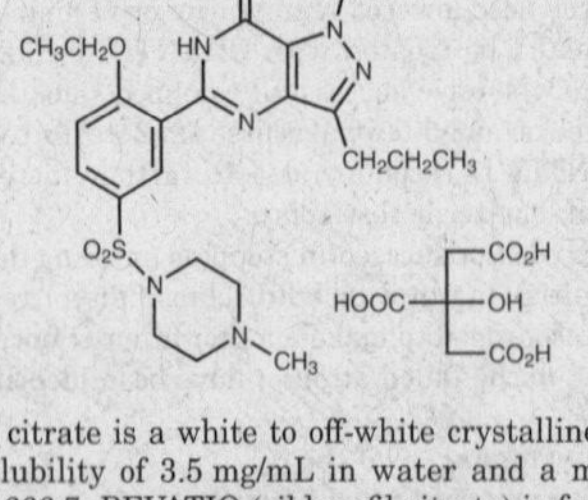

Sildenafil citrate is a white to off-white crystalline powder with a solubility of 3.5 mg/mL in water and a molecular weight of 666.7. REVATIO (sildenafil citrate) is formulated as white, film-coated round tablets equivalent to 20 mg of sildenafil for oral administration. In addition to the active ingredient, sildenafil citrate, each tablet contains the following inactive ingredients: microcrystalline cellulose, anhydrous dibasic calcium phosphate, croscarmellose sodium, magnesium stearate, hypromellose, titanium dioxide, lactose monohydrate, and triacetin.

CLINICAL PHARMACOLOGY

Mechanism of Action
Sildenafil is an inhibitor of cGMP specific phosphodiesterase type-5 (PDE5) in the smooth muscle of the pulmonary vasculature, where PDE5 is responsible for degradation of cGMP. Sildenafil, therefore, increases cGMP within pulmonary vascular smooth muscle cells resulting in relaxation. In patients with pulmonary hypertension, this can lead to vasodilation of the pulmonary vascular bed and, to a lesser degree, vasodilatation in the systemic circulation.

Studies *in vitro* have shown that sildenafil is selective for PDE5. Its effect is more potent on PDE5 than on other known phosphodiesterases (10-fold for PDE6, >80-fold for PDE1, >700-fold for PDE2, PDE3, PDE4, PDE7, PDE8, PDE9, PDE10, and PDE11). The approximately 4,000-fold selectivity for PDE5 versus PDE3 is important because PDE3 is involved in control of cardiac contractility. Sildenafil is only about 10-fold as potent for PDE5 compared to PDE6, an enzyme found in the retina and involved in the phototransduction pathway of the retina. This lower selectivity is thought to be the basis for abnormalities related to color vision observed with higher doses or plasma levels (see **Pharmacodynamics**).

In addition to pulmonary vascular smooth muscle and the corpus cavernosum, PDE5 is also found in other tissues including vascular and visceral smooth muscle and in platelets. The inhibition of PDE5 in these tissues by sildenafil may be the basis for the enhanced platelet anti-aggregatory activity of nitric oxide observed *in vitro*, and the mild peripheral arterial-venous dilatation *in vivo*.

Pharmacokinetics and Metabolism
Absorption and Distribution: REVATIO is rapidly absorbed after oral administration, with absolute bioavailability of about 40%. Maximum observed plasma concentrations are reached within 30 to 120 minutes (median 60 minutes) of oral dosing in the fasted state. When REVATIO is taken with a high-fat meal, the rate of absorption is reduced, with a mean delay in T_{max} of 60 minutes and a mean reduction in C_{max} of 29%. The mean steady state volume of distribution (Vss) for sildenafil is 105 L, indicating distribution into the tissues. Sildenafil and its major circulating N-desmethyl metabolite are both approximately 96% bound to plasma proteins. Protein binding is independent of total drug concentrations.

Metabolism and Excretion: Sildenafil is cleared predominantly by the CYP3A4 (major route) and cytochrome P450 2C9 (CYP2C9, minor route) hepatic microsomal isoenzymes. The major circulating metabolite results from N-desmethylation of sildenafil, and is, itself, further metabolized. This metabolite has a phosphodiesterase selectivity profile similar to sildenafil and an *in vitro* potency for PDE5 approximately 50% of the parent drug. In healthy volunteers, plasma concentrations of this metabolite are approximately 40% of those seen for sildenafil, so that the metabolite accounts for about 20% of sildenafil's pharmacologic effects. In patients with pulmonary arterial hypertension, however, the ratio of the metabolite to sildenafil is higher. Both sildenafil and the active metabolite have terminal half-lives of about 4 hours. The concomitant use of potent cytochrome P450 3A4 (CYP3A4) inhibitors (e.g., ritonavir ketoconazole, itraconazole) as well as the nonspecific CYP inhibitor, cimetidine, is associated with increased plasma levels of sildenafil (see **DOSAGE AND ADMINISTRATION and PRECAUTIONS/Drug Interactions**).

After either oral or intravenous administration, sildenafil is excreted as metabolites predominantly in the feces (approximately 80% of the administered oral dose) and to a lesser extent in the urine (approximately 13% of the administered oral dose).

Pharmacokinetics in Special Populations
Geriatrics: Healthy elderly volunteers (65 years or over) had a reduced clearance of sildenafil, with free plasma concentrations approximately 40% greater than those seen in healthy younger volunteers (18-45 years).

Renal Insufficiency: In volunteers with mild (CLcr =50-80 mL/min) and moderate (CLcr =30-49 mL/min) renal impairment, the pharmacokinetics of a single oral dose of sildenafil (50 mg) was not altered. In volunteers with severe (CLcr <30 mL/min) renal impairment, sildenafil clearance was reduced, resulting in approximately doubling of AUC and C_{max} compared to age-matched volunteers with no renal impairment.

Hepatic Insufficiency: In volunteers with hepatic cirrhosis (Child-Pugh class A and B), sildenafil clearance was reduced, resulting in increases in AUC (84%) and C_{max} (47%) compared to age-matched volunteers with no hepatic impairment. Patients with severe hepatic impairment (Child-Pugh class C) have not been studied.

Population pharmacokinetics
Age, gender, race, and renal and hepatic function were included as factors assessed in the population pharmacokinetic model to evaluate sildenafil pharmacokinetics in pulmonary arterial hypertension patients. The data set available for the population pharmacokinetic evaluation contained a wide range of demographic data and laboratory parameters associated with hepatic and renal function. None of these factors had a statistically significant impact on sildenafil pharmacokinetics in patients with pulmonary hypertension.

In patients with pulmonary hypertension, the average steady-state concentrations were 20-50% higher when compared to those of healthy volunteers. There was also a doubling of C_{min} levels compared to healthy volunteers. Both findings suggest a lower clearance and/or a higher oral bioavailability of sildenafil in patients with pulmonary hypertension compared to healthy volunteers.

Pharmacodynamics
Effects of REVATIO on Blood Pressure: Single oral doses of sildenafil (100 mg) administered to healthy volunteers produced decreases in supine blood pressure (mean maximum decrease in systolic/diastolic blood pressure of 8.4/5.5 mmHg). The decrease in blood pressure was most notable approximately 1-2 hours after dosing, and was not different from placebo at 8 hours. Similar effects on blood pressure were noted with 25 mg, 50 mg and 100 mg doses of sildenafil, therefore the effects are not related to dose or plasma levels within this dosage range. Larger effects were recorded among patients receiving concomitant nitrates (see **CONTRAINDICATIONS**).

Single oral doses of sildenafil up to 100 mg in healthy volunteers produced no clinically relevant effects on ECG. After chronic dosing of 80 mg t.i.d. to patients with pulmonary arterial hypertension, no clinically relevant effects on ECG were reported.

After chronic dosing of 80 mg t.i.d. sildenafil to healthy volunteers, the largest mean change from baseline in supine systolic and supine diastolic blood pressures was a decrease of 9.0 mmHg and 8.4 mmHg, respectively.

After chronic dosing of 80 mg t.i.d. sildenafil to patients with systemic hypertension, the mean change from baseline in systolic and diastolic blood pressures was a decrease of 9.4 mmHg and 9.1 mmHg, respectively.

After chronic dosing of 80 mg t.i.d. sildenafil to patients with pulmonary arterial hypertension, lesser reductions than above in systolic and diastolic blood pressures were observed (a decrease in both of 2 mmHg).

Effects of REVATIO on Vision: At single oral doses of 100 mg and 200 mg, transient dose-related impairment of color discrimination (blue/green) was detected using the Farnsworth-Munsell 100-hue test, with peak effects near the time of peak plasma levels. This finding is consistent with the inhibition of PDE6, which is involved in phototransduction in the retina. An evaluation of visual function at doses up to 200 mg revealed no effects of REVATIO on visual acuity, intraocular pressure, or pupillometry.

Clinical Studies
A randomized, double-blind, placebo-controlled study was conducted in 277 patients with pulmonary arterial hypertension (PAH, defined as a mean pulmonary artery pressure of ≥25 mmHg at rest with a pulmonary capillary wedge pressure <15 mmHg). Patients were predominantly functional classes II-III. Allowed background therapy included a combination of anticoagulation, digoxin, calcium channel blockers, diuretics or oxygen. The use of prostacyclin analogues, endothelin receptor antagonists, and arginine supplementation were not permitted. Subjects who had failed to respond to bosentan were also excluded. Patients with left ventricular ejection fraction <45% or left ventricular shortening fraction <0.2 also were not studied.

Patients were randomized to receive placebo (n=70) or REVATIO 20 mg (n=69), 40 mg (n=67) or 80 mg (n=71) t.i.d. for a period of 12 weeks. They had either primary pulmonary hypertension (63%), PAH associated with connective tissue disease (30%), or PAH following surgical repair of left-to-right congenital heart lesions (7%). The study population consisted of 25% men and 75% women with a mean age of 49 years (range: 18-81 years) and baseline 6-minute walk test distance between 100 and 450 meters.

The primary efficacy endpoint was the change from baseline at week 12 in 6-minute walk distance at least 4 hours after the last dose. Placebo-corrected mean increases in walk distance of 45-50 meters were observed with all doses of sildenafil. These increases were highly significantly different from placebo, but the dose groups were not different from each other (Figure 1). The improvement in walk distance was apparent after 4 weeks of treatment and was maintained at week 8 and week 12.

[See figure 1 at top of next page]

Pre-defined subpopulations in the pivotal study were also evaluated for efficacy, including patient differences in baseline walk distance, disease etiology, functional class, gender, age, and secondary hemodynamic parameters (Figure 2).

[See figure 2 at top of next page]

Patients on all REVATIO doses achieved a statistically significant reduction in mean pulmonary arterial pressure (mPAP) compared to those on placebo. Doses of 20 mg, 40 mg, and 80 mg t.i.d. produced a placebo-corrected decrease in mPAP of -2.7 mmHg, -3.0 mmHg, and -5.1 mmHg, respectively. There was no evidence of a difference in effect between sildenafil 20 mg t.i.d. and the higher doses tested. Data from other hemodynamic parameters can be found in Table 1. The relationship between these effects and improvements in 6-minute walk distance is unknown.

Table 1. Changes from Baseline to Week 12 in Hemodynamic Parameters at Sildenafil 20 mg t.i.d. Dose

PARAMETER [mean (95% CI)]	Placebo (N=65)*	Sildenafil 20 mg t.i.d. (N=65)*
PVR (dyn·s/cm^5)	49 (-54, 153)	-122 (-217, -27)
SVR (dyn·s/cm^5)	-78 (-197, 41)	-167 (-307, -26)
RAP (mmHg)	0.3 (-0.9, 1.5)	-0.8 (-1.9, 0.3)
CO (L/min)	-0.1 (-0.4, 0.2)	0.4 (0.1, 0.7)
HR (beats/min)	-1.3 (-4.1, 1.4)	-3.7 (-5.9, -1.4)

*The number of patients per treatment group varied slightly for each parameter due to missing assessments.

259 of the 277 treated patients entered a long-term, uncontrolled extension study. At the end of 1 year, 94% of these patients were still alive. Additionally, walk distance and functional class status appeared to be stable in patients taking sildenafil. Without a control group, these data must be interpreted cautiously.

INDICATIONS AND USAGE

REVATIO is indicated for the treatment of pulmonary arterial hypertension (WHO Group I) to improve exercise ability.

The efficacy of REVATIO has not been evaluated in patients currently on bosentan therapy.

CONTRAINDICATIONS

Consistent with its known effects on the nitric oxide/cGMP pathway (see **CLINICAL PHARMACOLOGY**), sildenafil was shown to potentiate the hypotensive effects of nitrates, and its administration to patients who are using organic nitrates, either regularly and/or intermittently, in any form is therefore contraindicated.

REVATIO is contraindicated in patients with a known hypersensitivity to any component of the tablet.

WARNINGS

The concomitant administration of the protease inhibitor ritonavir (a highly potent CYP3A4 inhibitor) substantially increases serum concentrations of sildenafil, therefore co-administration with REVATIO is not recommended (see **Drug Interactions** and **DOSAGE AND ADMINISTRATION**).

REVATIO has vasodilator properties, resulting in mild and transient decreases in blood pressure (see **PRECAUTIONS**). Prior to prescribing REVATIO, physicians should carefully consider whether their patients with certain underlying conditions could be adversely affected by such vasodilatory effects, for example patients with resting hypotension (BP <90/50), or with fluid depletion, severe left ventricular outflow obstruction, or autonomic dysfunction. Pulmonary vasodilators may significantly worsen the cardiovascular status of patients with pulmonary veno-occlusive disease (PVOD). Since there are no clinical data on administration of REVATIO to patients with veno-occlusive disease, administration of REVATIO to such patients is not recommended. Should signs of pulmonary edema occur when sildenafil is administered, the possibility of associated PVOD should be considered.

There is no controlled clinical data on the safety or efficacy of REVATIO in the following groups; if prescribed, this should be done with caution:

- Patients who have suffered a myocardial infarction, stroke, or life-threatening arrhythmia within the last 6 months;
- Patients with coronary artery disease causing unstable angina;
- Patients with hypertension (BP >170/110);
- Patients with retinitis pigmentosa (a minority of these patients have genetic disorders of retinal phosphodiesterases).
- Patients currently on bosentan therapy.

PRECAUTIONS

General

Before prescribing REVATIO, it is important to note the following:

- Caution is advised when phosphodiesterase type 5 (PDE5) inhibitors are co-administered with alpha-blockers. PDE5 inhibitors, including sildenafil, and alpha-adrenergic blocking agents are both vasodilators with blood pressure lowering effects. When vasodilators are used in combination, an additive effect on blood pressure may be anticipated. In some patients, concomitant use of these two drug classes can lower blood pressure significantly, leading to symptomatic hypotension. In the sildenafil interaction studies with alpha-blockers (see **Drug Interactions**), cases of symptomatic hypotension consisting of dizziness and lightheadedness were reported. No cases of syncope or fainting were reported during these interaction studies. Consideration should be given to the fact that safety of combined use of PDE5 inhibitors and alpha-blockers may be affected by other variables, including intravascular volume depletion and concomitant use of anti-hypertensive drugs.
- REVATIO should be used with caution in patients with anatomical deformation of the penis (such as angulation, cavernosal fibrosis or Peyronie's disease) or in patients who have conditions, which may predispose them to priapism (such as sickle cell anemia, multiple myeloma or leukemia). In the event of an erection that persists longer than 4 hours, the patient should seek immediate medical assistance. If priapism (painful erections greater than 6 hours in duration) is not treated immediately, penile tissue damage and permanent loss of potency could result.
- In humans, sildenafil has no effect on bleeding time when taken alone or with aspirin. *In vitro* studies with human platelets indicate that sildenafil potentiates the anti-aggregatory effect of sodium nitroprusside (a nitric oxide donor). The combination of heparin and sildenafil had an additive effect on bleeding time in the anesthetized rabbit, but this interaction has not been studied in humans.
- The incidence of epistaxis was higher in patients with PAH secondary to CTD (sildenafil 13%, placebo 0%) than in PPH patients (sildenafil 3%, placebo 2%). The incidence of epistaxis was also higher in sildenafil-treated patients with concomitant oral vitamin K antagonist (9% versus 2% in those not treated with concomitant vitamin K antagonist).
- The safety of REVATIO is unknown in patients with bleeding disorders and patients with active peptic ulceration.

Information for Patients

Physicians should discuss with patients the contraindication of REVATIO with regular and/or intermittent use of organic nitrates.

Sildenafil is also marketed as VIAGRA® for male erectile dysfunction.

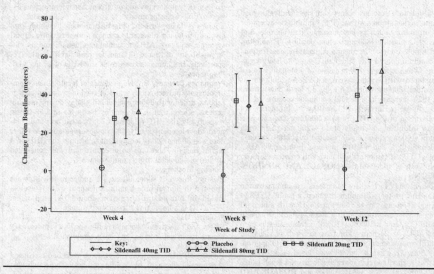

Figure 1: Change from Baseline in 6-Minute Walk Distance (meters): Mean (95% Confidence Interval)

Key:
- Sildenafil 40mg TID
- Placebo
- Sildenafil 80mg TID
- Sildenafil 20mg TID

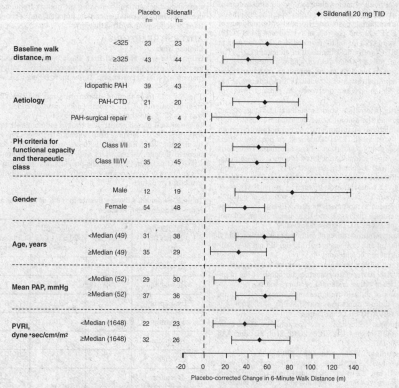

Figure 2: Placebo Corrected Change From Baseline in 6-Minute Walk Distance (meters) by study subpopulation: Mean (95% Confidence Interval)

Key: PAH = pulmonary arterial hypertension; CTD = connective tissue disease; PH, pulmonary hypertension; PAP = pulmonary arterial pressure; PVRI = pulmonary vascular resistance index; TID = three times daily.

Physicians should advise patients to seek immediate medical attention in the event of a sudden loss of vision in one or both eyes while taking all PDE5 inhibitors, including REVATIO. Such an event may be a sign of non-arteritic anterior ischemic optic neuropathy (NAION), a cause of decreased vision including permanent loss of vision, that has been reported rarely post-marketing in temporal association with the use of all PDE5 inhibitors when used in the treatment of male-erectile dysfunction. It is not possible to determine whether these events are related directly to the use of PDE5 inhibitors or to other factors. Physicians should also discuss with patients the increased risk of NAION in individuals who have already experienced NAION in one eye, including whether such individuals could be adversely affected by use of vasodilators, such as PDE5 inhibitors (see **ADVERSE REACTIONS**).

Physicians should advise patients to seek prompt medical attention in the event of sudden decrease or loss of hearing while taking all PDE5 inhibitors, including REVATIO. These events, which may be accompanied by tinnitus and dizziness, have been reported in temporal association to the intake of PDE5 inhibitors, including REVATIO. It is not possible to determine whether these events are related directly to the use of PDE5 inhibitors or to other factors (see **ADVERSE REACTIONS, Clinical Trials and Post-Marketing Experience**).

Drug Interactions

In PAH patients, the concomitant use of vitamin K antagonists and sildenafil resulted in a greater incidence of reports of bleeding (primarily epistaxis) versus placebo.

Effects of Other Drugs on REVATIO

In vitro studies: Sildenafil metabolism is principally mediated by the CYP3A4 (major route) and CYP2C9 (minor route) cytochrome P450 isoforms. Therefore, inhibitors of these isoenzymes may reduce sildenafil clearance and inducers of these isoenzymes may increase sildenafil clearance.

In vivo studies: Population pharmacokinetic analysis of clinical trial data indicated a reduction in sildenafil clearance and/or an increase of oral bioavailability when co-administered with CYP3A4 substrates and the combination of CYP3A4 substrates and beta-blockers. These were the only factors with a statistically significant impact on sildenafil pharmacokinetics.

Population data from patients in clinical trials indicated a reduction in sildenafil clearance when it was co-administered with CYP3A4 inhibitors. Sildenafil exposure without concomitant medication is shown to be 5-fold higher at a dose of 80 mg t.i.d. compared to its exposure at a dose of 20 mg t.i.d. This concentration range covers the same in-

Continued on next page

Revatio—Cont.

creased sildenafil exposure observed in specifically-designed drug interaction studies with CYP3A4 inhibitors (except for potent inhibitors such as ketoconazole, itraconazole, and ritonavir). Cimetidine (800 mg), a nonspecific CYP inhibitor, caused a 56% increase in plasma sildenafil concentrations when co-administered with sildenafil (50 mg) to healthy volunteers. When a single 100 mg dose of sildenafil was co-administered with erythromycin, a CYP3A4 inhibitor, at steady state (500 mg twice daily [b.i.d.] for 5 days), there was a 182% increase in sildenafil systemic exposure (AUC). In a study performed in healthy volunteers, co-administration of the HIV protease inhibitor saquinavir, a CYP3A4 inhibitor, at steady state (1200 mg t.i.d.) with sildenafil (100 mg single dose) resulted in a 140% increase in sildenafil C_{max} and a 210% increase in sildenafil AUC. Stronger CYP3A4 inhibitors will have still greater effects on plasma levels of sildenafil (see **DOSAGE AND ADMINISTRATION**).

In another study in healthy volunteers, co-administration with the HIV protease inhibitor ritonavir, a potent CYP3A4 inhibitor, at steady state (500 mg b.i.d.) with sildenafil (100 mg single dose) resulted in a 300% (4-fold) increase in sildenafil C_{max} and a 1000% (11-fold) increase in sildenafil plasma AUC. At 24 hours, the plasma levels of sildenafil were still approximately 200 ng/mL, compared to approximately 5 ng/mL when sildenafil was dosed alone. This is consistent with ritonavir's marked effects on a broad range of P450 substrates (see **WARNINGS** and **DOSAGE AND ADMINISTRATION**). Although the interaction between other protease inhibitors and REVATIO has not been studied, their concomitant use is expected to increase sildenafil levels.

In a study of healthy male volunteers, co-administration of sildenafil at steady state (80 mg t.i.d.) with the endothelin receptor antagonist bosentan (a moderate inducer of CYP3A4, CYP2C9 and possibly of cytochrome P450 2C19) at steady state (125 mg b.i.d.) resulted in a 63% decrease of sildenafil AUC and a 55% decrease in sildenafil C_{max}. The combination of both drugs did not lead to clinically significant changes in blood pressure (supine or standing). Concomitant administration of potent CYP3A4 inducers is expected to cause greater decreases in plasma levels of sildenafil.

In drug-drug interaction studies, sildenafil (25 mg, 50 mg, or 100 mg) and the alpha-blocker doxazosin (4 mg or 8 mg) were administered simultaneously to patients with benign prostatic hyperplasia (BPH) stabilized on doxazosin therapy. In these study populations, mean additional reductions of supine systolic and diastolic blood pressure of 7/7 mmHg, 9/5 mmHg, and 8/4 mmHg, respectively, were observed. Mean additional reductions of standing blood pressure of 6/6 mmHg, 11/4 mmHg, and 4/5 mmHg, respectively, were also observed. There were infrequent reports of patients who experienced symptomatic postural hypotension. These reports included dizziness and light-headedness, but not syncope (see **PRECAUTIONS: General**).

Concomitant administration of oral contraceptives (ethinyl estradiol 30 µg and levonorgestrel 150 µg) did not affect the pharmacokinetics of sildenafil.

Concomitant administration of a single 100 mg dose of sildenafil with 10 mg of atorvastatin did not alter the pharmacokinetics of either sildenafil or atorvastatin.

Single doses of antacid (magnesium hydroxide/aluminum hydroxide) did not affect the bioavailability of sildenafil.

Effects of REVATIO on Other Drugs

***In vitro* studies:** Sildenafil is a weak inhibitor of the cytochrome P450 isoforms 1A2, 2C9, 2C19, 2D6, 2E1 and 3A4 (IC50 >150 µM).

***In vivo* studies:** When sildenafil 100 mg oral was co-administered with amlodipine, 5 mg or 10 mg oral, to hypertensive patients, the mean additional reduction on supine blood pressure was 8 mmHg systolic and 7 mmHg diastolic. No significant interactions were shown with tolbutamide (250 mg) or warfarin (40 mg), both of which are metabolized by CYP2C9.

Sildenafil (50 mg) did not potentiate the increase in bleeding time caused by aspirin (150 mg).

Sildenafil (50 mg) did not potentiate the hypotensive effect of alcohol in healthy volunteers with mean maximum blood alcohol levels of 0.08%.

In healthy subjects, co-administration of 125 mg b.i.d. bosentan and 80 mg t.i.d. sildenafil resulted in a 63% decrease in AUC of sildenafil and a 50% increase in AUC of bosentan.

In a study of healthy volunteers, sildenafil (100 mg) did not affect the steady-state pharmacokinetics of the HIV protease inhibitors saquinavir and ritonavir, both of which are CYP3A4 substrates.

Sildenafil had no impact on the plasma levels of oral contraceptives (ethinyl estradiol 30 µg and levonorgestrel 150 µg).

Carcinogenesis, Mutagenesis, Impairment of Fertility

Sildenafil was not carcinogenic when administered to rats for up to 24 months at 60 mg/kg/day, a dose resulting in total systemic exposure (AUC) to unbound sildenafil and its major metabolite 33 and 37 times, for male and female rats respectively, the human exposure at the Recommended Human Dose (RHD) of 20 mg t.i.d. Sildenafil was not carcinogenic when administered to male and female mice for up to 21 and 18 months, respectively, at doses up to a maximally tolerated level of 10 mg/kg/day, a dose equivalent to the RHD on a mg/m^2 basis.

Sildenafil was negative in *in vitro* bacterial and Chinese hamster ovary cell assays to detect mutagenicity, and *in vitro* human lymphocytes and *in vivo* mouse micronucleus assays to detect clastogenicity.

There was no impairment of fertility in male or female rats given up to 60 mg sildenafil/kg/day, a dose producing a total systemic exposure (AUC) to unbound sildenafil and its major metabolite of 19 and 38 times for males and females, respectively, the human exposure at the RHD of 20 mg t.i.d.

Pregnancy

Pregnancy Category B. No evidence of teratogenicity, embryotoxicity or fetotoxicity was observed in pregnant rats or rabbits, dosed with 200 mg sildenafil/kg/day during organogenesis, a level that is, on a mg/m^2 basis, 32- and 68-times, respectively, the RHD of 20 mg t.i.d. In a rat pre- and postnatal development study, the no-observed-adverse-effect dose was 30 mg/kg/day (equivalent to 5-times the RHD on a mg/m^2 basis). There are no adequate and well-controlled studies of sildenafil in pregnant women.

Nursing Mothers

It is not known if sildenafil citrate and/or metabolites are excreted in human breast milk. Since many drugs are excreted in human milk, caution should be used when REVATIO is administered to nursing women.

Pediatric Use

Safety and Effectiveness of sildenafil in pediatric pulmonary hypertension patients has not been established.

Geriatric Use

Healthy elderly volunteers (65 years or over) had a reduced clearance of sildenafil, but studies did not include sufficient numbers of subjects to determine whether they respond differently from younger subjects. Other reported clinical experience has not identified differences in response between the elderly and younger pulmonary arterial hypertension patients. In general, dose selection for an elderly patient should be cautious, reflecting the greater frequency of decreased hepatic, renal, or cardiac function, and of concomitant disease or other drug therapy.

ADVERSE REACTIONS

Clinical Trials

Safety data were obtained from the pivotal study and an open-label extension study in 277 treated patients with pulmonary arterial hypertension. Doses up to 80 mg t.i.d. were studied.

The overall frequency of discontinuation in REVATIO-treated patients at the recommended dose of 20 mg t.i.d. was low (3%) and the same as placebo (3%).

In the pivotal placebo-controlled trial in pulmonary arterial hypertension, the adverse drug reactions that were reported by at least 3% of REVATIO patients treated at the recommended dosage (20 mg t.i.d.) and were more frequent in REVATIO patients than placebo patients, are shown in Table 2. Adverse events were generally transient and mild to moderate in nature.

Table 2. Sildenafil Adverse Events in ≥3% of Patients and More Frequent than Placebo

ADVERSE EVENT %	Placebo (n=70)	Sildenafil 20 mg t.i.d. (n=69)	Placebo Subtracted
Epistaxis	1	9	8
Headache	39	46	7
Dyspepsia	7	13	6
Flushing	4	10	6
Insomnia	1	7	6
Erythema	1	6	5
Dyspnea exacerbated	3	7	4
Rhinitis nos	0	4	4
Diarrhea nos	6	9	3
Myalgia	4	7	3
Pyrexia	3	6	3
Gastritis nos	0	3	3
Sinusitis	0	3	3
Paresthesia	0	3	3

At doses higher than the recommended 20 mg t.i.d. there was a greater incidence of some adverse events including flushing, diarrhea, myalgia and visual disturbances. Visual disturbances were identified as mild and transient, and were predominately color-tinge to vision, but also increased sensitivity to light or blurred vision.

In the pivotal study, the incidence of retinal hemorrhage at the recommended sildenafil 20 mg t.i.d. dose was 1.4% versus 0% placebo and for all sildenafil doses studied was 1.9% versus 0% placebo. The incidence of eye hemorrhage at both the recommended dose and at all doses studied was 1.4% for sildenafil versus 1.4% for placebo. The patients experiencing these events had risk factors for hemorrhage including concurrent anticoagulant therapy.

Post-Marketing Experience

In post-marketing experience with sildenafil citrate at doses indicated for male erectile dysfunction, serious cardiovascular, cerebrovascular, and vascular events, including myocardial infarction, sudden cardiac death, ventricular arrhythmia, cerebrovascular hemorrhage, transient ischemic attack, hypertension, pulmonary hemorrhage, and subarachnoid and intracerebral hemorrhages have been reported in temporal association with the use of the drug. Most, but not all, of these patients had preexisting cardiovascular risk factors. Many of these events were reported to occur during or shortly after sexual activity, and a few were reported to occur shortly after the use of sildenafil without sexual activity. Others were reported to have occurred hours to days after use concurrent with sexual activity. It is not possible to determine whether these events are related directly to sildenafil citrate, to sexual activity, to the patient's underlying cardiovascular disease, or to a combination of these or other factors.

When used to treat male-erectile dysfunction, non-arteritic anterior ischemic optic neuropathy (NAION), a cause of decreased vision including permanent loss of vision, has been reported rarely post-marketing in temporal association with the use of phosphodiesterase type 5 (PDE5) inhibitors, including sildenafil citrate. Most, but not all, of these patients had underlying anatomic or vascular risk factors for developing NAION, including but not necessarily limited to: low cup to disc ratio ("crowded disc"), age over 50, diabetes, hypertension, coronary artery disease, hyperlipidemia and smoking. It is not possible to determine whether these events are related directly to the use of PDE5 inhibitors, to the patient's underlying vascular risk factors or anatomical defects, to a combination of these factors, or to other factors (see **PRECAUTIONS/Information for Patients**).

Cases of sudden decrease or loss of hearing have been reported post-marketing in temporal association with the use of PDE5 inhibitors, including REVATIO. In some of the cases, medical conditions and other factors were reported that may have also played a role in the otologic adverse events. In many cases, medical follow-up information was limited. It is not possible to determine whether these reported events are related directly to the use of REVATIO, to the patient's underlying risk factors for hearing loss, a combination of these factors, or to other factors (see **PRECAUTIONS, Information for Patients**).

Other events:

The following list includes other adverse events that have been identified during post-marketing use of REVATIO. The list does not include adverse events that are reported from clinical trials and that are listed elsewhere in this section. These events have been chosen for inclusion either due to their seriousness, reporting frequency, lack of clear alternative causation, or a combination of these factors. Because these reactions were reported voluntarily from a population of uncertain size, it is not possible to reliably estimate their frequency or establish a causal relationship to drug exposure.

Nervous: seizure, seizure recurrence

OVERDOSAGE

In studies with healthy volunteers of single doses up to 800 mg, adverse events were similar to those seen at lower doses but rates were increased.

In cases of overdose, standard supportive measures should be adopted as required. Renal dialysis is not expected to accelerate clearance as sildenafil is highly bound to plasma proteins and it is not eliminated in the urine.

DOSAGE AND ADMINISTRATION

The recommended dose of REVATIO is 20 mg three times a day (t.i.d.). REVATIO tablets should be taken approximately 4-6 hours apart, with or without food. In the clinical trial no greater efficacy was achieved with the use of higher doses. Treatment with doses higher than 20 mg t.i.d. is not recommended. Dosages lower than 20 mg t.i.d. were not tested. Whether dosages lower than 20 mg t.i.d. are effective is not known.

In general, dose selection for elderly patients should be cautious, reflecting the greater frequency of decreased hepatic, renal, or cardiac function, and of concomitant disease or other drug therapy (see **CLINICAL PHARMACOLOGY**)

No dose adjustments are required for renal impaired patients (including severe renal impairment, creatinine clearance <30 mL/min), or for hepatic impaired patients (Child Pugh class A and B).

No dose adjustments are required for the co-administration of REVATIO with erythromycin or saquinavir.

Co-administration of REVATIO with CYP3A4 inducers (including bosentan; and more potent inducers such as barbiturates, carbamazepine, phenytoin, efavirenz, nevirapine, rifampin, rifabutin) may alter plasma levels of either or both medications. Dosage adjustments may be necessary (see **PRECAUTIONS: Drug Interactions**).

Co-administration of potent CYP3A4 inhibitors (e.g., ketoconazole, itraconazole, ritonavir) with REVATIO substantially increases serum concentrations of sildenafil and is therefore not recommended (see **WARNINGS** and **PRECAUTIONS: Drug Interactions**).

Sildenafil was shown to potentiate the hypotensive effects of nitrates and its administration in patients who use nitric oxide donors, or nitrates in any form, is therefore contraindicated.

HOW SUPPLIED

REVATIO (sildenafil citrate) is supplied as white, film-coated, round tablets containing sildenafil citrate equivalent to the nominally indicated amount of sildenafil as follows:

REVATIO Tablets

Package Configuration	Tablet Strength (mg)	NDC	Engraving on Tablet
Bottle of 90	20 mg	0069-4190-68	RVT20

Recommended Storage: Store at 25°C (77°F); excursions permitted to 15-30°C (59-86°F) [see USP Controlled Room Temperature].

Rx Only

Distributed by

Pfizer Labs

Division of Pfizer Inc, NY, NY 10017

LAB-0313-8.0   Revised October 2007

PATIENT INFORMATION

REVATIO® (re-VAH-tee-oh)

(sildenafil citrate) tablets

Read the Patient Information that comes with REVATIO before you start taking it and each time you get a refill. There may be new information. This leaflet does not take the place of talking with your doctor about your medical condition or treatment. If you have any questions about REVATIO, ask your doctor or pharmacist.

What is the most important information I should know about REVATIO (sildenafil citrate)?

• **Never take REVATIO with any nitrate medicines. Your blood pressure could drop quickly. It could fall to an unsafe level. Nitrate medicines include:**

  • **Medicines that treat chest pain (angina)**
  • **Nitroglycerin in any form**
  • **Isosorbide mononitrate or dinitrate**
  • **Street drugs called "poppers" (amyl nitrate or nitrite)**

Ask your doctor or pharmacist if you are not sure if you are taking a nitrate medicine.

What is REVATIO (sildenafil citrate)?

REVATIO is a prescription medicine used to treat **pulmonary arterial hypertension (PAH)**. REVATIO improves the ability to exercise. With PAH, the blood pressure in your lungs is too high. Your heart has to work hard to pump blood into your lungs.

REVATIO has **not** been studied

• in children under 18 years old
• in patients who are also taking a medicine called bosentan (Tracleer®)

REVATIO contains the same medicine as VIAGRA® (sildenafil citrate), which is used to treat erectile dysfunction (impotence).

Who should not take REVATIO (sildenafil citrate)?

Do not take REVATIO if you

• take nitrate medicines. See "**What is the most important information I should know about REVATIO?**"
• are allergic to sildenafil citrate or any other ingredient in REVATIO. See "**What are the ingredients in REVATIO?**" at the end of this leaflet.

What should I tell my doctor before taking REVATIO (sildenafil citrate)?

Tell your doctor about all of your medical conditions, including if you

• have had a heart attack, stroke, or irregular heartbeats in the last 6 months
• have chest pain (angina)
• have a disease called pulmonary veno-occlusive disease (PVOD)
• have high or low blood pressure or blood circulation problems
• have an eye problem called retinitis pigmentosa
• have or had loss of sight in one or both eyes
• have liver or kidney problems
• have any problem with the shape of your penis
• lose a large amount of body fluids (dehydration). This can happen if you are sick with a fever, vomiting, or diarrhea. Dehydration can also happen when you sweat a lot or don't drink enough liquids.
• have any blood cell problems such as cancer of blood cells or bone marrow or sickle cell anemia
• have a stomach ulcer or any bleeding problems
• are pregnant or planning to become pregnant. It is not known if REVATIO could harm your unborn baby.
• are breastfeeding. It is not known if REVATIO passes into your breast milk or if it could harm your baby.

Tell your doctor about all of the medicines you take, including prescription and non-prescription medicines, vitamins, and herbal products. REVATIO and certain other medicines can cause side effects if you take them together. The doses of some of your medicines may need to be adjusted while you take REVATIO.

Especially tell your doctor if you

• Take nitrate medicines. See "**What is the most important information I should know about REVATIO?**"
• Take ritonavir (Norvir®) or other medicines used to treat HIV infection
• Use ketoconazole (Nizoral®)

Know the medicines you take. Keep a list of your medicines and show it to your doctor and pharmacist when you get a new medicine.

How should I take REVATIO (sildenafil citrate)?

• Take REVATIO exactly as your doctor tells you.
• REVATIO is a tablet you take by mouth. Take a REVATIO tablet 3 times a day about 4 to 6 hours apart.

• Take REVATIO at the same times every day, with or without food.
• If you miss a dose, take it as soon as you remember. If it is close to your next dose, skip the missed dose, and take your next dose at the regular time.
• Do not take more than one dose of REVATIO at a time.
• Do not change your dose or stop taking REVATIO on your own. Talk to your doctor first.
• **If you take too much REVATIO, call your doctor or poison control center, or go to an emergency room.**

What are the possible side effects of REVATIO (sildenafil citrate)?

The following side effects were reported in patients taking REVATIO. Some of these were serious.

• **low blood pressure.** Low blood pressure may cause you to feel faint or dizzy. Lie down if you feel faint or dizzy.
• **more shortness of breath than usual.** Tell your doctor if you get more short of breath after you start REVATIO. More shortness of breath than usual may be due to your underlying medical condition.

The following side effects were reported rarely in patients taking sildenafil:

• **decreased eyesight or loss of sight in one or both eyes (NAION).** If you notice a sudden decrease or loss of eyesight, talk to your doctor right away. It is not possible to determine if these events are related to oral medicines for the treatment of erectile dysfunction, including sildenafil, or to other medical problems, or combination of these factors.
• **sudden decrease or loss of hearing.** If you notice a sudden decrease or loss of hearing, talk to your doctor right away. It is not possible to determine whether these events are related directly to this class of oral medicines, including sildenafil, or to other diseases or medications, to other factors, or to a combination of factors.
• **heart attack, stroke, irregular heartbeats, and death.** Most of these happened in men who already had heart problems.
• **erections that last several hours.** Tell your doctor right away if you have an erection that lasts more than 4 hours.

The most common side effects are nosebleed, headache, upset stomach, getting red or hot in the face (flushing), and trouble sleeping.

Tell your doctor if you have any side effect that bothers you or doesn't go away.

These are not all the possible side effects of REVATIO. For more information, ask your doctor or pharmacist.

How should I store REVATIO (sildenafil citrate)?

• Store REVATIO at room temperature, 59-86°F (15-30°C).
• **Keep REVATIO and all medicines away from children.**

General information about REVATIO (sildenafil citrate)

Medicines are sometimes prescribed for conditions that are not in the patient leaflet. Do not use REVATIO for a condition for which it was not prescribed. Do not give REVATIO to other people, even if they have the same symptoms you have. It could harm them.

This patient leaflet summarizes the most important information about REVATIO. If you would like more information about REVATIO:

• Ask your doctor or pharmacist for information about REVATIO that is written for health professionals.
• Go to **www.REVATIO.com** or call **1-800-879-3477.**

What are the ingredients in REVATIO (sildenafil citrate)?

Active ingredients: sildenafil citrate

Inactive ingredients: microcrystalline cellulose, anhydrous dibasic calcium phosphate, croscarmellose sodium, magnesium stearate, hypromellose, titanium dioxide, lactose monohydrate, and triacetin

Rx only

Distributed by

Pfizer Labs

Division of Pfizer Inc, NY, NY 10017

LAB-0335.3.0

December 2007

SUTENT®   ℞

(sunitinib malate) capsules, oral

Prescribing information for this product, which appears on pages 2546–2551 of the 2008 PDR, has been completely revised as follows. Please write "See Supplement A" next to the product heading.

HIGHLIGHTS OF PRESCRIBING INFORMATION

These highlights do not include all the information needed to use SUTENT safely and effectively. See full prescribing information for SUTENT.

SUTENT® (sunitinib malate) capsules, oral

Initial U.S. Approval: 2006

RECENT MAJOR CHANGES

Indications and Usage, Advanced Renal Cell Carcinoma (1.2)	2/2007
Warnings and Precautions, Left Ventricular Dysfunction (5.2)	2/2007
Warnings and Precautions, QT Interval Prolongation and Torsade de Pointes (5.3)	2/2007
Warnings and Precautions, Hypertension (5.4)	2/2007
Warnings and Precautions, Hemorrhagic Events (5.5)	2/2007
Warnings and Precautions, Hypothyroidism (5.6)	2/2007

INDICATIONS AND USAGE

SUTENT is a kinase inhibitor indicated for the treatment of:

• Gastrointestinal stromal tumor after disease progression on or intolerance to imatinib mesylate. (1.1)
• Advanced renal cell carcinoma. (1.2)

DOSAGE AND ADMINISTRATION

• 50 mg orally once daily, with or without food, 4 weeks on treatment followed by 2 weeks off. (2.1)
• Dose adjustments of 12.5 mg recommended based on individual safety and tolerability. (2.2)

DOSAGE FORMS AND STRENGTHS

• Capsules: 12.5 mg, 25 mg, 50 mg (3)

CONTRAINDICATIONS

• None (4)

WARNINGS AND PRECAUTIONS

• Women of childbearing potential should be advised of the potential hazard to the fetus and to avoid becoming pregnant. (5.1)
• Left ventricular ejection fraction declines to below the lower limit of normal have occurred. Monitor patients for signs and symptoms of congestive heart failure. (5.2)
• Prolonged QT intervals and Torsade de Pointes have been observed. Use with caution in patients at higher risk for developing QT interval prolongation. When using SUTENT, monitoring with on-treatment electrocardiograms and electrolytes should be considered. (5.3)
• Hypertension may occur. Monitor blood pressure and treat as needed. (5.4)
• Hemorrhagic events including tumor-related hemorrhage have occurred. Perform serial complete blood counts and physical examinations. (5.5)
• Hypothyroidism may occur. Patients with signs and symptoms suggestive of hypothyroidism should have laboratory monitoring of thyroid function performed and be treated as per standard medical practice. (5.6)
• Adrenal hemorrhage was observed in animal studies. Monitor adrenal function in case of stress such as surgery, trauma or severe infection. (5.7)

ADVERSE REACTIONS

• The most common adverse reactions (≥20%) are fatigue, asthenia, diarrhea, nausea, mucositis/stomatitis, vomiting, dyspepsia, abdominal pain, constipation, hypertension, rash, hand-foot syndrome, skin discoloration, altered taste, anorexia, and bleeding. (6)

To report SUSPECTED ADVERSE REACTIONS, contact Pfizer, Inc. at 1-800-438-1985 or FDA at 1-800-FDA-1088 or *www.fda.gov/medwatch*.

DRUG INTERACTIONS

• CYP3A4 Inhibitors: Consider dose reduction of SUTENT when administered with strong CYP3A4 inhibitors. (7.1)
• CYP3A4 Inducers: Consider dose increase of SUTENT when administered with CYP3A4 inducers. (7.2)

See 17 for PATIENT COUNSELING INFORMATION and FDA-approved patient labeling.

Revised: 10/2007

Continued on next page

Sutent—Cont.

13 NONCLINICAL TOXICOLOGY
13.1 Carcinogenesis, Mutagenesis, Impairment of Fertility
14 CLINICAL STUDIES
14.1 Gastrointestinal Stromal Tumor
14.2 Renal Cell Carcinoma
16 HOW SUPPLIED/STORAGE AND HANDLING
17 PATIENT COUNSELING INFORMATION
17.1 Gastrointestinal Disorders
17.2 Skin Effects
17.3 Other Common Events
17.4 Concomitant Medications
17.5 FDA-Approved Patient Labeling

* Sections or subsections omitted from the full prescribing information are not listed.

FULL PRESCRIBING INFORMATION:

1 INDICATIONS AND USAGE

1.1 Gastrointestinal Stromal Tumor

SUTENT is indicated for the treatment of gastrointestinal stromal tumor after disease progression on or intolerance to imatinib mesylate.

1.2 Advanced Renal Cell Carcinoma

SUTENT is indicated for the treatment of advanced renal cell carcinoma.

2 DOSAGE AND ADMINISTRATION

2.1 Recommended Dose

The recommended dose of SUTENT for gastrointestinal stromal tumor (GIST) and advanced renal cell carcinoma (RCC) is one 50 mg oral dose taken once daily, on a schedule of 4 weeks on treatment followed by 2 weeks off (Schedule 4/2). SUTENT may be taken with or without food.

2.2 Dose Modification

Dose increase or reduction of 12.5 mg increments is recommended based on individual safety and tolerability.

Strong CYP3A4 inhibitors such as ketoconazole may **increase** sunitinib plasma concentrations. Selection of an alternate concomitant medication with no or minimal enzyme inhibition potential is recommended. A dose reduction for SUTENT to a minimum of 37.5 mg daily should be considered if SUTENT must be co-administered with a strong CYP3A4 inhibitor *[see Drug Interactions (7.1) and Clinical Pharmacology (12.3)]*.

CYP3A4 inducers such as rifampin may **decrease** sunitinib plasma concentrations. Selection of an alternate concomitant medication with no or minimal enzyme induction potential is recommended. A dose increase for SUTENT to a maximum of 87.5 mg daily should be considered if SUTENT must be co-administered with a CYP3A4 inducer. If dose is increased, the patient should be monitored carefully for toxicity *[see Drug Interactions (7.2) and Clinical Pharmacology (12.3)]*.

3 DOSAGE FORMS AND STRENGTHS

12.5 mg capsules

Hard gelatin capsule with orange cap and orange body, printed with white ink "Pfizer" on the cap and "STN 12.5 mg" on the body.

25 mg capsules

Hard gelatin capsule with caramel cap and orange body, printed with white ink "Pfizer" on the cap and "STN 25 mg" on the body.

50 mg capsules

Hard gelatin capsule with caramel top and caramel body, printed with white ink "Pfizer" on the cap and "STN 50 mg" on the body.

4 CONTRAINDICATIONS

None

5 WARNINGS AND PRECAUTIONS

5.1 Pregnancy

Pregnancy Category D

As angiogenesis is a critical component of embryonic and fetal development, inhibition of angiogenesis following administration of SUTENT should be expected to result in adverse effects on pregnancy. There are no adequate and well-controlled studies of SUTENT in pregnant women. If the drug is used during pregnancy, or if the patient becomes pregnant while receiving this drug, the patient should be apprised of the potential hazard to the fetus. Women of childbearing potential should be advised to avoid becoming pregnant while receiving treatment with SUTENT.

Sunitinib was evaluated in pregnant rats (0.3, 1.5, 3.0, 5.0 mg/kg/day) and rabbits (0.5, 1, 5, 20 mg/kg/day) for effects on the embryo. Significant increases in the incidence of embryolethality and structural abnormalities were observed in rats at the dose of 5 mg/kg/day (approximately 5.5 times the systemic exposure [combined AUC of sunitinib + primary active metabolite] in patients administered the recommended daily doses [RDD]). Significantly increased embryolethality was observed in rabbits at 5 mg/kg/day while developmental effects were observed at ≥1 mg/kg/day (approximately 0.3 times the AUC in patients administered the RDD of 50 mg/day). Developmental effects consisted of fetal skeletal malformations of the ribs and vertebrae in rats. In rabbits, cleft lip was observed at 1 mg/kg/day and cleft lip and cleft palate were observed at 5 mg/kg/day (approximately 2.7 times the AUC in patients administered the RDD). Neither fetal loss nor malformations were observed in rats dosed at ≤3 mg/kg/day (approximately 2.3 times the AUC in patients administered the RDD).

5.2 Left Ventricular Dysfunction

In the presence of clinical manifestations of congestive heart failure (CHF), discontinuation of SUTENT is recommended. The dose of SUTENT should be interrupted and/or reduced in patients without clinical evidence of CHF but with an ejection fraction <50% and >20% below baseline.

More patients treated with SUTENT experienced decline in left ventricular ejection fraction (LVEF) than patients receiving either placebo or interferon-α (IFN-α). In GIST Study A, 22/209 patients (11%) on SUTENT and 3/102 patients (3%) on placebo had treatment-emergent LVEF values below the lower limit of normal (LLN). Nine of 22 GIST patients on SUTENT with LVEF changes recovered without intervention. Five patients had documented LVEF recovery following intervention (dose reduction: one patient; addition of antihypertensive or diuretic medications: four patients). Six patients went off study without documented recovery. Additionally, three patients on SUTENT had Grade 3 reductions in left ventricular systolic function to LVEF <40%; two of these patients died without receiving further study drug. No GIST patients on placebo had Grade 3 decreased LVEF. In GIST Study A, 1 patient on SUTENT and 1 patient on placebo died of diagnosed heart failure; 2 patients on SUTENT and 2 patients on placebo died of treatment-emergent cardiac arrest.

In the treatment-naïve MRCC study, 78/375 (21%) and 44/360 (12%) patients on SUTENT and IFN-α, respectively, had an LVEF value below the LLN. Thirteen patients on SUTENT (4%) and four on IFN-α (1%) experienced declines in LVEF of >20% from baseline and to below 50%. Left ventricular dysfunction was reported in three patients (1%) and CHF in one patient (<1%) who received SUTENT.

Patients who presented with cardiac events within 12 months prior to SUTENT administration, such as myocardial infarction (including severe/unstable angina), coronary/peripheral artery bypass graft, symptomatic CHF, cerebrovascular accident or transient ischemic attack, or pulmonary embolism were excluded from SUTENT clinical studies. It is unknown whether patients with these concomitant conditions may be at a higher risk of developing drug-related left ventricular dysfunction. Physicians are advised to weigh this risk against the potential benefits of the drug. **These patients should be carefully monitored for clinical signs and symptoms of CHF while receiving SUTENT. Baseline and periodic evaluations of LVEF should also be considered while the patient is receiving SUTENT. In patients without cardiac risk factors, a baseline evaluation of ejection fraction should be considered.**

5.3 QT Interval Prolongation and Torsade de Pointes

SUTENT has been shown to prolong the QT interval in a dose dependent manner, which may lead to an increased risk for ventricular arrhythmias including Torsade de Pointes. Torsade de Pointes has been observed in <0.1% of SUTENT-exposed patients.

SUTENT should be used with caution in patients with a history of QT interval prolongation, patients who are taking antiarrhythmics, or patients with relevant pre-existing cardiac disease, bradycardia, or electrolyte disturbances. When using SUTENT, periodic monitoring with on-treatment electrocardiograms and electrolytes (magnesium, potassium) should be considered. Concomitant treatment with strong CYP3A4 inhibitors, which may increase sunitinib plasma concentrations, should be used with caution and dose reduction of SUTENT should be considered *[see Dosage and Administration (2.2)]*.

5.4 Hypertension

Patients should be monitored for hypertension and treated as needed with standard anti-hypertensive therapy. In cases of severe hypertension, temporary suspension of SUTENT is recommended until hypertension is controlled.

Of patients receiving SUTENT for treatment-naïve MRCC, 111/375 patients (30%) receiving SUTENT compared with 13/360 patients (4%) on IFN-α experienced hypertension. Grade 3 hypertension was observed in 36/375 treatment-naïve MRCC patients (10%) on SUTENT compared to 1/360 patient (<1%) on IFN-α. While all-grade hypertension was similar in GIST patients on SUTENT compared to placebo, Grade 3 hypertension was reported in 9/202 GIST patients on SUTENT (4%), and none of the GIST patients on placebo. No Grade 4 hypertension was reported. SUTENT dosing was reduced or temporarily delayed for hypertension in 18/375 patients (5%) on the treatment-naive MRCC study. Two treatment-naïve MRCC patients, including one with malignant hypertension, and no GIST patients discontinued treatment due to hypertension. Severe hypertension (>200 mmHg systolic or 110 mmHg diastolic) occurred in 8/202 GIST patients on SUTENT (4%), 1/102 GIST patients on placebo (1%), and in 20/375 treatment-naïve MRCC patients (5%) on SUTENT and 2/360 patients (1%) on IFN-α.

5.5 Hemorrhagic Events

In patients receiving SUTENT for treatment-naïve MRCC, 112/375 patients (30%) had bleeding events compared with 27/360 patients (8%) receiving IFN-α. Bleeding events occurred in 37/202 patients (18%) receiving SUTENT in GIST Study A, compared to 17/102 patients (17%) receiving placebo. Epistaxis was the most common hemorrhagic adverse event reported. Less common bleeding events in GIST or MRCC patients included rectal, gingival, upper gastrointestinal, genital, and wound bleeding. In GIST Study A, 14/202 patients (7%) receiving SUTENT and 9/102 patients (9%) on placebo had Grade 3 or 4 bleeding events. In addition, one patient in Study A taking placebo had a fatal gastrointestinal bleeding event during Cycle 2. Most events in MRCC patients were Grade 1 or 2; there was one Grade 5 event of gastric bleed in a treatment-naïve patient.

Tumor-related hemorrhage has been observed in patients treated with SUTENT. These events may occur suddenly, and in the case of pulmonary tumors may present as severe and life-threatening hemoptysis or pulmonary hemorrhage. Fatal pulmonary hemorrhage occurred in 2 patients receiving SUTENT on a clinical trial of patients with metastatic non-small cell lung cancer (NSCLC). Both patients had squamous cell histology. SUTENT is not approved for use in patients with NSCLC. Treatment-emergent Grade 3 and 4 tumor hemorrhage occurred in 5/202 patients (3%) with GIST receiving SUTENT on Study A. Tumor hemorrhages were observed as early as Cycle 1 and as late as Cycle 6. One of these five patients received no further drug following tumor hemorrhage. None of the other four patients discontinued treatment or experienced dose delay due to tumor hemorrhage. No patients with GIST in the Study A placebo arm were observed to undergo intratumoral hemorrhage. Tumor hemorrhage has not been observed in patients with MRCC. Clinical assessment of these events should include serial complete blood counts (CBCs) and physical examinations.

Serious, sometimes fatal gastrointestinal complications including gastrointestinal perforation, have occurred rarely in patients with intra-abdominal malignancies treated with SUTENT.

5.6 Hypothyroidism

Baseline laboratory measurement of thyroid function is recommended and patients with hypothyroidism should be treated as per standard medical practice prior to the start of SUTENT treatment. All patients should be observed closely for signs and symptoms of hypothyroidism on SUTENT treatment. Patients with signs or symptoms suggestive of hypothyroidism should have laboratory monitoring of thyroid function performed and be treated as per standard medical practice.

Treatment-emergent acquired hypothyroidism was noted in eight GIST patients (4%) on SUTENT versus one (1%) on placebo. Hypothyroidism was reported as an adverse reaction in eleven patients (3%) on SUTENT in the treatment-naïve MRCC study and in one patient (<1%) in the IFN-α arm. An additional seven patients (2%) with no prior history of hypothyroidism were started on thyroid replacement therapy while on study.

5.7 Adrenal Function

Physicians prescribing SUTENT are advised to monitor for adrenal insufficiency in patients who experience stress such as surgery, trauma or severe infection.

Adrenal toxicity was noted in non-clinical repeat dose studies of 14 days to 9 months in rats and monkeys at plasma exposures as low as 0.7 times the AUC observed in clinical studies. Histological changes of the adrenal gland were characterized as hemorrhage, necrosis, congestion, hypertrophy and inflammation. In clinical studies, CT/MRI obtained in 336 patients after exposure to one or more cycles of SUTENT demonstrated no evidence of adrenal hemorrhage or necrosis. ACTH stimulation testing was performed in approximately 400 patients across multiple clinical trials of SUTENT. Among patients with normal baseline ACTH stimulation testing, one patient developed consistently abnormal test results during treatment that are unexplained and may be related to treatment with SUTENT. Eleven additional patients with normal baseline testing had abnormalities in the final test performed, with peak cortisol levels of 12-16.4 mcg/dL (normal >18 mcg/dL) following stimulation. None of these patients were reported to have clinical evidence of adrenal insufficiency.

5.8 Laboratory Tests

CBCs with platelet count and serum chemistries including phosphate should be performed at the beginning of each treatment cycle for patients receiving treatment with SUTENT.

6 ADVERSE REACTIONS

The data described below reflect exposure to SUTENT in 577 patients who participated in a placebo-controlled trial (n=202) for the treatment of GIST or an active-controlled trial (n=375) for the treatment of MRCC. In these two studies, 225 patients were exposed to SUTENT for at least 6 months and 16 were exposed for greater than one year. The population was 23 - 87 years of age and 69% male and 31% female. The race distribution was 92% White, 3% Asian, 2% Black and 3% not reported. The patients received a starting oral dose of 50 mg daily on Schedule 4/2 in repeated cycles. The most common adverse reactions (≥20%) in patients with GIST or MRCC are fatigue, asthenia, diarrhea, nausea, mucositis/stomatitis, vomiting, dyspepsia, abdominal pain, constipation, hypertension, rash, hand-foot syndrome, skin discoloration, altered taste, anorexia, and bleeding. The potentially serious adverse reactions of left ventricular dysfunction, QT interval prolongation, hemorrhage, hypertension, and adrenal function are discussed in *Warnings and Precautions (5)*. Other adverse reactions occurring in GIST and MRCC studies are described below.

Because clinical trials are conducted under widely varying conditions, adverse reaction rates observed in the clinical trials of a drug cannot be directly compared to rates in the clinical trials of another drug and may not reflect the rates observed in practice.

6.1 Adverse Reactions in GIST Study A

Median duration of blinded study treatment was two cycles for patients on SUTENT (mean 3.0, range 1-9) and one cycle (mean 1.8, range 1-6) for patients on placebo. Dose reductions occurred in 23 patients (11%) on SUTENT and none on placebo. Dose interruptions occurred in 59 patients (29%) on SUTENT and 31 patients (30%) on placebo. The rates of treatment-emergent, non-fatal adverse reactions resulting in permanent discontinuation were 7% and 6% in the SUTENT and placebo groups, respectively.

Most treatment-emergent adverse reactions in both study arms were Grade 1 or 2 in severity. Grade 3 or 4 treatment-emergent adverse reactions were reported in 56% versus 51% of patients on SUTENT versus placebo. Table 1 compares the incidence of common (≥10%) treatment-emergent adverse reactions for patients receiving SUTENT and reported more commonly in patients receiving SUTENT than in patients receiving placebo.

[See table 1 above]

Oral pain other than mucositis/stomatitis occurred in 12 patients (6%) on SUTENT versus 3 (3%) on placebo. Hair color changes occurred in 15 patients (7%) on SUTENT versus 4 (4%) on placebo. Alopecia was observed in 10 patients (5%) on SUTENT versus 2 (2%) on placebo.

Table 2 provides common (≥10%) treatment-emergent laboratory abnormalities.

[See table 2 above]

6.2 Adverse Reactions in the Treatment-Naïve MRCC Study

The as-treated patient population for the interim safety analysis of the treatment-naive MRCC study included 735 patients, 375 randomized to SUTENT and 360 randomized to IFN-α. The median duration of treatment was 5.6 months (range: 0.4-15.6) for SUTENT treatment and 4.1 months (range: 0.1-13.7) on IFN-α treatment. Dose reductions occurred in 121 patients (32%) on SUTENT and 77 patients (21%) on IFN-α. Dose interruptions occurred in 142 patients (38%) on SUTENT and 115 patients (32%) on IFN-α. The rates of treatment-emergent, non-fatal adverse reactions resulting in permanent discontinuation were 9% and 12% in the SUTENT and IFN-α groups, respectively. Most treatment-emergent adverse reactions in both study arms were Grade 1 or 2 in severity. Grade 3 or 4 treatment-emergent adverse reactions were reported in 67% versus 51% of patients on SUTENT versus IFN-α, respectively. Table 3 compares the incidence of common (≥10%) treatment-emergent adverse reactions for patients receiving SUTENT versus IFN-α.

[See table 3 at top of next page]

Treatment-emergent Grade 3/4 laboratory abnormalities are presented in Table 4.

[See table 4 at top of page 193]

6.3 Venous Thromboembolic Events

Seven patients (3%) on SUTENT and none on placebo in GIST Study A experienced venous thromboembolic events; five of the seven were Grade 3 deep venous thrombosis (DVT), and two were Grade 1 or 2. Four of these seven GIST patients discontinued treatment following first observation of DVT.

Eight (2%) patients receiving SUTENT for treatment-naïve MRCC had venous thromboembolic events reported. Four (1%) of these patients had pulmonary embolism, one was Grade 3 and three were Grade 4, and four (1%) patients had DVT, including one Grade 3. One patient was permanently withdrawn from SUTENT due to pulmonary embolism; dose interruption occurred in two patients with pulmonary embolism and one with DVT. In treatment-naïve MRCC patients receiving IFN-α, six (2%) venous thromboembolic events occurred; one patient (<1%) experienced a Grade 3 DVT and five patients (1%) had pulmonary embolism, one Grade 1 and four with Grade 4.

6.4 Reversible Posterior Leukoencephalopathy Syndrome

There have been rare (<1%) reports of subjects presenting with seizures and radiological evidence of reversible posterior leukoencephalopathy syndrome (RPLS). None of these subjects had a fatal outcome to the event. Patients with seizures and signs/symptoms consistent with RPLS, such as hypertension, headache, decreased alertness, altered mental functioning, and visual loss, including cortical blindness should be controlled with medical management including control of hypertension. Temporary suspension of SUTENT is recommended; following resolution, treatment may be resumed at the discretion of the treating physician.

6.5 Pancreatic and Hepatic Function

If symptoms of pancreatitis or hepatic failure are present, patients should have SUTENT discontinued. Pancreatitis was observed in 5 (1%) patients receiving SUTENT for treatment-naïve MRCC compared to 1 (<1%) patient receiving IFN-α. Hepatic failure was observed in <1% of solid tumor patients treated with SUTENT.

6.6 Post-marketing Experience

The following adverse reactions have been identified during post-approval use of SUTENT. Because these reactions are reported voluntarily from a population of uncertain size, it is not always possible to reliably estimate their frequency or establish a causal relationship to drug exposure.

Cases of serious infection (with or without neutropenia), in some cases with fatal outcome, have been reported.

Rare cases of myopathy and/or rhabdomyolysis, some with acute renal failure, have been reported. Most of these patients had pre-existing risk factors and/or were receiving concomitant medications known to be associated with these adverse reactions. Patients with signs or symptoms of muscle toxicity should be managed as per standard medical practice.

7 DRUG INTERACTIONS

7.1 CYP3A4 Inhibitors

Strong CYP3A4 inhibitors such as ketoconazole may **increase** sunitinib plasma concentrations. Selection of an alternate concomitant medication with no or minimal enzyme inhibition potential is recommended. Concurrent administration of SUTENT with the strong CYP3A4 inhibitor, ketoconazole, resulted in 49% and 51% increases in the combined (sunitinib + primary active metabolite) C_{max} and $AUC_{0-\infty}$ values, respectively, after a single dose of SUTENT in healthy volunteers. Co-administration of SUTENT with strong inhibitors of the CYP3A4 family (e.g., ketoconazole, itraconazole, clarithromycin, atazanavir, indinavir, nefazodone, nelfinavir, ritonavir, saquinavir, telithromycin, voriconazole) may increase sunitinib concentrations. Grapefruit may also increase plasma concentrations of sunitinib. A dose reduction for SUTENT should be considered when it must be co-administered with strong CYP3A4 inhibitors *[see Dosage and Administration (2.2)]*.

7.2 CYP3A4 Inducers

CYP3A4 inducers such as rifampin may **decrease** sunitinib plasma concentrations. Selection of an alternate concomitant medication with no or minimal enzyme induction potential is recommended. Concurrent administration of SUTENT with the strong CYP3A4 inducer, rifampin, resulted in a 23% and 46% reduction in the combined (sunitinib + primary active metabolite) C_{max} and $AUC_{0-\infty}$ values, respectively, after a single dose of SUTENT in healthy volunteers. Co-administration of SUTENT with inducers of the CYP3A4 family (e.g., dexamethasone, phenytoin, carbamazepine, rifampin, rifabutin, rifapentin, phenobarbital, St. John's Wort) may decrease sunitinib concentrations. St. John's Wort may decrease sunitinib plasma concentrations unpredictably. Patients receiving SUTENT should not take St. John's Wort concomitantly. A dose increase for SUTENT should be considered when it must be co-administered with CYP3A4 inducers *[see Dosage and Administration (2.2)]*.

7.3 In Vitro Studies of CYP Inhibition and Induction

In vitro studies indicated that sunitinib does not induce or inhibit major CYP enzymes. The *in vitro* studies in human liver microsomes and hepatocytes of the activity of CYP isoforms CYP1A2, CYP2A6, CYP2B6, CYP2C8, CYP2C9, CYP2C19, CYP2D6, CYP2E1, CYP3A4/5, and CYP4A9/11 indicated that sunitinib and its primary active metabolite are unlikely to have any clinically relevant drug-drug interactions with drugs that may be metabolized by these enzymes.

8 USE IN SPECIFIC POPULATIONS

8.1 Pregnancy

Pregnancy Category D *[see Warnings and Precautions (5.1)]*.

8.3 Nursing Mothers

Sunitinib and its metabolites are excreted in rat milk. In lactating female rats administered 15 mg/kg, sunitinib and its metabolites were extensively excreted in milk at concentrations up to 12-fold higher than in plasma. It is not known whether sunitinib or its primary active metabolite are excreted in human milk. Because drugs are commonly ex-

Continued on next page

Table 1. Adverse Reactions Reported in Study A in at Least 10% of GIST Patients who Received SUTENT and More Commonly Than in Patients Given Placebo*

Adverse Reaction, n (%)	GIST			
	SUTENT (n=202)		Placebo (n=102)	
	All Grades	Grade 3/4	All Grades	Grade 3/4
Any		114 (56)		52 (51)
Gastrointestinal				
Diarrhea	81 (40)	9 (4)	27 (27)	0 (0)
Mucositis/stomatitis	58 (29)	2 (1)	18 (18)	2 (2)
Constipation	41 (20)	0 (0)	14 (14)	2 (2)
Cardiac				
Hypertension	31 (15)	9 (4)	11 (11)	0 (0)
Dermatology				
Skin Discoloration	61 (30)	0 (0)	23 (23)	0 (0)
Rash	28 (14)	2 (1)	9 (9)	0 (0)
Hand-foot syndrome	28 (14)	9 (4)	10 (10)	3 (3)
Neurology				
Altered taste	42 (21)	0 (0)	12 (12)	0 (0)
Musculoskeletal				
Myalgia/limb pain	28 (14)	1 (1)	9 (9)	1 (1)
Metabolism/Nutrition				
Anorexia[a]	67 (33)	1 (1)	30 (29)	5 (5)
Asthenia	45 (22)	10 (5)	11 (11)	3 (3)

* Common Terminology Criteria for Adverse Events (CTCAE), Version 3.0
[a] Includes decreased appetite

Table 2. Laboratory Abnormalities Reported in Study A in at Least 10% of GIST Patients Who Received SUTENT or Placebo*

Laboratory Parameter, n (%)	GIST			
	SUTENT (n=202)		Placebo (n=102)	
	All Grades*	Grade 3/4*[a]	All Grades*	Grade 3/4*[b]
Any		68 (34)		22 (22)
Gastrointestinal				
AST/ALT	78 (39)	3 (2)	23 (23)	1 (1)
Lipase	50 (25)	20 (10)	17 (17)	7 (7)
Alkaline phosphatase	48 (24)	7 (4)	21 (21)	4 (4)
Amylase	35 (17)	10 (5)	12 (12)	3 (3)
Total bilirubin	32 (16)	2 (1)	8 (8)	0 (0)
Indirect bilirubin	20 (10)	0 (0)	4 (4)	0 (0)
Cardiac				
Decreased LVEF	22 (11)	2 (1)	3 (3)	0 (0)
Renal/Metabolic				
Creatinine	25 (12)	1 (1)	7 (7)	0 (0)
Potassium decreased	24 (12)	1 (1)	4 (4)	0 (0)
Sodium increased	20 (10)	0 (0)	4 (4)	1 (1)
Hematology				
Neutrophils	107 (53)	20 (10)	4 (4)	0 (0)
Lymphocytes	76 (38)	0 (0)	16 (16)	0 (0)
Platelets	76 (38)	10 (5)	4 (4)	0 (0)
Hemoglobin	52 (26)	6 (3)	22 (22)	2 (2)

LVEF=Left ventricular ejection fraction
* Common Terminology Criteria for Adverse Events (CTCAE), Version 3.0
[a] Grade 4 laboratory abnormalities in patients on SUTENT included alkaline phosphatase (1%), lipase (2%), creatinine (1%), potassium decreased (1%), neutrophils (2%), hemoglobin (2%), and platelets (1%).
[b] Grade 4 laboratory abnormalities in patients on placebo included amylase (1%), lipase (1%) and hemoglobin (2%).

Sutent—Cont.

creted in human milk and because of the potential for serious adverse reactions in nursing infants, a decision should be made whether to discontinue nursing or to discontinue the drug taking into account the importance of the drug to the mother [see Nonclinical Toxicology (13.1)].

8.4 Pediatric Use

The safety and efficacy of SUTENT in pediatric patients have not been studied in clinical trials.

Physeal dysplasia was observed in Cynomolgus monkeys with open growth plates treated for ≥ 3 months (3 month dosing 2, 6, 12 mg/kg/day; 8 cycles of dosing 0.3, 1.5, 6.0 mg/kg/day) with sunitinib at doses that were > 0.4 times the RDD based on systemic exposure (AUC). In developing rats treated continuously for 3 months (1.5, 5.0 and 15.0 mg/kg) or 5 cycles (0.3, 1.5, and 6.0 mg/kg/day), bone abnormalities consisted of thickening of the epiphyseal cartilage of the femur and an increase of fracture of the tibia at doses ≥ 5 mg/kg (approximately 10 times the RDD based on AUC). Additionally, caries of the teeth were observed in rats at >5 mg/kg. The incidence and severity of physeal dysplasia were dose-related and were reversible upon cessation of treatment however findings in the teeth were not. A no effect level was not observed in monkeys treated continuously for 3 months, but was 1.5 mg/kg/day when treated intermittently for 8 cycles. In rats the no effect level in bones was ≤ 2 mg/kg/day.

8.5 Geriatric Use

Of 825 GIST and MRCC patients who received SUTENT on clinical studies, 277 (34%) were 65 and over. No overall differences in safety or effectiveness were observed between younger and older patients.

8.6 Hepatic Impairment

No dose adjustment is required when administering SUTENT to patients with Child-Pugh Class A or B hepatic impairment. Sunitinib and its primary metabolite are primarily metabolized by the liver. Systemic exposures after a single dose of SUTENT were similar in subjects with mild or moderate (Child-Pugh Class A and B) hepatic impairment compared to subjects with normal hepatic function. SUTENT was not studied in subjects with severe (Child-Pugh Class C) hepatic impairment. Studies in cancer patients have excluded patients with ALT or AST >2.5 × ULN or, if due to liver metastases, >5.0 × ULN.

10 OVERDOSAGE

Treatment of overdose with SUTENT should consist of general supportive measures. There is no specific antidote for overdosage with SUTENT. If indicated, elimination of unabsorbed drug should be achieved by emesis or gastric lavage. No overdose of SUTENT was reported in completed clinical studies. In non-clinical studies mortality was observed following as few as 5 daily doses of 500 mg/kg (3000 mg/m^2) in rats. At this dose, signs of toxicity included impaired muscle coordination, head shakes, hypoactivity, ocular discharge, piloerection and gastrointestinal distress. Mortality and similar signs of toxicity were observed at lower doses when administered for longer durations.

11 DESCRIPTION

SUTENT, an oral multi-kinase inhibitor, is the malate salt of sunitinib. Sunitinib malate is described chemically as Butanedioic acid, hydroxy-, (2S)-, compound with N-[2-(diethylamino)ethyl]-5-[(Z)-(5-fluoro-1,2-dihydro-2-oxo-3H-indol-3-ylidine)methyl]-2,4-dimethyl-1H-pyrrole-3-carboxamide (1:1). The molecular formula is $C_{22}H_{27}FN_4O_2 \cdot C_4H_6O_5$ and the molecular weight is 532.6 Daltons.
The chemical structure of sunitinib malate is:

Sunitinib malate is a yellow to orange powder with a pKa of 8.95. The solubility of sunitinib malate in aqueous media over the range pH 1.2 to pH 6.8 is in excess of 25 mg/mL. The log of the distribution coefficient (octanol/water) at pH 7 is 5.2.
SUTENT (sunitinib malate) capsules are supplied as printed hard shell capsules containing sunitinib malate equivalent to 12.5 mg, 25 mg or 50 mg of sunitinib together with mannitol, croscarmellose sodium, povidone (K-25) and magnesium stearate as inactive ingredients.
The orange gelatin capsule shells contain titanium dioxide, and red iron oxide. The caramel gelatin capsule shells also contain yellow iron oxide and black iron oxide. The printing ink contains shellac, propylene glycol, sodium hydroxide, povidone and titanium dioxide.

12 CLINICAL PHARMACOLOGY

12.1 Mechanism of Action

Sunitinib is a small molecule that inhibits multiple receptor tyrosine kinases (RTKs), some of which are implicated in tumor growth, pathologic angiogenesis, and metastatic progression of cancer. Sunitinib was evaluated for its inhibitory activity against a variety of kinases (>80 kinases) and was identified as an inhibitor of platelet-derived growth factor

Table 3. Adverse Reactions Reported in at Least 10% of Patients with MRCC Who Received SUTENT or IFN-α*

Adverse Reaction	Treatment-Naïve MRCC			
	SUTENT (n=375)		IFN-α (n=360)	
	All Grades	Grade 3/4[a]	All Grades	Grade 3/4[b]
Any	370 (99)	250 (67)	354 (98)	184 (51)
Constitutional				
Fatigue	218 (58)	35 (9)	199 (55)	50 (14)
Asthenia	79 (21)	27 (7)	85 (24)	20 (6)
Fever	62 (17)	3 (1)	129 (36)	0 (0)
Weight decreased	45 (12)	0 (0)	54 (15)	2 (1)
Chills	42 (11)	3 (1)	108 (30)	0 (0)
Gastrointestinal				
Diarrhea	218 (58)	22 (6)	72 (20)	0 (0)
Nausea	183 (49)	16 (4)	136 (38)	5 (1)
Mucositis/stomatitis	162 (43)	12 (3)	14 (4)	2 (<1)
Vomiting	105 (28)	15 (4)	51 (14)	3 (1)
Dyspepsia	105 (28)	4 (1)	14 (4)	0 (0)
Abdominal pain[c]	83 (22)	10 (3)	42 (12)	5 (1)
Constipation	60 (16)	0 (0)	44 (12)	1 (<1)
Dry mouth	45 (12)	0 (0)	26 (7)	1 (<1)
GERD/reflux esophagitis	42 (11)	0 (0)	3 (1)	0 (0)
Flatulence	39 (10)	0 (0)	8 (2)	0 (0)
Oral pain	38 (10)	0 (0)	2 (1)	0 (0)
Glossodynia	37 (10)	0 (0)	2 (1)	0 (0)
Cardiac				
Hypertension	111 (30)	36 (10)	13 (4)	1 (<1)
Edema, peripheral	42 (11)	2 (1)	15 (4)	2 (1)
Dermatology				
Rash	103 (27)	3 (1)	40 (11)	2 (1)
Hand-foot syndrome	78 (21)	20 (5)	3 (1)	0 (0)
Skin discoloration/ yellow skin	72 (19)	0 (0)	0 (0)	0 (0)
Dry skin	67 (18)	1 (<1)	23 (6)	0 (0)
Hair color changes	56 (16)	0 (0)	1 (<1)	0 (0)
Neurology				
Altered taste[d]	166 (44)	1 (<1)	52 (14)	0 (0)
Headache	68 (18)	3 (1)	61 (17)	0 (0)
Dizziness	28 (7)	1 (<1)	42 (12)	1 (<1)
Musculoskeletal				
Back pain	70 (19)	13 (3)	44 (13)	6 (2)
Arthralgia	69 (18)	5 (1)	60 (17)	1 (<1)
Pain in extremity/ limb discomfort	65 (17)	6 (2)	28 (8)	4 (1)
Respiratory				
Cough	64 (18)	2 (1)	45 (12)	0 (0)
Dyspnea	58 (15)	15 (4)	65 (18)	14 (4)
Metabolism/Nutrition				
Anorexia[e]	142 (38)	6 (2)	145 (40)	7 (2)
Dehydration	30 (8)	8 (2)	17 (5)	2 (1)
Hemorrhage/Bleeding				
Bleeding, all sites	112 (30)	10 (3)[f]	27 (8)	2 (1)
Psychiatric				
Insomnia	42 (11)	1 (<1)	31 (9)	0 (0)
Depression[g]	29 (8)	0 (0)	47 (12)	5 (1)

* Common Terminology Criteria for Adverse Events (CTCAE), Version 3.0
[a] Grade 4 ARs in patients on SUTENT included back pain (1%), arthralgia (<1%), asthenia (<1%), dehydration (<1%), fatigue (<1%), limb pain (<1%) and rash (<1%).
[b] Grade 4 ARs in patients on IFN-α included dyspnea (1%), fatigue (1%) and depression (<1%).
[c] Includes flank pain
[d] Includes ageusia, hypogeusia and dysgeusia
[e] Includes decreased appetite
[f] Includes one patient with Grade 5 gastric hemorrhage
[g] Includes depressed mood

receptors (PDGFRα and PDGFRβ), vascular endothelial growth factor receptors (VEGFR1, VEGFR2 and VEGFR3), stem cell factor receptor (KIT), Fms-like tyrosine kinase-3 (FLT3), colony stimulating factor receptor Type 1 (CSF-1R), and the glial cell-line derived neurotrophic factor receptor (RET). Sunitinib inhibition of the activity of these RTKs has been demonstrated in biochemical and cellular assays, and inhibition of function has been demonstrated in cell proliferation assays. The primary metabolite exhibits similar potency compared to sunitinib in biochemical and cellular assays.

Sunitinib inhibited the phosphorylation of multiple RTKs (PDGFRβ, VEGFR2, KIT) in tumor xenografts expressing RTK targets in vivo and demonstrated inhibition of tumor growth or tumor regression and/or inhibited metastases in some experimental models of cancer. Sunitinib demonstrated the ability to inhibit growth of tumor cells expressing dysregulated target RTKs (PDGFR, RET, or KIT) in vitro and to inhibit PDGFRβ- and VEGFR2-dependent tumor angiogenesis in vivo.

12.3 Pharmacokinetics

The pharmacokinetics of sunitinib and sunitinib malate have been evaluated in 135 healthy volunteers and in 266 patients with solid tumors.
Maximum plasma concentrations (C_{max}) of sunitinib are generally observed between 6 and 12 hours (T_{max}) following

oral administration. Food has no effect on the bioavailability of sunitinib. SUTENT may be taken with or without food.
Binding of sunitinib and its primary active metabolite to human plasma protein in vitro was 95% and 90%, respectively, with no concentration dependence in the range of 100 – 4000 ng/mL. The apparent volume of distribution (Vd/F) for sunitinib was 2230 L. In the dosing range of 25 - 100 mg, the area under the plasma concentration-time curve (AUC) and C_{max} increase proportionally with dose. Sunitinib is metabolized primarily by the cytochrome P450 enzyme, CYP3A4, to produce its primary active metabolite, which is further metabolized by CYP3A4. The primary active metabolite comprises 23 to 37% of the total exposure. Elimination is primarily via feces. In a human mass balance study of [14C]sunitinib, 61% of the dose was eliminated in feces, with renal elimination accounting for 16% of the administered dose. Sunitinib and its primary active metabolite were the major drug-related compounds identified in plasma, urine, and feces, representing 91.5%, 86.4% and 73.8% of radioactivity in pooled samples, respectively. Minor metabolites were identified in urine and feces but generally not found in plasma. Total oral clearance (CL/F) ranged from 34 to 62 L/hr with an inter-patient variability of 40%. Following administration of a single oral dose in healthy volunteers, the terminal half-lives of sunitinib and its pri-

mary active metabolite are approximately 40 to 60 hours and 80 to 110 hours, respectively. With repeated daily administration, sunitinib accumulates 3- to 4-fold while the primary metabolite accumulates 7- to 10-fold. Steady-state concentrations of sunitinib and its primary active metabolite are achieved within 10 to 14 days. By Day 14, combined plasma concentrations of sunitinib and its active metabolite ranged from 62.9 – 101 ng/mL. No significant changes in the pharmacokinetics of sunitinib or the primary active metabolite were observed with repeated daily administration or with repeated cycles in the dosing regimens tested.

The pharmacokinetics were similar in healthy volunteers and in the solid tumor patient populations tested, including patients with GIST and MRCC.

Pharmacokinetics in Special Populations

Population pharmacokinetic analyses of demographic data indicate that there are no clinically relevant effects of age, body weight, creatinine clearance, race, gender, or ECOG score on the pharmacokinetics of SUTENT or the primary active metabolite.

Pediatric Use: The pharmacokinetics of SUTENT have not been evaluated in pediatric patients.

Renal Insufficiency: No clinical studies of SUTENT were conducted in patients with impaired renal function. Studies that were conducted excluded patients with serum creatinine > 2.0 × ULN. Population pharmacokinetic analyses have shown that sunitinib pharmacokinetics were unaltered in patients with calculated creatinine clearances in the range of 42 –347 mL/min.

Hepatic Insufficiency: Systemic exposures after a single dose of SUTENT were similar in subjects with mild (Child-Pugh Class A) or moderate (Child-Pugh Class B) hepatic impairment compared to subjects with normal hepatic function.

12.4   Cardiac Electrophysiology
See Warnings and Precautions (5.3).

13   NONCLINICAL TOXICOLOGY

13.1   Carcinogenesis, Mutagenesis, Impairment of Fertility

Although definitive carcinogenicity studies with sunitinib have not been performed, carcinoma and hyperplasia of the Brunner's gland of the duodenum have been observed at the highest dose tested in H2ras transgenic mice administered doses of 0, 10, 25, 75, or 200 mg/kg/day for 28 days. Sunitinib did not cause genetic damage when tested in *in vitro* assays (bacterial mutation [AMES Assay], human lymphocyte chromosome aberration) and an *in vivo* rat bone marrow micronucleus test.

Effects on the female reproductive system were identified in a 3-month repeat dose monkey study (2, 6, 12 mg/kg/day), where ovarian changes (decreased follicular development) were noted at 12 mg/kg/day (approximately 5.1 times the AUC in patients administered the RDD), while uterine changes (endometrial atrophy) were noted at ≥2 mg/kg/day (approximately 0.4 times the AUC in patients administered the RDD). With the addition of vaginal atrophy, the uterine and ovarian effects were reproduced at 6 mg/kg/day in the 9-month monkey study (0.3, 1.5 and 6 mg/kg/day administered daily for 28 days followed by a 14 day respite; the 6 mg/kg dose produced a mean AUC that was approximately 0.8 times the AUC in patients administered the RDD). A no effect level was not identified in the 3 month study; 1.5 mg/kg/day represents a no effect level in monkeys administered sunitinib for 9 months.

Although fertility was not affected in rats, SUTENT may impair fertility in humans. In female rats, no fertility effects were observed at doses of ≤5.0 mg/kg/day [(0.5, 1.5, 5.0 mg/kg/day) administered for 21 days up to gestational day 7; the 5.0 mg/kg dose produced an AUC that was approximately 5 times the AUC in patients administered the RDD], however significant embryolethality was observed at the 5.0 mg/kg dose. No reproductive effects were observed in male rats dosed (1, 3 or 10 mg/kg/day) for 58 days prior to mating with untreated females. Fertility, copulation, conception indices, and sperm evaluation (morphology, concentration, and motility) were unaffected by sunitinib at doses ≤10 mg/kg/day (the 10 mg/kg/day dose produced a mean AUC that was approximately 25.8 times the AUC in patients administered the RDD).

14   CLINICAL STUDIES

The clinical safety and efficacy of SUTENT have been studied in patients with gastrointestinal stromal tumor (GIST) after progression on or intolerance to imatinib mesylate, and in patients with metastatic renal cell carcinoma (MRCC).

14.1   Gastrointestinal Stromal Tumor
Study A

Study A was a two-arm, international, randomized, double-blind, placebo-controlled trial of SUTENT in patients with GIST who had disease progression during prior imatinib mesylate (imatinib) treatment or who were intolerant of imatinib. The objective was to compare Time-to-Tumor Progression (TTP) in patients receiving SUTENT plus best supportive care versus patients receiving placebo plus best supportive care. Other objectives included Progression-Free Survival (PFS), Objective Response Rate (ORR), and Overall Survival (OS). Patients were randomized (2:1) to receive either 50 mg SUTENT or placebo orally, once daily, on Schedule 4/2 until disease progression or withdrawal from the study for another reason. Treatment was unblinded at the time of disease progression. Patients randomized to placebo were then offered crossover to open-label SUTENT, and patients randomized to SUTENT were permitted to continue treatment per investigator judgment.

Table 4. Laboratory Abnormalities Reported in at Least 10% of Treatment-Naïve MRCC Patients Who Received SUTENT or IFN-α

Laboratory Parameter, n (%)	Treatment-Naïve MRCC			
	SUTENT (n=375)		IFN-α (n=360)	
	All Grades*	Grade 3/4*[a]	All Grades*	Grade 3/4*[b]
Gastrointestinal				
AST	195 (52)	6 (2)	124 (34)	6 (2)
ALT	171 (46)	10 (3)	140 (39)	6 (2)
Lipase	196 (52)	60 (16)	153 (43)	23 (6)
Alkaline phosphatase	156 (42)	7 (2)	126 (35)	6 (2)
Amylase	118 (31)	19 (5)	101 (28)	8 (2)
Total bilirubin	72 (19)	3 (1)	6 (2)	0 (0)
Indirect bilirubin	46 (12)	4 (1)	3 (1)	0 (0)
Renal/Metabolic				
Creatinine	246 (66)	1 (<1)	175 (49)	1 (<1)
Uric acid	155 (41)	43 (12)	112 (31)	29 (8)
Creatine kinase	152 (41)	1 (<1)	35 (10)	2 (1)
Phosphorus	134 (36)	17 (5)	115 (32)	22 (6)
Calcium decreased	132 (35)	1 (<1)	133 (37)	0 (0)
Glucose decreased	73 (19)	0 (0)	54 (15)	1 (<1)
Albumin	68 (18)	3 (1)	67 (19)	0 (0)
Glucose increased	58 (15)	10 (3)	49 (14)	20 (6)
Sodium decreased	51 (14)	18 (5)	41 (11)	9 (3)
Potassium increased	42 (11)	7 (2)	54 (15)	13 (4)
Sodium increased	40 (11)	0 (0)	35 (10)	0 (0)
Hematology				
Neutrophils	271 (72)	44 (12)	166 (46)	24 (7)
Hemoglobin	266 (71)	11 (3)	232 (64)	16 (4)
Platelets	244 (65)	30 (8)	77 (21)	0 (0)
Lymphocytes	223 (59)	44 (12)	227 (63)	79 (22)
Leukocytes	292 (78)	19 (5)	202 (56)	8 (2)

* Common Terminology Criteria for Adverse Events (CTCAE), Version 3.0
[a] Grade 4 laboratory abnormalities in patients on SUTENT included uric acid (12%), lipase (3%), amylase (1%), neutrophils (1%), ALT (<1%), calcium decreased (<1%), phosphorous (<1%), potassium increased (<1%), sodium decreased (<1%) and hemoglobin (<1%).
[b] Grade 4 laboratory abnormalities in patients on IFN-α included uric acid (8%), lipase (1%), amylase (<1%), calcium increased (<1%), glucose decreased (<1%), potassium increased (<1%) and hemoglobin (<1%).

Table 5. GIST Efficacy Results from Study A (interim analysis)

Efficacy Parameter	SUTENT (n=207)	Placebo (n=105)	P-value (log-rank test)	HR (95% CI)
Time to Tumor Progression[a] [median, weeks (95% CI)]	27.3 (16.0, 32.1)	6.4 (4.4, 10.0)	<0.0001*	0.33 (0.23, 0.47)
Progression-free Survival[b] [median, weeks (95% CI)]	24.1 (11.1, 28.3)	6.0 (4.4, 9.9)	<0.0001*	0.33 (0.24, 0.47)
Objective Response Rate (PR) [%, (95% CI)]	6.8 (3.7, 11.1)	0	0.006[c]	

CI=Confidence interval, HR=Hazard ratio, PR=Partial response
* A comparison is considered statistically significant if the p-value is < 0.0042 (O'Brien Fleming stopping boundary)
[a] Time from randomization to progression; deaths prior to documented progression were censored at time of last radiographic evaluation
[b] Time from randomization to progression or death due to any cause
[c] Pearson chi-square test

The intent-to-treat (ITT) population included 312 patients. Two-hundred seven (207) patients were randomized to the SUTENT arm, and 105 patients were randomized to the placebo arm. Demographics were comparable between the SUTENT and placebo groups with regard to age (69% vs 72% <65 years for SUTENT vs. placebo, respectively), gender (Male: 64% vs. 61%), race (White: (88% both arms, Asian: 5% both arms, Black: 4% both arms, remainder not reported), and Performance Status (ECOG 0: 44% vs. 46%, ECOG 1: 55% vs. 52%, and ECOG 2: 1 vs. 2%). Prior treatment included surgery (94% vs. 93%) and radiotherapy (8% vs. 15%). Outcome of prior imatinib treatment was also comparable between arms with intolerance (4% vs. 4%), progression within 6 months of starting treatment (17% vs. 16%), or progression beyond 6 months (78% vs. 80%) balanced.

A planned interim efficacy and safety analysis was performed after 149 TTP events had occurred. There was a statistically significant advantage for SUTENT over placebo in TTP and progression-free survival. OS data were not mature at the time of the interim analysis. Efficacy results are summarized in Table 5 and the Kaplan-Meier curve for TTP is in Figure 1.

[See table 5 above]
[See figure 1 at top of next column]

Study B

Study B was an open-label, multi-center, single-arm, dose-escalation study conducted in patients with GIST following progression on or intolerance to imatinib. Following identification of the recommended Phase 2 regimen (50 mg once daily on Schedule 4/2), 55 patients in this study received the 50 mg dose of SUTENT on treatment Schedule 4/2. Partial responses were observed in 5 of 55 patients [9.1% PR rate, 95% CI (3.0, 20.0)].

14.2   Renal Cell Carcinoma
Treatment-Naïve MRCC

A multi-center, international randomized study comparing single-agent SUTENT with IFN-α was conducted in patients with treatment-naïve MRCC. The objective was to

Figure 1: Kaplan-Meier Curve of TTP in Study A (Intent-to-Treat Population)

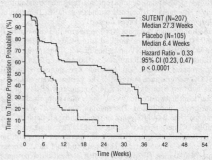

SUTENT (N=207) Median 27.3 Weeks
Placebo (N=105) Median 6.4 Weeks
Hazard Ratio = 0.33 95% CI (0.23, 0.47) p < 0.0001

compare Progression-Free Survival (PFS) in patients receiving SUTENT versus patients receiving IFN-α. Other endpoints included Objective Response Rate (ORR), Overall Survival (OS) and safety. Seven hundred fifty (750) patients were randomized (1:1) to receive either 50 mg SUTENT once daily on Schedule 4/2 or to receive IFN-α administered subcutaneously at 9 MIU three times a week. Patients were treated until disease progression or withdrawal from the study.

The ITT population for this interim analysis included 750 patients, 375 randomized to SUTENT and 375 randomized to IFN-α. Demographics were comparable between the SUTENT and IFN-α groups with regard to age (59% vs. 67% <65 years for SUTENT vs. IFN-α, respectively), gender (Male: 71% vs. 72%), race (White: 94% vs. 91%, Asian: 2% vs. 3%, Black: 1% vs. 2%, remainder not reported), and Performance Status (ECOG 0: 62% vs. 61%, ECOG 1: 38% each

Continued on next page

Table 6. Treatment-Naïve MRCC Efficacy Results (interim analysis)

Efficacy Parameter	SUTENT (n=375)	IFN-α (n=375)	P-value (log-rank test)	HR (95% CI)
Progression-Free Survival[a] [median, weeks (95% CI)]	47.3 (42.6, 50.7)	22.0 (16.4, 24.0)	<0.000001[b]	0.415 (0.320, 0.539)
Objective Response Rate[a] [%, (95% CI)]	27.5 (23.0, 32.3)	5.3 (3.3, 8.1)	<0.001[c]	NA

CI=Confidence interval, NA=Not applicable
[a] Assessed by blinded core radiology laboratory; 90 patients' scans had not been read at time of analysis
[b] A comparison is considered statistically significant if the p-value is < 0.0042 (O'Brien Fleming stopping boundary)
[c] Pearson Chi-square test

Sutent—Cont.

arm, ECOG 2: 0 vs. 1%). Prior treatment included nephrectomy (91% vs. 89%) and radiotherapy (14% each arm). The most common site of metastases present at screening was the lung (78% vs. 80%, respectively), followed by the lymph nodes (58% vs. 53%, respectively) and bone (30% each arm); the majority of the patients had multiple (2 or more) metastatic sites at baseline (80% vs. 77%, respectively).

A planned interim analysis showed a statistically significant advantage for SUTENT over IFN-α in the endpoint of PFS (see Table 6 and Figure 2). In the pre-specified stratification factors of LDH (>1.5 ULN vs. ≤1.5 ULN), ECOG performance status (0 vs. 1), and prior nephrectomy (yes vs. no), the hazard ratio favored SUTENT over IFN-α. The ORR was higher in the SUTENT arm (see Table 6). OS data were not mature at the time of the interim analysis.

[See table 6 above]

Figure 2. Kaplan-Meier Curve of PFS in Treatment-Naïve MRCC Study (Intent-to-Treat Population)

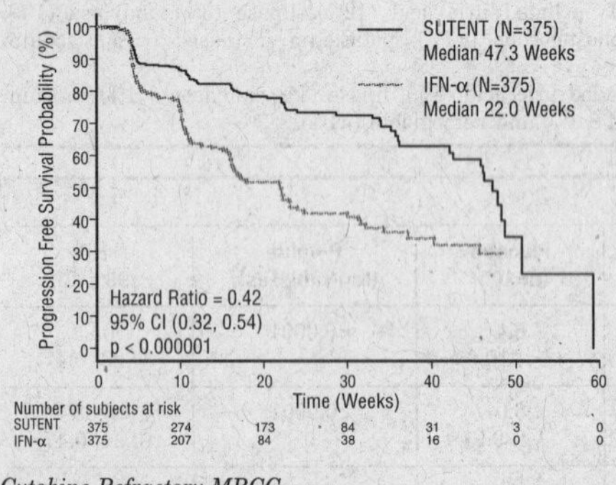
SUTENT (N=375)
Median 47.3 Weeks
IFN-α (N=375)
Median 22.0 Weeks
Progression Free Survival Probability (%)
Hazard Ratio = 0.42
95% CI (0.32, 0.54)
p < 0.000001
Time (Weeks)
Number of subjects at risk
SUTENT 375 274 173 84 31 3 0
IFN-α 375 207 84 38 16 0 0

Cytokine-Refractory MRCC

The use of single agent SUTENT in the treatment of cytokine-refractory MRCC was investigated in two single-arm, multi-center studies. All patients enrolled into these studies experienced failure of prior cytokine-based therapy. In Study 1, failure of prior cytokine therapy was based on radiographic evidence of disease progression defined by RECIST or World Health Organization (WHO) criteria during or within 9 months of completion of 1 cytokine therapy treatment (IFN-α, interleukin-2, or IFN-α plus interleukin-2; patients who were treated with IFN-α alone must have received treatment for at least 28 days). In Study 2, failure of prior cytokine therapy was defined as disease progression or unacceptable treatment-related toxicity. The endpoint for both studies was ORR. Duration of Response (DR) was also evaluated.

One hundred six patients (106) were enrolled into Study 1, and 63 patients were enrolled into Study 2. Patients received 50 mg SUTENT on Schedule 4/2. Therapy was continued until the patients met withdrawal criteria or had progressive disease. The baseline age, gender, race and ECOG performance statuses of the patients were comparable between Studies 1 and 2. Approximately 86-94% of patients in the two studies were White. Men comprised 65% of the pooled population. The median age was 57 years and ranged from 24 to 87 years in the studies. All patients had an ECOG performance status <2 at the screening visit.

The baseline malignancy and prior treatment history of the patients were comparable between Studies 1 and 2. Across the two studies, 95% of the pooled population of patients had at least some component of clear-cell histology. All patients in Study 1 were required to have a histological clear-cell component. Most patients enrolled in the studies (97% of the pooled population) had undergone nephrectomy; prior nephrectomy was required for patients enrolled in Study 1. All patients had received one previous cytokine regimen. Metastatic disease present at the time of study entry included lung metastases in 81% of patients. Liver metastases were more common in Study 1 (27% vs. 16% in Study 2) and bone metastases were more common in Study 2 (51% vs. 25% in Study 1); 52% of patients in the pooled population had at least 3 metastatic sites. Patients with known brain metastases or leptomeningeal disease were excluded from both studies.

The ORR and DR data from Studies 1 and 2 are provided in Table 7. There were 36 PRs in Study 1 as assessed by a core radiology laboratory for an ORR of 34.0% (95% CI 25.0, 43.8). There were 23 PRs in Study 2 as assessed by the investigators for an ORR of 36.5% (95% CI 24.7, 49.6). The majority (>90%) of objective disease responses were observed during the first four cycles; the latest reported response was observed in Cycle 10. DR data from Study 1 is premature as only 9 of 36 patients (25%) responding to treatment had experienced disease progression or died at the time of the data cutoff.

Table 7. Cytokine-Refractory MRCC Efficacy Results

Efficacy Parameter	Study 1 (N=106)	Study 2 (N=63)
Objective Response Rate [%, (95% CI)]	34.0[a] (25.0, 43.8)	36.5[b] (24.7, 49.6)
Duration of Response (DR) [median, weeks (95% CI)]	* (42.0, **)	54[b] (34.3, 70.1)

CI=Confidence interval
* Median DR has not yet been reached
**Data not mature enough to determine upper confidence limit
[a] Assessed by blinded core radiology laboratory
[b] Assessed by investigators

16 HOW SUPPLIED/STORAGE AND HANDLING

12.5 mg Capsules
Hard gelatin capsule with orange cap and orange body, printed with white ink "Pfizer" on the cap, "STN 12.5 mg" on the body; available in:
Bottles of 28: NDC 0069-0550-38
Bottles of 30: NDC 0069-0550-30
25 mg Capsules
Hard gelatin capsule with caramel cap and orange body, printed with white ink "Pfizer" on the cap, "STN 25 mg" on the body; available in:
Bottles of 28: NDC 0069-0770-38
Bottles of 30: NDC 0069-0770-30
50 mg Capsules
Hard gelatin capsule with caramel cap and caramel body, printed with white ink "Pfizer" on the cap, "STN 50 mg" on the body; available in:
Bottles of 28: NDC 0069-0980-38
Bottles of 30: NDC 0069-0980-30
Store at 25°C (77°F); excursions permitted to 15-30°C (59-86°F) [see USP Controlled Room Temperature].

17 PATIENT COUNSELING INFORMATION

See 17.5 for FDA-Approved Patient Labeling.

17.1 Gastrointestinal Disorders

Gastrointestinal disorders such as diarrhea, nausea, stomatitis, dyspepsia, and vomiting were the most commonly reported gastrointestinal events occurring in patients who received SUTENT. Supportive care for gastrointestinal adverse events requiring treatment may include anti-emetic or anti-diarrheal medication.

17.2 Skin Effects

Skin discoloration possibly due to the drug color (yellow) occurred in approximately one third of patients. Patients should be advised that depigmentation of the hair or skin may occur during treatment with SUTENT. Other possible dermatologic effects may include dryness, thickness or cracking of skin, blister or rash on the palms of the hands and soles of the feet.

17.3 Other Common Events

Other commonly reported adverse events included fatigue, high blood pressure, bleeding, swelling, mouth pain/irritation and taste disturbance.

17.4 Concomitant Medications

Patients should be advised to inform their health care providers of all concomitant medications, including over-the-counter medications and dietary supplements *[see Drug Interactions (7)]*.

17.5 FDA-Approved Patient Labeling

PATIENT INFORMATION

SUTENT (su TENT)

Read the patient information leaflet that comes with SUTENT before you start taking it. Read the leaflet each time you get a refill. There may be new information. This leaflet does not replace talking with your doctor about your condition or treatment. If you have any questions about SUTENT, ask your doctor or pharmacist.

What is the most important information I should know about SUTENT?

- **SUTENT may harm an unborn baby (cause birth defects).** Do not become pregnant. If you do become pregnant, tell your doctor right away. Stop taking SUTENT.

What is SUTENT?

SUTENT is a medicine that treats 2 kinds of cancer.

1. **GIST (gastrointestinal stromal tumor).** This is a rare cancer of the stomach, bowel, or esophagus. SUTENT is used when the medicine Gleevec® (imatinib mesylate) did not stop the cancer from growing OR when you cannot take Gleevec®.
2. **Advanced kidney cancer** (advanced renal cell carcinoma or RCC).

SUTENT may slow or stop the growth of cancer. It may help shrink tumors.

SUTENT has not been studied in children.

What should I tell my doctor before taking SUTENT?

Tell your doctor about all your medical conditions. **Be sure to tell your doctor if you:**

- are pregnant, could be pregnant, or plan to get pregnant. SUTENT may harm an unborn baby.
- are breast-feeding. Do not breast-feed while you are being treated with SUTENT.
- have any heart problems
- have high blood pressure
- have kidney function problems (other than cancer)
- have liver problems
- have any bleeding problem
- have seizures

SUTENT and other medicines

Tell your doctor about all your medicines. Include **prescription medicines**, over-the-counter drugs, vitamins, and herbal products. Some medicines can react with SUTENT and cause serious side effects.

Especially tell your doctor if you take:

- St. John's Wort. ***Do not take St. John's Wort while taking SUTENT.***
- Dexamethasone (a steroid)
- Medicine for:
  - tuberculosis (TB)
  - infections (antibiotics)
  - depression
  - seizures (epilepsy)
  - fungal infections (antifungals)
  - HIV (AIDS)

Keep a list of your medicines. Show it to your doctor or pharmacist. Talk with your doctor before starting any new medicines.

What are possible side effects of SUTENT?

Possible serious side effects include:

- **Heart Problems.** Tell your doctor if you feel very tired, are short of breath, or have swollen feet and ankles.
- **Rare life-threatening events:** hole in stomach or bowel wall (perforation) or bleeding from the tumor. Both of these side effects could cause symptoms such as painful, swollen abdomen, vomiting blood, and black, sticky stools. Your doctor can tell you other symptoms to watch for.
- **Increased blood pressure.** Your doctor may check your blood pressure. You may need treatment for high blood pressure.

Common side effects:

- Feeling tired
- Diarrhea, nausea, vomiting, mouth sores, upset stomach, abdominal pain, and constipation. Talk with your doctor about ways to handle these problems.
- The medicine in SUTENT is yellow, so it may make your skin look yellow. Your skin and hair may get lighter.
- Your skin may become dry, get thicker, or crack. You may get blisters or a rash on the palms of your hands and soles of your feet.
- Taste changes
- Swelling
- Loss of appetite
- High blood pressure
- Bleeding, such as nosebleeds or bleeding from cuts. Call your doctor if you have any swelling or bleeding.

There are other side effects. For a more complete list, ask your cancer specialist nurse or doctor.

How should I take SUTENT?

- SUTENT comes in 12.5 mg, 25 mg, and 50 mg capsules you take by mouth. Do not open the capsules.
- Take SUTENT once a day with or without food.
- Take it exactly the way your doctor tells you.
- Do not drink grapefruit juice or eat grapefruit. They may change the amount of SUTENT in your body.
- Dosing cycle:
  - Take SUTENT for 4 weeks (28 days) THEN
  - Stop for 2 weeks (14 days)
  - Repeat this cycle as long as your doctor tells you
- Your doctor may check your blood before each dosing cycle.
- If you miss a dose, take it as soon as you remember. Do not take it if it is close to your next dose. Just take the next dose at your regular time. Do not take more than 1 dose of SUTENT at a time. Tell your doctor or nurse about the missed dose.
- Call your doctor right away, if you take too much SUTENT.

How do I store SUTENT?

- Keep SUTENT and all medicines out of the reach of children.
- Store SUTENT at room temperature.

General information about SUTENT

Doctors can prescribe medicines for conditions that are not in this patient information leaflet. Use SUTENT only for what your doctor prescribed. Do not give it to other people, even if they have the same symptoms you have. It may harm them.

This leaflet gives the most important information about SUTENT. For more information about SUTENT, talk with your doctor or pharmacist. You can visit our website at www.SUTENT.com.

What is in SUTENT?

Active ingredient: sunitinib malate

Inactive ingredients: mannitol, croscarmellose sodium, povidone (K-25), magnesium stearate **Orange gelatin capsule shell:** titanium dioxide, red iron oxide **Caramel gelatin capsule shell:** yellow iron oxide, black iron oxide **Printing ink:** shellac, propylene glycol, sodium hydroxide, povidone, titanium dioxide

Gleevec® is a registered trademark of Novartis Pharmaceuticals Corp

Rx only

LAB-0317-8.0

Distributed by:
Pfizer Labs
Division of Pfizer Inc
New York, NY 10017

VIAGRA® ℞

[*vī-ă-gra*]

(sildenafil citrate)

Tablets

Prescribing information for this product, which appears on pages 2562–2566 of the 2008 PDR, has been completely revised as follows. Please write "See Supplement A" next to the product heading.

DESCRIPTION

VIAGRA®, an oral therapy for erectile dysfunction, is the citrate salt of sildenafil, a selective inhibitor of cyclic guanosine monophosphate (cGMP)-specific phosphodiesterase type 5 (PDE5).

Sildenafil citrate is designated chemically as 1-[[3-(6,7-dihydro-1-methyl-7-oxo-3-propyl-1*H*-pyrazolo[4,3-*d*]pyrimidin-5-yl)-4-ethoxyphenyl]sulfonyl]-4-methylpiperazine citrate and has the following structural formula:

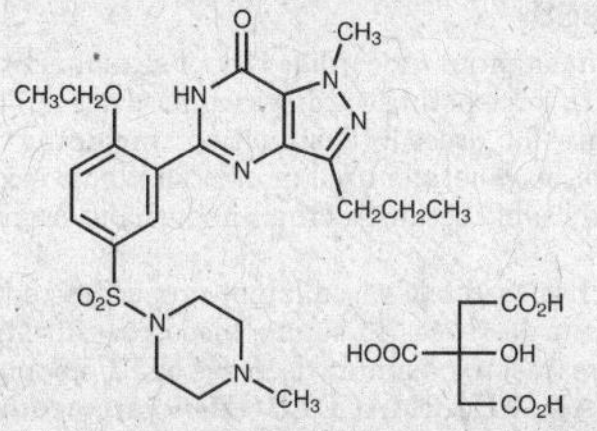

Sildenafil citrate is a white to off-white crystalline powder with a solubility of 3.5 mg/mL in water and a molecular weight of 666.7. VIAGRA (sildenafil citrate) is formulated as blue, film-coated rounded-diamond-shaped tablets equivalent to 25 mg, 50 mg and 100 mg of sildenafil for oral administration. In addition to the active ingredient, sildenafil citrate, each tablet contains the following inactive ingredients: microcrystalline cellulose, anhydrous dibasic calcium phosphate, croscarmellose sodium, magnesium stearate, hypromellose, titanium dioxide, lactose, triacetin, and FD & C Blue #2 aluminum lake.

CLINICAL PHARMACOLOGY

Mechanism of Action

The physiologic mechanism of erection of the penis involves release of nitric oxide (NO) in the corpus cavernosum during sexual stimulation. NO then activates the enzyme guanylate cyclase, which results in increased levels of cyclic guanosine monophosphate (cGMP), producing smooth muscle relaxation in the corpus cavernosum and allowing inflow of blood. Sildenafil has no direct relaxant effect on isolated human corpus cavernosum, but enhances the effect of nitric oxide (NO) by inhibiting phosphodiesterase type 5 (PDE5), which is responsible for degradation of cGMP in the corpus cavernosum. When sexual stimulation causes local release of NO, inhibition of PDE5 by sildenafil causes increased levels of cGMP in the corpus cavernosum, resulting in smooth muscle relaxation and inflow of blood to the corpus cavernosum. Sildenafil at recommended doses has no effect in the absence of sexual stimulation.

Studies *in vitro* have shown that sildenafil is selective for PDE5. Its effect is more potent on PDE5 than on other known phosphodiesterases (10-fold for PDE6, >80-fold for PDE1, >700-fold for PDE2, PDE3, PDE4, PDE7, PDE8, PDE9, PDE10, and PDE11). The approximately 4,000-fold selectivity for PDE5 versus PDE3 is important because PDE3 is involved in control of cardiac contractility. Sildenafil is only about 10-fold as potent for PDE5 compared to PDE6, an enzyme found in the retina which is involved in the phototransduction pathway of the retina. This lower selectivity is thought to be the basis for abnormalities related to color vision observed with higher doses or plasma levels (see **Pharmacodynamics**).

In addition to human corpus cavernosum smooth muscle, PDE5 is also found in lower concentrations in other tissues including platelets, vascular and visceral smooth muscle, and skeletal muscle. The inhibition of PDE5 in these tissues by sildenafil may be the basis for the enhanced platelet antiaggregatory activity of nitric oxide observed *in vitro*, an inhibition of platelet thrombus formation *in vivo* and peripheral arterial-venous dilatation *in vivo*.

TABLE 1. HEMODYNAMIC DATA IN PATIENTS WITH STABLE ISCHEMIC HEART DISEASE AFTER IV ADMINISTRATION OF 40 MG SILDENAFIL

Means ± SD	At rest				After 4 minutes of exercise			
	n	Baseline (B2)	n	Sildenafil (D1)	n	Baseline	n	Sildenafil
PAOP (mmHg)	8	8.1 ± 5.1	8	6.5 ± 4.3	8	36.0 ± 13.7	8	27.8 ± 15.3
Mean PAP (mmHg)	8	16.7 ± 4	8	12.1 ± 3.9	8	39.4 ± 12.9	8	31.7 ± 13.2
Mean RAP (mmHg)	7	5.7 ± 3.7	8	4.1 ± 3.7	-	-	-	-
Systolic SAP (mmHg)	8	150.4 ± 12.4	8	140.6 ± 16.5	8	199.5 ± 37.4	8	187.8 ± 30.0
Diastolic SAP (mmHg)	8	73.6 ± 7.8	8	65.9 ± 10	8	84.6 ± 9.7	8	79.5 ± 9.4
Cardiac output (L/min)	8	5.6 ± 0.9	8	5.2 ± 1.1	8	11.5 ± 2.4	8	10.2 ± 3.5
Heart rate (bpm)	8	67 ± 11.1	8	66.9 ± 12	8	101.9 ± 11.6	8	99.0 ± 20.4

Pharmacokinetics and Metabolism

VIAGRA is rapidly absorbed after oral administration, with absolute bioavailability of about 40%. Its pharmacokinetics are dose-proportional over the recommended dose range. It is eliminated predominantly by hepatic metabolism (mainly cytochrome P450 3A4) and is converted to an active metabolite with properties similar to the parent, sildenafil. The concomitant use of potent cytochrome P450 3A4 inhibitors (e.g., erythromycin, ketoconazole, itraconazole) as well as the nonspecific CYP inhibitor, cimetidine, is associated with increased plasma levels of sildenafil (see **DOSAGE AND ADMINISTRATION**). Both sildenafil and the metabolite have terminal half lives of about 4 hours.

Mean sildenafil plasma concentrations measured after the administration of a single oral dose of 100 mg to healthy male volunteers is depicted below:

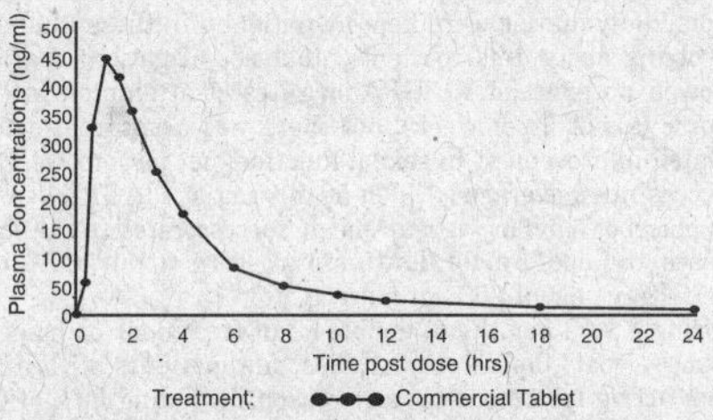

Figure 1: Mean Sildenafil Plasma Concentrations in Healthy Male Volunteers.

Absorption and Distribution: VIAGRA is rapidly absorbed. Maximum observed plasma concentrations are reached within 30 to 120 minutes (median 60 minutes) of oral dosing in the fasted state. When VIAGRA is taken with a high fat meal, the rate of absorption is reduced, with a mean delay in T_{max} of 60 minutes and a mean reduction in C_{max} of 29%. The mean steady state volume of distribution (Vss) for sildenafil is 105 L, indicating distribution into the tissues. Sildenafil and its major circulating N-desmethyl metabolite are both approximately 96% bound to plasma proteins. Protein binding is independent of total drug concentrations.

Based upon measurements of sildenafil in semen of healthy volunteers 90 minutes after dosing, less than 0.001% of the administered dose may appear in the semen of patients.

Metabolism and Excretion: Sildenafil is cleared predominantly by the CYP3A4 (major route) and CYP2C9 (minor route) hepatic microsomal isoenzymes. The major circulating metabolite results from N-desmethylation of sildenafil, and is itself further metabolized. This metabolite has a PDE selectivity profile similar to sildenafil and an *in vitro* potency for PDE5 approximately 50% of the parent drug. Plasma concentrations of this metabolite are approximately 40% of those seen for sildenafil, so that the metabolite accounts for about 20% of sildenafil's pharmacologic effects. After either oral or intravenous administration, sildenafil is excreted as metabolites predominantly in the feces (approximately 80% of administered oral dose) and to a lesser extent in the urine (approximately 13% of the administered oral dose). Similar values for pharmacokinetic parameters were seen in normal volunteers and in the patient population, using a population pharmacokinetic approach.

Pharmacokinetics in Special Populations

Geriatrics: Healthy elderly volunteers (65 years or over) had a reduced clearance of sildenafil, with free plasma concentrations approximately 40% greater than those seen in healthy younger volunteers (18-45 years).

Renal Insufficiency: In volunteers with mild (CLcr=50-80 mL/min) and moderate (CLcr=30-49 mL/min) renal impairment, the pharmacokinetics of a single oral dose of VIAGRA (50 mg) were not altered. In volunteers with severe (CLcr=<30 mL/min) renal impairment, sildenafil clearance was reduced, resulting in approximately doubling of AUC and C_{max} compared to age-matched volunteers with no renal impairment.

Hepatic Insufficiency: In volunteers with hepatic cirrhosis (Child-Pugh A and B), sildenafil clearance was reduced, resulting in increases in AUC (84%) and C_{max} (47%) compared to age-matched volunteers with no hepatic impairment.

Therefore, age >65, hepatic impairment and severe renal impairment are associated with increased plasma levels of sildenafil. A starting oral dose of 25 mg should be considered in those patients (see **DOSAGE AND ADMINISTRATION**).

Pharmacodynamics

Effects of VIAGRA on Erectile Response: In eight double-blind, placebo-controlled crossover studies of patients with either organic or psychogenic erectile dysfunction, sexual stimulation resulted in improved erections, as assessed by an objective measurement of hardness and duration of erections (RigiScan®), after VIAGRA administration compared with placebo. Most studies assessed the efficacy of VIAGRA approximately 60 minutes post dose. The erectile response, as assessed by RigiScan®, generally increased with increasing sildenafil dose and plasma concentration. The time course of effect was examined in one study, showing an effect for up to 4 hours but the response was diminished compared to 2 hours.

Effects of VIAGRA on Blood Pressure: Single oral doses of sildenafil (100 mg) administered to healthy volunteers produced decreases in supine blood pressure (mean maximum decrease in systolic/diastolic blood pressure of 8.4/5.5 mmHg). The decrease in blood pressure was most notable approximately 1-2 hours after dosing, and was not different than placebo at 8 hours. Similar effects on blood pressure were noted with 25 mg, 50 mg and 100 mg of VIAGRA, therefore the effects are not related to dose or plasma levels within this dosage range. Larger effects were recorded among patients receiving concomitant nitrates (see **CONTRAINDICATIONS**).

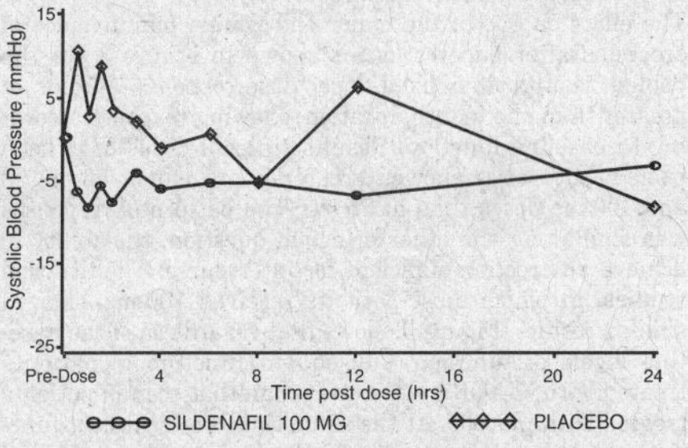

Figure 2: Mean Change from Baseline in Sitting Systolic Blood Pressure. Healthy Volunteers.

Effects of VIAGRA on Cardiac Parameters: Single oral doses of sildenafil up to 100 mg produced no clinically relevant changes in the ECGs of normal male volunteers.

Studies have produced relevant data on the effects of VIAGRA on cardiac output. In one small, open-label, uncontrolled, pilot study, eight patients with stable ischemic heart disease underwent Swan-Ganz catheterization. A total dose of 40 mg sildenafil was administered by four intravenous infusions.

The results from this pilot study are shown in Table 1; the mean resting systolic and diastolic blood pressures decreased by 7% and 10% compared to baseline in these patients. Mean resting values for right atrial pressure, pulmonary artery pressure, pulmonary artery occluded pressure and cardiac output decreased by 28%, 28%, 20% and 7% respectively. Even though this total dosage produced plasma sildenafil concentrations which were approximately 2 to 5 times higher than the mean maximum plasma concentrations following a single oral dose of 100 mg in healthy male volunteers, the hemodynamic response to exercise was preserved in these patients.

[See table 1 above]

In a double-blind study, 144 patients with erectile dysfunction and chronic stable angina limited by exercise, not receiving chronic oral nitrates, were randomized to a single dose of placebo or VIAGRA 100 mg 1 hour prior to exercise testing. The primary endpoint was time to limiting angina in the evaluable cohort. The mean times (adjusted for baseline) to onset of limiting angina were 423.6 and 403.7 seconds for sildenafil (N=70) and placebo, respectively. These results demonstrated that the effect of VIAGRA on the primary endpoint was statistically non-inferior to placebo.

Continued on next page

Viagra—Cont.

Effects of VIAGRA on Vision: At single oral doses of 100 mg and 200 mg, transient dose-related impairment of color discrimination (blue/green) was detected using the Farnsworth-Munsell 100-hue test, with peak effects near the time of peak plasma levels. This finding is consistent with the inhibition of PDE6, which is involved in phototransduction in the retina. An evaluation of visual function at doses up to twice the maximum recommended dose revealed no effects of VIAGRA on visual acuity, intraocular pressure, or pupillometry.

Clinical Studies

In clinical studies, VIAGRA was assessed for its effect on the ability of men with erectile dysfunction (ED) to engage in sexual activity and in many cases specifically on the ability to achieve and maintain an erection sufficient for satisfactory sexual activity. VIAGRA was evaluated primarily at doses of 25 mg, 50 mg and 100 mg in 21 randomized, double-blind, placebo-controlled trials of up to 6 months in duration, using a variety of study designs (fixed dose, titration, parallel, crossover). VIAGRA was administered to more than 3,000 patients aged 19 to 87 years, with ED of various etiologies (organic, psychogenic, mixed) with a mean duration of 5 years. VIAGRA demonstrated statistically significant improvement compared to placebo in all 21 studies. The studies that established benefit demonstrated improvements in success rates for sexual intercourse compared with placebo.

The effectiveness of VIAGRA was evaluated in most studies using several assessment instruments. The primary measure in the principal studies was a sexual function questionnaire (the International Index of Erectile Function - IIEF) administered during a 4-week treatment-free run-in period, at baseline, at follow-up visits, and at the end of double-blind, placebo-controlled, at-home treatment. Two of the questions from the IIEF served as primary study endpoints; categorical responses were elicited to questions about (1) the ability to achieve erections sufficient for sexual intercourse and (2) the maintenance of erections after penetration. The patient addressed both questions at the final visit for the last 4 weeks of the study. The possible categorical responses to these questions were (0) no attempted intercourse, (1) never or almost never, (2) a few times, (3) sometimes, (4) most times, and (5) almost always or always. Also collected as part of the IIEF was information about other aspects of sexual function, including information on erectile function, orgasm, desire, satisfaction with intercourse, and overall sexual satisfaction. Sexual function data were also recorded by patients in a daily diary. In addition, patients were asked a global efficacy question and an optional partner questionnaire was administered.

The effect on one of the major end points, maintenance of erections after penetration, is shown in Figure 3, for the pooled results of 5 fixed-dose, dose-response studies of greater than one month duration, showing response according to baseline function. Results with all doses have been pooled, but scores showed greater improvement at the 50 and 100 mg doses than at 25 mg. The pattern of responses was similar for the other principal question, the ability to achieve an erection sufficient for intercourse. The titration studies, in which most patients received 100 mg, showed similar results. Figure 3 shows that regardless of the baseline levels of function, subsequent function in patients treated with VIAGRA was better than that seen in patients treated with placebo. At the same time, on-treatment function was better in treated patients who were less impaired at baseline.

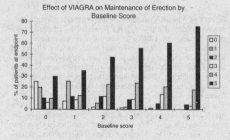

Effect of VIAGRA on Maintenance of Erection by Baseline Score

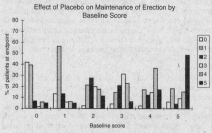

Effect of Placebo on Maintenance of Erection by Baseline Score

Figure 3. Effect of VIAGRA and Placebo on Maintenance of Erection by Baseline Score.

The frequency of patients reporting improvement of erections in response to a global question in four of the randomized, double-blind, parallel, placebo-controlled fixed dose studies (1797 patients) of 12 to 24 weeks duration is shown in Figure 4. These patients had erectile dysfunction at baseline that was characterized by median categorical scores of 2 (a few times) on principal IIEF questions. Erectile dysfunction was attributed to organic (58%; generally not characterized, but including diabetes and excluding spinal cord injury), psychogenic (17%), or mixed (24%) etiologies. Sixty-three percent, 74%, and 82% of the patients on 25 mg, 50 mg and 100 mg of VIAGRA, respectively, reported an improvement in their erections, compared to 24% on placebo. In the titration studies (n=644) (with most patients eventually receiving 100 mg), results were similar.

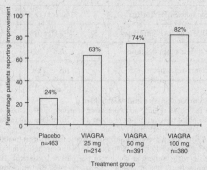

Overall treatment p<0.0001

Figure 4. Percentage of Patients Reporting an Improvement in Erections.

The patients in studies had varying degrees of ED. One-third to one-half of the subjects in these studies reported successful intercourse at least once during a 4-week, treatment-free run-in period.

In many of the studies, of both fixed dose and titration designs, daily diaries were kept by patients. In these studies, involving about 1600 patients, analyses of patient diaries showed no effect of VIAGRA on rates of attempted intercourse (about 2 per week), but there was clear treatment-related improvement in sexual function: per patient weekly success rates averaged 1.3 on 50-100 mg of VIAGRA vs 0.4 on placebo; similarly, group mean success rates (total successes divided by total attempts) were about 66% on VIAGRA vs about 20% on placebo.

During 3 to 6 months of double-blind treatment or longer-term (1 year), open-label studies, few patients withdrew from active treatment for any reason, including lack of effectiveness. At the end of the long-term study, 88% of patients reported that VIAGRA improved their erections.

Men with untreated ED had relatively low baseline scores for all aspects of sexual function measured (again using a 5-point scale) in the IIEF. VIAGRA improved these aspects of sexual function: frequency, firmness and maintenance of erections; frequency of orgasm; frequency and level of desire; frequency, satisfaction and enjoyment of intercourse; and overall relationship satisfaction.

One randomized, double-blind, flexible-dose, placebo-controlled study included only patients with erectile dysfunction attributed to complications of diabetes mellitus (n=268). As in the other titration studies, patients were started on 50 mg and allowed to adjust the dose up to 100 mg or down to 25 mg of VIAGRA; all patients, however, were receiving 50 mg or 100 mg at the end of the study. There were highly statistically significant improvements on the two principal IIEF questions (frequency of successful penetration during sexual activity and maintenance of erections after penetration) on VIAGRA compared to placebo. On a global improvement question, 57% of VIAGRA patients reported improved erections versus 10% on placebo. Diary data indicated that on VIAGRA, 48% of intercourse attempts were successful versus 12% on placebo.

One randomized, double-blind, placebo-controlled, crossover, flexible-dose (up to 100 mg) study of patients with erectile dysfunction resulting from spinal cord injury (n=178) was conducted. The changes from baseline in scoring on the two end point questions (frequency of successful penetration during sexual activity and maintenance of erections after penetration) were highly statistically significantly in favor of VIAGRA. On a global improvement question, 83% of patients reported improved erections on VIAGRA versus 12% on placebo. Diary data indicated that on VIAGRA, 59% of attempts at sexual intercourse were successful compared to 13% on placebo.

Across all trials, VIAGRA improved the erections of 43% of radical prostatectomy patients compared to 15% on placebo. Subgroup analyses of responses to a global improvement question in patients with psychogenic etiology in two fixed-dose studies (total n=179) and two titration studies (total n=149) showed 84% of VIAGRA patients reported improvement in erections compared with 26% of placebo. The changes from baseline in scoring on the two end point questions (frequency of successful penetration during sexual activity and maintenance of erections after penetration) were highly statistically significantly in favor of VIAGRA. Diary data in two of the studies (n=178) showed rates of successful intercourse per attempt of 70% for VIAGRA and 29% for placebo.

A review of population subgroups demonstrated efficacy regardless of baseline severity, etiology, race and age. VIAGRA was effective in a broad range of ED patients, including those with a history of coronary artery disease, hypertension, other cardiac disease, peripheral vascular disease, diabetes mellitus, depression, coronary artery bypass graft (CABG), radical prostatectomy, transurethral resection of the prostate (TURP) and spinal cord injury, and in patients taking antidepressants/antipsychotics and antihypertensives/diuretics.

Analysis of the safety database showed no apparent difference in the side effect profile in patients taking VIAGRA with and without antihypertensive medication. This analysis was performed retrospectively, and was not powered to detect any pre-specified difference in adverse reactions.

INDICATION AND USAGE

VIAGRA is indicated for the treatment of erectile dysfunction.

CONTRAINDICATIONS

Consistent with its known effects on the nitric oxide/cGMP pathway (see **CLINICAL PHARMACOLOGY**), VIAGRA was shown to potentiate the hypotensive effects of nitrates, and its administration to patients who are using organic nitrates, either regularly and/or intermittently, in any form is therefore contraindicated.

After patients have taken VIAGRA, it is unknown when nitrates, if necessary, can be safely administered. Based on the pharmacokinetic profile of a single 100 mg oral dose given to healthy normal volunteers, the plasma levels of sildenafil at 24 hours post dose are approximately 2 ng/mL (compared to peak plasma levels of approximately 440 ng/mL) (see **CLINICAL PHARMACOLOGY: Pharmacokinetics and Metabolism**). In the following patients: age >65, hepatic impairment (e.g., cirrhosis), severe renal impairment (e.g., creatinine clearance <30 mL/min), and concomitant use of potent cytochrome P450 3A4 inhibitors (erythromycin), plasma levels of sildenafil at 24 hours post dose have been found to be 3 to 8 times higher than those seen in healthy volunteers. Although plasma levels of sildenafil at 24 hours post dose are much lower than at peak concentration, it is unknown whether nitrates can be safely coadministered at this time point.

VIAGRA is contraindicated in patients with a known hypersensitivity to any component of the tablet.

WARNINGS

There is a potential for cardiac risk of sexual activity in patients with preexisting cardiovascular disease. Therefore, treatments for erectile dysfunction, including VIAGRA, should not be generally used in men for whom sexual activity is inadvisable because of their underlying cardiovascular status.

VIAGRA has systemic vasodilatory properties that resulted in transient decreases in supine blood pressure in healthy volunteers (mean maximum decrease of 8.4/5.5 mmHg), (see **CLINICAL PHARMACOLOGY: Pharmacodynamics**). While this normally would be expected to be of little consequence in most patients, prior to prescribing VIAGRA, physicians should carefully consider whether their patients with underlying cardiovascular disease could be affected adversely by such vasodilatory effects, especially in combination with sexual activity.

Patients with the following underlying conditions can be particularly sensitive to the actions of vasodilators including VIAGRA – those with left ventricular outflow obstruction (e.g. aortic stenosis, idiopathic hypertrophic subaortic stenosis) and those with severely impaired autonomic control of blood pressure.

There is no controlled clinical data on the safety or efficacy of VIAGRA in the following groups; if prescribed, this should be done with caution.
• Patients who have suffered a myocardial infarction, stroke, or life-threatening arrhythmia within the last 6 months;
• Patients with resting hypotension (BP <90/50) or hypertension (BP >170/110);
• Patients with cardiac failure or coronary artery disease causing unstable angina;
• Patients with retinitis pigmentosa (a minority of these patients have genetic disorders of retinal phosphodiesterases).

Prolonged erection greater than 4 hours and priapism (painful erections greater than 6 hours in duration) have been reported infrequently since market approval of VIAGRA. In the event of an erection that persists longer than 4 hours, the patient should seek immediate medical assistance. If priapism is not treated immediately, penile tissue damage and permanent loss of potency could result.

The concomitant administration of the protease inhibitor ritonavir substantially increases serum concentrations of sildenafil (**11-fold increase in AUC**). If VIAGRA is prescribed to patients taking ritonavir, caution should be used. Data from subjects exposed to high systemic levels of sildenafil are limited. Visual disturbances occurred more commonly at higher levels of sildenafil exposure. Decreased blood pressure, syncope, and prolonged erection were reported in some healthy volunteers exposed to high doses of sildenafil (200-800 mg). To decrease the chance of adverse events in patients taking ritonavir, a decrease in sildenafil dosage is recommended (see **Drug Interactions, ADVERSE REACTIONS** and **DOSAGE AND ADMINISTRATION**).

PRECAUTIONS

General

The evaluation of erectile dysfunction should include a determination of potential underlying causes and the identification of appropriate treatment following a complete medical assessment.

Before prescribing VIAGRA, it is important to note the following:

Caution is advised when Phosphodiesterase Type 5 (PDE5) inhibitors are co-administered with alpha-blockers. PDE5 inhibitors, including VIAGRA, and alpha-adrenergic blocking agents are both vasodilators with blood pressure lowering effects. When vasodilators are used in combination, an additive effect on blood pressure may be anticipated. In some patients, concomitant use of these two drug classes can lower blood pressure significantly (see Drug Interactions) leading to symptomatic hypotension (e.g. dizziness, lightheadedness, fainting).

Consideration should be given to the following:

- Patients should be stable on alpha-blocker therapy prior to initiating a PDE5 inhibitor. Patients who demonstrate hemodynamic instability on alpha-blocker therapy alone are at increased risk of symptomatic hypotension with concomitant use of PDE5 inhibitors.

- In those patients who are stable on alpha-blocker therapy, PDE5 inhibitors should be initiated at the lowest dose.

- In those patients already taking an optimized dose of a PDE5 inhibitor, alpha-blocker therapy should be initiated at the lowest dose. Stepwise increase in alpha-blocker dose may be associated with further lowering of blood pressure when taking a PDE5 inhibitor.

- Safety of combined use of PDE5 inhibitors and alpha-blockers may be affected by other variables, including intravascular volume depletion and other anti-hypertensive drugs.

Viagra has systemic vasodilatory properties and may augment the blood pressure lowering effect of other anti-hypertensive medications.

Patients on multiple antihypertensive medications were included in the pivotal clinical trials for VIAGRA. In a separate drug interaction study, when amlodipine, 5 mg or 10 mg, and VIAGRA, 100 mg were orally administered concomitantly to hypertensive patients mean additional blood pressure reduction of 8 mmHg systolic and 7 mmHg diastolic were noted (see **Drug Interactions**).

The safety of VIAGRA is unknown in patients with bleeding disorders and patients with active peptic ulceration. VIAGRA should be used with caution in patients with anatomical deformation of the penis (such as angulation, cavernosal fibrosis or Peyronie's disease), or in patients who have conditions which may predispose them to priapism (such as sickle cell anemia, multiple myeloma, or leukemia).

The safety and efficacy of combinations of VIAGRA with other treatments for erectile dysfunction have not been studied. Therefore, the use of such combinations is not recommended.

In humans, VIAGRA has no effect on bleeding time when taken alone or with aspirin. *In vitro* studies with human platelets indicate that sildenafil potentiates the antiaggregatory effect of sodium nitroprusside (a nitric oxide donor). The combination of heparin and VIAGRA had an additive effect on bleeding time in the anesthetized rabbit, but this interaction has not been studied in humans.

Information for Patients

Physicians should discuss with patients the contraindication of VIAGRA with regular and/or intermittent use of organic nitrates.

Physicians should advise patients of the potential for VIAGRA to augment the blood pressure lowering effect of alpha-blockers and anti-hypertensive medications. Concomitant administration of VIAGRA and an alpha-blocker may lead to symptomatic hypotension in some patients. Therefore, when VIAGRA is co-administered with alpha-blockers, patients should be stable on alpha-blocker therapy prior to initiating VIAGRA treatment and VIAGRA should be initiated at the lowest dose.

Physicians should discuss with patients the potential cardiac risk of sexual activity in patients with preexisting cardiovascular risk factors. Patients who experience symptoms (e.g., angina pectoris, dizziness, nausea) upon initiation of sexual activity should be advised to refrain from further activity and should discuss the episode with their physician. Physicians should advise patients to stop use of all PDE5 inhibitors, including VIAGRA, and seek medical attention in the event of a sudden loss of vision in one or both eyes. Such an event may be a sign of non-arteritic anterior ischemic optic neuropathy (NAION), a cause of decreased vision including permanent loss of vision, that has been reported rarely post-marketing in temporal association with the use of all PDE5 inhibitors. It is not possible to determine whether these events are related directly to the use of PDE5 inhibitors or to other factors. Physicians should also discuss with patients the increased risk of NAION in individuals who have already experienced NAION in one eye, including whether such individuals could be adversely affected by use of vasodilators, such as PDE5 inhibitors (see **POST-MARKETING EXPERIENCE/Special Senses**).

Physicians should advise patients to stop taking PDE5 inhibitors, including VIAGRA, and seek prompt medical attention in the event of sudden decrease or loss of hearing. These events, which may be accompanied by tinnitus and dizziness, have been reported in temporal association to the intake of PDE5 inhibitors, including VIAGRA. It is not possible to determine whether these events are related directly to the use of PDE5 inhibitors or to other factors (see AD-

VERSE REACTIONS, CLINICAL TRIALS and POST-MARKETING EXPERIENCE).

Physicians should warn patients that prolonged erections greater than 4 hours and priapism (painful erections greater than 6 hours in duration) have been reported infrequently since market approval of VIAGRA. In the event of an erection that persists longer than 4 hours, the patient should seek immediate medical assistance. If priapism is not treated immediately, penile tissue damage and permanent loss of potency may result.

The use of VIAGRA offers no protection against sexually transmitted diseases. Counseling of patients about the protective measures necessary to guard against sexually transmitted diseases, including the Human Immunodeficiency Virus (HIV), may be considered.

Drug Interactions

Effects of Other Drugs on VIAGRA

In vitro studies: Sildenafil metabolism is principally mediated by the cytochrome P450 (CYP) isoforms 3A4 (major route) and 2C9 (minor route). Therefore, inhibitors of these isoenzymes may reduce sildenafil clearance.

In vivo studies: Cimetidine (800 mg), a nonspecific CYP inhibitor, caused a 56% increase in plasma sildenafil concentrations when coadministered with VIAGRA (50 mg) to healthy volunteers.

When a single 100 mg dose of VIAGRA was administered with erythromycin, a specific CYP3A4 inhibitor, at steady state (500 mg bid for 5 days), there was a 182% increase in sildenafil systemic exposure (AUC). In addition, in a study performed in healthy male volunteers, coadministration of the HIV protease inhibitor saquinavir, also a CYP3A4 inhibitor, at steady state (1200 mg tid) with VIAGRA (100 mg single dose) resulted in a 140% increase in sildenafil C_{max} and a 210% increase in sildenafil AUC. VIAGRA had no effect on saquinavir pharmacokinetics. Stronger CYP3A4 inhibitors such as ketoconazole or itraconazole would be expected to have still greater effects, and population data from patients in clinical trials did indicate a reduction in sildenafil clearance when it was coadministered with CYP3A4 inhibitors (such as ketoconazole, erythromycin, or cimetidine) (see **DOSAGE AND ADMINISTRATION**).

In another study in healthy male volunteers, coadministration with the HIV protease inhibitor ritonavir, which is a highly potent P450 inhibitor, at steady state (500 mg bid) with VIAGRA (100 mg single dose) resulted in a 300% (4-fold) increase in sildenafil C_{max} and a 1000% (11-fold) increase in sildenafil plasma AUC. At 24 hours the plasma levels of sildenafil were still approximately 200 ng/mL, compared to approximately 5 ng/mL when sildenafil was dosed alone. This is consistent with ritonavir's marked effects on a broad range of P450 substrates. VIAGRA had no effect on ritonavir pharmacokinetics (see **DOSAGE AND ADMINISTRATION**).

Although the interaction between other protease inhibitors and sildenafil has not been studied, their concomitant use is expected to increase sildenafil levels.

In a study of healthy male volunteers, co-administration of sildenafil at steady state (80 mg t.i.d.) with endothelin receptor antagonist bosentan (a moderate inducer of CYP3A4, CYP2C9 and possibly of cytochrome P450 2C19) at steady state (125 mg b.i.d.) resulted in a 63% decrease of sildenafil AUC and a 55% decrease in sildenafil C_{max}. Concomitant administration of strong CYP3A4 inducers, such as rifampin, is expected to cause greater decreases in plasma levels of sildenafil.

Single doses of antacid (magnesium hydroxide/aluminum hydroxide) did not affect the bioavailability of VIAGRA.

Pharmacokinetic data from patients in clinical trials showed no effect on sildenafil pharmacokinetics of CYP2C9 inhibitors (such as tolbutamide, warfarin), CYP2D6 inhibitors (such as selective serotonin reuptake inhibitors, tricyclic antidepressants), thiazide and related diuretics, ACE inhibitors, and calcium channel blockers. The AUC of the active metabolite, N-desmethyl sildenafil, was increased 62% by loop and potassium-sparing diuretics and 102% by nonspecific beta-blockers. These effects on the metabolite are not expected to be of clinical consequence.

Effects of VIAGRA on Other Drugs

In vitro studies: Sildenafil is a weak inhibitor of the cytochrome P450 isoforms 1A2, 2C9, 2C19, 2D6, 2E1 and 3A4 (IC50 >150 µM). Given sildenafil peak plasma concentrations of approximately 1 µM after recommended doses, it is unlikely that VIAGRA will alter the clearance of substrates of these isoenzymes.

In vivo studies: Three double-blind, placebo-controlled, randomized, two-way crossover studies were conducted to assess the interaction of VIAGRA with doxazosin, an alpha-adrenergic blocking agent.

In the first study, a single oral dose of VIAGRA 100 mg or matching placebo was administered in a 2-period crossover design to 4 generally healthy males with benign prostatic hyperplasia (BPH). Following at least 14 consecutive daily doses of doxazosin, VIAGRA 100 mg or matching placebo was administered simultaneously with doxazosin. Following a review of the data from these first 4 subjects (details provided below), the VIAGRA dose was reduced to 25 mg. Thereafter, 17 subjects were treated with VIAGRA 25 mg or matching placebo in combination with doxazosin 4 mg (15 subjects) or doxazosin 8mg (2 subjects). The mean subject age was 66.5 years.

For the 17 subjects who received VIAGRA 25 mg and matching placebo, the placebo-subtracted mean maximum decreases from baseline (95% CI) in systolic blood pressure were as follows:

Placebo-subtracted mean maximum decrease in systolic blood pressure (mm Hg)	VIAGRA 25 mg
Supine	7.4 (-0.9, 15.7)
Standing	6.0 (-0.8, 12.8)

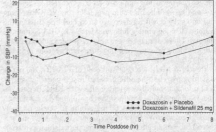

Figure 5: Mean Standing Systolic Blood Pressure Change from Baseline

Blood pressure was measured immediately pre-dose and at 15, 30, 45 minutes, and 1, 1.5, 2, 2.5, 3, 4, 6 and 8 hours after VIAGRA or matching placebo. Outliers were defined as subjects with a standing systolic blood pressure of <85 mmHg or a decrease from baseline in standing systolic blood pressure of >30 mmHg at one or more timepoints. There were no subjects treated with VIAGRA 25 mg who had a standing SBP < 85mmHg. There were three subjects with a decrease from baseline in standing systolic BP >30mmHg following VIAGRA 25 mg, one subject with a decrease from baseline in standing systolic BP > 30 mmHg following placebo and two subjects with a decrease from baseline in standing systolic BP > 30 mmHg following both VIAGRA and placebo. No severe adverse events potentially related to blood pressure effects were reported in this group. Of the four subjects who received VIAGRA 100 mg in the first part of this study, a severe adverse event related to blood pressure effect was reported in one patient (postural hypotension that began 35 minutes after dosing with VIAGRA with symptoms lasting for 8 hours), and mild adverse events potentially related to blood pressure effects were reported in two others (dizziness, headache and fatigue at 1 hour after dosing; and dizziness, lightheadedness and nausea at 4 hours after dosing). There were no reports of syncope among these patients. For these four subjects, the placebo-subtracted mean maximum decreases from baseline in supine and standing systolic blood pressures were 14.8 mmHg and 21.5 mmHg, respectively. Two of these subjects had a standing SBP < 85mmHg. Both of these subjects were protocol violators, one due to a low baseline standing SBP, and the other due to baseline orthostatic hypotension.

In the second study, a single oral dose of VIAGRA 50 mg or matching placebo was administered in a 2-period crossover design to 20 generally healthy males with BPH. Following at least 14 consecutive days of doxazosin, VIAGRA 50mg or matching placebo was administered simultaneously with doxazosin 4 mg (17 subjects) or with doxazosin 8 mg (3 subjects). The mean subject age in this study was 63.9 years. Twenty subjects received VIAGRA 50 mg, but only 19 subjects received matching placebo. One patient discontinued the study prematurely due to an adverse event of hypotension following dosing with VIAGRA 50 mg. This patient had been taking minoxidil, a potent vasodilator, during the study.

For the 19 subjects who received both VIAGRA and matching placebo, the placebo-subtracted mean maximum decreases from baseline (95% CI) in systolic blood pressure were as follows:

Placebo-subtracted mean maximum decrease in systolic blood pressure (mm Hg)	VIAGRA 50 mg (95% CI)
Supine	9.08 (5.48, 12.68)
Standing	11.62 (7.34, 15.90)

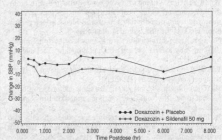

Figure 6: Mean Standing Systolic Blood Pressure Change from Baseline

Continued on next page

Viagra—Cont.

Blood pressure was measured after administration of VIAGRA at the same times as those specified for the first doxazosin study. There were two subjects who had a standing SBP of < 85 mmHg. In these two subjects, hypotension was reported as a moderately severe adverse event, beginning at approximately 1 hour after administration of VIAGRA 50 mg and resolving after approximately 7.5 hours. There was one subject with a decrease from baseline in standing systolic BP >30mmHg following VIAGRA 50 mg and one subject with a decrease from baseline in standing systolic BP > 30 mmHg following both VIAGRA 50 mg and placebo. There were no severe adverse events potentially related to blood pressure and no episodes of syncope reported in this study.

In the third study, a single oral dose of VIAGRA 100 mg or matching placebo was administered in a 3-period crossover design to 20 generally healthy males with BPH. In dose period 1, subjects were administered open-label doxazosin and a single dose of VIAGRA 50 mg simultaneously, after at least 14 consecutive days of doxazosin. If a subject did not successfully complete this first dosing period, he was discontinued from the study. Subjects who had successfully completed the previous doxazosin interaction study (using VIAGRA 50 mg), including no significant hemodynamic adverse events, were allowed to skip dose period 1. Treatment with doxazosin continued for at least 7 days after dose period 1. Thereafter, VIAGRA 100mg or matching placebo was administered simultaneously with doxazosin 4 mg (14 subjects) or doxazosin 8 mg (6 subjects) in standard crossover fashion. The mean subject age in this study was 66.4 years. Twenty-five subjects were screened. Two were discontinued after study period 1: one failed to meet pre-dose screening qualifications and the other experienced symptomatic hypotension as a moderately severe adverse event 30 minutes after dosing with open-label VIAGRA 50 mg. Of the twenty subjects who were ultimately assigned to treatment, a total of 13 subjects successfully completed dose period 1, and seven had successfully completed the previous doxazosin study (using VIAGRA 50 mg).

For the 20 subjects who received VIAGRA 100 mg and matching placebo, the placebo-subtracted mean maximum decreases from baseline (95% CI) in systolic blood pressure were as follows:

Placebo-subtracted mean maximum decrease in systolic blood pressure (mm Hg)	VIAGRA 100 mg
Supine	7.9 (4.6, 11.1)
Standing	4.3 (-1.8,10.3)

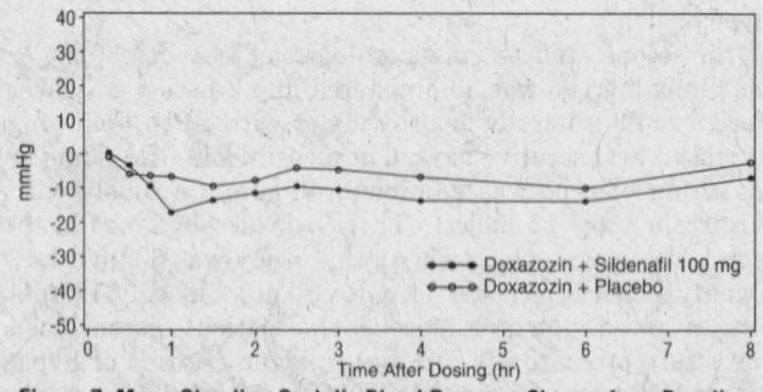

Figure 7: Mean Standing Systolic Blood Pressure Change from Baseline

Blood pressure was measured after administration of VIAGRA at the same times as those specified for the previous doxazosin studies. There were three subjects who had a standing SBP of < 85 mmHg. All three were taking VIAGRA 100 mg, and all three reported mild adverse events at the time of reductions in standing SBP, including vasodilation and lightheadedness. There were four subjects with a decrease from baseline in standing systolic BP >30mmHg following VIAGRA 100 mg, one subject with a decrease from baseline in standing systolic BP > 30 mmHg following placebo and one subject with a decrease from baseline in standing systolic BP > 30 mmHg following both VIAGRA and placebo. While there were no severe adverse events potentially related to blood pressure reported in this study, one subject reported moderate vasodilatation after both VIAGRA 50 mg and 100 mg. There were no episodes of syncope reported in this study.

When VIAGRA 100 mg oral was coadministered with amlodipine, 5 mg or 10 mg oral, to hypertensive patients, the mean additional reduction on supine blood pressure was 8 mmHg systolic and 7 mmHg diastolic.

No significant interactions were shown with tolbutamide (250 mg) or warfarin (40 mg), both of which are metabolized by CYP2C9.

VIAGRA (50 mg) did not potentiate the increase in bleeding time caused by aspirin (150 mg).

VIAGRA (50 mg) did not potentiate the hypotensive effect of alcohol in healthy volunteers with mean maximum blood alcohol levels of 0.08%.

In a study of healthy male volunteers, sildenafil (100 mg) did not affect the steady state pharmacokinetics of the HIV protease inhibitors, saquinavir and ritonavir, both of which are CYP3A4 substrates.

Sildenafil at steady state (80 mg t.i.d.) resulted in a 50% increase in AUC and a 42% increase in C_{max} of bosentan (125 mg b.i.d.).

Carcinogenesis, Mutagenesis, Impairment of Fertility

Sildenafil was not carcinogenic when administered to rats for 24 months at a dose resulting in total systemic drug exposure (AUCs) for unbound sildenafil and its major metabolite of 29- and 42-times, for male and female rats, respectively, the exposures observed in human males given the Maximum Recommended Human Dose (MRHD) of 100 mg. Sildenafil was not carcinogenic when administered to mice for 18-21 months at dosages up to the Maximum Tolerated Dose (MTD) of 10 mg/kg/day, approximately 0.6 times the MRHD on a mg/m^2 basis.

Sildenafil was negative in *in vitro* bacterial and Chinese hamster ovary cell assays to detect mutagenicity, and *in vitro* human lymphocytes and *in vivo* mouse micronucleus assays to detect clastogenicity.

There was no impairment of fertility in rats given sildenafil up to 60 mg/kg/day for 36 days to females and 102 days to males, a dose producing an AUC value of more than 25 times the human male AUC.

There was no effect on sperm motility or morphology after single 100 mg oral doses of VIAGRA in healthy volunteers.

Pregnancy, Nursing Mothers and Pediatric Use

VIAGRA is not indicated for use in newborns, children, or women.

Pregnancy Category B. No evidence of teratogenicity, embryotoxicity or fetotoxicity was observed in rats and rabbits which received up to 200 mg/kg/day during organogenesis. These doses represent, respectively, about 20 and 40 times the MRHD on a mg/m^2 basis in a 50 kg subject. In the rat pre- and postnatal development study, the no observed adverse effect dose was 30 mg/kg/day given for 36 days. In the nonpregnant rat the AUC at this dose was about 20 times human AUC. There are no adequate and well-controlled studies of sildenafil in pregnant women.

Geriatric Use: Healthy elderly volunteers (65 years or over) had a reduced clearance of sildenafil (see **CLINICAL PHARMACOLOGY: Pharmacokinetics in Special Populations**). Since higher plasma levels may increase both the efficacy and incidence of adverse events, a starting dose of 25 mg should be considered (see **DOSAGE AND ADMINISTRATION**).

ADVERSE REACTIONS

CLINICAL TRIALS:

VIAGRA was administered to over 3700 patients (aged 19-87 years) during pre-marketing clinical trials worldwide. Over 550 patients were treated for longer than one year.

In placebo-controlled clinical studies, the discontinuation rate due to adverse events for VIAGRA (2.5%) was not significantly different from placebo (2.3%). The adverse events were generally transient and mild to moderate in nature.

In trials of all designs, adverse events reported by patients receiving VIAGRA were generally similar. In fixed-dose studies, the incidence of some adverse events increased with dose. The nature of the adverse events in flexible-dose studies, which more closely reflect the recommended dosage regimen, was similar to that for fixed-dose studies.

When VIAGRA was taken as recommended (on an as-needed basis) in flexible-dose, placebo-controlled clinical trials, the following adverse events were reported:

TABLE 2. ADVERSE EVENTS REPORTED BY ≥2% OF PATIENTS TREATED WITH VIAGRA AND MORE FREQUENT ON DRUG THAN PLACEBO IN PRN FLEXIBLE-DOSE PHASE II/III STUDIES

Adverse Event	Percentage of Patients Reporting Event	
	VIAGRA N = 734	PLACEBO N = 725
Headache	16%	4%
Flushing	10%	1%
Dyspepsia	7%	2%
Nasal Congestion	4%	2%
Urinary Tract Infection	3%	2%
Abnormal Vision†	3%	0%
Diarrhea	3%	1%
Dizziness	2%	1%
Rash	2%	1%

† Abnormal Vision: Mild and transient, predominantly color tinge to vision, but also increased sensitivity to light or blurred vision. In these studies, only one patient discontinued due to abnormal vision.

Other adverse reactions occurred at a rate of >2%, but equally common on placebo: respiratory tract infection, back pain, flu syndrome, and arthralgia.

In fixed-dose studies, dyspepsia (17%) and abnormal vision (11%) were more common at 100 mg than at lower doses. At doses above the recommended dose range, adverse events were similar to those detailed above but generally were reported more frequently.

The following events occurred in <2% of patients in controlled clinical trials; a causal relationship to VIAGRA is uncertain. Reported events include those with a plausible relation to drug use; omitted are minor events and reports too imprecise to be meaningful:

Body as a whole: face edema, photosensitivity reaction, shock, asthenia, pain, chills, accidental fall, abdominal pain, allergic reaction, chest pain, accidental injury.

Cardiovascular: angina pectoris, AV block, migraine, syncope, tachycardia, palpitation, hypotension, postural hypotension, myocardial ischemia, cerebral thrombosis, cardiac arrest, heart failure, abnormal electrocardiogram, cardiomyopathy.

Digestive: vomiting, glossitis, colitis, dysphagia, gastritis, gastroenteritis, esophagitis, stomatitis, dry mouth, liver function tests abnormal, rectal hemorrhage, gingivitis.

Hemic and Lymphatic: anemia and leukopenia.

Metabolic and Nutritional: thirst, edema, gout, unstable diabetes, hyperglycemia, peripheral edema, hyperuricemia, hypoglycemic reaction, hypernatremia.

Musculoskeletal: arthritis, arthrosis, myalgia, tendon rupture, tenosynovitis, bone pain, myasthenia, synovitis.

Nervous: ataxia, hypertonia, neuralgia, neuropathy, paresthesia, tremor, vertigo, depression, insomnia, somnolence, abnormal dreams, reflexes decreased, hypesthesia.

Respiratory: asthma, dyspnea, laryngitis, pharyngitis, sinusitis, bronchitis, sputum increased, cough increased.

Skin and Appendages: urticaria, herpes simplex, pruritus, sweating, skin ulcer, contact dermatitis, exfoliative dermatitis.

Special Senses: sudden decrease or loss of hearing, mydriasis, conjunctivitis, photophobia, tinnitus, eye pain, ear pain, eye hemorrhage, cataract, dry eyes.

Urogenital: cystitis, nocturia, urinary frequency, breast enlargement, urinary incontinence, abnormal ejaculation, genital edema and anorgasmia.

POST-MARKETING EXPERIENCE:

Cardiovascular and cerebrovascular

Serious cardiovascular, cerebrovascular, and vascular events, including myocardial infarction, sudden cardiac death, ventricular arrhythmia, cerebrovascular hemorrhage, transient ischemic attack, hypertension, subarachnoid and intracerebral hemorrhages, and pulmonary hemorrhage have been reported post-marketing in temporal association with the use of VIAGRA. Most, but not all, of these patients had preexisting cardiovascular risk factors. Many of these events were reported to occur during or shortly after sexual activity, and a few were reported to occur shortly after the use of VIAGRA without sexual activity. Others were reported to have occurred hours to days after the use of VIAGRA and sexual activity. It is not possible to determine whether these events are related directly to VIAGRA, to sexual activity, to the patient's underlying cardiovascular disease, to a combination of these factors, or to other factors (see **WARNINGS** for further important cardiovascular information).

Special senses:

Cases of sudden decrease or loss of hearing have been reported postmarketing in temporal association with the use of PDE5 inhibitors, including VIAGRA. In some of the cases, medical conditions and other factors were reported that may have also played a role in the otologic adverse events. In many cases, medical follow-up information was limited. It is not possible to determine whether these reported events are related directly to the use of VIAGRA, to the patient's underlying risk factors for hearing loss, a combination of these factors, or to other factors (see **PRECAUTIONS, Information for Patients**).

Other Events

Other events reported post-marketing to have been observed in temporal association with VIAGRA and not listed in the clinical trial adverse reactions section above include:

Nervous: seizure, seizure recurrence, and anxiety.

Urogenital: prolonged erection, priapism (see **WARNINGS**), and hematuria.

Special Senses: diplopia, temporary vision loss/decreased vision, ocular redness or bloodshot appearance, ocular burning, ocular swelling/pressure, increased intraocular pressure, retinal vascular disease or bleeding, vitreous detachment/traction, paramacular edema and epistaxis.

Non-arteritic anterior ischemic optic neuropathy (NAION), a cause of decreased vision including permanent loss of vision, has been reported rarely post-marketing in temporal association with the use of phosphodiesterase type 5 (PDE5) inhibitors, including VIAGRA. Most, but not all, of these patients had underlying anatomic or vascular risk factors for developing NAION, including but not necessarily limited to: low cup to disc ratio ("crowded disc"), age over 50, diabetes, hypertension, coronary artery disease, hyperlipidemia and smoking. It is not possible to determine whether these events are related directly to the use of PDE5 inhibitors, to the patient's underlying vascular risk factors or anatomical defects, to a combination of these factors, or to other factors (see **PRECAUTIONS/Information for Patients**).

OVERDOSAGE

In studies with healthy volunteers of single doses up to 800 mg, adverse events were similar to those seen at lower doses but incidence rates were increased.

In cases of overdose, standard supportive measures should be adopted as required. Renal dialysis is not expected to accelerate clearance as sildenafil is highly bound to plasma proteins and it is not eliminated in the urine.

DOSAGE AND ADMINISTRATION

For most patients, the recommended dose is 50 mg taken, as needed, approximately 1 hour before sexual activity. However, VIAGRA may be taken anywhere from 4 hours to 0.5 hour before sexual activity. Based on effectiveness and toleration, the dose may be increased to a maximum recommended dose of 100 mg or decreased to 25 mg. The maximum recommended dosing frequency is once per day.

The following factors are associated with increased plasma levels of sildenafil: age >65 (40% increase in AUC), hepatic impairment (e.g., cirrhosis, 80%), severe renal impairment (creatinine clearance <30 mL/min, 100%), and concomitant use of potent cytochrome P450 3A4 inhibitors [ketoconazole, itraconazole, erythromycin (182%), saquinavir (210%)].

Since higher plasma levels may increase both the efficacy and incidence of adverse events, a starting dose of 25 mg should be considered in these patients.
Ritonavir greatly increased the systemic level of sildenafil in a study of healthy, non-HIV infected volunteers (11-fold increase in AUC, see **Drug Interactions**.) Based on these pharmacokinetic data, it is recommended not to exceed a maximum single dose of 25 mg of VIAGRA in a 48 hour period.
VIAGRA was shown to potentiate the hypotensive effects of nitrates and its administration in patients who use nitric oxide donors or nitrates in any form is therefore contraindicated.
When VIAGRA is co-administered with an alpha-blocker, patients should be stable on alpha-blocker therapy prior to initiating VIAGRA treatment and VIAGRA should be initiated at the lowest dose (see **Drug Interactions**).

HOW SUPPLIED

VIAGRA® (sildenafil citrate) is supplied as blue, film-coated, rounded-diamond-shaped tablets containing sildenafil citrate equivalent to the nominally indicated amount of sildenafil as follows:
[See table above]

	25 mg	50 mg	100 mg
Obverse	VGR25	VGR50	VGR100
Reverse	PFIZER	PFIZER	PFIZER
Bottle of 30	NDC-0069-4200-30	NDC-0069-4210-30	NDC-0069-4220-30
Bottle of 100	N/A	NDC-0069-4210-66	NDC-0069-4220-66

Recommended Storage: Store at 25°C (77°F); excursions permitted to 15-30°C (59-86°F) [see USP Controlled Room Temperature].
Rx only
Distributed by
Pfizer Labs
Division of Pfizer Inc., NY, NY 10017
LAB-0221-9.0 Revised February 2008

PATIENT SUMMARY OF INFORMATION ABOUT VIAGRA®

(sildenafil citrate) tablets

This summary contains important information about VIAGRA®. It is not meant to take the place of your doctor's instructions. Read this information carefully before you start taking VIAGRA. Ask your doctor or pharmacist if you do not understand any of this information or if you want to know more about VIAGRA.
This medicine can help many men when it is used as prescribed by their doctors. However, VIAGRA is not for everyone. It is intended for use only by men who have a condition called erectile dysfunction. **VIAGRA must never be used by men who are taking medicines that contain nitrates of any kind, at any time. This includes nitroglycerin. If you take VIAGRA with any nitrate medicine your blood pressure could suddenly drop to an unsafe or life threatening level.**

• WHAT IS VIAGRA?

VIAGRA is a pill used to treat erectile dysfunction (impotence) in men. It can help many men who have erectile dysfunction get and keep an erection when they become sexually excited (stimulated).
You will not get an erection just by taking this medicine. VIAGRA helps a man with erectile dysfunction get an erection only when he is sexually excited.

• HOW SEX AFFECTS THE BODY

When a man is sexually excited, the penis rapidly fills with more blood than usual. The penis then expands and hardens. This is called an erection. After the man is done having sex, this extra blood flows out of the penis back into the body. The erection goes away. If an erection lasts for a long time (more than 6 hours), it can permanently damage your penis. You should call a doctor immediately if you ever have a prolonged erection that lasts more than 4 hours.
Some conditions and medicines interfere with this natural erection process. The penis cannot fill with enough blood. The man cannot have an erection. This is called erectile dysfunction if it becomes a frequent problem.
During sex, your heart works harder. Therefore sexual activity may not be advisable for people who have heart problems. Before you start any treatment for erectile dysfunction, ask your doctor if your heart is healthy enough to handle the extra strain of having sex. If you have chest pains, dizziness or nausea during sex, stop having sex and immediately tell your doctor you have had this problem.

HOW VIAGRA WORKS

- VIAGRA enables many men with erectile dysfunction to respond to sexual stimulation. When a man is sexually excited, VIAGRA helps the penis fill with enough blood to cause an erection. After sex is over, the erection goes away.

• VIAGRA IS NOT FOR EVERYONE

As noted above (*How Sex Affects the Body*), ask your doctor if your heart is healthy enough for sexual activity.
If you take any medicines that contain nitrates – either regularly or as needed – you should never take VIAGRA. If you take VIAGRA with any nitrate medicine or recreational drug containing nitrates, your blood pressure could suddenly drop to an unsafe level. You could get dizzy, faint, or even have a heart attack or stroke. Nitrates are found in many prescription medicines that are used to treat angina (chest pain due to heart disease) such as:

- nitroglycerin (sprays, ointments, skin patches or pastes, and tablets that are swallowed or dissolved in the mouth)
- isosorbide mononitrate and isosorbide dinitrate (tablets that are swallowed, chewed, or dissolved in the mouth)

Nitrates are also found in recreational drugs such as amyl nitrate or nitrite ("poppers"). If you are not sure if any of your medicines contain nitrates, or if you do not understand what nitrates are, ask your doctor or pharmacist.
VIAGRA is only for patients with erectile dysfunction. VIAGRA is not for newborns, children, or women. Do not let anyone else take your VIAGRA. VIAGRA must be used only under a doctor's supervision.

• WHAT VIAGRA DOES NOT DO

- VIAGRA does not cure erectile dysfunction. It is a treatment for erectile dysfunction.
- VIAGRA does not protect you or your partner from getting sexually transmitted diseases, including HIV—the virus that causes AIDS.
- VIAGRA is not a hormone or an aphrodisiac.

• WHAT TO TELL YOUR DOCTOR BEFORE YOU BEGIN VIAGRA

Only your doctor can decide if VIAGRA is right for you. VIAGRA can cause mild, temporary lowering of your blood pressure. You will need to have a thorough medical exam to diagnose your erectile dysfunction and to find out if you can safely take VIAGRA alone or with your other medicines. Your doctor should determine if your heart is healthy enough to handle the extra strain of having sex.
Be sure to tell your doctor if you:

- have ever had any heart problems (e.g., angina, chest pain, heart failure, irregular heart beats, heart attack or narrowing of the aortic valve)
- have ever had a stroke
- have low or high blood pressure
- have ever had severe vision loss
- have a rare inherited eye disease called retinitis pigmentosa
- have ever had any kidney problems
- have ever had any liver problems
- have ever had any blood problems, including sickle cell anemia or leukemia
- are allergic to sildenafil or any of the other ingredients of VIAGRA tablets
- have a deformed penis, Peyronie's disease, or ever had an erection that lasted more than 4 hours
- have stomach ulcers or any types of bleeding problems
- are taking any other medicines

• VIAGRA AND OTHER MEDICINES

Some medicines can change the way VIAGRA works. Tell your doctor about **any medicines** you are taking. Do not start or stop taking any medicines before checking with your doctor or pharmacist. This includes prescription and nonprescription medicines or remedies:

- Remember, VIAGRA should never be used with medicines that contain nitrates (see *VIAGRA Is Not for Everyone*).
- If you are taking medicines called alpha-blockers for the treatment of high blood pressure or prostate problems, your blood pressure could suddenly drop. You could get dizzy or faint.
- If you are taking a protease inhibitor, your dose may be adjusted (please see *Finding the Right Dose for You*).
- VIAGRA should not be used with any other medical treatments that cause erections. These treatments include pills, medicines that are injected or inserted into the penis, implants or vacuum pumps.

• FINDING THE RIGHT DOSE FOR YOU

VIAGRA comes in different doses (25 mg, 50 mg and 100 mg). If you do not get the results you expect, talk with your doctor. You and your doctor can determine the dose that works best for you.

- Do not take more VIAGRA than your doctor prescribes.
- If you think you need a larger dose of VIAGRA, check with your doctor.
- VIAGRA should not be taken more than once a day.

Your doctor may prescribe a lower dose of VIAGRA in certain circumstances. For example:

- If you are older than age 65, or have serious liver or kidney problems, your doctor may start you at the lowest dose (25 mg) of VIAGRA.
- If you are taking protease inhibitors, such as for the treatment of HIV, your doctor may recommend a 25 mg dose and may limit you to a maximum single dose of 25 mg of VIAGRA in a 48 hour period.
- If you have prostate problems or high blood pressure for which you take medicines called alpha blockers, your doctor may start you on a lower dose of VIAGRA.

• HOW TO TAKE VIAGRA

Take VIAGRA about one hour before you plan to have sex. Beginning in about 30 minutes and for up to 4 hours, VIAGRA can help you get an erection if you are sexually excited. If you take VIAGRA after a high-fat meal (such as a cheeseburger and french fries), the medicine may take a little longer to start working. VIAGRA can help you get an erection when you are sexually excited. You will not get an erection just by taking the pill.

• POSSIBLE SIDE EFFECTS

Like all medicines, VIAGRA can cause some side effects. These effects are usually mild to moderate and usually don't last longer than a few hours. Some of these side effects are more likely to occur with higher doses. The most common side effects of VIAGRA are headache, flushing of the face, and upset stomach. Less common side effects that may occur are temporary changes in color vision (such as trouble telling the difference between blue and green objects or having a blue color tinge to them), eyes being more sensitive to light, or blurred vision.
In rare instances, men taking PDE5 inhibitors (oral erectile dysfunction medicines, including VIAGRA) reported a sudden decrease or loss of vision in one or both eyes. It is not possible to determine whether these events are related directly to these medicines, to other factors such as high blood pressure or diabetes, or to a combination of these. If you experience sudden decrease or loss of vision, stop taking PDE5 inhibitors, including VIAGRA, and call a doctor right away.
In rare instances, men have reported an erection that lasts many hours. You should call a doctor immediately if you ever have an erection that lasts more than 4 hours. If not treated right away, permanent damage to your penis could occur (see *How Sex Affects the Body*).
Sudden loss or decrease in hearing, sometimes with ringing in the ears and dizziness, has been rarely reported in people taking PDE5 inhibitors, including VIAGRA. It is not possible to determine whether these events are related directly to the PDE5 inhibitors, to other diseases or medications, to other factors, or to a combination of factors. If you experience these symptoms, stop taking VIAGRA and contact a doctor right away.
Heart attack, stroke, irregular heart beats, and death have been reported rarely in men taking VIAGRA. Most, but not all, of these men had heart problems before taking this medicine. It is not possible to determine whether these events were directly related to VIAGRA.
VIAGRA may cause other side effects besides those listed on this sheet. If you want more information or develop any side effects or symptoms you are concerned about, call your doctor.

• ACCIDENTAL OVERDOSE

In case of accidental overdose, call your doctor right away.

• STORING VIAGRA

Keep VIAGRA out of the reach of children. Keep VIAGRA in its original container. Store at 25°C (77°F); excursions permitted to 15-30°C (59-86°F) [see USP Controlled Room Temperature].

• FOR MORE INFORMATION ON VIAGRA

VIAGRA is a prescription medicine used to treat erectile dysfunction. Only your doctor can decide if it is right for you. This sheet is only a summary. If you have any questions or want more information about VIAGRA, talk with your doctor or pharmacist, visit www.viagra.com, or call 1-888-4VIAGRA.
Distributed by
Pfizer Labs
Division of Pfizer Inc, NY, NY 10017
LAB-0220-6.0
October 2007

Pharmacia & Upjohn

A Division of Pfizer
235 EAST 42ND STREET
NEW YORK, NY 10017-5755

For updates to the product information listed below, please check the Pfizer Web site, http://www.pfizerpro.com, or call (800) 438-1985. For complete product listing, please see the Manufacturers' Index.

For Medical Information, Contact:
(800) 438-1985
24 hours a day, seven days a week

Distribution:
1855 Shelby Oaks Drive North
Memphis, TN 38134
(901) 387-5200

Customer Service:
(800) 533-4535

DETROL® ℞

[*dē-trōl*]
tolterodine tartrate tablets

Prescribing information for this product, which appears on pages 2616–2619 of the 2008 PDR, has been completely revised as follows. Please write "See Supplement A" next to the product heading.

Continued on next page

Detrol—Cont.

DESCRIPTION

DETROL Tablets contain tolterodine tartrate. The active moiety, tolterodine, is a muscarinic receptor antagonist. The chemical name of tolterodine tartrate is (R)-2-[3-[bis(1-methylethyl)-amino]1-phenylpropyl]-4-methylphenol [R-(R*,R*)]-2,3dihydroxybutanedioate (1:1) (salt). The empirical formula of tolterodine tartrate is $C_{26}H_{37}NO_7$, and its molecular weight is 475.6. The structural formula of tolterodine tartrate is represented below:

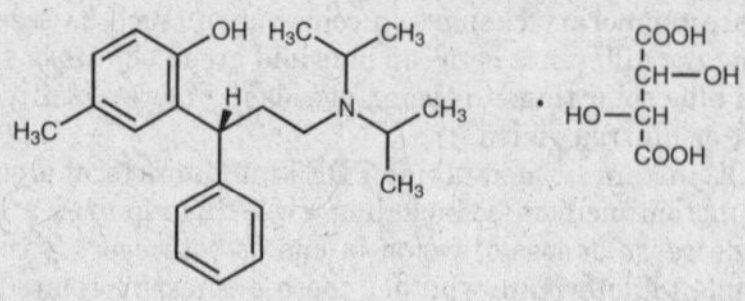

Tolterodine tartrate is a white, crystalline powder. The pKa value is 9.87 and the solubility in water is 12 mg/mL. It is soluble in methanol, slightly soluble in ethanol, and practically insoluble in toluene. The partition coefficient (Log D) between n-octanol and water is 1.83 at pH 7.3.

DETROL Tablets for oral administration contain 1 or 2 mg of tolterodine tartrate. The inactive ingredients are colloidal anhydrous silica, calcium hydrogen phosphate dihydrate, cellulose microcrystalline, hypromellose, magnesium stearate, sodium starch glycolate (pH 3.0 to 5.0), stearic acid, and titanium dioxide.

CLINICAL PHARMACOLOGY

Tolterodine is a competitive muscarinic receptor antagonist. Both urinary bladder contraction and salivation are mediated via cholinergic muscarinic receptors.

After oral administration, tolterodine is metabolized in the liver, resulting in the formation of the 5-hydroxymethyl derivative, a major pharmacologically active metabolite. The 5-hydroxymethyl metabolite, which exhibits an antimuscarinic activity similar to that of tolterodine, contributes significantly to the therapeutic effect. Both tolterodine and the 5-hydroxymethyl metabolite exhibit a high specificity for muscarinic receptors, since both show negligible activity or affinity for other neurotransmitter receptors and other potential cellular targets, such as calcium channels.

Tolterodine has a pronounced effect on bladder function. Effects on urodynamic parameters before and 1 and 5 hours after a single 6.4 mg dose of tolterodine immediate release were determined in healthy volunteers. The main effects of tolterodine at 1 and 5 hours were an increase in residual urine, reflecting an incomplete emptying of the bladder, and a decrease in detrusor pressure. These findings are consistent with an antimuscarinic action on the lower urinary tract.

Pharmacokinetics

Absorption: In a study with ^{14}C-tolterodine solution in healthy volunteers who received a 5-mg oral dose, at least 77% of the radiolabeled dose was absorbed. Tolterodine immediate release is rapidly absorbed, and maximum serum concentrations (C_{max}) typically occur within 1 to 2 hours after dose administration. C_{max} and area under the concentration-time curve (AUC) determined after dosage of tolterodine immediate release are dose-proportional over the range of 1 to 4 mg.

Effect of Food: Food intake increases the bioavailability of tolterodine (average increase 53%), but does not affect the levels of the 5-hydroxymethyl metabolite in extensive metabolizers. This change is not expected to be a safety concern and adjustment of dose is not needed.

Distribution: Tolterodine is highly bound to plasma proteins, primarily α_1-acid glycoprotein. Unbound concentrations of tolterodine average 3.7% ± 0.13% over the concentration range achieved in clinical studies. The 5-hydroxymethyl metabolite is not extensively protein bound, with unbound fraction concentrations averaging 36% ± 4.0%. The blood to serum ratio of tolterodine and the 5-hydroxymethyl metabolite averages 0.6 and 0.8, respectively, indicating that these compounds do not distribute extensively into erythrocytes. The volume of distribution of tolterodine following administration of a 1.28-mg intravenous dose is 113 ± 26.7 L.

Metabolism: Tolterodine is extensively metabolized by the liver following oral dosing. The primary metabolic route involves the oxidation of the 5-methyl group and is mediated by the cytochrome P450 2D6 (CYP2D6) and leads to the formation of a pharmacologically active 5-hydroxymethyl metabolite. Further metabolism leads to formation of the 5-carboxylic acid and *N*-dealkylated 5-carboxylic acid metabolites, which account for 51% ± 14% and 29% ± 6.3% of the metabolites recovered in the urine, respectively.

Variability in Metabolism: A subset (about 7%) of the population is devoid of CYP2D6, the enzyme responsible for the formation of the 5-hydroxymethyl metabolite of tolterodine. The identified pathway of metabolism for these individuals ("poor metabolizers") is dealkylation via cytochrome P450 3A4 (CYP3A4) to *N*-dealkylated tolterodine. The remainder of the population is referred to as "extensive metabolizers." Pharmacokinetic studies revealed that tolterodine is metabolized at a slower rate in poor metabolizers than in extensive metabolizers; this results in significantly higher serum concentrations of tolterodine and in negligible concentrations of the 5-hydroxymethyl metabolite.

Excretion: Following administration of a 5-mg oral dose of ^{14}C-tolterodine solution to healthy volunteers, 77% of radioactivity was recovered in urine and 17% was recovered in feces in 7 days. Less than 1% (<2.5% in poor metabolizers) of the dose was recovered as intact tolterodine, and 5% to 14% (<1% in poor metabolizers) was recovered as the active 5-hydroxymethyl metabolite.

A summary of mean (± standard deviation) pharmacokinetic parameters of tolterodine immediate release and the 5-hydroxymethyl metabolite in extensive (EM) and poor (PM) metabolizers is provided in Table 1. These data were obtained following single and multiple doses of tolterodine 4 mg administered twice daily to 16 healthy male volunteers (8 EM, 8 PM).

[See table 1 below]

Pharmacokinetics in Special Populations

Age: In Phase 1, multiple-dose studies in which tolterodine immediate release 4 mg (2 mg bid) was administered, serum concentrations of tolterodine and of the 5-hydroxymethyl metabolite were similar in healthy elderly volunteers (aged 64 through 80 years) and healthy young volunteers (aged less than 40 years). In another Phase 1 study, elderly volunteers (aged 71 through 81 years) were given tolterodine immediate release 2 or 4 mg (1 or 2 mg bid). Mean serum concentrations of tolterodine and the 5-hydroxymethyl metabolite in these elderly volunteers were approximately 20% and 50% higher, respectively, than reported in young healthy volunteers. However, no overall differences were observed in safety between older and younger patients on tolterodine in Phase 3, 12-week, controlled clinical studies; therefore, no tolterodine dosage adjustment for elderly patients is recommended (see **PRECAUTIONS, Geriatric Use**).

Pediatric: The pharmacokinetics of tolterodine have not been established in pediatric patients.

Gender: The pharmacokinetics of tolterodine immediate release and the 5-hydroxymethyl metabolite are not influenced by gender. Mean C_{max} of tolterodine (1.6 µg/L in males versus 2.2 µg/L in females) and the active 5-hydroxymethyl metabolite (2.2 µg/L in males versus 2.5 µg/L in females) are similar in males and females who were administered tolterodine immediate release 2 mg. Mean AUC values of tolterodine (6.7 µg·h/L in males versus 7.8 µg·h/L in females) and the 5-hydroxymethyl metabolite (10 µg·h/L in males versus 11 µg·h/L in females) are also similar. The elimination half-life of tolterodine for both males and females is 2.4 hours, and the half-life of the 5-hydroxymethyl metabolite is 3.0 hours in females and 3.3 hours in males.

Race: Pharmacokinetic differences due to race have not been established.

Renal Insufficiency: Renal impairment can significantly alter the disposition of tolterodine immediate release and its metabolites. In a study conducted in patients with creatinine clearance between 10 and 30 mL/min, tolterodine immediate release and the 5-hydroxymethyl metabolite levels were approximately 2–3 fold higher in patients with renal impairment than in healthy volunteers. Exposure levels of other metabolites of tolterodine (e.g., tolterodine acid, *N*-dealkylated tolterodine acid, *N*-dealkylated tolterodine, and *N*-dealkylated hydroxylated tolterodine) were significantly higher (10–30 fold) in renally impaired patients as compared to the healthy volunteers. The recommended dosage for patients with significantly reduced renal function is DETROL 1 mg twice daily (see **PRECAUTIONS, General** and **DOSAGE AND ADMINISTRATION**).

Hepatic Insufficiency: Liver impairment can significantly alter the disposition of tolterodine immediate release. In a study conducted in cirrhotic patients, the elimination half-life of tolterodine immediate release was longer in cirrhotic patients (mean, 7.8 hours) than in healthy, young, and elderly volunteers (mean, 2 to 4 hours). The clearance of orally administered tolterodine was substantially lower in cirrhotic patients (1.0 ± 1.7 L/h/kg) than in the healthy volunteers (5.7 ± 3.8 L/h/kg). The recommended dose for patients with significantly reduced hepatic function is DETROL 1 mg twice daily (see **PRECAUTIONS, General** and **DOSAGE AND ADMINISTRATION**).

Drug-Drug Interactions

Fluoxetine: Fluoxetine is a selective serotonin reuptake inhibitor and a potent inhibitor of CYP2D6 activity. In a study to assess the effect of fluoxetine on the pharmacokinetics of tolterodine immediate release and its metabolites, it was observed that fluoxetine significantly inhibited the metabolism of tolterodine immediate release in extensive metabolizers, resulting in a 4.8-fold increase in tolterodine AUC. There was a 52% decrease in C_{max} and a 20% decrease in AUC of the 5-hydroxymethyl metabolite. Fluoxetine thus alters the pharmacokinetics in patients who would otherwise be extensive metabolizers of tolterodine immediate release to resemble the pharmacokinetic profile in poor metabolizers. The sums of unbound serum concentrations of tolterodine immediate release and the 5-hydroxymethyl metabolite are only 25% higher during the interaction. No dose adjustment is required when DETROL and fluoxetine are coadministered.

Other Drugs Metabolized by Cytochrome P450 Isoenzymes: Tolterodine immediate release does not cause clinically significant interactions with other drugs metabolized by the major drug metabolizing CYP enzymes. *In vivo* drug-interaction data show that tolterodine immediate release does not result in clinically relevant inhibition of CYP1A2, 2D6, 2C9, 2C19, or 3A4 as evidenced by lack of influence on the marker drugs caffeine, debrisoquine, S-warfarin, and omeprazole. *In vitro* data show that tolterodine immediate release is a competitive inhibitor of CYP2D6 at high concentrations (Ki 1.05 µM), while tolterodine immediate release as well as the 5-hydroxymethyl metabolite are devoid of any significant inhibitory potential regarding the other isoenzymes.

CYP3A4 Inhibitors: The effect of 200 mg daily dose of ketoconazole on the pharmacokinetics of tolterodine immediate release was studied in 8 healthy volunteers, all of whom were poor metabolizers (see **Pharmacokinetics**, Variability in Metabolism for discussion of poor metabolizers). In the presence of ketoconazole, the mean C_{max} and AUC of tolterodine increased by 2 and 2.5 fold, respectively. Based on these findings, other potent CYP3A inhibitors such as other azole antifungals (eg, itraconazole, miconazole) or macrolide antibiotics (eg, erythromycin, clarithromycin) or cyclosporine or vinblastine may also lead to increases of tolterodine plasma concentrations (see **PRECAUTIONS** and **DOSAGE AND ADMINISTRATION**).

Warfarin: In healthy volunteers, coadministration of tolterodine immediate release 4 mg (2 mg bid) for 7 days and a single dose of warfarin 25 mg on day 4 had no effect on prothrombin time, Factor VII suppression, or on the pharmacokinetics of warfarin.

Oral Contraceptives: Tolterodine immediate release 4 mg (2 mg bid) had no effect on the pharmacokinetics of an oral contraceptive (ethinyl estradiol 30 µg/levonorgestrel 150 µg) as evidenced by the monitoring of ethinyl estradiol and levonorgestrel over a 2-month cycle in healthy female volunteers.

Diuretics: Coadministration of tolterodine immediate release up to 8 mg (4 mg bid) for up to 12 weeks with diuretic agents, such as indapamide, hydrochlorothiazide, triamterene, bendroflumethiazide, chlorothiazide, methylchlorothiazide, or furosemide, did not cause any adverse electrocardiographic (ECG) effects.

Cardiac Electrophysiology

The effect of 2 mg BID and 4 mg BID of tolterodine immediate release (IR) on the QT interval was evaluated in a 4-way crossover, double-blind, placebo- and active-controlled (moxifloxacin 400 mg QD) study in healthy male (N=25) and female (N=23) volunteers aged 18–55 years. Study subjects [approximately equal representation of CYP2D6 extensive metabolizers (EMs) and poor metabolizers (PMs)] completed sequential 4-day periods of dosing with moxifloxacin 400 mg QD, tolterodine 2 mg BID, tolterodine 4 mg BID, and placebo. The 4 mg BID dose of tolterodine IR (two times the highest recommended dose) was chosen because this dose results in tolterodine exposure similar to that observed upon coadministration of tolterodine 2 mg BID with potent CYP3A4 inhibitors in patients who are CYP2D6 poor metabolizers (see **PRECAUTIONS, Drug Interactions**). QT interval was measured over a 12-hour period following dosing, including the time of peak plasma concentration (T_{max}) of tolterodine and at steady state (Day 4 of dosing).

Table 2 summarizes the mean change from baseline to steady state in corrected QT interval (QTc) relative to placebo at the time of peak tolterodine (1 hour) and moxifloxacin (2 hour) concentrations. Both Fridericia's (QTcF) and a population-specific (QTcP) method were used to correct QT interval for heart rate. No single QT correction method is known to be more valid than others. QT interval was mea-

Table 1. Summary of Mean (±SD) Pharmacokinetic Parameters of Tolterodine and its Active Metabolite (5-hydroxymethyl metabolite) in Healthy Volunteers

	Tolterodine					5-Hydroxymethyl Metabolite			
Phenotype (CYP2D6)	t_{max} (h)	C_{max}* (µg/L)	C_{avg}* (µg/L)	$t_{1/2}$ (h)	CL/F (L/h)	t_{max} (h)	C_{max}* (µg/L)	C_{avg}* (µg/L)	$t_{1/2}$ (h)
Single-dose									
EM	1.6±1.5	1.6±1.2	0.50±0.35	2.0±0.7	534±697	1.8±1.4	1.8±0.7	0.62±0.26	3.1±0.7
PM	1.4±0.5	10±4.9	8.3±4.3	6.5±1.6	17±7.3	-†	-	-	-
Multiple-dose									
EM	1.2±0.5	2.6±2.8	0.58±0.54	2.2±0.4	415±377	1.2±0.5	2.4±1.3	0.92±0.46	2.9±0.4
PM	1.9±1.0	19±7.5	12±5.1	9.6±1.5	11±4.2	-	-	-	-

*Parameter was dose-normalized from 4 mg to 2 mg.
C_{max} = Maximum plasma concentration; t_{max} = Time of occurrence of C_{max}; C_{avg} = Average plasma concentration;
$t_{1/2}$ = Terminal elimination half-life; CL/F = Apparent oral clearance.
EM = Extensive metabolizers; PM = Poor metabolizers.
† - = not applicable.

sured manually and by machine, and data from both are presented. The mean increase of heart rate associated with a 4 mg/day dose of tolterodine in this study was 2.0 beats/minute and 6.3 beats/minute with 8 mg/day tolterodine. The change in heart rate with moxifloxacin was 0.5 beats/minute.
[See table 2 above]
The reason for the difference between machine and manual read of QT interval is unclear.
The QT effect of tolterodine immediate release tablets appeared greater for 8 mg/day (two times the therapeutic dose) compared to 4 mg/day. The effect of tolterodine 8 mg/day was not as large as that observed after four days of therapeutic dosing with the active control moxifloxacin. However, the confidence intervals overlapped.
Tolterodine's effect on QT interval was found to correlate with plasma concentration of tolterodine. There appeared to be a greater QTc interval increase in CYP2D6 poor metabolizers than in CYP2D6 extensive metabolizers after tolterodine treatment in this study.
This study was not designed to make direct statistical comparisons between drugs or dose levels. There has been no association of Torsade de Pointes in the international post-marketing experience with DETROL or DETROL LA (see **PRECAUTIONS, Patients with Congenital or Acquired QT Prolongation.**)

CLINICAL STUDIES

DETROL Tablets were evaluated for the treatment of overactive bladder with symptoms of urge urinary incontinence, urgency, and frequency in four randomized, double-blind, placebo-controlled, 12-week studies. A total of 853 patients received DETROL 2 mg twice daily and 685 patients received placebo. The majority of patients were Caucasian (95%) and female (78%), with a mean age of 60 years (range, 19 to 93 years). At study entry, nearly all patients perceived they had urgency and most patients had increased frequency of micturitions and urge incontinence. These characteristics were well balanced across treatment groups for the studies.
The efficacy endpoints for study 007 (see Table 3) included the change from baseline for:
• Number of incontinence episodes per week
• Number of micturitions per 24 hours (averaged over 7 days)
• Volume of urine voided per micturition (averaged over 2 days)
The efficacy endpoints for studies 008, 009, and 010 (see Table 4) were identical to the above endpoints with the exception that the number of incontinence episodes was per 24 hours (averaged over 7 days).
[See table 3 above]
[See table 4 above]

INDICATIONS AND USAGE

DETROL Tablets are indicated for the treatment of overactive bladder with symptoms of urge urinary incontinence, urgency, and frequency.

CONTRAINDICATIONS

DETROL Tablets are contraindicated in patients with urinary retention, gastric retention, or uncontrolled narrow-angle glaucoma. DETROL is also contraindicated in patients who have demonstrated hypersensitivity to the drug or its ingredients.

PRECAUTIONS
General
Risk of Urinary Retention and Gastric Retention: DETROL Tablets should be administered with caution to patients with clinically significant bladder outflow obstruction because of the risk of urinary retention and to patients with gastrointestinal obstructive disorders, such as pyloric stenosis, because of the risk of gastric retention (see **CONTRAINDICATIONS**).
Decreased Gastrointestinal Motility: DETROL, like other antimuscarinic drugs, should be used with caution in patients with decreased gastrointestinal motility.
Controlled Narrow-Angle Glaucoma: DETROL should be used with caution in patients being treated for narrow-angle glaucoma.
Reduced Hepatic and Renal Function: For patients with significantly reduced hepatic function or renal function, the recommended dose of DETROL is 1 mg twice daily (see **CLINICAL PHARMACOLOGY, Pharmacokinetics in Special Populations**).
Myasthenia Gravis: DETROL should be used with caution in patients with myasthenia gravis, a disease characterized by decreased cholinergic activity at the neuromuscular junction.

Patients with Congenital or Acquired QT Prolongation
In a study of the effect of tolterodine immediate release tablets on the QT interval (See **CLINICAL PHARMACOLOGY, Cardiac Electrophysiology**), the effect on the QT interval appeared greater for 8 mg/day (two times the therapeutic dose) compared to 4 mg/day and was more pronounced in CYP2D6 poor metabolizers (PM) than extensive metabolizers (EMs). The effect of tolterodine 8 mg/day was not as large as that observed after four days of therapeutic dosing with the active control moxifloxacin. However, the confidence intervals overlapped. These observations should be considered in clinical decisions to prescribe DETROL for patients with a known history of QT prolongation or patients who are taking Class IA (e.g., quinidine, procainamide) or Class III (e.g., amiodarone, sotalol) antiarrhythmic medications (see **PRECAUTIONS, Drug Interactions**).

Table 2. Mean (CI) change in QTc from baseline to steady state (Day 4 of dosing) at T_{max} (relative to placebo)

Drug/Dose	N	QTcF (msec) (manual)	QTcF (msec) (machine)	QTcP (msec) (manual)	QTcP (msec) (machine)
Tolterodine 2 mg BID[1]	48	5.01 (0.28, 9.74)	1.16 (-2.99, 5.30)	4.45 (-0.37, 9.26)	2.00 (-1.81, 5.81)
Tolterodine 4 mg BID[1]	48	11.84 (7.11, 16.58)	5.63 (1.48, 9.77)	10.31 (5.49, 15.12)	8.34 (4.53, 12.15)
Moxifloxacin 400 mg QD[2]	45	19.26[3] (15.49, 23.03)	8.90 (4.77, 13.03)	19.10[3] (15.32, 22.89)	9.29 (5.34, 13.24)

[1] At T_{max} of 1 hr; 95% Confidence Interval
[2] At T_{max} of 2 hr; 90% Confidence Interval
[3] The effect on QT interval with 4 days of moxifloxacin dosing in this QT trial may be greater than typically observed in QT trials of other drugs.

Table 3. 95% Confidence Intervals (CI) for the Difference between DETROL (2 mg bid) and Placebo for the Mean Change at Week 12 from Baseline in Study 007

	DETROL (SD) N=514	Placebo (SD) N=508	Difference (95% CI)
Number of Incontinence Episodes per Week			
Mean baseline	23.2	23.3	
Mean change from baseline	-10.6 (17)	-6.9 (15)	-3.7 (-5.7, -1.6)
Number of Micturitions per 24 Hours			
Mean baseline	11.1	11.3	
Mean change from baseline	-1.7 (3.3)	-1.2 (2.9)	-0.5* (-0.9, -0.1)
Volume Voided per Micturition (mL)			
Mean baseline	137	136	
Mean change from baseline	29 (47)	14 (41)	15* (9, 21)

SD = Standard Deviation.
*The difference between DETROL and placebo was statistically significant.

Table 4. 95% Confidence Intervals (CI) for the Difference between DETROL (2 mg bid) and Placebo for the Mean Change at Week 12 from Baseline in Studies 008, 009, 010

Study		DETROL (SD)	Placebo (SD)	Difference (95% CI)
Number of Incontinence Episodes per 24 Hours				
008	Number of patients	93	40	
	Mean baseline	2.9	3.3	
	Mean change from baseline	-1.3 (3.2)	-0.9 (1.5)	0.5 (-1.3,0.3)
009	Number of patients	116	55	
	Mean baseline	3.6	3.5	
	Mean change from baseline	-1.7 (2.5)	-1.3 (2.5)	-0.4 (-1.0,0.2)
010	Number of patients	90	50	
	Mean baseline	3.7	3.5	
	Mean change from baseline	-1.6 (2.4)	-1.1 (2.1)	-0.5 (-1.1,0.1)
Number of Micturitions per 24 Hours				
008	Number of patients	118	56	
	Mean baseline	11.5	11.7	
	Mean change from baseline	-2.7 (3.8)	-1.6 (3.6)	-1.2* (-2.0,-0.4)
009	Number of patients	128	64	
	Mean baseline	11.2	11.3	
	Mean change from baseline	-2.3 (2.1)	-1.4 (2.8)	-0.9* (-1.5,-0.3)
010	Number of patients	108	56	
	Mean baseline	11.6	11.6	
	Mean change from baseline	-1.7 (2.3)	-1.4 (2.8)	-0.38 (-1.1,0.3)
Volume Voided per Micturition (mL)				
008	Number of patients	118	56	
	Mean baseline	166	157	
	Mean change from baseline	38 (54)	6 (42)	32* (18,46)
009	Number of patients	129	64	
	Mean baseline	155	158	
	Mean change from baseline	36 (50)	10 (47)	26* (14,38)
010	Number of patients	108	56	
	Mean baseline	155	160	
	Mean change from baseline	31 (45)	13 (52)	18* (4,32)

SD = Standard Deviation.
*The difference between DETROL and placebo was statistically significant.

There has been no association of Torsade de Pointes in the international post-marketing experience with DETROL or DETROL LA.
Information for Patients
Patients should be informed that antimuscarinic agents such as DETROL may produce the following effects: blurred vision, dizziness, or drowsiness. Patients should be advised to exercise caution in decisions to engage in potentially dangerous activities until the drug's effects have been determined.
Drug Interactions
CYP3A4 Inhibitors: Ketoconazole, an inhibitor of the drug metabolizing enzyme CYP3A4, significantly increased plasma concentrations of tolterodine when coadministered to subjects who were poor metabolizers (see **CLINICAL PHARMACOLOGY**, Variability in Metabolism and **Drug-Drug Interactions**). For patients receiving ketoconazole or other potent CYP3A4 inhibitors such as other azole antifungals (e.g., itraconazole, miconazole) or macrolide antibiotics (e.g., erythromycin, clarithromycin) or cyclosporine or vinblastine, the recommended dose of DETROL is 1 mg twice daily (see **DOSAGE AND ADMINISTRATION**).
Drug-Laboratory-Test Interactions
Interactions between tolterodine and laboratory tests have not been studied.
Carcinogenesis, Mutagenesis, Impairment of Fertility
Carcinogenicity studies with tolterodine were conducted in mice and rats. At the maximum tolerated dose in mice (30 mg/kg/day), female rats (20 mg/kg/day), and male rats (30 mg/kg/day), AUC values obtained for tolterodine were 355, 291, and 462 µg·h/L, respectively. In comparison, the human AUC value for a 2-mg dose administered twice daily is estimated at 34 µg·h/L. Thus, tolterodine exposure in the

Continued on next page

Detrol—Cont.

carcinogenicity studies was 9- to 14-fold higher than expected in humans. No increase in tumors was found in either mice or rats.

No mutagenic effects of tolterodine were detected in a battery of *in vitro* tests, including bacterial mutation assays (Ames test) in 4 strains of *Salmonella typhimurium* and in 2 strains of *Escherichia coli*, a gene mutation assay in L5178Y mouse lymphoma cells, and chromosomal aberration tests in human lymphocytes. Tolterodine was also negative *in vivo* in the bone marrow micronucleus test in the mouse.

In female mice treated for 2 weeks before mating and during gestation with 20 mg/kg/day (corresponding to AUC value of about 500 µg·h/L), neither effects on reproductive performance or fertility were seen. Based on AUC values, the systemic exposure was about 15-fold higher in animals than in humans. In male mice, a dose of 30 mg/kg/day did not induce any adverse effects on fertility.

Pregnancy
Pregnancy Category C. At oral doses of 20 mg/kg/day (approximately 14 times the human exposure), no anomalies or malformations were observed in mice. When given at doses of 30 to 40 mg/kg/day, tolterodine has been shown to be embryolethal, reduce fetal weight, and increase the incidence of fetal abnormalities (cleft palate, digital abnormalities, intra-abdominal hemorrhage, and various skeletal abnormalities, primarily reduced ossification) in mice. At these doses, the AUC values were about 20- to 25-fold higher than in humans. Rabbits treated subcutaneously at a dose of 0.8 mg/kg/day achieved an AUC of 100 µg·h/L, which is about 3-fold higher than that resulting from the human dose. This dose did not result in any embryotoxicity or teratogenicity. There are no studies of tolterodine in pregnant women. Therefore, DETROL should be used during pregnancy only if the potential benefit for the mother justifies the potential risk to the fetus.

Nursing Mothers
Tolterodine is excreted into the milk in mice. Offspring of female mice treated with tolterodine 20 mg/kg/day during the lactation period had slightly reduced body weight gain. The offspring regained the weight during the maturation phase. It is not known whether tolterodine is excreted in human milk; therefore, DETROL should not be administered during nursing. A decision should be made whether to discontinue nursing or to discontinue DETROL in nursing mothers.

Pediatric Use
Efficacy in the pediatric population has not been demonstrated.

Two pediatric phase 3 randomized, placebo-controlled, double-blind, 12-week studies were conducted using tolterodine extended release (DETROL LA) capsules. A total of 710 pediatric patients (486 on DETROL LA and 224 on placebo) aged 5–10 years with urinary frequency and urge urinary incontinence were studied. The percentage of patients with urinary tract infections was higher in patients treated with DETROL LA (6.6%) compared to patients who received placebo (4.5%). Aggressive, abnormal and hyperactive behavior and attention disorders occurred in 2.9% of children treated with DETROL LA compared to 0.9% of children treated with placebo.

Geriatric Use
Of the 1120 patients who were treated in the four Phase 3, 12-week clinical studies of DETROL, 474 (42%) were 65 to 91 years of age. No overall differences in safety were observed between the older and younger patients (see **CLINICAL PHARMACOLOGY, Pharmacokinetics in Special Populations**).

ADVERSE REACTIONS

The Phase 2 and 3 clinical trial program for DETROL Tablets included 3071 patients who were treated with DETROL (N=2133) or placebo (N=938). The patients were treated with 1, 2, 4, or 8 mg/day for up to 12 months. No differences in the safety profile of tolterodine were identified based on age, gender, race, or metabolism.

The data described below reflect exposure to DETROL 2 mg bid in 986 patients and to placebo in 683 patients exposed for 12 weeks in five Phase 3, controlled clinical studies. Because clinical trials are conducted under widely varying conditions, adverse reaction rates observed in the clinical trials of a drug cannot be directly compared to rates in the clinical trials of another drug and may not reflect the rates observed in practice. The adverse reaction information from clinical trials does, however, provide a basis for identifying the adverse events that appear to be related to drug use and approximating rates.

Sixty-six percent of patients receiving DETROL 2 mg bid reported adverse events versus 56% of placebo patients. The most common adverse events reported by patients receiving DETROL were dry mouth, headache, constipation, vertigo/dizziness, and abdominal pain. Dry mouth, constipation, abnormal vision (accommodation abnormalities), urinary retention, and xerophthalmia are expected side effects of antimuscarinic agents.

Dry mouth was the most frequently reported adverse event for patients treated with DETROL 2 mg bid in the Phase 3 clinical studies, occurring in 34.8% of patients treated with DETROL and 9.8% of placebo-treated patients. One percent of patients treated with DETROL discontinued treatment due to dry mouth.

The frequency of discontinuation due to adverse events was highest during the first 4 weeks of treatment. Seven percent of patients treated with DETROL 2 mg bid discontinued treatment due to adverse events versus 6% of placebo patients. The most common adverse events leading to discontinuation of DETROL were dizziness and headache.

Three percent of patients treated with DETROL 2 mg bid reported a serious adverse event versus 4% of placebo patients. Significant ECG changes in QT and QTc have not been demonstrated in clinical-study patients treated with DETROL 2 mg bid. Table 5 lists the adverse events reported in 1% or more of the patients treated with DETROL 2 mg bid in the 12-week studies. The adverse events are reported regardless of causality.

[See table 5 below]

Post-marketing Surveillance
The following events have been reported in association with tolterodine use in worldwide post-marketing experience: *General:* anaphylactoid reactions, including angioedema; *Cardiovascular:* tachycardia, palpitations, peripheral edema; *Central/Peripheral Nervous:* confusion, disorientation, memory impairment, hallucinations.

Reports of aggravation of symptoms of dementia (e.g. confusion, disorientation, delusion) have been reported after tolterodine therapy was initiated in patients taking cholinesterase inhibitors for the treatment of dementia.

Because these spontaneously reported events are from the worldwide post-marketing experience, the frequency of events and the role of tolterodine in their causation cannot be reliably determined.

OVERDOSAGE

A 27-month-old child who ingested 5 to 7 DETROL Tablets 2 mg was treated with a suspension of activated charcoal and was hospitalized overnight with symptoms of dry mouth. The child fully recovered.

Management of Overdosage
Overdosage with DETROL can potentially result in severe central anticholinergic effects and should be treated accordingly.

ECG monitoring is recommended in the event of overdosage. In dogs, changes in the QT interval (slight prolongation of 10% to 20%) were observed at a suprapharmacologic dose of 4.5 mg/kg, which is about 68 times higher than the recommended human dose. In clinical trials of normal volunteers and patients, QT interval prolongation was observed with tolterodine immediate release at doses up to 8 mg (4 mg bid) and higher doses were not evaluated (see **PRECAUTIONS, Patients with Congenital** or **Acquired QT Prolongation**).

DOSAGE AND ADMINISTRATION

The initial recommended dose of DETROL Tablets is 2 mg twice daily. The dose may be lowered to 1 mg twice daily based on individual response and tolerability. For patients with significantly reduced hepatic or renal function or who are currently taking drugs that are potent inhibitors of CYP3A4, the recommended dose of DETROL is 1 mg twice daily (see **PRECAUTIONS, General** and **PRECAUTIONS, Drug Interactions**).

HOW SUPPLIED

DETROL Tablets 1 mg (white, round, biconvex, film-coated tablets engraved with arcs above and below the letters "TO") and **DETROL Tablets 2 mg** (white, round, biconvex, film-coated tablets engraved with arcs above and below the letters "DT") are supplied as follows:

Bottles of 60

1 mg	NDC 0009-4541-02
2 mg	NDC 0009-4544-02

Bottles of 500

1 mg	NDC 0009-4541-03
2 mg	NDC 0009-4544-03

Unit Dose Pack of 140

1 mg	NDC 0009-4541-01
2 mg	NDC 0009-4544-01

Store at 25°C (77°F); excursions permitted to 15–30°C (59–86°F) [see USP Controlled Room Temperature] (DTL).

Rx only

Distributed by:
Pharmacia & Upjohn Company
Division of Pfizer Inc, NY, NY 10017
LAB-0257-8.0
Revised March 2008

DETROL® LA   ℞
[dĕ-trŏl]
tolterodine tartrate
extended release capsules

Prescribing information for this product, which appears on pages 2619–2621 of the 2008 PDR, has been completely revised as follows. Please write "See Supplement A" next to the product heading.

DESCRIPTION

DETROL LA Capsules contain tolterodine tartrate. The active moiety, tolterodine, is a muscarinic receptor antagonist. The chemical name of tolterodine tartrate is (R)-N, N-diisopropyl-3-(2-hydroxy-5-methylphenyl)-3-phenylpropanamine L-hydrogen tartrate. The empirical formula of tolterodine tartrate is $C_{26}H_{37}NO_7$, and its molecular weight is 475.6. The structural formula of tolterodine tartrate is represented below.

Tolterodine tartrate is a white, crystalline powder. The pKa value is 9.87 and the solubility in water is 12 mg/mL. It is soluble in methanol, slightly soluble in ethanol, and practically insoluble in toluene. The partition coefficient (Log D) between n-octanol and water is 1.83 at pH 7.3.

DETROL LA for oral administration contains 2 mg or 4 mg of tolterodine tartrate. Inactive ingredients are sucrose, starch, hypromellose, ethylcellulose, medium chain triglycerides, oleic acid, gelatin, and FD&C Blue #2. The 2 mg capsules also contain yellow iron oxide. Both capsule strengths are imprinted with a pharmaceutical grade printing ink that contains shellac glaze, titanium dioxide, propylene glycol, and simethicone.

CLINICAL PHARMACOLOGY

Tolterodine is a competitive muscarinic receptor antagonist. Both urinary bladder contraction and salivation are mediated via cholinergic muscarinic receptors.

After oral administration, tolterodine is metabolized in the liver, resulting in the formation of the 5-hydroxymethyl derivative, a major pharmacologically active metabolite. The 5-hydroxymethyl metabolite, which exhibits an antimusca-

Table 5. Incidence* (%) of Adverse Events Exceeding Placebo Rate and Reported in >1% of Patients Treated with DETROL Tablets (2 mg bid) in 12-week, Phase 3 Clinical Studies

Body System	Adverse Event	% DETROL N=986	% Placebo N=683
Autonomic Nervous	accommodation abnormal	2	1
	dry mouth	35	10
General	chest pain	2	1
	fatigue	4	3
	headache	7	5
	influenza-like symptoms	3	2
Central/Peripheral Nervous	vertigo/dizziness	5	3
Gastrointestinal	abdominal pain	5	3
	constipation	7	4
	diarrhea	4	3
	dyspepsia	4	1
Urinary	dysuria	2	1
Skin/Appendages	dry skin	1	0
Musculoskeletal	arthralgia	2	1
Vision	xerophthalmia	3	2
Psychiatric	somnolence	3	2
Metabolic/Nutritional	weight gain	1	0
Resistance Mechanism	infection	1	0

* in nearest integer.

Table 1. Summary of Mean (±SD) Pharmacokinetic Parameters of Tolterodine Extended Release and its Active Metabolite (5-hydroxymethyl metabolite) in Healthy Volunteers

	Tolterodine				5-hydroxymethyl metabolite			
	t_{max}† (h)	C_{max} (μg/L)	C_{avg} (μg/L)	t½ (h)	t_{max}† (h)	C_{max} (μg/L)	C_{avg} (μg/L)	t½ (h)
Single dose 4 mg* EM	4(2–6)	1.3(0.8)	0.8(0.57)	8.4(3.2)	4(3–6)	1.6(0.5)	1.0(0.32)	8.8(5.9)
Multiple dose 4 mg EM	4(2–6)	3.4(4.9)	1.7(2.8)	6.9(3.5)	4(2–6)	2.7(0.90)	1.4(0.6)	9.9(4.0)
PM	4(3–6)	19(16)	13(11)	18(16)	—‡	—	—	—

* Parameter dose-normalized from 8 to 4 mg for the single-dose data.
C_{max} = Maximum serum concentration; t_{max} = Time of occurrence of C_{max};
C_{avg} = Average serum concentration; t½ = Terminal elimination half-life.
† Data presented as median (range).
‡ = not applicable.

Table 2: Mean (CI) change in QTc from baseline to steady state (Day 4 of dosing) at T_{max} (relative to placebo)

Drug/Dose	N	QTcF (msec) (manual)	QTcF (msec) (machine)	QTcP (msec) (manual)	QTcP (msec) (machine)
Tolterodine 2 mg BID[1]	48	5.01 (0.28, 9.74)	1.16 (-2.99, 5.30)	4.45 (-0.37, 9.26)	2.00 (-1.81, 5.81)
Tolterodine 4 mg BID[1]	48	11.84 (7.11, 16.58)	5.63 (1.48, 9.77)	10.31 (5.49, 15.12)	8.34 (4.53, 12.15)
Moxifloxacin 400 mg QD[2]	45	19.26[3] (15.49, 23.03)	8.90 (4.77, 13.03)	19.10[3] (15.32, 22.89)	9.29 (5.34, 13.24)

[1] At T_{max} of 1 hr; 95% Confidence Interval.
[2] At T_{max} of 2 hr; 90% Confidence Interval.
[3] The effect on QT interval with 4 days of moxifloxacin dosing in this QT trial may be greater than typically observed in QT trials of other drugs.

rinic activity similar to that of tolterodine, contributes significantly to the therapeutic effect. Both tolterodine and the 5-hydroxymethyl metabolite exhibit a high specificity for muscarinic receptors, since both show negligible activity or affinity for other neurotransmitter receptors and other potential cellular targets, such as calcium channels. Tolterodine has a pronounced effect on bladder function. Effects on urodynamic parameters before and 1 and 5 hours after a single 6.4-mg dose of tolterodine immediate release were determined in healthy volunteers. The main effects of tolterodine at 1 and 5 hours were an increase in residual urine, reflecting an incomplete emptying of the bladder, and a decrease in detrusor pressure. These findings are consistent with an antimuscarinic action on the lower urinary tract.

Pharmacokinetics

Absorption: In a study with ^{14}C-tolterodine solution in healthy volunteers who received a 5-mg oral dose, at least 77% of the radiolabeled dose was absorbed. C_{max} and area under the concentration-time curve (AUC) determined after dosage of tolterodine immediate release are dose-proportional over the range of 1 to 4 mg. Based on the sum of unbound serum concentrations of tolterodine and the 5-hydroxymethyl metabolite ("active moiety"), the AUC of tolterodine extended release 4 mg daily is equivalent to tolterodine immediate release 4 mg (2 mg bid). C_{max} and C_{min} levels of tolterodine extended release are about 75% and 150% of tolterodine immediate release, respectively. Maximum serum concentrations of tolterodine extended release are observed 2 to 6 hours after dose administration.

Effect of Food: There is no effect of food on the pharmacokinetics of tolterodine extended release.

Distribution: Tolterodine is highly bound to plasma proteins, primarily α_1-acid glycoprotein. Unbound concentrations of tolterodine average 3.7% ± 0.13% over the concentration range achieved in clinical studies. The 5-hydroxymethyl metabolite is not extensively protein bound, with unbound fraction concentrations averaging 36% ± 4.0%. The blood to serum ratio of tolterodine and the 5-hydroxymethyl metabolite averages 0.6 and 0.8, respectively, indicating that these compounds do not distribute extensively into erythrocytes. The volume of distribution of tolterodine following administration of a 1.28-mg intravenous dose is 113 ± 26.7 L.

Metabolism: Tolterodine is extensively metabolized by the liver following oral dosing. The primary metabolic route involves the oxidation of the 5-methyl group and is mediated by the cytochrome P450 2D6 (CYP2D6) and leads to the formation of a pharmacologically active 5-hydroxymethyl metabolite. Further metabolism leads to formation of the 5-carboxylic acid and *N*-dealkylated 5-carboxylic acid metabolites, which account for 51% ± 14% and 29% ± 6.3% of the metabolites recovered in the urine, respectively.

Variability in Metabolism: A subset (about 7%) of the Caucasian population is devoid of CYP2D6, the enzyme responsible for the formation of the 5-hydroxymethyl metabolite of tolterodine. The identified pathway of metabolism for these individuals ("poor metabolizers") is dealkylation via cytochrome P450 3A4 (CYP3A4) to *N*-dealkylated tolterodine. The remainder of the population is referred to as "extensive metabolizers." Pharmacokinetic studies revealed that tolterodine is metabolized at a slower rate in poor metabolizers than in extensive metabolizers; this results in significantly higher serum concentrations of tolterodine and in negligible concentrations of the 5-hydroxymethyl metabolite.

Excretion: Following administration of a 5-mg oral dose of ^{14}C-tolterodine solution to healthy volunteers, 77% of radioactivity was recovered in urine and 17% was recovered in feces in 7 days. Less than 1% (< 2.5% in poor metabolizers) of the dose was recovered as intact tolterodine, and 5% to 14% (<1% in poor metabolizers) was recovered as the active 5-hydroxymethyl metabolite.

A summary of mean (± standard deviation) pharmacokinetic parameters of tolterodine extended release and the 5-hydroxymethyl metabolite in extensive (EM) and poor (PM) metabolizers is provided in Table 1. These data were obtained following single and multiple doses of tolterodine extended release administered daily to 17 healthy male volunteers (13 EM, 4 PM).

[See table 1 above]

Pharmacokinetics in Special Populations

Age: In Phase 1, multiple-dose studies in which tolterodine immediate release 4 mg (2 mg bid) was administered, serum concentrations of tolterodine and of the 5-hydroxymethyl metabolite were similar in healthy elderly volunteers (aged 64 through 80 years) and healthy young volunteers (aged less than 40 years). In another Phase 1 study, elderly volunteers (aged 71 through 81 years) were given tolterodine immediate release 2 or 4 mg (1 or 2 mg bid). Mean serum concentrations of tolterodine and the 5-hydroxymethyl metabolite in these elderly volunteers were approximately 20% and 50% higher, respectively, than reported in young healthy volunteers. However, no overall differences were observed in safety between older and younger patients on tolterodine in the Phase 3, 12-week, controlled clinical studies; therefore, no tolterodine dosage adjustment for elderly patients is recommended (see **PRECAUTIONS, Geriatric Use**).

Pediatric: Efficacy in the pediatric population has not been demonstrated.

The pharmacokinetics of tolterodine extended release capsules have been evaluated in pediatric patients ranging in age from 11–15 years. The dose-plasma concentration relationship was linear over the range of doses assessed. Parent/metabolite ratios differed according to CYP2D6 metabolizer status: EMs had low serum concentrations of tolterodine and high concentrations of the active 5-hydroxymethyl metabolite, while PMs had high concentrations of tolterodine and negligible active metabolite concentrations.

Gender: The pharmacokinetics of tolterodine immediate release and the 5-hydroxymethyl metabolite are not influenced by gender. Mean C_{max} of tolterodine immediate release (1.6 μg/L in males versus 2.2 μg/L in females) and the active 5-hydroxymethyl metabolite (2.2 μg/L in males versus 2.5 μg/L in females) are similar in males and females who were administered tolterodine immediate release 2 mg. Mean AUC values of tolterodine (6.7 μg·h/L in males versus 7.8 μg·h/L in females) and the 5-hydroxymethyl metabolite (10 μg·h/L in males versus 11 μg·h/L in females) are also similar. The elimination half-life of tolterodine immediate release for both males and females is 2.4 hours, and the half-life of the 5-hydroxymethyl metabolite is 3.0 hours in females and 3.3 hours in males.

Race: Pharmacokinetic differences due to race have not been established.

Renal Insufficiency: Renal impairment can significantly alter the disposition of tolterodine immediate release and its metabolites. In a study conducted in patients with creatinine clearance between 10 and 30 mL/min, tolterodine immediate release and the 5-hydroxymethyl metabolite levels were approximately 2–3 fold higher in patients with renal impairment than in healthy volunteers. Exposure levels of other metabolites of tolterodine (e.g., tolterodine acid, *N*-dealkylated tolterodine acid, *N*-dealkylated tolterodine and *N*-dealkylated hydroxy tolterodine) were significantly higher (10–30 fold) in renally impaired patients as compared to the healthy volunteers. The recommended dose for patients with significantly reduced renal function is tolterodine 2 mg daily (see **PRECAUTIONS, General** and **DOSAGE AND ADMINISTRATION**).

Hepatic Insufficiency: Liver impairment can significantly alter the disposition of tolterodine immediate release. In a study of tolterodine immediate release conducted in cirrhotic patients, the elimination half-life of tolterodine immediate release was longer in cirrhotic patients (mean, 7.8 hours) than in healthy, young, and elderly volunteers (mean, 2 to 4 hours). The clearance of orally administered tolterodine immediate release was substantially lower in cirrhotic patients (1.0 ± 1.7 L/h/kg) than in the healthy volunteers (5.7 ± 3.8 L/h/kg). The recommended dose for patients with significantly reduced hepatic function is tolterodine 2 mg daily (see **PRECAUTIONS, General** and **DOSAGE AND ADMINISTRATION**).

Drug-Drug Interactions

Fluoxetine: Fluoxetine is a selective serotonin reuptake inhibitor and a potent inhibitor of CYP2D6 activity. In a study to assess the effect of fluoxetine on the pharmacokinetics of tolterodine immediate release and its metabolites, it was observed that fluoxetine significantly inhibited the metabolism of tolterodine immediate release in extensive metabolizers, resulting in a 4.8-fold increase in tolterodine AUC. There was a 52% decrease in C_{max} and a 20% decrease in AUC of the 5-hydroxymethyl metabolite. Fluoxetine thus alters the pharmacokinetics in patients who would otherwise be extensive metabolizers of tolterodine immediate release to resemble the pharmacokinetic profile in poor metabolizers. The sums of unbound serum concentrations of tolterodine immediate release and the 5-hydroxymethyl metabolite are only 25% higher during the interaction. No dose adjustment is required when tolterodine and fluoxetine are coadministered.

Other Drugs Metabolized by Cytochrome P450 Isoenzymes: Tolterodine immediate release does not cause clinically significant interactions with other drugs metabolized by the major drug metabolizing CYP enzymes. *In vivo* drug-interaction data show that tolterodine immediate release does not result in clinically relevant inhibition of CYP1A2, 2D6, 2C9, 2C19, or 3A4 as evidenced by lack of influence on the marker drugs caffeine, debrisoquine, S-warfarin, and omeprazole. *In vitro* data show that tolterodine immediate release is a competitive inhibitor of CYP2D6 at high concentrations (Ki 1.05 μM), while tolterodine immediate release as well as the 5-hydroxymethyl metabolite are devoid of any significant inhibitory potential regarding the other isoenzymes.

CYP3A4 Inhibitors: The effect of a 200-mg daily dose of ketoconazole on the pharmacokinetics of tolterodine immediate release was studied in 8 healthy volunteers, all of whom were poor metabolizers (see **Pharmacokinetics**, Variability in Metabolism for discussion of poor metabolizers). In the presence of ketoconazole, the mean C_{max} and AUC of tolterodine increased by 2 and 2.5 fold, respectively. Based on these findings, other potent CYP3A4 inhibitors such as other azole antifungals (eg, itraconazole, miconazole) or macrolide antibiotics (eg, erythromycin, clarithromycin) or cyclosporine or vinblastine may also lead to increases of tolterodine plasma concentrations (see **PRECAUTIONS** and **DOSAGE AND ADMINISTRATION**).

Warfarin: In healthy volunteers, coadministration of tolterodine immediate release 4 mg (2 mg bid) for 7 days and a single dose of warfarin 25 mg on day 4 had no effect on prothrombin time, Factor VII suppression, or on the pharmacokinetics of warfarin.

Oral Contraceptives: Tolterodine immediate release 4 mg (2 mg bid) had no effect on the pharmacokinetics of an oral contraceptive (ethinyl estradiol 30 μg/levonorgestrel 150 μg) as evidenced by the monitoring of ethinyl estradiol and levonorgestrel over a 2-month period in healthy female volunteers.

Diuretics: Coadministration of tolterodine immediate release up to 8 mg (4 mg bid) for up to 12 weeks with diuretic agents, such as indapamide, hydrochlorothiazide, triamterene, bendroflumethiazide, chlorothiazide, methylchlorothiazide, or furosemide, did not cause any adverse electrocardiographic (ECG) effects.

Cardiac Electrophysiology

The effect of 2 mg BID and 4 mg BID of Detrol immediate release (tolterodine IR) tablets on the QT interval was evaluated in a 4-way crossover, double-blind, placebo- and active-controlled (moxifloxacin 400 mg QD) study in healthy male (N=25) and female (N=23) volunteers aged 18–55 years. Study subjects [approximately equal representation

Continued on next page

Detrol LA—Cont.

of CYP2D6 extensive metabolizers (EMs) and poor metabolizers (PMs)] completed sequential 4-day periods of dosing with moxifloxacin 400 mg QD, tolterodine 2 mg BID, tolterodine 4 mg BID, and placebo. The 4 mg BID dose of tolterodine IR (two times the highest recommended dose) was chosen because this dose results in tolterodine exposure similar to that observed upon coadministration of tolterodine 2 mg BID with potent CYP3A4 inhibitors in patients who are CYP2D6 poor metabolizers (see **PRECAUTIONS, Drug Interactions**). QT interval was measured over a 12-hour period following dosing, including the time of peak plasma concentration (T_{max}) of tolterodine and at steady state (Day 4 of dosing).

Table 2 summarizes the mean change from baseline to steady state in corrected QT interval (QTc) relative to placebo at the time of peak tolterodine (1 hour) and moxifloxacin (2 hour) concentrations. Both Fridericia's (QTcF) and a population-specific (QTcP) method were used to correct QT interval for heart rate. No single QT correction method is known to be more valid than others. QT interval was measured manually and by machine, and data from both are presented. The mean increase of heart rate associated with a 4 mg/day dose of tolterodine in this study was 2.0 beats/minute and 6.3 beats/minute with 8 mg/day tolterodine. The change in heart rate with moxifloxacin was 0.5 beats/minute.

[See table 2 at top of previous page]

The reason for the difference between machine and manual read of QT interval is unclear.

The QT effect of tolterodine immediate release tablets appeared greater for 8 mg/day (two times the therapeutic dose) compared to 4 mg/day. The effect of tolterodine 8 mg/day was not as large as that observed after four days of therapeutic dosing with the active control moxifloxacin. However, the confidence intervals overlapped.

Tolterodine's effect on QT interval was found to correlate with plasma concentration of tolterodine. There appeared to be a greater QTc interval increase in CYP2D6 poor metabolizers than in CYP2D6 extensive metabolizers after tolterodine treatment in this study.

This study was not designed to make direct statistical comparisons between drugs or dose levels. There has been no association of Torsade de Pointes in the international post-marketing experience with DETROL or DETROL LA (see **PRECAUTIONS, Patients with Congenital or Acquired QT Prolongation**).

CLINICAL STUDIES

DETROL LA Capsules 2 mg were evaluated in 29 patients in a Phase 2 dose-effect study. DETROL LA 4 mg was evaluated for the treatment of overactive bladder with symptoms of urge urinary incontinence and frequency in a randomized, placebo-controlled, multicenter, double-blind, Phase 3, 12-week study. A total of 507 patients received DETROL LA 4 mg once daily in the morning and 508 received placebo. The majority of patients were Caucasian (95%) and female (81%), with a mean age of 61 years (range, 20 to 93 years). In the study, 642 patients (42%) were 65 to 93 years of age. The study included patients known to be responsive to tolterodine immediate release and other anticholinergic medications, however, 47% of patients never received prior pharmacotherapy for overactive bladder. At study entry, 97% of patients had at least 5 urge incontinence episodes per week and 91% of patients had 8 or more micturitions per day. The primary efficacy endpoint was change in mean number of incontinence episodes per week at week 12 from baseline. Secondary efficacy endpoints included change in mean number of micturitions per day and mean volume voided per micturition at week 12 from baseline.

[See table 3 above]

INDICATIONS AND USAGE

DETROL LA Capsules are once-daily extended release capsules indicated for the treatment of overactive bladder with symptoms of urge urinary incontinence, urgency, and frequency.

CONTRAINDICATIONS

DETROL LA Capsules are contraindicated in patients with urinary retention, gastric retention, or uncontrolled narrow-angle glaucoma. DETROL LA is also contraindicated in patients who have demonstrated hypersensitivity to the drug or its ingredients.

PRECAUTIONS

General

Risk of Urinary Retention and Gastric Retention: DETROL LA Capsules should be administered with caution to patients with clinically significant bladder outflow obstruction because of the risk of urinary retention and to patients with gastrointestinal obstructive disorders, such as pyloric stenosis, because of the risk of gastric retention (see **CONTRAINDICATIONS**).

Decreased Gastrointestinal Motility: DETROL LA, like other antimuscarinic drugs, should be used with caution in patients with decreased gastrointestinal motility.

Controlled Narrow-Angle Glaucoma: DETROL LA should be used with caution in patients being treated for narrow-angle glaucoma.

Reduced Hepatic and Renal Function: For patients with significantly reduced hepatic function or renal function, the recommended dose for DETROL LA is 2 mg daily (see

Table 3. 95% Confidence Intervals (CI) for the Difference between DETROL LA (4 mg daily) and Placebo for Mean Change at Week 12 from Baseline*

	DETROL LA (n=507)	Placebo (n=508)[†]	Treatment Difference, vs. Placebo (95% CI)
Number of incontinence episodes/week			
Mean Baseline	22.1	23.3	-4.8 [‡]
Mean Change from Baseline	-11.8 (SD 17.8)	-6.9 (SD 15.4)	(-6.9, -2.8)
Number of micturitions/day			
Mean Baseline	10.9	11.3	-0.6 [‡]
Mean Change from Baseline	-1.8 (SD 3.4)	-1.2 (SD 2.9)	(-1.0, -0.2)
Volume Voided per micturition (mL)			
Mean Baseline	141	136	20 [‡]
Mean Change from Baseline	34 (SD 51)	14 (SD 41)	(14, 26)

SD = Standard Deviation.
* Intent-to-treat analysis.
[†] 1 to 2 patients missing in placebo group for each efficacy parameter.
[‡] The difference between DETROL LA and placebo was statistically significant.

Table 4. Incidence* (%) of Adverse Events Exceeding Placebo Rate and Reported in ≥1% of Patients Treated with DETROL LA (4 mg daily) in a 12-week, Phase 3 Clinical Trial

Body System	Adverse Event	% DETROL LA n=505	% Placebo n=507
Autonomic Nervous	dry mouth	23	8
General	headache	6	4
	fatigue	2	1
Central/Peripheral Nervous	dizziness	2	1
Gastrointestinal	constipation	6	4
	abdominal pain	4	2
	dyspepsia	3	1
Vision	xerophthalmia	3	2
	vision abnormal	1	0
Psychiatric	somnolence	3	2
	anxiety	1	0
Respiratory	sinusitis	2	1
Urinary	dysuria	1	0

* in nearest integer.

CLINICAL PHARMACOLOGY, Pharmacokinetics in Special Populations).

Myasthenia Gravis: DETROL LA should be used with caution in patients with myasthenia gravis, a disease characterized by decreased cholinergic activity at the neuromuscular junction.

Patients with Congenital or Acquired QT Prolongation

In a study of the effect of tolterodine immediate release tablets on the QT interval (see **CLINICAL PHARMACOLOGY, Cardiac Electrophysiology**), the effect on the QT interval appeared greater for 8 mg/day (two times the therapeutic dose) compared to 4 mg/day and was more pronounced in CYP2D6 poor metabolizers (PM) than extensive metabolizers (EMs). The effect of tolterodine 8 mg/day was not as large as that observed after four days of therapeutic dosing with the active control moxifloxacin. However, the confidence intervals overlapped. These observations should be considered in clinical decisions to prescribe DETROL LA for patients with a known history of QT prolongation or patients who are taking Class IA (e.g., quinidine, procainamide) or Class III (e.g., amiodarone, sotalol) antiarrhythmic medications (see **PRECAUTIONS, Drug Interactions**). There has been no association of Torsade de Pointes in the international post-marketing experience with DETROL or DETROL LA.

Information for Patients

Patients should be informed that antimuscarinic agents such as DETROL LA may produce the following effects: blurred vision, dizziness, or drowsiness. Patients should be advised to exercise caution in decisions to engage in potentially dangerous activities until the drug's effects have been determined.

Drug Interactions

CYP3A4 Inhibitors: Ketoconazole, an inhibitor of the drug metabolizing enzyme CYP3A4, significantly increased plasma concentrations of tolterodine when coadministered to subjects who were poor metabolizers (see **CLINICAL PHARMACOLOGY**, Variability in Metabolism and **Drug-Drug Interactions**). For patients receiving ketoconazole or other potent CYP3A4 inhibitors such as other azole antifungals (e.g., itraconazole, miconazole) or macrolide antibiotics (eg, erythromycin, clarithromycin) or cyclosporine or vinblastine, the recommended dose of DETROL LA is 2 mg daily (see **DOSAGE AND ADMINISTRATION**).

Drug-Laboratory-Test Interactions

Interactions between tolterodine and laboratory tests have not been studied.

Carcinogenesis, Mutagenesis, Impairment of Fertility

Carcinogenicity studies with tolterodine immediate release were conducted in mice and rats. At the maximum tolerated dose in mice (30 mg/kg/day), female rats (20 mg/kg/day), and male rats (30 mg/kg/day), AUC values obtained for tolterodine were 355, 291, and 462 μg·h/L, respectively. In comparison, the human AUC value for a 2-mg dose administered twice daily is estimated at 34 μg·h/L. Thus, tolterodine exposure in the carcinogenicity studies was 9- to 14-fold higher than expected in humans. No increase in tumors was found in either mice or rats.

No mutagenic effects of tolterodine were detected in a battery of *in vitro* tests, including bacterial mutation assays (Ames test) in 4 strains of *Salmonella typhimurium* and in 2 strains of *Escherichia coli*, a gene mutation assay in L5178Y mouse lymphoma cells, and chromosomal aberration tests in human lymphocytes. Tolterodine was also negative *in vivo* in the bone marrow micronucleus test in the mouse.

In female mice treated for 2 weeks before mating and during gestation with 20 mg/kg/day (corresponding to AUC value of about 500 μg·h/L), neither effects on reproductive performance or fertility were seen. Based on AUC values, the systemic exposure was about 15-fold higher in animals than in humans. In male mice, a dose of 30 mg/kg/day did not induce any adverse effects on fertility.

Pregnancy

Pregnancy Category C. At oral doses of 20 mg/kg/day (approximately 14 times the human exposure), no anomalies or malformations were observed in mice. When given at doses of 30 to 40 mg/kg/day, tolterodine has been shown to be embryolethal and reduce fetal weight, and increase the incidence of fetal abnormalities (cleft palate, digital abnormalities, intra-abdominal hemorrhage, and various skeletal abnormalities, primarily reduced ossification) in mice. At these doses, the AUC values were about 20- to 25-fold higher than in humans. Rabbits treated subcutaneously at a dose of 0.8 mg/kg/day achieved an AUC of 100 μg·h/L, which is about 3-fold higher than that resulting from the human dose. This dose did not result in any embryotoxicity or teratogenicity. There are no studies of tolterodine in pregnant women. Therefore, DETROL LA should be used during

Bottles of 30	
2 mg Capsules	NDC 0009-5190-01
4 mg Capsules	NDC 0009-5191-01
Bottles of 90	
2 mg Capsules	NDC 0009-5190-02
4 mg Capsules	NDC 0009-5191-02
Bottles of 500	
2 mg Capsules	NDC 0009-5190-03
4 mg Capsules	NDC 0009-5191-03
Unit Dose Blisters	
2 mg Capsules	NDC 0009-5190-04
4 mg Capsules	NDC 0009-5191-04

pregnancy only if the potential benefit for the mother justifies the potential risk to the fetus.

Nursing Mothers

Tolterodine immediate release is excreted into the milk in mice. Offspring of female mice treated with tolterodine 20 mg/kg/day during the lactation period had slightly reduced body weight gain. The offspring regained the weight during the maturation phase. It is not known whether tolterodine is excreted in human milk; therefore, DETROL LA should not be administered during nursing. A decision should be made whether to discontinue nursing or to discontinue DETROL LA in nursing mothers.

Pediatric Use

Efficacy in the pediatric population has not been demonstrated.

A total of 710 pediatric patients (486 on DETROL LA, 224 on placebo) aged 5–10 with urinary frequency and urge incontinence were studied in two Phase 3 randomized, placebo-controlled, double-blind, 12-week studies. The percentage of patients with urinary tract infections was higher in patients treated with DETROL LA (6.6%) compared to patients who received placebo (4.5%). Aggressive, abnormal and hyperactive behavior and attention disorders occurred in 2.9% of children treated with DETROL LA compared to 0.9% of children treated with placebo.

Geriatric Use

No overall differences in safety were observed between the older and younger patients treated with tolterodine (see **CLINICAL PHARMACOLOGY, Pharmacokinetics in Special Populations**).

ADVERSE REACTIONS

The Phase 2 and 3 clinical trial program for DETROL LA Capsules included 1073 patients who were treated with DETROL LA (n=537) or placebo (n=536). The patients were treated with 2, 4, 6, or 8 mg/day for up to 15 months. Because clinical trials are conducted under widely varying conditions, adverse reaction rates observed in the clinical trials of a drug cannot be directly compared to rates in the clinical trials of another drug and may not reflect the rates observed in practice. The adverse reaction information from clinical trials does, however, provide a basis for identifying the adverse events that appear to be related to drug use and for approximating rates. The data described below reflect exposure to DETROL LA 4 mg once daily every morning in 505 patients and to placebo in 507 patients exposed for 12 weeks in the Phase 3, controlled clinical study.

Adverse events were reported in 52% (n=263) of patients receiving DETROL LA and in 49% (n=247) of patients receiving placebo. The most common adverse events reported by patients receiving DETROL LA were dry mouth, headache, constipation, and abdominal pain. Dry mouth was the most frequently reported adverse event for patients treated with DETROL LA occurring in 23.4% of patients treated with DETROL LA and 7.7% of placebo-treated patients. Dry mouth, constipation, abnormal vision (accommodation abnormalities), urinary retention, and dry eyes are expected side effects of antimuscarinic agents. A serious adverse event was reported by 1.4% (n=7) of patients receiving DETROL LA and by 3.6% (n=18) of patients receiving placebo.

The frequency of discontinuation due to adverse events was highest during the first 4 weeks of treatment. Similar percentages of patients treated with DETROL LA or placebo discontinued treatment due to adverse events. Treatment was discontinued due to adverse events and dry mouth was reported as an adverse event in 2.4% (n=12) of patients treated with DETROL LA and in 1.2% (n=6) of patients treated with placebo.

Table 4 lists the adverse events reported in 1% or more of patients treated with DETROL LA 4 mg once daily in the 12-week study. The adverse events were reported regardless of causality.

[See table 4 at top of previous page]

Post-marketing Surveillance

The following events have been reported in association with tolterodine use in worldwide post-marketing experience: *General:* anaphylactoid reactions, including angioedema; *Cardiovascular:* tachycardia, palpitations, peripheral edema; *Gastrointestinal:* diarrhea; *Central / Peripheral Nervous:* confusion, disorientation, memory impairment, hallucinations.

Reports of aggravation of symptoms of dementia (e.g. confusion, disorientation, delusion) have been reported after tolterodine therapy was initiated in patients taking cholinesterase inhibitors for the treatment of dementia.

Because these spontaneously reported events are from the worldwide post-marketing experience, the frequency of events and the role of tolterodine in their causation cannot be reliably determined.

OVERDOSAGE

A 27-month-old child who ingested 5 to 7 tolterodine immediate release tablets 2 mg was treated with a suspension of activated charcoal and was hospitalized overnight with symptoms of dry mouth. The child fully recovered.

Management of Overdosage

Overdosage with DETROL LA Capsules can potentially result in severe central anticholinergic effects and should be treated accordingly.

ECG monitoring is recommended in the event of overdosage. In dogs, changes in the QT interval (slight prolongation of 10% to 20%) were observed at a suprapharmacologic dose of 4.5 mg/kg, which is about 68 times higher than the recommended human dose. In clinical trials of normal volunteers and patients, QT interval prolongation was observed with tolterodine immediate release at doses up to 8 mg (4 mg bid) and higher doses were not evaluated (see **PRECAUTIONS, Patients with Congenital or Acquired QT Prolongation**).

DOSAGE AND ADMINISTRATION

The recommended dose of DETROL LA Capsules are 4 mg daily. DETROL LA should be taken once daily with liquids and swallowed whole. The dose may be lowered to 2 mg daily based on individual response and tolerability, however, limited efficacy data is available for DETROL LA 2 mg (see **CLINICAL STUDIES**).

For patients with significantly reduced hepatic or renal function or who are currently taking drugs that are potent inhibitors of CYP3A4, the recommended dose of DETROL LA is 2 mg daily (see **CLINICAL PHARMACOLOGY** and **PRECAUTIONS, Drug Interactions**).

HOW SUPPLIED

DETROL LA Capsules 2 mg are blue-green with symbol and 2 printed in white ink. DETROL LA Capsules 4 mg are blue with symbol and 4 printed in white ink. DETROL LA Capsules are supplied as follows:

[See table above]

Store at 25°C (77°F); excursions permitted to 15–30°C (59–86°F) [see USP Controlled Room Temperature]. Protect from light.

Rx only

Distributed by

Pharmacia & Upjohn Company

Division of Pfizer Inc, NY, NY 10017

LAB-0256-6.0

Revised March 2008

Purdue Pharma L.P.

ONE STAMFORD FORUM
STAMFORD, CT 06901-3431

For Medical Inquiries:
888-726-7535
Adverse Drug Experiences:
888-726-7535
Customer Service:
800-877-5666
FAX 800-877-3210

OXYCONTIN® Ⓒ Ⓡ

[*ŏks' ē-kŏn-tĭn*]

(OXYCODONE HCl CONTROLLED-RELEASE) TABLETS
10 mg 15 mg 20 mg 30 mg 40 mg 60 mg* 80 mg* 160 mg*

Prescribing information for this product, which appears on pages 2680–2685 of the 2008 PDR, has been completely revised as follows. Please write "See Supplement A" next to the product heading.

*** 60 mg, 80 mg, and 160 mg for use in opioid-tolerant patients only**

WARNING:

OxyContin is an opioid agonist and a Schedule II controlled substance with an abuse liability similar to morphine.

Oxycodone can be abused in a manner similar to other opioid agonists, legal or illicit. This should be considered when prescribing or dispensing OxyContin in situations where the physician or pharmacist is concerned about an increased risk of misuse, abuse, or diversion.

OxyContin Tablets are a controlled-release oral formulation of oxycodone hydrochloride indicated for the management of moderate to severe pain when a continuous, around-the-clock analgesic is needed for an extended period of time.

OxyContin Tablets are NOT intended for use as a prn analgesic.

OxyContin 60 mg, 80 mg, and 160 mg Tablets, or a single dose greater than 40 mg, ARE FOR USE IN OPIOID-TOLERANT PATIENTS ONLY. A single dose greater than 40 mg, or total daily doses greater than 80 mg, may cause fatal respiratory depression when administered to patients who are not tolerant to the respiratory depressant effects of opioids.

OxyContin TABLETS ARE TO BE SWALLOWED WHOLE AND ARE NOT TO BE BROKEN, CHEWED, OR CRUSHED. TAKING BROKEN, CHEWED, OR CRUSHED OxyContin TABLETS LEADS TO RAPID RELEASE AND ABSORPTION OF A POTENTIALLY FATAL DOSE OF OXYCODONE.

DESCRIPTION

OxyContin® (oxycodone hydrochloride controlled-release) Tablets are an opioid analgesic supplied in 10 mg, 15 mg, 20 mg, 30 mg, 40 mg, 60 mg, 80 mg, and 160 mg tablet strengths for oral administration. The tablet strengths describe the amount of oxycodone per tablet as the hydrochloride salt. The structural formula for oxycodone hydrochloride is as follows:

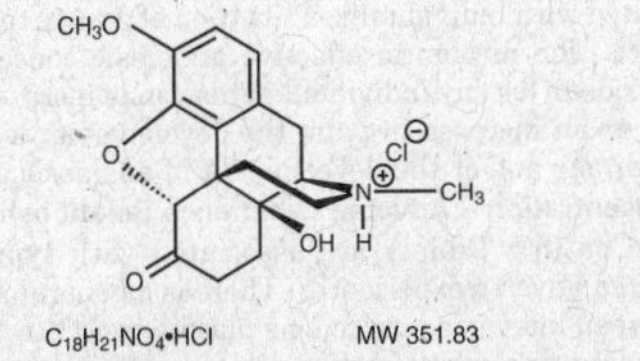

$C_{18}H_{21}NO_4$•HCl MW 351.83

The chemical formula is 4, 5α-epoxy-14-hydroxy-3-methoxy-17-methylmorphinan-6-one hydrochloride.

Oxycodone is a white, odorless crystalline powder derived from the opium alkaloid, thebaine. Oxycodone hydrochloride dissolves in water (1 g in 6 to 7 mL). It is slightly soluble in alcohol (octanol water partition coefficient 0.7). The tablets contain the following inactive ingredients: ammonio methacrylate copolymer, hypromellose, lactose, magnesium stearate, polyethylene glycol 400, povidone, sodium hydroxide, sorbic acid, stearyl alcohol, talc, titanium dioxide, and triacetin.

The 10 mg tablets also contain: hydroxypropyl cellulose.

The 15 mg tablets also contain: black iron oxide, yellow iron oxide, and red iron oxide.

The 20 mg tablets also contain: polysorbate 80 and red iron oxide.

The 30 mg tablets also contain: polysorbate 80, red iron oxide, yellow iron oxide, and black iron oxide.

The 40 mg tablets also contain: polysorbate 80 and yellow iron oxide.

The 60 mg tablets also contain: polysorbate 80 and FD&C Red No. 40 Aluminum Lake

The 80 mg tablets also contain: FD&C blue No. 2, hydroxypropyl cellulose, and yellow iron oxide.

The 160 mg tablets also contain: FD&C blue No. 2 and polysorbate 80.

CLINICAL PHARMACOLOGY

Oxycodone is a pure agonist opioid whose principal therapeutic action is analgesia. Other members of the class known as opioid agonists include substances such as morphine, hydromorphone, fentanyl, codeine, and hydrocodone. Pharmacological effects of opioid agonists include anxiolysis, euphoria, feelings of relaxation, respiratory depression, constipation, miosis, and cough suppression, as well as analgesia. Like all pure opioid agonist analgesics, with increasing doses there is increasing analgesia, unlike with mixed agonist/antagonists or non-opioid analgesics, where there is a limit to the analgesic effect with increasing doses. With pure opioid agonist analgesics, there is no defined maximum dose; the ceiling to analgesic effectiveness is imposed only by side effects, the more serious of which may include somnolence and respiratory depression.

Central Nervous System

The precise mechanism of the analgesic action is unknown. However, specific CNS opioid receptors for endogenous compounds with opioid-like activity have been identified throughout the brain and spinal cord and play a role in the analgesic effects of this drug.

Oxycodone produces respiratory depression by direct action on brain stem respiratory centers. The respiratory depression involves both a reduction in the responsiveness of the brain stem respiratory centers to increases in carbon dioxide tension and to electrical stimulation.

Oxycodone depresses the cough reflex by direct effect on the cough center in the medulla. Antitussive effects may occur with doses lower than those usually required for analgesia.

Oxycodone causes miosis, even in total darkness. Pinpoint pupils are a sign of opioid overdose but are not pathognomonic (e.g., pontine lesions of hemorrhagic or ischemic origin may produce similar findings). Marked mydriasis rather than miosis may be seen with hypoxia in the setting of OxyContin® overdose (See **OVERDOSAGE**).

Gastrointestinal Tract And Other Smooth Muscle

Oxycodone causes a reduction in motility associated with an increase in smooth muscle tone in the antrum of the stomach and duodenum. Digestion of food in the small intestine is delayed and propulsive contractions are decreased. Propulsive peristaltic waves in the colon are decreased, while tone may be increased to the point of spasm resulting in constipation. Other opioid-induced effects may include a reduction in gastric, biliary and pancreatic secretions, spasm of sphincter of Oddi, and transient elevations in serum amylase.

Continued on next page

OxyContin—Cont.

Cardiovascular System

Oxycodone may produce release of histamine with or without associated peripheral vasodilation. Manifestations of histamine release and/or peripheral vasodilation may include pruritus, flushing, red eyes, sweating, and/or orthostatic hypotension.

Concentration – Efficacy Relationships

Studies in normal volunteers and patients reveal predictable relationships between oxycodone dosage and plasma oxycodone concentrations, as well as between concentration and certain expected opioid effects, such as pupillary constriction, sedation, overall "drug effect", analgesia and feelings of "relaxation".

As with all opioids, the minimum effective plasma concentration for analgesia will vary widely among patients, especially among patients who have been previously treated with potent agonist opioids. As a result, patients must be treated with individualized titration of dosage to the desired effect. The minimum effective analgesic concentration of oxycodone for any individual patient may increase over time due to an increase in pain, the development of a new pain syndrome and/or the development of analgesic tolerance.

Concentration – Adverse Experience Relationships

OxyContin® Tablets are associated with typical opioid-related adverse experiences. There is a general relationship between increasing oxycodone plasma concentration and increasing frequency of dose-related opioid adverse experiences such as nausea, vomiting, CNS effects, and respiratory depression. In opioid-tolerant patients, the situation is altered by the development of tolerance to opioid-related side effects, and the relationship is not clinically relevant.

As with all opioids, the dose must be individualized (see **DOSAGE AND ADMINISTRATION**), because the effective analgesic dose for some patients will be too high to be tolerated by other patients.

PHARMACOKINETICS AND METABOLISM

The activity of OxyContin Tablets is primarily due to the parent drug oxycodone. OxyContin Tablets are designed to provide controlled delivery of oxycodone over 12 hours.

Breaking, chewing or crushing OxyContin Tablets eliminates the controlled delivery mechanism and results in the rapid release and absorption of a potentially fatal dose of oxycodone.

Oxycodone release from OxyContin Tablets is pH independent. Oxycodone is well absorbed from OxyContin Tablets with an oral bioavailability of 60% to 87%. The relative oral bioavailability of OxyContin to immediate-release oral dosage forms is 100%. Upon repeated dosing in normal volunteers in pharmacokinetic studies, steady-state levels were achieved within 24-36 hours. Dose proportionality and/or bioavailability has been established for the 10 mg, 20 mg, 40 mg, 80 mg, and 160 mg tablet strengths for both peak plasma levels (C_{max}) and extent of absorption (AUC). Oxycodone is extensively metabolized and eliminated primarily in the urine as both conjugated and unconjugated metabolites. The apparent elimination half-life of oxycodone following the administration of OxyContin® was 4.5 hours compared to 3.2 hours for immediate-release oxycodone.

Absorption

About 60% to 87% of an oral dose of oxycodone reaches the central compartment in comparison to a parenteral dose. This high oral bioavailability is due to low pre-systemic and/or first-pass metabolism. In normal volunteers, the t½ of absorption is 0.4 hours for immediate-release oral oxycodone. In contrast, OxyContin Tablets exhibit a biphasic absorption pattern with two apparent absorption half-lives of 0.6 and 6.9 hours, which describes the initial release of oxycodone from the tablet followed by a prolonged release.

Plasma Oxycodone by Time

Dose proportionality has been established for the 10 mg, 20 mg, 40 mg, and 80 mg tablet strengths for both peak plasma concentrations (C_{max}) and extent of absorption (AUC) (see Table 1 below). Another study established that the 160 mg tablet is bioequivalent to 2 × 80 mg tablets as well as to 4 × 40 mg for both peak plasma concentrations (C_{max}) and extent of absorption (AUC) (see Table 2 below). Given the short half-life of elimination of oxycodone from OxyContin®, steady-state plasma concentrations of oxycodone are achieved within 24-36 hours of initiation of dosing with OxyContin Tablets. In a study comparing 10 mg of OxyContin every 12 hours to 5 mg of immediate-release oxycodone every 6 hours, the two treatments were found to be equivalent for AUC and C_{max}, and similar for C_{min} (trough) concentrations.

[See figure at top of next column]

[See table 1 above]

[See table 2 above]

OxyContin® is NOT INDICATED FOR RECTAL ADMINISTRATION. Data from a study involving 21 normal volunteers show that OxyContin Tablets administered per rectum resulted in an AUC 39% greater and a C_{max} 9% higher than tablets administered by mouth. Therefore, there is an increased risk of adverse events with rectal administration.

Food Effects

Food has no significant effect on the extent of absorption of oxycodone from OxyContin. However, the peak plasma concentration of oxycodone increased by 25% when a OxyContin 160 mg Tablet was administered with a high-fat meal.

TABLE 1
Mean [% coefficient variation]

Regimen	Dosage Form	AUC (ng•hr/mL)†	C_{max} (ng/mL)	T_{max} (hrs)	Trough Conc. (ng/mL)
Single Dose	10 mg OxyContin	100.7 [26.6]	10.6 [20.1]	2.7 [44.1]	n.a.
	20 mg OxyContin	207.5 [35.9]	21.4 [36.6]	3.2 [57.9]	n.a.
	40 mg OxyContin	423.1 [33.3]	39.3 [34.0]	3.1 [77.4]	n.a.
	80 mg OxyContin*	1085.5 [32.3]	98.5 [32.1]	2.1 [52.3]	n.a.
Multiple Dose	10 mg OxyContin Tablets q12h	103.6 [38.6]	15.1 [31.0]	3.2 [69.5]	7.2 [48.1]
	5 mg immediate-release q6h	99.0 [36.2]	15.5 [28.8]	1.6 [49.7]	7.4 [50.9]

TABLE 2
Mean [% coefficient variation]

Regimen	Dosage Form	AUC_{∞} (ng•hr/mL)†	C_{max} (ng/mL)	T_{max} (hrs)	Trough Conc. (ng/mL)
Single Dose	4 × 40 mg OxyContin*	1935.3 [34.7]	152.0 [28.9]	2.56 [42.3]	n.a.
	2 × 80 mg OxyContin*	1859.3 [30.1]	153.4 [25.1]	2.78 [69.3]	n.a.
	1 × 160 mg OxyContin*	1856.4 [30.5]	156.4 [24.8]	2.54 [36.4]	n.a.

† for single-dose AUC = $AUC_{0\text{-}inf}$; for multiple-dose AUC = $AUC_{0\text{-}T}$
* data obtained while volunteers received naltrexone which can enhance absorption

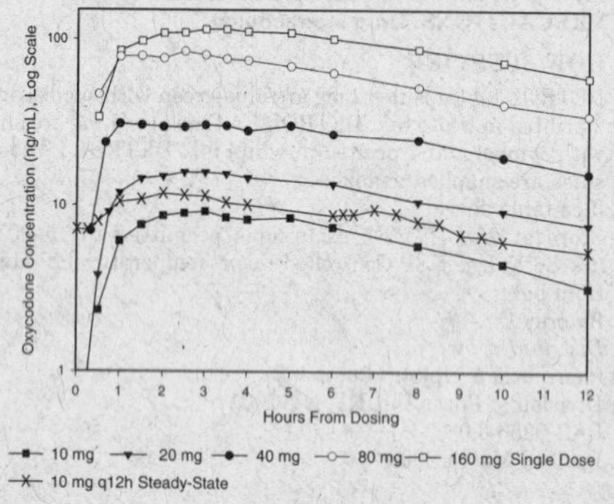

Distribution

Following intravenous administration, the volume of distribution (Vss) for oxycodone was 2.6 L/kg. Oxycodone binding to plasma protein at 37°C and a pH of 7.4 was about 45%. Once absorbed, oxycodone is distributed to skeletal muscle, liver, intestinal tract, lungs, spleen, and brain. Oxycodone has been found in breast milk (see **PRECAUTIONS**).

Metabolism

Oxycodone hydrochloride is extensively metabolized to noroxycodone, oxymorphone, noroxymorphone, and their glucuronides. The major circulating metabolite is noroxycodone with an AUC ratio of 0.6 relative to that of oxycodone. Noroxycodone is reported to be a considerably weaker analgesic than oxycodone. Oxymorphone, although possessing analgesic activity, is present in the plasma only in low concentrations. The correlation between oxymorphone concentrations and opioid effects was much less than that seen with oxycodone plasma concentrations. The analgesic activity profile of other metabolites is not known.

The formation of oxymorphone and noroxycodone is mediated by cytochrome P450 2D6 and cytochrome P450 3A4, respectively. In addition, noroxymorphone formation is mediated by both cytochrome P450 2D6 and cytochrome P450 3A4. Therefore, the formation of these metabolites can, in theory, be affected by other drugs (see **Drug-Drug Interactions**).

Excretion

Oxycodone and its metabolites are excreted primarily via the kidney. The amounts measured in the urine have been reported as follows: free oxycodone up to 19%; conjugated oxycodone up to 50%; free oxymorphone 0%; conjugated oxymorphone ≤ 14%; both free and conjugated noroxycodone have been found in the urine but not quantified. The total plasma clearance was 0.8 L/min for adults.

Special Populations

Elderly

The plasma concentrations of oxycodone are only nominally affected by age, being 15% greater in elderly as compared to young subjects.

Gender

Female subjects have, on average, plasma oxycodone concentrations up to 25% higher than males on a body weight adjusted basis. The reason for this difference is unknown.

Renal Impairment

Data from a pharmacokinetic study involving 13 patients with mild to severe renal dysfunction (creatinine clearance <60 mL/min) show peak plasma oxycodone and noroxycodone concentrations 50% and 20% higher, respectively, and AUC values for oxycodone, noroxycodone, and oxymorphone 60%, 50%, and 40% higher than normal subjects, respectively. This is accompanied by an increase in sedation but not by differences in respiratory rate, pupillary constriction, or several other measures of drug effect. There was an increase in t½ of elimination for oxycodone of only 1 hour (see **PRECAUTIONS**).

Hepatic Impairment

Data from a study involving 24 patients with mild to moderate hepatic dysfunction show peak plasma oxycodone and noroxycodone concentrations 50% and 20% higher, respectively, than normal subjects. AUC values are 95% and 65% higher, respectively. Oxymorphone peak plasma concentrations and AUC values are lower by 30% and 40%. These differences are accompanied by increases in some, but not other, drug effects. The t½ elimination for oxycodone increased by 2.3 hours (see **PRECAUTIONS**).

Drug-Drug Interactions (see PRECAUTIONS)

Oxycodone is metabolized in part by cytochrome P450 2D6 and cytochrome P450 3A4 and in theory can be affected by other drugs.

Oxycodone is metabolized in part by cytochrome P450 2D6 to oxymorphone which represents less than 15% of the total administered dose. This route of elimination may be blocked by a variety of drugs (e.g., certain cardiovascular drugs including amiodarone and quinidine as well as polycyclic antidepressants). However, in a study involving 10 subjects using quinidine, a known inhibitor of cytochrome P450 2D6, the pharmacodynamic effects of oxycodone were unchanged.

Pharmacodynamics

A single-dose, double-blind, placebo- and dose-controlled study was conducted using OxyContin® (10, 20, and 30 mg) in an analgesic pain model involving 182 patients with moderate to severe pain. Twenty and 30 mg of OxyContin were superior in reducing pain compared with placebo, and this difference was statistically significant. The onset of analgesic action with OxyContin occurred within 1 hour in most patients following oral administration.

CLINICAL TRIALS

A double-blind placebo-controlled, fixed-dose, parallel group, two-week study was conducted in 133 patients with chronic, moderate to severe pain, who were judged as having inadequate pain control with their current therapy. In this study, 20 mg OxyContin q12h but not 10 mg OxyContin q12h decreased pain compared with placebo, and this difference was statistically significant.

INDICATIONS AND USAGE

OxyContin Tablets are a controlled-release oral formulation of oxycodone hydrochloride indicated for the management of moderate to severe pain when a continuous, around-the-clock analgesic is needed for an extended period of time.

OxyContin is **NOT** intended for use as a prn analgesic.

Physicians should individualize treatment in every case, initiating therapy at the appropriate point along a progression from non-opioid analgesics, such as non-steroidal anti-inflammatory drugs and acetaminophen to opioids in a plan of pain management such as outlined by the World Health Organization, the Agency for Healthcare Research and Quality (formerly known as the Agency for HealthCare Policy and Research), the Federation of State Medical Boards Model Guidelines, or the American Pain Society.

OxyContin is not indicated for pain in the immediate postoperative period (the first 12-24 hours following surgery), or if the pain is mild, or not expected to persist for an extended period of time. OxyContin is only indicated for postoperative use if the patient is already receiving the drug prior to surgery or if the postoperative pain is expected to be moderate to severe and persist for an extended period of time. Physicians should individualize treatment, moving from parenteral to oral analgesics as appropriate. (See American Pain Society guidelines.)

CONTRAINDICATIONS

OxyContin® is contraindicated in patients with known hypersensitivity to oxycodone, or in any situation where opioids are contraindicated. This includes patients with significant respiratory depression (in unmonitored settings or the absence of resuscitative equipment), and patients with acute or severe bronchial asthma or hypercarbia. OxyContin is contraindicated in any patient who has or is suspected of having paralytic ileus.

WARNINGS

OXYCONTIN TABLETS ARE TO BE SWALLOWED WHOLE AND ARE NOT TO BE BROKEN, CHEWED, OR CRUSHED. TAKING BROKEN, CHEWED, OR CRUSHED OXYCONTIN TABLETS LEADS TO RAPID RELEASE AND ABSORPTION OF A POTENTIALLY FATAL DOSE OF OXYCODONE.

OxyContin 60 mg, 80 mg, and 160 mg Tablets, or a single dose greater than 40 mg, ARE FOR USE IN OPIOID-TOLERANT PATIENTS ONLY. A single dose greater than 40 mg, or total daily doses greater than 80 mg, may cause fatal respiratory depression when administered to patients who are not tolerant to the respiratory depressant effects of opioids.

Patients should be instructed against use by individuals other than the patient for whom it was prescribed, as such inappropriate use may have severe medical consequences, including death.

Misuse, Abuse and Diversion of Opioids

Oxycodone is an opioid agonist of the morphine-type. Such drugs are sought by drug abusers and people with addiction disorders and are subject to criminal diversion.

Oxycodone can be abused in a manner similar to other opioid agonists, legal or illicit. This should be considered when prescribing or dispensing OxyContin in situations where the physician or pharmacist is concerned about an increased risk of misuse, abuse, or diversion.

OxyContin has been reported as being abused by crushing, chewing, snorting, or injecting the dissolved product. These practices will result in the uncontrolled delivery of the opioid and pose a significant risk to the abuser that could result in overdose and death (see **WARNINGS** and **DRUG ABUSE AND ADDICTION**).

Concerns about abuse, addiction, and diversion should not prevent the proper management of pain.

Healthcare professionals should contact their State Professional Licensing Board, or State Controlled Substances Authority for information on how to prevent and detect abuse or diversion of this product.

Interactions with Alcohol and Drugs of Abuse

Oxycodone may be expected to have additive effects when used in conjunction with alcohol, other opioids, or illicit drugs that cause central nervous system depression.

DRUG ABUSE AND ADDICTION

OxyContin® contains oxycodone, which is a full mu-agonist opioid with an abuse liability similar to morphine and is a Schedule II controlled substance. Oxycodone, like morphine and other opioids used in analgesia, can be abused and is subject to criminal diversion.

Drug addiction is characterized by compulsive use, use for non-medical purposes, and continued use despite harm or risk of harm. There is a potential for drug addiction to develop following exposure to opioids, including oxycodone. Drug addiction is a treatable disease, utilizing a multidisciplinary approach, but relapse is common.

"Drug-seeking" behavior is very common in addicts and drug abusers. Drug-seeking tactics include emergency calls or visits near the end of office hours, refusal to undergo appropriate examination, testing or referral, repeated "loss" of prescriptions, tampering with prescriptions and reluctance to provide prior medical records or contact information for other treating physician(s). "Doctor shopping" to obtain additional prescriptions is common among drug abusers and people suffering from untreated addiction.

Abuse and addiction are separate and distinct from physical dependence and tolerance. Physicians should be aware that addiction may not be accompanied by concurrent tolerance and symptoms of physical dependence in all addicts. In addition, abuse of opioids can occur in the absence of true addiction and is characterized by misuse for non-medical purposes, often in combination with other psychoactive substances. OxyContin, like other opioids, has been diverted for non-medical use. Careful record-keeping of prescribing information, including quantity, frequency, and renewal requests is strongly advised.

Proper assessment of the patient, proper prescribing practices, periodic re-evaluation of therapy, and proper dispensing and storage are appropriate measures that help to limit abuse of opioid drugs.

OxyContin consists of a dual-polymer matrix, intended for oral use only. Abuse of the crushed tablet poses a hazard of overdose and death. This risk is increased with concurrent abuse of alcohol and other substances. With parenteral abuse, the tablet excipients, especially talc, can be expected to result in local tissue necrosis, infection, pulmonary granulomas, and increased risk of endocarditis and valvular heart injury. Parenteral drug abuse is commonly associated with transmission of infectious diseases such as hepatitis and HIV.

Respiratory Depression

Respiratory depression is the chief hazard from oxycodone, the active ingredient in OxyContin®, as with all opioid agonists. Respiratory depression is a particular problem in elderly or debilitated patients, usually following large initial doses in non-tolerant patients, or when opioids are given in conjunction with other agents that depress respiration.

Oxycodone should be used with extreme caution in patients with significant chronic obstructive pulmonary disease or

cor pulmonale, and in patients having a substantially decreased respiratory reserve, hypoxia, hypercapnia, or pre-existing respiratory depression. In such patients, even usual therapeutic doses of oxycodone may decrease respiratory drive to the point of apnea. In these patients alternative non-opioid analgesics should be considered, and opioids should be employed only under careful medical supervision at the lowest effective dose.

Head Injury

The respiratory depressant effects of opioids include carbon dioxide retention and secondary elevation of cerebrospinal fluid pressure, and may be markedly exaggerated in the presence of head injury, intracranial lesions, or other sources of pre-existing increased intracranial pressure. Oxycodone produces effects on pupillary response and consciousness which may obscure neurologic signs of further increases in intracranial pressure in patients with head injuries.

Hypotensive Effect

OxyContin may cause severe hypotension. There is an added risk to individuals whose ability to maintain blood pressure has been compromised by a depleted blood volume, or after concurrent administration with drugs such as phenothiazines or other agents which compromise vasomotor tone. Oxycodone may produce orthostatic hypotension in ambulatory patients. Oxycodone, like all opioid analgesics of the morphine-type, should be administered with caution to patients in circulatory shock, since vasodilation produced by the drug may further reduce cardiac output and blood pressure.

PRECAUTIONS

General

Opioid analgesics have a narrow therapeutic index in certain patient populations, especially when combined with CNS depressant drugs, and should be reserved for cases where the benefits of opioid analgesia outweigh the known risks of respiratory depression, altered mental state, and postural hypotension.

Use of OxyContin® is associated with increased potential risks and should be used only with caution in the following conditions: acute alcoholism; adrenocortical insufficiency (e.g., Addison's disease); CNS depression or coma; delirium tremens; debilitated patients; kyphoscoliosis associated with respiratory depression; myxedema or hypothyroidism; prostatic hypertrophy or urethral stricture; severe impairment of hepatic, pulmonary or renal function; and toxic psychosis.

The administration of oxycodone may obscure the diagnosis or clinical course in patients with acute abdominal conditions. Oxycodone may aggravate convulsions in patients with convulsive disorders, and all opioids may induce or aggravate seizures in some clinical settings.

Interactions with other CNS Depressants

OxyContin should be used with caution and started in a reduced dosage (1/3 to 1/2 of the usual dosage) in patients who are concurrently receiving other central nervous system depressants including sedatives or hypnotics, general anesthetics, phenothiazines, other tranquilizers, and alcohol. Interactive effects resulting in respiratory depression, hypotension, profound sedation, or coma may result if these drugs are taken in combination with the usual doses of OxyContin.

Interactions with Mixed Agonist/Antagonist Opioid Analgesics

Agonist/antagonist analgesics (i.e., pentazocine, nalbuphine, and butorphanol) should be administered with caution to a patient who has received or is receiving a course of therapy with a pure opioid agonist analgesic such as oxycodone. In this situation, mixed agonist/antagonist analgesics may reduce the analgesic effect of oxycodone and/or may precipitate withdrawal symptoms in these patients.

Ambulatory Surgery and Postoperative Use

OxyContin is not indicated for pre-emptive analgesia (administration pre-operatively for the management of postoperative pain).

OxyContin is not indicated for pain in the immediate postoperative period (the first 12 to 24 hours following surgery) for patients not previously taking the drug, because its safety in this setting has not been established.

OxyContin is not indicated for pain in the postoperative period if the pain is mild or not expected to persist for an extended period of time.

OxyContin is only indicated for postoperative use if the patient is already receiving the drug prior to surgery or if the postoperative pain is expected to be moderate to severe and persist for an extended period of time. Physicians should individualize treatment, moving from parenteral to oral analgesics as appropriate (See American Pain Society guidelines).

Patients who are already receiving OxyContin® Tablets as part of ongoing analgesic therapy may be safely continued on the drug if appropriate dosage adjustments are made considering the procedure, other drugs given, and the temporary changes in physiology caused by the surgical intervention (see **DOSAGE AND ADMINISTRATION**).

OxyContin and other morphine-like opioids have been shown to decrease bowel motility. Ileus is a common postoperative complication, especially after intra-abdominal surgery with opioid analgesia. Caution should be taken to monitor for decreased bowel motility in postoperative patients receiving opioids. Standard supportive therapy should be implemented.

Use in Pancreatic/Biliary Tract Disease

Oxycodone may cause spasm of the sphincter of Oddi and should be used with caution in patients with biliary tract disease, including acute pancreatitis. Opioids like oxycodone may cause increases in the serum amylase level.

Tolerance and Physical Dependence

Tolerance is the need for increasing doses of opioids to maintain a defined effect such as analgesia (in the absence of disease progression or other external factors). Physical dependence is manifested by withdrawal symptoms after abrupt discontinuation of a drug or upon administration of an antagonist. Physical dependence and tolerance are not unusual during chronic opioid therapy.

The opioid abstinence or withdrawal syndrome is characterized by some or all of the following: restlessness, lacrimation, rhinorrhea, yawning, perspiration, chills, myalgia, and mydriasis. Other symptoms also may develop, including: irritability, anxiety, backache, joint pain, weakness, abdominal cramps, insomnia, nausea, anorexia, vomiting, diarrhea, or increased blood pressure, respiratory rate, or heart rate.

In general, opioids should not be abruptly discontinued (see **DOSAGE AND ADMINISTRATION: Cessation of Therapy**).

Information for Patients/Caregivers

If clinically advisable, patients receiving OxyContin Tablets or their caregivers should be given the following information by the physician, nurse, pharmacist, or caregiver:

1. Patients should be aware that OxyContin Tablets contain oxycodone, which is a morphine-like substance.

2. Patients should be advised that OxyContin Tablets were designed to work properly only if swallowed whole. OxyContin Tablets will release all their contents at once if broken, chewed, or crushed, resulting in a risk of fatal overdose.

3. Patients should be advised to report episodes of breakthrough pain and adverse experiences occurring during therapy. Individualization of dosage is essential to make optimal use of this medication.

4. Patients should be advised not to adjust the dose of OxyContin® without consulting the prescribing professional.

5. Patients should be advised that OxyContin may impair mental and/or physical ability required for the performance of potentially hazardous tasks (e.g., driving, operating heavy machinery).

6. Patients should not combine OxyContin with alcohol or other central nervous system depressants (sleep aids, tranquilizers) except by the orders of the prescribing physician, because dangerous additive effects may occur, resulting in serious injury or death.

7. Women of childbearing potential who become, or are planning to become, pregnant should be advised to consult their physician regarding the effects of analgesics and other drug use during pregnancy on themselves and their unborn child.

8. Patients should be advised that OxyContin is a potential drug of abuse. They should protect it from theft, and it should never be given to anyone other than the individual for whom it was prescribed.

9. Patients should be advised that they may pass empty matrix "ghosts" (tablets) via colostomy or in the stool, and that this is of no concern since the active medication has already been absorbed.

10. Patients should be advised that if they have been receiving treatment with OxyContin for more than a few weeks and cessation of therapy is indicated, it may be appropriate to taper the OxyContin dose, rather than abruptly discontinue it, due to the risk of precipitating withdrawal symptoms. Their physician can provide a dose schedule to accomplish a gradual discontinuation of the medication.

11. Patients should be instructed to keep OxyContin in a secure place out of the reach of children. When OxyContin is no longer needed, the unused tablets should be destroyed by flushing down the toilet.

Use in Drug and Alcohol Addiction

OxyContin is an opioid with no approved use in the management of addictive disorders. Its proper usage in individuals with drug or alcohol dependence, either active or in remission is for the management of pain requiring opioid analgesia.

Drug-Drug Interactions

Opioid analgesics, including OxyContin®, may enhance the neuromuscular blocking action of skeletal muscle relaxants and produce an increased degree of respiratory depression. Oxycodone is metabolized in part by cytochrome P450 2D6 and cytochrome P450 3A4 and in theory can be affected by other drugs.

Oxycodone is metabolized in part to oxymorphone via cytochrome P450 2D6. While this pathway may be blocked by a variety of drugs (e.g., certain cardiovascular drugs including amiodarone and quinidine as well as polycyclic antidepressants), such blockade has not yet been shown to be of clinical significance with this agent. Clinicians should be aware of this possible interaction, however.

Use with CNS Depressants

OxyContin, like all opioid analgesics, should be started at 1/3 to 1/2 of the usual dosage in patients who are concurrently receiving other central nervous system depressants including sedatives or hypnotics, general anesthetics, phenothiazines, centrally acting anti-emetics, tranquilizers,

Continued on next page

OxyContin—Cont.

and alcohol because respiratory depression, hypotension, and profound sedation or coma may result. No specific interaction between oxycodone and monoamine oxidase inhibitors has been observed, but caution in the use of any opioid in patients taking this class of drugs is appropriate.

Carcinogenesis, Mutagenesis, Impairment of Fertility
Studies of oxycodone to evaluate its carcinogenic potential have not been conducted.

Oxycodone was not mutagenic in the following assays: Ames Salmonella and E. coli test with and without metabolic activation at doses of up to 5000 µg, chromosomal aberration test in human lymphocytes in the absence of metabolic activation at doses of up to 1500 µg/mL and with activation 48 hours after exposure at doses of up to 5000 µg/mL, and in the in vivo bone marrow micronucleus test in mice (at plasma levels of up to 48 µg/mL). Oxycodone was clastogenic in the human lymphocyte chromosomal assay in the presence of metabolic activation in the human chromosomal aberration test (at greater than or equal to 1250 µg/mL) at 24 but not 48 hours of exposure and in the mouse lymphoma assay at doses of 50 µg/mL or greater with metabolic activation and at 400 µg/mL or greater without metabolic activation.

Pregnancy
Teratogenic Effects - Category B: Reproduction studies have been performed in rats and rabbits by oral administration at doses up to 8 mg/kg and 125 mg/kg, respectively. These doses are 3 and 46 times a human dose of 160 mg/day, based on mg/kg basis. The results did not reveal evidence of harm to the fetus due to oxycodone. There are, however, no adequate and well-controlled studies in pregnant women. Because animal reproduction studies are not always predictive of human response, this drug should be used during pregnancy only if clearly needed.

Labor and Delivery
OxyContin® is not recommended for use in women during and immediately prior to labor and delivery because oral opioids may cause respiratory depression in the newborn. Neonates whose mothers have been taking oxycodone chronically may exhibit respiratory depression and/or withdrawal symptoms, either at birth and/or in the nursery.

Nursing Mothers
Low concentrations of oxycodone have been detected in breast milk. Withdrawal symptoms can occur in breast-feeding infants when maternal administration of an opioid analgesic is stopped. Ordinarily, nursing should not be undertaken while a patient is receiving OxyContin because of the possibility of sedation and/or respiratory depression in the infant.

Pediatric Use
Safety and effectiveness of OxyContin have not been established in pediatric patients below the age of 18. **It must be remembered that OxyContin Tablets cannot be crushed or divided for administration.**

Geriatric Use
In controlled pharmacokinetic studies in elderly subjects (greater than 65 years) the clearance of oxycodone appeared to be slightly reduced. Compared to young adults, the plasma concentrations of oxycodone were increased approximately 15% (see **PHARMACOKINETICS AND METABOLISM**). Of the total number of subjects (445) in clinical studies of OxyContin, 148 (33.3%) were age 65 and older (including those age 75 and older) while 40 (9.0%) were age 75 and older. In clinical trials with appropriate initiation of therapy and dose titration, no untoward or unexpected side effects were seen in the elderly patients who received OxyContin. Thus, the usual doses and dosing intervals are appropriate for these patients. As with all opioids, the starting dose should be reduced to 1/3 to 1/2 of the usual dosage in debilitated, non-tolerant patients. Respiratory depression is the chief hazard in elderly or debilitated patients, usually following large initial doses in non-tolerant patients, or when opioids are given in conjunction with other agents that depress respiration.

Laboratory Monitoring
Due to the broad range of plasma concentrations seen in clinical populations, the varying degrees of pain, and the development of tolerance, plasma oxycodone measurements are usually not helpful in clinical management. Plasma concentrations of the active drug substance may be of value in selected, unusual or complex cases.

Hepatic Impairment
A study of OxyContin in patients with hepatic impairment indicates greater plasma concentrations than those with normal function. The initiation of therapy at 1/3 to 1/2 the usual doses and careful dose titration is warranted.

Renal Impairment
In patients with renal impairment, as evidenced by decreased creatinine clearance (<60 mL/min), the concentrations of oxycodone in the plasma are approximately 50% higher than in subjects with normal renal function. Dose initiation should follow a conservative approach. Dosages should be adjusted according to the clinical situation.

Gender Differences
In pharmacokinetic studies, opioid-naive females demonstrate up to 25% higher average plasma concentrations and greater frequency of typical opioid adverse events than males, even after adjustment for body weight. The clinical relevance of a difference of this magnitude is low for a drug intended for chronic usage at individualized dosages, and there was no male/female difference detected for efficacy or adverse events in clinical trials.

ADVERSE REACTIONS

The safety of OxyContin® was evaluated in double-blind clinical trials involving 713 patients with moderate to severe pain of various etiologies. In open-label studies of cancer pain, 187 patients received OxyContin in total daily doses ranging from 20 mg to 640 mg per day. The average total daily dose was approximately 105 mg per day.

Serious adverse reactions which may be associated with OxyContin Tablet therapy in clinical use are those observed with other opioid analgesics, including respiratory depression, apnea, respiratory arrest, and (to an even lesser degree) circulatory depression, hypotension, or shock (see **OVERDOSAGE**).

The non-serious adverse events seen on initiation of therapy with OxyContin are typical opioid side effects. These events are dose-dependent, and their frequency depends upon the dose, the clinical setting, the patient's level of opioid tolerance, and host factors specific to the individual. They should be expected and managed as a part of opioid analgesia. The most frequent (>5%) include: constipation, nausea, somnolence, dizziness, vomiting, pruritus, headache, dry mouth, sweating, and asthenia.

In many cases the frequency of these events during initiation of therapy may be minimized by careful individualization of starting dosage, slow titration, and the avoidance of large swings in the plasma concentrations of the opioid. Many of these adverse events will cease or decrease in intensity as OxyContin therapy is continued and some degree of tolerance is developed.

Clinical trials comparing OxyContin with immediate-release oxycodone and placebo revealed a similar adverse event profile between OxyContin and immediate-release oxycodone. The most common adverse events (>5%) reported by patients at least once during therapy were:

TABLE 3

	OxyContin (n=227) (%)	Immediate-Release (n=225) (%)	Placebo (n=45) (%)
Constipation	(23)	(26)	(7)
Nausea	(23)	(27)	(11)
Somnolence	(23)	(24)	(4)
Dizziness	(13)	(16)	(9)
Pruritus	(13)	(12)	(2)
Vomiting	(12)	(14)	(7)
Headache	(7)	(8)	(7)
Dry Mouth	(6)	(7)	(2)
Asthenia	(6)	(7)	–
Sweating	(5)	(6)	(2)

The following adverse experiences were reported in OxyContin®-treated patients with an incidence between 1% and 5%. In descending order of frequency they were anorexia, nervousness, insomnia, fever, confusion, diarrhea, abdominal pain, dyspepsia, rash, anxiety, euphoria, dyspnea, postural hypotension, chills, twitching, gastritis, abnormal dreams, thought abnormalities, and hiccups.

The following adverse reactions occurred in less than 1% of patients involved in clinical trials or were reported in post-marketing experience.

Blood and lymphatic system disorders: lymphadenopathy

Cardiac disorders: palpitations (in the context of withdrawal)

Ear and labyrinth disorders: tinnitus

Endocrine disorders: syndrome of inappropriate antidiuretic hormone secretion (SIADH)

Eye disorders: abnormal vision

Gastrointestinal disorders: dysphagia, eructation, flatulence, gastrointestinal disorder, ileus, increased appetite, stomatitis

General disorders and administration site conditions: chest pain, edema, facial edema, malaise, pain, peripheral edema, thirst, withdrawal syndrome (with and without seizures)

Immune system disorders: anaphylactic or anaphylactoid reaction (symptoms of)

Infections and infestations: pharyngitis

Injury, poisoning and procedural complications: accidental injury

Investigations: hyponatremia, increased hepatic enzymes, ST depression

Metabolism and nutrition disorders: dehydration

Musculoskeletal and connective tissue disorders: neck pain

Nervous system disorders: abnormal gait, amnesia, hyperkinesia, hypertonia (muscular), hypesthesia, hypotonia, migraine, paresthesia, seizures, speech disorder, stupor, syncope, taste perversion, tremor, vertigo

Psychiatric disorders: agitation, depersonalization, depression, emotional lability, hallucination

Renal and urinary disorders: dysuria, hematuria, polyuria, urinary retention, urination impaired

Reproductive system and breast disorders: amenorrhea, decreased libido, impotence

Respiratory, thoracic and mediastinal disorders: cough increased, voice alteration

Skin and subcutaneous tissue disorders: dry skin, exfoliative dermatitis, urticaria

Vascular disorders: vasodilation

OVERDOSAGE

Acute overdosage with oxycodone can be manifested by respiratory depression, somnolence progressing to stupor or coma, skeletal muscle flaccidity, cold and clammy skin, constricted pupils, bradycardia, hypotension, and death.

Deaths due to overdose have been reported with abuse and misuse of OxyContin®, by ingesting, inhaling, or injecting the crushed tablets. Review of case reports has indicated that the risk of fatal overdose is further increased when OxyContin is abused concurrently with alcohol or other CNS depressants, including other opioids.

In the treatment of oxycodone overdosage, primary attention should be given to the re-establishment of a patent airway and institution of assisted or controlled ventilation. Supportive measures (including oxygen and vasopressors) should be employed in the management of circulatory shock and pulmonary edema accompanying overdose as indicated. Cardiac arrest or arrhythmias may require cardiac massage or defibrillation.

The pure opioid antagonists such as naloxone or nalmefene are specific antidotes against respiratory depression from opioid overdose. Opioid antagonists should not be administered in the absence of clinically significant respiratory or circulatory depression secondary to oxycodone overdose. In patients who are physically dependent on any opioid agonist including OxyContin, an abrupt or complete reversal of opioid effects may precipitate an acute abstinence syndrome. The severity of the withdrawal syndrome produced will depend on the degree of physical dependence and the dose of the antagonist administered. Please see the prescribing information for the specific opioid antagonist for details of their proper use.

DOSAGE AND ADMINISTRATION
General Principles
OXYCONTIN IS AN OPIOID AGONIST AND A SCHEDULE II CONTROLLED SUBSTANCE WITH AN ABUSE LIABILITY SIMILAR TO MORPHINE. OXYCODONE, LIKE MORPHINE AND OTHER OPIOIDS USED IN ANALGESIA, CAN BE ABUSED AND IS SUBJECT TO CRIMINAL DIVERSION.

OXYCONTIN TABLETS ARE TO BE SWALLOWED WHOLE AND ARE NOT TO BE BROKEN, CHEWED, OR CRUSHED. TAKING BROKEN, CHEWED, OR CRUSHED OXYCONTIN® TABLETS LEADS TO RAPID RELEASE AND ABSORPTION OF A POTENTIALLY FATAL DOSE OF OXYCODONE.

One OxyContin 160 mg tablet is comparable to two 80 mg tablets when taken on an empty stomach. With a high-fat meal, however, there is a 25% greater peak plasma concentration following one 160 mg tablet. Dietary caution should be taken when patients are initially titrated to 160 mg tablets (see DOSAGE AND ADMINISTRATION).

Patients should be started on the lowest appropriate dose (see **DOSAGE AND ADMINISTRATION: Initiation of Therapy**). In treating pain it is vital to assess the patient regularly and systematically. Therapy should also be regularly reviewed and adjusted based upon the patient's own reports of pain and side effects and the health professional's clinical judgment.

OxyContin Tablets are a controlled-release oral formulation of oxycodone hydrochloride indicated for the management of moderate to severe pain when a continuous, around-the-clock analgesic is needed for an extended period of time. The controlled-release nature of the formulation allows OxyContin to be effectively administered every 12 hours (see **CLINICAL PHARMACOLOGY; PHARMACOKINETICS AND METABOLISM**). While symmetric (same dose AM and PM), around-the-clock, q12h dosing is appropriate for the majority of patients, some patients may benefit from asymmetric (different dose given in AM than in PM) dosing, tailored to their pain pattern. It is usually appropriate to treat a patient with only one opioid for around-the-clock therapy.

Physicians should individualize treatment using a progressive plan of pain management such as outlined by the World Health Organization, the American Pain Society and the Federation of State Medical Boards Model Guidelines. Healthcare professionals should follow appropriate pain management principles of careful assessment and ongoing monitoring (see **BOXED WARNING**).

Initiation of Therapy
It is critical to initiate the dosing regimen for each patient individually, taking into account the patient's prior opioid and non-opioid analgesic treatment. Attention should be given to:

(1) the general condition and medical status of the patient;

(2) the daily dose, potency, and kind of the analgesic(s) the patient has been taking;

(3) the reliability of the conversion estimate used to calculate the dose of oxycodone;

(4) the patient's opioid exposure and opioid tolerance (if any);

(5) the **Special Instructions for OxyContin 60 mg, 80 mg, and 160 mg Tablets, or a Single Dose Greater Than 40 mg**; and

(6) the balance between pain control and adverse experiences.

Care should be taken to use low initial doses of OxyContin in patients who are not already opioid-tolerant, especially those who are receiving concurrent treatment with muscle relaxants, sedatives, or other CNS active medications (see **PRECAUTIONS: Drug-Drug Interactions**).

For initiation of OxyContin therapy for patients previously taking opioids, the conversion ratios from Foley, KM.

[NEJM, 1985; 313:84-95], found below, are a reasonable starting point, although not verified in well-controlled, multiple-dose trials.

Experience indicates a reasonable starting dose of OxyContin for patients who are taking non-opioid analgesics and require continuous around-the-clock therapy for an extended period of time is 10 mg q12h. If a non-opioid analgesic is being provided, it may be continued. OxyContin should be individually titrated to a dose that provides adequate analgesia and minimizes side effects.

1. Using standard conversion ratio estimates (see Table 4 below), multiply the mg/day of the previous opioids by the appropriate multiplication factors to obtain the equivalent total daily dose of oral oxycodone.
2. When converting from oxycodone, divide the 24-hour oxycodone dose in half to obtain the twice a day (q12h) dose of OxyContin.
3. Round down to a dose which is appropriate for the tablet strengths available.
4. Discontinue all other around-the-clock opioid drugs when OxyContin therapy is initiated.
5. No fixed conversion ratio is likely to be satisfactory in all patients, especially patients receiving large opioid doses. The recommended doses shown in Table 4 are only a starting point, and close observation and frequent titration are indicated until patients are stable on the new therapy.

TABLE 4
Multiplication Factors for Converting the Daily Dose of Prior Opioids to the Daily Dose of Oral Oxycodone*
(Mg/Day Prior Opioid × Factor = Mg/Day Oral Oxycodone)

	Oral Prior Opioid	Parenteral Prior Opioid
Oxycodone	1	—
Codeine	0.15	—
Hydrocodone	0.9	—
Hydromorphone	4	20
Levorphanol	7.5	15
Meperidine	0.1	0.4
Methadone	1.5	3
Morphine	0.5	3

*To be used only for conversion to oral oxycodone. For patients receiving high-dose parenteral opioids, a more conservative conversion is warranted. For example, for high-dose parenteral morphine, use 1.5 instead of 3 as a multiplication factor.

In all cases, supplemental analgesia should be made available in the form of a suitable short-acting analgesic.

OxyContin® can be safely used concomitantly with usual doses of non-opioid analgesics and analgesic adjuvants, provided care is taken to select a proper initial dose (see PRECAUTIONS).

Conversion from Transdermal Fentanyl to OxyContin
Eighteen hours following the removal of the transdermal fentanyl patch, OxyContin treatment can be initiated. Although there has been no systematic assessment of such conversion, a conservative oxycodone dose, approximately 10 mg q12h of OxyContin, should be initially substituted for each 25 μg/hr fentanyl transdermal patch. The patient should be followed closely for early titration, as there is very limited clinical experience with this conversion.

Managing Expected Opioid Adverse Experiences
Most patients receiving opioids, especially those who are opioid-naive, will experience side effects. Frequently the side effects from OxyContin are transient, but may require evaluation and management. Adverse events such as constipation should be anticipated and treated aggressively and prophylactically with a stimulant laxative and/or stool softener. Patients do not usually become tolerant to the constipating effects of opioids.

Other opioid-related side effects such as sedation and nausea are usually self-limited and often do not persist beyond the first few days. If nausea persists and is unacceptable to the patient, treatment with antiemetics or other modalities may relieve these symptoms and should be considered.

Patients receiving OxyContin® may pass an intact matrix "ghost" in the stool or via colostomy. These ghosts contain little or no residual oxycodone and are of no clinical consequence.

Individualization of Dosage
Once therapy is initiated, pain relief and other opioid effects should be frequently assessed. Patients should be titrated to adequate effect (generally mild or no pain with the regular use of no more than two doses of supplemental analgesia per 24 hours). Patients who experience breakthrough pain may require dosage adjustment or rescue medication. Because steady-state plasma concentrations are approximated within 24 to 36 hours, dosage adjustment may be carried out every 1 to 2 days. It is most appropriate to increase the q12h dose, not the dosing frequency. There is no clinical information on dosing intervals shorter than q12h. As a guideline, the total daily oxycodone dose usually can be increased by 25% to 50% of the current dose at each increase.

If signs of excessive opioid-related adverse experiences are observed, the next dose may be reduced. If this adjustment leads to inadequate analgesia, a supplemental dose of immediate-release oxycodone may be given. Alternatively, non-opioid analgesic adjuvants may be employed. Dose adjustments should be made to obtain an appropriate balance between pain relief and opioid-related adverse experiences.

If significant adverse events occur before the therapeutic goal of mild or no pain is achieved, the events should be treated aggressively. Once adverse events are under control, upward titration should continue to an acceptable level of pain control.

During periods of changing analgesic requirements, including initial titration, frequent contact is recommended between physician, other members of the healthcare team, the patient and the caregiver/family.

Special Instructions for OxyContin 60 mg, 80 mg, and 160 mg Tablets, or a Single Dose Greater Than 40 mg (for use in opioid-tolerant patients only)
OxyContin 60 mg, 80 mg, and 160 mg Tablets, or a single dose greater than 40 mg, are for use in opioid-tolerant patients only. A single daily dose greater than 40 mg, or total daily doses greater than 80 mg, may cause fatal respiratory depression when administered to patients who are not tolerant to the respiratory depressant effects of opioids. Patients should be instructed against use by individuals other than the patient for whom it was prescribed, as such inappropriate use may have severe medical consequences, including death.

One OxyContin® 160 mg tablet is comparable to two 80 mg tablets when taken on an empty stomach. With a high-fat meal, however, there is a 25% greater peak plasma concentration following one 160 mg tablet. Dietary caution should be taken when patients are initially titrated to 160 mg tablets.

Supplemental Analgesia
Most patients given around-the-clock therapy with controlled-release opioids may need to have immediate-release medication available for exacerbations of pain or to prevent pain that occurs predictably during certain patient activities (incident pain).

Maintenance of Therapy
The intent of the titration period is to establish a patient-specific q12h dose that will maintain adequate analgesia with acceptable side effects for as long as pain relief is necessary. Should pain recur then the dose can be incrementally increased to re-establish pain control. The method of therapy adjustment outlined above should be employed to re-establish pain control.

During chronic therapy, especially for non-cancer pain syndromes, the continued need for around-the-clock opioid therapy should be reassessed periodically (e.g., every 6 to 12 months) as appropriate.

Cessation of Therapy
When the patient no longer requires therapy with OxyContin Tablets, doses should be tapered gradually to prevent signs and symptoms of withdrawal in the physically dependent patient.

Conversion from OxyContin to Parenteral Opioids
To avoid overdose, conservative dose conversion ratios should be followed.

SAFETY AND HANDLING
OxyContin Tablets are solid dosage forms that contain oxycodone, which is a controlled substance. Like morphine, oxycodone is controlled under Schedule II of the Controlled Substances Act.

OxyContin has been targeted for theft and diversion by criminals. Healthcare professionals should contact their State Professional Licensing Board or State Controlled Substances Authority for information on how to prevent and detect abuse or diversion of this product.

HOW SUPPLIED
OxyContin® (oxycodone hydrochloride controlled-release) Tablets 10 mg are round, unscored, white-colored, convex tablets imprinted with OC on one side and 10 on the other. They are supplied as follows:
NDC 59011-100-10: child-resistant closure, opaque plastic bottles of 100
NDC 59011-100-20: unit dose packaging with 10 individually numbered tablets per card; two cards per glue end carton

OxyContin® (oxycodone hydrochloride controlled-release) Tablets 15 mg are round, unscored, gray-colored, convex tablets imprinted with OC on one side and 15 on the other. They are supplied as follows:
NDC 59011-815-10: child-resistant closure, opaque plastic bottles of 100

OxyContin® (oxycodone hydrochloride controlled-release) Tablets 20 mg are round, unscored, pink-colored, convex tablets imprinted with OC on one side and 20 on the other. They are supplied as follows:
NDC 59011-103-10: child-resistant closure, opaque plastic bottles of 100
NDC 59011-103-20: unit dose packaging with 10 individually numbered tablets per card; two cards per glue end carton

OxyContin® (oxycodone hydrochloride controlled-release) Tablets 30 mg are round, unscored, brown-colored, convex tablets imprinted with OC on one side and 30 on the other. They are supplied as follows:
NDC 59011-830-10: child-resistant closure, opaque plastic bottles of 100

OxyContin® (oxycodone hydrochloride controlled-release) Tablets 40 mg are round, unscored, yellow-colored, convex tablets imprinted with OC on one side and 40 on the other. They are supplied as follows:
NDC 59011-105-10: child-resistant closure, opaque plastic bottles of 100
NDC 59011-105-20: unit dose packaging with 10 individually numbered tablets per card; two cards per glue end carton

OxyContin® (oxycodone hydrochloride controlled-release) Tablets 60 mg are round, unscored, red-colored, convex tablets imprinted with OC on one side and 60 on the other. They are supplied as follows:
NDC 59011-860-10: child-resistant closure, opaque plastic bottles of 100

OxyContin® (oxycodone hydrochloride controlled-release) Tablets 80 mg are round, unscored, green-colored, convex tablets imprinted with OC on one side and 80 on the other. They are supplied as follows:
NDC 59011-107-10: child-resistant closure, opaque plastic bottles of 100
NDC 59011-107-20: unit dose packaging with 10 individually numbered tablets per card; two cards per glue end carton

OxyContin® (oxycodone hydrochloride controlled-release) Tablets 160 mg are caplet-shaped, unscored, blue-colored, convex tablets imprinted with OC on one side and 160 on the other. They are supplied as follows:
NDC 59011-109-10: child-resistant closure, opaque plastic bottles of 100
NDC 59011-109-20: unit dose packaging with 10 individually numbered tablets per card; two cards per glue end carton

Store at 25°C (77°F); excursions permitted between 15°-30°C (59°-86°F).
Dispense in tight, light-resistant container.
Healthcare professionals can telephone Purdue Pharma's Medical Services Department (1-888-726-7535) for information on this product.

CAUTION
DEA Order Form Required.
©2006, 2007, Purdue Pharma L.P.
Purdue Pharma L.P.
Stamford, CT 06901-3431
U.S. Patent Numbers 5,508,042 and 7,129,248
November 5, 2007
OT01343A
301371-0A

PATIENT INFORMATION

OXYCONTIN® Ⓒ
(Oxycodone HCl Controlled-Release) Tablets

> OxyContin® Tablets, 10 mg
> OxyContin® Tablets, 15 mg
> OxyContin® Tablets, 20 mg
> OxyContin® Tablets, 30 mg
> OxyContin® Tablets, 40 mg
> OxyContin® Tablets, 60 mg
> OxyContin® Tablets, 80 mg
> OxyContin® Tablets, 160 mg

Read this information carefully before you take OxyContin® (ox-e-CON-tin) tablets. Also read the information you get with your refills. There may be something new. This information does not take the place of talking with your doctor about your medical condition or your treatment. Only you and your doctor can decide if OxyContin is right for you. Share the important information in this leaflet with members of your household.

What Is The Most Important Information I Should Know About OxyContin®?
- Use OxyContin the way your doctor tells you to.
- Use OxyContin only for the condition for which it was prescribed.
- OxyContin is not for occasional ("as needed") use.
- **Swallow the tablets whole. Do not break, crush, dissolve, or chew them before swallowing.** OxyContin® works properly over 12 hours only when swallowed whole. **If a tablet is broken, crushed, dissolved, or chewed, the entire 12 hour dose will be absorbed into your body all at once. This can be dangerous, causing an overdose, and possibly death.**
- **Keep OxyContin® out of the reach of children.** Accidental overdose by a child is dangerous and may result in death.
- **Prevent theft and misuse.** OxyContin contains a narcotic painkiller that can be a target for people who abuse prescription medicines. Therefore, keep your tablets in a secure place, to protect them from theft. Never give them to anyone else. Selling or giving away this medicine is dangerous and against the law.

What is OxyContin®?
OxyContin® is a tablet that comes in several strengths and contains the medicine oxycodone (ox-e-KOE-done). This medicine is a painkiller like morphine. OxyContin treats moderate to severe pain that is expected to last for an extended period of time. Use OxyContin regularly during treatment. It contains enough medicine to last for up to twelve hours.

Who Should Not Take OxyContin®?
Do not take OxyContin® if
- your doctor did not prescribe OxyContin® for you.
- your pain is mild or will go away in a few days.
- your pain can be controlled by occasional use of other painkillers.
- you have severe asthma or severe lung problems.
- you have had a severe allergic reaction to codeine, hydrocodone, dihydrocodeine, or oxycodone (such as Tylox, Tylenol with Codeine, or Vicodin). A severe allergic reaction includes a severe rash, hives, breathing problems, or dizziness.
- you had surgery less than 12-24 hours ago and you were not taking OxyContin just before surgery.

Continued on next page

OxyContin—Cont.

Your doctor should know about all your medical conditions before deciding if OxyContin is right for you and what dose is best. Tell your doctor about all of your medical problems, especially the ones listed below:

- trouble breathing or lung problems
- head injury
- liver or kidney problems
- adrenal gland problems, such as Addison's disease
- convulsions or seizures
- alcoholism
- hallucinations or other severe mental problems
- past or present substance abuse or drug addiction

If any of these conditions apply to you, and you haven't told your doctor, then you should tell your doctor before taking OxyContin.

If you are pregnant or plan to become pregnant, talk with your doctor. OxyContin may not be right for you. **Tell your doctor if you are breast-feeding.** OxyContin will pass through the milk and may harm the baby.

Tell your doctor about all the medicines you take, including prescription and non-prescription medicines, vitamins, and herbal supplements. They may cause serious medical problems when taken with OxyContin, especially if they cause drowsiness.

How Should I Take OxyContin®?

- **Follow your doctor's directions exactly.** Your doctor may change your dose based on your reactions to the medicine. Do not change your dose unless your doctor tells you to change it. Do not take OxyContin more often than prescribed.
- **Swallow the tablets whole. Do not break, crush, dissolve, or chew before swallowing. If the tablets are not whole, your body will absorb too much medicine at one time. This can lead to serious problems, including overdose and death.**
- **If you miss a dose,** take it as soon as possible. If it is almost time for your next dose, skip the missed dose and go back to your regular dosing schedule. Do not take 2 doses at once unless your doctor tells you to.
- **In case of overdose,** call your local emergency number or Poison Control Center right away.
- **Review your pain regularly with your doctor** to determine if you still need OxyContin.
- **You may see tablets in your stools (bowel movements).** Do not be concerned. Your body has already absorbed the medicine.

If you continue to have pain or bothersome side effects, call your doctor.

Stopping OxyContin. Consult your doctor for instructions on how to stop this medicine slowly to avoid uncomfortable symptoms. You should not stop taking OxyContin all at once if you have been taking it for more than a few days.

After you stop taking OxyContin, flush the unused tablets down the toilet.

What Should I Avoid While Taking OxyContin®?

- **Do not drive, operate heavy machinery, or participate in any other possibly dangerous activities** until you know how you react to this medicine. OxyContin can make you sleepy.
- **Do not drink alcohol while using OxyContin. It may increase the chance of getting dangerous side effects.**
- **Do not take other medicines without your doctor's approval.** Other medicines include prescription and non-prescription medicines, vitamins, and supplements. Be especially careful about products that make you sleepy.

What are the Possible Side Effects of OxyContin®?

Call your doctor or get medical help right away if

- your breathing slows down
- you feel faint, dizzy, confused, or have any other unusual symptoms

Some of the common side effects of OxyContin® are nausea, vomiting, dizziness, drowsiness, constipation, itching, dry mouth, sweating, weakness, and headache. Some of these side effects may decrease with continued use.

There is a risk of abuse or addiction with narcotic painkillers. If you have abused drugs in the past, you may have a higher chance of developing abuse or addiction again while using OxyContin.

These are not all the possible side effects of OxyContin. For a complete list, ask your doctor or pharmacist.

General Advice About OxyContin

- Do not use OxyContin for conditions for which it was not prescribed.
- Do not give OxyContin to other people, even if they have the same symptoms you have. Sharing is illegal and may cause severe medical problems, including death.

This leaflet summarizes the most important information about OxyContin. If you would like more information, talk with your doctor. Also, you can ask your pharmacist or doctor for information about OxyContin that is written for health professionals.

Rx Only

©2006, 2007, Purdue Pharma L.P.

Purdue Pharma L.P.
Stamford, CT 06901-3431
November 5, 2007
OT01343A
301371-0A

Roche Laboratories Inc.
340 KINGSLAND STREET
NUTLEY, NJ 07110-1199
http://www.rocheusa.com

For Medical Information:
(24-hour service in emergencies), including routine inquiries, adverse drug events and product complaints:
Call: 1-800-526-6367
Fax: 1-800-532-3931 (product inquiries and complaints)
Fax: 973-562-3571 (adverse drug events)
Write: Professional Product Information
For Roche Patient Assistance Foundation Program
Call: 1-877-75-ROCHE (1-877-757-6243)
Write: Roche Patient Assistance Foundation
Order Fulfillment:
Call: 1-800-526-0625

TAMIFLU® ℞
[tă'-mĭ-flew]
(oseltamivir phosphate)
CAPSULES AND FOR ORAL SUSPENSION
℞ Only

Prescribing information for this product, which appears on pages 2753–2757 of the 2008 PDR, has been revised as follows. Please write "See Supplement A" next to the product heading.
The following subsections of **MICROBIOLOGY** *have been revised as follows:*

MICROBIOLOGY

Mechanism of Action

Oseltamivir phosphate is an ethyl ester prodrug requiring ester hydrolysis for conversion to the active form, oseltamivir carboxylate. Oseltamivir carboxylate is an inhibitor of influenza virus neuraminidase affecting release of viral particles.

Antiviral Activity

The antiviral activity of oseltamivir carboxylate against laboratory strains and clinical isolates of influenza virus was determined in cell culture assays. The concentrations of oseltamivir carboxylate required for inhibition of influenza virus were highly variable depending on the assay method used and the virus tested. The 50% and 90% effective concentrations (EC_{50} and EC_{90}) were in the range of 0.0008 μM to >35 μM and 0.004 μM to >100 μM, respectively (1 μM=0.284 μg/mL). The relationship between the antiviral activity in cell culture and the inhibition of influenza virus replication in humans has not been established.

Resistance

Influenza A virus isolates with reduced susceptibility to oseltamivir carboxylate have been recovered by serial passage of virus in cell culture in the presence of increasing concentrations of oseltamivir carboxylate. Genetic analysis of these isolates showed that reduced susceptibility to oseltamivir carboxylate is associated with mutations that result in amino acid changes in the viral neuraminidase or viral hemagglutinin or both. Resistance substitutions selected in cell culture in neuraminidase are I222T and H274Y in influenza A N1 and I222T and R292K in influenza A N2. Substitutions E119V, R292K and R305Q have been selected in avian influenza A neuraminidase N9. Substitutions A28T and R124M have been selected in the hemagglutinin of influenza A H3N2 and substitution H154Q in the hemagglutinin of a reassortant human/avian virus H1N9.

In clinical studies in the treatment of naturally acquired infection with influenza virus, 1.3% (4/301) of posttreatment isolates in adult patients and adolescents, and 8.6% (9/105) in pediatric patients aged 1 to 12 years showed emergence of influenza variants with decreased neuraminidase susceptibility in cell culture to oseltamivir carboxylate. Substitutions in influenza A neuraminidase resulting in decreased susceptibility were H274Y in neuraminidase N1 and E119V and R292K in neuraminidase N2. Insufficient information is available to fully characterize the risk of emergence of TAMIFLU resistance in clinical use.

In clinical studies of postexposure and seasonal prophylaxis, determination of resistance by population nucleotide sequence analysis was limited by the low overall incidence rate of influenza infection and prophylactic effect of TAMIFLU.

Cross-resistance

Cross-resistance between zanamivir-resistant influenza mutants and oseltamivir-resistant influenza mutants has been observed in cell culture. Due to limitations in the assays available to detect drug-induced shifts in virus susceptibility, an estimate of the incidence of oseltamivir resistance and possible cross-resistance to zanamivir in clinical isolates cannot be made. However, two of the three oseltamivir-induced substitutions (E119V, H274Y and R292K) in the viral neuraminidase from clinical isolates occur at the same amino acid residues as two of the three substitutions (E119G/A/D, R152K and R292K) observed in zanamivir-resistant virus.

The following subsection of **CLINICAL PHARMACOLOGY** *has been revised as follows:*

CLINICAL PHARMACOLOGY

Special Populations

Hepatic Impairment

In clinical studies oseltamivir carboxylate exposure was not altered in patients with mild or moderate hepatic impairment (see **PRECAUTIONS: Hepatic Impairment** and **DOSAGE AND ADMINISTRATION**).

The following subsections of **PRECAUTIONS** *have been revised as follows:*

PRECAUTIONS

Hepatic Impairment

The safety and pharmacokinetics in patients with severe hepatic impairment have not been evaluated (see **DOSAGE AND ADMINISTRATION**).

Neuropsychiatric Events

Influenza can be associated with a variety of neurologic and behavioral symptoms which can include events such as hallucinations, delirium, and abnormal behavior, in some cases resulting in fatal outcomes. These events may occur in the setting of encephalitis or encephalopathy but can occur without obvious severe disease.

There have been postmarketing reports (mostly from Japan) of delirium and abnormal behavior leading to injury, and in some cases resulting in fatal outcomes, in patients with influenza who were receiving TAMIFLU. Because these events were reported voluntarily during clinical practice, estimates of frequency cannot be made but they appear to be uncommon based on TAMIFLU usage data. These events were reported primarily among pediatric patients and often had an abrupt onset and rapid resolution. The contribution of TAMIFLU to these events has not been established. Patients with influenza should be closely monitored for signs of abnormal behavior. If neuropsychiatric symptoms occur, the risks and benefits of continuing treatment should be evaluated for each patient.

Information for Patients

A bottle of 13 g TAMIFLU for Oral Suspension contains approximately 11 g sorbitol. One dose of 75 mg TAMIFLU for Oral Suspension delivers 2 g sorbitol. For patients with hereditary fructose intolerance, this is above the daily maximum limit of sorbitol and may cause dyspepsia and diarrhea.

Drug Interactions

The concurrent use of TAMIFLU with live attenuated influenza vaccine (LAIV) intranasal has not been evaluated. However, because of the potential for interference between these products, LAIV should not be administered within 2 weeks before or 48 hours after administration of TAMIFLU, unless medically indicated. The concern about possible interference arises from the potential for antiviral drugs to inhibit replication of live vaccine virus. Trivalent inactivated influenza vaccine can be administered at any time relative to use of TAMIFLU.

Information derived from pharmacology and pharmacokinetic studies of oseltamivir suggests that clinically significant drug interactions are unlikely.

Oseltamivir is extensively converted to oseltamivir carboxylate by esterases, located predominantly in the liver. Drug interactions involving competition for esterases have not been extensively reported in literature. Low protein binding of oseltamivir and oseltamivir carboxylate reported in literature. Low protein binding of oseltamivir and oseltamivir carboxylate suggests that the probability of drug displacement interactions is low.

In vitro studies demonstrate that neither oseltamivir nor oseltamivir carboxylate is a good substrate for P450 mixed-function oxidases or for glucuronyl transferases.

Clinically important drug interactions involving competition for renal tubular secretion are unlikely due to the known safety margin for most of these drugs, the elimination characteristics of oseltamivir carboxylate (glomerular filtration and anionic tubular secretion) and the excretion capacity of these pathways. Coadministration of probenecid results in an approximate twofold increase in exposure to oseltamivir carboxylate due to a decrease in active anionic tubular secretion in the kidney. However, due to the safety margin of oseltamivir carboxylate, no dose adjustments are required when coadministering with probenecid.

No pharmacokinetic interactions have been observed when coadministering oseltamivir with amoxicillin, acetaminophen, cimetidine or with antacids (magnesium and aluminum hydroxides and calcium carbonates).

Carcinogenesis, Mutagenesis, and Impairment of Fertility

In 2-year carcinogenicity studies in mice and rats given daily oral doses of the pro-drug oseltamivir phosphate up to 400 mg/kg and 500 mg/kg, respectively, the pro-drug oseltamivir phosphate and the active form oseltamivir carboxylate induced no statistically significant increases in tumors over controls. The mean maximum daily exposures to the prodrug in mice and rats were approximately 130- and 320-fold, respectively, greater than those in humans at the proposed clinical dose based on AUC comparisons. The respective safety margins of the exposures to the active oseltamivir carboxylate were 15- and 50-fold.

The following subsection of **ADVERSE REACTIONS** *has been revised as follows:*

ADVERSE REACTIONS

Observed During Clinical Practice

The following adverse reactions have been identified during postmarketing use of TAMIFLU. Because these reactions are reported voluntarily from a population of uncertain size, it is not possible to reliably estimate their frequency or establish a causal relationship to TAMIFLU exposure.

Body as a Whole: Swelling of the face or tongue, allergy, anaphylactic/anaphylactoid reactions
Dermatologic: Dermatitis, rash, eczema, urticaria, erythema multiforme, Stevens-Johnson Syndrome, toxic epidermal necrolysis (see **PRECAUTIONS**)
Digestive: Hepatitis, liver function tests abnormal
Cardiac: Arrhythmia
Gastrointestinal disorders: Gastrointestinal bleeding, hemorrhagic colitis
Neurologic: Seizure
Metabolic: Aggravation of diabetes
Psychiatric: Delirium, including symptoms such as altered level of consciousness, confusion, abnormal behavior, delusions, hallucinations, agitation, anxiety, nightmares (see **PRECAUTIONS**)

The following subsection of **DOSAGE AND ADMINISTRATION** *has been revised as follows:*

DOSAGE AND ADMINISTRATION

Special Dosage Instructions

Hepatic Impairment

No dose adjustment is recommended for patients with mild or moderate hepatic impairment (Child-Pugh score ≤9) (see **CLINICAL PHARMACOLOGY: Pharmacokinetics: Special Populations**).

Distributed by: Roche Laboratories Inc., Nutley, New Jersey 07110

Licensor: Gilead Sciences, Inc., Foster City, California 94404

Revised: January 2008

Copyright © 1999-2008 by Roche Laboratories Inc. All rights reserved.

G.D. Searle & Co.

A Division of Pfizer
235 EAST 42ND STREET
NEW YORK, NY 10017-5755

For updates to the product information listed below, please check the Pfizer Web site, http://www.pfizerpro.com, or call (800) 438-1985. For complete product listing, please see the Manufacturers' Index.

For Medical Information, Contact:
(800) 438-1985
24 hours a day, seven days a week

Distribution:
1855 Shelby Oaks Drive North
Memphis, TN 38134
(901) 387-5200

Customer Service:
(800) 533-4535

CELEBREX® ℞

[*sĕ-lĕ-brĕks*]
celecoxib capsules

Prescribing information for this product, which appears on pages 3064–3069 of the 2008 PDR, has been completely revised as follows. Please write "See Supplement A" next to the product heading.

Cardiovascular Risk

- Celebrex may cause an increased risk of serious cardiovascular thrombotic events, myocardial infarction, and stroke, which can be fatal. All NSAIDs may have a similar risk. This risk may increase with duration of use. Patients with cardiovascular disease or risk factors for cardiovascular disease may be at greater risk (see **WARNINGS** and **CLINICAL STUDIES**).
- Celebrex is contraindicated for the treatment of perioperative pain in the setting of coronary artery bypass graft (CABG) surgery (see **WARNINGS**).

Gastrointestinal Risk

- NSAIDs, including Celebrex, cause an increased risk of serious gastrointestinal adverse events including bleeding, ulceration, and perforation of the stomach or intestines, which can be fatal. These events can occur at any time during use and without warning symptoms. Elderly patients are at greater risk for serious gastrointestinal events (see **WARNINGS**).

DESCRIPTION

Celebrex (celecoxib) is chemically designated as 4-[5-(4-methylphenyl)-3-(trifluoromethyl)-1H-pyrazol-1-yl] benzenesulfonamide and is a diaryl-substituted pyrazole. It has the following chemical structure:

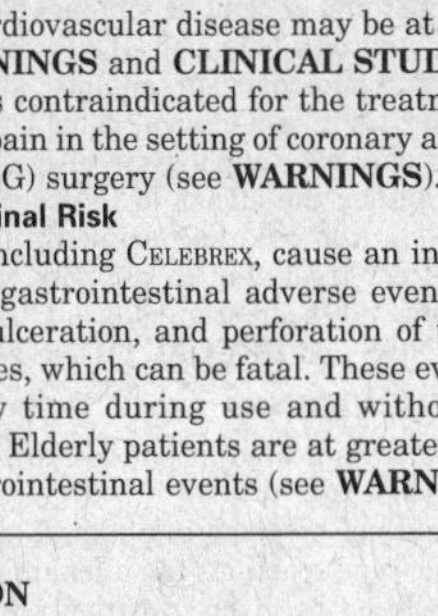

The empirical formula for celecoxib is $C_{17}H_{14}F_3N_3O_2S$, and the molecular weight is 381.38.

Celebrex oral capsules contain either 50 mg, 100 mg, 200 mg or 400 mg of celecoxib.

The inactive ingredients in Celebrex capsules include: croscarmellose sodium, edible inks, gelatin, lactose monohydrate, magnesium stearate, povidone and sodium lauryl sulfate.

CLINICAL PHARMACOLOGY

Mechanism of Action: Celebrex is a nonsteroidal anti-inflammatory drug that exhibits anti-inflammatory, analgesic, and antipyretic activities in animal models. The mechanism of action of Celebrex is believed to be due to inhibition of prostaglandin synthesis, primarily via inhibition of cyclooxygenase-2 (COX-2), and at therapeutic concentrations in humans, Celebrex does not inhibit the cyclooxygenase-1 (COX-1) isoenzyme. In animal colon tumor models, celecoxib reduced the incidence and multiplicity of tumors.

Platelets

In clinical trials using normal volunteers, Celebrex at single doses up to 800 mg and multiple doses of 600 mg twice daily for up to 7 days duration (higher than recommended therapeutic doses) had no effect on reduction of platelet aggregation or increase in bleeding time. Because of its lack of platelet effects, Celebrex is not a substitute for aspirin for cardiovascular prophylaxis. It is not known if there are any effects of Celebrex on platelets that may contribute to the increased risk of serious cardiovascular thrombotic adverse events associated with the use of Celebrex.

Fluid Retention

Inhibition of PGE2 synthesis may lead to sodium and water retention through increased reabsorption in the renal medullary thick ascending loop of Henle and perhaps other segments of the distal nephron. In the collecting ducts, PGE2 appears to inhibit water reabsorption by counteracting the action of antidiuretic hormone.

Pharmacokinetics:

Absorption

Peak plasma levels of celecoxib occur approximately 3 hrs after an oral dose. Under fasting conditions, both peak plasma levels (C_{max}) and area under the curve (AUC) are roughly dose proportional up to 200 mg BID; at higher doses there are less than proportional increases in C_{max} and AUC (see ***Food Effects***). Absolute bioavailability studies have not been conducted. With multiple dosing, steady state conditions are reached on or before Day 5.

The pharmacokinetic parameters of celecoxib in a group of healthy subjects are shown in Table 1.

Table 1
Summary of Single Dose (200 mg) Disposition Kinetics of Celecoxib in Healthy Subjects[1]

Mean (%CV) PK Parameter Values				
C_{max}, ng/mL	T_{max}, hr	Effective $t_{½}$, hr	V_{ss}/F, L	CL/F, L/hr
705 (38)	2.8 (37)	11.2 (31)	429 (34)	27.7 (28)

[1] Subjects under fasting conditions (n=36, 19-52 yrs.)

Food Effects

When Celebrex capsules were taken with a high fat meal, peak plasma levels were delayed for about 1 to 2 hours with an increase in total absorption (AUC) of 10% to 20%. Under fasting conditions, at doses above 200 mg, there is less than a proportional increase in C_{max} and AUC, which is thought to be due to the low solubility of the drug in aqueous media. Coadministration of Celebrex with an aluminum- and magnesium-containing antacid resulted in a reduction in plasma celecoxib concentrations with a decrease of 37% in C_{max} and 10% in AUC. Celebrex, at doses up to 200 mg BID can be administered without regard to timing of meals. Higher doses (400 mg BID) should be administered with food to improve absorption.

In healthy adult volunteers, the overall systemic exposure (AUC) of celecoxib was equivalent when celecoxib was administered as intact capsule or capsule contents sprinkled on applesauce. There were no significant alterations in C_{max}, T_{max} or $T_{½}$ after administration of capsule contents on applesauce.

Distribution

In healthy subjects, celecoxib is highly protein bound (~97%) within the clinical dose range. *In vitro* studies indicate that celecoxib binds primarily to albumin and, to a lesser extent, α_1-acid glycoprotein. The apparent volume of distribution at steady state (V_{ss}/F) is approximately 400 L, suggesting extensive distribution into the tissues. Celecoxib is not preferentially bound to red blood cells.

Metabolism

Celecoxib metabolism is primarily mediated via cytochrome P450 2C9. Three metabolites, a primary alcohol, the corresponding carboxylic acid and its glucuronide conjugate, have been identified in human plasma. These metabolites are inactive as COX-1 or COX-2 inhibitors. Patients who are known or suspected to be P450 2C9 poor metabolizers based on a previous history should be administered celecoxib with caution as they may have abnormally high plasma levels due to reduced metabolic clearance.

Excretion

Celecoxib is eliminated predominantly by hepatic metabolism with little (<3%) unchanged drug recovered in the urine and feces. Following a single oral dose of radiolabeled drug, approximately 57% of the dose was excreted in the feces and 27% was excreted into the urine. The primary metabolite in both urine and feces was the carboxylic acid metabolite (73% of dose) with low amounts of the glucuronide also appearing in the urine. It appears that the low solubility of the drug prolongs the absorption process making terminal half-life ($t_{½}$) determinations more variable. The effective half-life is approximately 11 hours under fasted conditions. The apparent plasma clearance (CL/F) is about 500 mL/min.

Special Populations

Geriatric: At steady state, elderly subjects (over 65 years old) had a 40% higher C_{max} and a 50% higher AUC compared to the young subjects. In elderly females, celecoxib C_{max} and AUC are higher than those for elderly males, but these increases are predominantly due to lower body weight in elderly females. Dose adjustment in the elderly is not generally necessary. However, for patients of less than 50 kg in body weight, initiate therapy at the lowest recommended dose.

Pediatric: The steady state pharmacokinetics of celecoxib administered as an investigational oral suspension was evaluated in 152 juvenile rheumatoid arthritis (JRA) patients 2 years to 17 years of age weighing ≥10 kg with pauciarticular or polyarticular course JRA and in patients with systemic onset JRA. Population pharmacokinetic analysis indicated that the oral clearance (unadjusted for body weight) of celecoxib increases less than proportionally to increasing weight, with 10 kg and 25 kg patients predicted to have 40% and 24% lower clearance, respectively, compared with a 70 kg adult RA patient.

Twice-daily administration of 50 mg capsules to JRA patients weighing ≥12 to ≤25 kg and 100 mg capsules to JRA patients weighing >25 kg should achieve plasma concentrations similar to those observed in a clinical trial that demonstrated the non-inferiority of celecoxib to naproxen 7.5 mg/kg twice daily (see **DOSAGE AND ADMINISTRATION**). Celecoxib has not been studied in JRA patients under the age of 2 years, in patients with body weight less than 10 kg (22 lbs), or beyond 24 weeks.

Race: Meta-analysis of pharmacokinetic studies has suggested an approximately 40% higher AUC of celecoxib in Blacks compared to Caucasians. The cause and clinical significance of this finding is unknown.

Hepatic Insufficiency: A pharmacokinetic study in subjects with mild (Child-Pugh Class A) and moderate (Child-Pugh Class B) hepatic impairment has shown that steady-state celecoxib AUC is increased about 40% and 180%, respectively, above that seen in healthy control subjects. Therefore, the daily recommended dose of Celebrex capsules should be reduced by approximately 50% in patients with moderate (Child-Pugh Class B) hepatic impairment. Patients with severe hepatic impairment (Child-Pugh Class C) have not been studied. The use of Celebrex in patients with severe hepatic impairment is not recommended (see **DOSAGE AND ADMINISTRATION**).

Renal Insufficiency: In a cross-study comparison, celecoxib AUC was approximately 40% lower in patients with chronic renal insufficiency (GFR 35-60 mL/min) than that seen in subjects with normal renal function. No significant relationship was found between GFR and celecoxib clearance. Patients with severe renal insufficiency have not been studied. Similar to other NSAIDs, Celebrex is not recommended in patients with severe renal insufficiency (see **WARNINGS – Advanced Renal Disease**).

Drug Interactions

Also see **PRECAUTIONS – Drug Interactions.**

General: Significant interactions may occur when celecoxib is administered together with drugs that inhibit P450 2C9. *In vitro* studies indicate that celecoxib is not an inhibitor of cytochrome P450 2C9, 2C19 or 3A4.

Clinical studies with celecoxib have identified potentially significant interactions with fluconazole and lithium. Experience with nonsteroidal anti-inflammatory drugs (NSAIDs) suggests the potential for interactions with furosemide and ACE inhibitors. The effects of celecoxib on the pharmacokinetics and/or pharmacodynamics of glyburide, ketoconazole, methotrexate, phenytoin, and tolbutamide have been studied *in vivo* and clinically important interactions have not been found.

CLINICAL STUDIES

Osteoarthritis (OA): Celebrex has demonstrated significant reduction in joint pain compared to placebo. Celebrex was evaluated for treatment of the signs and the symptoms of OA of the knee and hip in placebo- and active-controlled clinical trials of up to 12 weeks duration. In patients with OA, treatment with Celebrex 100 mg BID or 200 mg QD resulted in improvement in WOMAC (Western Ontario and McMaster Universities) osteoarthritis index, a composite of pain, stiffness, and functional measures in OA. In three 12-week studies of pain accompanying OA flare, Celebrex doses of 100 mg BID and 200 mg BID provided significant reduction of pain within 24-48 hours of initiation of dosing. At doses of 100 mg BID or 200 mg BID the effectiveness of Celebrex was shown to be similar to that of naproxen 500 mg BID. Doses of 200 mg BID provided no additional benefit above that seen with 100 mg BID. A total daily dose of 200 mg has been shown to be equally effective whether administered as 100 mg BID or 200 mg QD.

Rheumatoid Arthritis (RA): Celebrex has demonstrated significant reduction in joint tenderness/pain and joint

Continued on next page

Celebrex—Cont.

swelling compared to placebo. CELEBREX was evaluated for treatment of the signs and symptoms of RA in placebo- and active-controlled clinical trials of up to 24 weeks in duration. CELEBREX was shown to be superior to placebo in these studies, using the ACR20 Responder Index, a composite of clinical, laboratory, and functional measures in RA. CELEBREX doses of 100 mg BID and 200 mg BID were similar in effectiveness and both were comparable to naproxen 500 mg BID.

Although CELEBREX 100 mg BID and 200 mg BID provided similar overall effectiveness, some patients derived additional benefit from the 200 mg BID dose. Doses of 400 mg BID provided no additional benefit above that seen with 100-200 mg BID.

Juvenile Rheumatoid Arthritis (JRA): In a 12-week, randomized, double-blind active-controlled, parallel-group, multicenter, non-inferiority study, patients from 2 years to 17 years of age with pauciarticular, polyarticular course JRA or systemic onset JRA (with currently inactive systemic features), received one of the following treatments: celecoxib 3 mg/kg (to a maximum of 150 mg) twice daily; celecoxib 6 mg/kg (to a maximum of 300 mg) twice daily; or naproxen 7.5 mg/kg (to a maximum of 500 mg) twice daily. The response rates were based upon the JRA Definition of Improvement greater than or equal to 30% (JRA DOI 30) criterion, which is a composite of clinical, laboratory, and functional measures of JRA. The JRA DOI 30 response rates at week 12 were 69%, 80% and 67% in the celecoxib 3 mg/kg BID, celecoxib 6 mg/kg BID, and naproxen 7.5 mg/kg BID treatment groups, respectively.

The efficacy and safety of CELEBREX for JRA have not been studied beyond six months. The long-term cardiovascular toxicity in children exposed to CELEBREX has not been evaluated and it is unknown if the long-term risk may be similar to that seen in adults exposed to CELEBREX or other COX-2 selective and non-selective NSAIDS. (see **Boxed Warning, WARNINGS, and PRECAUTIONS**)

Analgesia, including primary dysmenorrhea: In acute analgesic models of post-oral surgery pain, post-orthopedic surgical pain, and primary dysmenorrhea, CELEBREX relieved pain that was rated by patients as moderate to severe. Single doses (see **DOSAGE AND ADMINISTRATION**) of CELEBREX provided pain relief within 60 minutes.

Ankylosing Spondylitis (AS): CELEBREX was evaluated in AS patients in two placebo- and active-controlled clinical trials of 6 and 12 weeks duration. CELEBREX at doses of 100 mg BID, 200 mg QD and 400 mg QD was shown to be statistically superior to placebo in these studies for all three co-primary efficacy measures assessing global pain intensity (Visual Analogue Scale), global disease activity (Visual Analogue Scale) and functional impairment (Bath Ankylosing Spondylitis Functional Index). In the 12-week study, there was no difference in the extent of improvement between the 200 mg and 400 mg celecoxib doses in a comparison of mean change from baseline, but there was a greater percentage of patients who responded to celecoxib 400 mg, 53%, than to celecoxib 200 mg, 44%, using the Assessment in Ankylosing Spondylitis response criteria (ASAS 20). The ASAS 20 defines a responder as improvement from baseline of at least 20% and an absolute improvement of at least 10 mm, on a 0 to 100 mm scale, in at least three of the four following domains: patient global, pain, Bath Ankylosing Spondylitis Functional Index, and inflammation. The responder analysis also demonstrated no change in the responder rates beyond 6 weeks.

Familial Adenomatous Polyposis (FAP): CELEBREX was evaluated to reduce the number of adenomatous colorectal polyps. A randomized double-blind placebo-controlled study was conducted in patients with FAP. The study population included 58 patients with a prior subtotal or total colectomy and 25 patients with an intact colon. Thirteen patients had the attenuated FAP phenotype.

One area in the rectum and up to four areas in the colon were identified at baseline for specific follow-up, and polyps were counted at baseline and following six months of treatment. The mean reduction in the number of colorectal polyps was 28% for CELEBREX 400 mg BID, 12% for CELEBREX 100 mg BID and 5% for placebo. The reduction in polyps observed with CELEBREX 400 mg BID was statistically superior to placebo at the six-month timepoint (p=0.003). (See Figure 1.)

[See figure 1 at top of next column]

Figure 1
Percent Change from Baseline in Number of Colorectal Polyps (FAP Patients)

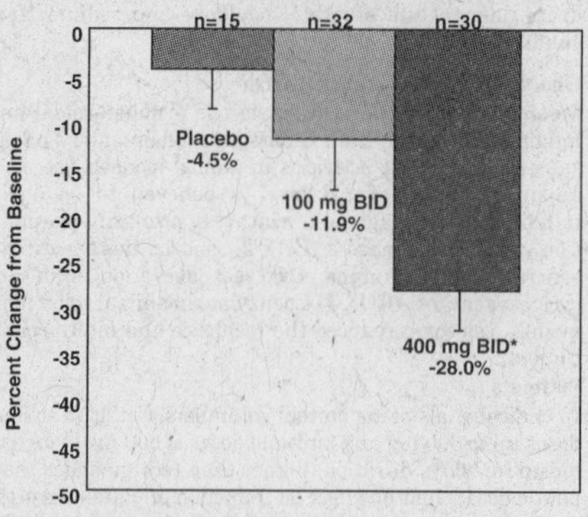

* p=0.003 versus placebo

Special Studies

Celecoxib Long-Term Arthritis Safety Study (CLASS)

The Celecoxib Long-Term Arthritis Safety Study (CLASS) was a prospective long-term safety outcome study conducted postmarketing in approximately 5,800 OA patients and 2,200 RA patients. Patients received CELEBREX 400 mg BID (4-fold and 2-fold the recommended OA and RA doses, respectively, and the approved dose for FAP), ibuprofen 800 mg TID or diclofenac 75 mg BID (common therapeutic doses). Median exposures for CELEBREX (n = 3,987) and diclofenac (n = 1,996) were 9 months while ibuprofen (n = 1,985) was 6 months. The primary endpoint of this outcome study was the incidence of *complicated ulcers* (gastrointestinal bleeding, perforation or obstruction). Patients were allowed to take concomitant low-dose (≤ 325 mg/day) aspirin (ASA) for cardiovascular prophylaxis (ASA subgroups: CELEBREX, n = 882; diclofenac, n = 445; ibuprofen, n = 412). Differences in the incidence of *complicated ulcers* between CELEBREX and the combined group of ibuprofen and diclofenac were not statistically significant.

Those patients on CELEBREX and concomitant low-dose ASA (N=882) experienced 4-fold higher rates of *complicated ulcers* compared to those not on ASA (N=3105). The Kaplan Meier rate for complicated ulcers at 9 months was 1.12% versus 0.32% for those on low dose ASA and those not on ASA, respectively (see **WARNINGS – Gastrointestinal (GI) Effects – Risk of GI Ulceration, Bleeding and Perforation**). The estimated cumulative rates at 9 months of *complicated and symptomatic ulcers* for patients treated with CELEBREX 400 mg BID are described in Table 2. Table 2 also displays results for patients less than or greater than 65 years of age. The difference in rates between CELEBREX alone and CELEBREX with ASA groups may be due to the higher risk for GI events in ASA users.

Table 2
***Complicated and Symptomatic Ulcer* Rates in Patients Taking CELEBREX 400 mg BID (Kaplan-Meier Rates at 9 months [%]) Based on Risk Factors**

	***Complicated and Symptomatic Ulcer* Rates**
All Patients	
Celebrex alone (n=3105)	0.78
Celebrex with ASA (n=882)	2.19
Patients <65 years	
Celebrex alone (n=2025)	0.47
Celebrex with ASA (n=403)	1.26
Patients ≥65 Years	
Celebrex alone (n=1080)	1.40
Celebrex with ASA (n=479)	3.06

In a small number of patients with a history of ulcer disease, the *complicated and symptomatic ulcer* rates in patients taking CELEBREX alone or CELEBREX with ASA were, respectively, 2.56% (n=243) and 6.85% (n=91) at 48 weeks. These results are to be expected in patients with a prior history of ulcer disease (see **WARNINGS – Gastrointestinal (GI) Effects – Risk of GI Ulceration, Bleeding, and Perforation** and **ADVERSE REACTIONS – Safety Data from CLASS Study – *Hematological Events***).

Cardiovascular safety outcomes were also evaluated in the CLASS trial. Kaplan-Meier cumulative rates for investigator-reported serious cardiovascular thromboembolic adverse events (including MI, pulmonary embolism, deep venous thrombosis, unstable angina, transient ischemic attacks, and ischemic cerebrovascular accidents) demonstrated no differences between the CELEBREX, diclofenac, or ibuprofen treatment groups. The cumulative rates in all patients at nine months for CELEBREX, diclofenac, and ibuprofen were 1.2%, 1.4%, and 1.1%, respectively. The cumulative rates in non-ASA users at nine months in each of the three treatment groups were less than 1%. The cumulative rates for myocardial infarction in non-ASA users at nine months in each of the three treatment groups were less than 0.2%. There was no placebo group in the CLASS trial, which limits the ability to determine whether the three drugs tested had no increased risk of CV events or if they all increased the risk to a similar degree.

Adenomatous Polyp Prevention Studies

Cardiovascular safety was evaluated in two randomized, double-blind, placebo-controlled, three-year studies involving patients with Sporadic Adenomatous Polyps treated with CELEBREX. The first of these studies was the APC (Prevention of Sporadic Colorectal Adenomas with Celecoxib) study, which compared CELEBREX 400 mg twice daily (N=671) and CELEBREX 200 mg twice daily (N=685) to placebo (N=679). Preliminary safety information from this trial demonstrated a dose-related increase in serious cardiovascular events (mainly myocardial infarction [MI]) at CELEBREX doses of 200 mg and 400 mg twice daily compared to placebo). The cumulative rates of serious cardiovascular thrombotic events began to differ between the CELEBREX treatment groups and placebo after approximately one year of treatment. There were 2.8 to 3.1 years of follow-up in the APC trial except those patients who died earlier. The relative risk (RR) for the composite endpoint of cardiovascular death, MI, or stroke was 3.4 (95% CI 1.4 – 8.5) for the higher dose and 2.5 (95% CI 1.0 – 6.4) for the lower dose of CELEBREX compared to placebo. The absolute risk for the composite endpoint was 3.0% for the higher dose of CELEBREX, 2.2% for the lower dose of CELEBREX, and 0.9% for placebo.

The second long-term study, PreSAP (Prevention of Colorectal Sporadic Adenomatous Polyps) compared CELEBREX 400 mg once daily to placebo. Preliminary safety information from this trial demonstrated no increased cardiovascular risk for the composite endpoint of cardiovascular death, MI or stroke. The reason for the differing results for CV events in the APC and PreSAP trials is not known.

Clinical trials of other COX-2 selective and nonselective NSAIDs of up to three-years duration have shown an increased risk of serious cardiovascular thrombotic events, myocardial infarction, and stroke, which can be fatal. As a result, all NSAIDs are considered potentially associated with this risk.

Endoscopic Studies

The correlation between findings of short-term endoscopic studies with CELEBREX and the relative incidence of clinically significant serious upper GI events with long-term use has not been established.

A randomized, double-blind study in 430 RA patients was conducted in which an endoscopic examination was performed at 6 months. The incidence of endoscopic ulcers in patients taking CELEBREX 200 mg twice daily was 4% vs. 15% for patients taking diclofenac SR 75 mg twice daily. However, CELEBREX was not statistically different than diclofenac for clinically relevant GI outcomes in the CLASS trial (see **Special Studies - *CLASS***).

The incidence of endoscopic ulcers was studied in two 12-week, placebo-controlled studies in 2157 OA and RA patients in whom baseline endoscopies revealed no ulcers. There was no dose relationship for the incidence of gastroduodenal ulcers and the dose of CELEBREX (50 mg to 400 mg twice daily). The incidence for naproxen 500 mg twice daily was 16.2 and 17.6% in the two studies, for placebo was 2.0 and 2.3%, and for all doses of CELEBREX the incidence ranged between 2.7%-5.9%. There have been no large, clinical outcome studies to compare clinically relevant GI outcomes with CELEBREX and naproxen.

In the endoscopic studies, approximately 11% of patients were taking aspirin (≤ 325 mg/day). In the CELEBREX groups, the endoscopic ulcer rate appeared to be higher in aspirin users than in non-users. However, the increased rate of ulcers in these aspirin users was less than the endoscopic ulcer rates observed in the active comparator groups, with or without aspirin.

Serious clinically significant upper GI bleeding has been observed in patients receiving CELEBREX in controlled and open-labeled trials (see **Special Studies - *CLASS*** and **WARNINGS – Gastrointestinal (GI) Effects – Risk of GI Ulceration, Bleeding and Perforation**).

INDICATIONS AND USAGE

Carefully consider the potential benefits and risks of CELEBREX and other treatment options before deciding to use CELEBREX. Use the lowest effective dose for the shortest duration consistent with individual patient treatment goals (see **WARNINGS**).

CELEBREX is indicated:

1) For relief of the signs and symptoms of osteoarthritis.

2) For relief of the signs and symptoms of rheumatoid arthritis in adults.

3) For relief of the signs and symptoms of juvenile rheumatoid arthritis in patients 2 years and older (**see CLINICAL STUDIES and ADVERSE REACTIONS - *Adverse Events from JRA Study***).

4) For the relief of signs and symptoms of ankylosing spondylitis.

5) For the management of acute pain in adults (see **CLINICAL STUDIES**).

6) For the treatment of primary dysmenorrhea.

7) To reduce the number of adenomatous colorectal polyps in familial adenomatous polyposis (FAP), as an adjunct to usual care (e.g., endoscopic surveillance, surgery). It is not known whether there is a clinical benefit from a reduction in the number of colorectal polyps in FAP patients. It is also not known whether the effects of CELEBREX treatment will persist after CELEBREX is discontinued. The efficacy and safety of CELEBREX treatment in patients with FAP beyond six months have not been studied (see **CLINICAL STUDIES, WARNINGS** and **PRECAUTIONS** sections).

CONTRAINDICATIONS

CELEBREX is contraindicated in patients with known hypersensitivity to celecoxib.

CELEBREX should not be given to patients who have demonstrated allergic-type reactions to sulfonamides.

CELEBREX should not be given to patients who have experienced asthma, urticaria, or allergic-type reactions after taking aspirin or other NSAIDs. Severe, rarely fatal, anaphylactic-like reactions to NSAIDs have been reported in such patients (see **WARNINGS — Anaphylactoid Reactions**, and **PRECAUTIONS — Preexisting Asthma**).

CELEBREX is contraindicated for the treatment of peri-operative pain in the setting of coronary artery bypass graft (CABG) surgery (see **WARNINGS**)

WARNINGS

Cardiovascular Effects

Cardiovascular Thrombotic Events

Chronic use of CELEBREX may cause an increased risk of serious adverse cardiovascular thrombotic events, myocardial infarction, and stroke, which can be fatal. In the APC trial, the relative risk for the composite endpoint of cardiovascular death, MI, or stroke was 3.4 (95% CI 1.4 – 8.5) for CELEBREX 400 mg twice daily and 2.5 (95% CI 1.0 – 6.4) for the CELEBREX 200 mg twice daily compared to placebo (see **Special Studies – *Adenomatous Polyp Studies*)**.

All NSAIDs, both COX-2 selective and nonselective, may have a similar risk. Patients with known CV disease or risk factors for CV disease may be at greater risk. To minimize the potential risk for an adverse CV event in patients treated with CELEBREX, the lowest effective dose should be used for the shortest duration possible. Physicians and patients should remain alert for the development of such events, even in the absence of previous CV symptoms. Patients should be informed about the signs and/or symptoms of serious CV toxicity and the steps to take if they occur.

There is no consistent evidence that concurrent use of aspirin mitigates the increased risk of serious CV thrombotic events associated with NSAID use. The concurrent use of aspirin and CELEBREX does increase the risk of serious GI events (see **GI WARNINGS - Risk of GI Ulceration, Bleeding, and Perforation**).

Two large, controlled, clinical trials of a different COX-2 selective NSAID for the treatment of pain in the first 10-14 days following CABG surgery found an increased incidence of myocardial infarction and stroke (see **CONTRAINDICATIONS**).

Hypertension

As with all NSAIDS, CELEBREX can lead to the onset of new hypertension or worsening of pre-existing hypertension, either of which may contribute to the increased incidence of CV events. Patients taking thiazides or loop diuretics may have impaired response to these therapies when taking NSAIDs. NSAIDs, including CELEBREX, should be used with caution in patients with hypertension. Blood pressure should be monitored closely during the initiation of therapy with CELEBREX and throughout the course of therapy. The rates of hypertension from the CLASS trial in the CELEBREX, ibuprofen and diclofenac treated patients were 2.4%, 4.2% and 2.5%, respectively (see **Special Studies - *CLASS***).

Congestive Heart Failure and Edema

Fluid retention and edema have been observed in some patients taking NSAIDs, including CELEBREX (see **ADVERSE REACTIONS**). In the CLASS study (see **Special Studies – CLASS**), the Kaplan-Meier cumulative rates at 9 months of peripheral edema in patients on CELEBREX 400 mg twice daily (4-fold and 2-fold the recommended OA and RA doses, respectively, and the approved dose for FAP), ibuprofen 800 mg three times daily and diclofenac 75 mg twice daily were 4.5%, 6.9% and 4.7%, respectively. CELEBREX should be used with caution in patients with fluid retention or heart failure.

Gastrointestinal (GI) Effects — Risk of GI Ulceration, Bleeding, and Perforation

NSAIDs, including CELEBREX, can cause serious gastrointestinal events including bleeding, ulceration, and perforation of the stomach, small intestine or large intestine, which can be fatal. These serious adverse events can occur at any time, with or without warning symptoms, in patients treated with NSAIDs. Only one in five patients who develop a serious upper GI adverse event on NSAID therapy is symptomatic. Complicated and symptomatic ulcer rates were 0.78% at nine months for all patients in the CLASS trial, and 2.19% for the subgroup on low dose ASA. Patients 65 years of age and older had an incidence of 1.40% at nine months, 3.06% when also taking ASA (see **Special Studies - *CLASS***). With longer duration of use of NSAIDs, there is a trend for increasing the likelihood of developing a serious GI event at some time during the course of therapy. However, even short-term therapy is not without risk.

NSAIDs should be prescribed with extreme caution in patients with a prior history of ulcer disease or gastrointestinal bleeding. Patients with a prior history of peptic ulcer disease and/or gastrointestinal bleeding who use NSAIDs have a greater than 10-fold increased risk for developing a GI bleed compared to patients with neither of these risk factors. Other factors that increase the risk of GI bleeding in patients treated with NSAIDs include concomitant use of oral corticosteroids or anticoagulants, longer duration of NSAID therapy, smoking, use of alcohol, older age, and poor general health status. Most spontaneous reports of fatal GI events are in elderly or debilitated patients and therefore special care should be taken in treating this population.

To minimize the potential risk for an adverse GI event, the lowest effective dose should be used for the shortest possible duration. Physicians and patients should remain alert for signs and symptoms of GI ulceration and bleeding during CELEBREX therapy and promptly initiate additional evaluation and treatment if a serious GI adverse event is suspected. For high-risk patients, alternate therapies that do not involve NSAIDs should be considered.

Renal Effects

Long-term administration of NSAIDs has resulted in renal papillary necrosis and other renal injury. Renal toxicity has also been seen in patients in whom renal prostaglandins have a compensatory role in the maintenance of renal perfusion. In these patients, administration of an NSAID may cause a dose-dependent reduction in prostaglandin formation and, secondarily, in renal blood flow, which may precipitate overt renal decompensation. Patients at greatest risk of this reaction are those with impaired renal function, heart failure, liver dysfunction, those taking diuretics and ACE inhibitors, angiotensin II receptor antagonists, and the elderly. Discontinuation of NSAID therapy is usually followed by recovery to the pretreatment state. Clinical trials with CELEBREX have shown renal effects similar to those observed with comparator NSAIDs.

Advanced Renal Disease

No information is available from controlled clinical studies regarding the use of CELEBREX in patients with advanced renal disease. Therefore, treatment with CELEBREX is not recommended in these patients with advanced renal disease. If CELEBREX therapy must be initiated, close monitoring of the patient's renal function is advisable.

Anaphylactoid Reactions

As with NSAIDs in general, anaphylactoid reactions have occurred in patients without known prior exposure to CELEBREX. In post-marketing experience, rare cases of anaphylactic reactions and angioedema have been reported in patients receiving CELEBREX. CELEBREX should not be given to patients with the aspirin triad. This symptom complex typically occurs in asthmatic patients who experience rhinitis with or without nasal polyps, or who exhibit severe, potentially fatal bronchospasm after taking aspirin or other NSAIDs (see **CONTRAINDICATIONS** and **PRECAUTIONS — Preexisting Asthma**). Emergency help should be sought in cases where an anaphylactoid reaction occurs.

Skin Reactions

CELEBREX is a sulfonamide and can cause serious skin adverse events such as exfoliative dermatitis, Stevens Johnson syndrome (SJS), and toxic epidermal necrolysis (TENS), which can be fatal. These serious events can occur without warning and in patients without prior known sulfa allergy. Patients should be informed about the signs and symptoms of serious skin manifestations and use of the drug should be discontinued at the first appearance of skin rash or any other sign of hypersensitivity.

Pregnancy

In late pregnancy CELEBREX should be avoided because it may cause premature closure of the ductus arteriosus (see **PRECAUTIONS – Pregnancy**).

Familial Adenomatous Polyposis (FAP): Treatment with CELEBREX in FAP has not been shown to reduce the risk of gastrointestinal cancer or the need for prophylactic colectomy or other FAP-related surgeries. Therefore, the usual care of FAP patients should not be altered because of the concurrent administration of CELEBREX. In particular, the frequency of routine endoscopic surveillance should not be decreased and prophylactic colectomy or other FAP-related surgeries should not be delayed.

PRECAUTIONS

General: CELEBREX cannot be expected to substitute for corticosteroids or to treat corticosteroid insufficiency. Abrupt discontinuation of corticosteroids may lead to exacerbation of corticosteroid-responsive illness. Patients on prolonged corticosteroid therapy should have their therapy tapered slowly if a decision is made to discontinue corticosteroids.

The concomitant use of CELEBREX with any dose of a non-aspirin NSAID should be avoided.

The pharmacological activity of CELEBREX in reducing inflammation, and possibly fever, may diminish the utility of these diagnostic signs in detecting infectious complications of presumed noninfectious, painful conditions.

Hepatic Effects: Borderline elevations of one or more liver associated enzymes may occur in up to 15% of patients taking NSAIDs, and notable elevations of ALT or AST (approximately 3 or more times the upper limit of normal) have been reported in approximately 1% of patients in clinical trials with NSAIDs. These laboratory abnormalities may progress, may remain unchanged, or may be transient with continuing therapy. Rare cases of severe hepatic reactions, including jaundice and fatal fulminant hepatitis, liver necrosis and hepatic failure (some with fatal outcome) have been reported with NSAIDs, including CELEBREX (see **ADVERSE REACTIONS – *post-marketing experience*)**. In controlled clinical trials of CELEBREX, the incidence of borderline elevations (greater than or equal to 1.2 times and less than 3 times the upper limit of normal) of liver associated enzymes was 6% for CELEBREX and 5% for placebo, and approximately 0.2% of patients taking CELEBREX and 0.3% of patients taking placebo had notable elevations of ALT and AST.

A patient with symptoms and/or signs suggesting liver dysfunction, or in whom an abnormal liver test has occurred, should be monitored carefully for evidence of the development of a more severe hepatic reaction while on therapy with CELEBREX. If clinical signs and symptoms consistent with liver disease develop, or if systemic manifestations occur (e.g., eosinophilia, rash, etc.), CELEBREX should be discontinued.

Hematological Effects: Anemia is sometimes seen in patients receiving CELEBREX. In controlled clinical trials the incidence of anemia was 0.6% with CELEBREX and 0.4% with placebo. Patients on long-term treatment with CELEBREX should have their hemoglobin or hematocrit checked if they exhibit any signs or symptoms of anemia or blood loss. CELEBREX does not generally affect platelet counts, prothrombin time (PT), or partial thromboplastin time (PTT), and does not inhibit platelet aggregation at indicated dosages (see **CLINICAL PHARMACOLOGY— Platelets**).

Systemic Onset Juvenile Rheumatoid Arthritis

CELEBREX should be used only with caution in pediatric patients with systemic onset JRA due to the risk for serious adverse reactions including disseminated intravascular coagulation.

Preexisting Asthma: Patients with asthma may have aspirin-sensitive asthma. The use of aspirin in patients with aspirin-sensitive asthma has been associated with severe bronchospasm, which can be fatal. Since cross reactivity, including bronchospasm, between aspirin and other nonsteroidal anti-inflammatory drugs has been reported in

such aspirin-sensitive patients, CELEBREX should not be administered to patients with this form of aspirin sensitivity and should be used with caution in patients with pre-existing asthma.

Information for Patients

Patients should be informed of the following information before initiating therapy with CELEBREX and periodically during the course of ongoing therapy. Patients should also be encouraged to read the NSAID Medication Guide that accompanies each prescription dispensed.

1. CELEBREX, like other NSAIDs, may cause serious CV side effects such as MI or stroke, which may result in hospitalization and even death. Although serious CV events can occur without warning symptoms, patients should be alert for the signs and symptoms of chest pain, shortness of breath, weakness, slurring of speech, and should ask for medical advice if they observe any of these signs or symptoms. Patients should be apprised of the importance of this follow-up (see **WARNINGS - Cardiovascular Effects**).

2. CELEBREX, like other NSAIDs, can cause gastrointestinal discomfort and, rarely, more serious side effects, such as ulcers and bleeding, which may result in hospitalization and even death. Although serious GI tract ulcerations and bleeding can occur without warning symptoms, patients should be alert for the signs and symptoms of ulcerations and bleeding, and should ask for medical advice when they observe any signs or symptoms that are indicative of these disorders, including epigastric pain, dyspepsia, melena, and hematemesis. Patients should be apprised of the importance of this follow-up (see **WARNINGS — Gastrointestinal (GI) Effects – Risk of Gastrointestinal Ulceration, Bleeding, and Perforation**).

3. Patients should be advised to stop the drug immediately if they develop any type of rash and contact their physicians as soon as possible. CELEBREX is a sulfonamide and can cause serious skin side effects such as exfoliative dermatitis, SJS, and TENS, which may result in hospitalizations and even death. These reactions can occur with all NSAIDs, even non-sulfonamides. Although serious skin reactions may occur without warning, patients should be alert for the signs and symptoms of skin rash and blisters, fever, or other signs of hypersensitivity such as itching, and should ask for medical advice when observing any indicative signs or symptoms. Patients with prior history of sulfa allergy should not take CELEBREX.

4. Patients should promptly report signs or symptoms of unexplained weight gain or edema to their physicians.

5. Patients should be informed of the warning signs and symptoms of hepatotoxicity (e.g., nausea, fatigue, lethargy, pruritus, jaundice, right upper quadrant tenderness, and "flu-like" symptoms). Patients should be instructed that they should stop therapy and seek immediate medical therapy if these signs and symptoms occur.

6. Patients should be informed of the signs and symptoms of an anaphylactoid reaction (e.g. difficulty breathing, swelling of the face or throat). Patients should be instructed to seek immediate emergency assistance if they develop any of these signs and symptoms (see **WARNINGS – Anaphylactoid Reactions**).

7. Patients should be informed that in late pregnancy CELEBREX should be avoided because it may cause premature closure of the ductus arteriosus.

8. Patients with familial adenomatous polyposis (FAP) should be informed that CELEBREX has not been shown to reduce colorectal, duodenal or other FAP-related cancers, or the need for endoscopic surveillance, prophylactic or other FAP-related surgery. Therefore, all patients with FAP should be instructed to continue their usual care while receiving CELEBREX.

Laboratory Tests: Because serious GI tract ulcerations and bleeding can occur without warning symptoms, physicians should monitor for signs or symptoms of GI bleeding. Patients on long-term treatment with NSAIDs, should have a CBC and a chemistry profile checked periodically. If abnormal liver tests or renal tests persist or worsen, CELEBREX should be discontinued.

In controlled clinical trials, elevated BUN occurred more frequently in patients receiving CELEBREX compared with patients on placebo. This laboratory abnormality was also seen in patients who received comparator NSAIDs in these studies. The clinical significance of this abnormality has not been established.

Drug Interactions

General: Celecoxib metabolism is predominantly mediated via cytochrome P450 2C9 in the liver. Co-administration of celecoxib with drugs that are known to inhibit 2C9 should be done with caution.

In vitro studies indicate that celecoxib, although not a substrate, is an inhibitor of cytochrome P450 2D6. Therefore, there is a potential for an *in vivo* drug interaction with drugs that are metabolized by P450 2D6.

ACE-inhibitors and Angiotensin II Antagonists: Reports suggest that NSAIDs may diminish the antihypertensive effect of Angiotensin Converting Enzyme (ACE) inhibitors and angiotensin II antagonists. This interaction should be given consideration in patients taking CELEBREX concomitantly with ACE-inhibitors and angiotensin II antagonists.

Continued on next page

Celebrex—Cont.

Aspirin: CELEBREX can be used with low-dose aspirin. However, concomitant administration of aspirin with CELEBREX increases the rate of GI ulceration or other complications, compared to use of CELEBREX alone (see **CLINICAL STUDIES — Special Studies — *CLASS*, WARNINGS – Gastrointestinal (GI) Effects – Risk of GI Ulceration, Bleeding, and Perforation**, and **WARNINGS – Cardiovascular Effects**). **Because of its lack of platelet effects, CELEBREX is not a substitute for aspirin for cardiovascular prophylaxis.**

Fluconazole: Concomitant administration of fluconazole at 200 mg QD resulted in a two-fold increase in celecoxib plasma concentration. This increase is due to the inhibition of celecoxib metabolism via P450 2C9 by fluconazole (see **Pharmacokinetics — Metabolism**). CELEBREX should be introduced at the lowest recommended dose in patients receiving fluconazole.

Furosemide: Clinical studies, as well as post marketing observations, have shown that NSAIDs can reduce the natriuretic effect of furosemide and thiazides in some patients. This response has been attributed to inhibition of renal prostaglandin synthesis.

Lithium: In a study conducted in healthy subjects, mean steady-state lithium plasma levels increased approximately 17% in subjects receiving lithium 450 mg BID with CELEBREX 200 mg BID as compared to subjects receiving lithium alone. Patients on lithium treatment should be closely monitored when CELEBREX is introduced or withdrawn.

Methotrexate: In an interaction study of rheumatoid arthritis patients taking methotrexate, CELEBREX did not have a significant effect on the pharmacokinetics of methotrexate.

Warfarin: Anticoagulant activity should be monitored, particularly in the first few days, after initiating or changing CELEBREX therapy in patients receiving warfarin or similar agents, since these patients are at an increased risk of bleeding complications. The effect of celecoxib on the anticoagulant effect of warfarin was studied in a group of healthy subjects receiving daily doses of 2-5 mg of warfarin. In these subjects, celecoxib did not alter the anticoagulant effect of warfarin as determined by prothrombin time. However, in post-marketing experience, serious bleeding events, some of which were fatal, have been reported, predominantly in the elderly, in association with increases in prothrombin time in patients receiving CELEBREX concurrently with warfarin.

Animal Toxicology

An increase in the incidence of background findings of spermatocele with or without secondary changes such as epididymal hypospermia as well as minimal to slight dilation of the seminiferous tubules was seen in the juvenile rat. These reproductive findings while apparently treatment-related did not increase in incidence or severity with dose and may indicate an exacerbation of a spontaneous condition. Similar reproductive findings were not observed in studies of juvenile or adult dogs or in adult rats treated with celecoxib. The clinical significance of this observation is unknown.

Carcinogenesis, mutagenesis, impairment of fertility: Celecoxib was not carcinogenic in rats given oral doses up to 200 mg/kg for males and 10 mg/kg for females (approximately 2- to 4-fold the human exposure as measured by the AUC_{0-24} at 200 mg BID) or in mice given oral doses up to 25 mg/kg for males and 50 mg/kg for females (approximately equal to human exposure as measured by the AUC_{0-24} at 200 mg BID) for two years.

Celecoxib was not mutagenic in an Ames test and a mutation assay in Chinese hamster ovary (CHO) cells, nor clastogenic in a chromosome aberration assay in CHO cells and an *in vivo* micronucleus test in rat bone marrow.

Celecoxib did not impair male and female fertility in rats at oral doses up to 600 mg/kg/day (approximately 11-fold human exposure at 200 mg BID based on the AUC_{0-24}).

Pregnancy

Teratogenic effects: Pregnancy Category C. Celecoxib at oral doses ≥150 mg/kg/day (approximately 2-fold human exposure at 200 mg BID as measured by AUC_{0-24}), caused an increased incidence of ventricular septal defects, a rare event, and fetal alterations, such as ribs fused, sternebrae fused and sternebrae misshapen when rabbits were treated throughout organogenesis. A dose-dependent increase in diaphragmatic hernias was observed when rats were given celecoxib at oral doses ≥30 mg/kg/day (approximately 6-fold human exposure based on the AUC_{0-24} at 200 mg BID) throughout organogenesis. There are no studies in pregnant women. CELEBREX should be used during pregnancy only if the potential benefit justifies the potential risk to the fetus.

Nonteratogenic effects: Celecoxib produced pre-implantation and post-implantation losses and reduced embryo/fetal survival in rats at oral dosages ≥50 mg/kg/day (approximately 6-fold human exposure based on the AUC_{0-24} at 200 mg BID). These changes are expected with inhibition of prostaglandin synthesis and are not the result of permanent alteration of female reproductive function, nor are they expected at clinical exposures. No studies have been conducted to evaluate the effect of celecoxib on the closure of the ductus arteriosus in humans. Therefore, use of CELEBREX during the third trimester of pregnancy should be avoided.

Labor and delivery: Celecoxib produced no evidence of delayed labor or parturition at oral doses up to 100 mg/kg in rats (approximately 7-fold human exposure as measured by the AUC_{0-24} at 200 mg BID). The effects of CELEBREX on labor and delivery in pregnant women are unknown.

Table 3
Adverse Events Occurring in ≥2% of CELEBREX Patients From CELEBREX Premarketing Controlled Arthritis Trials

	CELEBREX (100-200 mg BID or 200 mg QD) (n=4146)	Placebo (n=1864)	Naproxen 500 mg BID (n=1366)	Diclofenac 75 mg BID (n=387)	Ibuprofen 800 mg TID (n=345)
Gastrointestinal					
Abdominal pain	4.1%	2.8%	7.7%	9.0%	9.0%
Diarrhea	5.6%	3.8%	5.3%	9.3%	5.8%
Dyspepsia	8.8%	6.2%	12.2%	10.9%	12.8%
Flatulence	2.2%	1.0%	3.6%	4.1%	3.5%
Nausea	3.5%	4.2%	6.0%	3.4%	6.7%
Body as a whole					
Back pain	2.8%	3.6%	2.2%	2.6%	0.9%
Peripheral edema	2.1%	1.1%	2.1%	1.0%	3.5%
Injury-accidental	2.9%	2.3%	3.0%	2.6%	3.2%
Central and peripheral nervous system					
Dizziness	2.0%	1.7%	2.6%	1.3%	2.3%
Headache	15.8%	20.2%	14.5%	15.5%	15.4%
Psychiatric					
Insomnia	2.3%	2.3%	2.9%	1.3%	1.4%
Respiratory					
Pharyngitis	2.3%	1.1%	1.7%	1.6%	2.6%
Rhinitis	2.0%	1.3%	2.4%	2.3%	0.6%
Sinusitis	5.0%	4.3%	4.0%	5.4%	5.8%
Upper respiratory tract infection	8.1%	6.7%	9.9%	9.8%	9.9%
Skin					
Rash	2.2%	2.1%	2.1%	1.3%	1.2%

Nursing mothers: Celecoxib is excreted in the milk of lactating rats at concentrations similar to those in plasma. Limited data from one subject indicate that celecoxib is also excreted in human milk. Because many drugs are excreted in human milk and because of the potential for serious adverse reactions in nursing infants from CELEBREX, a decision should be made whether to discontinue nursing or to discontinue the drug, taking into account the importance of the drug to the mother.

Pediatric Use

CELEBREX is approved for relief of the signs and symptoms of Juvenile Rheumatoid Arthritis in patients 2 years and older. Safety and efficacy have not been studied beyond six months in children. The long-term cardiovascular toxicity in children exposed to CELEBREX has not been evaluated and it is unknown if long-term risks may be similar to that seen in adults exposed to CELEBREX or other COX-2 selective and non-selective NSAIDS. (see **Boxed Warning, WARNINGS, and CLINICAL STUDIES**)

The use of celecoxib in patients 2 years to 17 years of age with pauciarticular, polyarticular course JRA or in patients with systemic onset JRA was studied in a 12-week, double-blind, active controlled, pharmacokinetic, safety and efficacy study, with a 12-week open-label extension. Celecoxib has not been studied in patients under the age of 2 years, in patients with body weight less than 10 kg (22 lbs), and in patients with active systemic features. Patients with systemic onset JRA (without active systemic features) appear to be at risk for the development of abnormal coagulation laboratory tests. In some patients with systemic onset JRA, both celecoxib and naproxen were associated with mild prolongation of activated partial thromboplastin time (APTT) but not prothrombin time (PT). NSAIDs including celecoxib should be used only with caution in patients with systemic onset JRA, due to the risk of disseminated intravascular coagulation. Patients with systemic onset JRA should be monitored for the development of abnormal coagulation tests. (see **CLINICAL PHARMACOLOGY – *Pediatric*, CLINICAL STUDIES – *JRA*, PRECAUTIONS – *Systemic Onset JRA*, PRECAUTIONS - *Animal Toxicology*, ADVERSE REACTIONS - *Adverse events from JRA studies*, and DOSAGE and ADMINISTRATION - *JRA***).

Geriatric Use

Of the total number of patients who received CELEBREX in clinical trials, more than 3,300 were 65-74 years of age, while approximately 1,300 additional patients were 75 years and over. No substantial differences in effectiveness were observed between these subjects and younger subjects. In clinical studies comparing renal function as measured by the GFR, BUN and creatinine, and platelet function as measured by bleeding time and platelet aggregation, the results were not different between elderly and young volunteers. However, as with other NSAIDs, including those that selectively inhibit COX-2, there have been more spontaneous post-marketing reports of fatal GI events and acute renal failure in the elderly than in younger patients (see **WARNINGS – Gastrointestinal (GI) Effects – Risk of GI Ulceration, Bleeding, and Perforation**).

ADVERSE REACTIONS

Of the CELEBREX treated patients in the premarketing controlled clinical trials, approximately 4,250 were patients with OA, approximately 2,100 were patients with RA, and approximately 1,050 were patients with post-surgical pain. More than 8,500 patients have received a total daily dose of CELEBREX of 200 mg (100 mg BID or 200 mg QD) or more, including more than 400 treated at 800 mg (400 mg BID). Approximately 3,900 patients have received CELEBREX at these doses for 6 months or more; approximately 2,300 of these have received it for 1 year or more and 124 of these have received it for 2 years or more.

Adverse events from CELEBREX premarketing controlled arthritis trials: Table 3 lists all adverse events, regardless of causality, occurring in ≥2% of patients receiving CELEBREX from 12 controlled studies conducted in patients with OA or RA that included a placebo and/or a positive control group. Since these 12 trials were of different durations, and patients in the trials may not have been exposed for the same duration of time, these percentages do not capture cumulative rates of occurrence.

[See table 3 above]

In placebo- or active-controlled clinical trials, the discontinuation rate due to adverse events was 7.1% for patients receiving CELEBREX and 6.1% for patients receiving placebo. Among the most common reasons for discontinuation due to adverse events in the CELEBREX treatment groups were dyspepsia and abdominal pain (cited as reasons for discontinuation in 0.8% and 0.7% of CELEBREX patients, respectively). Among patients receiving placebo, 0.6% discontinued due to dyspepsia and 0.6% withdrew due to abdominal pain.

The following adverse events occurred in 0.1-1.9% of patients regardless of causality.

CELEBREX
(100-200 mg BID or 200 mg QD)

Gastrointestinal:	Constipation, diverticulitis, dysphagia, eructation, esophagitis, gastritis, gastroenteritis, gastroesophageal reflux, hemorrhoids, hiatal hernia, melena, dry mouth, stomatitis, tenesmus, tooth disorder, vomiting
Cardiovascular:	Aggravated hypertension, angina pectoris, coronary artery disorder, myocardial infarction
General:	Allergy aggravated, allergic reaction, asthenia, chest pain, cyst NOS, edema generalized, face edema, fatigue, fever, hot flushes, influenza-like symptoms, pain, peripheral pain
Resistance mechanism disorders:	Herpes simplex, herpes zoster, infection bacterial, infection fungal, infection soft tissue, infection viral, moniliasis, moniliasis genital, otitis media
Central, peripheral nervous system:	Leg cramps, hypertonia, hypoesthesia, migraine, neuralgia, neuropathy, paresthesia, vertigo
Female reproductive:	Breast fibroadenosis, breast neoplasm, breast pain, dysmenorrhea, menstrual disorder, vaginal hemorrhage, vaginitis
Male reproductive:	Prostatic disorder
Hearing and vestibular:	Deafness, ear abnormality, earache, tinnitus
Heart rate and rhythm:	Palpitation, tachycardia
Liver and biliary system:	Hepatic function abnormal, SGOT increased, SGPT increased
Metabolic and nutritional:	BUN increased, CPK increased, diabetes mellitus, hypercholesterolemia, hyperglycemia, hypokalemia, NPN increase, creatinine increased, alkaline phosphatase increased, weight increase
Musculoskeletal:	Arthralgia, arthrosis, bone disorder, fracture accidental, myalgia, neck stiffness, synovitis, tendinitis

Platelets (bleeding or clotting):	Ecchymosis, epistaxis, thrombocythemia
Psychiatric:	Anorexia, anxiety, appetite increased, depression, nervousness, somnolence
Hemic:	Anemia
Respiratory:	Bronchitis, bronchospasm, bronchospasm aggravated, coughing, dyspnea, laryngitis, pneumonia
Skin and appendages:	Alopecia, dermatitis, nail disorder, photosensitivity reaction, pruritus, rash erythematous, rash maculopapular, skin disorder, skin dry, sweating increased, urticaria
Application site disorders:	Cellulitis, dermatitis contact, injection site reaction, skin nodule
Special senses:	Taste perversion
Urinary system:	Albuminuria, cystitis, dysuria, hematuria, micturition frequency, renal calculus, urinary incontinence, urinary tract infection
Vision:	Blurred vision, cataract, conjunctivitis, eye pain, glaucoma

Other serious adverse reactions which occur rarely (estimated <0.1%), regardless of causality: The following serious adverse events have occurred rarely in patients taking CELEBREX. Cases reported only in the post-marketing experience are indicated in italics.

Cardiovascular:	Syncope, congestive heart failure, ventricular fibrillation, pulmonary embolism, cerebrovascular accident, peripheral gangrene, thrombophlebitis, *vasculitis, deep venous thrombosis*
Gastrointestinal:	Intestinal obstruction, intestinal perforation, gastrointestinal bleeding, colitis with bleeding, esophageal perforation, pancreatitis, ileus
Liver and biliary system:	Cholelithiasis, *hepatitis, jaundice, liver failure*
Hemic and lymphatic:	Thrombocytopenia, *agranulocytosis, aplastic anemia, pancytopenia, leukopenia*
Metabolic:	*Hypoglycemia, hyponatremia*
Nervous system:	Ataxia, suicide, *aseptic meningitis, ageusia, anosmia, fatal intracranial hemorrhage* (see PRECAUTIONS – Drug Interactions –*Warfarin*)
Renal:	Acute renal failure, *interstitial nephritis*
Skin:	*Erythema multiforme, exfoliative dermatitis, Stevens-Johnson syndrome, toxic epidermal necrolysis*
General:	Sepsis, sudden death, *anaphylactoid reaction, angioedema*

Adverse reactions from long-term, placebo-controlled polyp prevention studies: Exposure to CELEBREX in the APC and PreSAP trials was 400 to 800 mg daily for up to 3 years; see **Special Studies - *Adenomatous Polyp Prevention Studies.***

Some adverse reactions occurred in higher percentages of patients than in the arthritis pre-marketing trials (treatment durations up to 12 weeks; see ***Adverse events from CELEBREX premarketing controlled arthritis trials***). The adverse reactions for which these differences in patients treated with CELEBREX were greater as compared to the arthritis pre-marketing trials were as follows:

	CELEBREX (400-800 mg daily dose) (n=2285)	Placebo (n=1303)
Diarrhea	10.5%	7.0%
Gastroesophageal reflux disease	4.7%	3.1%
Nausea	6.8%	5.3%
Vomiting	3.2%	2.1%
Dyspnea	2.8%	1.6%
Hypertension	12.5%	9.8%

The following additional adverse reactions occurred in ≥0.1% and <1% of patients taking CELEBREX, at an incidence greater than placebo in the long-term polyp prevention studies and were either not reported during the controlled arthritis pre-marketing trials or occurred with greater frequency in the long-term, placebo-controlled polyp prevention studies:

Nervous system disorders:	Cerebral infarction
Eye disorders:	Vitreous floaters, conjunctival hemorrhage
Ear and labyrinth disorders:	Labyrinthitis
Cardiac disorders:	Angina unstable, aortic valve incompetence, sinus bradycardia, ventricular hypertrophy
Vascular disorders:	Deep vein thrombosis
Reproductive system and breast disorders:	Ovarian cyst
Investigations:	Blood potassium increased, blood sodium increased, blood testosterone decreased
Injury, poisoning and procedural complications:	Epicondylitis, tendon rupture

Safety Data from CLASS Study:

Hematological Events:

During this study (see **Special Studies – CLASS**), the incidence of clinically significant decreases in hemoglobin (>2 g/dL) confirmed by repeat testing was lower in patients on CELEBREX 400 mg BID (4-fold and 2-fold the recommended OA and RA doses, respectively, and the approved dose for FAP) compared to patients on either diclofenac 75 mg BID or ibuprofen 800 mg TID: 0.5%, 1.3% and 1.9%, respectively. The lower incidence of events with CELEBREX was maintained with or without ASA use (see **CLINICAL PHARMACOLOGY - Platelets**).

Withdrawals/Serious Adverse Events:

Kaplan-Meier cumulative rates at 9 months for withdrawals due to adverse events for CELEBREX, diclofenac and ibuprofen were 24%, 29%, and 26%, respectively. Rates for serious adverse events (i.e. those causing hospitalization or felt to be life threatening or otherwise medically significant) regardless of causality were not different across treatment groups, respectively, 8%, 7%, and 8%.

Adverse events from juvenile rheumatoid arthritis study: In a 12-week, double-blind, active-controlled study, 242 JRA patients 2 years to 17 years of age were treated with celecoxib or naproxen; 77 JRA patients were treated with celecoxib 3 mg/kg BID, 82 patients were treated with celecoxib 6 mg/kg BID, and 83 patients were treated with naproxen 7.5 mg/kg BID. The most commonly occurring (≥5%) adverse events in celecoxib treated patients were headache, fever (pyrexia), upper abdominal pain, cough, nasopharyngitis, abdominal pain, nausea, arthralgia, diarrhea and vomiting. The most commonly occurring (≥5%) adverse experiences for naproxen treated patients were headache, nausea, vomiting, fever, upper abdominal pain, diarrhea, cough, abdominal pain, and dizziness (Table 4). Compared with naproxen, celecoxib at doses of 3 and 6 mg/kg BID had no observable deleterious effect on growth and development during the course of the 12-week double-blind study. There was no substantial difference in the number of clinical exacerbations of uveitis or systemic features of JRA among treatment groups.

In a 12-week, open-label extension of the double-blind study described above, 202 JRA patients were treated with celecoxib 6 mg/kg BID. The incidence of adverse events was similar to that observed during the double-blind study; no unexpected adverse events of clinical importance emerged.

Table 4: Incidence of Adverse Events Occurring in ≥5% of JRA Patients in the Clinical Trial in Any Treatment Group by System Organ Class

System Organ Class/ Adverse Event Preferred Term	Celecoxib 3 mg/kg BID N=77	Celecoxib 6 mg/kg BID N=82	Naproxen 7.5 mg/kg BID N=83
Any Event, %	**64**	**70**	**72**
Eye Disorders	**5**	**5**	**5**
Gastrointestinal Disorders	**26**	**24**	**36**
Abdominal pain NOS	4	7	7
Abdominal pain upper	8	6	10
Vomiting NOS	3*	6	11
Diarrhea NOS	5	4	8
Nausea	7	4	11
General Disorders and Administration Site Conditions	**13**	**11**	**18**
Pyrexia	8	9	11
Infections and Infestations	**25**	**20**	**27**
Nasopharyngitis	5	6	5
Injury and Poisoning	**4**	**6**	**5**
Investigations*	**3**	**11**	**7**
Musculoskeletal, Connective Tissue and Bone Disorders	**8**	**10**	**17**
Arthralgia	3	7	4
Nervous System Disorders	**17**	**11**	**21**
Headache NOS	13	10	16
Dizziness (excluding vertigo)	1	1	7
Respiratory, Thoracic and Mediastinal Disorders	**8**	**15**	**15**
Cough	7	7	8
Skin & Subcutaneous Tissue Disorders	**10**	**7**	**18**

*Abnormal laboratory tests, which include: Prolonged activated partial thromboplastin time, Bacteriuria NOS present, Blood creatine phosphokinase increased, Blood culture positive, Blood glucose increased, Blood pressure increased, Blood uric acid increased, Hematocrit decreased, Hematuria present, Hemoglobin decreased, Liver function tests NOS abnormal, Proteinuria present, Transaminase NOS increased, Urine analysis abnormal NOS

Adverse events from ankylosing spondylitis studies: A total of 378 patients were treated with CELEBREX in placebo- and active-controlled ankylosing spondylitis studies. Doses up to 400 mg QD were studied. The types of adverse events reported in the ankylosing spondylitis studies were similar to those reported in the arthritis studies.

Adverse events from analgesia and dysmenorrhea studies: Approximately 1,700 patients were treated with CELEBREX in analgesia and dysmenorrhea studies. All patients in post-oral surgery pain studies received a single dose of study medication. Doses up to 600 mg/day of CELEBREX were studied in primary dysmenorrhea and post-orthopedic surgery pain studies. The types of adverse events in the analgesia and dysmenorrhea studies were similar to those reported in arthritis studies. The only additional adverse event reported was post-dental extraction alveolar osteitis (dry socket) in the post-oral surgery pain studies.

Adverse events from the controlled trial in familial adenomatous polyposis: The adverse event profile reported for the 83 patients with familial adenomatous polyposis enrolled in the randomized, controlled clinical trial was similar to that reported for patients in the arthritis controlled trials. Intestinal anastomotic ulceration was the only new adverse event reported in the FAP trial, regardless of causality, and was observed in 3 of 58 patients (one at 100 mg BID, and two at 400 mg BID) who had prior intestinal surgery.

OVERDOSAGE

No overdoses of CELEBREX were reported during clinical trials. Doses up to 2400 mg/day for up to 10 days in 12 patients did not result in serious toxicity. Symptoms following acute NSAID overdoses are usually limited to lethargy, drowsiness, nausea, vomiting, and epigastric pain, which are generally reversible with supportive care. Gastrointestinal bleeding can occur. Hypertension, acute renal failure, respiratory depression and coma may occur, but are rare. Anaphylactoid reactions have been reported with therapeutic ingestion of NSAIDs, and may occur following an overdose. Patients should be managed by symptomatic and supportive care following an NSAID overdose. There are no specific antidotes. No information is available regarding the removal of celecoxib by hemodialysis, but based on its high degree of plasma protein binding (>97%) dialysis is unlikely to be useful in overdose. Emesis and/or activated charcoal (60 to 100 g in adults, 1 to 2 g/kg in children) and/or osmotic cathartic may be indicated in patients seen within 4 hours of ingestion with symptoms or following a large overdose. Forced diuresis, alkalinization of urine, hemodialysis, or hemoperfusion may not be useful due to high protein binding.

DOSAGE AND ADMINISTRATION

Carefully consider the potential benefits and risks of CELEBREX and other treatment options before deciding to use CELEBREX. Use the lowest effective dose for the shortest duration consistent with individual patient treatment goals (see **WARNINGS**).

For osteoarthritis and rheumatoid arthritis, the lowest dose of CELEBREX should be sought for each patient. These doses can be given without regard to timing of meals.

Osteoarthritis: For relief of the signs and symptoms of osteoarthritis the recommended oral dose is 200 mg per day administered as a single dose or as 100 mg twice per day.

Rheumatoid arthritis: For relief of the signs and symptoms of rheumatoid arthritis the recommended oral dose is 100 to 200 mg twice per day.

Juvenile Rheumatoid Arthritis:

Pediatric Patients (2 years and older)	Dose
≥10 kg to ≤25 kg	50 mg capsule twice daily
>25 kg	100 mg capsule twice daily

Method of Administration

For patients who have difficulty swallowing capsules, the contents of a CELEBREX capsule can be added to applesauce. The entire capsule contents are carefully emptied onto a level teaspoon of cool or room temperature applesauce and

Continued on next page

Celebrex—Cont.

ingested immediately with water. The sprinkled capsule contents on applesauce are stable for up to 6 hours under refrigerated conditions (2-8° C/ 35-45° F).

Ankylosing Spondylitis (AS): For the management of the signs and symptoms of AS, the recommended dose of CELEBREX is 200 mg daily single (once per day) or divided (twice per day) doses. If no effect is observed after 6 weeks, a trial of 400 mg daily may be worthwhile. If no effect is observed after 6 weeks on 400 mg daily, a response is not likely and consideration should be given to alternate treatment options.

Management of Acute Pain and Treatment of Primary Dysmenorrhea: The recommended dose of CELEBREX is 400 mg initially, followed by an additional 200 mg dose if needed on the first day. On subsequent days, the recommended dose is 200 mg twice daily as needed.

Familial adenomatous polyposis (FAP): Usual medical care for FAP patients should be continued while on CELEBREX. To reduce the number of adenomatous colorectal polyps in patients with FAP, the recommended oral dose is 400 mg twice per day to be taken with food.

Special Populations

Hepatic insufficiency: The daily recommended dose of CELEBREX capsules in patients with moderate hepatic impairment (Child-Pugh Class B) should be reduced by approximately 50%. The use of CELEBREX in patients with severe hepatic impairment is not recommended (see **CLINICAL PHARMACOLOGY – Special Populations**).

HOW SUPPLIED

CELEBREX 50-mg capsules are white, with reverse printed white on red band of body and cap with markings of 7767 on the cap and 50 on the body, supplied as:

NDC Number	Size
0025-1515-01	bottle of 60

CELEBREX 100-mg capsules are white, reverse printed white on blue band of body and cap with markings of 7767 on the cap and 100 on the body, supplied as:

NDC Number	Size
0025-1520-31	bottle of 100
0025-1520-51	bottle of 500
0025-1520-34	carton of 100 unit dose

CELEBREX 200-mg capsules are white, with reverse printed white on gold band with markings of 7767 on the cap and 200 on the body, supplied as:

NDC Number	Size
0025-1525-31	bottle of 100
0025-1525-51	bottle of 500
0025-1525-34	carton of 100 unit dose

CELEBREX 400-mg capsules are white, with reverse printed white on green band with markings of 7767 on the cap and 400 on the body, supplied as:

NDC Number	Size
0025-1530-02	bottle of 60
0025-1530-01	carton of 100 unit dose

Store at 25°C (77°F); excursions permitted to 15-30°C (59-86°F) [see USP Controlled Room Temperature].

Rx only
Distributed by
G.D. Searle LLC
Division of Pfizer Inc, NY, NY 0017
LAB-0036-11
Revised January 2008

Medication Guide
for
Non-Steroidal Anti-Inflammatory Drugs (NSAIDs)
(See the end of this Medication Guide for a list of prescription NSAID medicines.)

What is the most important information I should know about medicines called Non-Steroidal Anti-Inflammatory Drugs (NSAIDs)?
NSAID medicines may increase the chance of a heart attack or stroke that can lead to death.
This chance increases:
• with longer use of NSAID medicines
• in people who have heart disease
NSAID medicines should never be used right before or after a heart surgery called a "coronary artery bypass graft (CABG)."
NSAID medicines can cause ulcers and bleeding in the stomach and intestines at any time during treatment. Ulcers and bleeding:
• can happen without warning symptoms
• may cause death
The chance of a person getting an ulcer or bleeding increases with:
• taking medicines called "corticosteroids" and "anticoagulants"
• longer use
• smoking
• drinking alcohol
• older age
• having poor health

NSAID medicines should only be used:
• exactly as prescribed
• at the lowest dose possible for your treatment
• for the shortest time needed

What are Non-Steroidal Anti-Inflammatory Drugs (NSAIDs)?
NSAID medicines are used to treat pain and redness, swelling, and heat (inflammation) from medical conditions such as:
• different types of arthritis
• menstrual cramps and other types of short-term pain

Who should not take a Non-Steroidal Anti-Inflammatory Drug (NSAID)?
Do not take an NSAID medicine:
• if you had an asthma attack, hives, or other allergic reaction with aspirin or any other NSAID medicine
• for pain right before or after heart bypass surgery

Tell your healthcare provider:
• about all of your medical conditions.
• about all of the medicines you take. NSAIDs and some other medicines can interact with each other and cause serious side effects. **Keep a list of your medicines to show to your healthcare provider and pharmacist.**
• if you are pregnant. **NSAID medicines should not be used by pregnant women late in their pregnancy.**
• if you are breastfeeding. **Talk to your doctor.**

What are the possible side effects of Non-Steroidal Anti-Inflammatory Drugs (NSAIDs)?

Serious side effects include:	Other side effects include:
• heart attack • stroke • high blood pressure • heart failure from body swelling (fluid retention) • kidney problems including kidney failure • bleeding and ulcers in the stomach and intestine • low red blood cells (anemia) • life-threatening skin reactions • life-threatening allergic reactions • liver problems including liver failure • asthma attacks in people who have asthma	• stomach pain • constipation • diarrhea • gas • heartburn • nausea • vomiting • dizziness

Get emergency help right away if you have any of the following symptoms:
• shortness of breath or trouble breathing
• chest pain
• weakness in one part or side of your body
• slurred speech
• swelling of the face or throat

Stop your NSAID medicine and call your healthcare provider right away if you have any of the following symptoms:
• nausea
• more tired or weaker than usual
• itching
• your skin or eyes look yellow
• stomach pain
• flu-like symptoms
• vomit blood
• there is blood in your bowel movement or it is black and sticky like tar
• skin rash or blisters with fever
• unusual weight gain
• swelling of the arms and legs, hands and feet
These are not all the side effects with NSAID medicines. Talk to your healthcare provider or pharmacist for more information about NSAID medicines.

Other information about Non-Steroidal Anti-Inflammatory Drugs (NSAIDs)
• Aspirin is an NSAID medicine but it does not increase the chance of a heart attack. Aspirin can cause bleeding in the brain, stomach, and intestines. Aspirin can also cause ulcers in the stomach and intestines.
• Some of these NSAID medicines are sold in lower doses without a prescription (over-the-counter). Talk to your healthcare provider before using over-the-counter NSAIDs for more than 10 days.

NSAID medicines that need a prescription

Generic Name	Tradename
Celecoxib	Celebrex
Diclofenac	Cataflam, Voltaren, Arthrotec (combined with misoprostol)
Diflunisal	Dolobid
Etodolac	Lodine, Lodine XL
Fenoprofen	Nalfon, Nalfon 200
Flurbiprofen	Ansaid
Ibuprofen	Motrin, Tab-Profen, Vicoprofen* (combined with hydrocodone), Combunox (combined with oxycodone)
Indomethacin	Indocin, Indocin SR, Indo-Lemmon, Indomethagan
Ketoprofen	Oruvail
Ketorolac	Toradol
Mefenamic Acid	Ponstel
Meloxicam	Mobic
Nabumetone	Relafen
Naproxen	Naprosyn, Anaprox, Anaprox DS, EC-Naproxyn, Naprelan, Naprapac (copackaged with lansoprazole)
Oxaprozin	Daypro
Piroxicam	Feldene
Sulindac	Clinoril
Tolmetin	Tolectin, Tolectin DS, Tolectin 600

* Vicoprofen contains the same dose of ibuprofen as over-the-counter (OTC) NSAIDs, and is usually used for less than 10 days to treat pain. The OTC NSAID label warns that long term continuous use may increase the risk of heart attack or stroke.

This Medication Guide has been approved by the U.S. Food and Drug Administration.

Shire US Inc.
725 CHESTERBROOK BOULEVARD
WAYNE, PA 19087

Direct Inquiries to:
Customer Service
(800) 828-2088
For Medical Information Contact:
(800) 828-2088

CARBATROL® ℞
[căr-bŏ'trōl]
(carbamazepine) Extended-Release Capsules
100 mg, 200 mg and 300 mg
Rx only

Prescribing information for this product, which appears on pages 3098–3101 of the 2008 PDR, has been completely revised as follows. Please write "See Supplement A" next to the product heading.

WARNING

SERIOUS DERMATOLOGIC REACTIONS AND HLA-B*1502 ALLELE
SERIOUS AND SOMETIMES FATAL DERMATOLOGIC REACTIONS, INCLUDING TOXIC EPIDERMAL NECROLYSIS (TEN) AND STEVENS-JOHNSON SYNDROME (SJS), HAVE BEEN REPORTED DURING TREATMENT WITH CARBAMAZEPINE. THESE REACTIONS ARE ESTIMATED TO OCCUR IN 1 TO 6 PER 10,000 NEW USERS IN COUNTRIES WITH MAINLY CAUCASIAN POPULATIONS, BUT THE RISK IN SOME ASIAN COUNTRIES IS ESTIMATED TO BE ABOUT 10 TIMES HIGHER. STUDIES IN PATIENTS OF CHINESE ANCESTRY HAVE FOUND A STRONG ASSOCIATION BETWEEN THE RISK OF DEVELOPING SJS/TEN AND THE PRESENCE OF HLA-B*1502, AN INHERITED ALLELIC VARIANT OF THE HLA-B GENE. HLA-B*1502 IS FOUND ALMOST EXCLUSIVELY IN PATIENTS WITH ANCESTRY ACROSS BROAD AREAS OF ASIA. PATIENTS WITH ANCESTRY IN GENETICALLY AT-RISK POPULATIONS SHOULD BE SCREENED FOR THE PRESENCE OF HLA-B*1502 PRIOR TO INITIATING TREATMENT WITH CARBATROL. PATIENTS TESTING POSITIVE FOR THE ALLELE SHOULD NOT BE TREATED WITH CARBATROL UNLESS THE BENEFIT CLEARLY OUTWEIGHS THE RISK (SEE WARNINGS AND PRECAUTIONS/LABORATORY TESTS).
APLASTIC ANEMIA AND AGRANULOCYTOSIS HAVE BEEN REPORTED IN ASSOCIATION WITH THE USE OF CARBAMAZEPINE. DATA FROM A POPULATION-BASED CASE-CONTROL STUDY DEMONSTRATE THAT THE RISK OF DEVELOPING THESE REACTIONS IS 5-8 TIMES GREATER THAN IN THE GENERAL POPULATION. HOWEVER, THE OVERALL RISK OF THESE REACTIONS IN THE UNTREATED GENERAL POPULATION IS LOW, APPROXIMATELY SIX PATIENTS PER ONE MILLION POPULATION PER YEAR FOR AGRANULOCYTOSIS AND TWO PATIENTS PER ONE MILLION POPULA-

TION PER YEAR FOR APLASTIC ANEMIA.
ALTHOUGH REPORTS OF TRANSIENT OR PERSISTENT DECREASED PLATELET OR WHITE BLOOD CELL COUNTS ARE NOT UNCOMMON IN ASSOCIATION WITH THE USE OF CARBAMAZEPINE, DATA ARE NOT AVAILABLE TO ESTIMATE ACCURATELY THEIR INCIDENCE OR OUTCOME. HOWEVER, THE VAST MAJORITY OF THE CASES OF LEUKOPENIA HAVE NOT PROGRESSED TO THE MORE SERIOUS CONDITIONS OF APLASTIC ANEMIA OR AGRANULOCYTOSIS.
BECAUSE OF THE VERY LOW INCIDENCE OF AGRANULOCYTOSIS AND APLASTIC ANEMIA, THE VAST MAJORITY OF MINOR HEMATOLOGIC CHANGES OBSERVED IN MONITORING OF PATIENTS ON CARBAMAZEPINE ARE UNLIKELY TO SIGNAL THE OCCURRENCE OF EITHER ABNORMALITY. NONETHELESS, COMPLETE PRETREATMENT HEMATOLOGICAL TESTING SHOULD BE OBTAINED AS A BASELINE. IF A PATIENT IN THE COURSE OF TREATMENT EXHIBITS LOW OR DECREASED WHITE BLOOD CELL OR PLATELET COUNTS, THE PATIENT SHOULD BE MONITORED CLOSELY. DISCONTINUATION OF THE DRUG SHOULD BE CONSIDERED IF ANY EVIDENCE OF SIGNIFICANT BONE MARROW DEPRESSION DEVELOPS.

Before prescribing Carbatrol, the physician should be thoroughly familiar with the details of this prescribing information, particularly regarding use with other drugs, especially those which accentuate toxicity potential.

DESCRIPTION

CARBATROL® is an anticonvulsant and specific analgesic for trigeminal neuralgia, available for oral administration as 100 mg, 200 mg and 300 mg extended-release capsules of Carbamazepine, USP. Carbamazepine is a white to off-white powder, practically insoluble in water and soluble in alcohol and in acetone. Its molecular weight is 236.27. Its chemical name is 5H-dibenz[b,f]azepine-5-carboxamide, and its structural formula is:

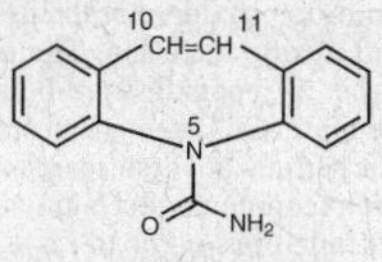

CARBAMAZEPINE

Carbatrol is a multi-component capsule formulation consisting of three different types of beads: immediate-release beads, extended-release beads, and enteric-release beads. The three bead types are combined in a specific ratio to provide twice daily dosing of Carbatrol.

Inactive ingredients: citric acid, colloidal silicon dioxide, lactose monohydrate, microcrystalline cellulose, polyethylene glycol, povidone, sodium lauryl sulfate, talc, triethyl citrate and other ingredients.

The 100 mg capsule shells contain gelatin-NF, FD&C Blue #2, Yellow Iron Oxide, and titanium dioxide and are imprinted with white ink; the 200 mg capsule shells contain gelatin-NF, FD&C Red #3, FD&C Yellow #6, Yellow Iron Oxide, FD&C Blue #2, and titanium dioxide, and are imprinted with white ink; and the 300 mg capsule shells contain gelatin-NF, FD&C Blue #2, FD&C Yellow #6, Red Iron Oxide, Yellow Iron Oxide, and titanium dioxide, and are imprinted with white ink.

CLINICAL PHARMACOLOGY

In controlled clinical trials, carbamazepine has been shown to be effective in the treatment of psychomotor and grand mal seizures, as well as trigeminal neuralgia.

Mechanism of Action

Carbamazepine has demonstrated anticonvulsant properties in rats and mice with electrically and chemically induced seizures. It appears to act by reducing polysynaptic responses and blocking the post-tetanic potentiation. Carbamazepine greatly reduces or abolishes pain induced by stimulation of the infraorbital nerve in cats and rats. It depresses thalamic potential and bulbar and polysynaptic reflexes, including the linguomandibular reflex in cats. Carbamazepine is chemically unrelated to other anticonvulsants or other drugs used to control the pain of trigeminal neuralgia. The mechanism of action remains unknown.

The principal metabolite of carbamazepine, carbamazepine-10,11-epoxide, has anticonvulsant activity as demonstrated in several *in vivo* animal models of seizures. Though clinical activity for the epoxide has been postulated, the significance of its activity with respect to the safety and efficacy of carbamazepine has not been established.

Pharmacokinetics

Carbamazepine (CBZ): Taken every 12 hours, carbamazepine extended-release capsules provide steady state plasma levels comparable to immediate-release carbamazepine tablets given every 6 hours, when administered at the same total mg daily dose.

Following a single 200 mg oral extended-release dose of carbamazepine, peak plasma concentration was 1.9 ± 0.3 μg/mL and the time to reach the peak was 19 ± 7 hours. Following chronic administration (800 mg every 12 hours), the peak levels were 11.0 ± 2.5 μg/mL and the time to reach the peak was 5.9 ± 1.8 hours. The pharmacokinetics of extended-release carbamazepine is linear over the single dose range of 200-800 mg.

Carbamazepine is 76% bound to plasma proteins. Carbamazepine is primarily metabolized in the liver. Cytochrome P450 3A4 was identified as the major isoform responsible for the formation of carbamazepine-10,11-epoxide. Since carbamazepine induces its own metabolism, the half-life is also variable. Following a single extended-release dose of carbamazepine, the average half-life range from 35-40 hours and 12-17 hours on repeated dosing. The apparent oral clearance following a single dose was 25 ± 5 mL/min and following multiple dosing was 80 ± 30 mL/min.

After oral administration of ^{14}C-carbamazepine, 72% of the administered radioactivity was found in the urine and 28% in the feces. This urinary radioactivity was composed largely of hydroxylated and conjugated metabolites, with only 3% of unchanged carbamazepine.

Carbamazepine-10,11-epoxide (CBZ-E): Carbamazepine-10,11-epoxide is considered to be an active metabolite of carbamazepine. Following a single 200 mg oral extended-release dose of carbamazepine, the peak plasma concentration of carbamazepine-10,11-epoxide was 0.11 ± 0.012 μg/mL and the time to reach the peak was 36 ± 6 hours. Following chronic administration of a extended-release dose of carbamazepine (800 mg every 12 hours), the peak levels of carbamazepine-10,11-epoxide were 2.2 ± 0.9 μg/mL and the time to reach the peak was 14 ± 8 hours. The plasma half-life of carbamazepine-10,11-epoxide following administration of carbamazepine is 34 ± 9 hours. Following a single oral dose of extended-release carbamazepine (200-800 mg) the AUC and C_{max} of carbamazepine-10,11-epoxide were less than 10% of carbamazepine. Following multiple dosing of extended-release carbamazepine (800-1600 mg daily for 14 days), the AUC and C_{max} of carbamazepine-10,11-epoxide were dose related, ranging from 15.7 μg.hr/mL and 1.5 μg/mL at 800 mg/day to 32.6 μg.hr/mL and 3.2 μg/mL at 1600 mg/day, respectively, and were less than 30% of carbamazepine. Carbamazepine-10,11-epoxide is 50% bound to plasma proteins.

Food Effect: A high fat meal diet increased the rate of absorption of a single 400 mg dose (mean T_{max} was reduced from 24 hours, in the fasting state, to 14 hours and C_{max} increased from 3.2 to 4.3 μg/mL) but not the extent (AUC) of absorption. The elimination half-life remains unchanged between fed and fasting state. The multiple dose study conducted in the fed state showed that the steady-state C_{max} values were within the therapeutic concentration range. The pharmacokinetic profile of extended-release carbamazepine was similar when given by sprinkling the beads over applesauce compared to the intact capsule administered in the fasted state.

Special Populations

Hepatic Dysfunction: The effect of hepatic impairment on the pharmacokinetics of carbamazepine is not known. However, given that carbamazepine is primarily metabolized in the liver, it is prudent to proceed with caution in patients with hepatic dysfunction.

Renal Dysfunction: The effect of renal impairment on the pharmacokinetics of carbamazepine is not known.

Gender: No difference in the mean AUC and C_{max} of carbamazepine and carbamazepine-10,11-epoxide was found between males and females.

Age: Carbamazepine is more rapidly metabolized to carbamazepine-10,11-epoxide in young children than adults. In children below the age of 15, there is an inverse relationship between CBZ-E/CBZ ratio and increasing age.

Race: No information is available on the effect of race on the pharmacokinetics of carbamazepine.

INDICATIONS AND USAGE

Epilepsy

Carbatrol is indicated for use as an anticonvulsant drug. Evidence supporting efficacy of carbamazepine as an anticonvulsant was derived from active drug-controlled studies that enrolled patients with the following seizure types:

1. Partial seizures with complex symptomatology (psychomotor, temporal lobe). Patients with these seizures appear to show greater improvements than those with other types.
2. Generalized tonic-clonic seizures (grand mal).
3. Mixed seizure patterns which include the above, or other partial or generalized seizures. Absence seizures (petit mal) do not appear to be controlled by carbamazepine (see PRECAUTIONS, General).

Trigeminal Neuralgia

Carbatrol is indicated in the treatment of the pain associated with true trigeminal neuralgia. Beneficial results have also been reported in glossopharyngeal neuralgia. This drug is not a simple analgesic and should not be used for the relief of trivial aches or pains.

CONTRAINDICATIONS

Carbamazepine should not be used in patients with a history of previous bone marrow depression, hypersensitivity to the drug, or known sensitivity to any of the tricyclic compounds, such as amitriptyline, desipramine, imipramine, protriptyline and nortriptyline. Likewise, on theoretical grounds its use with monoamine oxidase inhibitors is not recommended. Before administration of carbamazepine, MAO inhibitors should be discontinued for a minimum of 14 days, or longer if the clinical situation permits.

WARNINGS

Serious Dermatologic Reactions

Serious and sometimes fatal dermatologic reactions, including toxic epidermal necrolysis (TEN) and Stevens-Johnson syndrome (SJS), have been reported with carbamazepine treatment. The risk of these events is estimated to be about 1 to 6 per 10,000 new users in countries with mainly Caucasian populations. However, the risk in some Asian countries is estimated to be about 10 times higher. Carbatrol should be discontinued at the first sign of a rash, unless the rash is clearly not drug-related. If signs or symptoms suggest SJS/TEN, use of this drug should not be resumed and alternative therapy should be considered.

SJS/TEN and HLA-B*1502 Allele

Retrospective case-control studies have found that in patients of Chinese ancestry there is a strong association between the risk of developing SJS/TEN with carbamazepine treatment and the presence of an inherited variant of the HLA-B gene, HLA-B*1502. The occurrence of higher rates of these reactions in countries with higher frequencies of this allele suggests that the risk may be increased in allele-positive individuals of any ethnicity.

Across Asian populations, notable variation exists in the prevalence of HLA-B*1502. Greater than 15% of the population is reported positive in Hong Kong, Thailand, Malaysia, and parts of the Philippines, compared to about 10% in Taiwan and 4% in North China. South Asians, including Indians, appear to have intermediate prevalence of HLA-B*1502, averaging 2 to 4%, but higher in some groups. HLA-B*1502 is present in <1% of the population in Japan and Korea.

HLA-B*1502 is largely absent in individuals not of Asian origin (e.g., Caucasians, African-Americans, Hispanics, and Native Americans).

Prior to initiating Carbatrol therapy, testing for HLA-B*1502 should be performed in patients with ancestry in populations in which HLA-B*1502 may be present. In deciding which patients to screen, the rates provided above for the prevalence of HLA-B*1502 may offer a rough guide, keeping in mind the limitations of these figures due to wide variability in rates even within ethnic groups, the difficulty in ascertaining ethnic ancestry, and the likelihood of mixed ancestry. Carbatrol should not be used in patients positive for HLA-B*1502 unless the benefits clearly outweigh the risks. Tested patients who are found to be negative for the allele are thought to have a low risk of SJS/TEN (see **WARNINGS** and **PRECAUTIONS/Laboratory Tests**).

Over 90% of carbamazepine treated patients who will experience SJS/TEN have this reaction within the first few months of treatment. This information may be taken into consideration in determining the need for screening of genetically at-risk patients currently on Carbatrol.

The HLA-B*1502 allele has not been found to predict risk of less severe adverse cutaneous reactions from carbamazepine, such as anticonvulsant hypersensitivity syndrome or non-serious rash (maculopapular eruption [MPE]).

Limited evidence suggests that HLA-B*1502 may be a risk factor for the development of SJS/TEN in patients of Chinese ancestry taking other anti-epileptic drugs associated with SJS/TEN. Consideration should be given to avoiding use of other drugs associated with SJS/TEN in HLA-B*1502 positive patients, when alternative therapies are otherwise equally acceptable.

Application of HLA-B*1502 genotyping as a screening tool has important limitations and must never substitute for appropriate clinical vigilance and patient management. Many HLA-B*1502-positive Asian patients treated with carbamazepine will not develop SJS/TEN, and these reactions can still occur infrequently in HLA-B*1502-negative patients of any ethnicity. The role of other possible factors in the development of, and morbidity from, SJS/TEN, such as AED dose, compliance, concomitant medications, comorbidities, and the level of dermatologic monitoring have not been studied.

Patients should be made aware that Carbatrol contains carbamazepine and should not be used in combination with any other medications containing carbamazepine.

Usage in Pregnancy

Carbamazepine can cause fetal harm when administered to a pregnant woman.

Epidemiological data suggest that there may be an association between the use of carbamazepine during pregnancy and congenital malformations, including spina bifida. The prescribing physician will wish to weigh the benefits of therapy against the risks in treating or counseling women of childbearing potential. If this drug is used during pregnancy, or if the patient becomes pregnant while taking this drug, the patient should be apprised of the potential hazard to the fetus.

Retrospective case reviews suggest that, compared with monotherapy, there may be a higher prevalence of teratogenic effects associated with the use of anticonvulsants in combination therapy.

In humans, transplacental passage of carbamazepine is rapid (30-60 minutes), and the drug is accumulated in the fetal tissues, with higher levels found in liver and kidney than in brain and lung.

Carbamazepine has been shown to have adverse effects in reproduction studies in rats when given orally in dosages 10-25 times the maximum human daily dosage (MHDD) of 1200 mg on a mg/kg basis or 1.5-4 times the MHDD on a mg/m^2 basis. In rat teratology studies, 2 of 135 offspring showed kinked ribs at 250 mg/kg and 4 of 119 offspring at 650 mg/kg showed other anomalies (cleft palate, 1; talipes, 1; anophthalmos, 2). In reproduction studies in rats, nursing offspring demonstrated a lack of weight gain and an unkempt appearance at a maternal dosage level of 200 mg/kg.

Continued on next page

Carbatrol—Cont.

Antiepileptic drugs should not be discontinued abruptly in patients in whom the drug is administered to prevent major seizures because of the strong possibility of precipitating status epilepticus with attendant hypoxia and threat to life. In individual cases where the severity and frequency of the seizure disorder are such that removal of medication does not pose a serious threat to the patient, discontinuation of the drug may be considered prior to and during pregnancy, although it cannot be said with any confidence that even minor seizures do not pose some hazard to the developing embryo or fetus.

Tests to detect defects using current accepted procedures should be considered a part of routine prenatal care in child-bearing women receiving carbamazepine.

General

Patients with a history of adverse hematologic reaction to any drug may be particularly at risk of bone marrow depression.

In patients with seizure disorder, carbamazepine should not be discontinued abruptly because of the strong possibility of precipitating status epilepticus with attendant hypoxia and threat to life.

Carbamazepine has shown mild anticholinergic activity; therefore, patients with increased intraocular pressure should be closely observed during therapy.

Because of the relationship of the drug to other tricyclic compounds, the possibility of activation of a latent psychosis and, in elderly patients, of confusion or agitation should be considered.

Co-administration of carbamazepine and delavirdine may lead to loss of virologic response and possible resistance to PRESCRIPTOR or to the class of non-nucleoside reverse transcriptase inhibitors.

PRECAUTIONS

General

Before initiating therapy, a detailed history and physical examination should be made.

Carbamazepine should be used with caution in patients with a mixed seizure disorder that includes atypical absence seizures, since in these patients carbamazepine has been associated with increased frequency of generalized convulsions (see INDICATIONS AND USAGE).

Therapy should be prescribed only after critical benefit-to-risk appraisal in patients with a history of cardiac, hepatic, or renal damage; adverse hematologic reaction to other drugs; or interrupted courses of therapy with carbamazepine.

Information for Patients

Patients should be made aware of the early toxic signs and symptoms of a potential hematologic problem, such as fever, sore throat, rash, ulcers in the mouth, easy bruising, petechial or purpuric hemorrhage, and should be advised to report to the physician immediately if any such signs or symptoms appear.

Since dizziness and drowsiness may occur, patients should be cautioned about the hazards of operating machinery or automobiles or engaging in other potentially dangerous tasks. If necessary, the Carbatrol capsules can be opened and the contents sprinkled over food, such as a teaspoon of applesauce or other similar food products.

Carbatrol capsules or their contents should not be crushed or chewed. Carbatrol may interact with some drugs. Therefore, patients should be advised to report to their doctors the use of any other prescription or non-prescription medication or herbal products.

Laboratory Tests

For genetically at-risk patients [See WARNINGS], high-resolution 'HLA-B*1502 typing' is recommended. The test is positive if either one or two HLA-B*1502 alleles are detected and negative if no HLA-B*1502 alleles are detected. Complete pretreatment blood counts, including platelets and possibly reticulocytes and serum iron, should be obtained as a baseline. If a patient in the course of treatment exhibits low or decreased white blood cell or platelet counts, the patient should be monitored closely. Discontinuation of the drug should be considered if any evidence of significant bone marrow depression develops.

Baseline and periodic evaluations of liver function, particularly in patients with a history of liver disease, must be performed during treatment with this drug since liver damage may occur. The drug should be discontinued immediately in cases of aggravated liver dysfunction or active liver disease.

Baseline and periodic eye examinations, including slit-lamp, funduscopy, and tonometry, are recommended since many phenothiazines and related drugs have been shown to cause eye changes.

Baseline and periodic complete urinalysis and BUN determinations are recommended for patients treated with this agent because of observed renal dysfunction.

Increases in total cholesterol, LDL and HDL have been observed in some patients taking anticonvulsants. Therefore, periodic evaluation of these parameters is also recommended.

Monitoring of blood levels (see CLINICAL PHARMACOLOGY) has increased the efficacy and safety of anticonvulsants. This monitoring may be particularly useful in cases of dramatic increase in seizure frequency and for verification of compliance. In addition, measurement of drug serum levels may aid in determining the cause of toxicity when more than one medication is being used.

Thyroid function tests have been reported to show decreased values with carbamazepine administered alone.

Hyponatremia has been reported in association with carbamazepine use, either alone or in combination with other drugs.

Interference with some pregnancy tests has been reported.

Drug Interactions

Clinically meaningful drug interactions have occurred with concomitant medications and include, but are not limited to the following:

Agents Highly Bound to Plasma Protein:

Carbamazepine is not highly bound to plasma proteins; therefore, administration of Carbatrol® to a patient taking another drug that is highly protein bound should not cause increased free concentrations of the other drug.

Agents that Inhibits Cytochrome P450 Isoenzymes and/or Epoxide Hydrolase:

Carbamazepine is metabolized mainly by cytochrome P450 (CYP) 3A4 to the active carbamazepine 10,11-epoxide, which is further metabolized to the trans-diol by epoxide hydrolase. Therefore, the potential exists for interaction between carbamazepine and any agent that inhibits CYP3A4 and/or epoxide hydrolase. Agents that are CYP3A4 inhibitors that have been found, or are expected, to increase plasma levels of Carbatrol® are the following:

Acetazolamide, azole antifungals, cimetidine, clarithromycin[1], dalfopristin, danazol, delavirdine, diltiazem, erythromycin[1], fluoxetine, fluvoxamine, grapefruit juice, isoniazid, itraconazole, ketoconazole, loratadine, nefazadone, niacinamide, nicotinamide, protease inhibitors, propoxyphene, quinine, quinupristin, troleandomycin, valproate[1], verapamil, zileuton.

[1]also inhibits epoxide hydrolase resulting in increased levels of the active metabolite carbamazepine 10,11-epoxide

Thus, if a patient has been titrated to a stable dosage of Carbatrol®, and then begins a course of treatment with one of these CYP3A4 or epoxide hydrolase inhibitors, it is reasonable to expect that a dose reduction for Carbatrol® may be necessary.

Agents that Induce Cytochrome P450 Isoenzymes:

Carbamazepine is metabolized by CYP3A4. Therefore, the potential exists for interaction between carbamazepine and any agent that induces CYP3A4. Agents that are CYP inducers that have been found, or are expected, to decrease plasma levels of Carbatrol® are the following:

Cisplatin, doxorubicin HCL, felbamate, rifampin, phenobarbital, phenytoin[2], primidone, methsuximide, and theophylline

[2]Phenytoin plasma levels have also been reported to increase and decrease in the presence of carbamazepine, see below.

Thus, if a patient has been titrated to a stable dosage on Carbatrol®, and then begins a course of treatment with one of these CYP3A4 inducers, it is reasonable to expect that a dose increase for Carbatrol® may be necessary.

Agents with Decreased Levels in the Presence of Carbamazepine due to Induction of Cytochrome P450 Enzymes:

Carbamazepine is known to induce CYP1A2 and CYP3A4. Therefore, the potential exists for interaction between carbamazepine and any agent metabolized by one (or more) of these enzymes. Agents that have been found, or are expected to have decreased plasma levels in the presence of Carbatrol® due to induction of CYP enzymes are the following:

Acetaminophen, alprazolam, amitriptyline, bupropion, buspirone, citalopram, clobazam, clonazepam, clozapine, cyclosporin, delavirdine, desipramine, diazepam, dicumarol, doxycycline, ethosuximide, felbamate, felodipine, glucocorticoids, haloperidol, itraconazole, lamotrigine, levothyroxine, lorazepam, methadone, midazolam, mirtazapine, nortriptyline, olanzapine, oral contraceptives[3], oxcarbazepine, phenytoin[4], praziquantel, protease inhibitors, quetiapine, risperidone, theophylline, topiramate, tiagabine, tramadol, triazolam, trazodone[5], valproate, warfarin[6], ziprasidone, and zonisamide.

[3]Break through bleeding has been reported among patients receiving concomitant oral contraceptives and their reliability may be adversely affected.

[4]Phenytoin has also been reported to increase in the presence of carbamazepine. Careful monitoring of phenytoin plasma levels following co-medication with carbamazepine is advised.

[5]Following co-administration of carbamazepine 400mg/day with trazodone 100mg to 300mg daily, carbamazepine reduced trough plasma concentrations of trazodone (as well as meta-chlorophenylpiperazine [mCPP]) by 76 and 60% respectively, compared to precarbamazepine values.

[6]Warfarin's anticoagulant effect can be reduced in the presence of carbamazepine.

Thus, if a patient has been titrated to a stable dosage on one of the agents in this category, and then begins a course of treatment with Carbatrol®, it is reasonable to expect that a dose increase for the concomitant agent may be necessary.

Agents with Increased Levels in the Presence of Carbamazepine:

Carbatrol® increases the plasma levels of the following agents:

Clomipramine HCl, phenytoin[7], and primidone

[7]Phenytoin has also been reported to decrease in the presence of carbamazepine. Careful monitoring of phenytoin plasma levels following co-medication with carbamazepine is advised.

Thus, if a patient has been titrated to a stable dosage on one of the agents in this category, and then begins a course of the treatment with Carbatrol®, it is reasonable to expect that a dose decrease for the concomitant agent may be necessary.

Pharmacological/Pharmacodynamic Interactions with Carbamazepine:

Concomitant administration of carbamazepine and lithium may increase the risk of neurotoxic side effects.

Given the anticonvulsant properties of carbamazepine, Carbatrol® may reduce the thyroid function as has been reported with other anticonvulsants. Additionally, anti-malarial drugs, such as chloroquine and mefloquine, may antagonize the activity of carbamazepine.

Thus if a patient has been titrated to a stable dosage on one of the agents in this category, and then begins a course of treatment with Carbatrol®, it is reasonable to expect that a dose adjustment may be necessary.

Because of its primary CNS effect, caution should be used when Carbatrol® is taken with other centrally acting drugs and alcohol.

Carcinogenesis, Mutagenesis, Impairment of Fertility:

Administration of carbamazepine to Sprague-Dawley rats for two years in the diet at doses of 25, 75, and 250 mg/kg/day (low dose approximately 0.2 times the maximum human daily dose of 1200 mg on a mg/m^2 basis), resulted in a dose-related increase in the incidence of hepatocellular tumors in females and of benign interstitial cell adenomas in the testes of males.

Carbamazepine must, therefore, be considered to be carcinogenic in Sprague-Dawley rats. Bacterial and mammalian mutagenicity studies using carbamazepine produced negative results. The significance of these findings relative to the use of carbamazepine in humans is, at present, unknown.

Usage in Pregnancy

Pregnancy Category D (See WARNINGS)

Labor and Delivery

The effect of carbamazepine on human labor and delivery is unknown.

Nursing Mothers

Carbamazepine and its epoxide metabolite are transferred to breast milk and during lactation. The concentrations of carbamazepine and its epoxide metabolite are approximately 50% of the maternal plasma concentration. Because of the potential for serious adverse reactions in nursing infants from carbamazepine, a decision should be made whether to discontinue nursing or to discontinue the drug, taking into account the importance of the drug to the mother.

Pediatric Use

Substantial evidence of carbamazepine effectiveness for use in the management of children with epilepsy (see INDICATIONS for specific seizure types) is derived from clinical investigations performed in adults and from studies in several *in vitro* systems which support the conclusion that (1) the pathogenic mechanisms underlying seizure propagation are essentially identical in adults and children, and (2) the mechanism of action of carbamazepine in treating seizures is essentially identical in adults and children.

Taken as a whole, this information supports a conclusion that the generally acceptable therapeutic range of total carbamazepine in plasma (i.e., 4-12 µg/mL) is the same in children and adults.

The evidence assembled was primarily obtained from short-term use of carbamazepine. The safety of carbamazepine in children has been systematically studied up to 6 months. No longer term data from clinical trials is available.

Geriatric Use

No systematic studies in geriatric patients have been conducted.

ADVERSE REACTIONS

General: If adverse reactions are of such severity that the drug must be discontinued, the physician must be aware that abrupt discontinuation of any anticonvulsant drug in a responsive patient with epilepsy may lead to seizures or even status epilepticus with its life-threatening hazards.

The most severe adverse reactions previously observed with carbamazepine were reported in the hemopoietic system and skin (see BOX WARNING), and the cardiovascular system.

The most frequently observed adverse reactions, particularly during the initial phases of therapy, are dizziness, drowsiness, unsteadiness, nausea, and vomiting. To minimize the possibility of such reactions, therapy should be initiated at the lowest dosage recommended.

The following additional adverse reactions were previously reported with carbamazepine:

Hemopoietic System: Aplastic anemia, agranulocytosis, pancytopenia, bone marrow depression, thrombocytopenia, leukopenia, leukocytosis, eosinophilia, acute intermittent porphyria.

Skin: Toxic epidermal necrolysis (TEN) and Stevens-Johnson syndrome (SJS) (see BOXED WARNING), pruritic and erythematous rashes, urticaria, , photosensitivity reactions, alterations in skin pigmentation, exfoliative dermatitis, erythema multiforme and nodosum, purpura, aggravation of disseminated lupus erythematosus, alopecia, and diaphoresis. In certain cases, discontinuation of therapy may be necessary. Isolated cases of hirsutism have been reported, but a causal relationship is not clear.

Cardiovascular System: Congestive heart failure, edema, aggravation of hypertension, hypotension, syncope and collapse, aggravation of coronary artery disease, arrhythmias and AV block, thrombophlebitis, thromboembolism, and adenopathy or lymphadenopathy. Some of these cardiovascular complications have resulted in fatalities. Myocardial infarction has been associated with other tricyclic compounds.

Liver: Abnormalities in liver function tests, cholestatic and hepatocellular jaundice, hepatitis.

Respiratory System: Pulmonary hypersensitivity characterized by fever, dyspnea, pneumonitis, or pneumonia.

Genitourinary System: Urinary frequency, acute urinary retention, oliguria with elevated blood pressure, azotemia, renal failure, and impotence. Albuminuria, glycosuria, elevated BUN, and microscopic deposits in the urine have also been reported.

Testicular atrophy occurred in rats receiving carbamazepine orally from 4-52 weeks at dosage levels of 50-400 mg/kg/day. Additionally, rats receiving carbamazepine in the diet for 2 years at dosage levels of 25, 75, and 250 mg/kg/day had a dose-related incidence of testicular atrophy and aspermatogenesis. In dogs, it produced a brownish discoloration, presumably a metabolite, in the urinary bladder at dosage levels of 50 mg/kg/day and higher. Relevance of these findings to humans is unknown.

Nervous System: Dizziness, drowsiness, disturbances of coordination, confusion, headache, fatigue, blurred vision, visual hallucinations, transient diplopia, oculomotor disturbances, nystagmus, speech disturbances, abnormal involuntary movements, peripheral neuritis and paresthesias, depression with agitation, talkativeness, tinnitus, and hyperacusis.

There have been reports of associated paralysis and other symptoms of cerebral arterial insufficiency, but the exact relationship of these reactions to the drug has not been established.

Isolated cases of neuroleptic malignant syndrome have been reported with concomitant use of psychotropic drugs.

Digestive System: Nausea, vomiting, gastric distress and abdominal pain, diarrhea, constipation, anorexia, and dryness of the mouth and pharynx, including glossitis and stomatitis.

Eyes: Scattered punctate cortical lens opacities, as well as conjunctivitis, have been reported. Although a direct causal relationship has not been established, many phenothiazines and related drugs have been shown to cause eye changes.

Musculoskeletal System: Aching joints and muscles, and leg cramps.

Metabolism: Fever and chills, inappropriate antidiuretic hormone (ADH) secretion syndrome has been reported. Cases of frank water intoxication, with decreased serum sodium (hyponatremia) and confusion have been reported in association with carbamazepine use (see PRECAUTIONS, Laboratory Tests). Decreased levels of plasma calcium have been reported.

Other: Isolated cases of a lupus erythematosus-like syndrome have been reported. There have been occasional reports of elevated levels of cholesterol, HDL cholesterol, and triglycerides in patients taking anticonvulsants.

A case of aseptic meningitis, accompanied by myoclonus and peripheral eosinophilia, has been reported in a patient taking carbamazepine in combination with other medications. The patient was successfully dechallenged, and the meningitis reappeared upon rechallenge with carbamazepine.

DRUG ABUSE AND DEPENDENCE

No evidence of abuse potential has been associated with carbamazepine, nor is there evidence of psychological or physical dependence in humans.

OVERDOSAGE

Acute Toxicity

Lowest known lethal dose: adults, >60 g (39-year-old man). Highest known doses survived: adults, 30 g (31-year-old woman); children, 10 g (6-year-old boy); small children, 5 g (3-year-old girl).

Oral LD_{50} in animals (mg/kg): mice, 1100-3750; rats, 3850-4025; rabbits, 1500-2680; guinea pigs, 920.

Signs and Symptoms

The first signs and symptoms appear after 1-3 hours. Neuromuscular disturbances are the most prominent. Cardiovascular disorders are generally milder, and severe cardiac complications occur only when very high doses (>60 g) have been ingested.

Respiration: Irregular breathing, respiratory depression.

Cardiovascular System: Tachycardia, hypotension or hypertension, shock, conduction disorders.

Nervous System and Muscles: Impairment of consciousness ranging in severity to deep coma.

Convulsions, especially in small children. Motor restlessness, muscular twitching, tremor, athetoid movements, opisthotonos, ataxia, drowsiness, dizziness, mydriasis, nystagmus, adiadochokinesia, ballism, psychomotor disturbances, dysmetria. Initial hyperreflexia, followed by hyporeflexia.

Gastrointestinal Tract: Nausea, vomiting.

Kidneys and Bladder: Anuria or oliguria, urinary retention.

Laboratory Findings: Isolated instances of overdosage have included leukocytosis, reduced leukocyte count, glycosuria, and acetonuria. ECG may show dysrhythmias.

Combined Poisoning: When alcohol, tricyclic antidepressants, barbiturates, or hydantoins are taken at the same time, the signs and symptoms of acute poisoning with carbamazepine may be aggravated or modified.

Treatment

For the most up to date information on management of carbamazepine overdose, please contact the poison center for your area by calling 1-800-222-1222. The prognosis in cases of carbamazepine poisoning is generally favorable. Of 5,645 cases of carbamazepine exposures reported to US poison centers in 2002, a total of 8 deaths (0.14% mortality rate) occurred. Over 39% of the cases reported to these poison centers were managed safely at home with conservative care. Successful management of large or intentional carbamazepine exposures requires implementation of supportive care, frequent monitoring of serum drug concentrations, as well as aggressive but appropriate gastric decontamination.

Elimination of the Drug: The primary method for gastric decontamination of carbamazepine overdose is use of activated charcoal. For substantial recent ingestions, gastric lavage may also be considered. Administration of activated charcoal prior to hospital assessment has the potential to significantly reduce drug absorption. There is no specific antidote. In overdose, absorption of carbamazepine may be prolonged and delayed. More than one dose of activated charcoal may be beneficial in patients that have evidence of continued absorption (e.g., rising serum carbamazepine levels).

Measures to Accelerate Elimination: The data on use of dialysis to enhance elimination in carbamazepine is scarce. Dialysis, particularly high flux or high efficiency hemodialysis, may be considered in patients with severe carbamazepine poisoning associated with renal failure or in cases of status epilepticus, or where there are rising serum drug levels and worsening clinical status despite appropriate supportive care and gastric decontamination. For severe cases of carbamazepine overdose unresponsive to other measures, charcoal hemoperfusion may be used to enhance drug clearance.

Respiratory Depression: Keep the airways free; resort, if necessary, to endotracheal intubation, artificial respiration, and administration of oxygen.

Hypotension, Shock: Keep the patient's legs raised and administer a plasma expander. If blood pressure fails to rise despite measures taken to increase plasma volume, use of vasoactive substances should be considered.

Convulsions: Diazepam or barbiturates.

Warning: Diazepam or barbiturates may aggravate respiratory depression (especially in children), hypotension, and coma. However, barbiturates should not be used if drugs that inhibit monoamine oxidase have also been taken by the patient either in overdosage or in recent therapy (within 1 week).

Surveillance: Respiration, cardiac function (ECG monitoring), blood pressure, body temperature, pupillary reflexes, and kidney and bladder function should be monitored for several days.

Treatment of Blood Count Abnormalities: If evidence of significant bone marrow depression develops, the following recommendations are suggested: (1) stop the drug, (2) perform daily CBC, platelet, and reticulocyte counts, (3) do a bone marrow aspiration and trephine biopsy immediately and repeat with sufficient frequency to monitor recovery.

Special periodic studies might be helpful as follows: (1) white cell and platelet antibodies, (2) ^{59}Fe-ferrokinetic studies, (3) peripheral blood cell typing, (4) cytogenetic studies on marrow and peripheral blood, (5) bone marrow culture studies for colony-forming units, (6) hemoglobin electrophoresis for A_2 and F hemoglobin, and (7) serum folic acid and B_{12} levels.

A fully developed aplastic anemia will require appropriate, intensive monitoring and therapy, for which specialized consultation should be sought.

DOSAGE AND ADMINISTRATION

Monitoring of blood levels has increased the efficacy and safety of anticonvulsants (see PRECAUTIONS, Laboratory Tests). Dosage should be adjusted to the needs of the individual patients. A low initial daily dosage with gradual increase is advised. As soon as adequate control is achieved, the dosage may be reduced very gradually to the minimum effective level. The Carbatrol capsules may be opened and the beads sprinkled over food, such as a teaspoon of applesauce or other similar food products if this method of administration is preferred. Carbatrol capsules or their contents should not be crushed or chewed. Carbatrol can be taken with or without meals.

Carbatrol is an extended-release formulation for twice a day administration. When converting patients from immediate release carbamazepine to Carbatrol extended-release capsules, the same total daily mg dose of carbamazepine should be administered.

Epilepsy (see INDICATIONS AND USAGE)

Adults and children over 12 years of age. Initial: 200 mg twice daily. Increase at weekly intervals by adding up to 200 mg/day until the optimal response is obtained. Dosage generally should not exceed 1000 mg per day in children 12-15 years of age, and 1200 mg daily in patients above 15 years of age. Doses up to 1600 mg daily have been used in adults. **Maintenance:** Adjust dosage to the minimum effective level, usually 800-1200 mg daily.

Children under 12 years of age: Children taking total daily dosages of immediate-release carbamazepine of 400 mg or greater may be converted to the same total daily dosage of Carbatrol extended-release capsules, using a twice daily regimen. Ordinarily, optimal clinical response is achieved at daily doses below 35 mg/kg. If satisfactory clinical response has not been achieved, plasma levels should be measured to determine whether or not they are in the therapeutic range. No recommendation regarding the safety of Carbatrol for use at doses above 35 mg/kg/24 hours can be made.

Combination Therapy: Carbatrol may be used alone or with other anticonvulsants. When added to existing anticonvulsant therapy, the drug should be added gradually while the other anticonvulsants are maintained or gradually decreased, except phenytoin, which may have to be increased (see PRECAUTIONS, Drug Interactions, and Pregnancy Category D).

Trigeminal Neuralgia (see INDICATIONS AND USAGE)

Initial: On the first day, start with one 200 mg capsule. This daily dose may be increased by up to 200 mg/day every 12 hours only as needed to achieve freedom from pain. Do not exceed 1200 mg daily.

Maintenance: Control of pain can be maintained in most patients with 400-800 mg daily. However, some patients may be maintained on as little as 200 mg daily, while others may require as much as 1200 mg daily. At least once every 3 months throughout the treatment period, attempts should be made to reduce the dose to the minimum effective level or even to discontinue the drug.

HOW SUPPLIED

Carbatrol (carbamazepine) extended-release capsules is supplied in three dosage strengths.

100 mg-Two-piece hard gelatin capsule (bluish green opaque body and cap) printed with the Shire logo in white ink.

Supplied in bottles of 120 .... NDC 54092-171-12

200 mg-Two-piece hard gelatin capsule (light gray opaque body with bluish green opaque cap) printed with the Shire logo in white ink.

Supplied in bottles of 120 .... NDC 54092-172-12

300 mg-Two-piece hard gelatin capsule (black opaque body with bluish green opaque cap) printed with the Shire logo in white ink.

Supplied in bottles of 120 .... NDC 54092-173-12

Store at 25°C (77°F); excursions permitted to 15-30°C (59-86°F) [see USP controlled room temperature]. PROTECT FROM LIGHT AND MOISTURE.

Manufactured for:

Shire US Inc.

725 Chesterbrook Blvd, Wayne PA 19087

1-800-828-2088, Made in U.S.A. © 2005 Shire US Inc.

001724   172 1207 011   (Rev 12/2007)

VYVANSE™ ©II ℞

(lisdexamfetamine dimesylate)

Rx Only

Prescribing information for this product, which appears on pages 3115–3118 of the 2008 PDR, has been completely revised as follows. Please write "See Supplement A" next to the product heading.

AMPHETAMINES HAVE A HIGH POTENTIAL FOR ABUSE. ADMINISTRATION OF AMPHETAMINES FOR PROLONGED PERIODS OF TIME MAY LEAD TO DRUG DEPENDENCE. PARTICULAR ATTENTION SHOULD BE PAID TO THE POSSIBILITY OF SUBJECTS OBTAINING AMPHETAMINES FOR NON-THERAPEUTIC USE OR DISTRIBUTION TO OTHERS AND THE DRUGS SHOULD BE PRESCRIBED OR DISPENSED SPARINGLY.

MISUSE OF AMPHETAMINE MAY CAUSE SUDDEN DEATH AND SERIOUS CARDIOVASCULAR ADVERSE EVENTS.

DESCRIPTION

Vyvanse™ (lisdexamfetamine dimesylate) is designed as a capsule for once-a-day oral administration. The chemical designation for lisdexamfetamine dimesylate is (2S)-2,6-diamino-*N*-[(1*S*)-1-methyl-2-phenylethyl]hexanamide dimethanesulfonate. The molecular formula is $C_{15}H_{25}N_3O \bullet (CH_4O_3S)_2$, which corresponds to a molecular weight of 455.60. The chemical structure is:

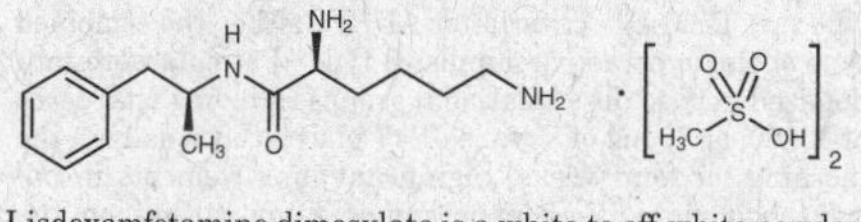

Lisdexamfetamine dimesylate is a white to off-white powder that is soluble in water (792 mg/mL). Vyvanse™ capsules contain 20 mg, 30 mg, 40 mg, 50 mg, 60 mg, and 70 mg of lisdexamfetamine dimesylate and the following inactive ingredients: microcrystalline cellulose, croscarmellose sodium, and magnesium stearate. The capsule shells contain gelatin, titanium dioxide, and one or more of the following: D&C Red #28, D&C Yellow #10, FD&C Blue #1, FD&C Green #3, and FD&C Red #40.

CLINICAL PHARMACOLOGY

Mechanism of Action and Pharmacology

Vyvanse™ is a prodrug of dextroamphetamine. After oral administration, lisdexamfetamine dimesylate is rapidly absorbed from the gastrointestinal tract and converted to dextroamphetamine, which is responsible for the drug's activity. Amphetamines are non-catecholamine sympathomimetic amines with CNS stimulant activity. The mode of therapeutic action in Attention-Deficit/Hyperactivity Disorder (ADHD) is not known. Amphetamines are thought to block the reuptake of norepinephrine and dopamine into the

Continued on next page

Vyvanse—Cont.

presynaptic neuron and increase the release of these monoamines into the extraneuronal space. The parent drug, lisdexamfetamine, does not bind to the sites responsible for the reuptake of norepinephrine and dopamine *in vitro*.

Pharmacokinetics

Pharmacokinetic studies of dextroamphetamine after oral administration of lisdexamfetamine dimesylate have been conducted in healthy adult and pediatric (6–12 yrs) patients with ADHD.

In 18 pediatric patients (6–12 yrs) with ADHD, the Tmax of dextroamphetamine was approximately 3.5 hours following single-dose oral administration of lisdexamfetamine dimesylate either 30 mg, 50 mg, or 70 mg after an 8-hour overnight fast. The Tmax of lisdexamfetamine dimesylate was approximately 1 hour. Linear pharmacokinetics of dextroamphetamine after single-dose oral administration of lisdexamfetamine dimesylate was established over the dose range of 30 mg to 70 mg in children aged 6 to 12 years.

There is no unexpected accumulation of dextroamphetamine AUC at steady state in healthy adults and no accumulation of lisdexamfetamine dimesylate after once-daily dosing for 7 consecutive days.

Food does not affect the observed AUC and Cmax of dextroamphetamine in healthy adults after single-dose oral administration of 70 mg of Vyvanse capsules but prolongs Tmax by approximately 1 hour (from 3.8 hrs at fasted state to 4.7 hrs after a high fat meal). After an 8-hour fast, the AUC for dextroamphetamine following oral administration of lisdexamfetamine dimesylate in solution and as intact capsules were equivalent.

Weight/Dose normalized AUC and Cmax were 22% and 12% lower, respectively, in adult females than in males on day 7 following a 70 mg/day dose of lisdexamfetamine for 7 days. Weight/Dose normalized AUC and Cmax values were the same in girls and boys following single doses of 30-70 mg.

Metabolism and Excretion

After oral administration, lisdexamfetamine dimesylate is rapidly absorbed from the gastrointestinal tract. Lisdexamfetamine dimesylate is converted to dextoamphetamine and L-lysine, which is believed to occur by first-pass intestinal and/or hepatic metabolism. Lisdexamfetamine is not metabolized by cytochrome P450 enzymes. Following the oral administration of a 70 mg dose of radiolabeled lisdexamfetamine dimesylate to 6 healthy subjects, approximately 96% of the oral dose radioactivity was recovered in the urine and only 0.3% recovered in the feces over a period of 120 hours. Of the radioactivity recovered in the urine 42% of the dose was related to amphetamine, 25% to hippuric acid, and 2% intact lisdexamfetamine. Plasma concentrations of unconverted lisdexamfetamine dimesylate are low and transient, generally becoming non-quantifiable by 8 hours after administration. The plasma elimination half-life of lisdexamfetamine typically averaged less than one hour in studies of lisdexamfetamine dimesylate in volunteers.

Dextroamphetamine is known to inhibit monoamine oxidase. The ability of dextroamphetamine and its metabolites to inhibit various P450 isozymes and other enzymes has not been adequately elucidated. *In vitro* experiments with human microsomes indicate minor inhibition of CYP2D6 by amphetamine and minor inhibition of CYP1A2, 2D6, and 3A4 by one or more metabolites, but there are no *in vivo* studies of p450 enzyme inhibition.

Special Populations

The pharmacokinetics of dextroamphetamine is similar in pediatric (6-12 years) and adolescent (13-17 years) ADHD patients, and healthy adult volunteers. Any differences in kinetics seen after oral administration are a result of differences in mg/kg dosing.

Gender

Systemic exposure to dextroamphetamine is similar for men and women given the same mg/kg dose.

Clinical Trials

A double-blind, randomized, placebo-controlled, parallel-group study was conducted in children aged 6–12 (N=290) who met DSM-IV® criteria for ADHD (either the combined type or the hyperactive-impulsive type). Patients were randomized to fixed dose treatment groups receiving final doses of 30, 50, or 70 mg of Vyvanse™ or placebo once daily in the morning for four weeks. Significant improvements in patient behavior, based upon investigator ratings on the ADHD Rating Scale (ADHD-RS), were observed at endpoint for all Vyvanse™ doses compared to patients who received placebo. Mean effects at all doses were fairly similar, although the highest dose (70 mg/day) was numerically superior to both lower doses (30 and 50 mg/day). The effects were maintained throughout the day based on parent ratings (Connor's Parent Rating Scale) in the morning (approximately 10 am), afternoon (approximately 2 pm), and early evening (approximately 6 pm).

A double-blind, placebo-controlled, randomized, crossover design, analog classroom study was conducted in children aged 6-12 (N=52) who met DSM-IV® criteria for ADHD (either the combined type or the hyperactive-impulsive type). Following a 3-week open-label dose titration with Adderall XR®, patients were randomly assigned to continue the same dose of Adderall XR® (10, 20, or 30 mg), Vyvanse™ (30, 50, and 70 mg), or placebo once daily in the morning for 1 week each treatment. A significant difference in patient behavior, based upon the average of investigator ratings on the Swanson, Kotkin, Agler, M.Flynn and Pelham (SKAMP)-Deportment scores across the 8 sessions of a 12 hour treatment day, was observed between patients who received Vyvanse™ compared to patients who received placebo. The drug effect was similar for all 8 sessions.

INDICATIONS AND USAGE

Vyvanse™ is indicated for the treatment of Attention-Deficit/Hyperactivity Disorder (ADHD).

The efficacy of Vyvanse™ in the treatment of ADHD was established on the basis of two controlled trials in children aged 6 to 12, who met DSM-IV® criteria for ADHD (see **CLINICAL TRIALS**).

A diagnosis of Attention-Deficit/Hyperactivity Disorder (ADHD; DSM-IV®) implies the presence of hyperactive-impulsive or inattentive symptoms that caused impairment and were present before age 7 years. The symptoms must cause clinically significant impairment, in social, academic, or occupational functioning, and be present in two or more settings, e.g., at school (or work) and at home. The symptoms must not be better accounted for by another mental disorder. For the Inattentive Type, at least six of the following symptoms must have persisted for at least 6 months: lack of attention to details/careless mistakes; lack of sustained attention; poor listener; failure to follow through on tasks; poor organization; avoids tasks requiring sustained mental effort; loses things; easily distracted; forgetful. For the Hyperactive-Impulsive Type, at least six of the following symptoms must have persisted for at least 6 months: fidgeting/squirming; leaving seat; inappropriate running/climbing; difficulty with quiet activities; "on the go"; excessive talking; blurting answers; can't wait turn; intrusive. The Combined Type requires both inattentive and hyperactive-impulsive criteria to be met.

Special Diagnostic Considerations: Specific etiology of this syndrome is unknown, and there is no single diagnostic test. Adequate diagnosis requires the use not only of medical but of special psychological, educational, and social resources. Learning may or may not be impaired. The diagnosis must be based upon a complete history and evaluation of the child and not solely on the presence of the required number of DSM-IV® characteristics.

Need for Comprehensive Treatment Program: Vyvanse™ is indicated as an integral part of a total treatment program for ADHD that may include other measures (psychological, educational, social) for patients with this syndrome. Drug treatment may not be indicated for all children with this syndrome. Stimulants are not intended for use in the child who exhibits symptoms secondary to environmental factors and/or other primary psychiatric disorders, including psychosis. Appropriate educational placement is essential and psychosocial intervention is often helpful. When remedial measures alone are insufficient, the decision to prescribe stimulant medication will depend upon the physician's assessment of the chronicity and severity of the child's symptoms.

Long-Term Use: The effectiveness of Vyvanse™ for long-term use, i.e., for more than 4 weeks, has not been systematically evaluated in controlled trials. Therefore, the physician who elects to use Vyvanse™ for extended periods should periodically re-evaluate the long-term usefulness of the drug for the individual patient.

CONTRAINDICATIONS

Advanced arteriosclerosis, symptomatic cardiovascular disease, moderate to severe hypertension, hyperthyroidism, known hypersensitivity or idiosyncrasy to the sympathomimetic amines, glaucoma.

Agitated states.

Patients with a history of drug abuse.

During or within 14 days following the administration of monoamine oxidase inhibitors (hypertensive crises may result).

WARNINGS

Serious Cardiovascular Events

Sudden Death and Pre-existing Structural Cardiac Abnormalities or Other Serious Heart Problems

Children and Adolescents

Sudden death has been reported in association with CNS stimulant treatment at usual doses in children and adolescents with structural cardiac abnormalities or other serious heart problems. Although some serious heart problems alone carry an increased risk of sudden death, stimulant products generally should not be used in children or adolescents with known serious structural cardiac abnormalities, cardiomyopathy, serious heart rhythm abnormalities, or other serious cardiac problems that may place them at increased vulnerability to the sympathomimetic effects of a stimulant drug (see **CONTRAINDICATIONS**).

Adults

Sudden deaths, stroke, and myocardial infarction have been reported in adults taking stimulant drugs at usual doses for ADHD. Although the role of stimulants in these adult cases is also unknown, adults have a greater likelihood than children of having serious structural cardiac abnormalities, cardiomyopathy, serious heart rhythm abnormalities, coronary artery disease, or other serious cardiac problems. Adults with such abnormalities should also generally not be treated with stimulant drugs (see **CONTRAINDICATIONS**).

Hypertension and other Cardiovascular Conditions

Stimulant medications cause a modest increase in average blood pressure (about 2-4 mmHg) and average heart rate (about 3-6 bpm), and individuals may have larger increases. While the mean changes alone would not be expected to have short-term consequences, all patients should be monitored for larger changes in heart rate and blood pressure. Caution is indicated in treating patients whose underlying medical conditions might be compromised by increases in blood pressure or heart rate, e.g., those with pre-existing hypertension, heart failure, recent myocardial infarction, or ventricular arrhythmia (see **CONTRAINDICATIONS**).

Assessing Cardiovascular Status in Patients being Treated with Stimulant Medications

Children, adolescents, or adults who are being considered for treatment with stimulant medications should have a careful history (including assessment for a family history of sudden death or ventricular arrhythmia) and physical exam to assess for the presence of cardiac disease, and should receive further cardiac evaluation if findings suggest such disease (e.g. electrocardiogram and echocardiogram). Patients who develop symptoms such as exertional chest pain, unexplained syncope, or other symptoms suggestive of cardiac disease during stimulant treatment should undergo a prompt cardiac evaluation.

Psychiatric Adverse Events

Pre-Existing Psychosis

Administration of stimulants may exacerbate symptoms of behavior disturbance and thought disorder in patients with pre-existing psychotic disorder.

Bipolar Illness

Particular care should be taken in using stimulants to treat ADHD patients with comorbid bipolar disorder because of concern for possible induction of mixed/manic episode in such patients. Prior to initiating treatment with a stimulant, patients with comorbid depressive symptoms should be adequately screened to determine if they are at risk for bipolar disorder; such screening should include a detailed psychiatric history, including a family history of suicide, bipolar disorder, and depression.

Emergence of New Psychotic or Manic Symptoms

Treatment emergent psychotic or manic symptoms, e.g., hallucinations, delusional thinking, or mania in children and adolescents without prior history of psychotic illness or mania can be caused by stimulants at usual doses. If such symptoms occur, consideration should be given to a possible causal role of the stimulant, and discontinuation of treatment may be appropriate. In a pooled analysis of multiple short-term, placebo-controlled studies, such symptoms occurred in about 0.1% (4 patients with events out of 3482 exposed to methylphenidate or amphetamine for several weeks at usual doses) of stimulant-treated patients compared to 0 in placebo-treated patients.

Aggression

Aggressive behavior or hostility is often observed in children and adolescents with ADHD, and has been reported in clinical trials and the postmarketing experience of some medications indicated for the treatment of ADHD. Although there is no systematic evidence that stimulants cause aggressive behavior or hostility, patients beginning treatment for ADHD should be monitored for the appearance of or worsening of aggressive behavior or hostility.

Long-Term Suppression of Growth

Careful follow-up of weight and height in children ages 7 to 10 years who were randomized to either methylphenidate or non-medication treatment groups over 14 months, as well as in naturalistic subgroups of newly methylphenidate-treated and non-medication treated children over 36 months (to the ages of 10 to 13 years), suggests that consistently medicated children (i.e., treatment for 7 days per week throughout the year) have a temporary slowing in growth rate (on average, a total of about 2 cm less growth in height and 2.7 kg less growth in weight over 3 years), without evidence of growth rebound during this period of development. In a controlled trial of amphetamine (d to l enantiomer ratio of 3:1) in adolescents, mean weight change from baseline within the initial 4 weeks of therapy was –1.1 lbs. and –2.8 lbs., respectively, for patients receiving 10 mg and 20 mg of amphetamine (d to l enantiomer ratio of 3:1). Higher doses were associated with greater weight loss within the initial 4 weeks of treatment. In a controlled trial of lisdexamfetamine in children ages 6 to 12 years, mean weight loss from baseline after 4 weeks of therapy was –0.9, –1.9, and –2.5 lb, respectively, for patients receiving 30 mg, 50 mg, and 70 mg of lisdexamfetamine, compared to a 1 lb weight gain for patients receiving placebo. Higher doses were associated with greater weight loss with 4 weeks of treatment. Careful follow-up for weight in children ages 6 to 12 years who received lisdexamfetamine over 12 months suggests that consistently medicated children (i.e., treatment for 7 days per week throughout the year) have a slowing in growth rate measured by body weight as demonstrated by an age- and sex-normalized mean change from baseline in percentile of -13.4 over 1 year (average percentile at baseline and 12 months, were 60.6 and 47.2, respectively). Therefore, growth should be monitored during treatment with stimulants, and patients who are not growing or gaining weight as expected may need to have their treatment interrupted.

Seizures

There is some clinical evidence that stimulants may lower the convulsive threshold in patients with prior history of seizure, in patients with prior EEG abnormalities in absence of seizures, and very rarely, in patients without a history of seizures and no prior EEG evidence of seizures. In the presence of seizures, the drug should be discontinued.

Visual Disturbance

Difficulties with accommodation and blurring of vision have been reported with stimulant treatment.

PRECAUTIONS

General: The least amount of Vyvanse™ feasible should be prescribed or dispensed at one time in order to minimize the possibility of overdosage. Vyvanse™ should be used with caution in patients who use other sympathomimetic drugs.

Tics: Amphetamines have been reported to exacerbate motor and phonic tics and Tourette's syndrome. Therefore, clinical evaluation for tics and Tourette's syndrome in children and their families should precede use of stimulant medications.

Information for Patients: Amphetamines may impair the ability of the patient to engage in potentially hazardous activities such as operating machinery or vehicles; the patient should therefore be cautioned accordingly.

Prescribers or other health professionals should inform patients, their families, and their caregivers about the benefits and risks associated with treatment with lisdexamfetamine and should counsel them in its appropriate use. A patient Medication Guide is available for Vyvanse™. The prescriber or health professional should instruct patients, their families, and their caregivers to read the Medication Guide and should assist them in understanding its contents. Patients should be given the opportunity to discuss the contents of the Medication Guide and to obtain answers to any questions they may have. The complete text of the Medication Guide is reprinted at the end of this document.

Drug Interactions:

Urinary acidifying agents—These agents (ammonium chloride, sodium acid phosphate, etc.) increase the concentration of the ionized species of the amphetamine molecule, thereby increasing urinary excretion. These agents lower blood levels and efficacy of amphetamines.

Adrenergic blockers—Adrenergic blockers are inhibited by amphetamines.

Antidepressants, tricyclic—Amphetamines may enhance the activity of tricyclic antidepressants or sympathomimetic agents; d-amphetamine with desipramine or protriptyline and possibly other tricyclics cause striking and sustained increases in the concentration of d-amphetamine in the brain; cardiovascular effects can be potentiated.

MAO inhibitors—MAOI antidepressants, as well as a metabolite of furazolidone, slow amphetamine metabolism. This slowing potentiates amphetamines, increasing their effect on the release of norepinephrine and other monoamines from adrenergic nerve endings; this can cause headaches and other signs of hypertensive crisis. A variety of toxic neurological effects and malignant hyperpyrexia can occur, sometimes with fatal results.

Antihistamines—Amphetamines may counteract the sedative effect of antihistamines.

Antihypertensives—Amphetamines may antagonize the hypotensive effects of antihypertensives.

Chlorpromazine—Chlorpromazine blocks dopamine and norepinephrine receptors, thus inhibiting the central stimulant effects of amphetamines and can be used to treat amphetamine poisoning.

Ethosuximide—Amphetamines may delay intestinal absorption of ethosuximide.

Haloperidol—Haloperidol blocks dopamine receptors, thus inhibiting the central stimulant effects of amphetamines.

Lithium carbonate—The anorectic and stimulatory effects of amphetamines may be inhibited by lithium carbonate.

Meperidine—Amphetamines potentiate the analgesic effect of meperidine.

Methenamine therapy—Urinary excretion of amphetamines is increased, and efficacy is reduced by acidifying agents used in methenamine therapy.

Norepinephrine—Amphetamines enhance the adrenergic effect of norepinephrine.

Phenobarbital—Amphetamines may delay intestinal absorption of phenobarbital; co-administration of phenobarbital may produce a synergistic anticonvulsant action.

Phenytoin—Amphetamines may delay intestinal absorption of phenytoin; co-administration of phenytoin may produce a synergistic anticonvulsant action.

Propoxyphene—In cases of propoxyphene overdosage, amphetamine CNS stimulation is potentiated and fatal convulsions can occur.

Veratrum alkaloids—Amphetamines inhibit the hypotensive effect of veratrum alkaloids.

Drug/Laboratory Test Interactions: Amphetamines can cause a significant elevation in plasma corticosteroid levels. This increase is greatest in the evening. Amphetamines may interfere with urinary steroid determinations.

Carcinogenesis/Mutagenesis and Impairment of Fertility: Carcinogenicity studies of lisdexamfetamine have not been performed.

No evidence of carcinogenicity was found in studies in which d, l-amphetamine (enantiomer ratio of 1:1) was administered to mice and rats in the diet for 2 years at doses of up to 30 mg/kg/day in male mice, 19 mg/kg/day in female mice, and 5 mg/kg/day in male and female rats.

Lisdexamfetamine dimesylate was not clastogenic in the mouse bone marrow micronucleus test *in vivo* and was negative when tested in the *E. coli* and *S. typhimurium* components of the Ames test and in the L5178Y/TK$^+$ mouse lymphoma assay *in vitro*.

Amphetamine (d to l enantiomer ratio of 3:1) did not adversely affect fertility or early embryonic development in the rat at doses of up to 20 mg/kg/day.

Pregnancy: Pregnancy Category C. Reproduction studies of lisdexamfetamine have not been performed.

Amphetamine (d to l enantiomer ratio of 3:1) had no apparent effects on embryofetal morphological development or survival when orally administered to pregnant rats and rab-

bits throughout the period of organogenesis at doses of up to 6 and 16 mg/kg/day, respectively. Fetal malformations and death have been reported in mice following parenteral administration of dextroamphetamine doses of 50 mg/kg/day or greater to pregnant animals. Administration of these doses was also associated with severe maternal toxicity.

A number of studies in rodents indicate that prenatal or early postnatal exposure to amphetamine (d- or d,l-) at doses similar to those used clinically can result in long term neurochemical and behavioral alterations. Reported behavioral effects include learning and memory deficits, altered locomotor activity, and changes in sexual function.

There are no adequate and well-controlled studies in pregnant women. There has been one report of severe congenital bony deformity, tracheo-esophageal fistula, and anal atresia (vater association) in a baby born to a woman who took dextroamphetamine sulfate with lovastatin during the first trimester of pregnancy. Amphetamines should be used during pregnancy only if the potential benefit justifies the potential risk to the fetus.

Nonteratogenic Effects: Infants born to mothers dependent on amphetamine have an increased risk of premature delivery and low birth weight. Also, these infants may experience symptoms of withdrawal as demonstrated by dysphoria, including agitation, and significant lassitude.

Usage in Nursing Mothers: Amphetamines are excreted in human milk. Mothers taking amphetamines should be advised to refrain from nursing.

Pediatric Use: Vyvanse™ is indicated for use in children aged 6 to 12 years.

A study was conducted in which juvenile rats received oral doses of 4, 10, or 40 mg/kg/day of lisdexamfetamine from day 7 to day 63 of age. These doses are approximately 0.3, 0.7, and 3 times the maximum recommended human daily dose of 70 mg on a mg/m² basis. Dose-related decreases in food consumption, bodyweight gain, and crown-rump length were seen; after a four week drug-free recovery period bodyweights and crown-rump lengths had significantly recovered in females but were still substantially reduced in males. Time to vaginal opening was delayed in females at the highest dose, but there were no drug effects on fertility when the animals were mated beginning on day 85 of age. In a study in which juvenile dogs received lisdexamfetamine for 6 months beginning at 10 weeks of age, decreased bodyweight gain was seen at all doses tested (2, 5, and 12 mg/kg/day, which are approximately 0.5, 1, and 3 times the maximum recommended human daily dose on a mg/m² basis). This effect partially or fully reversed during a four week drug-free recovery period.

Use in Children under Six Years of Age: Lisdexamfetamine dimesylate has not been studied in 3-5 year olds. Long-term effects of amphetamines in children have not been well established. Amphetamines are not recommended for use in children under 3 years of age.

Geriatric Use: Vyvanse™ has not been studied in the geriatric population.

ADVERSE EVENTS

The premarketing development program for Vyvanse™ included exposures in a total of 404 participants in clinical trials (348 pediatric patients and 56 healthy adult subjects). Of these, 348 pediatric patients (ages 6 to 12) were evaluated in two controlled clinical studies (one parallel-group and one crossover), one open-label extension study, and one single-dose clinical pharmacology study. The information included in this section is based on data from the 4-week parallel-group controlled clinical trial in pediatric patients with ADHD. Adverse reactions were assessed by collecting adverse events, results of physical examinations, vital signs, weights, laboratory analyses, and ECGs.

Adverse events during exposure were obtained primarily by general inquiry and recorded by clinical investigators using terminology of their own choosing. Consequently, it is not possible to provide a meaningful estimate of the proportion of individuals experiencing adverse events without first grouping similar types of events into a smaller number of standardized event categories. In the tables and listings that follow, MedRA terminology has been used to classify reported adverse events.

The stated frequencies of adverse events represent the proportion of individuals who experienced, at least once, a treatment-emergent adverse event of the type listed.

Adverse events associated with discontinuation of treatment: Ten percent (21/218) of Vyvanse™-treated patients discontinued due to adverse events compared to 1% (1/72) who received placebo. The most frequent adverse events leading to discontinuation and considered to be drug-related (i.e., leading to discontinuation in at least 1% of Vyvanse™-treated patients and at a rate at least twice that of placebo) were ECG voltage criteria for ventricular hypertrophy, tic, vomiting, psychomotor hyperactivity, insomnia, and rash (2/218 each; 1%).

Adverse events occurring in a controlled trial: Adverse events reported in a 4-week clinical trial in pediatric patients treated with Vyvanse™ or placebo are presented in the table below.

The prescriber should be aware that these figures cannot be used to predict the incidence of adverse events in the course of usual medical practice where patient characteristics and other factors differ from those which prevailed in the clinical trials. Similarly, the cited frequencies cannot be compared with figures obtained from other clinical investigations involving different treatments, uses, and investigators. The cited figures, however, do provide the prescribing

physician with some basis for estimating the relative contribution of drug and non-drug factors to the adverse event incidence rate in the population studied.

The following adverse events that occurred in at least 5% of the Vyvanse™ patients and at a rate twice that of the placebo group (Table 1): Upper abdominal pain, decreased appetite, dizziness, dry mouth, irritability, insomnia, nausea, vomiting, and decreased weight.

Table 1 Adverse Events Reported by 2% or More of Pediatric Patients Taking Vyvanse™ in a 4 Week Clinical Trial

Body System	Preferred Term	Vyvanse™ (n=218)	Placebo (n=72)
Gastrointestinal Disorders	Abdominal Pain Upper	12%	6%
	Dry Mouth	5%	0%
	Nausea	6%	3%
	Vomiting	9%	4%
General Disorder and Administration Site Conditions	Pyrexia	2%	1%
Investigations	Weight Decreased	9%	1%
Metabolism and Nutrition	Decreased Appetite	39%	4%
Nervous System Disorders	Dizziness	5%	0%
	Headache	12%	10%
	Somnolence	2%	1%
Psychiatric Disorders	Affect lability	3%	0%
	Initial Insomnia	4%	0%
	Insomnia	19%	3%
	Irritability	10%	0%
	Tic	2%	0%
Skin and Subcutaneous Tissue Disorders	Rash	3%	0%

Note: This table only includes those events for which the incidence in patients taking Vyvanse is greater than the incidence in patients taking placebo.

The following additional adverse reactions have been associated with the use of amphetamine, amphetamine (d to l enantiomer ratio of 3:1), or Vyvanse™:

Cardiovascular: Palpitations, tachycardia, elevation of blood pressure, sudden death, myocardial infarction. There have been isolated reports of cardiomyopathy associated with chronic amphetamine use.

Central Nervous System: Psychotic episodes at recommended doses, overstimulation, restlessness, dizziness, euphoria, dyskinesia, dysphoria, depression, tremor, headache, exacerbation of motor and phonic tics and Tourette's syndrome, seizures, stroke.

Gastrointestinal: Dryness of the mouth, unpleasant taste, diarrhea, constipation.

Allergic: Urticaria, hypersensitivity reactions including angioedema and anaphylaxis. Serious skin rashes, including Stevens Johnson Syndrome and toxic epidermal necrolysis have been reported.

Endocrine: Impotence, changes in libido.

DRUG ABUSE AND DEPENDENCE

Controlled Substance Class

Vyvanse™ is classified as a Schedule II controlled substance.

Amphetamines have been extensively abused. Tolerance, extreme psychological dependence, and severe social disability have occurred. There are reports of patients who have increased the dosage to levels many times higher than recommended. Abrupt cessation following prolonged high dosage administration results in extreme fatigue and mental depression; changes are also noted on the sleep EEG. Manifestations of chronic intoxication with amphetamines may include severe dermatoses, marked insomnia, irritability, hyperactivity, and personality changes. The most severe manifestation of chronic intoxication is psychosis, often clinically indistinguishable from schizophrenia.

Human Studies

In a human abuse liability study, when equivalent oral doses of 100 mg lisdexamfetamine dimesylate and 40 mg immediate release d-amphetamine sulfate were administered to individuals with a history of drug abuse, lisdexamfetamine 100 mg produced subjective responses on a scale of "Drug Liking Effects" "Amphetamine Effects", and "Stimulant Effects" that were significantly less than d-amphetamine immediate release 40 mg. However, oral administration of 150 mg lisdexamfetamine produced increases in positive subjective responses on these scales that were statistically indistinguishable from the positive subjective responses produced by 40 mg of oral immediate-release d-amphetamine and 200 mg of diethylpropion (C-IV).

Intravenous administration of 50 mg lisdexamfetamine to individuals with a history of drug abuse produced positive subjective responses on scales measuring "Drug Liking",

Continued on next page

Vyvanse—Cont.

"Euphoria", "Amphetamine Effects", and "Benzedrine Effects" that were greater than placebo but less than those produced by an equivalent dose (20 mg) of intravenous d-amphetamine.

Animal Studies

In animal studies, lisdexamfetamine produced behavioral effects qualitatively similar to those of the CNS stimulant d-amphetamine. In monkeys trained to self-administer cocaine, intravenous lisdexamfetamine maintained self-administration at a rate that was statistically less than that for cocaine, but greater than that of placebo.

OVERDOSAGE

Individual response to amphetamines varies widely. Toxic symptoms may occur idiosyncratically at low doses.

Symptoms: Manifestations of acute overdosage with amphetamines include restlessness, tremor, hyperreflexia, rapid respiration, confusion, assaultiveness, hallucinations, panic states, hyperpyrexia and rhabdomyolysis. Fatigue and depression usually follow the central nervous system stimulation. Cardiovascular effects include arrhythmias, hypertension or hypotension and circulatory collapse. Gastrointestinal symptoms include nausea, vomiting, diarrhea, and abdominal cramps. Fatal poisoning is usually preceded by convulsions and coma.

Treatment: Consult with a Certified Poison Control Center for up to date guidance and advice. Management of acute amphetamine intoxication is largely symptomatic and includes gastric lavage, administration of activated charcoal, administration of a cathartic and sedation. Experience with hemodialysis or peritoneal dialysis is inadequate to permit recommendation in this regard. Acidification of the urine increases amphetamine excretion, but is believed to increase risk of acute renal failure if myoglobinuria is present. If acute severe hypertension complicates amphetamine overdosage, administration of intravenous phentolamine has been suggested. However, a gradual drop in blood pressure will usually result when sufficient sedation has been achieved. Chlorpromazine antagonizes the central stimulant effects of amphetamines and can be used to treat amphetamine intoxication.

The prolonged release of Vyvanse™ in the body should be considered when treating patients with overdose.

DOSAGE AND ADMINISTRATION

Dosage should be individualized according to the therapeutic needs and response of the patient. Vyvanse™ should be administered at the lowest effective dosage.

In children with ADHD who are 6-12 years of age and are either starting treatment for the first time or switching from another medication, 30 mg once daily in the morning is the recommended dose. If the decision is made to increase the dose beyond 30 mg/day, daily dosage may be adjusted in increments of 10 mg or 20 mg and at approximately weekly intervals. When in the judgment of the clinician a lower initial dose is appropriate, patients may begin treatment with 20 mg once daily in the morning. The maximum recommended dose for children is 70 mg/day; doses greater than 70 mg/day of Vyvanse™ have not been studied in children. Amphetamines are not recommended for children under 3 years of age. Vyvanse™ has not been studied in children under 6 or over 12 years of age.

Vyvanse™ should be taken in the morning. Afternoon doses should be avoided because of the potential for insomnia.

Vyvanse™ may be taken with or without food.

Vyvanse™ capsules may be taken whole, or the capsule may be opened and the entire contents dissolved in a glass of water. If the patient is using the solution administration method, the solution should be consumed immediately; it should not be stored. The dose of a single capsule should not be divided. The contents of the entire capsule should be taken, and patients should not take anything less than one capsule per day.

Where possible, drug administration should be interrupted occasionally to determine if there is a recurrence of behavioral symptoms sufficient to require continued therapy.

HOW SUPPLIED

Vyvanse™ capsules 20 mg: ivory body/ivory cap (imprinted NRP104 20 mg), bottles of 100, NDC 59417-102-10
Vyvanse™ capsules 30 mg: white body/orange cap (imprinted NRP104 30 mg), bottles of 100, NDC 59417-103-10
Vyvanse™ capsules 40 mg: white body/blue green cap (imprinted NRP104 40 mg), bottles of 100, NDC 59417-104-10
Vyvanse™ capsules 50 mg: white body/blue cap (imprinted NRP104 50 mg), bottles of 100, NDC 59417-105-10
Vyvanse™ capsules 60 mg: aqua blue body/aqua blue cap (imprinted NRP104 60 mg), bottles of 100, NDC 59417-106-10
Vyvanse™ capsules 70 mg: blue body/orange cap (imprinted NRP104 70 mg), bottles of 100, NDC 59417-107-10
Dispense in a tight, light-resistant container as defined in the USP.

Store at 25° C (77° F). Excursions permitted to 15-30° C (59-86° F) [see USP Controlled Room Temperature]

ANIMAL TOXICOLOGY

Acute administration of high doses of amphetamine (d- or d,l-) has been shown to produce long-lasting neurotoxic effects, including irreversible nerve fiber damage, in rodents. The significance of these findings to humans is unknown.

Manufactured for: New River Pharmaceuticals Inc., Blacksburg, VA 24060. Made in USA.

Distributed by: Shire US Inc., Wayne, PA 19087

For more information call 1-800-828-2088, or visit www.vyvanse.com

Pharmacist: Medication Guide to be dispensed to patients

Vyvanse™ is a trademark of Shire LLC.

Copyright ©2007 New River Pharmaceuticals Inc.

Rev 08/07   XXXXXX

MEDICATION GUIDE

VYVANSE™

(lisdexamfetamine dimesylate) CII

Read the Medication Guide that comes with Vyvanse before you or your child starts taking it and each time you get a refill. There may be new information. This Medication Guide does not take the place of talking to your doctor about you or your child's treatment with Vyvanse.

What is the most important information I should know about Vyvanse?

Vyvanse is a stimulant medicine. The following have been reported with use of stimulant medicines.

1. Heart-related problems:

- **sudden death in patients who have heart problems or heart defects**
- **stroke and heart attack in adults**
- **increased blood pressure and heart rate**

Tell your doctor if you or your child have any heart problems, heart defects, high blood pressure, or a family history of these problems.

Your doctor should check you or your child carefully for heart problems before starting Vyvanse.

Your doctor should check you or your child's blood pressure and heart rate regularly during treatment with Vyvanse.

Call your doctor right away if you or your child has any signs of heart problems such as chest pain, shortness of breath, or fainting while taking Vyvanse.

2. Mental (Psychiatric) problems:

All Patients

- **new or worse behavior and thought problems**
- **new or worse bipolar illness**
- **new or worse aggressive behavior or hostility**

Children and Teenagers

- **new psychotic symptoms (such as hearing voices, believing things that are not true, are suspicious) or new manic symptoms**

Tell your doctor about any mental problems you or your child have, or about a family history of suicide, bipolar illness, or depression.

Call your doctor right away if you or your child have any new or worsening mental symptoms or problems while taking Vyvanse, especially seeing or hearing things that are not real, believing things that are not real, or are suspicious.

What Is Vyvanse?

Vyvanse is a central nervous system stimulant prescription medicine. It is used for the treatment of Attention-Deficit Hyperactivity Disorder (ADHD). Vyvanse may help increase attention and decrease impulsiveness and hyperactivity in patients with ADHD.

Vyvanse should be used as a part of a total treatment program for ADHD that may include counseling or other therapies.

Vyvanse is a federally controlled substance (CII) because it can be abused or lead to dependence. Keep Vyvanse in a safe place to prevent misuse and abuse. Selling or giving away Vyvanse may harm others, and is against the law.

Tell your doctor if you or your child have (or have a family history of) ever abused or been dependent on alcohol, prescription medicines or street drugs.

Who should not take Vyvanse?

Vyvanse should not be taken if you or your child:

- have heart disease or hardening of the arteries
- have moderate to severe high blood pressure
- have hyperthyroidism
- have an eye problem called glaucoma
- are very anxious, tense, or agitated
- have a history of drug abuse
- are taking or have taken within the past 14 days an anti-depression medicine called a monoamine oxidase inhibitor or MAOI.
- is sensitive to, allergic to, or had a reaction to other stimulant medicines

Vyvanse has not been studied in children less than 6 years old.

Vyvanse is not recommended for use in children less than 3 years old.

Vyvanse may not be right for you or your child. Before starting Vyvanse tell your or your child's doctor about all health conditions (or a family history of) including:

- heart problems, heart defects, high blood pressure
- mental problems including psychosis, mania, bipolar illness, or depression
- tics or Tourette's syndrome
- liver or kidney problems
- thyroid problems
- seizures or have had an abnormal brain wave test (EEG)

Tell your doctor if you or your child is pregnant, planning to become pregnant, or breastfeeding.

Can Vyvanse be taken with other medicines?

Tell your doctor about all of the medicines that you or your child take including prescription and nonprescription medicines, vitamins, and herbal supplements. Vyvanse and some medicines may interact with each other and cause serious side effects. Sometimes the doses of other medicines will need to be adjusted while taking Vyvanse.

Your doctor will decide whether Vyvanse can be taken with other medicines.

Especially tell your doctor if you or your child takes:

- anti-depression medicines including MAOIs
- anti-psychotic medicines
- lithium
- blood pressure medicines
- seizure medicines
- narcotic pain medicines

Know the medicines that you or your child takes. Keep a list of your medicines with you to show your doctor and pharmacist.

Do not start any new medicine while taking Vyvanse without talking to your doctor first.

How should Vyvanse be taken?

- **Take Vyvanse exactly as prescribed.** Vyvanse comes in 6 different strength capsules. Your doctor may adjust the dose until it is right for you or your child.
- Take Vyvanse once a day in the morning.
- Vyvanse can be taken with or without food.
- From time to time, your doctor may stop Vyvanse treatment for a while to check ADHD symptoms.
- Your doctor may do regular checks of the blood, heart, and blood pressure while taking Vyvanse. Children should have their height and weight checked often while taking Vyvanse. Vyvanse treatment may be stopped if a problem is found during these check-ups.
- If you or your child takes too much Vyvanse or overdoses, call your doctor or poison control center right away, or get emergency treatment.

What are possible side effects of Vyvanse?

See "What is the most important information I should know about Vyvanse?" for information on reported heart and mental problems.

Other serious side effects include:

- slowing of growth (height and weight) in children
- seizures, mainly in patients with a history of seizures
- eyesight changes or blurred vision

Common side effects include:

- upper belly pain
- dizziness
- irritability
- nausea
- weight loss
- decreased appetite
- dry mouth
- trouble sleeping
- vomiting

Vyvanse may affect you or your child's ability to drive or do other dangerous activities.

Talk to your doctor if you or your child has side effects that are bothersome or do not go away.

This is not a complete list of possible side effects. Ask your doctor or pharmacist for more information

How should I store Vyvanse?

- Store Vyvanse in a safe place at room temperature, 59 to 86° F (15 to 30° C). Protect from light.
- **Keep Vyvanse and all medicines out of the reach of children.**

General information about Vyvanse

Medicines are sometimes prescribed for purposes other than those listed in a Medication Guide. Do not use Vyvanse for a condition for which it was not prescribed. Do not give Vyvanse to other people, even if they have the same condition. It may harm them and it is against the law.

This Medication Guide summarizes the most important information about Vyvanse. If you would like more information, talk with your doctor. You can ask your doctor or pharmacist for information about Vyvanse that was written for healthcare professionals. For more information about Vyvanse, please contact Shire US Inc. at 1-800-828-2088 or visit www.vyvanse.com.

What are the ingredients in Vyvanse?

Active Ingredient: lisdexamfetamine dimesylate

Inactive Ingredients: microcrystalline cellulose, croscarmellose sodium, and magnesium stearate. The capsule shells contain gelatin, titanium dioxide, and one or more of the following: D&C Red #28, D&C Yellow #10, FC&C Blue #1, FD&C Green #3, and FC&C Red #40.

This Medication Guide has been approved by the U.S. Food and Drug Administration.

Rev 08/07

XXXXXX

To keep your **PDR** up to date
throughout the year, note these revisions
on the corresponding pages of the annual
volume. Simply write "See Supplement A"
next to the product heading.

Takeda Pharmaceuticals America, Inc.
ONE TAKEDA PARKWAY
DEERFIELD, IL 60015

Direct Inquiries to:
Sales and Ordering:
Customer Service
(877) 5 TAKEDA
(877) 582-5332
For Medical Information Contact:
General:
(877) TAKEDA 7
(877) 825-3327
Adverse Drug Experiences:
(877) TAKEDA 7
(877) 825-3327

ACTOPLUS MET®   ℞

[ak-TO-plus-mĕt]
**(pioglitazone hydrochloride and
metformin hydrochloride) tablets**

*Prescribing information for this product, which appears on
pages 3151–3156 of the 2008 PDR, has been completely revised as follows. Please write "See Supplement A" next to the
product heading.*

> **WARNING: CONGESTIVE HEART FAILURE**
>
> • Thiazolidinediones, including pioglitazone, which is a
> component of ACTOPLUS MET, cause or exacerbate
> congestive heart failure in some patients (see **WARN-
> INGS, *Pioglitazone hydrochloride*).** After initiation of
> ACTOPLUS MET, and after dose increases, observe
> patients carefully for signs and symptoms of heart
> failure (including excessive, rapid weight gain, dysp-
> nea, and/or edema). If these signs and symptoms de-
> velop, the heart failure should be managed according
> to the current standards of care. Furthermore, discon-
> tinuation or dose reduction of ACTOPLUS MET must
> be considered.
> • ACTOPLUS MET is not recommended in patients
> with symptomatic heart failure. Initiation of
> ACTOPLUS MET in patients with established NYHA
> Class III or IV heart failure is contraindicated (see
> **CONTRAINDICATIONS** and **WARNINGS,**
> ***Pioglitazone hydrochloride*).**

DESCRIPTION
ACTOPLUS MET® (pioglitazone hydrochloride and
metformin hydrochloride) tablets contain two oral antihyperglycemic drugs used in the management of type 2
diabetes: pioglitazone hydrochloride and metformin
hydrochloride. The concomitant use of pioglitazone and
metformin has been previously approved based on clinical
trials in patients with type 2 diabetes inadequately controlled on metformin. Additional efficacy and safety information about pioglitazone and metformin monotherapies
may be found in the prescribing information for each individual drug.
Pioglitazone hydrochloride is an oral antihyperglycemic
agent that acts primarily by decreasing insulin resistance.
Pioglitazone is used in the management of type 2 diabetes.
Pharmacological studies indicate that pioglitazone improves sensitivity to insulin in muscle and adipose tissue
and inhibits hepatic gluconeogenesis. Pioglitazone improves
glycemic control while reducing circulating insulin levels.
Pioglitazone [(±)-5-[[4-[2-(5-ethyl-2-pyridinyl)ethoxy]
phenyl]methyl]-2,4-] thiazolidinedione monohydrochloride
belongs to a different chemical class and has a different
pharmacological action than the sulfonylureas, biguanides,
or the α-glucosidase inhibitors. The molecule contains one
asymmetric center, and the synthetic compound is a racemate. The two enantiomers of pioglitazone interconvert *in
vivo*. The structural formula is as shown:

pioglitazone hydrochloride

Pioglitazone hydrochloride is an odorless white crystalline
powder that has a molecular formula of $C_{19}H_{20}N_2O_3S \cdot HCl$
and a molecular weight of 392.90. It is soluble in *N,N*-
dimethylformamide, slightly soluble in anhydrous ethanol,
very slightly soluble in acetone and acetonitrile, practically
insoluble in water, and insoluble in ether.
Metformin hydrochloride (*N,N*-dimethylimidodicarboni-
midic diamide hydrochloride) is not chemically or pharmacologically related to any other classes of oral antihyperglycemic agents. Metformin hydrochloride is a white
crystalline powder with a molecular formula of
$C_4H_{11}N_5 \cdot HCl$ and a molecular weight of 165.62. Metformin
hydrochloride is freely soluble in water and is practically
insoluble in acetone, ether, and chloroform. The pKa of
metformin is 12.4. The pH of a 1% aqueous solution of

metformin hydrochloride is 6.68. The structural formula is
as shown:

metformin hydrochloride

ACTOPLUS MET is available as a tablet for oral administration containing 15 mg pioglitazone hydrochloride (as the
base) with 500 mg metformin hydrochloride (15 mg/500 mg)
or 15 mg pioglitazone hydrochloride (as the base) with
850 mg metformin hydrochloride (15 mg/850 mg) formulated with the following excipients: povidone USP, microcrystalline cellulose NF, croscarmellose sodium NF, magnesium stearate NF, hypromellose 2910 USP, polyethylene
glycol 8000 NF, titanium dioxide USP, and talc USP.

CLINICAL PHARMACOLOGY
Mechanism of Action
ACTOPLUS MET
ACTOPLUS MET combines two antihyperglycemic agents
with different mechanisms of action to improve glycemic
control in patients with type 2 diabetes: pioglitazone
hydrochloride, a member of the thiazolidinedione class, and
metformin hydrochloride, a member of the biguanide class.
Thiazolidinediones are insulin-sensitizing agents that act
primarily by enhancing peripheral glucose utilization,
whereas biguanides act primarily by decreasing endogenous
hepatic glucose production.
Pioglitazone hydrochloride
Pioglitazone depends on the presence of insulin for its mechanism of action. Pioglitazone decreases insulin resistance in
the periphery and in the liver resulting in increased insulin-
dependent glucose disposal and decreased hepatic glucose
output. Unlike sulfonylureas, pioglitazone is not an insulin
secretagogue. Pioglitazone is a potent and highly selective
agonist for peroxisome proliferator-activated receptor-
gamma (PPARγ). PPAR receptors are found in tissues important for insulin action such as adipose tissue, skeletal
muscle, and liver. Activation of PPARγ nuclear receptors
modulates the transcription of a number of insulin responsive genes involved in the control of glucose and lipid
metabolism.
In animal models of diabetes, pioglitazone reduces the hyperglycemia, hyperinsulinemia, and hypertriglyceridemia
characteristic of insulin-resistant states such as type 2 diabetes. The metabolic changes produced by pioglitazone result in increased responsiveness of insulin-dependent tissues and are observed in numerous animal models of
insulin resistance.
Since pioglitazone enhances the effects of circulating insulin
(by decreasing insulin resistance), it does not lower blood
glucose in animal models that lack endogenous insulin.
Metformin hydrochloride
Metformin hydrochloride improves glucose tolerance in patients with type 2 diabetes, lowering both basal and postprandial plasma glucose. Metformin decreases hepatic glucose production, decreases intestinal absorption of glucose
and improves insulin sensitivity by increasing peripheral
glucose uptake and utilization. Unlike sulfonylureas,
metformin does not produce hypoglycemia in either patients
with type 2 diabetes or normal subjects (except in special
circumstances, see **PRECAUTIONS, General:** *Metformin
hydrochloride*) and does not cause hyperinsulinemia. With
metformin therapy, insulin secretion remains unchanged
while fasting insulin levels and day-long plasma insulin response may actually decrease.

Table 1. Mean (SD) Pharmacokinetic Parameters for ACTOPLUS MET®

Regimen	N	AUC(0-inf) (ng•h/mL)	N	C_{max} (ng/mL)	N	T_{max} (h)	N	$T_{\frac{1}{2}}$ (h)
pioglitazone HCl								
15 mg/500 mg ACTOPLUS MET®	51	5984 (1599)	63	585 (198)	63	1.83 (0.93)	51	8.69 (3.86)
15 mg ACTOS® and 500 mg Glucophage®	54	5810 (1472)	63	608 (204)	63	1.75 (0.90)	54	7.90 (3.08)
15 mg/850 mg ACTOPLUS MET®	52	5671 (1585)	60	569 (222)	60	1.89 (0.80)	52	7.19 (1.84)
15 mg ACTOS® and 850 mg Glucophage®	55	5957 (1680)	61	603 (239)	61	2.01 (1.54)	55	7.16 (1.85)
metformin HCl								
15 mg/500 mg ACTOPLUS MET®	59	7783 (2266)	63	1203 (325)	63	2.32 (0.88)	59	8.57 (14.30)
15 mg ACTOS® and 500 mg Glucophage®	59	7599 (2385)	63	1215 (329)	63	2.53 (0.95)	59	6.73 (5.87)
15 mg/850 mg ACTOPLUS MET®	47	11927 (3311)	60	1827 (536)	60	2.41 (0.91)	47	17.56 (20.08)
15 mg ACTOS® and 850 mg Glucophage®	52	11569 (3494)	61	1797 (525)	61	2.26 (0.85)	52	17.01 (18.09)

Pharmacokinetics and Drug Metabolism
Absorption and Bioavailability:
ACTOPLUS MET
In bioequivalence studies of ACTOPLUS MET 15 mg/
500 mg and 15 mg/850 mg, the area under the curve (AUC)
and maximum concentration (C_{max}) of both the pioglitazone
and the metformin component following a single dose of the
combination tablet were bioequivalent to ACTOS® 15 mg
concomitantly administered with Glucophage® (500 mg or
850 mg respectively) tablets under fasted conditions in
healthy subjects (**Table 1**).
[See table 1 above]
Administration of ACTOPLUS MET 15 mg/850 mg with
food resulted in no change in overall exposure of
pioglitazone. With metformin there was no change in AUC;
however mean peak serum concentration of metformin was
decreased by 28% when administered with food. A delayed
time to peak serum concentration was observed for both
components (1.9 hours for pioglitazone and 0.8 hours for
metformin) under fed conditions. These changes are not
likely to be clinically significant.
Pioglitazone hydrochloride
Following oral administration, in the fasting state,
pioglitazone is first measurable in serum within 30 minutes, with peak concentrations observed within 2 hours.
Food slightly delays the time to peak serum concentration
to 3 to 4 hours, but does not alter the extent of absorption.
Metformin hydrochloride
The absolute bioavailability of a 500 mg metformin tablet
given under fasting conditions is approximately 50% - 60%.
Studies using single oral doses of metformin tablets of
500 mg to 1500 mg, and 850 mg to 2550 mg, indicate that
there is a lack of dose proportionality with increasing doses,
which is due to decreased absorption rather than an alteration in elimination. Food decreases the extent of and
slightly delays the absorption of metformin, as shown by approximately a 40% lower mean peak plasma concentration,
a 25% lower AUC in plasma concentration versus time
curve, and a 35 minute prolongation of time to peak plasma
concentration following administration of a single 850 mg
tablet of metformin with food, compared to the same tablet
strength administered fasting. The clinical relevance of
these decreases is unknown.
Distribution:
Pioglitazone hydrochloride
The mean apparent volume of distribution (V/F) of
pioglitazone following single-dose administration is 0.63 ±
0.41 (mean ± SD) L/kg of body weight. Pioglitazone is extensively protein bound (> 99%) in human serum, principally to serum albumin. Pioglitazone also binds to other
serum proteins, but with lower affinity. Metabolites M-III
and M-IV also are extensively bound (> 98%) to serum
albumin.
Metformin hydrochloride
The apparent volume of distribution (V/F) of metformin following single oral doses of 850 mg averaged 654 ± 358 L.
Metformin is negligibly bound to plasma proteins.
Metformin partitions into erythrocytes, most likely as a
function of time. At usual clinical doses and dosing schedules of metformin, steady-state plasma concentrations of
metformin are reached within 24 - 48 hours and are generally <1 μg/mL. During controlled clinical trials, maximum
metformin plasma levels did not exceed 5 μg/mL, even at
maximum doses.
Metabolism, Elimination and Excretion:
Pioglitazone hydrochloride
Pioglitazone is extensively metabolized by hydroxylation
and oxidation; the metabolites also partly convert to glu-

Continued on next page

Actoplus Met—Cont.

curonide or sulfate conjugates. Metabolites M-II and M-IV (hydroxy derivatives of pioglitazone) and M-III (keto derivative of pioglitazone) are pharmacologically active in animal models of type 2 diabetes. In addition to pioglitazone, M-III and M-IV are the principal drug-related species found in human serum following multiple dosing. At steady-state, in both healthy volunteers and in patients with type 2 diabetes, pioglitazone comprises approximately 30% to 50% of the total peak serum concentrations and 20% to 25% of the total AUC.

In vitro data demonstrate that multiple CYP isoforms are involved in the metabolism of pioglitazone. The cytochrome P450 isoforms involved are CYP2C8 and, to a lesser degree, CYP3A4 with additional contributions from a variety of other isoforms including the mainly extrahepatic CYP1A1. *In vivo* studies of pioglitazone in combination with P450 inhibitors and substrates have been performed (see **PRECAUTIONS, Drug Interactions,** *Pioglitazone hydrochloride*). Urinary 6ß-hydroxycortisol/cortisol ratios measured in patients treated with pioglitazone showed that pioglitazone is not a strong CYP3A4 enzyme inducer.

Following oral administration, approximately 15% to 30% of the pioglitazone dose is recovered in the urine. Renal elimination of pioglitazone is negligible and the drug is excreted primarily as metabolites and their conjugates. It is presumed that most of the oral dose is excreted into the bile either unchanged or as metabolites and eliminated in the feces.

The mean serum half-life of pioglitazone and total pioglitazone ranges from 3 to 7 hours and 16 to 24 hours, respectively. Pioglitazone has an apparent clearance, CL/F, calculated to be 5 to 7 L/hr.

Metformin hydrochloride

Intravenous single-dose studies in normal subjects demonstrate that metformin is excreted unchanged in the urine and does not undergo hepatic metabolism (no metabolites have been identified in humans) nor biliary excretion. Renal clearance is approximately 3.5 times greater than creatinine clearance which indicates that tubular secretion is the major route of metformin elimination. Following oral administration, approximately 90% of the absorbed drug is eliminated via the renal route within the first 24 hours, with a plasma elimination half-life of approximately 6.2 hours. In blood, the elimination half-life is approximately 17.6 hours, suggesting that the erythrocyte mass may be a compartment of distribution.

Special Populations
Renal Insufficiency:
Pioglitazone hydrochloride

The serum elimination half-life of pioglitazone, M-III and M-IV remains unchanged in patients with moderate (creatinine clearance 30 to 60 mL/min) to severe (creatinine clearance < 30 mL/min) renal impairment when compared to normal subjects.

Metformin hydrochloride

In patients with decreased renal function (based on creatinine clearance), the plasma and blood half-life of metformin is prolonged and the renal clearance is decreased in proportion to the decrease in creatinine clearance (see **CONTRAINDICATIONS AND WARNINGS,** *Metformin hydrochloride*, also see GLUCOPHAGE® prescribing information, **CLINICAL PHARMACOLOGY, Pharmacokinetics**). Since metformin is contraindicated in patients with renal impairment, ACTOPLUS MET is also contraindicated in these patients.

Hepatic Insufficiency:
Pioglitazone hydrochloride

Compared with normal controls, subjects with impaired hepatic function (Child-Pugh Grade B/C) have an approximate 45% reduction in pioglitazone and total pioglitazone mean peak concentrations but no change in the mean AUC values.

Therapy with ACTOPLUS MET should not be initiated if the patient exhibits clinical evidence of active liver disease or serum transaminase levels (ALT) exceed 2.5 times the upper limit of normal (see **PRECAUTIONS, General:** *Pioglitazone hydrochloride*).

Metformin hydrochloride

No pharmacokinetic studies of metformin have been conducted in subjects with hepatic insufficiency.

Elderly:
Pioglitazone hydrochloride

In healthy elderly subjects, peak serum concentrations of pioglitazone and total pioglitazone are not significantly different, but AUC values are slightly higher and the terminal half-life values slightly longer than for younger subjects. These changes were not of a magnitude that would be considered clinically relevant.

Metformin hydrochloride

Limited data from controlled pharmacokinetic studies of metformin in healthy elderly subjects suggest that total plasma clearance is decreased, the half-life is prolonged, and C_{max} is increased, compared to healthy young subjects. From these data, it appears that the change in metformin pharmacokinetics with aging is primarily accounted for by a change in renal function (see GLUCOPHAGE® prescribing information, **CLINICAL PHARMACOLOGY, Special Populations, Geriatrics**).

ACTOPLUS MET treatment should not be initiated in patients ≥ 80 years of age unless measurement of creatinine clearance demonstrates that renal function is not reduced

(see **WARNINGS,** *Metformin hydrochloride* and **DOSAGE AND ADMINISTRATION**; also see GLUCOPHAGE® prescribing information).

Pediatrics:
Pioglitazone hydrochloride

Pharmacokinetic data in the pediatric population are not available.

Metformin hydrochloride

After administration of a single oral metformin 500 mg tablet with food, geometric mean metformin C_{max} and AUC differed less than 5% between pediatric type 2 diabetic patients (12 to 16 years of age) and gender- and weight-matched healthy adults (20 to 45 years of age), and all with normal renal function.

Gender:
Pioglitazone hydrochloride

As monotherapy and in combination with sulfonylurea, metformin, or insulin, pioglitazone improved glycemic control in both males and females. The mean C_{max} and AUC values were increased 20% to 60% in females. In controlled clinical trials, hemoglobin A1C (A1C) decreases from baseline were generally greater for females than for males (average mean difference in A1C 0.5%). Since therapy should be individualized for each patient to achieve glycemic control, no dose adjustment is recommended based on gender alone.

Metformin hydrochloride

Metformin pharmacokinetic parameters did not differ significantly between normal subjects and patients with type 2 diabetes when analyzed according to gender (males = 19, females = 16). Similarly, in controlled clinical studies in patients with type 2 diabetes, the antihyperglycemic effect of metformin was comparable in males and females.

Ethnicity:
Pioglitazone hydrochloride

Pharmacokinetic data among various ethnic groups are not available.

Metformin hydrochloride

No studies of metformin pharmacokinetic parameters according to race have been performed. In controlled clinical studies of metformin in patients with type 2 diabetes, the antihyperglycemic effect was comparable in whites (n=249), blacks (n=51), and Hispanics (n=24).

Drug-Drug Interactions
Co-administration of a single dose of metformin (1000 mg) and pioglitazone after 7 days of pioglitazone (45 mg) did not alter the pharmacokinetics of the single dose of metformin. Specific pharmacokinetic drug interaction studies with ACTOPLUS MET have not been performed, although such studies have been conducted with the individual pioglitazone and metformin components.

Pioglitazone hydrochloride

The following drugs were studied in healthy volunteers with co-administration of pioglitazone 45 mg once daily. Results are listed below:

Oral Contraceptives: Co-administration of pioglitazone (45 mg once daily) and an oral contraceptive (1 mg norethindrone plus 0.035 mg ethinyl estradiol once daily) for 21 days, resulted in 11% and 11-14% decrease in ethinyl estradiol AUC (0-24h) and C_{max} respectively. There were no significant changes in norethindrone AUC (0-24h) and C_{max}. In view of the high variability of ethinyl estradiol pharmacokinetics, the clinical significance of this finding is unknown.

Midazolam: Administration of pioglitazone for 15 days followed by a single 7.5 mg dose of midazolam syrup resulted in a 26% reduction in midazolam C_{max} and AUC.

Nifedipine ER: Co-administration of pioglitazone for 7 days with 30 mg nifedipine ER administered orally once daily for 4 days to male and female volunteers resulted in a ratio of least square mean (90% CI) values for unchanged nifedipine of 0.83 (0.73 - 0.95) for C_{max} and 0.88 (0.80 - 0.96) for AUC. In view of the high variability of nifedipine pharmacokinetics, the clinical significance of this finding is unknown.

Ketoconazole: Co-administration of pioglitazone for 7 days with ketoconazole 200 mg administered twice daily resulted in a ratio of least square mean (90% CI) values for unchanged pioglitazone of 1.14 (1.06 - 1.23) for C_{max}, 1.34 (1.26 - 1.41) for AUC and 1.87 (1.71 - 2.04) for C_{min}.

Atorvastatin Calcium: Co-administration of pioglitazone for 7 days with atorvastatin calcium (LIPITOR®) 80 mg once daily resulted in a ratio of least square mean (90% CI) values for unchanged pioglitazone of 0.69 (0.57 - 0.85) for C_{max}, 0.76 (0.65 - 0.88) for AUC and 0.96 (0.87 - 1.05) for C_{min}. For unchanged atorvastatin the ratio of least square mean (90% CI) values were 0.77 (0.66 - 0.90) for C_{max}, 0.86 (0.78 - 0.94) for AUC and 0.92 (0.82 - 1.02) for C_{min}.

Cytochrome P450: See **PRECAUTIONS, Drug Interactions,** *Pioglitazone hydrochloride*

Gemfibrozil: Concomitant administration of gemfibrozil (oral 600 mg twice daily), an inhibitor of CYP2C8, with pioglitazone (oral 30 mg) in 10 healthy volunteers pretreated for 2 days prior with gemfibrozil (oral 600 mg twice daily) resulted in pioglitazone exposure (AUC$_{0-24}$) being 226% of the pioglitazone exposure in the absence of gemfibrozil (see **PRECAUTIONS, Drug Interactions,** *Pioglitazone hydrochloride*).[1]

Rifampin: Concomitant administration of rifampin (oral 600 mg once daily), an inducer of CYP2C8 with pioglitazone (oral 30 mg) in 10 healthy volunteers pre-treated for 5 days prior with rifampin (oral 600 mg once daily) resulted in a decrease in the AUC of pioglitazone by 54% (see **PRECAUTIONS, Drug Interactions,** *Pioglitazone hydrochloride*).[2]

In other drug-drug interaction studies, pioglitazone had no significant effect on the pharmacokinetics of fexofenadine, glipizide, digoxin, warfarin, ranitidine HCl or theophylline.

Metformin hydrochloride

See **PRECAUTIONS, Drug Interactions,** *Metformin hydrochloride*

Pharmacodynamics and Clinical Effects
Pioglitazone hydrochloride

Clinical studies demonstrate that pioglitazone improves insulin sensitivity in insulin-resistant patients. Pioglitazone enhances cellular responsiveness to insulin, increases insulin-dependent glucose disposal, improves hepatic sensitivity to insulin, and improves dysfunctional glucose homeostasis. In patients with type 2 diabetes, the decreased insulin resistance produced by pioglitazone results in lower plasma glucose concentrations, lower plasma insulin levels, and lower A1C values. Based on results from an open-label extension study, the glucose-lowering effects of pioglitazone appear to persist for at least one year. In controlled clinical studies, pioglitazone in combination with metformin had an additive effect on glycemic control.

Patients with lipid abnormalities were included in placebo-controlled monotherapy clinical studies with pioglitazone. Overall, patients treated with pioglitazone had mean decreases in triglycerides, mean increases in HDL cholesterol, and no consistent mean changes in LDL cholesterol and total cholesterol compared to the placebo group. A similar pattern of results was seen in 16-week and 24-week combination therapy studies of pioglitazone with metformin.

Clinical Studies
There have been no clinical efficacy studies conducted with ACTOPLUS MET. However, the efficacy and safety of the separate components have been previously established and the co-administration of the separate components has been evaluated for efficacy and safety in two clinical studies. These clinical studies established an added benefit of pioglitazone in patients with inadequately controlled type 2 diabetes while on metformin therapy. Bioequivalence of ACTOPLUS MET with co-administered pioglitazone and metformin tablets was demonstrated for both ACTOPLUS MET strengths (see **CLINICAL PHARMACOLOGY, Pharmacokinetics and Drug Metabolism**).

Clinical Trials of Pioglitazone Add-on Therapy in Patients Not Adequately Controlled on Metformin
Two treatment-randomized, controlled clinical studies in patients with type 2 diabetes were conducted to evaluate the safety and efficacy of pioglitazone plus metformin. Both studies included patients receiving metformin, either alone or in combination with another antihyperglycemic agent, who had inadequate glycemic control. All other antihyperglycemic agents were discontinued prior to starting study treatment. In the first study, 328 patients received either 30 mg of pioglitazone or placebo once daily for 16 weeks in addition to their established metformin regimen. In the second study, 827 patients received either 30 mg or 45 mg of pioglitazone once daily for 24 weeks in addition to their established metformin regimen.

In the first study, the addition of pioglitazone 30 mg once daily to metformin treatment significantly reduced the mean A1C by 0.83% and the mean FPG by 37.7 mg/dL at Week 16 from that observed with metformin alone. In the second study, the mean reductions from Baseline at Week 24 in A1C were 0.80% and 1.01% for the 30 mg and 45 mg doses, respectively. Mean reductions from Baseline in FPG were 38.2 mg/dL and 50.7 mg/dL, respectively. Based on these reductions in A1C and FPG (**Table 2**), the addition of pioglitazone to metformin resulted in significant improvements in glycemic control irrespective of the metformin dose.

[See table 2 at top of next page]

INDICATIONS AND USAGE
ACTOPLUS MET is indicated as an adjunct to diet and exercise to improve glycemic control in patients with type 2 diabetes who are already treated with a combination of pioglitazone and metformin or whose diabetes is not adequately controlled with metformin alone, or for those patients who have initially responded to pioglitazone alone and require additional glycemic control.

Management of type 2 diabetes should also include nutritional counseling, weight reduction as needed, and exercise. These efforts are important not only in the primary treatment of type 2 diabetes, but also to maintain the efficacy of drug therapy.

CONTRAINDICATIONS
Initiation of ACTOPLUS MET in patients with established New York Heart Association (NYHA) Class III or IV heart failure is contraindicated (see **BOXED WARNING**).

In addition, ACTOPLUS MET is contraindicated in patients with:

1. Renal disease or renal dysfunction (e.g., as suggested by serum creatinine levels ≥ 1.5 mg/dL [males], ≥ 1.4 mg/dL [females], or abnormal creatinine clearance) which may also result from conditions such as cardiovascular collapse (shock), acute myocardial infarction, and septicemia (see **WARNINGS,** *Metformin hydrochloride* and **PRECAUTIONS, General:** *Metformin hydrochloride*).

2. Known hypersensitivity to pioglitazone, metformin or any other component of ACTOPLUS MET.

3. Acute or chronic metabolic acidosis, including diabetic ketoacidosis, with or without coma. Diabetic ketoacidosis should be treated with insulin.

ACTOPLUS MET should be temporarily discontinued in patients undergoing radiologic studies involving intravascular administration of iodinated contrast materials, because use of such products may result in acute alteration of renal function (see **PRECAUTIONS, General:** ***Metformin hydrochloride***).

WARNINGS

Metformin hydrochloride

Lactic Acidosis: Lactic acidosis is a rare, but serious, metabolic complication that can occur due to metformin accumulation during treatment with ACTOPLUS MET (pioglitazone hydrochloride and metformin hydrochloride) tablets; when it occurs, it is fatal in approximately 50% of cases. Lactic acidosis may also occur in association with a number of pathophysiologic conditions, including diabetes mellitus, and whenever there is significant tissue hypoperfusion and hypoxemia. Lactic acidosis is characterized by elevated blood lactate levels (> 5 mmol/L), decreased blood pH, electrolyte disturbances with an increased anion gap, and an increased lactate/pyruvate ratio. When metformin is implicated as the cause of lactic acidosis, metformin plasma levels > 5 µg/mL are generally found.

The reported incidence of lactic acidosis in patients receiving metformin hydrochloride is very low (approximately 0.03 cases/1000 patient-years, with approximately 0.015 fatal cases/1000 patient-years). In more than 20,000 patient-years exposure to metformin in clinical trials, there were no reports of lactic acidosis. Reported cases have occurred primarily in diabetic patients with significant renal insufficiency, including both intrinsic renal disease and renal hypoperfusion, often in the setting of multiple concomitant medical/surgical problems and multiple concomitant medications. Patients with congestive heart failure requiring pharmacologic management, in particular those with unstable or acute congestive heart failure who are at risk of hypoperfusion and hypoxemia, are at increased risk of lactic acidosis. The risk of lactic acidosis increases with the degree of renal dysfunction and the patient's age. The risk of lactic acidosis may, therefore, be significantly decreased by regular monitoring of renal function in patients taking metformin and by use of the minimum effective dose of metformin. In particular, treatment of the elderly should be accompanied by careful monitoring of renal function. Metformin treatment should not be initiated in patients ≥ 80 years of age unless measurement of creatinine clearance demonstrates that renal function is not reduced, as these patients are more susceptible to developing lactic acidosis. In addition, metformin should be promptly withheld in the presence of any condition associated with hypoxemia, dehydration, or sepsis. Because impaired hepatic function may significantly limit the ability to clear lactate, metformin should generally be avoided in patients with clinical or laboratory evidence of hepatic disease. Patients should be cautioned against excessive alcohol intake, either acute or chronic, when taking metformin, since alcohol potentiates the effects of metformin hydrochloride on lactate metabolism. In addition, metformin should be temporarily discontinued prior to any intravascular radiocontrast study and for any surgical procedure (see PRECAUTIONS, General: *Metformin hydrochloride*).

The onset of lactic acidosis often is subtle, and accompanied only by nonspecific symptoms such as malaise, myalgias, respiratory distress, increasing somnolence, and nonspecific abdominal distress. There may be associated hypothermia, hypotension, and resistant bradyarrhythmias with more marked acidosis. The patient and the patient's physician must be aware of the possible importance of such symptoms and the patient should be instructed to notify the physician immediately if they occur (see PRECAUTIONS, General: *Metformin hydrochloride*). Metformin should be withdrawn until the situation is clarified. Serum electrolytes, ketones, blood glucose, and, if indicated, blood pH, lactate levels, and even blood metformin levels may be useful. Once a patient is stabilized on any dose level of metformin, gastrointestinal symptoms, which are common during initiation of therapy, are unlikely to be drug related. Later occurrence of gastrointestinal symptoms could be due to lactic acidosis or other serious disease.

Levels of fasting venous plasma lactate above the upper limit of normal but less than 5 mmol/L in patients taking metformin do not necessarily indicate impending lactic acidosis and may be explainable by other mechanisms, such as poorly controlled diabetes or obesity, vigorous physical activity, or technical problems in sample handling (see PRECAUTIONS, General: *Metformin hydrochloride*).

Lactic acidosis should be suspected in any diabetic patient with metabolic acidosis lacking evidence of ketoacidosis (ketonuria and ketonemia).

Lactic acidosis is a medical emergency that must be treated in a hospital setting. In a patient with lactic acidosis who is taking metformin, the drug should be discontinued immediately and general supportive measures promptly instituted. Because metformin hydrochloride is dialyzable (with a clearance of up to 170 mL/min under good hemodynamic conditions), prompt hemodialysis is recommended to correct the acidosis and remove the accumulated metformin. Such management often results in prompt reversal of symptoms and recovery (see CONTRAINDICATIONS and PRECAUTIONS, General: *Metformin hydrochloride*).

Table 2. Glycemic Parameters in 16-Week and 24-Week Pioglitazone Hydrochloride + Metformin Hydrochloride Combination Studies

Parameter	Placebo + metformin	Pioglitazone 30 mg + metformin
16-Week Study		
A1C (%)	N=153	N=161
Baseline mean	9.77	9.92
Mean change from Baseline at 16 Weeks	0.19	-0.64*,†
Difference in change from placebo + metformin		-0.83
Responder rate (%) (a)	21.6	54.0
FPG (mg/dL)	N=157	N=165
Baseline mean	259.9	254.4
Mean change from Baseline at 16 Weeks	-5.2	-42.8*,†
Difference in change from placebo + metformin		-37.7
Responder rate (%) (b)	23.6	59.4
Parameter	**Pioglitazone 30 mg + metformin**	**Pioglitazone 45 mg + metformin**
24-Week Study		
A1C (%)	N=400	N=398
Baseline mean	9.88	9.81
Mean Change from Baseline at 24 Weeks	-0.80*	-1.01*
Responder rate (%) (a)	55.8	63.3
FPG (mg/dL)	N=398	N=399
Baseline mean	232.5	232.1
Mean Change from Baseline at 24 Weeks	-38.2*	-50.7*,‡
Responder rate (%) (b)	52.3	63.7

* significant change from Baseline p ≤ 0.050.
† significant difference from placebo plus metformin, p ≤ 0.050.
‡ significant difference from 30 mg pioglitazone, p ≤ 0.050.
(a) patients who achieved an A1C ≤ 6.1% or ≥ 0.6% decrease from Baseline.
(b) patients who achieved a decrease in FPG by ≥ 30 mg/dL.

Pioglitazone hydrochloride

Cardiac Failure and Other Cardiac Effects: Pioglitazone, like other thiazolidinediones, can cause fluid retention when used alone or in combination with other antihyperglycemic agents, including insulin. Fluid retention may lead to or exacerbate heart failure. Patients should be observed for signs and symptoms of heart failure. If these signs and symptoms develop, the heart failure should be managed according to current standards of care. Furthermore, discontinuation or dose reduction of pioglitazone must be considered. Patients with NYHA Class III and IV cardiac status were not studied during pre-approval clinical trials and pioglitazone is not recommended in these patients (see **BOXED WARNING** and **CONTRAINDICATIONS**).

In one 16-week U.S. double-blind, placebo-controlled clinical trial involving 566 patients with type 2 diabetes, pioglitazone at doses of 15 mg and 30 mg in combination with insulin was compared to insulin therapy alone. This trial included patients with long-standing diabetes and a high prevalence of pre-existing medical conditions as follows: arterial hypertension (57.2%), peripheral neuropathy (22.6%), coronary heart disease (19.6%), retinopathy (13.1%), myocardial infarction (8.8%), vascular disease (6.4%), angina pectoris (4.4%), stroke and/or transient ischemic attack (4.1%), and congestive heart failure (2.3%).

In this study two of the 191 patients receiving 15 mg pioglitazone plus insulin (1.1%) and two of the 188 patients receiving 30 mg pioglitazone plus insulin (1.1%) developed congestive heart failure compared with none of the 187 patients on insulin therapy alone. All four of these patients had previous histories of cardiovascular conditions including coronary artery disease, previous CABG procedures, and myocardial infarction. In a 24-week dose-controlled study in which pioglitazone was co-administered with insulin, 0.3% of patients (1/345) on 30 mg and 0.9% (3/345) of patients on 45 mg reported CHF as a serious adverse event. Analysis of data from these studies did not identify specific factors that predict increased risk of congestive heart failure on combination therapy with insulin.

In type 2 diabetes and congestive heart failure (systolic dysfunction)

A 24-week post-marketing safety study was performed to compare ACTOS (n=262) to glyburide (n=256) in uncontrolled diabetic patients (mean A1C 8.8% at baseline) with NYHA Class II and III heart failure and ejection fraction less than 40% (mean EF 30% at baseline). Over the course of the study, overnight hospitalization for congestive heart failure was reported in 9.9% of patients on ACTOS compared to 4.7% of patients on glyburide with a treatment difference observed from 6 weeks. This adverse event associated with ACTOS was more marked in patients using insulin at baseline and in patients over 64 years of age. No difference in cardiovascular mortality between the treatment groups was observed.

ACTOS should be initiated at the lowest approved dose if it is prescribed for patients with type 2 diabetes and systolic heart failure (NYHA Class II). If subsequent dose escalation is necessary, the dose should be increased gradually only after several months of treatment with careful monitoring for weight gain, edema, or signs and symptoms of CHF exacerbation.

Prospective Pioglitazone Clinical Trial In Macrovascular Events (PROactive)

In PROactive, 5238 patients with type 2 diabetes and a prior history of macrovascular disease were treated with ACTOS (n=2605), force-titrated up to 45 mg once daily, or placebo (n=2633) (see **ADVERSE REACTIONS**). The percentage of patients who had an event of serious heart failure was higher for patients treated with ACTOS (5.7%, n=149) than for patients treated with placebo (4.1%, n=108). The incidence of death subsequent to a report of serious heart failure was 1.5% (n=40) in patients treated with ACTOS and 1.4% (n=37) in placebo-treated patients. In patients treated with an insulin-containing regimen at baseline, the incidence of serious heart failure was 6.3% (n=54/864) with ACTOS and 5.2% (n=47/896) with placebo. For those patients treated with a sulfonylurea-containing regimen at baseline, the incidence of serious heart failure was 5.8% (n=94/1624) with ACTOS and 4.4% (n=71/1626) with placebo.

PRECAUTIONS

General: *Pioglitazone hydrochloride*

Pioglitazone exerts its antihyperglycemic effect only in the presence of insulin. Therefore, ACTOPLUS MET should not be used in patients with type 1 diabetes or for the treatment of diabetic ketoacidosis.

Hypoglycemia: Patients receiving pioglitazone in combination with insulin or oral hypoglycemic agents may be at risk for hypoglycemia, and a reduction in the dose of the concomitant agent may be necessary.

Cardiovascular: In U.S. placebo-controlled clinical trials that excluded patients with New York Heart Association (NYHA) Class III and IV cardiac status, the incidence of serious cardiac adverse events related to volume expansion was not increased in patients treated with pioglitazone as monotherapy or in combination with sulfonylureas or metformin vs. placebo-treated patients. In insulin combination studies, a small number of patients with a history of previously existing cardiac disease developed congestive heart failure when treated with pioglitazone in combination with insulin (see **WARNINGS, *Pioglitazone hydrochloride***). Patients with NYHA Class III and IV cardiac status were not studied in pre-approval pioglitazone clinical trials. Pioglitazone is not indicated in patients with NYHA Class III or IV cardiac status.

Continued on next page

Actoplus Met—Cont.

In postmarketing experience with pioglitazone, cases of congestive heart failure have been reported in patients both with and without previously known heart disease.

Edema: In all U.S. clinical trials with pioglitazone, edema was reported more frequently in patients treated with pioglitazone than in placebo-treated patients and appears to be dose related (see ADVERSE REACTIONS). In postmarketing experience, reports of initiation or worsening of edema have been received. Since thiazolidinediones, including pioglitazone, can cause fluid retention, which can exacerbate or lead to congestive heart failure, ACTOPLUS MET should be used with caution in patients at risk for heart failure. Patients should be monitored for signs and symptoms of heart failure (see BOXED WARNING, WARNINGS, *Pioglitazone hydrochloride,* and PRECAUTIONS, Information for Patients).

Weight Gain: Dose related weight gain was observed with pioglitazone alone and in combination with other hypoglycemic agents (Table 3). The mechanism of weight gain is unclear but probably involves a combination of fluid retention and fat accumulation.

[See table 3 below]

Ovulation: Therapy with pioglitazone, like other thiazolidinediones, may result in ovulation in some premenopausal anovulatory women. Thus, adequate contraception in premenopausal women should be recommended while taking ACTOPLUS MET. This possible effect has not been investigated in clinical studies so the frequency of this occurrence is not known.

Hematologic: Across all clinical studies with pioglitazone, mean hemoglobin values declined by 2% to 4% in patients treated with pioglitazone. These changes primarily occurred within the first 4 to 12 weeks of therapy and remained relatively constant thereafter. These changes may be related to increased plasma volume and have rarely been associated with any significant hematologic clinical effects (see ADVERSE REACTIONS, Laboratory Abnormalities). ACTOPLUS MET may cause decreases in hemoglobin and hematocrit.

Hepatic Effects: In pre-approval clinical studies worldwide, over 4500 subjects were treated with pioglitazone. In U.S. clinical studies, over 4700 patients with type 2 diabetes received pioglitazone. There was no evidence of drug-induced hepatotoxicity or elevation of ALT levels in the clinical studies.

During pre-approval placebo-controlled clinical trials in the U.S., a total of 4 of 1526 (0.26%) patients treated with pioglitazone and 2 of 793 (0.25%) placebo-treated patients had ALT values $\geq$ 3 times the upper limit of normal. The ALT elevations in patients treated with pioglitazone were reversible and were not clearly related to therapy with pioglitazone.

In postmarketing experience with pioglitazone, reports of hepatitis and of hepatic enzyme elevations to 3 or more times the upper limit of normal have been received. Very rarely, these reports have involved hepatic failure with and without fatal outcome, although causality has not been established.

Pending the availability of the results of additional large, long-term controlled clinical trials and additional postmarketing safety data on pioglitazone, it is recommended that patients treated with ACTOPLUS MET undergo periodic monitoring of liver enzymes.

Serum ALT (alanine aminotransferase) levels should be evaluated prior to the initiation of therapy with ACTOPLUS MET in all patients and periodically thereafter per the clinical judgment of the health care professional. Liver function tests should also be obtained for patients if symptoms suggestive of hepatic dysfunction occur, e.g., nausea, vomiting, abdominal pain, fatigue, anorexia, or dark urine. The decision whether to continue the patient on therapy with ACTOPLUS MET should be guided by clinical judgment pending laboratory evaluations. If jaundice is observed, drug therapy should be discontinued.

Therapy with ACTOPLUS MET should not be initiated if the patient exhibits clinical evidence of active liver disease or the ALT levels exceed 2.5 times the upper limit of normal.

Patients with mildly elevated liver enzymes (ALT levels at 1 to 2.5 times the upper limit of normal) at baseline or any time during therapy with ACTOPLUS MET should be evaluated to determine the cause of the liver enzyme elevation. Initiation or continuation of therapy with ACTOPLUS MET in patients with mildly elevated liver enzymes should proceed with caution and include appropriate clinical follow-up which may include more frequent liver enzyme monitoring. If serum transaminase levels are increased (ALT > 2.5 times the upper limit of normal), liver function tests should be evaluated more frequently until the levels return to normal or pretreatment values. If ALT levels exceed 3 times the upper limit of normal, the test should be repeated as soon as possible. If ALT levels remain > 3 times the upper limit of normal or if the patient is jaundiced, ACTOPLUS MET therapy should be discontinued.

Macular Edema: Macular edema has been reported in post-marketing experience in diabetic patients who were taking pioglitazone or another thiazolidinedione. Some patients presented with blurred vision or decreased visual acuity, but some patients appear to have been diagnosed on routine ophthalmologic examination. Some patients had peripheral edema at the time macular edema was diagnosed. Some patients had improvement in their macular edema after discontinuation of their thiazolidinedione. It is unknown whether or not there is a causal relationship between pioglitazone and macular edema. Patients with diabetes should have regular eye exams by an ophthalmologist, per the Standards of Care of the American Diabetes Association. Additionally, any diabetic who reports any kind of visual symptom should be promptly referred to an ophthalmologist, regardless of the patient's underlying medications or other physical findings (see ADVERSE REACTIONS).

Fractures: In a randomized trial (PROactive) in patients with type 2 diabetes (mean duration of diabetes 9.5 years), an increased incidence of bone fracture was noted in female patients taking pioglitazone. During a mean follow-up of 34.5 months, the incidence of bone fracture in females was 5.1% (44/870) for pioglitazone versus 2.5% (23/905) for placebo. This difference was noted after the first year of treatment and remained during the course of the study. The majority of fractures observed in female patients were nonvertebral fractures including lower limb and distal upper limb. No increase in fracture rates was observed in men treated with pioglitazone 1.7% (30/1735) versus placebo 2.1% (37/1728). The risk of fracture should be considered in the care of patients, especially female patients, treated with pioglitazone and attention should be given to assessing and maintaining bone health according to current standards of care.

General: *Metformin hydrochloride*

Monitoring of renal function: Metformin is known to be substantially excreted by the kidney, and the risk of metformin accumulation and lactic acidosis increases with the degree of impairment of renal function. Thus, patients with serum creatinine levels above the upper limit of normal for their age should not receive ACTOPLUS MET. In patients with advanced age, ACTOPLUS MET should be carefully titrated to establish the minimum dose for adequate glycemic effect, because aging is associated with reduced renal function. In elderly patients, particularly those $\geq$ 80 years of age, renal function should be monitored regularly and, generally, ACTOPLUS MET should not be titrated to the maximum dose of the metformin component (see WARNINGS, *Metformin hydrochloride* and DOSAGE AND ADMINISTRATION).

Before initiation of therapy with ACTOPLUS MET and at least annually thereafter, renal function should be assessed and verified as normal. In patients in whom development of renal dysfunction is anticipated, renal function should be assessed more frequently and ACTOPLUS MET discontinued if evidence of renal impairment is present.

Use of concomitant medications that may affect renal function or metformin disposition: Concomitant medication(s) that may affect renal function or result in significant hemodynamic change or may interfere with the disposition of metformin, such as cationic drugs that are eliminated by renal tubular secretion (see PRECAUTIONS, Drug Interactions, *Metformin hydrochloride*), should be used with caution.

Radiologic studies involving the use of intravascular iodinated contrast materials (for example, intravenous urogram, intravenous cholangiography, angiography, and computed tomography (CT) scans with intravascular contrast materials): Intravascular contrast studies with iodinated materials can lead to acute alteration of renal function and have been associated with lactic acidosis in patients receiving metformin (see CONTRAINDICATIONS). Therefore, in patients in whom any such study is planned, ACTOPLUS MET should be temporarily discontinued at the time of or prior to the procedure, and withheld for 48 hours subsequent to the procedure and reinstituted only after renal function has been re-evaluated and found to be normal.

Hypoxic states: Cardiovascular collapse (shock) from whatever cause, acute congestive heart failure, acute myocardial infarction and other conditions characterized by hypoxemia have been associated with lactic acidosis and may also cause prerenal azotemia. When such events occur in patients receiving ACTOPLUS MET therapy, the drug should be promptly discontinued.

Surgical procedures: Use of ACTOPLUS MET should be temporarily suspended for any surgical procedure (except minor procedures not associated with restricted intake of food and fluids) and should not be restarted until the patient's oral intake has resumed and renal function has been evaluated as normal.

Alcohol intake: Alcohol is known to potentiate the effect of metformin on lactate metabolism. Patients, therefore, should be warned against excessive alcohol intake, acute or chronic, while receiving ACTOPLUS MET.

Impaired hepatic function: Since impaired hepatic function has been associated with some cases of lactic acidosis, ACTOPLUS MET should generally be avoided in patients with clinical or laboratory evidence of hepatic disease.

Vitamin B_{12} levels: In controlled clinical trials of metformin at 29 weeks' duration, a decrease to subnormal levels of previously normal serum vitamin B_{12} levels, without clinical manifestations, was observed in approximately 7% of patients. Such decrease, possibly due to interference with B_{12} absorption from the B_{12}-intrinsic factor complex, is, however, very rarely associated with anemia and appears to be rapidly reversible with discontinuation of metformin or vitamin B_{12} supplementation. Measurement of hematologic parameters on an annual basis is advised in patients on ACTOPLUS MET and any apparent abnormalities should be appropriately investigated and managed (see PRECAUTIONS, General: *Metformin hydrochloride* and Laboratory Tests). Certain individuals (those with inadequate vitamin B_{12} or calcium intake or absorption) appear to be predisposed to developing subnormal vitamin B_{12} levels. In these patients, routine serum vitamin B_{12} measurements at two- to three-year intervals may be useful.

Change in clinical status of patients with previously controlled type 2 diabetes: A patient with type 2 diabetes previously well-controlled on ACTOPLUS MET who develops laboratory abnormalities or clinical illness (especially vague and poorly defined illness) should be evaluated promptly for evidence of ketoacidosis or lactic acidosis. Evaluation should include serum electrolytes and ketones, blood glucose and, if indicated, blood pH, lactate, pyruvate and metformin levels. If acidosis of either form occurs, ACTOPLUS MET must be stopped immediately and other appropriate corrective measures initiated (see WARNINGS, *Metformin hydrochloride*).

Hypoglycemia: Hypoglycemia does not occur in patients receiving metformin alone under usual circumstances of use, but could occur when caloric intake is deficient, when strenuous exercise is not compensated by caloric supplementation, or during concomitant use with hypoglycemic agents (such as sulfonylureas or insulin) or ethanol. Elderly, debilitated or malnourished patients and those with adrenal or pituitary insufficiency or alcohol intoxication are particularly susceptible to hypoglycemic effects. Hypoglycemia may be difficult to recognize in the elderly and in people who are taking beta-adrenergic blocking drugs.

Loss of control of blood glucose: When a patient stabilized on any diabetic regimen is exposed to stress such as fever, trauma, infection, or surgery, a temporary loss of glycemic control may occur. At such times, it may be necessary to withhold ACTOPLUS MET and temporarily administer insulin. ACTOPLUS MET may be reinstituted after the acute episode is resolved.

Laboratory Tests

FPG and A1C measurements should be performed periodically to monitor glycemic control and therapeutic response to ACTOPLUS MET.

Liver enzyme monitoring is recommended prior to initiation of therapy with ACTOPLUS MET in all patients and periodically thereafter per the clinical judgment of the health care professional (see PRECAUTIONS, General: *Pioglitazone hydrochloride* and ADVERSE REACTIONS, Serum Transaminase Levels).

Initial and periodic monitoring of hematologic parameters (e.g., hemoglobin/hematocrit and red blood cell indices) and renal function (serum creatinine) should be performed, at least on an annual basis. While megaloblastic anemia has rarely been seen with metformin therapy, if this is suspected, Vitamin B_{12} deficiency should be excluded.

Information for Patients

Patients should be instructed regarding the importance of adhering to dietary instructions, a regular exercise program, and regular testing of blood glucose and A1C. During periods of stress such as fever, trauma, infection, or surgery, medication requirements may change and patients should be reminded to seek medical advice promptly.

Table 3. Weight Changes (kg) from Baseline during Double-Blind Clinical Trials with Pioglitazone

		Control Group	pioglitazone 15 mg	pioglitazone 30 mg	pioglitazone 45 mg
		Median (25th/75th percentile)	Median (25th/75th percentile)	Median (25th/75th percentile)	Median (25th/75th percentile)
Monotherapy		-1.4 (-2.7/0.0) n=256	0.9 (-0.5/3.4) n=79	1.0 (-0.9/3.4) n=188	2.6 (0.2/5.4) n=79
Combination Therapy	Sulfonylurea	-0.5 (-1.8/0.7) n=187	2.0 (0.2/3.2) n=183	3.1 (1.1/5.4) n=528	4.1 (1.8/7.3) n=333
	Metformin	-1.4 (-3.2/0.3) n=160	N/A	0.9 (-0.3/3.2) n=567	1.8 (-0.9/5.0) n=407
	Insulin	0.2 (-1.4/1.4) n=182	2.3 (0.5/4.3) n=190	3.3 (0.9/6.3) n=522	4.1 (1.4/6.8) n=338

Note: Trial durations of 16 to 26 weeks

The risks of lactic acidosis, its symptoms and conditions that predispose to its development, as noted in the WARNINGS, *Metformin hydrochloride* and PRECAUTIONS, General: *Metformin hydrochloride* sections, should be explained to patients. Patients should be advised to discontinue ACTOPLUS MET immediately and to promptly notify their health care professional if unexplained hyperventilation, myalgia, malaise, unusual somnolence or other nonspecific symptoms occur. Gastrointestinal symptoms are common during initiation of metformin treatment and may occur during initiation of ACTOPLUS MET therapy; however, patients should consult with their physician if they develop unexplained symptoms. Although gastrointestinal symptoms that occur after stabilization are unlikely to be drug related, such an occurrence of symptoms should be evaluated to determine if it may be due to lactic acidosis or other serious disease.

Patients should be counseled against excessive alcohol intake, either acute or chronic, while receiving ACTOPLUS MET.

Patients who experience an unusually rapid increase in weight or edema or who develop shortness of breath or other symptoms of heart failure while on ACTOPLUS MET should immediately report these symptoms to their physician.

Patients should be told that blood tests for liver function will be performed prior to the start of therapy and periodically thereafter per the clinical judgment of the health care professional. Patients should be told to seek immediate medical advice for unexplained nausea, vomiting, abdominal pain, fatigue, anorexia, or dark urine.

Patients should be informed about the importance of regular testing of renal function and hematologic parameters when receiving treatment with ACTOPLUS MET.

Therapy with a thiazolidinedione, which is the active pioglitazone component of the ACTOPLUS MET tablet, may result in ovulation in some premenopausal anovulatory women. As a result, these patients may be at an increased risk for pregnancy while taking ACTOPLUS MET. Thus, adequate contraception in premenopausal women should be recommended. This possible effect has not been investigated in clinical studies so the frequency of this occurrence is not known.

Combination antihyperglycemic therapy may cause hypoglycemia. When initiating ACTOPLUS MET, the risks of hypoglycemia, its symptoms and treatment, and conditions that predispose to its development should be explained to patients.

Patients should be told to take ACTOPLUS MET as prescribed and instructed that any change in dosing should only be done if directed by their physician.

Drug Interactions
Pioglitazone hydrochloride
In vivo drug-drug interaction studies have suggested that pioglitazone may be a weak inducer of CYP450 isoform 3A4 substrate.

An enzyme inhibitor of CYP2C8 (such as gemfibrozil) may significantly increase the AUC of pioglitazone and an enzyme inducer of CYP2C8 (such as rifampin) may significantly decrease the AUC of pioglitazone. Therefore, if an inhibitor or inducer of CYP2C8 is started or stopped during treatment with pioglitazone, changes in diabetes treatment may be needed based on clinical response (see **CLINICAL PHARMACOLOGY, Drug-Drug Interactions,** *Pioglitazone hydrochloride*).

Metformin hydrochloride
Furosemide: A single-dose, metformin-furosemide drug interaction study in healthy subjects demonstrated that pharmacokinetic parameters of both compounds were affected by co-administration. Furosemide increased the metformin plasma and blood C_{max} by 22% and blood AUC by 15%, without any significant change in metformin renal clearance. When administered with metformin, the C_{max} and AUC of furosemide were 31% and 12% smaller, respectively, than when administered alone and the terminal half-life was decreased by 32%, without any significant change in furosemide renal clearance. No information is available about the interaction of metformin and furosemide when co-administered chronically.

Nifedipine: A single-dose, metformin-nifedipine drug interaction study in normal healthy volunteers demonstrated that co-administration of nifedipine increased plasma metformin C_{max} and AUC by 20% and 9%, respectively and increased the amount excreted in the urine. T_{max} and half-life were unaffected. Nifedipine appears to enhance the absorption of metformin. Metformin had minimal effects on nifedipine.

Cationic Drugs: Cationic drugs (e.g., amiloride, digoxin, morphine, procainamide, quinidine, quinine, ranitidine, triamterene, trimethoprim, and vancomycin) that are eliminated by renal tubular secretion theoretically have the potential for interaction with metformin by competing for common renal tubular transport systems. Such interaction between metformin and oral cimetidine has been observed in normal healthy volunteers in both single- and multiple-dose, metformin-cimetidine drug interaction studies with a 60% increase in peak metformin plasma and whole blood concentrations and a 40% increase in plasma and whole blood metformin AUC. There was no change in elimination half-life in the single-dose study. Metformin had no effect on cimetidine pharmacokinetics. Although such interactions remain theoretical (except for cimetidine), careful patient monitoring and dose adjustment of ACTOPLUS MET and/or the interfering drug is recommended in patients who are taking cationic medications that are excreted via the proximal renal tubular secretory system.

Other: Certain drugs tend to produce hyperglycemia and may lead to loss of glycemic control. These drugs include thiazides and other diuretics, corticosteroids, phenothiazines, thyroid products, estrogens, oral contraceptives, phenytoin, nicotinic acid, sympathomimetics, calcium channel blocking drugs, and isoniazid. When such drugs are administered to a patient receiving ACTOPLUS MET, the patient should be closely observed to maintain adequate glycemic control.

In healthy volunteers, the pharmacokinetics of metformin and propranolol and metformin and ibuprofen were not affected when co-administered in single-dose interaction studies.

Metformin is negligibly bound to plasma proteins and is therefore, less likely to interact with highly protein-bound drugs such as salicylates, sulfonamides, chloramphenicol and probenecid.

Carcinogenesis, Mutagenesis, Impairment of Fertility
ACTOPLUS MET
No animal studies have been conducted with ACTOPLUS MET. The following data are based on findings in studies performed with pioglitazone or metformin individually.

Pioglitazone hydrochloride
A two-year carcinogenicity study was conducted in male and female rats at oral doses up to 63 mg/kg (approximately 14 times the maximum recommended human oral dose of 45 mg based on mg/m². Drug-induced tumors were not observed in any organ except for the urinary bladder. Benign and/or malignant transitional cell neoplasms were observed in male rats at 4 mg/kg/day and above (approximately equal to the maximum recommended human oral dose based on mg/m². A two-year carcinogenicity study was conducted in male and female mice at oral doses up to 100 mg/kg/day (approximately 11 times the maximum recommended human oral dose based on mg/m². No drug-induced tumors were observed in any organ.

During prospective evaluation of urinary cytology involving more than 1800 patients receiving pioglitazone in clinical trials up to one year in duration, no new cases of bladder tumors were identified. In two 3-year studies in which pioglitazone was compared to placebo or glyburide, there were 16/3656 (0.44%) reports of bladder cancer in patients taking pioglitazone compared to 5/3679 (0.14%) in patients not taking pioglitazone. After excluding patients in whom exposure to study drug was less than one year at the time of diagnosis of bladder cancer, there were six (0.16%) cases on pioglitazone and two (0.05%) on placebo.

Pioglitazone HCl was not mutagenic in a battery of genetic toxicology studies, including the Ames bacterial assay, a mammalian cell forward gene mutation assay (CHO/HPRT and AS52/XPRT), an *in vitro* cytogenetics assay using CHL cells, an unscheduled DNA synthesis assay, and an *in vivo* micronucleus assay.

No adverse effects upon fertility were observed in male and female rats at oral doses up to 40 mg/kg pioglitazone HCl daily prior to and throughout mating and gestation (approximately 9 times the maximum recommended human oral dose based on mg/m².

Metformin hydrochloride
Long-term carcinogenicity studies have been performed in rats (dosing duration of 104 weeks) and mice (dosing duration of 91 weeks) at doses up to and including 900 mg/kg/day and 1500 mg/kg/day, respectively. These doses are both approximately four times a human daily dose of 2000 mg of the metformin component of ACTOPLUS MET based on body surface area comparisons. No evidence of carcinogenicity with metformin was found in either male or female mice. Similarly, there was no tumorigenic potential observed with metformin in male rats. There was, however, an increased incidence of benign stromal uterine polyps in female rats treated with 900 mg/kg/day.

There was no evidence of mutagenic potential of metformin in the following *in vitro* tests: Ames test (*S. typhimurium*), gene mutation test (mouse lymphoma cells), or chromosomal aberrations test (human lymphocytes). Results in the *in vivo* mouse micronucleus test were also negative.

Fertility of male or female rats was unaffected by metformin when administered at doses as high as 600 mg/kg/day, which is approximately three times the maximum recommended human daily dose of the metformin component of ACTOPLUS MET based on body surface area comparisons.

Animal Toxicology
Pioglitazone hydrochloride
Heart enlargement has been observed in mice (100 mg/kg), rats (4 mg/kg and above) and dogs (3 mg/kg) treated orally with the pioglitazone HCl component of ACTOPLUS MET (approximately 11, 1, and 2 times the maximum recommended human oral dose for mice, rats, and dogs, respectively, based on mg/m². In a one-year rat study, drug-related early death due to apparent heart dysfunction occurred at an oral dose of 160 mg/kg/day (approximately 35 times the maximum recommended human oral dose based on mg/m². Heart enlargement was seen in a 13-week study in monkeys at oral doses of 8.9 mg/kg and above (approximately 4 times the maximum recommended human oral dose based on mg/m², but not in a 52-week study at oral doses up to 32 mg/kg (approximately 13 times the maximum recommended human oral dose based on mg/m².

Pregnancy: Pregnancy Category C
ACTOPLUS MET
Because current information strongly suggests that abnormal blood glucose levels during pregnancy are associated with a higher incidence of congenital anomalies, as well as increased neonatal morbidity and mortality, most experts recommend that insulin be used during pregnancy to maintain blood glucose levels as close to normal as possible. ACTOPLUS MET should not be used during pregnancy unless the potential benefit justifies the potential risk to the fetus.

There are no adequate and well-controlled studies in pregnant women with ACTOPLUS MET or its individual components. No animal studies have been conducted with the combined products in ACTOPLUS MET. The following data are based on findings in studies performed with pioglitazone or metformin individually.

Pioglitazone hydrochloride
Pioglitazone was not teratogenic in rats at oral doses up to 80 mg/kg or in rabbits given up to 160 mg/kg during organogenesis (approximately 17 and 40 times the maximum recommended human oral dose based on mg/m², respectively). Delayed parturition and embryotoxicity (as evidenced by increased postimplantation losses, delayed development and reduced fetal weights) were observed in rats at oral doses of 40 mg/kg/day and above (approximately 10 times the maximum recommended human oral dose based on mg/m². No functional or behavioral toxicity was observed in offspring of rats. In rabbits, embryotoxicity was observed at an oral dose of 160 mg/kg (approximately 40 times the maximum recommended human oral dose based on mg/m². Delayed postnatal development, attributed to decreased body weight, was observed in offspring of rats at oral doses of 10 mg/kg and above during late gestation and lactation periods (approximately 2 times the maximum recommended human oral dose based on mg/m².

Metformin hydrochloride
Metformin was not teratogenic in rats and rabbits at doses up to 600 mg/kg/day. This represents an exposure of about two and six times a human daily dose of 2000 mg based on body surface area comparisons for rats and rabbits, respectively. Determination of fetal concentrations demonstrated a partial placental barrier to metformin.

Nursing Mothers
No studies have been conducted with the combined components of ACTOPLUS MET. In studies performed with the individual components, both pioglitazone and metformin are secreted in the milk of lactating rats. It is not known whether pioglitazone and/or metformin is secreted in human milk. Because many drugs are excreted in human milk, ACTOPLUS MET should not be administered to a breastfeeding woman. If ACTOPLUS MET is discontinued, and if diet alone is inadequate for controlling blood glucose, insulin therapy should be considered.

Pediatric Use
Safety and effectiveness of ACTOPLUS MET in pediatric patients have not been established.

Elderly Use
Pioglitazone hydrochloride
Approximately 500 patients in placebo-controlled clinical trials of pioglitazone were 65 and over. No significant differences in effectiveness and safety were observed between these patients and younger patients.

Metformin hydrochloride
Controlled clinical studies of metformin did not include sufficient numbers of elderly patients to determine whether they respond differently from younger patients, although other reported clinical experience has not identified differences in responses between the elderly and young patients. Metformin is known to be substantially excreted by the kidney and because the risk of serious adverse reactions to the drug is greater in patients with impaired renal function, ACTOPLUS MET should only be used in patients with normal renal function (see **CONTRAINDICATIONS, WARNINGS,** *Metformin hydrochloride* and **CLINICAL PHARMACOLOGY, Special Populations**). Because aging is associated with reduced renal function, ACTOPLUS MET should be used with caution as age increases. Care should be taken in dose selection and should be based on careful and regular monitoring of renal function. Generally, elderly patients should not be titrated to the maximum dose of ACTOPLUS MET (see **WARNINGS,** *Metformin hydrochloride* and **DOSAGE AND ADMINISTRATION**).

ADVERSE REACTIONS

Over 8500 patients with type 2 diabetes have been treated with pioglitazone in randomized, double-blind, controlled clinical trials. This includes 2605 high-risk patients with type 2 diabetes treated with pioglitazone from the PROactive clinical trial. Over 6000 patients have been treated for 6 months or longer, and over 4500 patients for one year or longer. Over 3000 patients have received pioglitazone for at least 2 years.

The most common adverse events reported in at least 5% of patients in the controlled 16-week clinical trial between placebo plus metformin and pioglitazone 30 mg plus metformin were upper respiratory tract infection (15.6% and 15.5%), diarrhea (6.3% and 4.8%), combined edema/peripheral edema (2.5% and 6.0%) and headache (1.9% and 6.0%), respectively.

The incidence and type of adverse events reported in at least 5% of patients in any combined treatment group from the 24-week study comparing pioglitazone 30 mg plus metformin and pioglitazone 45 mg plus metformin are shown in Table 4; the rate of adverse events resulting in study discontinuation between the two treatment groups was 7.8% and 7.7%, respectively.

Continued on next page

Actoplus Met—Cont.

[See table 4 at right]

Most clinical adverse events were similar between groups treated with pioglitazone in combination with metformin and those treated with pioglitazone monotherapy. Other adverse events reported in at least 5% of patients in controlled clinical trials between placebo and pioglitazone monotherapy included myalgia (2.7% and 5.4%), tooth disorder (2.3% and 5.3%), diabetes mellitus aggravated (8.1% and 5.1%) and pharyngitis (0.8% and 5.1%), respectively.

In U.S. double-blind studies, anemia was reported in ≤ 2% of patients treated with pioglitazone plus metformin (see **PRECAUTIONS, General:** *Pioglitazone hydrochloride*).

In monotherapy studies, edema was reported for 4.8% (with doses from 7.5 mg to 45 mg) of patients treated with pioglitazone versus 1.2% of placebo-treated patients. Most of these events were considered mild or moderate in intensity (see **PRECAUTIONS, General:** *Pioglitazone hydrochloride*).

Prospective Pioglitazone Clinical Trial In Macrovascular Events (PROactive)

In PROactive, 5238 patients with type 2 diabetes and a prior history of macrovascular disease were treated with ACTOS (n=2605), force-titrated up to 45 mg daily, or placebo (n=2633), in addition to standard of care. Almost all subjects (95%) were receiving cardiovascular medications (beta blockers, ACE inhibitors, ARBs, calcium channel blockers, nitrates, diuretics, aspirin, statins, fibrates). Patients had a mean age of 61.8 years, mean duration of diabetes 9.5 years, and mean A1C 8.1%. Average duration of follow-up was 34.5 months. The primary objective of this trial was to examine the effect of ACTOS on mortality and macrovascular morbidity in patients with type 2 diabetes mellitus who were at high risk for macrovascular events. The primary efficacy variable was the time to the first occurrence of any event in the cardiovascular composite endpoint (see table 5 below). Although there was no statistically significant difference between ACTOS and placebo for the 3-year incidence of a first event within this composite, there was no increase in mortality or in total macrovascular events with ACTOS.

[See table 5 at right]

Postmarketing reports of new onset or worsening diabetic macular edema with decreased visual acuity have also been received (see **PRECAUTIONS, General:** *Pioglitazone hydrochloride*).

Laboratory Abnormalities

Hematologic: Pioglitazone may cause decreases in hemoglobin and hematocrit. The fall in hemoglobin and hematocrit with pioglitazone appears to be dose related. Across all clinical studies, mean hemoglobin values declined by 2% to 4% in patients treated with pioglitazone. These changes generally occurred within the first 4 to 12 weeks of therapy and remained relatively stable thereafter. These changes may be related to increased plasma volume associated with pioglitazone therapy and have rarely been associated with any significant hematologic clinical effects (see **PRECAUTIONS, General:** *Pioglitazone hydrochloride*).

In controlled clinical trials of metformin at 29 weeks' duration, a decrease to subnormal levels of previously normal serum vitamin B$_{12}$ levels, without clinical manifestations, was observed in approximately 7% of patients. Such decrease, possibly due to interference with B$_{12}$ absorption from the B$_{12}$-intrinsic factor complex, is, however, very rarely associated with anemia and appears to be rapidly reversible with discontinuation of metformin or vitamin B$_{12}$ supplementation (see **PRECAUTIONS, General:** *Metformin hydrochloride*).

Serum Transaminase Levels: During all clinical studies in the U.S., 14 of 4780 (0.30%) patients treated with pioglitazone had ALT values ≥ 3 times the upper limit of normal during treatment. All patients with follow-up values had reversible elevations in ALT. In the population of patients treated with pioglitazone, mean values for bilirubin, AST, ALT, alkaline phosphatase, and GGT were decreased at the final visit compared with baseline. Fewer than 0.9% of patients treated with pioglitazone were withdrawn from clinical trials in the U.S. due to abnormal liver function tests.

In pre-approval clinical trials, there were no cases of idiosyncratic drug reactions leading to hepatic failure (see **PRECAUTIONS, General:** *Pioglitazone hydrochloride*).

CPK Levels: During required laboratory testing in clinical trials with pioglitazone, sporadic, transient elevations in creatine phosphokinase levels (CPK) were observed. An isolated elevation to greater than 10 times the upper limit of normal was noted in 9 patients (values of 2150 to 11400 IU/L). Six of these patients continued to receive pioglitazone, two patients had completed receiving study medication at the time of the elevated value and one patient discontinued study medication due to the elevation. These elevations resolved without any apparent clinical sequelae. The relationship of these events to pioglitazone therapy is unknown.

OVERDOSAGE

Pioglitazone hydrochloride

During controlled clinical trials, one case of overdose with pioglitazone was reported. A male patient took 120 mg per day for four days, then 180 mg per day for seven days. The patient denied any clinical symptoms during this period.

In the event of overdosage, appropriate supportive treatment should be initiated according to patient's clinical signs and symptoms.

Metformin hydrochloride

Overdose of metformin hydrochloride has occurred, including ingestion of amounts greater than 50 grams. Hypoglycemia was reported in approximately 10% of cases, but no causal association with metformin hydrochloride has been established. Lactic acidosis has been reported in approximately 32% of metformin overdose cases (see **WARNINGS,** *Metformin hydrochloride*). Metformin is dialyzable with a clearance of up to 170 mL/min under good hemodynamic conditions. Therefore, hemodialysis may be useful for removal of accumulated metformin from patients in whom metformin overdosage is suspected.

DOSAGE AND ADMINISTRATION

General

The use of antihyperglycemic therapy in the management of type 2 diabetes should be individualized on the basis of effectiveness and tolerability while not exceeding the maximum recommended daily dose of pioglitazone 45 mg and metformin 2550 mg.

Dosage Recommendations

Selecting the starting dose of ACTOPLUS MET should be based on the patient's current regimen of pioglitazone and/or metformin. After initiation of ACTOPLUS MET or with dose increase, patients should be carefully monitored for adverse events related to fluid retention (see **BOXED WARNING** and **WARNINGS,** *Pioglitazone hydrochloride*). ACTOPLUS MET should be given in divided daily doses with meals to reduce the gastrointestinal side effects associated with metformin.

Starting dose for patients inadequately controlled on metformin monotherapy

Based on the usual starting dose of pioglitazone (15-30 mg daily), ACTOPLUS MET may be initiated at either the 15 mg/500 mg or 15 mg/850 mg tablet strength once or twice daily, and gradually titrated after assessing adequacy of therapeutic response.

Starting dose for patients who initially responded to pioglitazone monotherapy and require additional glycemic control

Based on the usual starting doses of metformin (500 mg twice daily or 850 mg daily), ACTOPLUS MET may be initiated at either the 15 mg/500 mg twice daily or 15 mg/850 mg tablet strength once daily, and gradually titrated after assessing adequacy of therapeutic response.

Starting dose for patients switching from combination therapy of pioglitazone plus metformin as separate tablets

ACTOPLUS MET may be initiated with either the 15 mg/500 mg or 15 mg/850 mg tablet strengths based on the dose of pioglitazone and metformin already being taken.

No studies have been performed specifically examining the safety and efficacy of ACTOPLUS MET in patients previously treated with other oral hypoglycemic agents and switched to ACTOPLUS MET. Any change in therapy of type 2 diabetes should be undertaken with care and appropriate monitoring as changes in glycemic control can occur. Sufficient time should be given to assess adequacy of therapeutic response. Ideally, the response to therapy should be evaluated using A1C, which is a better indicator of long-term glycemic control than FPG alone. A1C reflects glycemia over the past two to three months. In clinical use, it is recommended that patients be treated with ACTOPLUS MET for a period of time adequate to evaluate change in A1C (8-12 weeks) unless glycemic control as measured by FPG deteriorates.

Special Patient Populations

ACTOPLUS MET is not recommended for use in pregnancy or for use in pediatric patients.

The initial and maintenance dosing of ACTOPLUS MET should be conservative in patients with advanced age, due to the potential for decreased renal function in this population. Any dosage adjustment should be based on a careful assessment of renal function. Generally, elderly, debilitated, and malnourished patients should not be titrated to the maximum dose of ACTOPLUS MET. Monitoring of renal function is necessary to aid in prevention of metformin-associated lactic acidosis, particularly in the elderly (see **WARNINGS,** *Metformin hydrochloride* and **PRECAUTIONS, General:** *Metformin hydrochloride*).

Therapy with ACTOPLUS MET should not be initiated if the patient exhibits clinical evidence of active liver disease or increased serum transaminase levels (ALT greater than 2.5 times the upper limit of normal) at start of therapy (see **PRECAUTIONS, General:** *Pioglitazone hydrochloride* and **CLINICAL PHARMACOLOGY, Special Populations, Hepatic Insufficiency**). Liver enzyme monitoring is recommended in all patients prior to initiation of therapy with ACTOPLUS MET and periodically thereafter (see **PRECAUTIONS, General:** *Pioglitazone hydrochloride* and **PRECAUTIONS, Laboratory Tests**).

Maximum Recommended Dose

ACTOPLUS MET tablets are available as a 15 mg pioglitazone plus 500 mg metformin or a 15 mg pioglitazone plus 850 mg metformin formulation for oral administration. The maximum recommended dose for pioglitazone is 45 mg daily. The maximum recommended daily dose for metformin is 2550 mg in adults.

HOW SUPPLIED

ACTOPLUS MET is available in 15 mg pioglitazone hydrochloride (as the base)/500 mg metformin hydrochloride and 15 mg pioglitazone hydrochloride (as the base)/850 mg metformin hydrochloride tablets as follows:

15 mg/500 mg tablet: white to off-white, oblong, film-coated tablet with "4833M" on one side, and "15/500" on the other, available in:

Table 4. Adverse Events That Occurred in ≥ 5% of Patients in Any Treatment Group During the 24-Week Study

Adverse Event Preferred Term	Pioglitazone 30 mg + metformin N=411 n (%)	Pioglitazone 45 mg + metformin N=416 n (%)
Upper Respiratory Tract Infection	51 (12.4)	56 (13.5)
Diarrhea	24 (5.8)	20 (4.8)
Nausea	24 (5.8)	15 (3.6)
Headache	19 (4.6)	22 (5.3)
Urinary Tract Infection	24 (5.8)	22 (5.3)
Sinusitis	18 (4.4)	21 (5.0)
Dizziness	22 (5.4)	20 (4.8)
Edema Lower Limb	12 (2.9)	47 (11.3)
Weight Increased	12 (2.9)	28 (6.7)

Table 5.

Number of First and Total Events for Each Component within the Cardiovascular Composite Endpoint

Cardiovascular Events	Placebo N=2633		ACTOS N=2605	
	First Events (N)	Total events (N)	First Events (N)	Total events (N)
Any event	572	900	514	803
All-cause mortality	122	186	110	177
Non-fatal MI	118	157	105	131
Stroke	96	119	76	92
ACS	63	78	42	65
Cardiac intervention	101	240	101	195
Major leg amputation	15	28	9	28
Leg revascularization	57	92	71	115

Bottles of 60	NDC 64764-155-60
Bottles of 180	NDC 64764-155-18

15 mg/850 mg tablet: white to off-white, oblong, film-coated tablet with "4833M" on one side, and "15/850" on the other, available in:

Bottles of 60	NDC 64764-158-60
Bottles of 180	NDC 64764-158-18

STORAGE

Store at 25°C (77°F); excursions permitted to 15-30°C (59-86°F) [see USP Controlled Room Temperature]. Keep container tightly closed, and protect from moisture and humidity.

REFERENCES

1. Deng, LJ, et al. Effect of gemfibrozil on the pharmacokinetics of pioglitazone. *Eur J Clin Pharmacol* 2005; 61: 831-836, Table 1.
2. Jaakkola, T, et al. Effect of rifampicin on the pharmacokinetics of pioglitazone. *Brit J Clin Pharmacol* 2006; 61:1 70-78.

Rx only

ACTOS® and ACTOPLUS MET® are trademarks of Takeda Pharmaceutical Company Limited and used under license by Takeda Pharmaceuticals America, Inc.

GLUCOPHAGE® is a registered trademark of Merck Sante S.A.S., an associate of Merck KGaA of Darmstadt, Germany. Licensed to Bristol-Myers Squibb Company.

Distributed by:
Takeda Pharmaceuticals America, Inc.
Deerfield, IL 60015
©2005 Takeda Pharmaceuticals America, Inc.
05-1139 Revised: September, 2007
L-PIOM-0907-7

ACTOS® ℞

[ăk'tōs]

(pioglitazone hydrochloride) Tablets

Prescribing information for this product, which appears on pages 3156–3161 of the 2008 PDR, has been completely revised as follows. Please write "See Supplement A" next to the product heading.

> **WARNING: CONGESTIVE HEART FAILURE**
>
> - Thiazolidinediones, including ACTOS, cause or exacerbate congestive heart failure in some patients (see **WARNINGS**). After initiation of ACTOS, and after dose increases, observe patients carefully for signs and symptoms of heart failure (including excessive, rapid weight gain, dyspnea, and/or edema). If these signs and symptoms develop, the heart failure should be managed according to the current standards of care. Furthermore, discontinuation or dose reduction of ACTOS must be considered.
> - ACTOS is not recommended in patients with symptomatic heart failure. Initiation of ACTOS in patients with established NYHA Class III or IV heart failure is contraindicated (see **CONTRAINDICATIONS** and **WARNINGS**).

DESCRIPTION

ACTOS (pioglitazone hydrochloride) is an oral antidiabetic agent that acts primarily by decreasing insulin resistance. ACTOS is used in the management of type 2 diabetes mellitus (also known as non-insulin-dependent diabetes mellitus [NIDDM] or adult-onset diabetes). Pharmacological studies indicate that ACTOS improves sensitivity to insulin in muscle and adipose tissue and inhibits hepatic gluconeogenesis. ACTOS improves glycemic control while reducing circulating insulin levels.

Pioglitazone [(±)-5-[[4-[2-(5-ethyl-2-pyridinyl)ethoxy] phenyl]methyl]-2,4-] thiazolidinedione monohydrochloride belongs to a different chemical class and has a different pharmacological action than the sulfonylureas, metformin, or the α-glucosidase inhibitors. The molecule contains one asymmetric carbon, and the compound is synthesized and used as the racemic mixture. The two enantiomers of pioglitazone interconvert *in vivo*. No differences were found in the pharmacologic activity between the two enantiomers. The structural formula is as shown:

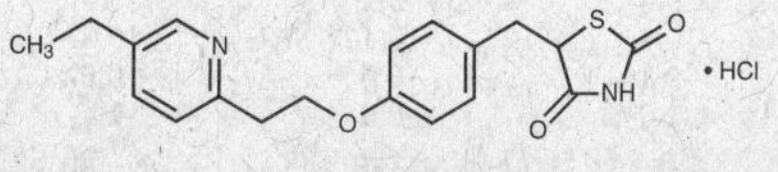

Pioglitazone hydrochloride is an odorless white crystalline powder that has a molecular formula of $C_{19}H_{20}N_2O_3S \cdot HCl$ and a molecular weight of 392.90 daltons. It is soluble in *N,N*-dimethylformamide, slightly soluble in anhydrous ethanol, very slightly soluble in acetone and acetonitrile, practically insoluble in water, and insoluble in ether.

ACTOS is available as a tablet for oral administration containing 15 mg, 30 mg, or 45 mg of pioglitazone (as the base) formulated with the following excipients: lactose monohydrate NF, hydroxypropylcellulose NF, carboxymethylcellulose calcium NF, and magnesium stearate NF.

CLINICAL PHARMACOLOGY

Mechanism of Action

ACTOS is a thiazolidinedione antidiabetic agent that depends on the presence of insulin for its mechanism of action. ACTOS decreases insulin resistance in the periphery and in the liver resulting in increased insulin-dependent glucose disposal and decreased hepatic glucose output. Unlike sulfonylureas, pioglitazone is not an insulin secretagogue. Pioglitazone is a potent agonist for peroxisome proliferator-activated receptor-gamma (PPARγ). PPAR receptors are found in tissues important for insulin action such as adipose tissue, skeletal muscle, and liver. Activation of PPARγ nuclear receptors modulates the transcription of a number of insulin responsive genes involved in the control of glucose and lipid metabolism.

In animal models of diabetes, pioglitazone reduces the hyperglycemia, hyperinsulinemia, and hypertriglyceridemia characteristic of insulin-resistant states such as type 2 diabetes.The metabolic changes produced by pioglitazone result in increased responsiveness of insulin-dependent tissues and are observed in numerous animal models of insulin resistance.

Since pioglitazone enhances the effects of circulating insulin (by decreasing insulin resistance), it does not lower blood glucose in animal models that lack endogenous insulin.

Pharmacokinetics and Drug Metabolism

Serum concentrations of total pioglitazone (pioglitazone plus active metabolites) remain elevated 24 hours after once daily dosing. Steady-state serum concentrations of both pioglitazone and total pioglitazone are achieved within 7 days. At steady-state, two of the pharmacologically active metabolites of pioglitazone, Metabolites III (M-III) and IV (M-IV), reach serum concentrations equal to or greater than pioglitazone. In both healthy volunteers and in patients with type 2 diabetes, pioglitazone comprises approximately 30% to 50% of the peak total pioglitazone serum concentrations and 20% to 25% of the total area under the serum concentration-time curve (AUC).

Maximum serum concentration (C_{max}), AUC, and trough serum concentrations (C_{min}) for both pioglitazone and total pioglitazone increase proportionally at doses of 15 mg and 30 mg per day. There is a slightly less than proportional increase for pioglitazone and total pioglitazone at a dose of 60 mg per day.

Absorption: Following oral administration, in the fasting state, pioglitazone is first measurable in serum within 30 minutes, with peak concentrations observed within 2 hours. Food slightly delays the time to peak serum concentration to 3 to 4 hours, but does not alter the extent of absorption.

Distribution: The mean apparent volume of distribution (Vd/F) of pioglitazone following single-dose administration is 0.63 ± 0.41 (mean ± SD) L/kg of body weight. Pioglitazone is extensively protein bound (> 99%) in human serum, principally to serum albumin. Pioglitazone also binds to other serum proteins, but with lower affinity. Metabolites M-III and M-IV also are extensively bound (> 98%) to serum albumin.

Metabolism: Pioglitazone is extensively metabolized by hydroxylation and oxidation; the metabolites also partly convert to glucuronide or sulfate conjugates. Metabolites M-II and M-IV (hydroxy derivatives of pioglitazone) and M-III (keto derivative of pioglitazone) are pharmacologically active in animal models of type 2 diabetes. In addition to pioglitazone, M-III and M-IV are the principal drug-related species found in human serum following multiple dosing. At steady-state, in both healthy volunteers and in patients with type 2 diabetes, pioglitazone comprises approximately 30% to 50% of the total peak serum concentrations and 20% to 25% of the total AUC.

In vitro data demonstrate that multiple CYP isoforms are involved in the metabolism of pioglitazone. The cytochrome P450 isoforms involved are CYP2C8 and, to a lesser degree, CYP3A4 with additional contributions from a variety of other isoforms including the mainly extrahepatic CYP1A1. *In vivo* studies of pioglitazone in combination with P450 inhibitors and substrates have been performed (see **Drug Interactions**). Urinary 6β-hydroxycortisol/cortisol ratios measured in patients treated with ACTOS showed that pioglitazone is not a strong CYP3A4 enzyme inducer.

Excretion and Elimination: Following oral administration, approximately 15% to 30% of the pioglitazone dose is recovered in the urine. Renal elimination of pioglitazone is negligible, and the drug is excreted primarily as metabolites and their conjugates. It is presumed that most of the oral dose is excreted into the bile either unchanged or as metabolites and eliminated in the feces.

The mean serum half-life of pioglitazone and total pioglitazone ranges from 3 to 7 hours and 16 to 24 hours, respectively. Pioglitazone has an apparent clearance, CL/F, calculated to be 5 to 7 L/hr.

Special Populations

Renal Insufficiency: The serum elimination half-life of pioglitazone, M-III, and M-IV remains unchanged in patients with moderate (creatinine clearance 30 to 60 mL/min) to severe (creatinine clearance < 30 mL/min) renal impairment when compared to normal subjects. No dose adjustment in patients with renal dysfunction is recommended (see **DOSAGE AND ADMINISTRATION**).

Hepatic Insufficiency: Compared with normal controls, subjects with impaired hepatic function (Child-Pugh Grade B/C) have an approximate 45% reduction in pioglitazone and total pioglitazone mean peak concentrations but no change in the mean AUC values.

ACTOS therapy should not be initiated if the patient exhibits clinical evidence of active liver disease or serum transaminase levels (ALT) exceed 2.5 times the upper limit of normal (see **PRECAUTIONS**, Hepatic Effects).

Elderly: In healthy elderly subjects, peak serum concentrations of pioglitazone and total pioglitazone are not significantly different, but AUC values are slightly higher and the terminal half-life values slightly longer than for younger subjects. These changes were not of a magnitude that would be considered clinically relevant.

Pediatrics: Pharmacokinetic data in the pediatric population are not available.

Gender: The mean C_{max} and AUC values were increased 20% to 60% in females. As monotherapy and in combination with sulfonylurea, metformin, or insulin, ACTOS improved glycemic control in both males and females. In controlled clinical trials, hemoglobin A_{1c} (HbA_{1c}) decreases from baseline were generally greater for females than for males (average mean difference in HbA_{1c} 0.5%). Since therapy should be individualized for each patient to achieve glycemic control, no dose adjustment is recommended based on gender alone.

Ethnicity: Pharmacokinetic data among various ethnic groups are not available.

Drug-Drug Interactions

The following drugs were studied in healthy volunteers with a co-administration of ACTOS 45 mg once daily. Listed below are the results:

Oral Contraceptives: Co-administration of ACTOS (45 mg once daily) and an oral contraceptive (1 mg norethindrone plus 0.035 mg ethinyl estradiol once daily) for 21 days, resulted in 11% and 11-14% decrease in ethinyl estradiol AUC (0-24h) and C_{max} respectively. There were no significant changes in norethindrone AUC (0-24h) and C_{max}. In view of the high variability of ethinyl estradiol pharmacokinetics, the clinical significance of this finding is unknown.

Fexofenadine HCl: Co-administration of ACTOS for 7 days with 60 mg fexofenadine administered orally twice daily resulted in no significant effect on pioglitazone pharmacokinetics. ACTOS had no significant effect on fexofenadine pharmacokinetics.

Glipizide: Co-administration of ACTOS and 5 mg glipizide administered orally once daily for 7 days did not alter the steady-state pharmacokinetics of glipizide.

Digoxin: Co-administration of ACTOS with 0.25 mg digoxin administered orally once daily for 7 days did not alter the steady-state pharmacokinetics of digoxin.

Warfarin: Co-administration of ACTOS for 7 days with warfarin did not alter the steady-state pharmacokinetics of warfarin. ACTOS has no clinically significant effect on prothrombin time when administered to patients receiving chronic warfarin therapy.

Metformin: Co-administration of a single dose of metformin (1000 mg) and ACTOS after 7 days of ACTOS did not alter the pharmacokinetics of the single dose of metformin.

Midazolam: Administration of ACTOS for 15 days followed by a single 7.5 mg dose of midazolam syrup resulted in a 26% reduction in midazolam C_{max} and AUC.

Ranitidine HCl: Co-administration of ACTOS for 7 days with ranitidine administered orally twice daily for either 4 or 7 days resulted in no significant effect on pioglitazone pharmacokinetics. ACTOS showed no significant effect on ranitidine pharmacokinetics.

Nifedipine ER: Co-administration of ACTOS for 7 days with 30 mg nifedipine ER administered orally once daily for 4 days to male and female volunteers resulted in least square mean (90% CI) values for unchanged nifedipine of 0.83 (0.73 - 0.95) for C_{max} and 0.88 (0.80 - 0.96) for AUC. In view of the high variability of nifedipine pharmacokinetics, the clinical significance of this finding is unknown.

Ketoconazole: Co-administration of ACTOS for 7 days with ketoconazole 200 mg administered twice daily resulted in least square mean (90% CI) values for unchanged pioglitazone of 1.14 (1.06 - 1.23) for C_{max}, 1.34 (1.26 - 1.41) for AUC and 1.87 (1.71 - 2.04) for C_{min}.

Atorvastatin Calcium: Co-administration of ACTOS for 7 days with atorvastatin calcium (LIPITOR®) 80 mg once daily resulted in least square mean (90% CI) values for unchanged pioglitazone of 0.69 (0.57 - 0.85) for C_{max}, 0.76 (0.65 - 0.88) for AUC and 0.96 (0.87 - 1.05) for C_{min}. For unchanged atorvastatin the least square mean (90% CI) values were 0.77 (0.66 - 0.90) for C_{max}, 0.86 (0.78 - 0.94) for AUC and 0.92 (0.82 - 1.02) for C_{min}.

Theophylline: Co-administration of ACTOS for 7 days with theophylline 400 mg administered twice daily resulted in no change in the pharmacokinetics of either drug.

Cytochrome P450: See **PRECAUTIONS**

Gemfibrozil: Concomitant administration of gemfibrozil (oral 600 mg twice daily), an inhibitor of CYP2C8, with pioglitazone (oral 30 mg) in 10 healthy volunteers pre-treated for 2 days prior with gemfibrozil (oral 600 mg twice daily) resulted in pioglitazone exposure (AUC_{0-24}) being 226% of the pioglitazone exposure in the absence of gemfibrozil (see **PRECAUTIONS**).[1]

Rifampin: Concomitant administration of rifampin (oral 600 mg once daily), an inducer of CYP2C8 with pioglitazone (oral 30 mg) in 10 healthy volunteers pre-treated for 5 days prior with rifampin (oral 600 mg once daily) resulted in a decrease in the AUC of pioglitazone by 54% (see **PRECAUTIONS**).[2]

Pharmacodynamics and Clinical Effects

Clinical studies demonstrate that ACTOS improves insulin sensitivity in insulin-resistant patients. ACTOS enhances cellular responsiveness to insulin, increases insulin-dependent glucose disposal, improves hepatic sensitivity to insulin, and improves dysfunctional glucose homeostasis. In patients with type 2 diabetes, the decreased insulin resistance produced by ACTOS results in lower plasma glucose concentrations, lower plasma insulin levels, and lower

Continued on next page

Actos—Cont.

HbA$_{1c}$ values. Based on results from an open-label extension study, the glucose lowering effects of ACTOS appear to persist for at least one year. In controlled clinical trials, ACTOS in combination with sulfonylurea, metformin, or insulin had an additive effect on glycemic control.

Patients with lipid abnormalities were included in clinical trials with ACTOS. Overall, patients treated with ACTOS had mean decreases in triglycerides, mean increases in HDL cholesterol, and no consistent mean changes in LDL and total cholesterol.

In a 26-week, placebo-controlled, dose-ranging study, mean triglyceride levels decreased in the 15 mg, 30 mg, and 45 mg ACTOS dose groups compared to a mean increase in the placebo group. Mean HDL levels increased to a greater extent in patients treated with ACTOS than in the placebo-treated patients. There were no consistent differences for LDL and total cholesterol in patients treated with ACTOS compared to placebo (**Table 1**).

[See table 1 above]

In the two other monotherapy studies (24 weeks and 16 weeks) and in combination therapy studies with sulfonylurea (24 weeks and 16 weeks) and metformin (24 weeks and 16 weeks), the results were generally consistent with the data above. In placebo-controlled trials, the placebo-corrected mean changes from baseline decreased 5% to 26% for triglycerides and increased 6% to 13% for HDL in patients treated with ACTOS. A similar pattern of results was seen in 24-week combination therapy studies of ACTOS with sulfonylurea or metformin.

In a combination therapy study with insulin (16 weeks), the placebo-corrected mean percent change from baseline in triglyceride values for patients treated with ACTOS was also decreased. A placebo-corrected mean change from baseline in LDL cholesterol of 7% was observed for the 15 mg dose group. Similar results to those noted above for HDL and total cholesterol were observed. A similar pattern of results was seen in a 24-week combination therapy study with ACTOS with insulin.

Clinical Studies

Monotherapy

In the U.S., three randomized, double-blind, placebo-controlled trials with durations from 16 to 26 weeks were conducted to evaluate the use of ACTOS as monotherapy in patients with type 2 diabetes. These studies examined ACTOS at doses up to 45 mg or placebo once daily in 865 patients.

In a 26-week, dose-ranging study, 408 patients with type 2 diabetes were randomized to receive 7.5 mg, 15 mg, 30 mg, or 45 mg of ACTOS, or placebo once daily. Therapy with any previous antidiabetic agent was discontinued 8 weeks prior to the double-blind period. Treatment with 15 mg, 30 mg, and 45 mg of ACTOS produced statistically significant improvements in HbA$_{1c}$ and fasting plasma glucose (FPG) at endpoint compared to placebo (**Figure 1, Table 2**).

Figure 1 shows the time course for changes in FPG and HbA$_{1c}$ for the entire study population in this 26-week study.

[See figure 1 above]

Table 2 shows HbA$_{1c}$ and FPG values for the entire study population.

[See table 2 above]

The study population included patients not previously treated with antidiabetic medication (naïve; 31%) and patients who were receiving antidiabetic medication at the time of study enrollment (previously treated; 69%). The data for the naïve and previously-treated patient subsets are shown in Table 3. All patients entered an 8 week washout/run-in period prior to double-blind treatment. This run-in period was associated with little change in HbA$_{1c}$ and FPG values from screening to baseline for the naïve patients; however, for the previously-treated group, washout from previous antidiabetic medication resulted in deterioration of glycemic control and increases in HbA$_{1c}$ and FPG. Although most patients in the previously-treated group had a decrease from baseline in HbA$_{1c}$ and FPG with ACTOS, in many cases the values did not return to screening levels by the end of the study. The study design did not permit the evaluation of patients who switched directly to ACTOS from another antidiabetic agent.

[See table 3 above]

In a 24-week, placebo-controlled study, 260 patients with type 2 diabetes were randomized to one of two forced-titration ACTOS treatment groups or a mock titration placebo group. Therapy with any previous antidiabetic agent was discontinued 6 weeks prior to the double-blind period. In one ACTOS treatment group, patients received an initial dose of 7.5 mg once daily. After four weeks, the dose was increased to 15 mg once daily and after another four weeks, the dose was increased to 30 mg once daily for the remainder of the study (16 weeks). In the second ACTOS treatment group, patients received an initial dose of 15 mg once daily and were titrated to 30 mg once daily and 45 mg once daily in a similar manner. Treatment with ACTOS, as described, produced statistically significant improvements in HbA$_{1c}$ and FPG at endpoint compared to placebo (**Table 4**).

[See table 4 at top of next page]

For patients who had not been previously treated with antidiabetic medication (24%), mean values at screening were 10.1% for HbA$_{1c}$ and 238 mg/dL for FPG. At baseline, mean HbA$_{1c}$ was 10.2% and mean FPG was 243 mg/dL. Compared with placebo, treatment with ACTOS titrated to a final dose of 30 mg and 45 mg resulted in reductions from baseline in

mean HbA$_{1c}$ of 2.3% and 2.6% and mean FPG of 63 mg/dL and 95 mg/dL, respectively. For patients who had been previously treated with antidiabetic medication (76%), this medication was discontinued at screening. Mean values at screening were 9.4% for HbA$_{1c}$ and 216 mg/dL for FPG. At baseline, mean HbA$_{1c}$ was 10.7% and mean FPG was 290 mg/dL. Compared with placebo, treatment with ACTOS titrated to a final dose of 30 mg and 45 mg resulted in re-

ductions from baseline in mean HbA$_{1c}$ of 1.3% and 1.4% and mean FPG of 55 mg/dL and 60 mg/dL, respectively. For many previously-treated patients, HbA$_{1c}$ and FPG had not returned to screening levels by the end of the study.

In a 16-week study, 197 patients with type 2 diabetes were randomized to treatment with 30 mg of ACTOS or placebo once daily. Therapy with any previous antidiabetic agent was discontinued 6 weeks prior to the double-blind period.

Table 1   Lipids in a 26-Week Placebo-Controlled Monotherapy Dose-Ranging Study

	Placebo	ACTOS 15 mg Once Daily	ACTOS 30 mg Once Daily	ACTOS 45 mg Once Daily
Triglycerides (mg/dL)	N=79	N=79	N=84	N=77
Baseline (mean)	262.8	283.8	261.1	259.7
Percent change from baseline (mean)	4.8%	-9.0%	-9.6%	-9.3%
HDL Cholesterol (mg/dL)	N=79	N=79	N=83	N=77
Baseline (mean)	41.7	40.4	40.8	40.7
Percent change from baseline (mean)	8.1%	14.1%	12.2%	19.1%
LDL Cholesterol (mg/dL)	N=65	N=63	N=74	N=62
Baseline (mean)	138.8	131.9	135.6	126.8
Percent change from baseline (mean)	4.8%	7.2%	5.2%	6.0%
Total Cholesterol (mg/dL)	N=79	N=79	N=84	N=77
Baseline (mean)	224.6	220.0	222.7	213.7
Percent change from baseline (mean)	4.4%	4.6%	3.3%	6.4%

Figure 1   Mean Change from Baseline for FPG and HbA$_{1c}$ in a 26-Week Placebo-Controlled Dose-Ranging Study

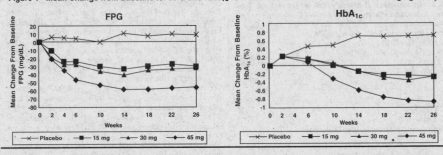

Table 2   Glycemic Parameters in a 26-Week Placebo-Controlled Dose-Ranging Study

	Placebo	ACTOS 15 mg Once Daily	ACTOS 30 mg Once Daily	ACTOS 45 mg Once Daily
Total Population				
HbA$_{1c}$ (%)	N=79	N=79	N=85	N=76
Baseline (mean)	10.4	10.2	10.2	10.3
Change from baseline (adjusted mean[+])	0.7	-0.3	-0.3	-0.9
Difference from placebo (adjusted mean[+])		-1.0*	-1.0*	-1.6*
FPG (mg/dL)	N=79	N=79	N=84	N=77
Baseline (mean)	268	267	269	276
Change from baseline (adjusted mean[+])	9	-30	-32	-56
Difference from placebo (adjusted mean[+])		-39*	-41*	-65*

[+] Adjusted for baseline, pooled center, and pooled center by treatment interaction
*p $\leq$ 0.050 vs. placebo

Table 3   Glycemic Parameters in a 26-Week Placebo-Controlled Dose-Ranging Study

	Placebo	ACTOS 15 mg Once Daily	ACTOS 30 mg Once Daily	ACTOS 45 mg Once Daily
Naïve to Therapy				
HbA$_{1c}$ (%)	N=25	N=26	N=26	N=21
Screening (mean)	9.3	10.0	9.5	9.8
Baseline (mean)	9.0	9.9	9.3	10.0
Change from baseline (adjusted mean*)	0.6	-0.8	-0.6	-1.9
Difference from placebo (adjusted mean*)		-1.4	-1.3	-2.6
FPG (mg/dL)	N=25	N=26	N=26	N=21
Screening (mean)	223	245	239	239
Baseline (mean)	229	251	225	235
Change from baseline (adjusted mean*)	16	-37	-41	-64
Difference from placebo (adjusted mean*)		-52	-56	-80
Previously Treated				
HbA$_{1c}$ (%)	N=54	N=53	N=59	N=55
Screening (mean)	9.3	9.0	9.1	9.0
Baseline (mean)	10.9	10.4	10.4	10.6
Change from baseline (adjusted mean*)	0.8	-0.1	-0.0	-0.6
Difference from placebo (adjusted mean*)		-1.0	-0.9	-1.4
FPG (mg/dL)	N=54	N=53	N=58	N=56
Screening (mean)	222	209	230	215
Baseline (mean)	285	275	286	292
Change from baseline (adjusted mean*)	4	-32	-27	-55
Difference from placebo (adjusted mean*)		-36	-31	-59

*Adjusted for baseline and pooled center

Treatment with 30 mg of ACTOS produced statistically significant improvements in HbA_{1c} and FPG at endpoint compared to placebo **(Table 5)**.

[See table 5 above]

For patients who had not been previously treated with antidiabetic medication (40%), mean values at screening were 10.3% for HbA_{1c} and 240 mg/dL for FPG. At baseline, mean HbA_{1c} was 10.4% and mean FPG was 254 mg/dL. Compared with placebo, treatment with ACTOS 30 mg resulted in reductions from baseline in mean HbA_{1c} of 1.0% and mean FPG of 62 mg/dL. For patients who had been previously treated with antidiabetic medication (60%), this medication was discontinued at screening. Mean values at screening were 9.4% for HbA_{1c} and 216 mg/dL for FPG. At baseline, mean HbA_{1c} was 10.6% and mean FPG was 287 mg/dL. Compared with placebo, treatment with ACTOS 30 mg resulted in reductions from baseline in mean HbA_{1c} of 1.3% and mean FPG of 46 mg/dL. For many previously-treated patients, HbA_{1c} and FPG had not returned to screening levels by the end of the study.

Combination Therapy

Three 16-week, randomized, double-blind, placebo-controlled clinical studies and three 24-week, randomized, double-blind, dose-controlled clinical studies were conducted to evaluate the effects of ACTOS on glycemic control in patients with type 2 diabetes who were inadequately controlled ($HbA_{1c} \geq 8\%$) despite current therapy with a sulfonylurea, metformin, or insulin. Previous diabetes treatment may have been monotherapy or combination therapy.

ACTOS Plus Sulfonylurea Studies

Two clinical studies were conducted with ACTOS in combination with a sulfonylurea. Both studies included patients with type 2 diabetes on a sulfonylurea, either alone or in combination with another antidiabetic agent. All other antidiabetic agents were withdrawn prior to starting study treatment. In the first study, 560 patients were randomized to receive 15 mg or 30 mg of ACTOS or placebo once daily for 16 weeks in addition to their current sulfonylurea regimen. When compared to placebo at Week 16, the addition of ACTOS to the sulfonylurea significantly reduced the mean HbA_{1c} by 0.9% and 1.3% and mean FPG by 39 mg/dL and 58 mg/dL for the 15 mg and 30 mg doses, respectively.

In the second study, 702 patients were randomized to receive 30 mg or 45 mg of ACTOS once daily for 24 weeks in addition to their current sulfonylurea regimen. The mean reductions from baseline at Week 24 in HbA_{1c} were 1.55% and 1.67% for the 30 mg and 45 mg doses, respectively. Mean reductions from baseline in FPG were 51.5 mg/dL and 56.1 mg/dL.

The therapeutic effect of ACTOS in combination with sulfonylurea was observed in patients regardless of whether the patients were receiving low, medium, or high doses of sulfonylurea.

ACTOS Plus Metformin Studies

Two clinical studies were conducted with ACTOS in combination with metformin. Both studies included patients with type 2 diabetes on metformin, either alone or in combination with another antidiabetic agent. All other antidiabetic agents were withdrawn prior to starting study treatment. In the first study, 328 patients were randomized to receive either 30 mg of ACTOS or placebo once daily for 16 weeks in addition to their current metformin regimen. When compared to placebo at Week 16, the addition of ACTOS to metformin significantly reduced the mean HbA_{1c} by 0.8% and decreased the mean FPG by 38 mg/dL.

In the second study, 827 patients were randomized to receive either 30 mg or 45 mg of ACTOS once daily for 24 weeks in addition to their current metformin regimen. The mean reductions from baseline at Week 24 in HbA_{1c} were 0.80% and 1.01% for the 30 mg and 45 mg doses, respectively. Mean reductions from baseline in FPG were 38.2 mg/dL and 50.7 mg/dL.

The therapeutic effect of ACTOS in combination with metformin was observed in patients regardless of whether the patients were receiving lower or higher doses of metformin.

ACTOS Plus Insulin Studies

Two clinical studies were conducted with ACTOS in combination with insulin. Both studies included patients with type 2 diabetes on insulin, either alone or in combination with another antidiabetic agent. All other antidiabetic agents were withdrawn prior to starting study treatment. In the first study, 566 patients receiving a median of 60.5 units per day of insulin were randomized to receive either 15 mg or 30 mg of ACTOS or placebo once daily for 16 weeks in addition to their insulin regimen. When compared to placebo at Week 16, the addition of ACTOS to insulin significantly reduced both HbA_{1c} by 0.7% and 1.0% and FPG by 35 mg/dL and 49 mg/dL for the 15 mg and 30 mg dose, respectively.

In the second study, 690 patients receiving a median of 60.0 units per day of insulin received either 30 mg or 45 mg of ACTOS once daily for 24 weeks in addition to their current insulin regimen. The mean reductions from baseline at Week 24 in HbA_{1c} were 1.17% and 1.46% for the 30 mg and 45 mg doses, respectively. Mean reductions from baseline in FPG were 31.9 mg/dL and 45.8 mg/dL. Improved glycemic control was accompanied by mean decreases from baseline in insulin dose requirements of 6.0% and 9.4% per day for the 30 mg and 45 mg dose, respectively.

The therapeutic effect of ACTOS in combination with insulin was observed in patients regardless of whether the patients were receiving lower or higher doses of insulin.

Table 4 Glycemic Parameters in a 24-Week Placebo-Controlled Forced-Titration Study

	Placebo	ACTOS 30 mg+ Once Daily	ACTOS 45 mg+ Once Daily
Total Population			
HbA_{1c} (%)	N=83	N=85	N=85
Baseline (mean)	10.8	10.3	10.8
Change from baseline (adjusted mean++)	0.9	-0.6	-0.6
Difference from placebo (adjusted mean++)		-1.5*	-1.5*
FPG (mg/dL)	N=78	N=82	N=85
Baseline (mean)	279	268	281
Change from baseline (adjusted mean++)	18	-44	-50
Difference from placebo (adjusted mean++)		-62*	-68*

\+ Final dose in forced titration

++ Adjusted for baseline, pooled center, and pooled center by treatment interaction

* $p \leq 0.050$ vs. placebo

Table 5 Glycemic Parameters in a 16-Week Placebo-Controlled Study

	Placebo	ACTOS 30 mg Once Daily
Total Population		
HbA_{1c} (%)	N=93	N=100
Baseline (mean)	10.3	10.5
Change from baseline (adjusted mean+)	0.8	-0.6
Difference from placebo (adjusted mean+)		-1.4*
FPG (mg/dL)	N=91	N=99
Baseline (mean)	270	273
Change from baseline (adjusted mean+)	8	-50
Difference from placebo (adjusted mean+)		-58*

\+ Adjusted for baseline, pooled center, and pooled center by treatment interaction

* $p \leq 0.050$ vs. placebo

INDICATIONS AND USAGE

ACTOS is indicated as an adjunct to diet and exercise to improve glycemic control in patients with type 2 diabetes (non-insulin-dependent diabetes mellitus, NIDDM). ACTOS is indicated for monotherapy. ACTOS is also indicated for use in combination with a sulfonylurea, metformin, or insulin when diet and exercise plus the single agent do not result in adequate glycemic control.

Management of type 2 diabetes should also include nutritional counseling, weight reduction as needed, and exercise. These efforts are important not only in the primary treatment of type 2 diabetes, but also to maintain the efficacy of drug therapy.

CONTRAINDICATIONS

Initiation of ACTOS in patients with established New York Heart Association (NYHA) Class III or IV heart failure is contraindicated (see **BOXED WARNING**).

ACTOS is contraindicated in patients with known hypersensitivity to this product or any of its components.

WARNINGS

Cardiac Failure and Other Cardiac Effects

ACTOS, like other thiazolidinediones, can cause fluid retention when used alone or in combination with other antidiabetic agents, including insulin. Fluid retention may lead to or exacerbate heart failure. Patients should be observed for signs and symptoms of heart failure. If these signs and symptoms develop, the heart failure should be managed according to current standards of care. Furthermore, discontinuation or dose reduction of ACTOS must be considered (see **BOXED WARNING**). Patients with NYHA Class III and IV cardiac status were not studied during pre-approval clinical trials and ACTOS is not recommended in these patients (see **BOXED WARNING** and **CONTRAINDICATIONS**).

In one 16-week, U.S. double-blind, placebo-controlled clinical trial involving 566 patients with type 2 diabetes, ACTOS at doses of 15 mg and 30 mg in combination with insulin was compared to insulin therapy alone. This trial included patients with long-standing diabetes and a high prevalence of pre-existing medical conditions as follows: arterial hypertension (57.2%), peripheral neuropathy (22.6%), coronary heart disease (19.6%), retinopathy (13.1%), myocardial infarction (8.8%), vascular disease (6.4%), angina pectoris (4.4%), stroke and/or transient ischemic attack (4.1%), and congestive heart failure (2.3%).

In this study, two of the 191 patients receiving 15 mg ACTOS plus insulin (1.1%) and two of the 188 patients receiving 30 mg ACTOS plus insulin (1.1%) developed congestive heart failure compared with none of the 187 patients on insulin therapy alone. All four of these patients had previous histories of cardiovascular conditions including coronary artery disease, previous CABG procedures, and myocardial infarction. In a 24-week, dose-controlled study in which ACTOS was coadministered with insulin, 0.3% of patients (1/345) on 30 mg and 0.9% (3/345) of patients on 45 mg reported CHF as a serious adverse event.

Analysis of data from these studies did not identify specific factors that predict increased risk of congestive heart failure on combination therapy with insulin.

In type 2 diabetes and congestive heart failure (systolic dysfunction)

A 24-week post-marketing safety study was performed to compare ACTOS (n=262) to glyburide (n=256) in uncontrolled diabetic patients (mean HbA_{1c} 8.8% at baseline) with NYHA Class II and III heart failure and ejection fraction less than 40% (mean EF 30% at baseline). Over the course of the study, overnight hospitalization for congestive heart failure was reported in 9.9% of patients on ACTOS compared to 4.7% of patients on glyburide with a treatment difference observed from 6 weeks. This adverse event associated with ACTOS was more marked in patients using insulin at baseline and in patients over 64 years of age. No difference in cardiovascular mortality between the treatment groups was observed.

ACTOS should be initiated at the lowest approved dose if it is prescribed for patients with type 2 diabetes and systolic heart failure (NYHA Class II). If subsequent dose escalation is necessary, the dose should be increased gradually only after several months of treatment with careful monitoring for weight gain, edema, or signs and symptoms of CHF exacerbation.

Prospective Pioglitazone Clinical Trial In Macrovascular Events (PROactive)

In PROactive, 5238 patients with type 2 diabetes and a prior history of macrovascular disease were treated with ACTOS (n=2605), force-titrated up to 45 mg once daily, or placebo (n=2633) (see **ADVERSE REACTIONS**). The percentage of patients who had an event of serious heart failure was higher for patients treated with ACTOS (5.7%, n=149) than for patients treated with placebo (4.1%, n=108). The incidence of death subsequent to a report of serious heart failure was 1.5% (n=40) in patients treated with ACTOS and 1.4% (n=37) in placebo-treated patients. In patients treated with an insulin-containing regimen at baseline, the incidence of serious heart failure was 6.3% (n=54/864) with ACTOS and 5.2% (n=47/896) with placebo. For those patients treated with a sulfonylurea-containing regimen at baseline, the incidence of serious heart failure was 5.8% (n=94/1624) with ACTOS and 4.4% (n=71/1626) with placebo.

PRECAUTIONS

General

ACTOS exerts its antihyperglycemic effect only in the presence of insulin. Therefore, ACTOS should not be used in patients with type 1 diabetes or for the treatment of diabetic ketoacidosis.

Hypoglycemia: Patients receiving ACTOS in combination with insulin or oral hypoglycemic agents may be at risk for hypoglycemia, and a reduction in the dose of the concomitant agent may be necessary.

Cardiovascular: In U.S. placebo-controlled clinical trials that excluded patients with New York Heart Association (NYHA) Class III and IV cardiac status, the incidence of serious cardiac adverse events related to volume expansion was not increased in patients treated with ACTOS as monotherapy or in combination with sulfonylureas or metformin vs. placebo-treated patients. In insulin combination studies, a small number of patients with a history of previously existing cardiac disease developed congestive heart failure when treated with ACTOS in combination with insulin (see **WARNINGS**). Patients with NYHA Class III and IV cardiac status were not studied in these ACTOS clinical trials. ACTOS is not indicated in patients with NYHA Class III or IV cardiac status.

In postmarketing experience with ACTOS, cases of congestive heart failure have been reported in patients both with and without previously known heart disease.

Continued on next page

Actos—Cont.

Edema: ACTOS should be used with caution in patients with edema. In all U.S. clinical trials, edema was reported more frequently in patients treated with ACTOS than in placebo-treated patients and appears to be dose related (see **ADVERSE REACTIONS**). In postmarketing experience, reports of initiation or worsening of edema have been received. Since thiazolidinediones, including ACTOS, can cause fluid retention, which can exacerbate or lead to congestive heart failure, ACTOS should be used with caution in patients at risk for heart failure. Patients should be monitored for signs and symptoms of heart failure (see **BOXED WARNING, WARNINGS**, and **PRECAUTIONS, Information for Patients**).

Weight Gain: Dose related weight gain was seen with ACTOS alone and in combination with other hypoglycemic agents (**Table 6**). The mechanism of weight gain is unclear but probably involves a combination of fluid retention and fat accumulation.

[See table 6 below]

Ovulation: Therapy with ACTOS, like other thiazolidinediones, may result in ovulation in some premenopausal anovulatory women. As a result, these patients may be at an increased risk for pregnancy while taking ACTOS. Thus, adequate contraception in premenopausal women should be recommended. This possible effect has not been investigated in clinical studies so the frequency of this occurrence is not known.

Hematologic: ACTOS may cause decreases in hemoglobin and hematocrit. Across all clinical studies, mean hemoglobin values declined by 2% to 4% in patients treated with ACTOS. These changes primarily occurred within the first 4 to 12 weeks of therapy and remained relatively constant thereafter. These changes may be related to increased plasma volume and have rarely been associated with any significant hematologic clinical effects (see **ADVERSE REACTIONS, Laboratory Abnormalities**).

Hepatic Effects: In pre-approval clinical studies worldwide, over 4500 subjects were treated with ACTOS. In U.S. clinical studies, over 4700 patients with type 2 diabetes received ACTOS. There was no evidence of drug-induced hepatotoxicity or elevation of ALT levels in the clinical studies. During pre-approval placebo-controlled clinical trials in the U.S., a total of 4 of 1526 (0.26%) patients treated with ACTOS and 2 of 793 (0.25%) placebo-treated patients had ALT values ≥ 3 times the upper limit of normal. The ALT elevations in patients treated with ACTOS were reversible and were not clearly related to therapy with ACTOS.

In postmarketing experience with ACTOS, reports of hepatitis and of hepatic enzyme elevations to 3 or more times the upper limit of normal have been received. Very rarely, these reports have involved hepatic failure with and without fatal outcome, although causality has not been established.

Pending the availability of the results of additional large, long-term controlled clinical trials and additional postmarketing safety data, it is recommended that patients treated with ACTOS undergo periodic monitoring of liver enzymes.

Serum ALT (alanine aminotransferase) levels should be evaluated prior to the initiation of therapy with ACTOS in all patients and periodically thereafter per the clinical judgment of the health care professional. Liver function tests should also be obtained for patients if symptoms suggestive of hepatic dysfunction occur, e.g., nausea, vomiting, abdominal pain, fatigue, anorexia, or dark urine. The decision whether to continue the patient on therapy with ACTOS should be guided by clinical judgment pending laboratory evaluations. If jaundice is observed, drug therapy should be discontinued.

Therapy with ACTOS should not be initiated if the patient exhibits clinical evidence of active liver disease or the ALT levels exceed 2.5 times the upper limit of normal. Patients with mildly elevated liver enzymes (ALT levels at 1 to 2.5 times the upper limit of normal) at baseline or any time during therapy with ACTOS should be evaluated to determine the cause of the liver enzyme elevation. Initiation or continuation of therapy with ACTOS in patients with mildly elevated liver enzymes should proceed with caution and include appropriate clinical follow-up which may include more frequent liver enzyme monitoring. If serum transaminase levels are increased (ALT > 2.5 times the upper limit of normal), liver function tests should be evaluated more frequently until the levels return to normal or pretreatment values. If ALT levels exceed 3 times the upper limit of normal, the test should be repeated as soon as possible. If ALT levels remain > 3 times the upper limit of normal or if the patient is jaundiced, ACTOS therapy should be discontinued.

Macular Edema: Macular edema has been reported in post-marketing experience in diabetic patients who were taking pioglitazone or another thiazolidinedione. Some patients presented with blurred vision or decreased visual acuity, but some patients appear to have been diagnosed on routine ophthalmologic examination. Some patients had peripheral edema at the time macular edema was diagnosed. Some patients had improvement in their macular edema after discontinuation of their thiazolidinedione. It is unknown whether or not there is a causal relationship between pioglitazone and macular edema. Patients with diabetes should have regular eye examinations by an ophthalmologist, per the Standards of Care of the American Diabetes Association. Additionally, any diabetic who reports any kind of visual symptom should be promptly referred to an ophthalmologist, regardless of the patient's underlying medications or other physical findings (see **ADVERSE REACTIONS**).

Fractures: In a randomized trial (PROactive) in patients with type 2 diabetes (mean duration of diabetes 9.5 years), an increased incidence of bone fracture was noted in female patients taking pioglitazone. During a mean follow-up of 34.5 months, the incidence of bone fracture in females was 5.1% (44/870) for pioglitazone versus 2.5% (23/905) for placebo. This difference was noted after the first year of treatment and remained during the course of the study. The majority of fractures observed in female patients were nonvertebral fractures including lower limb and distal upper limb. No increase in fracture rates was observed in men treated with pioglitazone 1.7% (30/1735) versus placebo 2.1% (37/1728). The risk of fracture should be considered in the care of patients, especially female patients, treated with pioglitazone and attention should be given to assessing and maintaining bone health according to current standards of care.

Laboratory Tests

FPG and HbA_{1c} measurements should be performed periodically to monitor glycemic control and the therapeutic response to ACTOS.

Liver enzyme monitoring is recommended prior to initiation of therapy with ACTOS in all patients and periodically thereafter per the clinical judgment of the health care professional (see **PRECAUTIONS, General**, Hepatic Effects and **ADVERSE REACTIONS, Serum Transaminase Levels**).

Information for Patients

It is important to instruct patients to adhere to dietary instructions and to have blood glucose and glycosylated hemoglobin tested regularly. During periods of stress such as fever, trauma, infection, or surgery, medication requirements may change and patients should be reminded to seek medical advice promptly.

Patients who experience an unusually rapid increase in weight or edema or who develop shortness of breath or other symptoms of heart failure while on ACTOS should immediately report these symptoms to their physician.

Patients should be told that blood tests for liver function will be performed prior to the start of therapy and periodically thereafter per the clinical judgment of the health care professional. Patients should be told to seek immediate medical advice for unexplained nausea, vomiting, abdominal pain, fatigue, anorexia, or dark urine.

Patients should be told to take ACTOS once daily. ACTOS can be taken with or without meals. If a dose is missed on one day, the dose should not be doubled the following day.

When using combination therapy with insulin or oral hypoglycemic agents, the risks of hypoglycemia, its symptoms and treatment, and conditions that predispose to its development should be explained to patients and their family members.

Therapy with ACTOS, like other thiazolidinediones, may result in ovulation in some premenopausal anovulatory women. As a result, these patients may be at an increased risk for pregnancy while taking ACTOS. Thus, adequate contraception in premenopausal women should be recommended. This possible effect has not been investigated in clinical studies so the frequency of this occurrence is not known.

Drug Interactions

In vivo drug-drug interaction studies have suggested that pioglitazone may be a weak inducer of CYP 450 isoform 3A4 substrate (see **CLINICAL PHARMACOLOGY, Metabolism** and **Drug-Drug Interactions**).

An enzyme inhibitor of CYP2C8 (such as gemfibrozil) may significantly increase the AUC of pioglitazone and an enzyme inducer of CYP2C8 (such as rifampin) may significantly decrease the AUC of pioglitazone. Therefore, if an inhibitor or inducer of CYP2C8 is started or stopped during treatment with pioglitazone, changes in diabetes treatment may be needed based on clinical response (see **CLINICAL PHARMACOLOGY, Drug-Drug Interactions**).

Carcinogenesis, Mutagenesis, Impairment of Fertility

A two-year carcinogenicity study was conducted in male and female rats at oral doses up to 63 mg/kg (approximately 14 times the maximum recommended human oral dose of 45 mg based on mg/m^2). Drug-induced tumors were not observed in any organ except for the urinary bladder. Benign and/or malignant transitional cell neoplasms were observed in male rats at 4 mg/kg/day and above (approximately equal to the maximum recommended human oral dose based on mg/m^2). A two-year carcinogenicity study was conducted in male and female mice at oral doses up to 100 mg/kg/day (approximately 11 times the maximum recommended human oral dose based on mg/m^2). No drug-induced tumors were observed in any organ.

During prospective evaluation of urinary cytology involving more than 1800 patients receiving ACTOS in clinical trials up to one year in duration, no new cases of bladder tumors were identified. In two 3-year studies in which pioglitazone was compared to placebo or glyburide, there were 16/3656 (0.44%) reports of bladder cancer in patients taking pioglitazone compared to 5/3679 (0.14%) in patients not taking pioglitazone. After excluding patients in whom exposure to study drug was less than one year at the time of diagnosis of bladder cancer, there were six (0.16%) cases on pioglitazone and two (0.05%) on placebo.

Pioglitazone HCl was not mutagenic in a battery of genetic toxicology studies, including the Ames bacterial assay, a mammalian cell forward gene mutation assay (CHO/HPRT and AS52/XPRT), an *in vitro* cytogenetics assay using CHL cells, an unscheduled DNA synthesis assay, and an *in vivo* micronucleus assay.

No adverse effects upon fertility were observed in male and female rats at oral doses up to 40 mg/kg pioglitazone HCl daily prior to and throughout mating and gestation (approximately 9 times the maximum recommended human oral dose based on mg/m^2).

Animal Toxicology

Heart enlargement has been observed in mice (100 mg/kg), rats (4 mg/kg and above) and dogs (3 mg/kg) treated orally with pioglitazone HCl (approximately 11, 1, and 2 times the maximum recommended human oral dose for mice, rats, and dogs, respectively, based on mg/m^2). In a one-year rat study, drug-related early death due to apparent heart dysfunction occurred at an oral dose of 160 mg/kg/day (approximately 35 times the maximum recommended human oral dose based on mg/m^2). Heart enlargement was seen in a 13-week study in monkeys at oral doses of 8.9 mg/kg and above (approximately 4 times the maximum recommended human oral dose based on mg/m^2), but not in a 52-week study at oral doses up to 32 mg/kg (approximately 13 times the maximum recommended human oral dose based on mg/m^2).

Pregnancy

Pregnancy Category C. Pioglitazone was not teratogenic in rats at oral doses up to 80 mg/kg or in rabbits given up to 160 mg/kg during organogenesis (approximately 17 and 40 times the maximum recommended human oral dose based on mg/m^2, respectively). Delayed parturition and embryotoxicity (as evidenced by increased postimplantation losses, delayed development and reduced fetal weights) were observed in rats at oral doses of 40 mg/kg/day and above (approximately 10 times the maximum recommended human oral dose based on mg/m^2). No functional or behavioral toxicity was observed in offspring of rats. In rabbits, embryotoxicity was observed at an oral dose of 160 mg/kg (approximately 40 times the maximum recommended human oral dose based on mg/m^2). Delayed postnatal development, attributed to decreased body weight, was observed in offspring of rats at oral doses of 10 mg/kg and above during late gestation and lactation periods (approximately 2 times the maximum recommended human oral dose based on mg/m^2).

There are no adequate and well-controlled studies in pregnant women. ACTOS should be used during pregnancy only if the potential benefit justifies the potential risk to the fetus.

Because current information strongly suggests that abnormal blood glucose levels during pregnancy are associated with a higher incidence of congenital anomalies, as well as increased neonatal morbidity and mortality, most experts recommend that insulin be used during pregnancy to maintain blood glucose levels as close to normal as possible.

Nursing Mothers

Pioglitazone is secreted in the milk of lactating rats. It is not known whether ACTOS is secreted in human milk. Because many drugs are excreted in human milk, ACTOS should not be administered to a breastfeeding woman.

Table 6 Weight Changes (kg) from Baseline during Double-Blind Clinical Trials with ACTOS

		Control Group (Placebo)	ACTOS 15 mg	ACTOS 30 mg	ACTOS 45 mg
		Median (25th / 75th percentile)	Median (25th / 75th percentile)	Median (25th / 75th percentile)	Median (25th / 75th percentile)
Monotherapy		-1.4 (-2.7/0.0) n=256	0.9 (-0.5/3.4) n=79	1.0 (-0.9/3.4) n=188	2.6 (0.2/5.4) n=79
Combination Therapy	Sulfonylurea	-0.5 (-1.8/0.7) n=187	2.0 (0.2/3.2) n=183	3.1 (1.1/5.4) n=528	4.1 (1.8/7.3) n=333
	Metformin	-1.4 (-3.2/0.3) n=160	N/A	0.9 (-0.3/3.2) n=567	1.8 (-0.9/5.0) n=407
	Insulin	0.2 (-1.4/1.4) n=182	2.3 (0.5/4.3) n=190	3.3 (0.9/6.3) n=522	4.1 (1.4/6.8) n=338

Note: Trial durations of 16 to 26 weeks

Pediatric Use

Safety and effectiveness of ACTOS in pediatric patients have not been established.

Elderly Use

Approximately 500 patients in placebo-controlled clinical trials of ACTOS were 65 and over. No significant differences in effectiveness and safety were observed between these patients and younger patients.

ADVERSE REACTIONS

Over 8500 patients with type 2 diabetes have been treated with ACTOS in randomized, double-blind, controlled clinical trials. This includes 2605 high-risk patients with type 2 diabetes treated with ACTOS from the PROactive clinical trial. Over 6000 patients have been treated for 6 months or longer, and over 4500 patients for one year or longer. Over 3000 patients have received ACTOS for at least 2 years.

The overall incidence and types of adverse events reported in placebo-controlled clinical trials of ACTOS monotherapy at doses of 7.5 mg, 15 mg, 30 mg, or 45 mg once daily are shown in Table 7.

[See table 7 above]

For most clinical adverse events the incidence was similar for groups treated with ACTOS monotherapy and those treated in combination with sulfonylureas, metformin, and insulin. There was an increase in the occurrence of edema in the patients treated with ACTOS and insulin compared to insulin alone.

In a 16-week, placebo-controlled ACTOS plus insulin trial (n=379), 10 patients treated with ACTOS plus insulin developed dyspnea and also, at some point during their therapy, developed either weight change or edema. Seven of these 10 patients received diuretics to treat these symptoms. This was not reported in the insulin plus placebo group.

The incidence of withdrawals from placebo-controlled clinical trials due to an adverse event other than hyperglycemia was similar for patients treated with placebo (2.8%) or ACTOS (3.3%).

In controlled combination therapy studies with either a sulfonylurea or insulin, mild to moderate hypoglycemia, which appears to be dose related, was reported (see **PRECAUTIONS, General**, Hypoglycemia and **DOSAGE and ADMINISTRATION, Combination Therapy**).

In U.S. double-blind studies, anemia was reported in ≤ 2% of patients treated with ACTOS plus sulfonylurea, metformin or insulin (see **PRECAUTIONS, General**, Hematologic).

In monotherapy studies, edema was reported for 4.8% (with doses from 7.5 mg to 45 mg) of patients treated with ACTOS versus 1.2% of placebo-treated patients. In combination therapy studies, edema was reported for 7.2% of patients treated with ACTOS and sulfonylureas compared to 2.1% of patients on sulfonylureas alone. In combination therapy studies with metformin, edema was reported in 6.0% of patients on combination therapy compared to 2.5% of patients on metformin alone. In combination therapy studies with insulin, edema was reported in 15.3% of patients on combination therapy compared to 7.0% of patients on insulin alone. Most of these events were considered mild or moderate in intensity (see **PRECAUTIONS, General**, Edema).

In one 16-week clinical trial of insulin plus ACTOS combination therapy, more patients developed congestive heart failure on combination therapy (1.1%) compared to none on insulin alone (see **WARNINGS, Cardiac Failure and Other Cardiac Effects**).

Prospective Pioglitazone Clinical Trial In Macrovascular Events (PROactive)

In PROactive, 5238 patients with type 2 diabetes and a prior history of macrovascular disease were treated with ACTOS (n=2605), force-titrated up to 45 mg daily or placebo (n=2633) in addition to standard of care. Almost all subjects (95%) were receiving cardiovascular medications (beta blockers, ACE inhibitors, ARBs, calcium channel blockers, nitrates, diuretics, aspirin, statins, fibrates). Patients had a mean age of 61.8 years, mean duration of diabetes 9.5 years, and mean HbA_{1c} 8.1%. Average duration of follow-up was 34.5 months. The primary objective of this trial was to examine the effect of ACTOS on mortality and macrovascular morbidity in patients with type 2 diabetes mellitus who were at high risk for macrovascular events. The primary efficacy variable was the time to the first occurrence of any event in the cardiovascular composite endpoint (see **Table 8** below). Although there was no statistically significant difference between ACTOS and placebo for the 3-year incidence of a first event within this composite, there was no increase in mortality or in total macrovascular events with ACTOS.

[See table 8 above]

Postmarketing reports of new onset or worsening diabetic macular edema with decreased visual acuity have also been received (see **PRECAUTIONS, General**, Macular Edema).

Laboratory Abnormalities

Hematologic: ACTOS may cause decreases in hemoglobin and hematocrit. The fall in hemoglobin and hematocrit with ACTOS appears to be dose related. Across all clinical studies, mean hemoglobin values declined by 2% to 4% in patients treated with ACTOS. These changes generally occurred within the first 4 to 12 weeks of therapy and remained relatively stable thereafter. These changes may be related to increased plasma volume associated with ACTOS therapy and have rarely been associated with any significant hematologic clinical effects.

Serum Transaminase Levels: During all clinical studies in the U.S., 14 of 4780 (0.30%) patients treated with ACTOS had ALT values ≥ 3 times the upper limit of normal during

treatment. All patients with follow-up values had reversible elevations in ALT. In the population of patients treated with ACTOS, mean values for bilirubin, AST, ALT, alkaline phosphatase, and GGT were decreased at the final visit compared with baseline. Fewer than 0.9% of patients treated with ACTOS were withdrawn from clinical trials in the U.S. due to abnormal liver function tests.

In pre-approval clinical trials, there were no cases of idiosyncratic drug reactions leading to hepatic failure (see **PRECAUTIONS, General**, Hepatic Effects).

CPK Levels: During required laboratory testing in clinical trials, sporadic, transient elevations in creatine phosphokinase levels (CPK) were observed. An isolated elevation to greater than 10 times the upper limit of normal was noted in 9 patients (values of 2150 to 11400 IU/L). Six of these patients continued to receive ACTOS, two patients had completed receiving study medication at the time of the elevated value and one patient discontinued study medication due to the elevation. These elevations resolved without any apparent clinical sequelae. The relationship of these events to ACTOS therapy is unknown.

OVERDOSAGE

During controlled clinical trials, one case of overdose with ACTOS was reported. A male patient took 120 mg per day for four days, then 180 mg per day for seven days. The patient denied any clinical symptoms during this period.

In the event of overdosage, appropriate supportive treatment should be initiated according to patient's clinical signs and symptoms.

DOSAGE AND ADMINISTRATION

ACTOS should be taken once daily without regard to meals. The management of antidiabetic therapy should be individualized. Ideally, the response to therapy should be evaluated using HbA_{1c} which is a better indicator of long-term glycemic control than FPG alone. HbA_{1c} reflects glycemia over the past two to three months. In clinical use, it is recommended that patients be treated with ACTOS for a period of time adequate to evaluate change in HbA_{1c} (three months) unless glycemic control deteriorates. After initiation of ACTOS or with dose increase, patients should be carefully monitored for adverse events related to fluid retention (see **BOXED WARNING** and **WARNINGS**).

Monotherapy

ACTOS monotherapy in patients not adequately controlled with diet and exercise may be initiated at 15 mg or 30 mg once daily. For patients who respond inadequately to the initial dose of ACTOS, the dose can be increased in increments up to 45 mg once daily. For patients not responding adequately to monotherapy, combination therapy should be considered.

Combination Therapy

Sulfonylureas: ACTOS in combination with a sulfonylurea may be initiated at 15 mg or 30 mg once daily. The current sulfonylurea dose can be continued upon initiation of ACTOS therapy. If patients report hypoglycemia, the dose of the sulfonylurea should be decreased.

Metformin: ACTOS in combination with metformin may be initiated at 15 mg or 30 mg once daily. The current metformin dose can be continued upon initiation of ACTOS therapy. It is unlikely that the dose of metformin will require adjustment due to hypoglycemia during combination therapy with ACTOS.

Insulin: ACTOS in combination with insulin may be initiated at 15 mg or 30 mg once daily. The current insulin dose can be continued upon initiation of ACTOS therapy. In patients receiving ACTOS and insulin, the insulin dose can be decreased by 10% to 25% if the patient reports hypoglycemia or if plasma glucose concentrations decrease to less than 100 mg/dL. Further adjustments should be individualized based on glucose-lowering response.

Maximum Recommended Dose

The dose of ACTOS should not exceed 45 mg once daily in monotherapy or in combination with sulfonylurea, metformin, or insulin.

Dose adjustment in patients with renal insufficiency is not recommended (see **CLINICAL PHARMACOLOGY, Pharmacokinetics and Drug Metabolism**).

Therapy with ACTOS should not be initiated if the patient exhibits clinical evidence of active liver disease or increased serum transaminase levels (ALT greater than 2.5 times the upper limit of normal) at start of therapy (see **PRECAUTIONS, General**, Hepatic Effects and **CLINICAL PHARMACOLOGY, Special Populations**, Hepatic Insufficiency).

Liver enzyme monitoring is recommended in all patients prior to initiation of therapy with ACTOS and periodically thereafter (see **PRECAUTIONS, General**, Hepatic Effects).

There are no data on the use of ACTOS in patients under 18 years of age; therefore, use of ACTOS in pediatric patients is not recommended.

No data are available on the use of ACTOS in combination with another thiazolidinedione.

HOW SUPPLIED

ACTOS is available in 15 mg, 30 mg, and 45 mg tablets as follows:

15 mg Tablet: white to off-white, round, convex, non-scored tablet with "ACTOS" on one side, and "15" on the other, available in:

NDC 64764-151-04 Bottles of 30
NDC 64764-151-05 Bottles of 90
NDC 64764-151-06 Bottles of 500

30 mg Tablet: white to off-white, round, flat, non-scored tablet with "ACTOS" on one side, and "30" on the other, available in:

NDC 64764-301-14 Bottles of 30
NDC 64764-301-15 Bottles of 90
NDC 64764-301-16 Bottles of 500

45 mg Tablet: white to off-white, round, flat, non-scored tablet with "ACTOS" on one side, and "45" on the other, available in:

NDC 64764-451-24 Bottles of 30

Table 7 Placebo-Controlled Clinical Studies of ACTOS Monotherapy: Adverse Events Reported at a Frequency ≥ 5% of Patients Treated with ACTOS

(% of Patients)		
	Placebo N=259	ACTOS N=606
Upper Respiratory Tract Infection	8.5	13.2
Headache	6.9	9.1
Sinusitis	4.6	6.3
Myalgia	2.7	5.4
Tooth Disorder	2.3	5.3
Diabetes Mellitus Aggravated	8.1	5.1
Pharyngitis	0.8	5.1

Table 8 Number of First and Total Events for Each Component Within the Cardiovascular Composite Endpoint

Cardiovascular Events	Placebo N=2633		ACTOS N=2605	
	First Events (N)	Total Events (N)	First Events (N)	Total Events (N)
Any event	572	900	514	803
All-cause mortality	122	186	110	177
Non-fatal MI	118	157	105	131
Stroke	96	119	76	92
ACS	63	78	42	65
Cardiac intervention	101	240	101	195
Major leg amputation	15	28	9	28
Leg revascularization	57	92	71	115

Continued on next page

Actos—Cont.

NDC 64764-451-25 Bottles of 90
NDC 64764-451-26 Bottles of 500

STORAGE
Store at 25°C (77°F); excursions permitted to 15-30°C (59-86°F) [see USP Controlled Room Temperature]. Keep container tightly closed, and protect from moisture and humidity.

REFERENCES

1. Deng, LJ, et al. Effect of gemfibrozil on the pharmacokinetics of pioglitazone. *Eur J Clin Pharmacol* 2005; 61: 831-836, Table 1.
2. Jaakkola, T, et al. Effect of rifampicin on the pharmacokinetics of pioglitazone. *Brit J Clin Pharmacol* 2006; 61:1 70-78.

Rx only
Manufactured by:
Takeda Pharmaceutical Company Limited
Osaka, Japan
Marketed by:
Takeda Pharmaceuticals America, Inc.
One Takeda Parkway
Deerfield, IL 60015
ACTOS® is a registered trademark of Takeda Pharmaceutical Company Limited and used under license by Takeda Pharmaceuticals America, Inc.
All other trademark names are the property of their respective owners.
© 1999, 2006 Takeda Pharmaceuticals America, Inc.
05-1141 Revised: September, 2007
L-PIO-0907-14

DUETACT™   ℞
[doo-et'-ăct]
(pioglitazone hydrochloride and glimepiride) tablets

Prescribing information for this product, which appears on pages 3163-3169 of the 2008 PDR, has been completely revised as follows. Please write "See Supplement A" next to the product heading.

> **WARNING: CONGESTIVE HEART FAILURE**
>
> • Thiazolidinediones, including pioglitazone, which is a component of DUETACT, cause or exacerbate congestive heart failure in some patients (see **WARNINGS**, *Pioglitazone hydrochloride*). After initiation of DUETACT, observe patients carefully for signs and symptoms of heart failure (including excessive, rapid weight gain, dyspnea, and/or edema). If these signs and symptoms develop, the heart failure should be managed according to the current standards of care. Furthermore, discontinuation of DUETACT must be considered.
>
> • DUETACT is not recommended in patients with symptomatic heart failure. Initiation of DUETACT in patients with established NYHA Class III or IV heart failure is contraindicated (see **CONTRAINDICATIONS** and **WARNINGS**, *Pioglitazone hydrochloride*).

DESCRIPTION
DUETACT™ (pioglitazone hydrochloride and glimepiride) tablets contain two oral antihyperglycemic agents used in the management of type 2 diabetes: pioglitazone hydrochloride and glimepiride. The concomitant use of pioglitazone and a sulfonylurea, the class of drugs that includes glimepiride, has been previously approved based on clinical trials in patients with type 2 diabetes inadequately controlled on a sulfonylurea. Additional efficacy and safety information about pioglitazone and glimepiride monotherapies may be found in the prescribing information for each individual drug.
Pioglitazone hydrochloride is an oral antihyperglycemic agent that acts primarily by decreasing insulin resistance. Pioglitazone is used in the management of type 2 diabetes. Pharmacological studies indicate that pioglitazone improves sensitivity to insulin in muscle and adipose tissue and inhibits hepatic gluconeogenesis. Pioglitazone improves glycemic control while reducing circulating insulin levels. Pioglitazone (±)-5-[[4-[2-(5-ethyl-2-pyridinyl)ethoxy] phenyl]methyl]-2,4-thiazolidinedione monohydrochloride belongs to a different chemical class and has a different pharmacological action than the sulfonylureas, biguanides, or the α-glucosidase inhibitors. The molecule contains one asymmetric center, and the synthetic compound is a racemate. The two enantiomers of pioglitazone interconvert *in vivo*. The structural formula is as shown:

pioglitazone hydrochloride

Pioglitazone hydrochloride is an odorless, white crystalline powder that has a molecular formula of $C_{19}H_{20}N_2O_3S \cdot HCl$ and a molecular weight of 392.90. It is soluble in *N,N*-dimethylformamide, slightly soluble in anhydrous ethanol, very slightly soluble in acetone and acetonitrile, practically insoluble in water, and insoluble in ether.

Table 1. Mean (SD) Pharmacokinetic Parameters for DUETACT

Regimen		N	AUC(0–inf) (ng·h/mL)	N	C_{max} (ng/mL)	N	T_{max} (h)	N	$T_{1/2}$ (h)
30 mg/2 mg DUETACT	pioglitazone	58	11414 (2704)	66	910 (336)	66	1.81 (1.11)	65	14.02 (6.23)
	glimepiride	62	651 (239)	66	156 (52.5)	66	1.39 (0.29)	63	7.05 (4.32)
30 mg pioglitazone + 2 mg glimepiride tablets	pioglitazone	58	11496 (2926)	66	975 (367)	66	1.48 (1.13)	65	12.71 (5.60)
	glimepiride	62	635 (240)	66	165 (53.1)	66	1.36 (0.35)	63	5.54 (4.21)
30 mg/4 mg DUETACT	pioglitazone	55	11119 (3399)	67	1062 (333)	67	1.53 (0.81)	67	10.88 (4.71)
	glimepiride	64	1645 (576)	67	319 (95.3)	67	1.45 (0.39)	64	10.52 (3.49)
30 mg pioglitazone + 4 mg glimepiride tablets	pioglitazone	55	10674 (2895)	67	1026 (346)	67	1.52 (1.95)	67	12.21 (6.30)
	glimepiride	64	1590 (554)	67	313 (97.8)	67	1.76 (1.13)	64	9.07 (3.47)

Glimepiride 1-[[p-[2-(3-ethyl-4-methyl-2-oxo-3-pyrroline-1-carboxamido)ethyl]phenyl]sulfonyl]-3-(*trans*-4-methyl-cyclohexyl)-urea is an oral blood glucose-lowering drug of the sulfonylurea class and is used in the management of type 2 diabetes. The molecule is the trans-isomer with respect to the cyclohexyl substituents. The chemical structure is as shown:

glimepiride

Glimepiride is a white to yellowish-white crystalline, odorless, to practically odorless powder, that has a molecular formula of $C_{24}H_{34}N_4O_5S$ and a molecular weight of 490.62. It is soluble in dimethylsulfoxide, slightly soluble in acetone, very slightly soluble in acetonitrile and methanol, and practically insoluble in water.
DUETACT is available as a tablet for oral administration containing 30 mg pioglitazone hydrochloride (as the base) with 2 mg glimepiride (30 mg/2 mg) or 30 mg pioglitazone hydrochloride (as the base) with 4 mg glimepiride (30 mg/4 mg) formulated with the following excipients: croscarmellose sodium NF, lactose monohydrate NF, magnesium stearate NF, hydroxypropyl cellulose NF, polysorbate 80 NF, and microcrystalline cellulose NF.

CLINICAL PHARMACOLOGY
Mechanism of Action
DUETACT
DUETACT combines two antihyperglycemic agents with different mechanisms of action to improve glycemic control in patients with type 2 diabetes: pioglitazone hydrochloride, a member of the thiazolidinedione class, and glimepiride, a member of the sulfonylurea class. Thiazolidinediones are insulin-sensitizing agents that act primarily by enhancing peripheral glucose utilization, whereas sulfonylureas are insulin secretogogues that act primarily by stimulating release of insulin from functioning pancreatic beta cells.
Pioglitazone hydrochloride
Pioglitazone depends on the presence of insulin for its mechanism of action. Pioglitazone decreases insulin resistance in the periphery and in the liver resulting in increased insulin-dependent glucose disposal and decreased hepatic glucose output. Pioglitazone is a potent and highly selective agonist for peroxisome proliferator-activated receptor-gamma (PPARγ). PPAR receptors are found in tissues important for insulin action such as adipose tissue, skeletal muscle, and liver. Activation of PPARγ nuclear receptors modulates the transcription of a number of insulin responsive genes involved in the control of glucose and lipid metabolism.
In animal models of diabetes, pioglitazone reduces the hyperglycemia, hyperinsulinemia, and hypertriglyceridemia characteristic of insulin-resistant states such as type 2 diabetes. The metabolic changes produced by pioglitazone result in increased responsiveness of insulin-dependent tissues and are observed in numerous animal models of insulin resistance.
Since pioglitazone enhances the effects of circulating insulin (by decreasing insulin resistance), it does not lower blood glucose in animal models that lack endogenous insulin.
Glimepiride
The primary mechanism of action of glimepiride in lowering blood glucose appears to be dependent on stimulating the release of insulin from functioning pancreatic beta cells. In addition, extrapancreatic effects may also play a role in the activity of sulfonylureas such as glimepiride. This is supported by both preclinical and clinical studies demonstrating that glimepiride administration can lead to increased sensitivity of peripheral tissues to insulin. These findings are consistent with the results of a long-term, randomized, placebo-controlled trial in which glimepiride therapy improved postprandial insulin/C-peptide responses and overall glycemic control without producing clinically meaningful increases in fasting insulin/C-peptide levels. However, as with other sulfonylureas, the mechanism by which glimepiride lowers blood glucose during long-term administration has not been clearly established.

Pharmacokinetics and Drug Metabolism
Absorption and Bioavailability:
DUETACT
Bioequivalence studies were conducted following a single dose of the DUETACT 30 mg/2 mg and 30 mg/4 mg tablets and concomitant administration of ACTOS (30 mg) and glimepiride (2 mg or 4 mg) under fasting conditions in healthy subjects.
Based on the area under the curve (AUC) and maximum concentration (C_{max}) of both pioglitazone and glimepiride, DUETACT 30 mg/2 mg and 30 mg/4 mg were bioequivalent to ACTOS 30 mg concomitantly administered with glimepiride (2 mg or 4 mg, respectively) (**Table 1**).
[See table 1 above]
Food did not change the systemic exposures of glimepiride or pioglitazone following administration of DUETACT. The presence of food did not significantly alter the time to peak serum concentration of glimepiride or pioglitazone or peak exposure (C_{max}) of pioglitazone. However, for glimepiride, there was a 22% increase in C_{max} when DUETACT was administered with food.
Pioglitazone hydrochloride
Following oral administration, in the fasting state, pioglitazone is first measurable in serum within 30 minutes, with peak concentrations observed within 2 hours.
Glimepiride
After oral administration, glimepiride is completely (100%) absorbed from the GI tract. Studies with single oral doses in normal subjects and with multiple oral doses in patients with type 2 diabetes have shown significant absorption of glimepiride within 1 hour after administration and C_{max} at 2 to 3 hours.
Distribution:
Pioglitazone hydrochloride
The mean apparent volume of distribution (Vd/F) of pioglitazone following single-dose administration is 0.63 ± 0.41 (mean ± SD) L/kg of body weight. Pioglitazone is extensively protein bound (> 99%) in human serum, principally to serum albumin. Pioglitazone also binds to other serum proteins, but with lower affinity. Metabolites M-III and M-IV also are extensively bound (> 98%) to serum albumin.
Glimepiride
After intravenous (IV) dosing in normal subjects, Vd/F was 8.8 L (113 mL/kg), and the total body clearance (CL) was 47.8 mL/min. Protein binding was greater than 99.5%.
Metabolism:
Pioglitazone hydrochloride
Pioglitazone is extensively metabolized by hydroxylation and oxidation; the metabolites also partly convert to glucuronide or sulfate conjugates. Metabolites M-II and M-IV (hydroxy derivatives of pioglitazone) and M-III (keto derivative of pioglitazone) are pharmacologically active in animal models of type 2 diabetes. In addition to pioglitazone, M-III and M-IV are the principal drug-related species found in human serum following multiple dosing. At steady-state, in both healthy volunteers and in patients with type 2 diabe-

tes, pioglitazone comprises approximately 30% to 50% of the total peak serum concentrations and 20% to 25% of the total AUC.

In vitro data demonstrate that multiple CYP isoforms are involved in the metabolism of pioglitazone. The cytochrome P450 isoforms involved are CYP2C8 and, to a lesser degree, CYP3A4 with additional contributions from a variety of other isoforms including the mainly extrahepatic CYP1A1. *In vivo* studies of pioglitazone in combination with P450 inhibitors and substrates have been performed (see **PRECAUTIONS, Drug Interactions,** *Pioglitazone hydrochloride*). Urinary 6β-hydroxycortisol/cortisol ratios measured in patients treated with pioglitazone showed that pioglitazone is not a strong CYP3A4 enzyme inducer.

Glimepiride

Glimepiride is completely metabolized by oxidative biotransformation after either an IV or oral dose. The major metabolites are the cyclohexyl hydroxy methyl derivative (M1) and the carboxyl derivative (M2). CYP2C9 has been shown to be involved in the biotransformation of glimepiride to M1. M1 is further metabolized to M2 by one or several cytosolic enzymes. M1, but not M2, possesses about 1/3 of the pharmacological activity as compared to its parent in an animal model; however, whether the glucose-lowering effect of M1 is clinically meaningful is not clear.

Excretion and Elimination:

Pioglitazone hydrochloride

Following oral administration, approximately 15% to 30% of the pioglitazone dose is recovered in the urine. Renal elimination of pioglitazone is negligible and the drug is excreted primarily as metabolites and their conjugates. It is presumed that most of the oral dose is excreted into the bile either unchanged or as metabolites and eliminated in the feces.

The mean serum half-life of pioglitazone and total pioglitazone ranges from 3 to 7 hours and 16 to 24 hours, respectively. Pioglitazone has an apparent clearance, CL/f, calculated to be 5 to 7 L/hr.

Glimepiride

When ^{14}C-glimepiride was given orally, approximately 60% of the total radioactivity was recovered in the urine in 7 days and M1 (predominant) and M2 accounted for 80-90% of that recovered in the urine. Approximately 40% of the total radioactivity was recovered in feces and M1 and M2 (predominant) accounted for about 70% of that recovered in feces. No parent drug was recovered from urine or feces. After IV dosing in patients, no significant biliary excretion of glimepiride or its M1 metabolite has been observed.

Special Populations

Renal Insufficiency:

Pioglitazone hydrochloride

The serum elimination half-life of pioglitazone, M-III and M-IV remains unchanged in patients with moderate (creatinine clearance 30 to 60 mL/min) to severe (creatinine clearance < 30 mL/min) renal impairment when compared to normal subjects. No dose adjustment in patients with renal dysfunction is recommended.

Glimepiride

A single-dose, open-label study was conducted in 15 patients with renal impairment. Glimepiride (3 mg) was administered to 3 groups of patients with different levels of mean creatinine clearance (CLcr); (Group I, CLcr = 77.7 mL/min, n = 5), (Group II, CLcr = 27.7 mL/min, n = 3), and (Group III, CLcr = 9.4 mL/min, n = 7). Glimepiride was found to be well tolerated in all 3 groups. The results showed that glimepiride serum levels decreased as renal function decreased. However, M1 and M2 serum levels (mean AUC values) increased 2.3 and 8.6 times from Group I to Group III. The apparent terminal half-life ($T_{1/2}$) for glimepiride did not change, while the half-lives for M1 and M2 increased as renal function decreased. Mean urinary excretion of M1 plus M2 as percent of dose, however, decreased (44.4%, 21.9%, and 9.3% for Groups I to III).

A multiple-dose titration study was also conducted in 16 patients with type 2 diabetes and with renal impairment using doses ranging from 1-8 mg daily for 3 months. The results were consistent with those observed after single doses. All patients with a CLcr less than 22 mL/min had adequate control of their glucose levels with a dosage regimen of only 1 mg daily. The results from this study suggested that a starting dose of 1 mg glimepiride may be given to patients with type 2 diabetes and kidney disease, and the dose may be titrated based on fasting blood glucose levels (see **DOSAGE AND ADMINISTRATION, Special Patient Populations**).

Hepatic Insufficiency:

Pioglitazone hydrochloride

Compared with normal controls, subjects with impaired hepatic function (Child-Pugh Grade B/C) have an approximate 45% reduction in pioglitazone and total pioglitazone mean peak concentrations but no change in the mean AUC values. Therapy with DUETACT should not be initiated if the patient exhibits clinical evidence of active liver disease or serum transaminase levels (ALT) exceed 2.5 times the upper limit of normal (see **PRECAUTIONS, General: *Pioglitazone hydrochloride,*** Hepatic Effects).

Glimepiride

No studies were performed in patients with hepatic insufficiency.

Elderly:

Pioglitazone hydrochloride

In healthy elderly subjects, peak serum concentrations of pioglitazone and total pioglitazone are not significantly different, but AUC values are slightly higher and the terminal half-life values slightly longer than for younger subjects. These changes were not of a magnitude that would be considered clinically relevant.

Glimepiride

Comparison of glimepiride pharmacokinetics in patients with type 2 diabetes ≤ 65 years and those > 65 years was performed in a study using a dosing regimen of 6 mg daily. There were no significant differences in glimepiride pharmacokinetics between the two age groups. The mean AUC at steady-state for the older patients was about 13% lower than that for the younger patients; the mean weight-adjusted clearance for the older patients was about 11% higher than that for the younger patients.

Pediatrics:

No pharmacokinetic studies of DUETACT were performed in pediatric patients.

Gender:

Pioglitazone hydrochloride

As monotherapy and in combination with sulfonylurea, metformin, or insulin, pioglitazone improved glycemic control in both males and females. The mean C_{max} and AUC values were increased 20% to 60% in females. In controlled clinical trials, hemoglobin A1C (A1C) decreases from baseline were generally greater for females than for males (average mean difference in A1C 0.5%). Since therapy should be individualized for each patient to achieve glycemic control, no dose adjustment is recommended based on gender alone.

Glimepiride

There were no differences between males and females in the pharmacokinetics of glimepiride when adjustment was made for differences in body weight.

Ethnicity:

Pioglitazone hydrochloride

Pharmacokinetic data among various ethnic groups are not available.

Glimepiride

No pharmacokinetic studies to assess the effects of race have been performed, but in placebo-controlled studies of glimepiride in patients with type 2 diabetes, the antihyperglycemic effect was comparable in whites (n = 536), blacks (n = 63), and Hispanics (n = 63).

Other Populations:

Glimepiride

There were no important differences in glimepiride metabolism in subjects identified as phenotypically different drug-metabolizers by their metabolism of sparteine. The pharmacokinetics of glimepiride in morbidly obese patients were similar to those in the normal weight group, except for a lower C_{max} and AUC. However, since neither C_{max} nor AUC values were normalized for body surface area, the lower values of C_{max} and AUC for the obese patients were likely the result of their excess weight and not due to a difference in the kinetics of glimepiride.

Drug-Drug Interactions

Co-administration of pioglitazone (45 mg) and a sulfonylurea (5 mg glipizide) administered orally once daily for 7 days did not alter the steady-state pharmacokinetics of glipizide. Glimepiride and glipizide have similar metabolic pathways and are mediated by CYP2C9; therefore, drug-drug interaction between pioglitazone and glimepiride is considered unlikely. Specific pharmacokinetic drug interaction studies with DUETACT have not been performed, although such studies have been conducted with the individual pioglitazone and glimepiride components.

Pioglitazone hydrochloride

The following drugs were studied in healthy volunteers with co-administration of pioglitazone 45 mg once daily. Results are listed below:

Oral Contraceptives: Co-administration of pioglitazone (45 mg once daily) and an oral contraceptive (1 mg norethindrone plus 0.035 mg ethinyl estradiol once daily) for 21 days, resulted in 11% and 11-14% decrease in ethinyl estradiol AUC (0-24h) and C_{max} respectively. There were no significant changes in norethindrone AUC (0-24h) and C_{max}. In view of the high variability of ethinyl estradiol pharmacokinetics, the clinical significance of this finding is unknown.

Midazolam: Administration of pioglitazone for 15 days followed by a single 7.5 mg dose of midazolam syrup resulted in a 26% reduction in midazolam C_{max} and AUC.

Nifedipine ER: Co-administration of pioglitazone for 7 days with 30 mg nifedipine ER administered orally once daily for 4 days to male and female volunteers resulted in a ratio of least square mean (90% CI) values for unchanged nifedipine of 0.83 (0.73 - 0.95) for C_{max} and 0.88 (0.80 - 0.96) for AUC. In view of the high variability of nifedipine pharmacokinetics, the clinical significance of this finding is unknown.

Ketoconazole: Co-administration of pioglitazone for 7 days with ketoconazole 200 mg administered twice daily resulted in a ratio of least square mean (90% CI) values for unchanged pioglitazone of 1.14 (1.06 - 1.23) for C_{max}, 1.34 (1.26 - 1.41) for AUC and 1.87 (1.71 - 2.04) for C_{min}.

Atorvastatin Calcium: Co-administration of pioglitazone for 7 days with atorvastatin calcium (LIPITOR®) 80 mg once daily resulted in a ratio of least square mean (90% CI) values for unchanged pioglitazone of 0.69 (0.57 - 0.85) for C_{max}, 0.76 (0.65 - 0.88) for AUC and 0.96 (0.87 - 1.05) for C_{min}. For unchanged atorvastatin, the ratio of least square mean (90% CI) values were 0.77 (0.66 - 0.90) for C_{max}, 0.86 (0.78 - 0.94) for AUC and 0.92 (0.82 - 1.02) for C_{min}.

Cytochrome P450: See **PRECAUTIONS, Drug Interactions,** *Pioglitazone hydrochloride*

Gemfibrozil: Concomitant administration of gemfibrozil (oral 600 mg twice daily), an inhibitor of CYP2C8, with pioglitazone (oral 30 mg) in 10 healthy volunteers pre-treated for 2 days prior with gemfibrozil (oral 600 mg twice daily) resulted in pioglitazone exposure (AUC_{0-24}) being 226% of the pioglitazone exposure in the absence of gemfibrozil (see **PRECAUTIONS, Drug Interactions,** *Pioglitazone hydrochloride*).[1]

Rifampin: Concomitant administration of rifampin (oral 600 mg once daily), an inducer of CYP2C8 with pioglitazone (oral 30 mg) in 10 healthy volunteers pre-treated for 5 days prior with rifampin (oral 600 mg once daily) resulted in a decrease in the AUC of pioglitazone by 54% (see **PRECAUTIONS, Drug Interactions,** *Pioglitazone hydrochloride*).[2]

In other drug-drug interaction studies, pioglitazone had no significant effect on the pharmacokinetics of fexofenadine, metformin, digoxin, warfarin, ranitidine, or theophylline.

Glimepiride

The hypoglycemic action of sulfonylureas may be potentiated by certain drugs, including nonsteroidal anti-inflammatory drugs and other drugs that are highly protein bound, such as salicylates, sulfonamides, chloramphenicol, coumarins, probenecid, monoamine oxidase inhibitors, and beta adrenergic blocking agents. Due to the potential drug interaction between these drugs and glimepiride, the patient should be observed closely for hypoglycemia when these drugs are co-administered. Conversely, when these drugs are withdrawn, the patient should be observed closely for loss of glycemic control.

Certain drugs tend to produce hyperglycemia and may lead to loss of control. These drugs include the thiazides and other diuretics, corticosteroids, phenothiazines, thyroid products, estrogens, oral contraceptives, phenytoin, nicotinic acid, sympathomimetics, and isoniazid. Due to the potential drug interaction between these drugs and glimepiride, the patient should be observed closely for loss of glycemic control when these drugs are co-administered. Conversely, when these drugs are withdrawn, the patient should be observed closely for hypoglycemia.

Aspirin: Co-administration of aspirin (1 g three times daily) and glimepiride led to a 34% decrease in the mean glimepiride AUC and, therefore, a 34% increase in the mean CL/f. The mean C_{max} had a decrease of 4%. Blood glucose and serum C-peptide concentrations were unaffected and no hypoglycemic symptoms were reported. Pooled data from clinical trials showed no evidence of clinically significant adverse interactions with uncontrolled concurrent administration of aspirin and other salicylates.

Cimetidine/Ranitidine: Co-administration of either cimetidine (800 mg once daily) or ranitidine (150 mg twice daily) with a single 4-mg oral dose of glimepiride did not significantly alter the absorption and disposition of glimepiride, and no differences were seen in hypoglycemic symptomatology. Pooled data from clinical trials showed no evidence of clinically significant adverse interactions with uncontrolled concurrent administration of H2-receptor antagonists.

Propranolol: Concomitant administration of propranolol (40 mg three times daily) and glimepiride significantly increased C_{max}, AUC, and $T_{1/2}$ of glimepiride by 23%, 22%, and 15%, respectively, and it decreased CL/f by 18%. The recovery of M1 and M2 from urine, however, did not change. The pharmacodynamic responses to glimepiride were nearly identical in normal subjects receiving propranolol and placebo. Pooled data from clinical trials in patients with type 2 diabetes showed no evidence of clinically significant adverse interactions with uncontrolled concurrent administration of beta-blockers. However, if beta-blockers are used, caution should be exercised and patients should be warned about the potential for hypoglycemia.

Warfarin: Concomitant administration of glimepiride (4 mg once daily) did not alter the pharmacokinetic characteristics of R- and S-warfarin enantiomers following administration of a single dose (25 mg) of racemic warfarin to healthy subjects. No changes were observed in warfarin plasma protein binding. Glimepiride treatment did result in a slight, but statistically significant, decrease in the pharmacodynamic response to warfarin. The reductions in mean area under the prothrombin time (PT) curve and maximum PT values during glimepiride treatment were very small (3.3% and 9.9%, respectively) and are unlikely to be clinically important.

Ramipril: The responses of serum glucose, insulin, C-peptide, and plasma glucagon to 2 mg glimepiride were unaffected by co-administration of ramipril (an ACE inhibitor) 5 mg once daily in normal subjects. No hypoglycemic symptoms were reported. Pooled data from clinical trials in patients with type 2 diabetes showed no evidence of clinically significant adverse interactions with uncontrolled concurrent administration of ACE inhibitors.

Miconazole: A potential interaction between oral miconazole and oral hypoglycemic agents leading to severe hypoglycemia has been reported. Whether this interaction also occurs with the intravenous, topical, or vaginal preparations of miconazole is not known. There is a potential interaction of glimepiride with inhibitors (e.g. fluconazole) and inducers (e.g. rifampicin) of cytochrome P450 2C9.

Although no specific interaction studies were performed with glimepiride, pooled data from clinical trials showed no evidence of clinically significant adverse interactions with uncontrolled concurrent administration of calcium-channel blockers, estrogens, fibrates, NSAIDS, HMG CoA reductase inhibitors, sulfonamides, or thyroid hormone.

Continued on next page

Duetact—Cont.

Pharmacodynamics and Clinical Effects

Pioglitazone hydrochloride

Clinical studies demonstrate that pioglitazone improves insulin sensitivity in insulin-resistant patients. Pioglitazone enhances cellular responsiveness to insulin, increases insulin-dependent glucose disposal, improves hepatic sensitivity to insulin, and improves dysfunctional glucose homeostasis. In patients with type 2 diabetes, the decreased insulin resistance produced by pioglitazone results in lower plasma glucose concentrations, lower plasma insulin levels, and lower A1C values. Based on results from an open-label extension study, the glucose-lowering effects of pioglitazone appear to persist for at least one year. In controlled clinical studies, pioglitazone in combination with a sulfonylurea had an additive effect on glycemic control.

Patients with lipid abnormalities were included in placebo-controlled monotherapy clinical studies with pioglitazone. Overall, patients treated with pioglitazone had mean decreases in triglycerides, mean increases in HDL cholesterol, and no consistent mean changes in LDL cholesterol and total cholesterol compared to the placebo group. A similar pattern of results was seen in 16-week and 24-week combination therapy studies of pioglitazone with a sulfonylurea.

Glimepiride

A mild glucose-lowering effect first appeared following single oral doses as low as 0.5-0.6 mg in healthy subjects. The time required to reach the maximum effect (i.e., minimum blood glucose level [T_{min}]) was about 2 to 3 hours. In patients with type 2 diabetes, both fasting and 2-hour postprandial glucose levels were significantly lower with glimepiride (1, 2, 4, and 8 mg once daily) than with placebo after 14 days of oral dosing. The glucose-lowering effect in all active treatment groups was maintained over 24 hours. In larger dose-ranging studies, blood glucose and A1C were found to respond in a dose-dependent manner over the range of 1 to 4 mg/day of glimepiride. Some patients, particularly those with higher fasting plasma glucose (FPG) levels, may benefit from doses of glimepiride up to 8 mg once daily. No difference in response was found when glimepiride was administered once or twice daily.

In two 14-week, placebo-controlled studies in 720 subjects, the average net reduction in A1C for patients treated with 8 mg of glimepiride once daily was 2.0% in absolute units compared with placebo-treated patients. In a long-term, randomized, placebo-controlled study of patients with type 2 diabetes unresponsive to dietary management, glimepiride therapy improved postprandial insulin/C-peptide responses, and 75% of patients achieved and maintained control of blood glucose and A1C. Efficacy results were not affected by age, gender, weight, or race. In long-term extension trials with previously-treated patients, no meaningful deterioration in mean fasting plasma glucose (FPG) or A1C levels was seen after 2 1/2 years of glimepiride therapy.

Glimepiride therapy is effective in controlling blood glucose without deleterious changes in the plasma lipoprotein profiles of patients treated for type 2 diabetes.

Clinical Studies

There have been no clinical efficacy studies conducted with DUETACT. However, the efficacy and safety of the separate components have been previously established. The co-administration of pioglitazone and a sulfonylurea, including glimepiride, has been evaluated for efficacy and safety in two clinical studies. These clinical studies established an added-benefit of pioglitazone in glycemic control of patients with inadequately controlled type 2 diabetes while on sulfonylurea therapy. Bioequivalence of DUETACT with co-administered pioglitazone and glimepiride tablets was demonstrated at the 30 mg/2 mg and 30 mg/4 mg dosage strengths (see **CLINICAL PHARMACOLOGY, Pharmacokinetics and Drug Metabolism, Absorption and Bioavailability**).

Clinical Studies of Pioglitazone Add-On Therapy in Patients Not Adequately Controlled on a Sulfonylurea

Two treatment-randomized, controlled clinical studies in patients with type 2 diabetes were conducted to evaluate the safety and efficacy of pioglitazone plus a sulfonylurea. Both studies included patients receiving a sulfonylurea, either alone or in combination with another antihyperglycemic agent, who had inadequate glycemic control. Excluding the sulfonylurea agent, all other antihyperglycemic agents were discontinued prior to starting study treatment. In the first study, 560 patients were randomized to receive 15 mg or 30 mg of pioglitazone or placebo once daily in addition to their current sulfonylurea regimen for 16 weeks. In the second study, 702 patients were randomized to receive 30 mg or 45 mg of pioglitazone once daily in addition to their current sulfonylurea regimen for 24 weeks.

In the first study, the addition of pioglitazone 15 mg or 30 mg once daily to treatment with a sulfonylurea after 16 weeks significantly reduced the mean A1C by 0.88% and 1.28% and the mean FPG by 39.4 mg/dL and 57.9 mg/dL, respectively, from that observed with sulfonylurea treatment alone. In the second study, the mean reductions from baseline at Week 24 in A1C were 1.55% and 1.67% for the 30 mg and 45 mg doses, respectively. Mean reductions from baseline in FPG were 51.5 mg/dL and 56.1 mg/dL, respectively. Based on these reductions in A1C and FPG (**Table 2**), the addition of pioglitazone to sulfonylurea resulted in significant improvements in glycemic control irrespective of the sulfonylurea dosage.

[See table 2 above]

Table 2. Glycemic Parameters in 16-Week and 24-Week Pioglitazone Hydrochloride + Sulfonylurea Combination Studies

Parameter	Placebo + sulfonylurea	Pioglitazone 15 mg + sulfonylurea	Pioglitazone 30 mg + sulfonylurea
16-Week Study			
A1C (%)	N=181	N=176	N=182
Baseline mean	9.86	10.01	9.93
Mean change from baseline at 16 weeks	0.06	-0.82*†	-1.22*†
Difference in change from placebo + sulfonylurea		-0.88	-1.28
Responder rate (%) (a)	23.8	56.8	74.2
FPG (mg/dL)	N=182	N=179	N=186
Baseline mean	236	246.8	238.9
Mean change from baseline at 16 weeks	5.6	-33.8*†	-52.3*†
Difference in change from placebo + sulfonylurea		-39.4	-57.9
Responder rate (%) (b)	22.0	55.3	67.7

Parameter	Pioglitazone 30 mg + sulfonylurea	Pioglitazone 45 mg + sulfonylurea
24-Week Study		
A1C (%)	N=340	N=332
Baseline mean	9.77	9.85
Mean change from baseline at 24 weeks	-1.55*	-1.67*
Responder rate (%) (a)	77.4	79.5
FPG (mg/dL)	N=338	N=329
Baseline mean	214.4	217.2
Mean change from baseline at 24 weeks	-51.5*	-56.1*
Responder rate (%) (b)	63.6	71.1

* significant change from baseline p ≤ 0.050
† significant difference from placebo plus sulfonylurea, p ≤ 0.050
(a) patients who achieved an A1C ≤ 6.1% or ≥ 0.6% decrease from baseline
(b) patients who achieved a decrease in FPG by ≥ 30 mg/dL

[See table above]

INDICATIONS AND USAGE

DUETACT is indicated as an adjunct to diet and exercise as a once-daily combination therapy to improve glycemic control in patients with type 2 diabetes who are already treated with a combination of pioglitazone and a sulfonylurea or whose diabetes is not adequately controlled with a sulfonylurea alone, or for those patients who have initially responded to pioglitazone alone and require additional glycemic control.

Management of type 2 diabetes should also include nutritional counseling, weight reduction as needed, and exercise. These efforts are important not only in the primary treatment of type 2 diabetes, but also to maintain the efficacy of drug therapy.

CONTRAINDICATIONS

Initiation of DUETACT in patients with established New York Heart Association (NYHA) Class III or IV heart failure is contraindicated (see **BOXED WARNING**).

In addition, DUETACT is contraindicated in patients with:
1. Known hypersensitivity to pioglitazone, glimepiride or any other component of DUETACT.
2. Diabetic ketoacidosis, with or without coma. This condition should be treated with insulin.

WARNINGS

Glimepiride

SPECIAL WARNING ON INCREASED RISK OF CARDIOVASCULAR MORTALITY

The administration of oral hypoglycemic drugs has been reported to be associated with increased cardiovascular mortality as compared to treatment with diet alone or diet plus insulin. This warning is based on the study conducted by the University Group Diabetes Program (UGDP), a long-term, prospective clinical trial designed to evaluate the effectiveness of glucose-lowering drugs in preventing or delaying vascular complications in patients with non-insulin-dependent diabetes. The study involved 823 patients who were randomly assigned to one of four treatment groups (Diabetes, 19 supp. 2: 747–830, 1970).

UGDP reported that patients treated for 5 to 8 years with diet plus a fixed dose of tolbutamide (1.5 grams per day) had a rate of cardiovascular mortality approximately 2-1/2 times that of patients treated with diet alone. A significant increase in total mortality was not observed, but the use of tolbutamide was discontinued based on the increase in cardiovascular mortality, thus limiting the opportunity for the study to show an increase in overall mortality. Despite controversy regarding the interpretation of these results, the findings of the UGDP study provide an adequate basis for this warning. The patient should be informed of the potential risks and advantages of glimepiride tablets and of alternative modes of therapy.

Although only one drug in the sulfonylurea class (tolbutamide) was included in this study, it is prudent from a safety standpoint to consider that this warning may also apply to other oral hypoglycemic drugs in this class, in view of their close similarities in mode of action and chemical structure.

Pioglitazone hydrochloride

Cardiac Failure and Other Cardiac Effects

Pioglitazone, like other thiazolidinediones, can cause fluid retention when used alone or in combination with other antidiabetic agents, including insulin. Fluid retention may lead to or exacerbate heart failure. Patients should be observed for signs and symptoms of heart failure. If these signs and symptoms develop, the heart failure should be managed according to current standards of care. Furthermore, discontinuation or dose reduction of pioglitazone must be considered. Patients with NYHA Class III and IV cardiac status were not studied during pre-approval clinical trials and pioglitazone is not recommended in these patients (see **BOXED WARNING** and **CONTRAINDICATIONS**).

In one 16-week U.S. double-blind, placebo-controlled clinical trial involving 566 patients with type 2 diabetes, pioglitazone at doses of 15 mg and 30 mg in combination with insulin was compared to insulin therapy alone. This trial included patients with long-standing diabetes and a high prevalence of pre-existing medical conditions as follows: arterial hypertension (57.2%), peripheral neuropathy (22.6%), coronary heart disease (19.6%), retinopathy (13.1%), myocardial infarction (8.8%), vascular disease (6.4%), angina pectoris (4.4%), stroke and/or transient ischemic attack (4.1%), and congestive heart failure (2.3%). In this study, two of the 191 patients receiving 15 mg pioglitazone plus insulin (1.1%) and two of the 188 patients receiving 30 mg pioglitazone plus insulin (1.1%) developed congestive heart failure compared with none of the 187 patients on insulin therapy alone. All four of these patients had previous histories of cardiovascular conditions including coronary artery disease, previous CABG procedures, and myocardial infarction. In a 24-week dose-controlled study in which pioglitazone was coadministered with insulin, 0.3% of patients (1/345) on 30 mg and 0.9% (3/345) of patients on 45 mg reported CHF as a serious adverse event. Analysis of data from these studies did not identify specific factors that predict increased risk of congestive heart failure on combination therapy with insulin.

In type 2 diabetes and congestive heart failure (systolic dysfunction)

A 24-week post-marketing safety study was performed to compare pioglitazone (n=262) to glyburide (n=256) in uncontrolled diabetic patients (mean A1C 8.8% at baseline) with NYHA Class II and III heart failure and ejection fraction less than 40% (mean EF 30% at baseline). Over the course of the study, overnight hospitalization for congestive heart failure was reported in 9.9% of patients on pioglitazone compared to 4.7% of patients on glyburide with a treatment difference observed from 6 weeks. This adverse event associated with pioglitazone was more marked in patients using insulin at baseline and in patients over 64 years of age. No difference in cardiovascular mortality between the treatment groups was observed.

Pioglitazone should be initiated at the lowest approved dose if it is prescribed for patients with type 2 diabetes and systolic heart failure (NYHA Class II). If subsequent dose escalation is necessary, the dose should be increased gradually only after several months of treatment with careful monitoring for weight gain, edema, or signs and symptoms of CHF exacerbation (see **DOSAGE AND ADMINISTRATION, Special Patient Populations**).

Prospective Pioglitazone Clinical Trial In Macrovascular Events (PROactive)

In PROactive, 5238 patients with type 2 diabetes and a prior history of macrovascular disease were treated with ACTOS (n=2605), force-titrated up to 45 mg once daily, or placebo (n=2633) (see **ADVERSE REACTIONS**). The percentage of patients who had an event of serious heart failure was higher for patients treated with ACTOS (5.7%, n=149) than for patients treated with placebo (4.1%, n=108). The incidence of death subsequent to a report of serious heart failure was 1.5% (n=40) in patients treated with ACTOS and 1.4% (n=37) in placebo-treated patients. In patients treated with an insulin-containing regimen at baseline, the incidence of serious heart failure was 6.3% (n=54/864) with ACTOS and 5.2% (n=47/896) with placebo. For those patients treated with a sulfonylurea-containing regimen at baseline, the incidence of serious heart failure was 5.8% (n=94/1624) with ACTOS and 4.4% (n=71/1626) with placebo.

Table 3. Weight Changes (kg) from Baseline During Double-Blind Clinical Trials with Pioglitazone

		Control Group (Placebo)	pioglitazone 15 mg	pioglitazone 30 mg	pioglitazone 45 mg
		Median ($25^{th}/75^{th}$ percentile)	Median ($25^{th}/75^{th}$ percentile)	Median ($25^{th}/75^{th}$ percentile)	Median ($25^{th}/75^{th}$ percentile)
Monotherapy		-1.4 (-2.7/0.0) n=256	0.9 (-0.5/3.4) n=79	1.0 (-0.9/3.4) n=188	2.6 (0.2/5.4) n=79
Combination Therapy	**Sulfonylurea**	-0.5 (-1.8/0.7) n=187	2.0 (0.2/3.2) n=183	3.1 (1.1/5.4) n=528	4.1 (1.8/7.3) n=333
	Metformin	-1.4 (-3.2/0.3) n=160	N/A	0.9 (-0.3/3.2) n=567	1.8 (-0.9/5.0) n=407
	Insulin	0.2 (-1.4/1.4) n=182	2.3 (0.5/4.3) n=190	3.3 (0.9/6.3) n=522	4.1 (1.4/6.8) n=338

Note: Trial durations of 16 to 26 weeks

PRECAUTIONS

General: ***Pioglitazone hydrochloride***

Pioglitazone exerts its antihyperglycemic effect only in the presence of insulin. Therefore, DUETACT should not be used in patients with type 1 diabetes or for the treatment of diabetic ketoacidosis.

Hypoglycemia: Patients receiving pioglitazone in combination with insulin or oral hypoglycemic agents may be at risk for hypoglycemia, and a reduction in the dose of the concomitant agent may be necessary.

Cardiovascular: In U.S. placebo-controlled clinical trials that excluded patients with New York Heart Association (NYHA) Class III and IV cardiac status, the incidence of serious cardiac adverse events related to volume expansion was not increased in patients treated with pioglitazone as monotherapy or in combination with sulfonylureas or metformin vs. placebo-treated patients. In insulin combination studies, a small number of patients with a history of previously existing cardiac disease developed congestive heart failure when treated with pioglitazone in combination with insulin (see **WARNINGS, *Pioglitazone hydrochloride*, Cardiac Failure and Other Cardiac Effects**). Patients with NYHA Class III and IV cardiac status were not studied in pre-approval pioglitazone clinical trials. Pioglitazone is not indicated in patients with NYHA Class III or IV cardiac status.

In postmarketing experience with pioglitazone, cases of congestive heart failure have been reported in patients both with and without previously known heart disease.

Edema: In all U.S. clinical trials with pioglitazone, edema was reported more frequently in patients treated with pioglitazone than in placebo-treated patients and appears to be dose related (see **ADVERSE REACTIONS,** *Pioglitazone hydrochloride*). In postmarketing experience, reports of initiation or worsening of edema have been received. Since thiazolidinediones, including pioglitazone, can cause fluid retention, which can exacerbate or lead to congestive heart failure, DUETACT should be used with caution in patients at risk for heart failure. Patients should be monitored for signs and symptoms of heart failure (see **BOXED WARNING, WARNINGS, *Pioglitazone hydrochloride* and PRECAUTIONS, Information for Patients**).

Weight Gain: Dose related weight gain was observed with pioglitazone alone and in combination with other hypoglycemic agents **(Table 3)**. The mechanism of weight gain is unclear but probably involves a combination of fluid retention and fat accumulation.

[See table 3 above]

Ovulation: Therapy with pioglitazone, like other thiazolidinediones, may result in ovulation in some premenopausal anovulatory women. Thus, adequate contraception in premenopausal women should be recommended while taking DUETACT. This possible effect has not been investigated in clinical studies so the frequency of this occurrence is not known.

Hematologic: Across all clinical studies with pioglitazone, mean hemoglobin values declined by 2% to 4% in patients treated with pioglitazone. These changes primarily occurred within the first 4 to 12 weeks of therapy and remained relatively constant thereafter. These changes may be related to increased plasma volume and have rarely been associated with any significant hematologic clinical effects (see **ADVERSE REACTIONS, Laboratory Abnormalities,** *Pioglitazone hydrochloride,* Hematologic). DUETACT may cause decreases in hemoglobin and hematocrit.

Hepatic Effects: In pre-approval clinical studies worldwide, over 4500 subjects were treated with pioglitazone. In U.S. clinical studies, over 4700 patients with type 2 diabetes received pioglitazone. There was no evidence of drug-induced hepatotoxicity or elevation of ALT levels in the clinical studies.

During pre-approval placebo-controlled clinical trials in the U.S., a total of 4 of 1526 (0.26%) patients treated with pioglitazone and 2 of 793 (0.25%) placebo-treated patients had ALT values $\geq$ 3 times the upper limit of normal. The ALT elevations in patients treated with pioglitazone were reversible and were not clearly related to therapy with pioglitazone.

In postmarketing experience with pioglitazone, reports of hepatitis and of hepatic enzyme elevations to 3 or more times the upper limit of normal have been received. Very rarely, these reports have involved hepatic failure with and without fatal outcome, although causality has not been established.

Pending the availability of the results of additional large, long-term controlled clinical trials and additional postmarketing safety data on pioglitazone, it is recommended that patients treated with DUETACT undergo periodic monitoring of liver enzymes.

Serum ALT (alanine aminotransferase) levels should be evaluated prior to the initiation of therapy with DUETACT in all patients and periodically thereafter per the clinical judgment of the health care professional. Liver function tests should also be obtained for patients if symptoms suggestive of hepatic dysfunction occur, e.g., nausea, vomiting, abdominal pain, fatigue, anorexia, or dark urine. The decision whether to continue the patient on therapy with DUETACT should be guided by clinical judgment pending laboratory evaluations. If jaundice is observed, drug therapy should be discontinued.

Therapy with DUETACT should not be initiated if the patient exhibits clinical evidence of active liver disease or the ALT levels exceed 2.5 times the upper limit of normal. Patients with mildly elevated liver enzymes (ALT levels at 1 to 2.5 times the upper limit of normal) at baseline or any time during therapy with DUETACT should be evaluated to determine the cause of the liver enzyme elevation. Initiation or continuation of therapy with DUETACT in patients with mildly elevated liver enzymes should proceed with caution and include appropriate clinical follow-up which may include more frequent liver enzyme monitoring. If serum transaminase levels are increased (ALT > 2.5 times the upper limit of normal), liver function tests should be evaluated more frequently until the levels return to normal or pretreatment values. If ALT levels exceed 3 times the upper limit of normal, the test should be repeated as soon as possible. If ALT levels remain > 3 times the upper limit of normal or if the patient is jaundiced, DUETACT therapy should be discontinued.

Macular Edema: Macular edema has been reported in post-marketing experience in diabetic patients who were taking pioglitazone or another thiazolidinedione. Some patients presented with blurred vision or decreased visual acuity, but some patients appear to have been diagnosed on routine ophthalmologic examination. Some patients had peripheral edema at the time macular edema was diagnosed. Some patients had improvement in their macular edema after discontinuation of their thiazolidinedione. It is unknown whether or not there is a causal relationship between pioglitazone and macular edema. Patients with diabetes should have regular eye exams by an ophthalmologist, per the Standards of Care of the American Diabetes Association. Additionally, any diabetic who reports any kind of visual symptom should be promptly referred to an ophthalmologist, regardless of the patient's underlying medications or other physical findings (see **ADVERSE REACTIONS**).

Fractures: In a randomized trial (PROactive) in patients with type 2 diabetes (mean duration of diabetes 9.5 years), an increased incidence of bone fracture was noted in female patients taking pioglitazone. During a mean follow-up of 34.5 months, the incidence of bone fracture in females was 5.1% (44/870) for pioglitazone versus 2.5% (23/905) for placebo. This difference was noted after the first year of treatment and remained during the course of the study. The majority of fractures observed in female patients were nonvertebral fractures including lower limb and distal upper limb. No increase in fracture rates was observed in men treated with pioglitazone 1.7% (30/1735) versus placebo 2.1% (37/1728). The risk of fracture should be considered in the care of patients, especially female patients, treated with pioglitazone and attention should be given to assessing and maintaining bone health according to current standards of care.

General: ***Glimepiride***

Hypoglycemia: All sulfonylurea drugs are capable of producing severe hypoglycemia. Proper patient selection, dosage, and instructions are important to avoid hypoglycemic episodes. Patients with impaired renal function may be more sensitive to the glucose-lowering effect of glimepiride. A starting dose of 1 mg of glimepiride once daily followed by appropriate dose titration is recommended in those patients (see **DOSAGE AND ADMINISTRATION, Special Patient Populations**). Debilitated or malnourished patients, and those with adrenal, pituitary, or hepatic insufficiency are particularly susceptible to the hypoglycemic action of glucose-lowering drugs. Hypoglycemia may be difficult to recognize in the elderly and in people who are taking beta-adrenergic blocking drugs or other sympatholytic agents. Hypoglycemia is more likely to occur when caloric intake is deficient, after severe or prolonged exercise, when alcohol is ingested, or when more than one glucose-lowering drug is used. Combined use of glimepiride with insulin or metformin may increase the potential for hypoglycemia.

Loss of control of blood glucose: When a patient stabilized on any diabetic regimen is exposed to stress such as fever, trauma, infection, or surgery, a loss of control may occur. The effectiveness of any oral hypoglycemic drug, including DUETACT, in lowering blood glucose to a desired level decreases in many patients over a period of time, which may be due to progression of the severity of the diabetes or to diminished responsiveness to the drug.

Laboratory Tests

FPG and A1C measurements should be performed periodically to monitor glycemic control and therapeutic response to DUETACT.

Liver enzyme monitoring is recommended prior to initiation of therapy with DUETACT in all patients and periodically thereafter per the clinical judgment of the health care professional (see **PRECAUTIONS, General: *Pioglitazone hydrochloride,*** Hepatic Effects and **ADVERSE REACTIONS, Laboratory Abnormalities,** *Pioglitazone hydrochloride*, Serum Transaminase Levels).

Information for Patients

Patients should be instructed regarding the importance of adhering to dietary instructions, a regular exercise program, and regular testing of blood glucose and A1C. During periods of stress such as fever, trauma, infection, or surgery, medication requirements may change and patients should be reminded to seek medical advice promptly. Patients should also be informed of the potential risks and advantages of DUETACT and of alternative modes of therapy.

Prior to initiation of DUETACT therapy, the risks of hypoglycemia, its symptoms and treatment, and conditions that predispose to its development should be explained to patients and responsible family members (see **PRECAUTIONS, General: *Pioglitazone hydrochloride* and *Glimepiride*,** Hypoglycemia). Combination therapy of DUETACT with other antihyperglycemic agents may also cause hypoglycemia.

Patients who experience an unusually rapid increase in weight or edema or who develop shortness of breath or other symptoms of heart failure while on DUETACT should immediately report these symptoms to their physician.

Patients should be told that blood tests for liver function will be performed prior to the start of therapy and periodically thereafter per the clinical judgment of the health care professional. Patients should be told to seek immediate medical advice for unexplained nausea, vomiting, abdominal pain, fatigue, anorexia, or dark urine.

Therapy with a thiazolidinedione, including the active pioglitazone component of the DUETACT tablet, may result in ovulation in some premenopausal anovulatory women. As a result, these patients may be at an increased risk for pregnancy while taking DUETACT. This possible effect has not been investigated in clinical studies so the frequency of this occurrence is not known. Thus, adequate contraception in premenopausal women should be recommended. Patients who become pregnant while on DUETACT or are planning a pregnancy should be advised to discuss with their physician a regimen appropriate for maintaining adequate glycemic control (see **PRECAUTIONS, Pregnancy: Pregnancy Category C**).

Patients should be told to take a single dose of DUETACT once daily with the first main meal and instructed that any change in dosing should be made only if directed by their physician (see **DOSAGE AND ADMINISTRATION, Maximum Recommended Dose**).

Drug Interactions

Pioglitazone hydrochloride

In vivo drug-drug interaction studies have suggested that pioglitazone may be a weak inducer of CYP 450 isoform 3A4 substrate.

Continued on next page

Duetact—Cont.

An enzyme inhibitor of CYP2C8 (such as gemfibrozil) may significantly increase the AUC of pioglitazone and an enzyme inducer of CYP2C8 (such as rifampin) may significantly decrease the AUC of pioglitazone. Therefore, if an inhibitor or inducer of CYP2C8 is started or stopped during treatment with pioglitazone, changes in diabetes treatment may be needed based on clinical response (see **CLINICAL PHARMACOLOGY, Drug-Drug Interactions,** *Pioglitazone hydrochloride*).

Glimepiride

(See **CLINICAL PHARMACOLOGY, Drug-Drug Interactions,** *Glimepiride*)

Carcinogenesis, Mutagenesis, Impairment of Fertility

DUETACT

No animal studies have been conducted with DUETACT. The following data are based on findings in studies performed with pioglitazone or glimepiride individually.

Pioglitazone hydrochloride

A two-year carcinogenicity study was conducted in male and female rats at oral doses up to 63 mg/kg (approximately 14 times the maximum recommended human oral dose of 45 mg based on mg/m^2). Drug-induced tumors were not observed in any organ except for the urinary bladder. Benign and/or malignant transitional cell neoplasms were observed in male rats at 4 mg/kg/day and above (approximately equal to the maximum recommended human oral dose based on mg/m^2). A two-year carcinogenicity study was conducted in male and female mice at oral doses up to 100 mg/kg/day (approximately 11 times the maximum recommended human oral dose based on mg/m^2). No drug-induced tumors were observed in any organ.

During prospective evaluation of urinary cytology involving more than 1800 patients receiving pioglitazone in clinical trials up to one year in duration, no new cases of bladder tumors were identified. In two 3 year studies in which pioglitazone was compared to placebo or glyburide, there were 16/3656 (0.44%) reports of bladder cancer in patients taking pioglitazone compared to 5/3679 (0.14%) in patients not taking pioglitazone. After excluding patients in whom exposure to study drug was less than one year at the time of diagnosis of bladder cancer, there were six cases (0.16%) on pioglitazone and two (0.05%) on placebo.

Pioglitazone hydrochloride was not mutagenic in a battery of genetic toxicology studies, including the Ames bacterial assay, a mammalian cell forward gene mutation assay (CHO/HPRT and AS52/XPRT), an *in vitro* cytogenetics assay using CHL cells, an unscheduled DNA synthesis assay, and an *in vivo* micronucleus assay.

No adverse effects upon fertility were observed in male and female rats at oral doses up to 40 mg/kg pioglitazone hydrochloride daily prior to and throughout mating and gestation (approximately 9 times the maximum recommended human oral dose based on mg/m^2).

Glimepiride

Studies in rats at doses of up to 5000 ppm in complete feed (approximately 340 times the maximum recommended human dose, based on surface area) for 30 months showed no evidence of carcinogenesis. In mice, administration of glimepiride for 24 months resulted in an increase in benign pancreatic adenoma formation which was dose related and is thought to be the result of chronic pancreatic stimulation. The no-effect dose for adenoma formation in mice in this study was 320 ppm in complete feed, or 46-54 mg/kg body weight/day. This is about 35 times the maximum human recommended dose of 8 mg once daily based on surface area.

Glimepiride was non-mutagenic in a battery of *in vitro* and *in vivo* mutagenicity studies (Ames test, somatic cell mutation, chromosomal aberration, unscheduled DNA synthesis, mouse micronucleus test).

There was no effect of glimepiride on male mouse fertility in animals exposed up to 2500 mg/kg body weight (>1,700 times the maximum recommended human dose based on surface area). Glimepiride had no effect on the fertility of male and female rats administered up to 4000 mg/kg body weight (approximately 4,000 times the maximum recommended human dose based on surface area).

Animal Toxicology

Pioglitazone hydrochloride

Heart enlargement has been observed in mice (100 mg/kg), rats (4 mg/kg and above) and dogs (3 mg/kg) treated orally with pioglitazone hydrochloride (approximately 11, 1, and 2 times the maximum recommended human oral dose for mice, rats, and dogs, respectively, based on mg/m^2). In a one-year rat study, drug-related early death due to apparent heart dysfunction occurred at an oral dose of 160 mg/kg/day (approximately 35 times the maximum recommended human oral dose based on mg/m^2). Heart enlargement was seen in a 13-week study in monkeys at oral doses of 8.9 mg/kg and above (approximately 4 times the maximum recommended human oral dose based on mg/m^2), but not in a 52-week study at oral doses up to 32 mg/kg (approximately 13 times the maximum recommended human oral dose based on mg/m^2).

Glimepiride

Reduced serum glucose values and degranulation of the pancreatic beta cells were observed in beagle dogs exposed to 320 mg glimepiride/kg/day for 12 months (approximately 1,000 times the recommended human dose based on surface area). No evidence of tumor formation was observed in any organ. One female and one male dog developed bilateral subcapsular cataracts. Non-GLP studies indicated that glimepiride was unlikely to exacerbate cataract formation. Evaluation of the co-cataractogenic potential of glimepiride in several diabetic and cataract rat models was negative and there was no adverse effect of glimepiride on bovine ocular lens metabolism in organ culture.

Pregnancy: Pregnancy Category C

DUETACT

Because current information strongly suggests that abnormal blood glucose levels during pregnancy are associated with a higher incidence of congenital anomalies, as well as increased neonatal morbidity and mortality, most experts recommend that insulin be used during pregnancy to maintain blood glucose levels as close to normal as possible. DUETACT should not be used during pregnancy unless the potential benefit justifies the potential risk to the fetus.

There are no adequate and well-controlled studies in pregnant women with DUETACT or its individual components. No animal studies have been conducted with the combined products in DUETACT. The following data are based on findings in studies performed with pioglitazone or glimepiride individually.

Pioglitazone hydrochloride

Pioglitazone was not teratogenic in rats at oral doses up to 80 mg/kg or in rabbits given up to 160 mg/kg during organogenesis (approximately 17 and 40 times the maximum recommended human oral dose based on mg/m^2, respectively). Delayed parturition and embryotoxicity (as evidenced by increased postimplantation losses, delayed development and reduced fetal weights) were observed in rats at oral doses of 40 mg/kg/day and above (approximately 10 times the maximum recommended human oral dose based on mg/m^2). No functional or behavioral toxicity was observed in offspring of rats. In rabbits, embryotoxicity was observed at an oral dose of 160 mg/kg (approximately 40 times the maximum recommended human oral dose based on mg/m^2). Delayed postnatal development, attributed to decreased body weight, was observed in offspring of rats at oral doses of 10 mg/kg and above during late gestation and lactation periods (approximately 2 times the maximum recommended human oral dose based on mg/m^2).

Glimepiride

Teratogenic Effects: Glimepiride did not produce teratogenic effects in rats exposed orally up to 4000 mg/kg body weight (approximately 4000 times the maximum recommended human dose based on surface area) or in rabbits exposed up to 32 mg/kg body weight (approximately 60 times the maximum recommended human dose based on surface area). Glimepiride has been shown to be associated with intrauterine fetal death in rats when given in doses as low as 50 times the human dose based on surface area and in rabbits when given in doses as low as 0.1 times the human dose based on surface area. This fetotoxicity, observed only at doses inducing maternal hypoglycemia, has been similarly noted with other sulfonylureas, and is believed to be directly related to the pharmacologic (hypoglycemic) action of glimepiride.

Nonteratogenic Effects: In some studies in rats, offspring of dams exposed to high levels of glimepiride during pregnancy and lactation developed skeletal deformities consisting of shortening, thickening, and bending of the humerus during the postnatal period. Significant concentrations of glimepiride were observed in the serum and breast milk of the dams as well as in the serum of the pups. These skeletal deformations were determined to be the result of nursing from mothers exposed to glimepiride.

Prolonged severe hypoglycemia (4 to 10 days) has been reported in neonates born to mothers who were receiving a sulfonylurea drug at the time of delivery. This has been reported more frequently with the use of agents with prolonged half-lives. Patients who are planning a pregnancy should consult their physician, and it is recommended that they change over to insulin for the entire course of pregnancy and lactation.

Nursing Mothers

No studies have been conducted with the combined components of DUETACT. In studies performed with the individual components, pioglitazone was secreted in the milk of lactating rats and significant concentrations of glimepiride were observed in the serum and breast milk of the dams and serum of the pups. It is not known whether pioglitazone or glimepiride are secreted in human milk. However, other sulfonylureas are excreted in human milk. Because the potential for hypoglycemia in nursing infants may exist, and because of the effects on nursing animals, DUETACT should not be administered to a woman breastfeeding. If DUETACT is discontinued, and if diet alone is inadequate for controlling blood glucose, insulin therapy should be considered (see **PRECAUTIONS, Pregnancy: Pregnancy Category C,** *Glimepiride*, Nonteratogenic Effects).

Pediatric Use

Safety and effectiveness of DUETACT in pediatric patients have not been established.

Elderly Use

Pioglitazone hydrochloride

Approximately 500 patients in placebo-controlled clinical trials of pioglitazone were 65 and over. No significant differences in effectiveness and safety were observed between these patients and younger patients.

Glimepiride

In U.S. clinical studies of glimepiride, 608 of 1986 patients were 65 and over. No overall differences in safety or effectiveness were observed between these subjects and younger subjects, but greater sensitivity of some older individuals cannot be ruled out.

Comparison of glimepiride pharmacokinetics in patients with type 2 diabetes ≤ 65 years (n=49) and those > 65 years (n=42) was performed in a study using a dosing regimen of 6 mg daily. There were no significant differences in glimepiride pharmacokinetics between the two age groups (see **CLINICAL PHARMACOLOGY, Special Populations, Elderly:** *Glimepiride*).

Glimepiride is known to be substantially excreted by the kidney, and the risk of toxic reactions to this drug may be greater in patients with impaired renal function. Because elderly patients are more likely to have decreased renal function, care should be taken in dose selection, and it may be useful to monitor renal function.

Elderly patients are particularly susceptible to hypoglycemic action of glucose-lowering drugs. In elderly, debilitated, or malnourished patients, or in patients with renal and hepatic insufficiency, the initial dosing, dose increments, and maintenance dosage should be conservative based upon blood glucose levels prior to and after initiation of treatment to avoid hypoglycemic reactions. Hypoglycemia may be difficult to recognize in the elderly and in people who are taking beta-adrenergic blocking drugs or other sympatholytic agents (see **CLINICAL PHARMACOLOGY, Special Populations, Renal Insufficiency:** *Glimepiride*; **PRECAUTIONS, General:** ***Glimepiride***, Hypoglycemia and **DOSAGE AND ADMINISTRATION, Special Patient Populations**).

ADVERSE REACTIONS

The adverse events reported in at least 5% of patients in the controlled 16-week clinical studies between placebo plus a sulfonylurea and pioglitazone (15 mg and 30 mg combined) plus sulfonylurea-treatment arms were upper respiratory tract infection (15.5% and 16.6%), accidental injury (8.6% and 3.5%) and combined edema/peripheral edema (2.1% and 7.2%), respectively.

The incidence and type of adverse events reported in at least 5% of patients in any combined treatment group from the 24-week study comparing pioglitazone 30 mg plus a sulfonylurea and pioglitazone 45 mg plus a sulfonylurea are shown in Table 4; the rate of adverse events resulting in study discontinuation between the two treatment groups was 6.0% and 9.7%, respectively.

Table 4. Adverse Events That Occurred in ≥ 5% of Patients in Any Treatment Group During the 24-Week Study

Adverse Event	Pioglitazone 30 mg + sulfonylurea N=351 n (%)	Pioglitazone 45 mg + sulfonylurea N=351 n (%)
Hypoglycemia	47 (13.4)	55 (15.7)
Upper Respiratory Tract Infection	43 (12.3)	52 (14.8)
Weight Increased	32 (9.1)	47 (13.4)
Edema Lower Limb	20 (5.7)	43 (12.3)
Headache	25 (7.1)	14 (4.0)
Urinary Tract Infection	20 (5.7)	24 (6.8)
Diarrhea	21 (6.0)	15 (4.3)
Nausea	18 (5.1)	14 (4.0)
Pain in Limb	19 (5.4)	14 (4.0)

In U.S. double-blind studies, anemia was reported in ≤ 2% of patients treated with pioglitazone plus a sulfonylurea (see **PRECAUTIONS, General:** ***Pioglitazone hydrochloride***).

Pioglitazone hydrochloride

Over 8500 patients with type 2 diabetes have been treated with pioglitazone in randomized, double-blind, controlled clinical trials. This includes 2605 high-risk patients with type 2 diabetes treated with pioglitazone from the PROactive clinical trial. Over 6000 patients have been treated for 6 months or longer, and over 4500 patients for one year or longer. Over 3000 patients have received pioglitazone for at least 2 years.

Most clinical adverse events were similar between groups treated with pioglitazone in combination with a sulfonylurea and those treated with pioglitazone monotherapy. Other adverse events reported in at least 5% of patients in controlled clinical studies between placebo and pioglitazone monotherapy included myalgia (2.7% and 5.4%), tooth disorder (2.3% and 5.3%), diabetes mellitus aggravated (8.1% and 5.1%) and pharyngitis (0.8% and 5.1%), respectively.

In monotherapy studies, edema was reported for 4.8% (with doses from 7.5 mg to 45 mg) of patients treated with pioglitazone versus 1.2% of placebo-treated patients. Most of these events were considered mild or moderate in intensity (see **PRECAUTIONS, General:** ***Pioglitazone hydrochloride,*** Edema).

Prospective Pioglitazone Clinical Trial In Macrovascular Events (PROactive)

In PROactive, 5238 patients with type 2 diabetes and a prior history of macrovascular disease were treated with

ACTOS (n=2605), force-titrated up to 45 mg daily, or placebo (n=2633), in addition to standard of care. Almost all subjects (95%) were receiving cardiovascular medications (beta blockers, ACE inhibitors, ARBs, calcium channel blockers, nitrates, diuretics, aspirin, statins, fibrates). Patients had a mean age of 61.8 years, mean duration of diabetes 9.5 years, and mean A1C 8.1%. Average duration of follow-up was 34.5 months. The primary objective of this trial was to examine the effect of ACTOS on mortality and macrovascular morbidity in patients with type 2 diabetes mellitus who were at high risk for macrovascular events. The primary efficacy variable was the time to the first occurrence of any event in the cardiovascular composite endpoint (see table 5 below). Although there was no statistically significant difference between ACTOS and placebo for the 3-year incidence of a first event within this composite, there was no increase in mortality or in total macrovascular events with ACTOS.

[See table 5 above]

Postmarketing reports of new onset or worsening diabetic macular edema with decreased visual acuity have also been received (see **PRECAUTIONS, General:** *Pioglitazone hydrochloride*).

Glimepiride

Adverse events that occurred in controlled clinical trials with placebo and glimepiride monotherapy, other than hypoglycemia, headache and nausea, also included dizziness (0.3% and 1.7%) and asthenia (1.0% and 1.6%), respectively.

Gastrointestinal Reactions: Vomiting, gastrointestinal pain, and diarrhea have been reported with glimepiride, but the incidence in placebo-controlled trials was less than 1%. In rare cases, there may be an elevation of liver enzyme levels. In isolated instances, impairment of liver function (e.g. with cholestasis and jaundice), as well as hepatitis, which may also lead to liver failure have been reported with sulfonylureas, including glimepiride.

Dermatologic Reactions: Allergic skin reactions, e.g., pruritus, erythema, urticaria, and morbilliform or maculopapular eruptions, occur in less than 1% of glimepiride-treated patients. These may be transient and may disappear despite continued use of glimepiride. If those hypersensitivity reactions persist or worsen, the drug should be discontinued. Porphyria cutanea tarda, photosensitivity reactions, and allergic vasculitis have been reported with sulfonylureas.

Metabolic Reactions: Hepatic porphyria reactions and disulfiram-like reactions have been reported with sulfonylureas; however, no cases have yet been reported with glimepiride tablets. Cases of hyponatremia have been reported with glimepiride and all other sulfonylureas, most often in patients who are on other medications or have medical conditions known to cause hyponatremia or increase release of antidiuretic hormone. The syndrome of inappropriate antidiuretic hormone (SIADH) secretion has been reported with certain other sulfonylureas, and it has been suggested that these sulfonylureas may augment the peripheral (antidiuretic) action of ADH and/or increase release of ADH.

Hematologic Reactions: Leukopenia, agranulocytosis, thrombocytopenia, hemolytic anemia, aplastic anemia, and pancytopenia have been reported with sulfonylureas.

Other Reactions: Changes in accommodation and/or blurred vision may occur with the use of glimepiride. In placebo-controlled trials of glimepiride, the incidence of blurred vision with placebo was 0.7%, and with glimepiride, 0.4%. This is thought to be due to changes in blood glucose, and may be more pronounced when treatment is initiated. This condition is also seen in untreated diabetic patients, and may actually be reduced by treatment.

Laboratory Abnormalities

Pioglitazone hydrochloride

Hematologic: Pioglitazone may cause decreases in hemoglobin and hematocrit. The fall in hemoglobin and hematocrit with pioglitazone appears to be dose related. Across all clinical studies, mean hemoglobin values declined by 2% to 4% in patients treated with pioglitazone. These changes generally occurred within the first 4 to 12 weeks of therapy and remained relatively stable thereafter. These changes may be related to increased plasma volume associated with pioglitazone therapy and have rarely been associated with any significant hematologic clinical effects (see **PRECAUTIONS, General:** *Pioglitazone hydrochloride*, Hematologic).

Serum Transaminase Levels: During all clinical studies in the U.S., 14 of 4780 (0.30%) patients treated with pioglitazone had ALT values ≥ 3 times the upper limit of normal during treatment. All patients with follow-up values had reversible elevations in ALT. In the population of patients treated with pioglitazone, mean values for bilirubin, AST, ALT, alkaline phosphatase, and GGT were decreased at the final visit compared with baseline. Fewer than 0.9% of patients treated with pioglitazone were withdrawn from clinical trials in the U.S. due to abnormal liver function tests.

In pre-approval clinical trials, there were no cases of idiosyncratic drug reactions leading to hepatic failure (see **PRECAUTIONS, General:** *Pioglitazone hydrochloride*, Hepatic Effects).

CPK Levels: During required laboratory testing in clinical trials with pioglitazone, sporadic, transient elevations in creatine phosphokinase levels (CPK) were observed. An isolated elevation to greater than 10 times the upper limit of normal was noted in 9 patients (values of 2150 to 11400 IU/L). Six of these patients continued to receive pioglitazone, two patients had completed receiving study

Table 5.

Number of First and Total Events for Each Component within the Cardiovascular Composite Endpoint				
	Placebo N=2633		ACTOS N=2605	
Cardiovascular Events	First Events (N)	Total events (N)	First Events (N)	Total events (N)
Any event	572	900	514	803
All-cause mortality	122	186	110	177
Non-fatal MI	118	157	105	131
Stroke	96	119	76	92
ACS	63	78	42	65
Cardiac intervention	101	240	101	195
Major leg amputation	15	28	9	28
Leg revascularization	57	92	71	115

medication at the time of the elevated value and one patient discontinued study medication due to the elevation. These elevations resolved without any apparent clinical sequelae. The relationship of these events to pioglitazone therapy is unknown.

OVERDOSAGE

Pioglitazone hydrochloride

During controlled clinical trials, one case of overdose with pioglitazone was reported. A male patient took 120 mg per day for four days, then 180 mg per day for seven days. The patient denied any clinical symptoms during this period.

In the event of overdosage, appropriate supportive treatment should be initiated according to patient's clinical signs and symptoms.

Glimepiride

Overdosage of sulfonylureas, including glimepiride, can produce hypoglycemia. Mild hypoglycemic symptoms without loss of consciousness or neurologic findings should be treated aggressively with oral glucose and adjustments in drug dosage and/or meal patterns. Close monitoring should continue until the physician is assured that the patient is out of danger. Severe hypoglycemic reactions with coma, seizure, or other neurological impairment occur infrequently, but constitute medical emergencies requiring immediate hospitalization. If hypoglycemic coma is diagnosed or suspected, the patient should be given a rapid intravenous injection of concentrated (50%) glucose solution. This should be followed by a continuous infusion of a more dilute (10%) glucose solution at a rate that will maintain the blood glucose at a level above 100 mg/dL. Patients should be closely monitored for a minimum of 24 to 48 hours, because hypoglycemia may recur after apparent clinical recovery.

DOSAGE AND ADMINISTRATION

General

The use of antihyperglycemic therapy in the management of type 2 diabetes should be individualized on the basis of effectiveness and tolerability. Failure to follow an appropriate dosage regimen may precipitate hypoglycemia.

Dosage Recommendations

Selecting the starting dose of DUETACT should be based on the patient's current regimen of pioglitazone and/or sulfonylurea. Those patients who may be more sensitive to antihyperglycemic drugs should be monitored carefully during dose adjustment. After initiation of DUETACT, patients should be carefully monitored for adverse events related to fluid retention (see **BOXED WARNING** and **WARNINGS, Pioglitazone hydrochloride**). It is recommended that a single dose of DUETACT be administered once daily with the first main meal.

Starting dose for patients currently on glimepiride monotherapy

Based on the usual starting dose of pioglitazone (15 mg or 30 mg daily), DUETACT may be initiated at 30 mg/2 mg or 30 mg/4 mg tablet strengths once daily, and adjusted after assessing adequacy of therapeutic response.

For patients with type 2 diabetes and systolic dysfunction, see **DOSAGE AND ADMINISTRATION, Special Patient Populations**.

Starting dose for patients currently on pioglitazone monotherapy

Based on the usual starting doses of glimepiride (1 mg or 2 mg once daily), and pioglitazone 15 mg or 30 mg, DUETACT may be initiated at 30 mg/2 mg once daily, and adjusted after assessing adequacy of therapeutic response. For patients who are not currently on glimepiride and may be more sensitive to hypoglycemia, see **DOSAGE AND ADMINISTRATION, Special Patient Populations**.

Starting dose for patients switching from combination therapy of pioglitazone plus glimepiride as separate tablets

DUETACT may be initiated with 30 mg/2 mg or 30 mg/4 mg tablet strengths based on the dose of pioglitazone and glimepiride already being taken. Patients who are not controlled with 15 mg of pioglitazone in combination with glimepiride should be carefully monitored when switched to DUETACT.

Starting dose for patients currently on a different sulfonylurea monotherapy or switching from combination therapy of pioglitazone plus a different sulfonylurea (e.g. glyburide, glipizide, chlorpropamide, tolbutamide, acetohexamide)

No exact dosage relationship exists between glimepiride and the other sulfonylurea agents. Therefore, based on the maximum starting dose of 2 mg glimepiride, DUETACT should be limited initially to a starting dose of 30 mg/2 mg once daily, and adjusted after assessing adequacy of therapeutic response.

Any change in diabetic therapy should be undertaken with care and appropriate monitoring as changes in glycemic control can occur. Patients should be observed carefully for hypoglycemia (1-2 weeks) when being transferred to DUETACT, especially from longer half-life sulfonylureas (e.g. chlorpropamide) due to potential overlapping of drug effect.

Sufficient time should be given to assess adequacy of therapeutic response. Ideally, the response to therapy should be evaluated using A1C, which is a better indicator of longterm glycemic control than FPG alone. A1C reflects glycemia over the past two to three months. In clinical use, it is recommended that patients be treated with DUETACT for a period of time adequate to evaluate change in A1C (8-12 weeks) unless glycemic control as measured by FPG deteriorates.

Special Patient Populations

DUETACT is not recommended for use in pregnancy, nursing mothers or for use in pediatric patients.

In elderly, debilitated, or malnourished patients, or in patients with renal or hepatic insufficiency, the initial dosing, dose increments, and maintenance dosage of DUETACT should be conservative to avoid hypoglycemic reactions. These patients should be started at 1 mg of glimepiride prior to prescribing DUETACT. During initiation of DUETACT therapy and any subsequent dose adjustment, patients should be observed carefully for hypoglycemia (see **PRECAUTIONS, General: Glimepiride**, Hypoglycemia).

Therapy with DUETACT should not be initiated if the patient exhibits clinical evidence of active liver disease or increased serum transaminase levels (ALT greater than 2.5 times the upper limit of normal) at start of therapy (see **PRECAUTIONS, General: Pioglitazone hydrochloride**, Hepatic Effects and **CLINICAL PHARMACOLOGY, Special Populations, Hepatic Insufficiency**: *Pioglitazone hydrochloride*). Liver enzyme monitoring is recommended in all patients prior to initiation of therapy with DUETACT and periodically thereafter (see **PRECAUTIONS, General: Pioglitazone hydrochloride**, Hepatic Effects and **PRECAUTIONS, Laboratory Tests**).

The lowest approved dose of DUETACT therapy should be prescribed to patients with type 2 diabetes and systolic dysfunction only after titration from 15 mg to 30 mg of pioglitazone has been safely tolerated. If subsequent dose adjustment is necessary, patients should be carefully monitored for weight gain, edema, or signs and symptoms of CHF exacerbation (see **WARNINGS, Pioglitazone Hydrochloride**, Cardiac Failure and Other Cardiac Effects).

Maximum Recommended Dose

DUETACT tablets are available as a 30 mg pioglitazone plus 2 mg glimepiride or a 30 mg pioglitazone plus 4 mg glimepiride formulation for oral administration. The maximum recommended daily dose for pioglitazone is 45 mg and the maximum recommended daily dose for glimepiride is 8 mg.

DUETACT should therefore not be given more than once daily at any of the tablet strengths.

HOW SUPPLIED

DUETACT is available in 30 mg pioglitazone plus 2 mg glimepiride or 30 mg pioglitazone plus 4 mg glimepiride tablets as follows:

30 mg/2 mg tablet: white to off-white, round, convex, uncoated tablet, debossed with 30/2 on one side and 4833G on the other, available in:

Continued on next page

Duetact—Cont.

NDC 64764-302-30 Bottles of 30
NDC 64764-302-90 Bottles of 90
30 mg/4 mg tablet: white to off-white, round, convex, uncoated tablet, debossed with 30/4 on one side and 4833G on the other, available in:
NDC 64764-304-30 Bottles of 30
NDC 64764-304-90 Bottles of 90

STORAGE

Store at 25°C (77°F); excursions permitted to 15-30°C (59-86°F) [see USP Controlled Room Temperature]. Keep container tightly closed and protect from moisture and humidity.

REFERENCES

1. Deng, LJ, et al. Effect of gemfibrozil on the pharmacokinetics of pioglitazone. Eur J Clin Pharmacol 2005; 61: 831-836, Table 1.
2. Jaakkola, T, et al. Effect of rifampicin on the pharmacokinetics of pioglitazone. Br J Clin Pharmacol 2006; 61:1 70-78.

HUMAN OPHTHALMOLOGY DATA

Glimepiride

Ophthalmic examinations were carried out in over 500 subjects during long-term studies using the methodology of Taylor and West and Laties et al. No significant differences were seen between glimepiride and glyburide in the number of subjects with clinically important changes in visual acuity, intraocular tension, or in any of the five lens-related variables examined.

Ophthalmic examinations were carried out during long-term studies using the method of Chylack et al. No significant or clinically meaningful differences were seen between glimepiride and glipizide with respect to cataract progression by subjective LOCS II grading and objective image analysis systems, visual acuity, intraocular pressure, and general ophthalmic examination.

Rx only

ACTOS® and DUETACT™ are trademarks of Takeda Pharmaceutical Company Limited and used under license by Takeda Pharmaceuticals America, Inc.

Distributed by:
Takeda Pharmaceuticals America, Inc.
Deerfield, IL 60015
© 2006 Takeda Pharmaceuticals America, Inc.
Item No.: 05-1142 Revised: October, 2007
L-PIOSU-1007-7

UCB, Inc.

1950 LAKE PARK DRIVE
SMYRNA, GA 30080

Direct Inquiries to:
UCB, Inc.
1950 Lake Park Drive
Smyrna, GA 30080
(800) 477-7877
For Medical Information Contact:
Medical Affairs Department
(866) 822-0068
FAX: 770-970-8859

KEPPRA® ℞

[kepp-ruh]
(levetiracetam)
250 mg, 500 mg, 750 mg, and 1000 mg tablets
100 mg/mL oral solution
Rx only

Prescribing information for this product, which appears on pages 3249–3256 of the 2008 PDR, has been completely revised as follows. Please write "See Supplement A" next to the product heading.

DESCRIPTION

KEPPRA is an antiepileptic drug available as 250 mg (blue), 500 mg (yellow), 750 mg (orange), and 1000 mg (white) tablets and as a clear, colorless, grape-flavored liquid (100 mg/mL) for oral administration.

The chemical name of levetiracetam, a single enantiomer, is (-)-(S)-α-ethyl-2-oxo-1-pyrrolidine acetamide, its molecular formula is $C_8H_{14}N_2O_2$ and its molecular weight is 170.21. Levetiracetam is chemically unrelated to existing antiepileptic drugs (AEDs). It has the following structural formula:

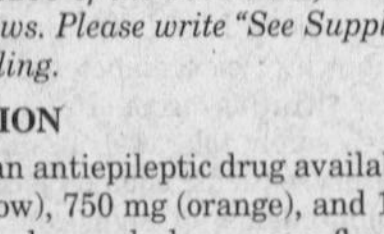

Levetiracetam is a white to off-white crystalline powder with a faint odor and a bitter taste. It is very soluble in water (104.0 g/100 mL). It is freely soluble in chloroform (65.3 g/100 mL) and in methanol (53.6 g/100 mL), soluble in ethanol (16.5 g/100 mL), sparingly soluble in acetonitrile (5.7 g/100 mL) and practically insoluble in n-hexane. (Solubility limits are expressed as g/100 mL solvent.)

KEPPRA tablets contain the labeled amount of levetiracetam. Inactive ingredients: colloidal silicon dioxide, croscarmellose sodium, magnesium stearate, polyethylene glycol 3350, polyethylene glycol 6000, polyvinyl alcohol, talc, titanium dioxide, and additional agents listed below:

250 mg tablets: FD&C Blue #2/indigo carmine aluminum lake
500 mg tablets: iron oxide yellow
750 mg tablets: FD&C yellow #6/sunset yellow FCF aluminum lake, iron oxide red

KEPPRA oral solution contains 100 mg of levetiracetam per mL. Inactive ingredients: ammonium glycyrrhizinate, citric acid monohydrate, glycerin, maltitol solution, methylparaben, potassium acesulfame, propylparaben, purified water, sodium citrate dihydrate and natural and artificial flavor.

CLINICAL PHARMACOLOGY

Mechanism Of Action

The precise mechanism(s) by which levetiracetam exerts its antiepileptic effect is unknown. The antiepileptic activity of levetiracetam was assessed in a number of animal models of epileptic seizures. Levetiracetam did not inhibit single seizures induced by maximal stimulation with electrical current or different chemoconvulsants and showed only minimal activity in submaximal stimulation and in threshold tests. Protection was observed, however, against secondarily generalized activity from focal seizures induced by pilocarpine and kainic acid, two chemoconvulsants that induce seizures that mimic some features of human complex partial seizures with secondary generalization. Levetiracetam also displayed inhibitory properties in the kindling model in rats, another model of human complex partial seizures, both during kindling development and in the fully kindled state. The predictive value of these animal models for specific types of human epilepsy is uncertain.

In vitro and *in vivo* recordings of epileptiform activity from the hippocampus have shown that levetiracetam inhibits burst firing without affecting normal neuronal excitability, suggesting that levetiracetam may selectively prevent hypersynchronization of epileptiform burst firing and propagation of seizure activity.

Levetiracetam at concentrations of up to 10 μM did not demonstrate binding affinity for a variety of known receptors, such as those associated with benzodiazepines, GABA (gamma-aminobutyric acid), glycine, NMDA (N-methyl-D-aspartate), re-uptake sites, and second messenger systems. Furthermore, *in vitro* studies have failed to find an effect of levetiracetam on neuronal voltage-gated sodium or T-type calcium currents and levetiracetam does not appear to directly facilitate GABAergic neurotransmission. However, *in vitro* studies have demonstrated that levetiracetam opposes the activity of negative modulators of GABA- and glycine-gated currents and partially inhibits N-type calcium currents in neuronal cells.

A saturable and stereoselective neuronal binding site in rat brain tissue has been described for levetiracetam. Experimental data indicate that this binding site is the synaptic vesicle protein SV2A, thought to be involved in the regulation of vesicle exocytosis. Although the molecular significance of levetiracetam binding to synaptic vesicle protein SV2A is not understood, levetiracetam and related analogs showed a rank order of affinity for SV2A which correlated with the potency of their antiseizure activity in audiogenic seizure-prone mice. These findings suggest that the interaction of levetiracetam with the SV2A protein may contribute to the antiepileptic mechanism of action of the drug.

Pharmacokinetics

The pharmacokinetics of levetiracetam have been studied in healthy adult subjects, adults and pediatric patients with epilepsy, elderly subjects and subjects with renal and hepatic impairment.

Overview

Levetiracetam is rapidly and almost completely absorbed after oral administration. Levetiracetam tablets and oral solution are bioequivalent. The pharmacokinetics are linear and time-invariant, with low intra- and inter-subject variability. The extent of bioavailability of levetiracetam is not affected by food. Levetiracetam is not significantly protein-bound (<10% bound) and its volume of distribution is close to the volume of intracellular and extracellular water. Sixty-six percent (66%) of the dose is renally excreted unchanged. The major metabolic pathway of levetiracetam (24% of dose) is an enzymatic hydrolysis of the acetamide group. It is not liver cytochrome P450 dependent. The metabolites have no known pharmacological activity and are renally excreted. Plasma half-life of levetiracetam across studies is approximately 6-8 hours. It is increased in the elderly (primarily due to impaired renal clearance) and in subjects with renal impairment.

Absorption And Distribution

Absorption of levetiracetam is rapid, with peak plasma concentrations occurring in about an hour following oral administration in fasted subjects. The oral bioavailability of levetiracetam tablets is 100% and the tablets and oral solution are bioequivalent in rate and extent of absorption. Food does not affect the extent of absorption of levetiracetam but it decreases C_{max} by 20% and delays T_{max} by 1.5 hours. The pharmacokinetics of levetiracetam are linear over the dose range of 500-5000 mg. Steady state is achieved after 2 days of multiple twice-daily dosing. Levetiracetam and its major metabolite are less than 10% bound to plasma proteins; clinically significant interactions with other drugs through competition for protein binding sites are therefore unlikely.

Metabolism

Levetiracetam is not extensively metabolized in humans. The major metabolic pathway is the enzymatic hydrolysis of the acetamide group, which produces the carboxylic acid metabolite, ucb L057 (24% of dose) and is not dependent on any liver cytochrome P450 isoenzymes. The major metabolite is inactive in animal seizure models. Two minor metabolites were identified as the product of hydroxylation of the 2-oxo-pyrrolidine ring (2% of dose) and opening of the 2-oxo-pyrrolidine ring in position 5 (1% of dose). There is no enantiomeric interconversion of levetiracetam or its major metabolite.

Elimination

Levetiracetam plasma half-life in adults is 7 ± 1 hour and is unaffected by either dose or repeated administration. Levetiracetam is eliminated from the systemic circulation by renal excretion as unchanged drug which represents 66% of administered dose. The total body clearance is 0.96 mL/min/kg and the renal clearance is 0.6 mL/min/kg. The mechanism of excretion is glomerular filtration with subsequent partial tubular reabsorption. The metabolite ucb L057 is excreted by glomerular filtration and active tubular secretion with a renal clearance of 4 mL/min/kg. Levetiracetam elimination is correlated to creatinine clearance. Levetiracetam clearance is reduced in patients with impaired renal function (see Special Populations, Renal Impairment and DOSAGE AND ADMINISTRATION, Adult Patients With Impaired Renal Function).

Pharmacokinetic Interactions

In vitro data on metabolic interactions indicate that levetiracetam is unlikely to produce, or be subject to, pharmacokinetic interactions. Levetiracetam and its major metabolite, at concentrations well above C_{max} levels achieved within the therapeutic dose range, are neither inhibitors of, nor high affinity substrates for, human liver cytochrome P450 isoforms, epoxide hydrolase or UDP-glucuronidation enzymes. In addition, levetiracetam does not affect the *in vitro* glucuronidation of valproic acid.

Potential pharmacokinetic interactions of or with levetiracetam were assessed in clinical pharmacokinetic studies (phenytoin, valproate, warfarin, digoxin, oral contraceptive, probenecid) and through pharmacokinetic screening in the placebo-controlled clinical studies in epilepsy patients (see PRECAUTIONS, Drug Interactions).

Special Populations

Elderly

Pharmacokinetics of levetiracetam were evaluated in 16 elderly subjects (age 61-88 years) with creatinine clearance ranging from 30 to 74 mL/min. Following oral administration of twice-daily dosing for 10 days, total body clearance decreased by 38% and the half-life was 2.5 hours longer in the elderly compared to healthy adults. This is most likely due to the decrease in renal function in these subjects.

Pediatric Patients

Pharmacokinetics of levetiracetam were evaluated in 24 pediatric patients (age 6-12 years) after single dose (20 mg/kg). The body weight adjusted apparent clearance of levetiracetam was approximately 40% higher than in adults.

A repeat dose pharmacokinetic study was conducted in pediatric patients (age 4-12 years) at doses of 20 mg/kg/day, 40 mg/kg/day, and 60 mg/kg/day. The evaluation of the pharmacokinetic profile of levetiracetam and its metabolite (ucb L057) in 14 pediatric patients demonstrated rapid absorption of levetiracetam at all doses with a T_{max} of about 1 hour and a $t_{1/2}$ of 5 hours across the three dosing levels. The pharmacokinetics of levetiracetam in children was linear between 20 to 60 mg/kg/day. The potential interaction of levetiracetam with other AEDs was also evaluated in these patients (see PRECAUTIONS, Drug Interactions). Levetiracetam had no significant effect on the plasma concentrations of carbamazepine, valproic acid, topiramate or lamotrigine. However, there was about a 22% increase of apparent clearance of levetiracetam when it was co-administered with an enzyme-inducing AED (e.g. carbamazepine). Population pharmacokinetic analysis showed that body weight was significantly correlated to clearance of levetiracetam in pediatric patients; clearance increased with an increase in body weight.

Gender

Levetiracetam C_{max} and AUC were 20% higher in women (N=11) compared to men (N=12). However, clearances adjusted for body weight were comparable.

Race

Formal pharmacokinetic studies of the effects of race have not been conducted. Cross study comparisons involving Caucasians (N=12) and Asians (N=12), however, show that pharmacokinetics of levetiracetam were comparable between the two races. Because levetiracetam is primarily renally excreted and there are no important racial differences in creatinine clearance, pharmacokinetic differences due to race are not expected.

Renal Impairment

The disposition of levetiracetam was studied in adult subjects with varying degrees of renal function. Total body clearance of levetiracetam is reduced in patients with impaired renal function by 40% in the mild group (CLcr = 50-80 mL/min), 50% in the moderate group (CLcr = 30-50 mL/min) and 60% in the severe renal impairment group (CLcr <30 mL/min). Clearance of levetiracetam is correlated with creatinine clearance.

In anuric (end stage renal disease) patients, the total body clearance decreased 70% compared to normal subjects (CLcr >80mL/min). Approximately 50% of the pool of levetiracetam in the body is removed during a standard 4-hour hemodialysis procedure.

Dosage should be reduced in patients with impaired renal function receiving levetiracetam, and supplemental doses should be given to patients after dialysis (see PRECAUTIONS and DOSAGE AND ADMINISTRATION, Adult Patients With Impaired Renal Function).

Hepatic Impairment

In subjects with mild (Child-Pugh A) to moderate (Child-Pugh B) hepatic impairment, the pharmacokinetics of levetiracetam were unchanged. In patients with severe hepatic impairment (Child-Pugh C), total body clearance was 50% that of normal subjects, but decreased renal clearance accounted for most of the decrease. No dose adjustment is needed for patients with hepatic impairment.

CLINICAL STUDIES

In the following studies, statistical significance versus placebo indicates a p value < 0.05.

Effectiveness In Partial Onset Seizures In Adults With Epilepsy

The effectiveness of KEPPRA as adjunctive therapy (added to other antiepileptic drugs) in adults was established in three multicenter, randomized, double-blind, placebo-controlled clinical studies in patients who had refractory partial onset seizures with or without secondary generalization. The tablet formulation was used in all these studies. In these studies, 904 patients were randomized to placebo, 1000 mg, 2000 mg, or 3000 mg/day. Patients enrolled in Study 1 or Study 2 had refractory partial onset seizures for at least two years and had taken two or more classical AEDs. Patients enrolled in Study 3 had refractory partial onset seizures for at least 1 year and had taken one classical AED. At the time of the study, patients were taking a stable dose regimen of at least one and could take a maximum of two AEDs. During the baseline period, patients had to have experienced at least two partial onset seizures during each 4-week period.

Study 1

Study 1 was a double-blind, placebo-controlled, parallel-group study conducted at 41 sites in the United States comparing KEPPRA 1000 mg/day (N=97), KEPPRA 3000 mg/day (N=101), and placebo (N=95) given in equally divided doses twice daily. After a prospective baseline period of 12 weeks, patients were randomized to one of the three treatment groups described above. The 18-week treatment period consisted of a 6-week titration period, followed by a 12-week fixed dose evaluation period, during which concomitant AED regimens were held constant. The primary measure of effectiveness was a between group comparison of the percent reduction in weekly partial seizure frequency relative to placebo over the entire randomized treatment period (titration + evaluation period). Secondary outcome variables included the responder rate (incidence of patients with ≥50% reduction from baseline in partial onset seizure frequency). The results of the analysis of Study 1 are displayed in Table 1.

Table 1: Reduction In Mean Over Placebo In Weekly Frequency Of Partial Onset Seizures In Study 1

	Placebo (N=95)	KEPPRA 1000 mg/day (N=97)	KEPPRA 3000 mg/day (N=101)
Percent reduction in partial seizure frequency over placebo	–	26.1%*	30.1%*

*statistically significant versus placebo

The percentage of patients (y-axis) who achieved ≥50% reduction in weekly seizure rates from baseline in partial onset seizure frequency over the entire randomized treatment period (titration + evaluation period) within the three treatment groups (x-axis) is presented in Figure 1.

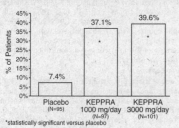

Figure 1: Responder Rate (≥50% Reduction From Baseline) In Study 1

*statistically significant versus placebo

Study 2

Study 2 was a double-blind, placebo-controlled, crossover study conducted at 62 centers in Europe comparing KEPPRA 1000 mg/day (N=106), KEPPRA 2000 mg/day (N=105), and placebo (N=111) given in equally divided doses twice daily.

The first period of the study (Period A) was designed to be analyzed as a parallel-group study. After a prospective baseline period of up to 12 weeks, patients were randomized to one of the three treatment groups described above. The 16-week treatment period consisted of the 4-week titration period followed by a 12-week fixed dose evaluation period, during which concomitant AED regimens were held constant.

The primary measure of effectiveness was a between group comparison of the percent reduction in weekly partial seizure frequency relative to placebo over the entire randomized treatment period (titration + evaluation period). Secondary outcome variables included the responder rate (incidence of patients with ≥50% reduction from baseline in partial onset seizure frequency). The results of the analysis of Period A are displayed in Table 2.

Table 2: Reduction In Mean Over Placebo In Weekly Frequency Of Partial Onset Seizures In Study 2: Period A

	Placebo (N=111)	KEPPRA 1000 mg/day (N=106)	KEPPRA 2000 mg/day (N=105)
Percent reduction in partial seizure frequency over placebo	–	17.1%*	21.4%*

*statistically significant versus placebo

The percentage of patients (y-axis) who achieved ≥50% reduction in weekly seizure rates from baseline in partial onset seizure frequency over the entire randomized treatment period (titration + evaluation period) within the three treatment groups (x-axis) is presented in Figure 2.

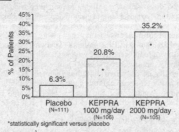

Figure 2: Responder Rate (≥50% Reduction From Baseline) In Study 2: Period A

*statistically significant versus placebo

The comparison of KEPPRA 2000 mg/day to KEPPRA 1000 mg/day for responder rate was statistically significant (P=0.02). Analysis of the trial as a cross-over yielded similar results.

Study 3

Study 3 was a double-blind, placebo-controlled, parallel-group study conducted at 47 centers in Europe comparing KEPPRA 3000 mg/day (N=180) and placebo (N=104) in patients with refractory partial onset seizures, with or without secondary generalization, receiving only one concomitant AED. Study drug was given in two divided doses. After a prospective baseline period of 12 weeks, patients were randomized to one of two treatment groups described above. The 16-week treatment period consisted of a 4-week titration period, followed by a 12-week fixed dose evaluation period, during which concomitant AED doses were held constant. The primary measure of effectiveness was a between group comparison of the percent reduction in weekly seizure frequency relative to placebo over the entire randomized treatment period (titration + evaluation period). Secondary outcome variables included the responder rate (incidence of patients with ≥50% reduction from baseline in partial onset seizure frequency). Table 3 displays the results of the analysis of Study 3.

Table 3: Reduction In Mean Over Placebo In Weekly Frequency Of Partial Onset Seizures In Study 3

	Placebo (N=104)	KEPPRA 3000 mg/day (N=180)
Percent reduction in partial seizure frequency over placebo	–	23.0%*

*statistically significant versus placebo

The percentage of patients (y-axis) who achieved ≥50% reduction in weekly seizure rates from baseline in partial onset seizure frequency over the entire randomized treatment period (titration + evaluation period) within the two treatment groups (x-axis) is presented in Figure 3.
[See figure 3 at top of next column]

Effectiveness In Partial Onset Seizures In Pediatric Patients With Epilepsy

The effectiveness of KEPPRA as adjunctive therapy (added to other antiepileptic drugs) in pediatric patients was established in one multicenter, randomized double-blind, placebo-controlled study, conducted at 60 sites in North America, in children 4 to 16 years of age with partial seizures uncontrolled by standard antiepileptic drugs (AEDs). Eligible patients on a stable dose of 1-2 AEDs, who still experienced at least 4 partial onset seizures during the 4 weeks prior to screening, as well as at least 4 partial onset seizures in each of the two 4-week baseline periods, were randomized to receive either KEPPRA or placebo. The en-

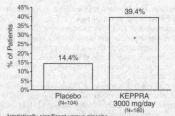

Figure 3: Responder Rate (≥50% Reduction From Baseline) In Study 3

*statistically significant versus placebo

rolled population included 198 patients (KEPPRA N=101, placebo N=97) with refractory partial onset seizures, whether or not secondarily generalized. The study consisted of an 8-week baseline period and 4-week titration period followed by a 10-week evaluation period. Dosing was initiated at a dose of 20 mg/kg/day in two divided doses. During the treatment period, KEPPRA doses were adjusted in 20 mg/kg/day increments, at 2-week intervals to the target dose of 60 mg/kg/day. The primary measure of effectiveness was a between group comparison of the percent reduction in weekly partial seizure frequency relative to placebo over the entire 14-week randomized treatment period (titration + evaluation period). Secondary outcome variables included the responder rate (incidence of patients with ≥ 50% reduction from baseline in partial onset seizure frequency per week). Table 4 displays the results of this study.

Table 4: Reduction In Mean Over Placebo In Weekly Frequency Of Partial Onset Seizures

	Placebo (N=97)	KEPPRA (N=101)
Percent reduction in partial seizure frequency over placebo	–	26.8%*

*statistically significant versus placebo

The percentage of patients (y-axis) who achieved ≥ 50% reduction in weekly seizure rates from baseline in partial onset seizure frequency over the entire randomized treatment period (titration + evaluation period) within the two treatment groups (x-axis) is presented in Figure 4.

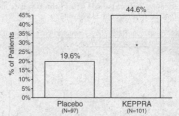

Figure 4: Responder Rate (≥50% Reduction From Baseline)

*statistically significant versus placebo

Effectiveness In Myoclonic Seizures In Patients ≥12 Years Of Age With Juvenile Myoclonic Epilepsy (JME)

The effectiveness of KEPPRA as adjunctive therapy (added to other antiepileptic drugs) in patients 12 years of age and older with juvenile myoclonic epilepsy (JME) experiencing myoclonic seizures was established in one multicenter, randomized, double-blind, placebo-controlled study, conducted at 37 sites in 14 countries. Of the 120 patients enrolled, 113 had a diagnosis of confirmed or suspected JME. Eligible patients on a stable dose of 1 antiepileptic drug (AED) experiencing one or more myoclonic seizures per day for at least 8 days during the prospective 8-week baseline period were randomized to either KEPPRA or placebo (KEPPRA N=60, placebo N=60). Patients were titrated over 4 weeks to a target dose of 3000 mg/day and treated at a stable dose of 3000 mg/day over 12 weeks (evaluation period). Study drug was given in 2 divided doses.

The primary measure of effectiveness was the proportion of patients with at least 50% reduction in the number of days per week with one or more myoclonic seizures during the treatment period (titration + evaluation periods) as compared to baseline. Table 5 displays the results for the 113 patients with JME in this study.

Table 5: Responder Rate (≥50% Reduction From Baseline) In Myoclonic Seizure Days Per Week for Patients with JME

	Placebo (N=59)	KEPPRA (N=54)
Percentage of responders	23.7%	60.4%*

*statistically significant versus placebo

Continued on next page

Keppra—Cont.

Effectiveness For Primary Generalized Tonic-Clonic Seizures In Patients ≥6 Years Of Age

The effectiveness of KEPPRA as adjunctive therapy (added to other antiepileptic drugs) in patients 6 years of age and older with idiopathic generalized epilepsy experiencing primary generalized tonic-clonic (PGTC) seizures was established in one multicenter, randomized, double-blind, placebo-controlled study, conducted at 50 sites in 8 countries. Eligible patients on a stable dose of 1 or 2 antiepileptic drugs (AEDs) experiencing at least 3 PGTC seizures during the 8-week combined baseline period (at least one PGTC seizure during the 4 weeks prior to the prospective baseline period and at least one PGTC seizure during the 4-week prospective baseline period) were randomized to either KEPPRA or placebo. The 8-week combined baseline period is referred to as "baseline" in the remainder of this section. The population included 164 patients (KEPPRA N=80, placebo N=84) with idiopathic generalized epilepsy (predominately juvenile myoclonic epilepsy, juvenile absence epilepsy, childhood absence epilepsy, or epilepsy with Grand Mal seizures on awakening) experiencing primary generalized tonic-clonic seizures. Each of these syndromes of idiopathic generalized epilepsy was well represented in this patient population. Patients were titrated over 4 weeks to a target dose of 3000 mg/day for adults or a pediatric target dose of 60 mg/kg/day and treated at a stable dose of 3000 mg/day (or 60 mg/kg/day for children) over 20 weeks (evaluation period). Study drug was given in 2 equally divided doses per day.

The primary measure of effectiveness was the percent reduction from baseline in weekly PGTC seizure frequency for KEPPRA and placebo treatment groups over the treatment period (titration + evaluation periods). There was a statistically significant decrease from baseline in PGTC frequency in the KEPPRA-treated patients compared to the placebo-treated patients.

Table 6: Median Percent Reduction From Baseline In PGTC Seizure Frequency Per Week

	Placebo (N=84)	KEPPRA (N=78)
Percent reduction in PGTC seizure frequency	44.6%	77.6%*

*statistically significant versus placebo

The percentage of patients (y-axis) who achieved ≥50% reduction in weekly seizure rates from baseline in PGTC seizure frequency over the entire randomized treatment period (titration + evaluation period) within the two treatment groups (x-axis) is presented in Figure 5.

Figure 5: Responder Rate (≥50% Reduction From Baseline) In PGTC Seizure Frequency Per Week

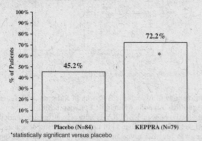

*statistically significant versus placebo

INDICATIONS AND USAGE

KEPPRA is indicated as adjunctive therapy in the treatment of partial onset seizures in adults and children 4 years of age and older with epilepsy.

KEPPRA is indicated as adjunctive therapy in the treatment of myoclonic seizures in adults and adolescents 12 years of age and older with juvenile myoclonic epilepsy.

KEPPRA is indicated as adjunctive therapy in the treatment of primary generalized tonic-clonic seizures in adults and children 6 years of age and older with idiopathic generalized epilepsy.

CONTRAINDICATIONS

This product should not be administered to patients who have previously exhibited hypersensitivity to levetiracetam or any of the inactive ingredients in KEPPRA tablets or oral solution.

WARNINGS

Neuropsychiatric Adverse Events

Partial Onset Seizures

Adults

In adults experiencing partial onset seizures, KEPPRA use is associated with the occurrence of central nervous system adverse events that can be classified into the following categories: 1) somnolence and fatigue, 2) coordination difficulties, and 3) behavioral abnormalities.

In controlled trials of adult patients with epilepsy experiencing partial onset seizures, 14.8% of KEPPRA-treated patients reported somnolence, compared to 8.4% of placebo patients. There was no clear dose response up to 3000 mg/day. In a study where there was no titration, about 45% of pa-

tients receiving 4000 mg/day reported somnolence. The somnolence was considered serious in 0.3% of the treated patients, compared to 0% in the placebo group. About 3% of KEPPRA-treated patients discontinued treatment due to somnolence, compared to 0.7% of placebo patients. In 1.4% of treated patients and in 0.9% of placebo patients the dose was reduced, while 0.3% of the treated patients were hospitalized due to somnolence.

In controlled trials of adult patients with epilepsy experiencing partial onset seizures, 14.7% of treated patients reported asthenia, compared to 9.1% of placebo patients. Treatment was discontinued in 0.8% of treated patients as compared to 0.5% of placebo patients. In 0.5% of treated patients and in 0.2% of placebo patients the dose was reduced.

A total of 3.4% of KEPPRA-treated patients experienced coordination difficulties, (reported as either ataxia, abnormal gait, or incoordination) compared to 1.6% of placebo patients. A total of 0.4% of patients in controlled trials discontinued KEPPRA treatment due to ataxia, compared to 0% of placebo patients. In 0.7% of treated patients and in 0.2% of placebo patients the dose was reduced due to coordination difficulties, while one of the treated patients was hospitalized due to worsening of pre-existing ataxia.

Somnolence, asthenia and coordination difficulties occurred most frequently within the first 4 weeks of treatment.

In controlled trials of patients with epilepsy experiencing partial onset seizures, 5 (0.7%) of KEPPRA-treated patients experienced psychotic symptoms compared to 1 (0.2%) placebo patient. Two (0.3%) KEPPRA-treated patients were hospitalized and their treatment was discontinued. Both events, reported as psychosis, developed within the first week of treatment and resolved within 1 to 2 weeks following treatment discontinuation. Two other events, reported as hallucinations, occurred after 1-5 months and resolved within 2-7 days while the patients remained on treatment. In one patient experiencing psychotic depression occurring within a month, symptoms resolved within 45 days while the patient continued treatment.

A total of 13.3% of KEPPRA patients experienced other behavioral symptoms (reported as aggression, agitation, anger, anxiety, apathy, depersonalization, depression, emotional lability, hostility, irritability, etc.) compared to 6.2% of placebo patients. Approximately half of these patients reported these events within the first 4 weeks. A total of 1.7% of treated patients discontinued treatment due to these events, compared to 0.2% of placebo patients. The treatment dose was reduced in 0.8% of treated patients and in 0.5% of placebo patients. A total of 0.8% of treated patients had a serious behavioral event (compared to 0.2% of placebo patients) and were hospitalized.

In addition, 4 (0.5%) of treated patients attempted suicide compared to 0% of placebo patients. One of these patients completed suicide. In the other 3 patients, the events did not lead to discontinuation or dose reduction. The events occurred after patients had been treated for between 4 weeks and 6 months (see PRECAUTIONS, Information For Patients).

Pediatric Patients

In pediatric patients experiencing partial onset seizures, KEPPRA is associated with somnolence, fatigue, and behavioral abnormalities.

In the double-blind, controlled trial in children with epilepsy experiencing partial onset seizures, 22.8% of KEPPRA-treated patients experienced somnolence, compared to 11.3% of placebo patients. The design of the study prevented accurately assessing dose-response effects. No patient discontinued treatment for somnolence. In about 3.0% of KEPPRA-treated patients and in 3.1% of placebo patients the dose was reduced as a result of somnolence.

Asthenia was reported in 8.9% of KEPPRA-treated patients, compared to 3.1% of placebo patients. No patient discontinued treatment for asthenia, but asthenia led to a dose reduction in 3.0% of KEPPRA-treated patients compared to 0% of placebo patients.

A total of 37.6% of the KEPPRA-treated patients experienced behavioral symptoms (reported as agitation, anxiety, apathy, depersonalization, depression, emotional lability, hostility, hyperkinesia, nervousness, neurosis, and personality disorder), compared to 18.6% of placebo patients. Hostility was reported in 11.9% of KEPPRA-treated patients, compared to 6.2% of placebo patients. Nervousness was reported in 9.9% of KEPPRA-treated patients, compared to 2.1% of placebo patients. Depression was reported in 3.0% of KEPPRA-treated patients, compared to 1.0% of placebo patients.

One KEPPRA-treated patient experienced suicidal ideation (see PRECAUTIONS, Information For Patients).

A total of 3.0% of KEPPRA-treated patients discontinued treatment due to psychotic and nonpsychotic adverse events, compared to 4.1% of placebo patients. Overall, 10.9% of KEPPRA-treated patients experienced behavioral symptoms associated with discontinuation or dose reduction, compared to 6.2% of placebo patients.

Myoclonic Seizures

During clinical development, the number of patients with myoclonic seizures exposed to KEPPRA was considerably smaller than the number with partial seizures. Therefore, under-reporting of certain adverse events was more likely to occur in the myoclonic seizure population. In adult and adolescent patients experiencing myoclonic seizures, KEPPRA is associated with somnolence and behavioral abnormalities. It is expected that the events seen in partial seizure patients would occur in patients with JME.

In the double-blind, controlled trial in adults and adolescents with juvenile myoclonic epilepsy experiencing myo-

clonic seizures, 11.7% of KEPPRA-treated patients experienced somnolence compared to 1.7% of placebo patients. No patient discontinued treatment as a result of somnolence. In 1.7% of KEPPRA-treated patients and in 0% of placebo patients the dose was reduced as a result of somnolence.

Non-psychotic behavioral disorders (reported as aggression and irritability) occurred in 5% of the KEPPRA-treated patients compared to 0% of placebo patients. Non-psychotic mood disorders (reported as depressed mood, depression, and mood swings) occurred in 6.7% of KEPPRA-treated patients compared to 3.3% of placebo patients. A total of 5.0% of KEPPRA-treated patients had a reduction in dose or discontinued treatment due to behavioral or psychiatric events (reported as anxiety, depressed mood, depression, irritability, and nervousness), compared to 1.7% of placebo patients.

Primary Generalized Tonic-Clonic Seizures

During clinical development, the number of patients with primary generalized tonic-clonic epilepsy exposed to KEPPRA was considerably smaller than the number with partial epilepsy, described above. As in the partial seizure patients, behavioral symptoms appeared to be associated with KEPPRA treatment. Gait disorders and somnolence were also described in the study in primary generalized seizures, but with no difference between placebo and KEPPRA treatment groups and no appreciable discontinuations. Although it may be expected that drug related events seen in partial seizure patients would be seen in primary generalized epilepsy patients (e.g. somnolence and gait disturbance), these events may not have been observed because of the smaller sample size.

In patients 6 years of age and older experiencing primary generalized tonic-clonic seizures, KEPPRA is associated with behavioral abnormalities.

In the double-blind, controlled trial in patients with idiopathic generalized epilepsy experiencing primary generalized tonic-clonic seizures, irritability was the most frequently reported psychiatric adverse event occurring in 6.3% of KEPPRA-treated patients compared to 2.4% of placebo patients. Additionally, non-psychotic behavioral disorders (reported as abnormal behavior, aggression, conduct disorder, and irritability) occurred in 11.4% of the KEPPRA-treated patients compared to 3.6% of placebo patients. Of the KEPPRA-treated patients experiencing non-psychotic behavioral disorders, one patient discontinued treatment due to aggression. Non-psychotic mood disorders (reported as anger, apathy, depression, mood altered, mood swings, negativism, suicidal ideation (see PRECAUTIONS, Information For Patients), and tearfulness) occurred in 12.7% of KEPPRA-treated patients compared to 8.3% of placebo patients. No KEPPRA-treated patients discontinued or had a dose reduction as a result of these events. One KEPPRA-treated patient experienced suicidal ideation (see PRECAUTIONS, Information For Patients). One patient experienced delusional behavior that required the lowering of the dose of KEPPRA.

In a long-term open label study that examined patients with various forms of primary generalized epilepsy, along with the non-psychotic behavioral disorders, 2 of 192 patients studied exhibited psychotic-like behavior. Behavior in one case was characterized by auditory hallucinations and suicidal thoughts and led to KEPPRA discontinuation. The other case was described as worsening of pre-existent schizophrenia and did not lead to drug discontinuation.

Withdrawal Seizures

Antiepileptic drugs, including KEPPRA, should be withdrawn gradually to minimize the potential of increased seizure frequency.

PRECAUTIONS

Hematologic Abnormalities

Partial Onset Seizures

Adults

Minor, but statistically significant, decreases compared to placebo in total mean RBC count ($0.03 \times 10^6/mm^3$), mean hemoglobin (0.09 g/dL), and mean hematocrit (0.38%), were seen in KEPPRA-treated patients in controlled trials.

A total of 3.2% of treated and 1.8% of placebo patients had at least one possibly significant ($\leq 2.8 \times 10^9/L$) decreased WBC, and 2.4% of treated and 1.4% of placebo patients had at least one possibly significant ($\leq 1.0 \times 10^9/L$) decreased neutrophil count. Of the treated patients with a low neutrophil count, all but one rose towards or to baseline with continued treatment. No patient was discontinued secondary to low neutrophil counts.

Pediatric Patients

Minor, but statistically significant, decreases in WBC and neutrophil counts were seen in KEPPRA-treated patients as compared to placebo. The mean decreases from baseline in the KEPPRA-treated group were $-0.4 \times 10^9/L$ and $-0.3 \times 10^9/L$, respectively, whereas there were small increases in the placebo group. Mean relative lymphocyte counts increased by 1.7% in KEPPRA-treated patients, compared to a decrease of 4% in placebo patients (statistically significant).

In the well-controlled trial, more KEPPRA-treated patients had a possibly clinically significant abnormally low WBC value (3.0% KEPPRA-treated versus 0% placebo), however, there was no apparent difference between treatment groups with respect to neutrophil count (5.0% KEPPRA-treated versus 4.2% placebo). No patient was discontinued secondary to low WBC or neutrophil counts.

Juvenile Myoclonic Epilepsy

Although there were no obvious hematologic abnormalities observed in patients with JME, the limited number of patients makes any conclusion tentative. The data from the partial seizure patients should be considered to be relevant for JME patients.

Hepatic Abnormalities

There were no meaningful changes in mean liver function tests (LFT) in controlled trials in adult or pediatric patients; lesser LFT abnormalities were similar in drug and placebo treated patients in controlled trials (1.4%). No adult or pediatric patients were discontinued from controlled trials for LFT abnormalities except for 1 (0.07%) adult epilepsy patient receiving open treatment.

Information For Patients

Patients should be instructed to take KEPPRA only as prescribed.

Patients should be advised to notify their physician if they become pregnant or intend to become pregnant during therapy.

Patients should be advised that KEPPRA may cause dizziness and somnolence. Accordingly, patients should be advised not to drive or operate machinery or engage in other hazardous activities until they have gained sufficient experience on KEPPRA to gauge whether it adversely affects their performance of these activities.

Patients should be advised that KEPPRA may cause changes in behavior (e.g. aggression, agitation, anger, anxiety, apathy, depression, hostility, and irritability) and in rare cases patients may experience psychotic symptoms.

Patients should be advised to immediately report any symptoms of depression and/or suicidal ideation to their prescribing physician as suicide, suicide attempt and suicidal ideation have been reported in patients treated with levetiracetam.

Physicians should advise patients and caregivers to read the patient information leaflet which appears as the last section of the labeling.

Laboratory Tests

Although most laboratory tests are not systematically altered with KEPPRA treatment, there have been relatively infrequent abnormalities seen in hematologic parameters and liver function tests.

Drug Interactions

In vitro data on metabolic interactions indicate that KEPPRA is unlikely to produce, or be subject to, pharmacokinetic interactions. Levetiracetam and its major metabolite, at concentrations well above C_{max} levels achieved within the therapeutic dose range, are neither inhibitors of nor high affinity substrates for human liver cytochrome P450 isoforms, epoxide hydrolase or UDP-glucuronidation enzymes. In addition, levetiracetam does not affect the *in vitro* glucuronidation of valproic acid.

Levetiracetam circulates largely unbound (<10% bound) to plasma proteins; clinically significant interactions with other drugs through competition for protein binding sites are therefore unlikely.

Potential pharmacokinetic interactions were assessed in clinical pharmacokinetic studies (phenytoin, valproate, oral contraceptive, digoxin, warfarin, probenecid) and through pharmacokinetic screening in the placebo-controlled clinical studies in epilepsy patients.

Drug-Drug Interactions Between KEPPRA And Other Antiepileptic Drugs (AEDs)

Phenytoin

KEPPRA (3000 mg daily) had no effect on the pharmacokinetic disposition of phenytoin in patients with refractory epilepsy. Pharmacokinetics of levetiracetam were also not affected by phenytoin.

Valproate

KEPPRA (1500 mg twice daily) did not alter the pharmacokinetics of valproate in healthy volunteers. Valproate 500 mg twice daily did not modify the rate or extent of levetiracetam absorption or its plasma clearance or urinary excretion. There also was no effect on exposure to and the excretion of the primary metabolite, ucb L057.

Potential drug interactions between KEPPRA and other AEDs (carbamazepine, gabapentin, lamotrigine, phenobarbital, phenytoin, primidone and valproate) were also assessed by evaluating the serum concentrations of levetiracetam and these AEDs during placebo-controlled clinical studies. These data indicate that levetiracetam does not influence the plasma concentration of other AEDs and that these AEDs do not influence the pharmacokinetics of levetiracetam.

Effect Of AEDs In Pediatric Patients

There was about a 22% increase of apparent total body clearance of levetiracetam when it was co-administered with enzyme-inducing AEDs. Dose adjustment is not recommended. Levetiracetam had no effect on plasma concentrations of carbamazepine, valproate, topiramate, or lamotrigine.

Other Drug Interactions

Oral Contraceptives

KEPPRA (500 mg twice daily) did not influence the pharmacokinetics of an oral contraceptive containing 0.03 mg ethinyl estradiol and 0.15 mg levonorgestrel, or of the luteinizing hormone and progesterone levels, indicating that impairment of contraceptive efficacy is unlikely. Coadministration of this oral contraceptive did not influence the pharmacokinetics of levetiracetam.

Digoxin

KEPPRA (1000 mg twice daily) did not influence the pharmacokinetics and pharmacodynamics (ECG) of digoxin given as a 0.25 mg dose every day. Coadministration of digoxin did not influence the pharmacokinetics of levetiracetam.

Warfarin

KEPPRA (1000 mg twice daily) did not influence the pharmacokinetics of R and S warfarin. Prothrombin time was not affected by levetiracetam. Coadministration of warfarin did not affect the pharmacokinetics of levetiracetam.

Probenecid

Probenecid, a renal tubular secretion blocking agent, administered at a dose of 500 mg four times a day, did not change the pharmacokinetics of levetiracetam 1000 mg twice daily. C^{ss}_{max} of the metabolite, ucb L057, was approximately doubled in the presence of probenecid while the fraction of drug excreted unchanged in the urine remained the same. Renal clearance of ucb L057 in the presence of probenecid decreased 60%, probably related to competitive inhibition of tubular secretion of ucb L057. The effect of KEPPRA on probenecid was not studied.

Carcinogenesis, Mutagenesis, Impairment Of Fertility

Carcinogenesis

Rats were dosed with levetiracetam in the diet for 104 weeks at doses of 50, 300 and 1800 mg/kg/day. The highest dose corresponds to 6 times the maximum recommended daily human dose (MRHD) of 3000 mg on a mg/m^2 basis and it also provided systemic exposure (AUC) approximately 6 times that achieved in humans receiving the MRHD. There was no evidence of carcinogenicity. A study was conducted in which mice received levetiracetam in the diet for 80 weeks at doses of 60, 240 and 960 mg/kg/day (high dose is equivalent to 2 times the MRHD on a mg/m^2 or exposure basis). Although no evidence for carcinogenicity was seen, the potential for a carcinogenic response has not been fully evaluated in that species because adequate doses have not been studied.

Mutagenesis

Levetiracetam was not mutagenic in the Ames test or in mammalian cells *in vitro* in the Chinese hamster ovary/HGPRT locus assay. It was not clastogenic in an *in vitro* analysis of metaphase chromosomes obtained from Chinese hamster ovary cells or in an *in vivo* mouse micronucleus assay. The hydrolysis product and major human metabolite of levetiracetam (ucb L057) was not mutagenic in the Ames test or the *in vitro* mouse lymphoma assay.

Impairment Of Fertility

No adverse effects on male or female fertility or reproductive performance were observed in rats at doses up to 1800 mg/kg/day (approximately 6 times the maximum recommended human dose on a mg/m^2 or exposure basis).

Pregnancy

Pregnancy Category C

In animal studies, levetiracetam produced evidence of developmental toxicity at doses similar to or greater than human therapeutic doses.

Administration to female rats throughout pregnancy and lactation was associated with increased incidences of minor fetal skeletal abnormalities and retarded offspring growth pre- and/or postnatally at doses ≥350 mg/kg/day (approximately equivalent to the maximum recommended human dose of 3000 mg [MRHD] on a mg/m^2 basis) and with increased pup mortality and offspring behavioral alterations at a dose of 1800 mg/kg/day (6 times the MRHD on a mg/m^2 basis). The developmental no effect dose was 70 mg/kg/day (0.2 times the MRHD on a mg/m^2 basis). There was no overt maternal toxicity at the doses used in this study.

Treatment of pregnant rabbits during the period of organogenesis resulted in increased embryofetal mortality and increased incidences of minor fetal skeletal abnormalities at doses ≥600 mg/kg/day (approximately 4 times MRHD on a mg/m^2 basis) and in decreased fetal weights and increased incidences of fetal malformations at a dose of 1800 mg/kg/day (12 times the MRHD on a mg/m^2 basis). The developmental no effect dose was 200 mg/kg/day (1.3 times the MRHD on a mg/m^2 basis). Maternal toxicity was also observed at 1800 mg/kg/day.

When pregnant rats were treated during the period of organogenesis, fetal weights were decreased and the incidence of fetal skeletal variations was increased at a dose of 3600 mg/kg/day (12 times the MRHD). 1200 mg/kg/day (4 times the MRHD) was a developmental no effect dose. There was no evidence of maternal toxicity in this study.

Treatment of rats during the last third of gestation and throughout lactation produced no adverse developmental or maternal effects at doses of up to 1800 mg/kg/day (6 times the MRHD on a mg/m^2 basis).

There are no adequate and well-controlled studies in pregnant women. KEPPRA should be used during pregnancy only if the potential benefit justifies the potential risk to the fetus.

KEPPRA Pregnancy Registry

UCB, Inc. has established the KEPPRA Pregnancy Registry to advance scientific knowledge about safety and outcomes associated with pregnant women being treated with KEPPRA. To ensure broad program access and reach, either a healthcare provider or the patient can initiate enrollment in the KEPPRA Pregnancy Registry by calling (888) 537-7734 (toll free). Patients may also enroll in the North American Antiepileptic Drug Pregnancy Registry by calling (888) 233-2334 (toll free).

Labor And Delivery

The effect of KEPPRA on labor and delivery in humans is unknown.

Nursing Mothers

Levetiracetam is excreted in breast milk. Because of the potential for serious adverse reactions in nursing infants from KEPPRA, a decision should be made whether to discontinue nursing or discontinue the drug, taking into account the importance of the drug to the mother.

Pediatric Use

Safety and effectiveness in patients below 4 years of age have not been established.

Studies of levetiracetam in juvenile rats (dosing from day 4 through day 52 of age) and dogs (dosing from week 3 through week 7 of age) at doses of up to 1800 mg/kg/day (approximately 7 and 24 times, respectively, the maximum recommended pediatric dose of 60 mg/kg/day on a mg/m^2 basis) did not indicate a potential for age-specific toxicity.

Geriatric Use

Of the total number of subjects in clinical studies of levetiracetam, 347 were 65 and over. No overall differences in safety were observed between these subjects and younger subjects. There were insufficient numbers of elderly subjects in controlled trials of epilepsy to adequately assess the effectiveness of KEPPRA in these patients.

A study in 16 elderly subjects (age 61-88 years) with oral administration of single dose and multiple twice-daily doses for 10 days showed no pharmacokinetic differences related to age alone.

Levetiracetam is known to be substantially excreted by the kidney, and the risk of adverse reactions to this drug may be greater in patients with impaired renal function. Because elderly patients are more likely to have decreased renal function, care should be taken in dose selection, and it may be useful to monitor renal function.

Use In Patients With Impaired Renal Function

Clearance of levetiracetam is decreased in patients with renal impairment and is correlated with creatinine clearance. Caution should be taken in dosing patients with moderate and severe renal impairment and in patients undergoing hemodialysis. The dosage should be reduced in patients with impaired renal function receiving KEPPRA and supplemental doses should be given to patients after dialysis (see CLINICAL PHARMACOLOGY and DOSAGE AND ADMINISTRATION, Adult Patients With Impaired Renal Function).

ADVERSE REACTIONS

The prescriber should be aware that the adverse event incidence figures in the following tables, obtained when KEPPRA was added to concurrent AED therapy, cannot be used to predict the frequency of adverse experiences in the course of usual medical practice where patient characteristics and other factors may differ from those prevailing during clinical studies. Similarly, the cited frequencies cannot be directly compared with figures obtained from other clinical investigations involving different treatments, uses, or investigators. An inspection of these frequencies, however, does provide the prescriber with one basis to estimate the relative contribution of drug and non-drug factors to the adverse event incidences in the population studied.

Partial Onset Seizures

In well-controlled clinical studies in adults with partial onset seizures, the most frequently reported adverse events associated with the use of KEPPRA in combination with other AEDs, not seen at an equivalent frequency among placebo-treated patients, were somnolence, asthenia, infection and dizziness. In the well-controlled pediatric clinical study in children 4 to 16 years of age with partial onset seizures, the adverse events most frequently reported with the use of KEPPRA in combination with other AEDs, not seen at an equivalent frequency among placebo-treated patients, were somnolence, accidental injury, hostility, nervousness, and asthenia.

Table 7 lists treatment-emergent adverse events that occurred in at least 1% of adult epilepsy patients treated with KEPPRA participating in placebo-controlled studies and were numerically more common than in patients treated with placebo. Table 8 lists treatment-emergent adverse events that occurred in at least 2% of pediatric epilepsy patients (ages 4-16 years) treated with KEPPRA participating in the placebo-controlled study and were numerically more common than in pediatric patients treated with placebo. In these studies, either KEPPRA or placebo was added to concurrent AED therapy. Adverse events were usually mild to moderate in intensity.

Table 7: Incidence (%) Of Treatment-Emergent Adverse Events In Placebo-Controlled, Add-On Studies In Adults Experiencing Partial Onset Seizures By Body System (Adverse Events Occurred In At Least 1% Of KEPPRA-Treated Patients And Occurred More Frequently Than Placebo-Treated Patients)

Body System/ Adverse Event	KEPPRA (N=769) %	Placebo (N=439) %
Body as a Whole		
Asthenia	15	9
Headache	14	13
Infection	13	8
Pain	7	6
Digestive System		
Anorexia	3	2

Continued on next page

Keppra—Cont.

Nervous System		
Somnolence	15	8
Dizziness	9	4
Depression	4	2
Nervousness	4	2
Ataxia	3	1
Vertigo	3	1
Amnesia	2	1
Anxiety	2	1
Hostility	2	1
Paresthesia	2	1
Emotional Lability	2	0
Respiratory System		
Pharyngitis	6	4
Rhinitis	4	3
Cough Increased	2	1
Sinusitis	2	1
Special Senses		
Diplopia	2	1

Other events reported by at least 1% of adult KEPPRA-treated patients but as or more frequent in the placebo group were the following: abdominal pain, accidental injury, amblyopia, arthralgia, back pain, bronchitis, chest pain, confusion, constipation, convulsion, diarrhea, drug level increased, dyspepsia, ecchymosis, fever, flu syndrome, fungal infection, gastroenteritis, gingivitis, grand mal convulsion, insomnia, nausea, otitis media, rash, thinking abnormal, tremor, urinary tract infection, vomiting and weight gain.

Table 8: Incidence (%) Of Treatment-Emergent Adverse Events In A Placebo-Controlled, Add-On Study In Pediatric Patients Ages 4-16 Years Experiencing Partial Onset Seizures By Body System (Adverse Events Occurred In At Least 2% Of KEPPRA-Treated Patients And Occurred More Frequently Than Placebo-Treated Patients)

Body System/ Adverse Event	KEPPRA (N=101) %	Placebo (N=97) %
Body as a Whole		
Accidental Injury	17	10
Asthenia	9	3
Pain	6	3
Flu Syndrome	3	2
Face Edema	2	1
Neck Pain	2	1
Viral Infection	2	1
Digestive System		
Vomiting	15	13
Anorexia	13	8
Diarrhea	8	7
Gastroenteritis	4	2
Constipation	3	1
Hemic and Lymphatic System		
Ecchymosis	4	1
Metabolic and Nutritional		
Dehydration	2	1
Nervous System		
Somnolence	23	11
Hostility	12	6
Nervousness	10	2
Personality Disorder	8	7
Dizziness	7	2
Emotional Lability	6	4
Agitation	6	1
Depression	3	1
Vertigo	3	1
Reflexes Increased	2	1
Confusion	2	0
Respiratory System		
Rhinitis	13	8
Cough Increased	11	7
Pharyngitis	10	8
Asthma	2	1
Skin and Appendages		
Pruritus	2	0
Skin Discoloration	2	0
Vesiculobullous Rash	2	0
Special Senses		
Conjunctivitis	3	2
Amblyopia	2	0
Ear Pain	2	0
Urogenital System		
Albuminuria	4	0
Urine Abnormality	2	1

Other events occurring in at least 2% of pediatric KEPPRA-treated patients but as or more frequent in the placebo group were the following: abdominal pain, allergic reaction, ataxia, convulsion, epistaxis, fever, headache, hyperkinesia, infection, insomnia, nausea, otitis media, rash, sinusitis, status epilepticus (not otherwise specified), thinking abnormal, tremor, and urinary incontinence.

Myoclonic Seizures

Although the pattern of adverse events in this study seems somewhat different from that seen in patients with partial seizures, this is likely due to the much smaller number of patients in this study compared to partial seizure studies. The adverse event pattern for patients with JME is expected to be essentially the same as for patients with partial seizures.

In the well-controlled clinical study that included both adolescent (12 to 16 years of age) and adult patients with myoclonic seizures, the most frequently reported adverse events associated with the use of KEPPRA in combination with other AEDs, not seen at an equivalent frequency among placebo-treated patients, were somnolence, neck pain, and pharyngitis.

Table 9 lists treatment-emergent adverse events that occurred in at least 5% of juvenile myoclonic epilepsy patients experiencing myoclonic seizures treated with KEPPRA and were numerically more common than in patients treated with placebo. In this study, either KEPPRA or placebo was added to concurrent AED therapy. Adverse events were usually mild to moderate in intensity.

Table 9: Incidence (%) Of Treatment-Emergent Adverse Events In A Placebo-Controlled, Add-On Study In Patients 12 Years Of Age And Older With Myoclonic Seizures By Body System (Adverse Events Occurred In At Least 5% Of KEPPRA-Treated Patients And Occurred More Frequently Than Placebo-Treated Patients)

Body System / MedDRA preferred term	KEPPRA (N=60) %	Placebo (N=60) %
Ear and labyrinth disorders		
Vertigo	5	3
Infections and infestations		
Pharyngitis	7	0
Influenza	5	2
Musculoskeletal and connective tissue disorders		
Neck pain	8	2

Nervous system disorders		
Somnolence	12	2
Psychiatric disorders		
Depression	5	2

Other events occurring in at least 5% of KEPPRA-treated patients with myoclonic seizures but as or more frequent in the placebo group were the following: fatigue and headache.

Primary Generalized Tonic-Clonic Seizures

Although the pattern of adverse events in this study seems somewhat different from that seen in patients with partial seizures, this is likely due to the much smaller number of patients in this study compared to partial seizure studies. The adverse event pattern for patients with PGTC seizures is expected to be essentially the same as for patients with partial seizures.

In the well-controlled clinical study that included patients 4 years of age and older with primary generalized tonic-clonic (PGTC) seizures, the most frequently reported adverse event associated with the use of KEPPRA in combination with other AEDs, not seen at an equivalent frequency among placebo-treated patients, was nasopharyngitis.

Table 10 lists treatment-emergent adverse events that occurred in at least 5% of idiopathic generalized epilepsy patients experiencing PGTC seizures treated with KEPPRA and were numerically more common than in patients treated with placebo. In this study, either KEPPRA or placebo was added to concurrent AED therapy. Adverse events were usually mild to moderate in intensity.

Table 10: Incidence (%) Of Treatment-Emergent Adverse Events In A Placebo-Controlled, Add-On Study In Patients 4 Years Of Age And Older With PGTC Seizures By MedDRA System Organ Class (Adverse Events Occurred In At Least 5% Of KEPPRA-Treated Patients And Occurred More Frequently Than Placebo-Treated Patients)

MedDRA System Organ Class/ Preferred Term	KEPPRA (N=79) %	Placebo (N=84) %
Gastrointestinal disorders		
Diarrhea	8	7
General disorders and administration site conditions		
Fatigue	10	8
Infections and infestations		
Nasopharyngitis	14	5
Psychiatric disorders		
Irritability	6	2
Mood swings	5	1

Other events occurring in at least 5% of KEPPRA-treated patients with PGTC seizures but as or more frequent in the placebo group were the following: dizziness, headache, influenza, and somnolence.

Time Course Of Onset Of Adverse Events For Partial Onset Seizures

Of the most frequently reported adverse events in adults experiencing partial onset seizures, asthenia, somnolence and dizziness appeared to occur predominantly during the first 4 weeks of treatment with KEPPRA.

Discontinuation Or Dose Reduction In Well-Controlled Clinical Studies

Partial Onset Seizures

In well-controlled adult clinical studies, 15.0% of patients receiving KEPPRA and 11.6% receiving placebo either discontinued or had a dose reduction as a result of an adverse event. Table 11 lists the most common (>1%) adverse events that resulted in discontinuation or dose reduction.

Table 11: Adverse Events That Most Commonly Resulted In Discontinuation Or Dose Reduction In Placebo-Controlled Studies In Adult Patients Experiencing Partial Onset Seizures

	Number (%)	
	KEPPRA (N=769)	Placebo (N=439)
Asthenia	10 (1.3%)	3 (0.7%)
Convulsion	23 (3.0%)	15 (3.4%)
Dizziness	11 (1.4%)	0

Rash	0	5 (1.1%)
Somnolence	34 (4.4%)	7 (1.6%)

In the well-controlled pediatric clinical study, 16.8% of patients receiving KEPPRA and 20.6% receiving placebo either discontinued or had a dose reduction as a result of an adverse event. The adverse events most commonly associated (≥3% in patients receiving KEPPRA) with discontinuation or dose reduction in the well-controlled study are presented in Table 12.

Table 12: Adverse Events Most Commonly Associated With Discontinuation Or Dose Reduction In The Placebo-Controlled Study In Pediatric Patients Ages 4-16 Years Experiencing Partial Onset Seizures

	Number (%)	
	KEPPRA (N=101)	Placebo (N=97)
Asthenia	3 (3.0%)	0
Hostility	7 (6.9%)	2 (2.1%)
Somnolence	3 (3.0%)	3 (3.1%)

Myoclonic Seizures
In the placebo-controlled study, 8.3% of patients receiving KEPPRA and 1.7% receiving placebo either discontinued or had a dose reduction as a result of an adverse event. The adverse events that led to discontinuation or dose reduction in the well-controlled study are presented in Table 13.

Table 13: Adverse Events That Resulted In Discontinuation Or Dose Reduction In The Placebo-Controlled Study In Patients With Juvenile Myoclonic Epilepsy

Body System/ MedDRA preferred term	KEPPRA (N=60) n (%)	Placebo (N=60) n (%)
Anxiety	2 (3.3%)	1 (1.7%)
Depressed mood	1 (1.7%)	0
Depression	1 (1.7%)	0
Diplopia	1 (1.7%)	0
Hypersomnia	1 (1.7%)	0
Insomnia	1 (1.7%)	0
Irritability	1 (1.7%)	0
Nervousness	1 (1.7%)	0
Somnolence	1 (1.7%)	0

Primary Generalized Tonic-Clonic Seizures
In the placebo-controlled study, 5.1% of patients receiving KEPPRA and 8.3% receiving placebo either discontinued or had a dose reduction during the treatment period as a result of a treatment-emergent adverse event.
This study was too small to adequately characterize the adverse events leading to discontinuation. It is expected that the adverse events that would lead to discontinuation in this population would be similar to those resulting in discontinuation in other epilepsy trials (see tables 11-13).
Comparison Of Gender, Age And Race
The overall adverse experience profile of KEPPRA was similar between females and males. There are insufficient data to support a statement regarding the distribution of adverse experience reports by age and race.
Postmarketing Experience
In addition to the adverse experiences listed above, the following have been reported in patients receiving marketed KEPPRA worldwide. The listing is alphabetized: abnormal liver function test, hepatic failure, hepatitis, leukopenia, neutropenia, pancreatitis, pancytopenia (with bone marrow suppression identified in some of these cases), thrombocytopenia, and weight loss. Alopecia has been reported with KEPPRA use; recovery was observed in majority of cases where KEPPRA was discontinued. There have been reports of suicidal behavior (including completed suicide, suicide attempt and suicidal ideation) with marketed KEPPRA (see PRECAUTIONS, Information For Patients). These adverse experiences have not been listed above, and data are insufficient to support an estimate of their incidence or to establish causation.

DRUG ABUSE AND DEPENDENCE

The abuse and dependence potential of KEPPRA has not been evaluated in human studies.

OVERDOSAGE

Signs, Symptoms And Laboratory Findings Of Acute Overdosage In Humans
The highest known dose of KEPPRA received in the clinical development program was 6000 mg/day. Other than drowsiness, there were no adverse events in the few known cases

of overdose in clinical trials. Cases of somnolence, agitation, aggression, depressed level of consciousness, respiratory depression and coma were observed with KEPPRA overdoses in postmarketing use.
Treatment Or Management Of Overdose
There is no specific antidote for overdose with KEPPRA. If indicated, elimination of unabsorbed drug should be attempted by emesis or gastric lavage; usual precautions should be observed to maintain airway. General supportive care of the patient is indicated including monitoring of vital signs and observation of the patient's clinical status. A Certified Poison Control Center should be contacted for up to date information on the management of overdose with KEPPRA.
Hemodialysis
Standard hemodialysis procedures result in significant clearance of levetiracetam (approximately 50% in 4 hours) and should be considered in cases of overdose. Although hemodialysis has not been performed in the few known cases of overdose, it may be indicated by the patient's clinical state or in patients with significant renal impairment.

DOSAGE AND ADMINISTRATION

KEPPRA is indicated as adjunctive treatment of partial onset seizures in adults and children 4 years of age and older with epilepsy.
KEPPRA is indicated as adjunctive therapy in the treatment of myoclonic seizures in adults and adolescents 12 years of age and older with juvenile myoclonic epilepsy.
KEPPRA is indicated as adjunctive therapy in the treatment of primary generalized tonic-clonic seizures in adults and children 6 years of age and older with idiopathic generalized epilepsy.
Partial Onset Seizures
Adults 16 Years And Older
In clinical trials, daily doses of 1000 mg, 2000 mg, and 3000 mg, given as twice-daily dosing, were shown to be effective. Although in some studies there was a tendency toward greater response with higher dose (see CLINICAL STUDIES), a consistent increase in response with increased dose has not been shown.
Treatment should be initiated with a daily dose of 1000 mg/day, given as twice-daily dosing (500 mg BID). Additional dosing increments may be given (1000 mg/day additional every 2 weeks) to a maximum recommended daily dose of 3000 mg. Doses greater than 3000 mg/day have been used in open-label studies for periods of 6 months and longer. There is no evidence that doses greater than 3000 mg/day confer additional benefit.
Pediatric Patients Ages 4 To <16 Years
Treatment should be initiated with a daily dose of 20 mg/kg in 2 divided doses (10 mg/kg BID). The daily dose should be increased every 2 weeks by increments of 20 mg/kg to the recommended daily dose of 60 mg/kg (30 mg/kg BID). If a patient cannot tolerate a daily dose of 60 mg/kg, the daily dose may be reduced. In the clinical trial, the mean daily dose was 52 mg/kg. Patients with body weight ≤ 20 kg should be dosed with oral solution. Patients with body weight above 20 kg can be dosed with either tablets or oral solution. Table 14 below provides a guideline for tablet dosing based on weight during titration to 60 mg/kg/day. Only whole tablets should be administered.
KEPPRA is given orally with or without food.

Table 14: KEPPRA Tablet Weight-Based Dosing Guide For Children

Patient Weight	Daily Dose		
	20 mg/kg/day (BID dosing)	40 mg/kg/day (BID dosing)	60 mg/kg/day (BID dosing)
20.1-40 kg	500 mg/day (1 × 250 mg tablet BID)	1000 mg/day (1 × 500 mg tablet BID)	1500 mg/day (1 × 750 mg tablet BID)
>40 kg	1000 mg/day (1 × 500 mg tablet BID)	2000 mg/day (2 × 500 mg tablets BID)	3000 mg/day (2 × 750 mg tablets BID)

The following calculation should be used to determine the appropriate daily dose of oral solution for pediatric patients based on a daily dose of 20 mg/kg/day, 40 mg/kg/day or 60 mg/kg/day:

$$\text{Total daily dose (mL/day)} = \frac{\text{Daily dose (mg/kg/day)} \times \text{patient weight (kg)}}{100 \text{ mg/mL}}$$

A household teaspoon or tablespoon is not an adequate measuring device. It is recommended that a calibrated measuring device be obtained and used. Healthcare providers should recommend a device that can measure and deliver the prescribed dose accurately, and provide instructions for measuring the dosage.
Myoclonic Seizures In Patients 12 Years Of Age And Older With Juvenile Myoclonic Epilepsy
Treatment should be initiated with a dose of 1000 mg/day, given as twice-daily dosing (500 mg BID). Dosage should be increased by 1000 mg/day every 2 weeks to the recommended daily dose of 3000 mg. The effectiveness of doses lower than 3000 mg/day has not been studied.
Primary Generalized Tonic-Clonic Seizures
Adults 16 Years And Older
Treatment should be initiated with a dose of 1000 mg/day, given as twice-daily dosing (500 mg BID). Dosage should be

increased by 1000 mg/day every 2 weeks to the recommended daily dose of 3000 mg. The effectiveness of doses lower than 3000 mg/day has not been adequately studied.
Pediatric Patients Ages 6 To <16 Years
Treatment should be initiated with a daily dose of 20 mg/kg in 2 divided doses (10 mg/kg BID). The daily dose should be increased every 2 weeks by increments of 20 mg/kg to the recommended daily dose of 60 mg/kg (30 mg/kg BID). The effectiveness of doses lower than 60 mg/kg/day has not been adequately studied. Patients with body weight ≤ 20 kg should be dosed with oral solution. Patients with body weight above 20 kg can be dosed with either tablets or oral solution. See Table 14 for tablet dosing based on weight during titration to 60 mg/kg/day. Only whole tablets should be administered.
Adult Patients With Impaired Renal Function
KEPPRA dosing must be individualized according to the patient's renal function status. Recommended doses and adjustment for dose for adults are shown in Table 15. To use this dosing table, an estimate of the patient's creatinine clearance (CLcr) in mL/min is needed. CLcr in mL/min may be estimated from serum creatinine (mg/dL) determination using the following formula:

$$CLcr = \frac{[140 - \text{age (years)}] \times \text{weight (kg)}}{72 \times \text{serum creatinine (mg/dL)}} \quad (\times 0.85 \text{ for female patients})$$

Table 15: Dosing Adjustment Regimen For Adult Patients With Impaired Renal Function

Group	Creatinine Clearance (mL/min)	Dosage (mg)	Frequency
Normal	> 80	500 to 1,500	Every 12 h
Mild	50 – 80	500 to 1,000	Every 12 h
Moderate	30 – 50	250 to 750	Every 12 h
Severe	< 30	250 to 500	Every 12 h
ESRD patients using dialysis	—	500 to 1,000	[1]Every 24 h

[1] Following dialysis, a 250 to 500 mg supplemental dose is recommended.

HOW SUPPLIED

KEPPRA 250 mg tablets are blue, oblong-shaped, scored, film-coated tablets debossed with "ucb 250" on one side. They are supplied in white HDPE bottles containing 120 tablets (NDC 50474-594-40).
KEPPRA 500 mg tablets are yellow, oblong-shaped, scored, film-coated tablets debossed with "ucb 500" on one side. They are supplied in white HDPE bottles containing 120 tablets (NDC 50474-595-40).
KEPPRA 750 mg tablets are orange, oblong-shaped, scored, film-coated tablets debossed with "ucb 750" on one side. They are supplied in white HDPE bottles containing 120 tablets (NDC 50474-596-40).
KEPPRA 1000 mg tablets are white, oblong-shaped, scored, film-coated tablets debossed with "ucb 1000" on one side. They are supplied in white HDPE bottles containing 60 tablets (NDC 50474-597-66).
KEPPRA 100 mg/mL oral solution is a clear, colorless, grape-flavored liquid. It is supplied in 16 fl. oz. white HDPE bottles (NDC 50474-001-48).
Storage
Store at 25°C (77°F); excursions permitted to 15-30°C (59-86°F) [see USP Controlled Room Temperature].
For Medical Information
Contact: Medical Affairs Department
Phone: (866) 822-0068
Fax: (770) 970-8859
KEPPRA Tablets and KEPPRA Oral Solution
Manufactured for
UCB, Inc.
Smyrna, GA 30080
KEPPRA is a registered trademark of the UCB Group of companies
© 2008, UCB, Inc., Smyrna, GA 30080. All rights reserved.
Printed in the U.S.A.
Rev. 26E 02/2008

PATIENT INFORMATION

KEPPRA® (pronounced KEPP-ruh) (levetiracetam) 250 mg, 500 mg, 750 mg, and 1000 mg tablets and 100 mg/mL oral solution
Read the Patient Information that comes with KEPPRA before you start using it and each time you get a refill. There may be new information. This leaflet does not take the place of talking with your healthcare provider about your condition or your treatment.
Before taking your medicine, make sure you have received the correct medicine. Compare the name above with the name on your bottle and the appearance of your medicine with the description of KEPPRA provided below. Contact your pharmacist immediately if you believe a dispensing error may have occurred.
250 mg KEPPRA tablets are blue, oblong-shaped, scored, film-coated tablets marked with "ucb 250" on one side.

Continued on next page

Keppra—Cont.

500 mg KEPPRA tablets are yellow, oblong-shaped, scored, film-coated tablets marked with "ucb 500" on one side.
750 mg KEPPRA tablets are orange, oblong-shaped, scored, film-coated tablets marked with "ucb 750" on one side.
1000 mg KEPPRA tablets are white, oblong-shaped, scored, film-coated tablets marked with "ucb 1000" on one side.
KEPPRA oral solution is a clear, colorless, grape-flavored liquid.

What is KEPPRA?
KEPPRA is a medicine taken by mouth that is used with other medicines to treat:
- partial onset seizures in patients 4 years of age and older with epilepsy
- myoclonic seizures in patients 12 years of age and older with juvenile myoclonic epilepsy
- primary generalized tonic-clonic seizures in adults and children 6 years of age and older with idiopathic generalized epilepsy.

Who should not take KEPPRA?
Do not take KEPPRA if you are allergic to any of its ingredients. The active ingredient is levetiracetam. See the end of this leaflet for a list of all the ingredients in KEPPRA.

What should I tell my healthcare provider before starting KEPPRA?
Tell your healthcare provider about all of your medical conditions, including if you:
- **have kidney disease.** You may need a lower dose of KEPPRA.
- **are pregnant or planning to become pregnant.** It is not known if KEPPRA can harm your unborn baby. If you use KEPPRA while you are pregnant, ask your healthcare provider about being in the KEPPRA Pregnancy Registry. You can join this registry by calling (888) 537-7734 (toll free). You may also join the North American Antiepileptic Drug Pregnancy Registry by calling (888) 233-2334 (toll free).
- **are breast feeding.** KEPPRA can pass into your milk and may harm your baby. You should choose to either take KEPPRA or breast feed, but not both.
Tell your healthcare provider about all the medicines you take, including prescription, nonprescription, vitamins, and herbal supplements.
Know the medicines you take. Keep a list of them to show your healthcare provider and pharmacist each time you get a new medicine.

How should I take KEPPRA?
- Take KEPPRA exactly as prescribed. KEPPRA is usually taken twice a day. Once in the morning and once at night. Take KEPPRA at the same times each day.
- Your healthcare provider may start you on a lower dose of KEPPRA and increase it as your body gets used to the medicine.
- Take KEPPRA with or without food. Swallow the tablets whole. Do not chew or crush tablets. Use the KEPPRA oral solution if you cannot swallow tablets. Use a medicine dropper or medicine cup to measure KEPPRA oral solution. Do not use a teaspoon. Ask your pharmacist for a medicine dropper or medicine cup to help you measure KEPPRA. If your healthcare provider has given you KEPPRA oral solution for your child, be sure to ask your pharmacist for a medicine syringe to help you measure the correct amount of KEPPRA oral solution. Ask your pharmacist for instructions on how to properly use the medicine syringe or dosing device that has been provided to you.
- If you miss a dose of KEPPRA, do not double your next dose to make up for the missed dose. If it has only been a few hours since your missed dose, take KEPPRA as soon as you remember then return to your regular schedule. If it is almost time for the next dose, skip the missed dose and resume your regular schedule. Talk with your healthcare provider for more detailed instructions.
- If you take too much KEPPRA or overdose, call your local Poison Control Center or emergency room right away.
- Do not stop taking KEPPRA or any other seizure medicine unless your healthcare provider told you to. Stopping a seizure medicine all at once can cause seizures that will not stop (status epilepticus), a very serious problem.
- Tell your healthcare provider if your seizures get worse or if you have any new types of seizures.

What should I avoid while taking KEPPRA?
Do not drive, operate machinery or do other dangerous activities until you know how KEPPRA affects you. KEPPRA may make you dizzy or sleepy.

What are the possible side effects of KEPPRA?
Adults
KEPPRA may cause the following serious problems in adults. Call your healthcare provider right away if you get any of the following symptoms:
- extreme sleepiness, tiredness, and weakness
- problems with muscle coordination (problems walking and moving)
- mood and behavior changes such as aggression, agitation, anger, anxiety, apathy, mood swings, depression, hostility, and irritability. A few people may get psychotic symptoms such as hallucinations (seeing or hearing things that are really not there), delusions (false or strange thoughts or beliefs) and unusual behavior.
- thoughts of suicide (thoughts of killing yourself)
The most common side effects with KEPPRA in adults are:
- sleepiness
- weakness

- dizziness
- infection
These side effects could happen at any time but happen most often within the first four weeks of treatment except for infection.
Children
KEPPRA may cause the following serious problems in children. Call your child's healthcare provider right away if they get any of the following symptoms:
- extreme sleepiness, tiredness, and weakness
- mood and behavior changes such as aggression, agitation, anger, anxiety, apathy, depression, hostility, and irritability
- thoughts of suicide
The most common side effects with KEPPRA in children, in addition to those seen in adults are:
- sleepiness
- accidental injury
- hostility
- irritability
- weakness
These side effects could happen at any time.
These are not all the side effects of KEPPRA. For more information, ask your healthcare provider or pharmacist. If you get any side effects that concern you, call your healthcare provider.

How should I store KEPPRA?
- Store KEPPRA at room temperature away from heat and light.
- **Keep KEPPRA and all medicines out of the reach of children.**

General information about KEPPRA.
Medicines are sometimes prescribed for conditions other than those described in patient information leaflets. Do not use KEPPRA for a condition for which it was not prescribed. Do not give your KEPPRA to other people, even if they have the same symptoms that you have. It may harm them.
This leaflet summarizes the most important information about KEPPRA. If you would like more information, talk with your healthcare provider. You can ask your healthcare provider or pharmacist for information about KEPPRA that is written for healthcare professionals. You can also get information about KEPPRA at www.keppra.com.

What are the ingredients of KEPPRA?
KEPPRA tablets contain the labeled amount of levetiracetam. Inactive ingredients: colloidal silicon dioxide, croscarmellose sodium, magnesium stearate, polyethylene glycol 3350, polyethylene glycol 6000, polyvinyl alcohol, talc, titanium dioxide, and additional agents listed below:
250 mg tablets: FD&C Blue #2/indigo carmine aluminum lake
500 mg tablets: iron oxide yellow
750 mg tablets: FD&C yellow #6/sunset yellow FCF aluminum lake, iron oxide red
KEPPRA oral solution contains 100 mg of levetiracetam per mL. Inactive ingredients: ammonium glycyrrhizinate, citric acid monohydrate, glycerin, maltitol solution, methylparaben, potassium acesulfame, propylparaben, purified water, sodium citrate dihydrate and natural and artificial flavor. KEPPRA does not contain lactose or gluten. KEPPRA oral solution does contain carbohydrates. The liquid is dye-free.

Rx Only
This patient leaflet has been approved by the US Food and Drug Administration.
Distributed by
UCB, Inc.
Smyrna, GA 30080

KEPPRA® INJECTION   ℞

[kepp-ruh]
(levetiracetam)
Injection for Intravenous Use
Initial U.S. Approval: 1999

Prescribing information for this product, which appears on pages 3256–3259 of the 2008 PDR, has been completely revised as follows. Please write "See Supplement A" next to the product heading.
HIGHLIGHTS OF PRESCRIBING INFORMATION
These highlights do not include all the information needed to use KEPPRA® injection safely and effectively. See full prescribing information for KEPPRA® injection.
------------RECENT MAJOR CHANGES-------------
Indications and Usage, Myoclonic Seizures (**1.2**)   [09/2007]
Dosage and Administration (**2.2**)   [09/2007]
Warnings and Precautions (**5.1,5.3**)   [09/2007]
-------------INDICATIONS AND USAGE-------------
KEPPRA injection is an antiepileptic drug indicated for:
Partial Onset Seizures (1.1)
- Adjunct therapy in adults (≥16 years of age) when oral administration of KEPPRA is temporarily not feasible.
Myoclonic Seizures in Patients with Juvenile Myoclonic Epilepsy (1.2)
- Adjunct therapy in adults (≥16 years of age) with juvenile myoclonic epilepsy when oral administration of KEPPRA is temporarily not feasible.
----------DOSAGE AND ADMINISTRATION----------
KEPPRA injection should be diluted in 100 mL of a compatible diluent and administered intravenously as a 15-minute infusion (**2.1**).
Initial Exposure (2.2):
- **Partial Onset Seizures:**   1000 mg/day, given as twice-daily dosing (500 mg twice daily), increased as needed

and as tolerated in increments of 1000 mg/day additional every 2 weeks to a maximum recommended daily dose of 3000 mg.
- **Myoclonic Seizures in Patients with Juvenile Myoclonic Epilepsy:**   1000 mg/day, given as twice-daily dosing (500 mg twice daily), increased by 1000 mg/day every 2 weeks to the recommended daily dose of 3000 mg.
Replacement Therapy (2.3):
When switching from oral KEPPRA, the initial total daily intravenous dosage of KEPPRA should be equivalent to the total daily dosage and frequency of oral KEPPRA. At the end of the intravenous treatment period, the patient may be switched to KEPPRA oral administration at the equivalent daily dosage and frequency of the intravenous administration.
See full prescribing information for dosing instructions (**2.5**), adult patients with impaired renal function (**2.6**), and compatibility and stability (**2.7**).
--------DOSAGE FORMS AND STRENGTHS--------
- 500 mg/5 mL single-use vial (**3**)
-----------------CONTRAINDICATIONS---------------
- None (**4**)
----------WARNINGS AND PRECAUTIONS----------
- **Neuropsychiatric Adverse Reactions:** Including: 1) Somnolence and fatigue, 2) Coordination difficulties and 3) Behavioral Abnormalities (e.g., psychotic symptoms, suicide ideation, and other abnormalities). (**5.1**)
- **Withdrawal Seizures:**   lKEPPRA must be gradually withdrawn. (**5.2**)
----------------ADVERSE REACTIONS----------------
- Most common adverse reactions (difference in incidence rate is ≥5% between KEPPRA-treated patients and placebo-treated patients and occurred more frequently in KEPPRA-treated patients) include: somnolence, asthenia, infection, and dizziness (**6.1**).
- Important behavioral adverse reactions (incidence of KEPPRA-treated patients > placebo-treated patients, but <5%) include depression, nervousness, anxiety, and emotional lability (**6.1**).
To report SUSPECTED ADVERSE REACTIONS, contact UCB, Inc. at 866-822-0068 or FDA at 1-800-FDA-1088 or www.fda.gov/medwatch
----------USE IN SPECIFIC POPULATIONS----------
- To enroll in the KEPPRA Pregnancy Registry call 888-537-7734 (toll free). To enroll in the North American Antiepileptic Drug Pregnancy Registry call (888) 233-2334 (toll free). (**8.1**)
- A dose adjustment is recommended for patients with impaired renal function, based on the patient's estimated creatinine clearance (**8.6**).
See 17 for PATIENT COUNSELING INFORMATION
Revised: [02/2008]

FULL PRESCRIBING INFORMATION: CONTENTS*

*Sections or subsections omitted from the Full Prescribing Information are not listed.

FULL PRESCRIBING INFORMATION

1 INDICATIONS AND USAGE

KEPPRA injection is an alternative for adult patients (16 years and older) when oral administration is temporarily not feasible.

1.1 Partial Onset Seizures

KEPPRA is indicated as adjunctive therapy in the treatment of partial onset seizures in adults with epilepsy.

1.2 Myoclonic Seizures in Patients with Juvenile Myoclonic Epilepsy

KEPPRA is indicated as adjunctive therapy in the treatment of myoclonic seizures in adults with juvenile myoclonic epilepsy.

2 DOSAGE AND ADMINISTRATION

2.1 General Information

KEPPRA injection is for intravenous use only and must be diluted prior to administration. KEPPRA injection (500 mg/5 mL) should be diluted in 100 mL of a compatible diluent [*see Dosage and Administration (2.7)*] and administered intravenously as a 15-minute IV infusion.

Product with particulate matter or discoloration should not be used.

Any unused portion of the KEPPRA injection vial contents should be discarded.

2.2 Initial Exposure to KEPPRA

KEPPRA can be initiated with either intravenous or oral administration.

Partial Onset Seizures

In clinical trials of oral KEPPRA, daily doses of 1000 mg, 2000 mg, and 3000 mg, given as twice-daily dosing, were shown to be effective. Although in some studies there was a tendency toward greater response with higher dose [*see Clinical Studies (14.1)*], a consistent increase in response with increased dose has not been shown.

Treatment should be initiated with a daily dose of 1000 mg/day, given as twice-daily dosing (500 mg twice daily). Additional dosing increments may be given (1000 mg/day additional every 2 weeks) to a maximum recommended daily dose of 3000 mg. Doses greater than 3000 mg/day have been used in open-label studies with KEPPRA tablets for periods of 6 months and longer. There is no evidence that doses greater than 3000 mg/day confer additional benefit.

Myoclonic Seizures in Patients with Juvenile Myoclonic Epilepsy

Treatment should be initiated with a dose of 1000 mg/day, given as twice-daily dosing (500 mg twice daily). Dosage should be increased by 1000 mg/day every 2 weeks to the recommended daily dose of 3000 mg. The effectiveness of doses lower than 3000 mg/day has not been studied.

2.3 Replacement Therapy

When switching from oral KEPPRA, the initial total daily intravenous dosage of KEPPRA should be equivalent to the total daily dosage and frequency of oral KEPPRA and should be administered as a 15-minute intravenous infusion following dilution in 100 mL of a compatible diluent.

2.4 Switching to Oral Dosing

At the end of the intravenous treatment period, the patient may be switched to KEPPRA oral administration at the equivalent daily dosage and frequency of the intravenous administration.

2.5 Dosing Instructions

KEPPRA injection is for intravenous use only and must be diluted prior to administration. One vial of KEPPRA injection contains 500 mg levetiracetam (500 mg/5 mL). See Table 1 for the recommended preparation and administration of KEPPRA injection to achieve a dose of 500 mg, 1000 mg, or 1500 mg.

Table 1: Preparation and Administration of KEPPRA Injection

Dose	Withdraw Volume	Volume of Diluent	Infusion Time
500 mg	5 mL (5 mL vial)	100 mL	15 minutes
1000 mg	10 mL (two 5 mL vials)	100 mL	15 minutes
1500 mg	15 mL (three 5 mL vials)	100 mL	15 minutes

For example, to prepare a 1000 mg dose, dilute 10 mL of KEPPRA injection in 100 mL of a compatible diluent [*see Dosage and Administration (2.7)*] and administer intravenously as a 15-minute infusion.

2.6 Adult Patients with Impaired Renal Function

KEPPRA dosing must be individualized according to the patient's renal function status. Recommended doses and adjustment for dose for adults are shown in Table 2. To use this dosing table, an estimate of the patient's creatinine clearance (CLcr) in mL/min is needed. CLcr in mL/min may be estimated from serum creatinine (mg/dL) determination using the following formula:

[See table above]

$$CLcr = \frac{[140\text{-age (years)}] \times \text{weight (kg)}}{72 \times \text{serum creatinine (mg/dL)}} \times {}^{1}0.85$$

[1] For female patients

Table 2: Dosing Adjustment Regimen for Adult Patients with Impaired Renal Function

Group	Creatinine Clearance (mL/min)	Dosage (mg)	Frequency
Normal	> 80	500 to 1,500	Every 12 h
Mild	50 – 80	500 to 1,000	Every 12 h
Moderate	30 – 50	250 to 750	Every 12 h
Severe	< 30	250 to 500	Every 12 h
ESRD patients using dialysis	----	500 to 1,000	[1]Every 24 h

[1] Following dialysis, a 250 to 500 mg supplemental dose is recommended.

2.7 Compatibility and Stability

KEPPRA injection was found to be physically compatible and chemically stable when mixed with the following diluents and antiepileptic drugs for at least 24 hours and stored in polyvinyl chloride (PVC) bags at controlled room temperature 15-30°C (59-86°F).

Diluents

Sodium chloride (0.9%) injection, USP
Lactated Ringer's injection
Dextrose 5% injection, USP

Other Antiepileptic Drugs

Lorazepam
Diazepam
Valproate sodium

There is no data to support the physical compatibility of KEPPRA injection with antiepileptic drugs that are not listed above.

Parenteral drug products should be inspected visually for particulate matter and discoloration prior to administration whenever solution and container permit.

3 DOSAGE FORMS AND STRENGTHS

One vial of KEPPRA injection contains 500 mg levetiracetam (500 mg/5 mL).

4 CONTRAINDICATIONS

None

5 WARNINGS AND PRECAUTIONS

5.1 Neuropsychiatric Adverse Reactions

Partial Onset Seizures

In some adults experiencing partial onset seizures, KEPPRA causes the occurrence of central nervous system adverse reactions that can be classified into the following categories: 1) somnolence and fatigue, 2) coordination difficulties, and 3) behavioral abnormalities.

In controlled trials of adult patients with epilepsy experiencing partial onset seizures, 14.8% of KEPPRA-treated patients reported somnolence, compared to 8.4% of placebo patients. There was no clear dose response up to 3000 mg/day. In a study where there was no titration, about 45% of patients receiving 4000 mg/day reported somnolence. The somnolence was considered serious in 0.3% of the treated patients, compared to 0% in the placebo group. About 3% of KEPPRA-treated patients discontinued treatment due to somnolence, compared to 0.7% of placebo patients. In 1.4% of treated patients and in 0.9% of placebo patients the dose was reduced, while 0.3% of the treated patients were hospitalized due to somnolence.

In controlled trials of adult patients with epilepsy experiencing partial onset seizures, 14.7% of treated patients reported asthenia, compared to 9.1% of placebo patients. Treatment was discontinued in 0.8% of treated patients as compared to 0.5% of placebo patients. In 0.5% of treated patients and in 0.2% of placebo patients the dose was reduced.

A total of 3.4% of KEPPRA-treated patients experienced coordination difficulties, (reported as either ataxia, abnormal gait, or incoordination) compared to 1.6% of placebo patients. A total of 0.4% of patients in controlled trials discontinued KEPPRA treatment due to ataxia, compared to 0% of placebo patients. In 0.7% of treated patients and in 0.2% of placebo patients the dose was reduced due to coordination difficulties, while one of the treated patients was hospitalized due to worsening of pre-existing ataxia.

Somnolence, asthenia and coordination difficulties occurred most frequently within the first 4 weeks of treatment.

In controlled trials of patients with epilepsy experiencing partial onset seizures, 5 (0.7%) of KEPPRA-treated patients experienced psychotic symptoms compared to 1 (0.2%) placebo patient. Two (0.3%) KEPPRA-treated patients were hospitalized and their treatment was discontinued. Both events, reported as psychosis, developed within the first week of treatment and resolved within 1 to 2 weeks following treatment discontinuation. Two other events, reported as hallucinations, occurred after 1-5 months and resolved within 2-7 days while the patients remained on treatment. In one patient experiencing psychotic depression occurring within a month, symptoms resolved within 45 days while the patient continued treatment.

A total of 13.3% of KEPPRA patients experienced other behavioral symptoms (reported as aggression, agitation, anger, anxiety, apathy, depersonalization, depression, emotional lability, hostility, irritability, etc.) compared to 6.2% of placebo patients. Approximately half of these patients reported these events within the first 4 weeks. A total of 1.7% of treated patients discontinued treatment due to these events, compared to 0.2% of placebo patients. The treatment dose was reduced in 0.8% of treated patients and in 0.5% of placebo patients. A total of 0.8% of treated patients had a serious behavioral event (compared to 0.2% of placebo patients) and were hospitalized.

In addition, 4 (0.5%) of treated patients attempted suicide compared to 0% of placebo patients. One of these patients completed suicide. In the other 3 patients, the events did not lead to discontinuation or dose reduction. The events occurred after patients had been treated for between 4 weeks and 6 months [*see Patient Counseling Information (17)*].

Myoclonic Seizures

During clinical development, the number of patients with myoclonic seizures exposed to KEPPRA was considerably smaller than the number with partial seizures. Therefore, under-reporting of certain adverse reactions was more likely to occur in the myoclonic seizure population. In some patients experiencing myoclonic seizures, KEPPRA causes somnolence and behavioral abnormalities. It is expected that the events seen in partial seizure patients would occur in patients with JME.

In the double-blind, controlled trial in patients with juvenile myoclonic epilepsy experiencing myoclonic seizures, 11.7% of KEPPRA-treated patients experienced somnolence compared to 1.7% of placebo patients. No patient discontinued treatment as a result of somnolence. In 1.7% of KEPPRA-treated patients and in 0% of placebo patients the dose was reduced as a result of somnolence.

Non-psychotic behavioral disorders (reported as aggression and irritability) occurred in 5% of the KEPPRA-treated patients compared to 0% of placebo patients. Non-psychotic mood disorders (reported as depressed mood, depression, and mood swings) occurred in 6.7% of KEPPRA-treated patients compared to 3.3% of placebo patients. A total of 5.0% of KEPPRA-treated patients had a reduction in dose or discontinued treatment due to behavioral or psychiatric events (reported as anxiety, depressed mood, depression, irritability, and nervousness), compared to 1.7% of placebo patients.

5.2 Withdrawal Seizures

Antiepileptic drugs, including KEPPRA, should be withdrawn gradually to minimize the potential of increased seizure frequency.

5.3 Hematologic Abnormalities

Partial Onset Seizures

Minor, but statistically significant, decreases compared to placebo in total mean RBC count (0.03×10^6 /mm^3), mean hemoglobin (0.09 g/dL), and mean hematocrit (0.38%), were seen in KEPPRA-treated patients in controlled trials.

A total of 3.2% of treated and 1.8% of placebo patients had at least one possibly significant ($\leq 2.8 \times 10^9$ /L) decreased WBC, and 2.4% of treated and 1.4% of placebo patients had at least one possibly significant ($\leq 1.0 \times 10^9$ /L) decreased neutrophil count. Of the treated patients with a low neutrophil count, all but one rose towards or to baseline with continued treatment. No patient was discontinued secondary to low neutrophil counts.

Juvenile Myoclonic Epilepsy

Although there were no obvious hematologic abnormalities observed in patients with JME, the limited number of patients makes any conclusion tentative. The data from the partial seizure patients should be considered to be relevant for JME patients.

5.4 Hepatic Abnormalities

There were no meaningful changes in mean liver function tests (LFT) in controlled trials in adult patients; lesser LFT abnormalities were similar in drug and placebo treated patients in controlled trials (1.4%). No patients were discontinued from controlled trials for LFT abnormalities except for 1 (0.07%) adult epilepsy patient receiving open treatment.

5.5 Laboratory Tests

Although most laboratory tests are not systematically altered with KEPPRA treatment, there have been relatively infrequent abnormalities seen in hematologic parameters and liver function tests.

6 ADVERSE REACTIONS

6.1 Clinical Studies Experience

Because clinical trials are conducted under widely varying conditions, adverse reaction rates observed in the clinical trials of a drug cannot be directly compared to rates in the clinical trials of another drug and may not reflect the rates observed in practice.

The adverse reactions that result from KEPPRA injection use include all of those reported for KEPPRA tablets and oral solution. Equivalent doses of intravenous (IV) levetiracetam and oral levetiracetam result in equivalent C_{max}, C_{min}, and total systemic exposure to levetiracetam when the IV levetiracetam is administered as a 15 minute infusion.

Continued on next page

Keppra Injection—Cont.

The prescriber should be aware that the adverse reaction incidence figures in the following tables, obtained when KEPPRA was added to concurrent AED therapy, cannot be used to predict the frequency of adverse experiences in the course of usual medical practice where patient characteristics and other factors may differ from those prevailing during clinical studies. Similarly, the cited frequencies cannot be directly compared with figures obtained from other clinical investigations involving different treatments, uses, or investigators. An inspection of these frequencies, however, does provide the prescriber with one basis to estimate the relative contribution of drug and non-drug factors to the adverse reaction incidences in the population studied.

Partial Onset Seizures

In well-controlled clinical studies using KEPPRA tablets in adults with partial onset seizures, the most frequently reported adverse reactions in patients receiving KEPPRA in combination with other AEDs, not seen at an equivalent frequency among placebo-treated patients, were somnolence, asthenia, infection and dizziness.

Of the most frequently reported adverse reactions in placebo-controlled studies using KEPPRA tablets in adults experiencing partial onset seizures, asthenia, somnolence and dizziness appeared to occur predominantly during the first 4 weeks of treatment with KEPPRA.

Table 3 lists treatment-emergent adverse reactions that occurred in at least 1% of adult epilepsy patients treated with KEPPRA tablets participating in placebo-controlled studies and were numerically more common than in patients treated with placebo. In these studies, either KEPPRA or placebo was added to concurrent AED therapy. Adverse reactions were usually mild to moderate in intensity.

Table 3: Incidence (%) Of Treatment-Emergent Adverse Reactions In Placebo-Controlled, Add-On Studies In Adults Experiencing Partial Onset Seizures By Body System (Adverse Reactions Occurred In At Least 1% Of KEPPRA-Treated Patients And Occurred More Frequently Than Placebo-Treated Patients)

Body System/ Adverse Reaction	KEPPRA (N=769) %	Placebo (N=439) %
Body as a Whole		
Asthenia	15	9
Headache	14	13
Infection	13	8
Pain	7	6
Digestive System		
Anorexia	3	2
Nervous System		
Somnolence	15	8
Dizziness	9	4
Depression	4	2
Nervousness	4	2
Ataxia	3	1
Vertigo	3	1
Amnesia	2	1
Anxiety	2	1
Hostility	2	1
Paresthesia	2	1
Emotional Lability	2	0
Respiratory System		
Pharyngitis	6	4
Rhinitis	4	3
Cough Increased	2	1
Sinusitis	2	1
Special Senses		
Diplopia	2	1

Myoclonic Seizures

Although the pattern of adverse reactions in this study seems somewhat different from that seen in patients with partial seizures, this is likely due to the much smaller number of patients in this study compared to partial seizure studies. The adverse reaction pattern for patients with JME is expected to be essentially the same as for patients with partial seizures.

In the well-controlled clinical study using KEPPRA tablets in patients with myoclonic seizures, the most frequently reported adverse reactions in patients using KEPPRA in combination with other AEDs, not seen at an equivalent frequency among placebo-treated patients, were somnolence, neck pain, and pharyngitis.

Table 4 lists treatment-emergent adverse reactions that occurred in at least 5% of juvenile myoclonic epilepsy patients experiencing myoclonic seizures treated with KEPPRA tablets and were numerically more common than in patients treated with placebo. In this study, either KEPPRA or placebo was added to concurrent AED therapy. Adverse reactions were usually mild to moderate in intensity.

Table 4: Incidence (%) Of Treatment-Emergent Adverse Reactions In A Placebo-Controlled, Add-On Study In Patients With Myoclonic Seizures By Body System (Adverse Reactions Occurred In At Least 5% Of KEPPRA-Treated Patients And Occurred More Frequently Than Placebo-Treated Patients)

Body System/ Adverse Reaction	KEPPRA (N=60) %	Placebo (N=60) %
Ear and labyrinth disorders		
Vertigo	5	3
Infections and infestations		
Pharyngitis	7	0
Influenza	5	2
Musculoskeletal and connective tissue disorders		
Neck pain	8	2
Nervous system disorders		
Somnolence	12	2
Psychiatric disorders		
Depression	5	2

Discontinuation Or Dose Reduction In Well-Controlled Clinical Studies

Partial Onset Seizures: In well-controlled adult clinical studies using KEPPRA tablets, 15.0% of patients receiving KEPPRA and 11.6% receiving placebo either discontinued or had a dose reduction as a result of an adverse event. Table 5 lists the most common (>1%) adverse reactions that resulted in discontinuation or dose reduction and that occurred more frequently in KEPPRA-treated patients than in placebo-treated patients.

Table 5: Adverse Reactions That Most Commonly Resulted In Discontinuation Or Dose Reduction That Occurred More Frequently in KEPPRA-Treated Patients In Placebo-Controlled Studies In Adult Patients Experiencing Partial Onset Seizures

Adverse Reaction	KEPPRA (N=769) n %	Placebo (N=439) n %
Asthenia	10 (1.3%)	3 (0.7%)
Dizziness	11 (1.4%)	0
Somnolence	34 (4.4%)	7 (1.6%)

Myoclonic Seizures: In the placebo-controlled study using KEPPRA tablets, 8.3% of patients receiving KEPPRA and 1.7% receiving placebo either discontinued or had a dose reduction as a result of an adverse event. The adverse reactions that led to discontinuation or dose reduction in the well-controlled study and that occurred more frequently in KEPPRA-treated patients than in placebo-treated patients are presented in Table 6.

Table 6: Adverse Reactions That Resulted In Discontinuation Or Dose Reduction That Occurred More Frequently in KEPPRA-Treated Patients In The Placebo-Controlled Study In Patients With Juvenile Myoclonic Epilepsy

Adverse Reaction	KEPPRA (N=60) n %	Placebo (N=60) n %
Anxiety	2 (3.3%)	1 (1.7%)
Depressed mood	1 (1.7%)	0
Depression	1 (1.7%)	0
Diplopia	1 (1.7%)	0
Hypersomnia	1 (1.7%)	0
Insomnia	1 (1.7%)	0
Irritability	1 (1.7%)	0
Nervousness	1 (1.7%)	0
Somnolence	1 (1.7%)	0

Comparison Of Gender, Age And Race

The overall adverse experience profile of KEPPRA was similar between females and males. There are insufficient data to support a statement regarding the distribution of adverse experience reports by age and race.

6.2   Postmarketing Experience

The following adverse events have been identified during postapproval use of KEPPRA. Because these events are reported voluntarily from a population of uncertain size, it is not always possible to reliably estimate their frequency or establish a casual relationship to drug exposure.

In addition to the adverse reactions listed above [*see Adverse Reactions (6.1)*], the following adverse events have been reported in patients receiving marketed KEPPRA worldwide. The listing is alphabetized: abnormal liver function test, hepatic failure, hepatitis, leukopenia, neutropenia, pancreatitis, pancytopenia (with bone marrow suppression identified in some of these cases), thrombocytopenia and weight loss. Alopecia has been reported with KEPPRA use; recovery was observed in majority of cases where KEPPRA was discontinued. There have been reports of suicidal behavior (including completed suicide, suicide attempt and suicidal ideation) with marketed KEPPRA [*see Patient Counseling Information (17)*].

7   DRUG INTERACTIONS

7.1   General Information

In vitro data on metabolic interactions indicate that KEPPRA is unlikely to produce, or be subject to, pharmacokinetic interactions. Levetiracetam and its major metabolite, at concentrations well above C_{max} levels achieved within the therapeutic dose range, are neither inhibitors of nor high affinity substrates for human liver cytochrome P450 isoforms, epoxide hydrolase or UDP-glucuronidation enzymes. In addition, levetiracetam does not affect the *in vitro* glucuronidation of valproic acid.

Levetiracetam circulates largely unbound (<10% bound) to plasma proteins; clinically significant interactions with other drugs through competition for protein binding sites are therefore unlikely.

Potential pharmacokinetic interactions were assessed in clinical pharmacokinetic studies (phenytoin, valproate, oral contraceptive, digoxin, warfarin, probenecid) and through pharmacokinetic screening in the placebo-controlled clinical studies in epilepsy patients.

7.2   Phenytoin

KEPPRA (3000 mg daily) had no effect on the pharmacokinetic disposition of phenytoin in patients with refractory epilepsy. Pharmacokinetics of levetiracetam were also not affected by phenytoin.

7.3   Valproate

KEPPRA (1500 mg twice daily) did not alter the pharmacokinetics of valproate in healthy volunteers. Valproate 500 mg twice daily did not modify the rate or extent of levetiracetam absorption or its plasma clearance or urinary excretion. There also was no effect on exposure to and the excretion of the primary metabolite, ucb L057.

7.4   Other Antiepileptic Drugs

Potential drug interactions between KEPPRA and other AEDs (carbamazepine, gabapentin, lamotrigine, phenobarbital, phenytoin, primidone and valproate) were also assessed by evaluating the serum concentrations of levetiracetam and these AEDs during placebo-controlled clinical studies. These data indicate that levetiracetam does not influence the plasma concentration of other AEDs and that these AEDs do not influence the pharmacokinetics of levetiracetam.

7.5   Oral Contraceptives

KEPPRA (500 mg twice daily) did not influence the pharmacokinetics of an oral contraceptive containing 0.03 mg ethinyl estradiol and 0.15 mg levonorgestrel, or of the luteinizing hormone and progesterone levels, indicating that impairment of contraceptive efficacy is unlikely. Coadministration of this oral contraceptive did not influence the pharmacokinetics of levetiracetam.

7.6   Digoxin

KEPPRA (1000 mg twice daily) did not influence the pharmacokinetics and pharmacodynamics (ECG) of digoxin given as a 0.25 mg dose every day. Coadministration of digoxin did not influence the pharmacokinetics of levetiracetam.

7.7   Warfarin

KEPPRA (1000 mg twice daily) did not influence the pharmacokinetics of R and S warfarin. Prothrombin time was not affected by levetiracetam. Coadministration of warfarin did not affect the pharmacokinetics of levetiracetam.

7.8   Probenecid

Probenecid, a renal tubular secretion blocking agent, administered at a dose of 500 mg four times a day, did not change the pharmacokinetics of levetiracetam 1000 mg twice daily. C^{ss}_{max} of the metabolite, ucb L057, was approximately doubled in the presence of probenecid while the fraction of drug excreted unchanged in the urine remained the same. Renal clearance of ucb L057 in the presence of probenecid decreased 60%, probably related to competitive inhibition of tubular secretion of ucb L057. The effect of KEPPRA on probenecid was not studied.

8 USE IN SPECIFIC POPULATIONS

8.1 Pregnancy

Pregnancy Category C: There are no adequate and well-controlled studies in pregnant women. In animal studies, levetiracetam produced evidence of developmental toxicity, including teratogenic effects, at doses similar to or greater than human therapeutic doses. KEPPRA should be used during pregnancy only if the potential benefit justifies the potential risk to the fetus.

Administration to female rats throughout pregnancy and lactation led to increased incidences of minor fetal skeletal abnormalities and retarded offspring growth pre- and/or postnatally at doses ≥350 mg/kg/day (approximately equivalent to the maximum recommended human dose of 3000 mg [MRHD] on a mg/m^2 basis) and with increased pup mortality and offspring behavioral alterations at a dose of 1800 mg/kg/day (6 times the MRHD on a mg/m^2 basis). The developmental no effect dose was 70 mg/kg/day (0.2 times the MRHD on a mg/m^2 basis). There was no overt maternal toxicity at the doses used in this study.

Treatment of pregnant rabbits during the period of organogenesis resulted in increased embryofetal mortality and increased incidences of minor fetal skeletal abnormalities at doses ≥600 mg/kg/day (approximately 4 times MRHD on a mg/m^2 basis) and in decreased fetal weights and increased incidences of fetal malformations at a dose of 1800 mg/kg/day (12 times the MRHD on a mg/m^2 basis). The developmental no effect dose was 200 mg/kg/day (1.3 times the MRHD on a mg/m^2 basis). Maternal toxicity was also observed at 1800 mg/kg/day.

When pregnant rats were treated during the period of organogenesis, fetal weights were decreased and the incidence of fetal skeletal variations was increased at a dose of 3600 mg/kg/day (12 times the MRHD). 1200 mg/kg/day (4 times the MRHD) was a developmental no effect dose. There was no evidence of maternal toxicity in this study.

Treatment of rats during the last third of gestation and throughout lactation produced no adverse developmental or maternal effects at doses of up to 1800 mg/kg/day (6 times the MRHD on a mg/m^2 basis).

KEPPRA Pregnancy Registry

UCB, Inc. has established the KEPPRA Pregnancy Registry to advance scientific knowledge about safety and outcomes in pregnant women being treated with KEPPRA. To ensure broad program access and reach, either a healthcare provider or the patient can initiate enrollment in the KEPPRA Pregnancy Registry by calling (888) 537-7734 (toll free). Patients may also enroll in the North American Antiepileptic Drug Pregnancy Registry by calling (888) 233-2334 (toll free).

8.2 Labor And Delivery

The effect of KEPPRA on labor and delivery in humans is unknown.

8.3 Nursing Mothers

Levetiracetam is excreted in breast milk. Because of the potential for serious adverse reactions in nursing infants from KEPPRA, a decision should be made whether to discontinue nursing or discontinue the drug, taking into account the importance of the drug to the mother.

8.4 Pediatric Use

Safety and effectiveness of KEPPRA injection in patients below the age of 16 years have not been established.

8.5 Geriatric Use

Of the total number of subjects in clinical studies of levetiracetam, 347 were 65 and over. No overall differences in safety were observed between these subjects and younger subjects. There were insufficient numbers of elderly subjects in controlled trials of epilepsy to adequately assess the effectiveness of KEPPRA in these patients.

A study in 16 elderly subjects (age 61-88 years) with oral administration of single dose and multiple twice-daily doses for 10 days showed no pharmacokinetic differences related to age alone.

Levetiracetam is known to be substantially excreted by the kidney, and the risk of adverse reactions to this drug may be greater in patients with impaired renal function. Because elderly patients are more likely to have decreased renal function, care should be taken in dose selection, and it may be useful to monitor renal function.

8.6 Use in Patients with Impaired Renal Function

Clearance of levetiracetam is decreased in patients with renal impairment and is correlated with creatinine clearance. Caution should be taken in dosing patients with moderate and severe renal impairment and in patients undergoing hemodialysis. The dosage should be reduced in patients with impaired renal function receiving KEPPRA and supplemental doses should be given to patients after dialysis [*see Clinical Pharmacology (12.3)* and *Dosage and Administration (2.6)*].

9 DRUG ABUSE AND DEPENDENCE

The abuse and dependence potential of KEPPRA has not been evaluated in human studies.

10 OVERDOSAGE

Signs, Symptoms and Laboratory Findings of Acute Overdosage in Humans

The highest known dose of oral KEPPRA received in the clinical development program was 6000 mg/day. Other than drowsiness, there were no adverse reactions in the few known cases of overdose in clinical trials. Cases of somnolence, agitation, aggression, depressed level of consciousness, respiratory depression and coma were observed with KEPPRA overdoses in postmarketing use.

Treatment or Management of Overdose

There is no specific antidote for overdose with KEPPRA. If indicated, elimination of unabsorbed drug should be attempted by emesis or gastric lavage; usual precautions should be observed to maintain airway. General supportive care of the patient is indicated including monitoring of vital signs and observation of the patient's clinical status. A Certified Poison Control Center should be contacted for up to date information on the management of overdose with KEPPRA.

Hemodialysis

Standard hemodialysis procedures result in significant clearance of levetiracetam (approximately 50% in 4 hours) and should be considered in cases of overdose. Although hemodialysis has not been performed in the few known cases of overdose, it may be indicated by the patient's clinical state or in patients with significant renal impairment.

11 DESCRIPTION

KEPPRA injection is an antiepileptic drug available as a clear, colorless, sterile solution (100 mg/mL) for intravenous administration.

The chemical name of levetiracetam, a single enantiomer, is (-)-(S)-α-ethyl-2-oxo-1-pyrrolidine acetamide, its molecular formula is $C_8H_{14}N_2O_2$ and its molecular weight is 170.21. Levetiracetam is chemically unrelated to existing antiepileptic drugs (AEDs). It has the following structural formula:

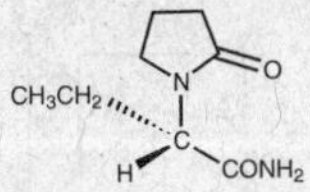

Levetiracetam is a white to off-white crystalline powder with a faint odor and a bitter taste. It is very soluble in water (104.0 g/100 mL). It is freely soluble in chloroform (65.3 g/100 mL) and in methanol (53.6 g/100 mL), soluble in ethanol (16.5 g/100 mL), sparingly soluble in acetonitrile (5.7 g/100 mL) and practically insoluble in n-hexane. (Solubility limits are expressed as g/100 mL solvent.)

KEPPRA injection contains 100 mg of levetiracetam per mL. It is supplied in single-use 5 mL vials containing 500 mg levetiracetam, water for injection, 45 mg sodium chloride, and buffered at approximately pH 5.5 with glacial acetic acid and 8.2 mg sodium acetate trihydrate. KEPPRA injection must be diluted prior to intravenous infusion [*see Dosage and Administration (2.1)*].

12 CLINICAL PHARMACOLOGY

12.1 Mechanism of Action

The precise mechanism(s) by which levetiracetam exerts its antiepileptic effect is unknown. The antiepileptic activity of levetiracetam was assessed in a number of animal models of epileptic seizures. Levetiracetam did not inhibit single seizures induced by maximal stimulation with electrical current or different chemoconvulsants and showed only minimal activity in submaximal stimulation and in threshold tests. Protection was observed, however, against secondarily generalized activity from focal seizures induced by pilocarpine and kainic acid, two chemoconvulsants that induce seizures that mimic some features of human complex partial seizures with secondary generalization. Levetiracetam also displayed inhibitory properties in the kindling model in rats, another model of human complex partial seizures, both during kindling development and in the fully kindled state. The predictive value of these animal models for specific types of human epilepsy is uncertain.

In vitro and *in vivo* recordings of epileptiform activity from the hippocampus have shown that levetiracetam inhibits burst firing without affecting normal neuronal excitability, suggesting that levetiracetam may selectively prevent hypersynchronization of epileptiform burst firing and propagation of seizure activity.

Levetiracetam at concentrations of up to 10 μM did not demonstrate binding affinity for a variety of known receptors, such as those associated with benzodiazepines, GABA (gamma-aminobutyric acid), glycine, NMDA (N-methyl-D-aspartate), re-uptake sites, and second messenger systems. Furthermore, *in vitro* studies have failed to find an effect of levetiracetam on neuronal voltage-gated sodium or T-type calcium currents and levetiracetam does not appear to directly facilitate GABAergic neurotransmission. However, *in vitro* studies have demonstrated that levetiracetam opposes the activity of negative modulators of GABA- and glycine-gated currents and partially inhibits N-type calcium currents in neuronal cells.

A saturable and stereoselective neuronal binding site in rat brain tissue has been described for levetiracetam. Experimental data indicate that this binding site is the synaptic vesicle protein SV2A, thought to be involved in the regulation of vesicle exocytosis. Although the molecular significance of levetiracetam binding to synaptic vesicle protein SV2A is not understood, levetiracetam and related analogs showed a rank order of affinity for SV2A which correlated with the potency of their antiseizure activity in audiogenic seizure-prone mice. These findings suggest that the interaction of levetiracetam with the SV2A protein may contribute to the antiepileptic mechanism of action of the drug.

12.3 Pharmacokinetics

Equivalent doses of intravenous (IV) levetiracetam and oral levetiracetam result in equivalent C_{max}, C_{min}, and total systemic exposure to levetiracetam when the IV levetiracetam is administered as a 15 minute infusion.

The pharmacokinetics of levetiracetam have been studied in healthy adult subjects, adults and pediatric patients with epilepsy, elderly subjects and subjects with renal and hepatic impairment.

Overview

Levetiracetam is rapidly and almost completely absorbed after oral administration. Levetiracetam injection and tablets are bioequivalent. The pharmacokinetics of levetiracetam are linear and time-invariant, with low intra- and inter-subject variability. Levetiracetam is not significantly protein-bound (<10% bound) and its volume of distribution is close to the volume of intracellular and extracellular water. Sixty-six percent (66%) of the dose is renally excreted unchanged. The major metabolic pathway of levetiracetam (24% of dose) is an enzymatic hydrolysis of the acetamide group. It is not liver cytochrome P450 dependent. The metabolites have no known pharmacological activity and are renally excreted. Plasma half-life of levetiracetam across studies is approximately 6-8 hours. It is increased in the elderly (primarily due to impaired renal clearance) and in subjects with renal impairment.

Distribution

The equivalence of levetiracetam injection and the oral formulation was demonstrated in a bioavailability study of 17 healthy volunteers. In this study, levetiracetam 1500 mg was diluted in 100 mL 0.9% sterile saline solution and was infused over 15 minutes. The selected infusion rate provided plasma concentrations of levetiracetam at the end of the infusion period similar to those achieved at T_{max} after an equivalent oral dose. It is demonstrated that levetiracetam 1500 mg intravenous infusion is equivalent to levetiracetam 3 × 500 mg oral tablets. The time independent pharmacokinetic profile of levetiracetam was demonstrated following 1500 mg intravenous infusion for 4 days with BID dosing. The $AUC_{(0-12)}$ at steady-state was equivalent to AUC_{inf} following an equivalent single dose.

Levetiracetam and its major metabolite are less than 10% bound to plasma proteins; clinically significant interactions with other drugs through competition for protein binding sites are therefore unlikely.

Metabolism

Levetiracetam is not extensively metabolized in humans. The major metabolic pathway is the enzymatic hydrolysis of the acetamide group, which produces the carboxylic acid metabolite, ucb L057 (24% of dose) and is not dependent on any liver cytochrome P450 isoenzymes. The major metabolite is inactive in animal seizure models. Two minor metabolites were identified as the product of hydroxylation of the 2-oxo-pyrrolidine ring (2% of dose) and opening of the 2-oxo-pyrrolidine ring in position 5 (1% of dose). There is no enantiomeric interconversion of levetiracetam or its major metabolite.

Elimination

Levetiracetam plasma half-life in adults is 7 ± 1 hour and is unaffected by either dose, route of administration or repeated administration. Levetiracetam is eliminated from the systemic circulation by renal excretion as unchanged drug which represents 66% of administered dose. The total body clearance is 0.96 mL/min/kg and the renal clearance is 0.6 mL/min/kg. The mechanism of excretion is glomerular filtration with subsequent partial tubular reabsorption. The metabolite ucb L057 is excreted by glomerular filtration and active tubular secretion with a renal clearance of 4 mL/min/kg. Levetiracetam elimination is correlated to creatinine clearance. Levetiracetam clearance is reduced in patients with impaired renal function [*see Use in Specific Populations (8.6)* and *Dosage and Administration (2.6)*].

Pharmacokinetic Interactions

In vitro data on metabolic interactions indicate that levetiracetam is unlikely to produce, or be subject to, pharmacokinetic interactions. Levetiracetam and its major metabolite, at concentrations well above C_{max} levels achieved within the therapeutic dose range, are neither inhibitors of, nor high affinity substrates for, human liver cytochrome P450 isoforms, epoxide hydrolase or UDP-glucuronidation enzymes. In addition, levetiracetam does not affect the *in vitro* glucuronidation of valproic acid.

Potential pharmacokinetic interactions of or with levetiracetam were assessed in clinical pharmacokinetic studies (phenytoin, valproate, warfarin, digoxin, oral contraceptive, probenecid) and through pharmacokinetic screening in the placebo-controlled clinical studies in epilepsy patients [*see Drug Interactions (7)*].

Special Populations

Elderly: Pharmacokinetics of levetiracetam were evaluated in 16 elderly subjects (age 61-88 years) with creatinine clearance ranging from 30 to 74 mL/min. Following oral administration of twice-daily dosing for 10 days, total body clearance decreased by 38% and the half-life was 2.5 hours longer in the elderly compared to healthy adults. This is most likely due to the decrease in renal function in these subjects.

Pediatric Patients: Safety and effectiveness of KEPPRA injection in patients below the age of 16 years have not been established.

Gender: Levetiracetam C_{max} and AUC were 20% higher in women (N=11) compared to men (N=12). However, clearances adjusted for body weight were comparable.

Continued on next page

Keppra Injection—Cont.

Race: Formal pharmacokinetic studies of the effects of race have not been conducted. Cross study comparisons involving Caucasians (N=12) and Asians (N=12), however, show that pharmacokinetics of levetiracetam were comparable between the two races. Because levetiracetam is primarily renally excreted and there are no important racial differences in creatinine clearance, pharmacokinetic differences due to race are not expected.

Renal Impairment: The disposition of levetiracetam was studied in adult subjects with varying degrees of renal function. Total body clearance of levetiracetam is reduced in patients with impaired renal function by 40% in the mild group (CLcr = 50-80 mL/min), 50% in the moderate group (CLcr = 30-50 mL/min) and 60% in the severe renal impairment group (CLcr <30 mL/min). Clearance of levetiracetam is correlated with creatinine clearance.

In anuric (end stage renal disease) patients, the total body clearance decreased 70% compared to normal subjects (CLcr >80mL/min). Approximately 50% of the pool of levetiracetam in the body is removed during a standard 4 hour hemodialysis procedure.

Dosage should be reduced in patients with impaired renal function receiving levetiracetam, and supplemental doses should be given to patients after dialysis [*see Dosage and Administration (2.6)*].

Hepatic Impairment: In subjects with mild (Child-Pugh A) to moderate (Child-Pugh B) hepatic impairment, the pharmacokinetics of levetiracetam were unchanged. In patients with severe hepatic impairment (Child-Pugh C), total body clearance was 50% that of normal subjects, but decreased renal clearance accounted for most of the decrease. No dose adjustment is needed for patients with hepatic impairment.

13 NONCLINICAL TOXICOLOGY

13.1 Carcinogenesis, Mutagenesis, Impairment of Fertility

Carcinogenesis

Rats were dosed with levetiracetam in the diet for 104 weeks at doses of 50, 300 and 1800 mg/kg/day. The highest dose corresponds to 6 times the maximum recommended daily human dose (MRHD) of 3000 mg on a mg/m^2 basis and it also provided systemic exposure (AUC) approximately 6 times that achieved in humans receiving the MRHD. There was no evidence of carcinogenicity. A study was conducted in which mice received levetiracetam in the diet for 80 weeks at doses of 60, 240 and 960 mg/kg/day (high dose is equivalent to 2 times the MRHD on a mg/m^2 or exposure basis). Although no evidence for carcinogenicity was seen, the potential for a carcinogenic response has not been fully evaluated in that species because adequate doses have not been studied.

Mutagenesis

Levetiracetam was not mutagenic in the Ames test or in mammalian cells *in vitro* in the Chinese hamster ovary/HGPRT locus assay. It was not clastogenic in an *in vitro* analysis of metaphase chromosomes obtained from Chinese hamster ovary cells or in an *in vivo* mouse micronucleus assay. The hydrolysis product and major human metabolite of levetiracetam (ucb L057) was not mutagenic in the Ames test or the *in vitro* mouse lymphoma assay.

Impairment of Fertility

No adverse effects on male or female fertility or reproductive performance were observed in rats at doses up to 1800 mg/kg/day (approximately 6 times the maximum recommended human dose on a mg/m^2 or exposure basis).

13.2 Animal Toxicology and/or Pharmacology

In animal studies, levetiracetam produced evidence of developmental toxicity at doses similar to or greater than human therapeutic doses.

14 CLINICAL STUDIES

14.1 Partial Onset Seizures

Effectiveness in Partial Onset Seizures in Adults with Epilepsy

The effectiveness of KEPPRA as adjunctive therapy (added to other antiepileptic drugs) in adults was established in three multicenter, randomized, double-blind, placebo-controlled clinical studies in patients who had refractory partial onset seizures with or without secondary generalization. The tablet formulation was used in all these studies. In these studies, 904 patients were randomized to placebo, 1000 mg, 2000 mg, or 3000 mg/day. Patients enrolled in Study 1 or Study 2 had refractory partial onset seizures for at least two years and had taken two or more classical AEDs. Patients enrolled in Study 3 had refractory partial onset seizures for at least 1 year and had taken one classical AED. At the time of the study, patients were taking a stable dose regimen of at least one and could take a maximum of two AEDs. During the baseline period, patients had to have experienced at least two partial onset seizures during each 4-week period.

The criteria for statistical significance in all studies was a p<0.05.

Study 1: Study 1 was a double-blind, placebo-controlled, parallel-group study conducted at 41 sites in the United States comparing KEPPRA 1000 mg/day (N=97), KEPPRA 3000 mg/day (N=101), and placebo (N=95) given in equally divided doses twice daily. After a prospective baseline period of 12 weeks, patients were randomized to one of the three treatment groups described above. The 18-week treatment period consisted of a 6-week titration period, followed by a 12-week fixed dose evaluation period, during which concomitant AED regimens were held constant. The primary measure of effectiveness was a between group comparison of the percent reduction in weekly partial seizure frequency relative to placebo over the entire randomized treatment period (titration + evaluation period). Secondary outcome variables included the responder rate (incidence of patients with ≥50% reduction from baseline in partial onset seizure frequency). The results of the analysis of Study 1 are displayed in Table 7.

Table 7: Reduction in Mean over Placebo in Weekly Frequency of Partial Onset Seizures in Study 1

	Placebo (N=95)	KEPPRA 1000 mg/day (N=97)	KEPPRA 3000 mg/day (N=101)
Percent reduction in partial seizure frequency over placebo	–	26.1%*	30.1%*

**Statistically significant versus placebo*

The percentage of patients (y-axis) who achieved ≥50% reduction in weekly seizure rates from baseline in partial onset seizure frequency over the entire randomized treatment period (titration + evaluation period) within the three treatment groups (x-axis) is presented in Figure 1.

Figure 1: Responder Rate (≥50% Reduction from Baseline) in Study 1

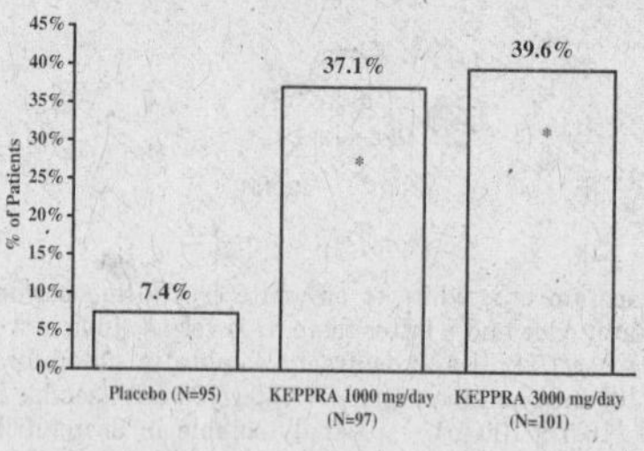

* *Statistically significant versus placebo*

Study 2: Study 2 was a double-blind, placebo-controlled, crossover study conducted at 62 centers in Europe comparing KEPPRA 1000 mg/day (N=106), KEPPRA 2000 mg/day (N=105), and placebo (N=111) given in equally divided doses twice daily.

The first period of the study (Period A) was designed to be analyzed as a parallel-group study. After a prospective baseline period of up to 12 weeks, patients were randomized to one of the three treatment groups described above. The 16-week treatment period consisted of the 4-week titration period followed by a 12-week fixed dose evaluation period, during which concomitant AED regimens were held constant. The primary measure of effectiveness was a between group comparison of the percent reduction in weekly partial seizure frequency relative to placebo over the entire randomized treatment period (titration + evaluation period). Secondary outcome variables included the responder rate (incidence of patients with ≥50% reduction from baseline in partial onset seizure frequency). The results of the analysis of Period A are displayed in Table 8.

Table 8: Reduction in Mean Over Placebo in Weekly Frequency of Partial Onset Seizures in Study 2: Period A

	Placebo (N=111)	KEPPRA 1000 mg/day (N=106)	KEPPRA 2000 mg/day (N=105)
Percent reduction in partial seizure frequency over placebo	–	17.1%*	21.4%*

**Statistically significant versus placebo*

The percentage of patients (y-axis) who achieved ≥50% reduction in weekly seizure rates from baseline in partial onset seizure frequency over the entire randomized treatment period (titration + evaluation period) within the three treatment groups (x-axis) is presented in Figure 2.

[See figure 2 at top of next column]

Figure 2: Responder Rate (≥50% Reduction from Baseline) in Study 2: Period A

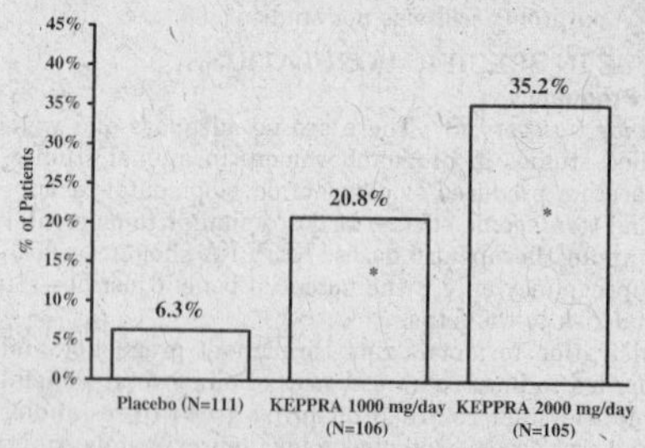

* *Statistically significant versus placebo*

The comparison of KEPPRA 2000 mg/day to KEPPRA 1000 mg/day for responder rate was statistically significant (P=0.02). Analysis of the trial as a cross-over yielded similar results.

Study 3: Study 3 was a double-blind, placebo-controlled, parallel-group study conducted at 47 centers in Europe comparing KEPPRA 3000 mg/day (N=180) and placebo (N=104) in patients with refractory partial onset seizures, with or without secondary generalization, receiving only one concomitant AED. Study drug was given in two divided doses. After a prospective baseline period of 12 weeks, patients were randomized to one of two treatment groups described above. The 16-week treatment period consisted of a 4-week titration period, followed by a 12-week fixed dose evaluation period, during which concomitant AED doses were held constant. The primary measure of effectiveness was a between group comparison of the percent reduction in weekly seizure frequency relative to placebo over the entire randomized treatment period (titration + evaluation period). Secondary outcome variables included the responder rate (incidence of patients with ≥50% reduction from baseline in partial onset seizure frequency). Table 9 displays the results of the analysis of Study 3.

Table 9: Reduction in Mean over Placebo in Weekly Frequency of Partial Onset Seizures in Study 3

	Placebo (N=104)	KEPPRA 3000 mg/day (N=180)
Percent reduction in partial seizure frequency over placebo	–	23.0%*

**Statistically significant versus placebo*

The percentage of patients (y-axis) who achieved ≥50% reduction in weekly seizure rates from baseline in partial onset seizure frequency over the entire randomized treatment period (titration + evaluation period) within the two treatment groups (x-axis) is presented in Figure 3.

Figure 3: Responder Rate (≥50% Reduction from Baseline) in Study 3

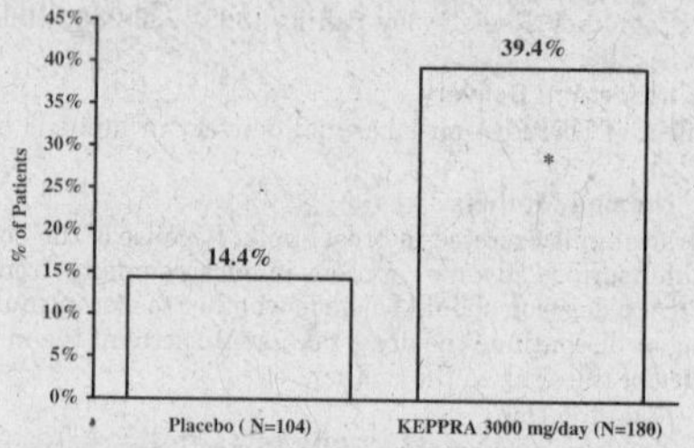

* *Statistically significant versus placebo*

14.2 Myoclonic Seizures in Patients with Juvenile Myoclonic Epilepsy

Effectiveness in Myoclonic Seizures in Patients with Juvenile Myoclonic Epilepsy (JME)

The effectiveness of KEPPRA as adjunctive therapy (added to other antiepileptic drugs) in patients with juvenile myoclonic epilepsy (JME) experiencing myoclonic seizures was established in one multicenter, randomized, double-blind, placebo-controlled study, conducted at 37 sites in 14 countries. Of the 120 patients enrolled, 113 had a diagnosis of confirmed or suspected JME. Eligible patients on a stable dose of 1 antiepileptic drug (AED) experiencing one or more myoclonic seizures per day for at least 8 days during the prospective 8-week baseline period were randomized to either KEPPRA or placebo (KEPPRA N=60, placebo N=60). Patients were titrated over 4 weeks to a target dose of 3000 mg/day and treated at a stable dose of 3000 mg/day over 12 weeks (evaluation period). Study drug was given in 2 divided doses.

The primary measure of effectiveness was the proportion of patients with at least 50% reduction in the number of days per week with one or more myoclonic seizures during the treatment period (titration + evaluation periods) as compared to baseline. Table 10 displays the results for the 113 patients with JME in this study.

Table 10: Responder Rate (≥50% Reduction from Baseline) in Myoclonic Seizure Days Per Week for Patients with JME

	Placebo (N=59)	KEPPRA (N=54)
Percentage of responders	23.7%	60.4%*

**Statistically significant versus placebo*

16 HOW SUPPLIED/STORAGE AND HANDLING

16.1 How Supplied

KEPPRA (levetiracetam) 500 mg/5 mL injection is a clear, colorless, sterile solution. It is supplied in single-use 5 mL vials, available in cartons of 10 vials (NDC 50474-002-63).

16.2 Storage

Store at 25°C (77°F); excursions permitted to 15-30°C (59-86°F) [see USP Controlled Room Temperature].

17 PATIENT COUNSELING INFORMATION

Patients should be advised to notify their physician if they are pregnant prior to therapy.

Patients should be advised that KEPPRA may cause dizziness and somnolence. Accordingly, patients should be advised not to drive or operate heavy machinery or engage in other hazardous activities until they have gained sufficient experience on KEPPRA to gauge whether it adversely affects their performance of these activities.

Patients should be advised that Keppra may cause changes in behavior (e.g. aggression, agitation, anger, anxiety, apathy, depression, hostility, and irritability) and in rare cases patients may experience psychotic symptoms.

Patients should be advised to immediately report any symptoms of depression and/or suicidal ideation to their prescribing physician as suicide, suicide attempt and suicidal ideation have been reported in patients treated with levetiracetam.

KEPPRA injection manufactured for
UCB, Inc.
Smyrna, GA 30080

Validus Pharmaceuticals

119 CHERRY HILL ROAD, SUITE 310
PARSIPPANY, NJ 07054

Direct Inquiries to:
Customer Care Center
Phone: 1-866-9VALIDUS
Phone: (973)-265-2777
Fax: (973)-265-2770
info@validuspharma.com

EQUETRO™ ℞

[ē-kwĕ-trō]
(carbamazepine)
Extended-Release Capsules
100 mg, 200 mg and 300 mg
Rx only

Prescribing Information

Prescribing information for this product, which appears on pages 3106–3109 of the 2008 PDR, has been completely revised as follows. Please write "See Supplement A" next to the product heading.

WARNING

SERIOUS DERMATOLOGIC REACTIONS AND HLA-B*1502 ALLELE

SERIOUS AND SOMETIMES FATAL DERMATOLOGIC REACTIONS, INCLUDING TOXIC EPIDERMAL NECROLYSIS (TEN) AND STEVENS-JOHNSON SYNDROME (SJS), HAVE BEEN REPORTED DURING TREATMENT WITH CARBAMAZEPINE. THESE REACTIONS ARE ESTIMATED TO OCCUR IN 1 TO 6 PER 10,000 NEW USERS IN COUNTRIES WITH MAINLY CAUCASIAN POPULATIONS, BUT THE RISK IN SOME ASIAN COUNTRIES IS ESTIMATED TO BE ABOUT 10 TIMES HIGHER. STUDIES IN PATIENTS OF CHINESE ANCESTRY HAVE FOUND A STRONG ASSOCIATION BETWEEN THE RISK OF DEVELOPING SJS/TEN AND THE PRESENCE OF HLA-B*1502, AN INHERITED ALLELIC VARIANT OF THE HLA-B GENE. HLA-B*1502 IS FOUND ALMOST EXCLUSIVELY IN PATIENTS WITH ANCESTRY ACROSS BROAD AREAS OF ASIA. PATIENTS WITH ANCESTRY IN GENETICALLY AT-RISK POPULATIONS SHOULD BE SCREENED FOR THE PRESENCE OF HLA-B*1502 PRIOR TO INITIATING TREATMENT WITH EQUETRO™. PATIENTS TESTING POSITIVE FOR THE ALLELE SHOULD NOT BE TREATED WITH EQUETRO™ UNLESS THE BENEFIT CLEARLY OUTWEIGHS THE RISK (see WARNINGS and PRECAUTIONS, Laboratory Tests).

APLASTIC ANEMIA AND AGRANULOCYTOSIS HAVE BEEN REPORTED IN ASSOCIATION WITH THE USE OF CARBAMAZEPINE. DATA FROM A POPULATION-BASED CASE-CONTROL STUDY DEMONSTRATE THAT THE RISK OF DEVELOPING THESE REACTIONS IS 5-8 TIMES GREATER THAN IN THE GENERAL POPULATION. HOWEVER, THE OVERALL RISK OF THESE REACTIONS IN THE UNTREATED GENERAL POPULATION IS LOW, APPROXIMATELY SIX PATIENTS PER ONE MILLION POPULATION PER YEAR FOR AGRANULOCYTOSIS AND TWO PATIENTS PER ONE MILLION POPULATION PER YEAR FOR APLASTIC ANEMIA.

ALTHOUGH REPORTS OF TRANSIENT OR PERSISTENT DECREASED PLATELET OR WHITE BLOOD CELL COUNTS ARE NOT UNCOMMON IN ASSOCIATION WITH THE USE OF CARBAMAZEPINE, DATA ARE NOT AVAILABLE TO ESTIMATE ACCURATELY THEIR INCIDENCE OR OUTCOME. HOWEVER, THE VAST MAJORITY OF THE CASES OF LEUKOPENIA HAVE NOT PROGRESSED TO THE MORE SERIOUS CONDITIONS OF APLASTIC ANEMIA OR AGRANULOCYTOSIS.

BECAUSE OF THE VERY LOW INCIDENCE OF AGRANULOCYTOSIS AND APLASTIC ANEMIA, THE VAST MAJORITY OF MINOR HEMATOLOGIC CHANGES OBSERVED IN MONITORING OF PATIENTS ON CARBAMAZEPINE ARE UNLIKELY TO SIGNAL THE OCCURRENCE OF EITHER ABNORMALITY. NONETHELESS, COMPLETE PRETREATMENT HEMATOLOGICAL TESTING SHOULD BE OBTAINED AS A BASELINE. IF A PATIENT IN THE COURSE OF TREATMENT EXHIBITS LOW OR DECREASED WHITE BLOOD CELL OR PLATELET COUNTS, THE PATIENT SHOULD BE MONITORED CLOSELY. DISCONTINUATION OF THE DRUG SHOULD BE CONSIDERED IF ANY EVIDENCE OF SIGNIFICANT BONE MARROW DEPRESSION DEVELOPS.

Before prescribing EQUETRO™, the physician should be thoroughly familiar with the details of this prescribing information, particularly regarding use with other drugs, especially those which accentuate toxicity potential.

DESCRIPTION

EQUETRO™ is available for oral administration as 100 mg, 200 mg, and 300 mg extended-release capsules of carbamazepine, USP. Carbamazepine is a white to off-white powder, practically insoluble in water and soluble in alcohol and in acetone. Its molecular weight is 236.27. Its chemical name is 5H-dibenz[b,f]azepine-5-carboxamide, and its structural formula is:

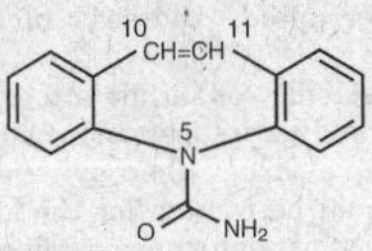

CARBAMAZEPINE

EQUETRO™ is a multi-component capsule formulation consisting of three different types of beads: immediate-release beads, extended-release beads, and enteric-release beads. The three bead types are combined in a specific ratio to provide twice-daily dosing of EQUETRO™.

Inactive ingredients: citric acid, colloidal silicon dioxide, lactose monohydrate, microcrystalline cellulose, polyethylene glycol, povidone, sodium lauryl sulfate, talc, triethyl citrate, and other ingredients.

The 100 mg capsule shells contain gelatin-NF, FD&C Blue #2, Yellow Iron Oxide, and Titanium Dioxide, and are imprinted with white ink; the 200 mg capsule shells contain gelatin-NF, Yellow Iron Oxide, FD&C Blue #2, and Titanium Dioxide, and are imprinted with white ink; and the 300 mg capsule shells contain gelatin-NF, FD&C Blue #2, Yellow Iron Oxide, and Titanium Dioxide, and are imprinted with white ink.

CLINICAL PHARMACOLOGY

In controlled clinical trials, carbamazepine has been shown to be effective in the treatment of Bipolar I Disorder.

Mechanism of Action

The mechanism(s) of action of carbamazepine in the treatment of bipolar disorder has not been elucidated. Although numerous pharmacological effects of carbamazepine have been described in the published literature (e.g., modulation of ion channels [sodium and calcium], receptor-mediated neurotransmission [GABAergic, glutamatergic, and monoaminergic], and intracellular signaling pathways in experimental preparations), the contribution of these effects to the efficacy of carbamazepine in bipolar disorder is unknown.

Pharmacokinetics

Carbamazepine (CBZ): Following a single 200 mg oral extended-release dose of carbamazepine, peak plasma concentration was 1.9 ± 0.3 μg/mL and the time to reach the peak was 19 ± 7 hours. Following repeat dose administration (800 mg every 12 hours), the peak levels were 11.0 ± 2.5 μg/mL and the time to reach the peak was 5.9 ± 1.8 hours. The pharmacokinetics of extended-release carbamazepine is linear over the single dose range of 200-800 mg.

Carbamazepine is 76% bound to plasma proteins. Carbamazepine is primarily metabolized in the liver. Cytochrome P450 3A4 was identified as the major isoform responsible for the formation of carbamazepine-10,11-epoxide. Since carbamazepine induces its own metabolism, the half-life is also variable. The average half-life ranged from 35 to 40 hours following a single extended-release dose of carbamazepine and from 12 to 17 hours following repeated dosing. The apparent oral clearance was 25 ± 5 mL/min following a single dose and 80 ± 30 mL/min following multiple dosing.

After oral administration of ^{14}C-carbamazepine, 72% of the administered radioactivity was found in the urine and 28% was found in the feces. This urinary radioactivity was composed largely of hydroxylated and conjugated metabolites, with only 3% of unchanged carbamazepine.

Carbamazepine-10,11-epoxide (CBZ-E): Carbamazepine-10,11-epoxide is considered to be an active metabolite of carbamazepine. Following a single 200 mg oral extended-release dose of carbamazepine, the peak plasma concentration of carbamazepine-10,11-epoxide was 0.11 ± 0.012 μg/mL and the time to reach the peak was 36 ± 6 hours. Following chronic administration of an extended-release dose of carbamazepine (800 mg every 12 hours), the peak levels of carbamazepine-10,11-epoxide were 2.2 ± 0.9 μg/mL and the time to reach the peak was 14 ± 8 hours. The plasma half-life of carbamazepine-10,11-epoxide following administration of carbamazepine is 34 ± 9 hours. Following a single oral dose of extended-release carbamazepine (200-800 mg) the AUC and C_{max} of carbamazepine-10,11-epoxide were less than 10% of carbamazepine. Following multiple dosing of extended-release carbamazepine (800-1600 mg daily for 14 days), the AUC and C_{max} of carbamazepine-10,11-epoxide were dose-related, ranging from 15.7 μg.hr/mL and 1.5 μg/mL at 800 mg/day to 32.6 μg.hr/mL and 3.2 μg/mL at 1600 mg/day, respectively, and were less than 30% those of carbamazepine. Carbamazepine-10,11-epoxide is 50% bound to plasma proteins.

Food Effect: A high-fat meal diet increased the rate of absorption of a single 400 mg dose (mean T_{max} was reduced from 24 hours, in the fasting state, to 14 hours, and C_{max} increased from 3.2 to 4.3 μg/mL) but not the extent (AUC) of absorption. The elimination half-life remained unchanged between fed and fasting state. The multiple-dose study conducted in the fed state showed that the steady-state C_{max} values were within the therapeutic concentration range. The pharmacokinetic profile of extended-release carbamazepine was similar when given by sprinkling the beads over applesauce compared to the intact capsule administered in the fasted state.

Special Populations

Hepatic Dysfunction: The effect of hepatic impairment on the pharmacokinetics of carbamazepine is not known. However, given that carbamazepine is primarily metabolized in the liver, it is prudent to proceed with caution in patients with hepatic dysfunction.

Renal Dysfunction: The effect of renal impairment on the pharmacokinetics of carbamazepine is not known.

Gender: No difference in the mean AUC and C_{max} of carbamazepine and carbamazepine-10,11-epoxide was found between males and females.

Age: Carbamazepine is more rapidly metabolized to carbamazepine-10,11-epoxide in young children than in adults. In children below the age of 15, there is an inverse relationship between CBZ-E/CBZ ratio and increasing age. The safety and effectiveness of EQUETRO™ in pediatric and adolescent patients have not been established.

Race: No information is available on the effect of race on the pharmacokinetics of carbamazepine.

CLINICAL STUDIES

The effectiveness of EQUETRO™ in the acute treatment of manic and mixed symptoms in patients with Bipolar I Disorder was established in 2 (3-week) multicenter, randomized, double-blind, flexible-dose, placebo-controlled studies in adult patients who met the DSM-IV criteria for Bipolar I Disorder with manic or mixed episode. In both studies, patients were titrated to a dose range from 400 mg/day to 1600 mg/day, given in divided doses, twice daily. The mean carbamazepine ER dose during the last week was 952 mg/day in the first study, and 726 mg/day in the second.

The primary rating instrument used for assessing manic symptoms in these trials was the Young Mania Rating Scale (YMRS), an 11-item clinician-rated scale traditionally used to assess the degree of manic symptomatology in a range from 0 (no manic features) to 60 (maximum score). The primary outcome in these trials was change from baseline in the YMRS total score.

EQUETRO™ was significantly more effective than placebo in reduction of the YMRS total score for both studies.

INDICATIONS AND USAGE

EQUETRO™ is indicated for the treatment of acute manic and mixed episodes associated with Bipolar I Disorder.

A manic episode is a distinct period of abnormally and persistently elevated, expansive, or irritable mood. A mixed episode is characterized by the criteria for a manic episode in conjunction with those for a major depressive episode (depressed mood, loss of interest or pleasure in nearly all activities).

The efficacy of EQUETRO™ in acute mania was established in 2 placebo-controlled, double-blind, 3-week studies in patients meeting DSM-IV criteria for Bipolar I Disorder who currently displayed an acute manic or mixed episode (see **CLINICAL PHARMACOLOGY**).

The effectiveness of EQUETRO™ for longer-term use and for prophylactic use in mania has not been systematically evaluated in controlled clinical trials. Therefore, physicians who elect to use EQUETRO™ for extended periods should periodically re-evaluate the long-term risks and benefits of the drug for the individual patient (see **DOSAGE AND ADMINISTRATION**).

CONTRAINDICATIONS

Carbamazepine should not be used in patients with a history of previous bone marrow depression, hypersensitivity to the drug, or known sensitivity to any of the tricyclic compounds, such as amitriptyline, desipramine, imipramine, protriptyline, and nortriptyline. Likewise, on theoretical grounds its use with monoamine oxidase inhibitors is not recommended. Before administration of carbamazepine, MAO inhibitors should be discontinued for a minimum of 14 days, or longer if the clinical situation permits.

WARNINGS

Serious Dermatologic Reactions

Serious and sometimes fatal dermatologic reactions, including toxic epidermal necrolysis (TEN) and Stevens-Johnson

Continued on next page

Equetro—Cont.

syndrome (SJS), have been reported with carbamazepine treatment. The risk of these events is estimated to be about 1 to 6 per 10,000 new users in countries with mainly Caucasian populations. However, the risk in some Asian countries is estimated to be about 10 times higher. EQUETRO™ should be discontinued at the first sign of a rash, unless the rash is clearly not drug-related. If signs or symptoms suggest SJS/TEN, use of this drug should not be resumed and alternative therapy should be considered.

SJS/TEN and HLA-B*1502 Allele

Retrospective case-control studies have found that in patients of Chinese ancestry there is a strong association between the risk of developing SJS/TEN with carbamazepine treatment and the presence of an inherited variant of the HLA-B gene, HLA-B*1502. The occurrence of higher rates of these reactions in countries with higher frequencies of this allele suggests that the risk may be increased in allele-positive individuals of any ethnicity.

Across Asian populations, notable variation exists in the prevalence of HLA-B*1502. Greater than 15% of the population is reported positive in Hong Kong, Thailand, Malaysia, and parts of the Philippines, compared to about 10% in Taiwan and 4% in North China. South Asians, including Indians, appear to have intermediate prevalence of HLA-B*1502, averaging 2 to 4%, but higher in some groups. HLA-B*1502 is present in <1% of the population in Japan and Korea.

HLA-B*1502 is largely absent in individuals not of Asian origin (e.g., Caucasians, African-Americans, Hispanics, and Native Americans).

Prior to initiating EQUETRO™ therapy, testing for HLA-B*1502 should be performed in patients with ancestry in populations in which HLA-B*1502 may be present. In deciding which patients to screen, the rates provided above for the prevalence of HLA-B*1502 may offer a rough guide, keeping in mind the limitations of these figures due to wide variability in rates even within ethnic groups, the difficulty in ascertaining ethnic ancestry, and the likelihood of mixed ancestry. EQUETRO™ should not be used in patients positive for HLA-B*1502 unless the benefits clearly outweigh the risks. Tested patients who are found to be negative for the allele are thought to have a low risk of SJS/TEN (see **WARNINGS** and **PRECAUTIONS, Laboratory Tests**).

Over 90% of carbamazepine-treated patients who will experience SJS/TEN have this reaction within the first few months of treatment. This information may be taken into consideration in determining the need for screening of genetically at-risk patients currently on EQUETRO™.

The HLA-B*1502 allele has not been found to predict risk of less severe adverse cutaneous reactions from carbamazepine, such as anticonvulsant hypersensitivity syndrome or non-serious rash (maculopapular eruption [MPE]).

Limited evidence suggests that HLA-B*1502 may be a risk factor for the development SJS/TEN in patients of Chinese ancestry other anti-epileptic drugs associated with SJS/TEN. Consideration should be given to avoiding use of other drugs associated with SJS/TEN in HLA-B*1502-positive patients when alternative therapies are otherwise equally acceptable.

Application of HLA-B*1502 genotyping as a screening tool has important limitations and must never substitute for appropriate clinical vigilance and patient management. Many HLA-B*1502-positive Asian patients treated with carbamazepine will not develop SJS/TEN, and these reactions can still occur infrequently in HLA-B*1502-negative patients of any ethnicity. The role of other possible factors in the development of, and morbidity from, SJS/TEN, such as AED dose, compliance, concomitant medications, comorbidities, and the level of dermatologic monitoring, has not been studied.

Patients should be made aware that EQUETRO™ contains carbamazepine and should not be used in combination with any other medications containing carbamazepine.

Usage in Pregnancy

Carbamazepine can cause fetal harm when administered to a pregnant woman.

Epidemiological data suggest that there may be an association between the use of carbamazepine during pregnancy and congenital malformations, including spina bifida. The prescribing physician will wish to weigh the benefits of therapy against the risks in treating or counseling women of childbearing potential. If this drug is used during pregnancy, or if the patient becomes pregnant while taking this drug, the patient should be apprised of the potential hazard to the fetus.

Retrospective case reviews suggest that, compared with monotherapy, there may be a higher prevalence of teratogenic effects associated with the use of anticonvulsants in combination therapy.

In humans, transplacental passage of carbamazepine is rapid (30-60 minutes), and the drug is accumulated in the fetal tissues, with higher levels found in liver and kidney than in brain and lung.

Carbamazepine has been shown to have adverse effects in reproduction studies in rats when given orally in dosages 10-25 times a human daily dosage of 1200 mg on a mg/kg basis or 1.5-4 times the human daily dosage on a mg/m^2 basis. In rat teratology studies, 2 of 135 offspring showed kinked ribs at 250 mg/kg, and 4 of 119 offspring showed other anomalies at 650 mg/kg (cleft palate, 1; talipes, 1; anophthalmos, 2). In reproduction studies in rats, nursing offspring demonstrated a lack of weight gain and an unkempt appearance at a maternal dosage level of 200 mg/kg.

Tests to detect defects using current accepted procedures should be considered a part of routine prenatal care in childbearing women receiving carbamazepine.

General

Patients with a history of adverse hematologic reaction to any drug may be particularly at risk of bone marrow depression.

In patients with seizure disorder, carbamazepine should not be discontinued abruptly because of the strong possibility of precipitating status epilepticus with attendant hypoxia and threat to life.

Carbamazepine has shown mild anticholinergic activity; therefore, patients with increased intraocular pressure should be closely observed during therapy.

Because of the relationship of the drug to other tricyclic compounds, the possibility of activation of a latent psychosis and, in elderly patients, of confusion or agitation should be considered.

Co-administration of carbamazepine and delavirdine may lead to loss of virologic response and possible resistance to RESCRIPTOR or to the class of non-nucleoside reverse transcriptase inhibitors.

PRECAUTIONS

General

Before initiating therapy, a detailed history and physical examination should be made.

Therapy should be prescribed only after critical benefit-to-risk appraisal in patients with a history of cardiac, hepatic, or renal damage; adverse hematologic reaction to other drugs; or interrupted courses of therapy with carbamazepine.

Suicide: The possibility of suicide attempt is inherent in Bipolar Disorder, and close supervision of high-risk patients should accompany drug therapy. Prescriptions for EQUETRO™ should be written for the smallest quantity consistent with good patient management in order to reduce the risk of overdose.

Information for Patients

Patients should be made aware of the early toxic signs and symptoms of a potential hematologic problem, such as fever, sore throat, rash, ulcers in the mouth, easy bruising, and petechial or purpuric hemorrhage, and should be advised to report to the physician immediately if any such signs or symptoms appear.

Since dizziness and drowsiness may occur, patients should be cautioned about the hazards of operating machinery or automobiles or engaging in other potentially dangerous tasks.

If necessary, the EQUETRO™ capsules can be opened and the contents sprinkled over food, such as a teaspoon of applesauce or other similar food products. EQUETRO™ capsules or their contents should not be crushed or chewed. EQUETRO™ may interact with some drugs. Therefore, patients should be advised to report to their doctors the use of any other prescription or non-prescription medication or herbal products.

Laboratory Tests

For genetically at-risk patients [see **WARNINGS**], high-resolution 'HLA-B*1502 typing' is recommended. The test is positive if either one or two HLA-B*1502 alleles are detected and negative if no HLA-B*1502 alleles are detected.

Complete pretreatment blood counts, including platelets and possibly reticulocytes and serum iron, should be obtained as a baseline. If a patient in the course of treatment exhibits low or decreased white blood cell or platelet counts, the patient should be monitored closely. Discontinuation of the drug should be considered if any evidence of significant bone marrow depression develops.

Baseline and periodic evaluations of liver function, particularly in patients with a history of liver disease, must be performed during treatment with this drug, since liver damage may occur. The drug should be discontinued immediately in cases of aggravated liver dysfunction or active liver disease.

Baseline and periodic eye examinations, including slit-lamp examination, funduscopy, and tonometry, are recommended, since many phenothiazines and related drugs have been shown to cause eye changes.

Baseline and periodic complete urinalysis and BUN determinations are recommended for patients treated with this agent because of observed renal dysfunction.

Increases in total cholesterol, LDL, and HDL have been observed in some patients taking anticonvulsants. Therefore, periodic evaluation of these parameters is also recommended.

Monitoring of blood levels (see **CLINICAL PHARMACOLOGY**) may be useful for verification of drug compliance, assessing safety, and determining the cause of toxicity, including when more than one medication is being used.

Thyroid function tests have been reported to show decreased values with carbamazepine administered alone.

Hyponatremia has been reported in association with carbamazepine use, either alone or in combination with other drugs.

Interference with some pregnancy tests has been reported.

Drug Interactions

Clinically meaningful drug interactions have occurred with concomitant medications and include, but are not limited to, the following:

Agents Highly Bound to Plasma Protein: Carbamazepine is not highly bound to plasma proteins; therefore, administration of EQUETRO™ to a patient taking another drug that is highly protein-bound should not cause increased free concentrations of the other drug.

Agents that Inhibit Cytochrome P450 Isoenzymes and/or Epoxide Hydrolase: Carbamazepine is metabolized mainly by cytochrome P450 (CYP) 3A4 to the active carbamazepine 10,11-epoxide, which is further metabolized to the trans-diol by epoxide hydrolase. Therefore, the potential exists for interaction between carbamazepine and any agent that inhibits CYP3A4 and/or epoxide hydrolase. Agents that are CYP3A4 inhibitors that have been found, or are expected, to increase plasma levels of EQUETRO™ are the following:

Acetazolamide, azole antifungals, cimetidine, clarithromycin[1], dalfopristin, danazol, delavirdine, diltiazem, erythromycin[1], fluoxetine, fluvoxamine, grapefruit juice, isoniazid, itraconazole, ketoconazole, loratadine, nefazodone, niacinamide, nicotinamide, protease inhibitors, propoxyphene, quinine, quinupristin, troleandomycin, valproate[1], verapamil, zileuton.

[1] Also inhibits epoxide hydrolase, resulting in increased levels of the active metabolite carbamazepine 10,11-epoxide.

Thus, if a patient has been titrated to a stable dosage of EQUETRO™, and then begins a course of treatment with one of these CYP3A4 or epoxide hydrolase inhibitors, it is reasonable to expect that a dose reduction for EQUETRO™ may be necessary.

Agents that Induce Cytochrome P450 Isoenzymes: Carbamazepine is metabolized by CYP3A4. Therefore, the potential exists for interaction between carbamazepine and any agent that induces CYP3A4. Agents that are CYP inducers that have been found, or are expected, to decrease plasma levels of EQUETRO™ are the following:

Cisplatin, doxorubicin HCl, felbamate, rifampin, phenobarbital, phenytoin[2] primidone, methsuximide, and theophylline

[2] Phenytoin plasma levels have also been reported to increase and decrease in the presence of carbamazepine; see below.

Thus, if a patient has been titrated to a stable dosage on EQUETRO™, and then begins a course of treatment with one of these CYP3A4 inducers, it is reasonable to expect that a dose increase for EQUETRO™ may be necessary.

Agents with Decreased Levels in the Presence of Carbamazepine Due to Induction of Cytochrome P450 Enzymes: Carbamazepine is known to induce CYP1A2 and CYP3A4. Therefore, the potential exists for interaction between carbamazepine and any agent metabolized by one (or more) of these enzymes. Agents that have been found, or are expected, to have decreased plasma levels in the presence of EQUETRO™ due to induction of CYP enzymes are the following:

Acetaminophen, alprazolam, amitriptyline, bupropion, buspirone, citalopram, clobazam, clonazepam, clozapine, cyclosporin, delavirdine, desipramine, diazepam, dicumarol, doxycycline, ethosuximide, felbamate, felodipine, glucocorticoids, haloperidol, itraconazole, lamotrigine, levothyroxine, lorazepam, methadone, midazolam, mirtazapine, nortriptyline, olanzapine, oral contraceptives[3], oxcarbazepine, phenytoin[4], praziquantel, protease inhibitors, quetiapine, risperidone, theophylline, topiramate, tiagabine, tramadol, triazolam, trazodone[5], valproate, warfarin[6], ziprasidone, and zonisamide.

[3] Breakthrough bleeding has been reported among patients receiving concomitant oral contraceptives, and their reliability may be adversely affected.

[4] Phenytoin has also been reported to increase in the presence of carbamazepine. Careful monitoring of phenytoin plasma levels following co-medication with carbamazepine is advised.

[5] Following co-administration of carbamazepine 400 mg/day with trazodone 100 mg to 300 mg daily, carbamazepine reduced the plasma concentration of trazodone (as well as meta-chlorophenylpiperazine [mCPP]) by 76% and 60% respectively, compared to pre-carbamazepine values.

[6] Warfarin's anticoagulant effect can be reduced in the presence of carbamazepine.

Thus, if a patient has been titrated to a stable dosage on one of the agents in this category, and then begins a course of treatment with EQUETRO™, it is reasonable to expect that a dose increase for the concomitant agent may be necessary.

Agents with Increased Levels in the Presence of Carbamazepine: EQUETRO™ increases the plasma levels of the following agents:

Clomipramine HCl, phenytoin[7], and primidone

[7] Phenytoin has also been reported to decrease in the presence of carbamazepine. Careful monitoring of phenytoin plasma levels following co-medication with carbamazepine is advised.

Thus, if a patient has been titrated to a stable dosage on one of the agents in this category, and then begins a course of the treatment with EQUETRO™, it is reasonable to expect that a dose decrease for the concomitant agent may be necessary.

Pharmacological/Pharmacodynamic Interactions with Carbamazepine: Concomitant administration of carbamazepine and lithium may increase the risk of neurotoxic side effects.

Given the anticonvulsant properties of carbamazepine, EQUETRO™ may reduce the thyroid function, as has been reported with other anticonvulsants. Additionally, antimalarial drugs, such as chloroquine and mefloquine, may antagonize the activity of carbamazepine.

Thus, if a patient has been titrated to a stable dosage on one of the agents in this category and then begins a course of treatment with EQUETRO™, it is reasonable to expect that a dose adjustment may be necessary.

Because of its primary CNS effect, caution should be used when EQUETRO™ is taken with other centrally acting drugs and alcohol.

Carcinogenesis, Mutagenesis, Impairment of Fertility: Administration of carbamazepine to Sprague-Dawley rats for 2 years in the diet at doses of 25, 75, and 250 mg/kg/day (low dose approximately 0.2 times the human daily dose of 1200 mg on a mg/m² basis) resulted in a dose-related increase in the incidence of hepatocellular tumors in females and of benign interstitial cell adenomas in the testes of males.

Carbamazepine must, therefore, be considered to be carcinogenic in Sprague-Dawley rats. Bacterial and mammalian mutagenicity studies using carbamazepine produced negative results. The significance of these findings relative to the use of carbamazepine in humans is, at present, unknown.

Usage in Pregnancy: Pregnancy Category D (see **WARNINGS**).

Labor and Delivery: The effect of carbamazepine on human labor and delivery is unknown.

Nursing Mothers: Carbamazepine and its epoxide metabolite are transferred to breast milk during lactation. Because of the potential for serious adverse reactions in nursing infants from carbamazepine, a decision should be made whether to discontinue nursing or to discontinue the drug, taking into account the importance of the drug to the mother.

Pediatric Use: The safety and effectiveness of EQUETRO™ in pediatric and adolescent patients have not been established.

Geriatric Use: No systematic studies in geriatric patients have been conducted.

ADVERSE REACTIONS
General

The most severe adverse reactions previously observed with carbamazepine were reported in the hemopoietic system and skin (see **BOXED WARNING**), and in the cardiovascular system.

The most frequently observed adverse reactions, particularly during the initial phases of therapy, are dizziness, drowsiness, unsteadiness, nausea, and vomiting. To minimize the possibility of such reactions, therapy should be initiated at the lowest dosage recommended.

The most commonly observed adverse experiences (5% and at least twice placebo) seen in association with the use of EQUETRO™ (400 to 1600 mg/day, dose adjusted in 200 mg daily increments in week 1 in Bipolar I Disorder in the double-blind, placebo-controlled trials of 3 weeks' duration) are included in Table 1 below:

Table 1. Most Common Adverse Events Reported in Double-Blind, Placebo Controlled Trials (Incidence ≥5% and at least twice Placebo)

Adverse Events	EQUETRO™ (N = 251)	Placebo (N = 248)
DIZZINESS	44%	12%
SOMNOLENCE	32%	13%
NAUSEA	29%	10%
VOMITING	18%	3%
ATAXIA	15%	0%
PRURITUS	8%	2%
DRY MOUTH	8%	3%
AMBLYOPIA*	6%	2%
SPEECH DISORDER	6%	0%

*Reported as blurred vision

EQUETRO™ and placebo-treated patients from two of the double-blind, placebo-controlled studies were enrolled in a 6-month open-label study. Table 2 below summarizes the most common adverse events with an incidence of 5% or more.

Table 2. Most Common Adverse Events Reported in Open Label Trials (Incidence ≥5%)

Body As A Whole	% events reported
Headache	22%
Infection	12%
Pain	12%
Asthenia	8%
Accidental Injury	7%
Chest Pain	5%
Back Pain	5%
Digestive	
Diarrhea	10%
Dyspepsia	10%
Nausea	10%
Constipation	5%
Nervous System	
Dizziness	16%
Somnolence	12%
Amnesia^	8%
Anxiety	7%
Depression*	7%
Manic Depressive Reaction	7%
Ataxia	5%
Skin Appendages	
Rash	13%
Pruritus	5%

^ Amnesia includes poor memory, forgetful, and memory disturbance.
* Depression includes suicidal ideation.

Other significant adverse events seen in less than 5% of patients include: Suicide Attempt, Manic Reaction, Insomnia, Nervousness, Depersonalization and Extrapyramidal Symptoms, Infections (Fungal, Viral, Bacterial), Pharyngitis, Rhinitis, Sinusitis, Bronchitis, Urinary Tract Infection, Leukopenia and Lymphadenopathy, Liver Function Tests Abnormal, Edema, Peripheral Edema, Allergic Reaction, Photosensitivity Reaction, Alopecia, Diplopia, and Ear Pain. The following additional adverse reactions were previously reported with carbamazepine:

Hemopoietic System: Aplastic anemia, agranulocytosis, pancytopenia, bone marrow depression, thrombocytopenia, leukopenia, leukocytosis, eosinophilia, acute intermittent porphyria.

Skin: Toxic epidermal necrolysis (TEN) and Stevens-Johnson syndrome (SJS) (see **BOXED WARNING**), pruritic and erythematous rashes, urticaria, photosensitivity reactions, alterations in skin pigmentation, exfoliative dermatitis, erythema multiforme and nodosum, purpura, aggravation of disseminated lupus erythematosus, alopecia, and diaphoresis. In certain cases, discontinuation of therapy may be necessary. Isolated cases of hirsutism have been reported, but a causal relationship is not clear.

Cardiovascular System: Congestive heart failure, edema, aggravation of hypertension, hypotension, syncope and collapse, aggravation of coronary artery disease, arrhythmias and AV block, thrombophlebitis, thromboembolism, and adenopathy or lymphadenopathy. Some of these cardiovascular complications have resulted in fatalities. Myocardial infarction has been associated with other tricyclic compounds.

Liver: Abnormalities in liver function tests, cholestatic and hepatocellular jaundice, hepatitis.

Respiratory System: Pulmonary hypersensitivity characterized by fever, dyspnea, pneumonitis, or pneumonia.

Genitourinary System: Urinary frequency, acute urinary retention, oliguria with elevated blood pressure, azotemia, renal failure, and impotence. Albuminuria, glycosuria, elevated BUN, and microscopic deposits in the urine have also been reported.

Testicular atrophy occurred in rats receiving carbamazepine orally from 4-52 weeks at dosage levels of 50-400 mg/kg/day. Additionally, rats receiving carbamazepine in the diet for 2 years at dosage levels of 25, 75, and 250 mg/kg/day had a dose-related incidence of testicular atrophy and aspermatogenesis. In dogs, it produced a brownish discoloration, presumably a metabolite, in the urinary bladder at dosage levels of 50 mg/kg/day and higher. Relevance of these findings to humans is unknown.

Nervous System: Dizziness, drowsiness, disturbances of coordination, confusion, headache, fatigue, blurred vision, visual hallucinations, transient diplopia, oculomotor disturbances, nystagmus, speech disturbances, abnormal involuntary movements, peripheral neuritis and paresthesias, depression with agitation, talkativeness, tinnitus, and hyperacusis.

There have been reports of associated paralysis and other symptoms of cerebral arterial insufficiency, but the exact relationship of these reactions to the drug has not been established.

Isolated cases of neuroleptic malignant syndrome have been reported with concomitant use of psychotropic drugs.

Digestive System: Nausea, vomiting, gastric distress and abdominal pain, diarrhea, constipation, anorexia, and dryness of the mouth and pharynx, including glossitis and stomatitis.

Eyes: Scattered punctate cortical lens opacities, as well as conjunctivitis, have been reported. Although a direct causal relationship has not been established, many phenothiazines and related drugs have been shown to cause eye changes.

Musculoskeletal System: Aching joints and muscles, and leg cramps.

Metabolism: Fever and chills and inappropriate antidiuretic hormone (ADH) secretion syndrome have been reported. Cases of frank water intoxication, with decreased serum sodium (hyponatremia) and confusion, have been reported in association with carbamazepine use (see **PRECAUTIONS, Laboratory Tests**). Decreased levels of plasma calcium have been reported.

Other: Isolated cases of a lupus erythematosus-like syndrome have been reported. There have been occasional reports of elevated levels of cholesterol, HDL cholesterol, and triglycerides in patients taking anticonvulsants.

A case of aseptic meningitis, accompanied by myoclonus and peripheral eosinophilia, has been reported in a patient taking carbamazepine in combination with other medications. The patient was successfully dechallenged, and the meningitis reappeared upon rechallenge with carbamazepine.

DRUG ABUSE AND DEPENDENCE

No evidence of abuse potential has been associated with carbamazepine, nor is there evidence of psychological or physical dependence in humans.

OVERDOSAGE
Acute Toxicity

Lowest known lethal dose: adults, >60 g (39-year-old man). Highest known doses survived: adults, 30 g (31-year-old woman); children, 10 g (6-year-old boy); small children, 5 g (3-year-old girl).

Oral LD₅₀ in animals (mg/kg): mice, 1100-3750; rats, 3850-4025; rabbits, 1500-2680; guinea pigs, 920.

Signs and Symptoms

The first signs and symptoms appear after 1-3 hours. Neuromuscular disturbances are the most prominent. Cardiovascular disorders are generally milder, and severe cardiac complications occur only when very high doses (>60 g) have been ingested.

Respiration: Irregular breathing, respiratory depression.

Cardiovascular System: Tachycardia, hypotension or hypertension, shock, conduction disorders.

Nervous System and Muscles: Impairment of consciousness ranging in severity to deep coma. Convulsions, especially in small children. Motor restlessness, muscular twitching, tremor, athetoid movements, opisthotonos, ataxia, drowsiness, dizziness, mydriasis, nystagmus, adiadochokinesia, ballism, psychomotor disturbances, dysmetria. Initial hyperreflexia, followed by hyporeflexia.

Gastrointestinal Tract: Nausea, vomiting.

Kidneys and Bladder: Anuria or oliguria, urinary retention.

Laboratory Findings: Isolated instances of overdosage have included leukocytosis, reduced leukocyte count, glycosuria, and acetonuria. ECG may show dysrhythmias.

Combined Poisoning: When alcohol, tricyclic antidepressants, barbiturates, or hydantoins are taken at the same time, the signs and symptoms of acute poisoning with carbamazepine may be aggravated or modified.

Treatment

For the most up to date information on management of carbamazepine overdose, please contact the poison center for your area by calling 1-800-222-1222. The prognosis in cases of carbamazepine poisoning is generally favorable. Of 5,645 cases of carbamazepine exposures reported to US poison centers in 2002, a total of 8 deaths (0.14% mortality rate) occurred. Over 39% of the cases reported to these poison centers were managed safely at home with conservative care. Successful management of large or intentional carbamazepine exposures requires implementation of supportive care, frequent monitoring of serum drug concentrations, and aggressive but appropriate gastric decontamination.

Elimination of the Drug: The primary method for gastric decontamination of carbamazepine overdose is use of activated charcoal. For substantial recent ingestions, gastric lavage may also be considered. Administration of activated charcoal prior to hospital assessment has the potential to significantly reduce drug absorption. There is no specific antidote. In overdose, absorption of carbamazepine may be prolonged and delayed. More than one dose of activated charcoal may be beneficial in patients who have evidence of continued absorption (e.g., rising serum carbamazepine levels).

Measures to Accelerate Elimination: The data on use of dialysis to enhance elimination in carbamazepine is scarce. Dialysis, particularly high-flux or high-efficiency hemodialysis, may be considered in patients with severe carbamazepine poisoning associated with renal failure or in cases of status epilepticus, or where there are rising serum drug levels and worsening clinical status despite appropriate supportive care and gastric decontamination. For severe cases of carbamazepine overdose unresponsive to other measures, charcoal hemoperfusion may be used to enhance drug clearance.

Continued on next page

Equetro—Cont.

Respiratory Depression: Keep the airways free; resort, if necessary, to endotracheal intubation, artificial respiration, and administration of oxygen.

Hypotension, Shock: Keep the patient's legs raised and administer a plasma expander. If blood pressure fails to rise despite measures taken to increase plasma volume, use of vasoactive substances should be considered.

Convulsions: Diazepam or barbiturates.

Warning: Diazepam or barbiturates may aggravate respiratory depression (especially in children), hypotension, and coma. However, barbiturates should not be used if drugs that inhibit monoamine oxidase have also been taken by the patient either in overdosage or in recent therapy (within 1 week).

Surveillance: Respiration, cardiac function (ECG monitoring), blood pressure, body temperature, pupillary reflexes, and kidney and bladder function should be monitored for several days.

Treatment of Blood Count Abnormalities: If evidence of significant bone marrow depression develops, the following recommendations are suggested: (1) stop the drug, (2) perform daily CBC, platelet, and reticulocyte counts, (3) do a bone marrow aspiration and trephine biopsy immediately and repeat with sufficient frequency to monitor recovery.

Special periodic studies might be helpful, as follows: (1) white cell and platelet antibodies, (2) ^{59}Fe-ferrokinetic studies, (3) peripheral blood cell typing, (4) cytogenetic studies on marrow and peripheral blood, (5) bone marrow culture studies for colony-forming units, (6) hemoglobin electrophoresis for A_2 and F hemoglobin, and (7) serum folic acid and B_{12} levels.

A fully developed aplastic anemia will require appropriate, intensive monitoring and therapy, for which specialized consultation should be sought.

DOSAGE AND ADMINISTRATION

The recommended initial dose of EQUETRO™ is 400 mg/day given in divided doses, twice daily. The dose should be adjusted in 200 mg daily increments to achieve optimal clinical response. Doses higher than 1600 mg/day have not been studied.

Monitoring of blood levels (see **PRECAUTIONS, Laboratory Tests**) may be useful for verification of drug compliance, assessing safety, and determining the cause of toxicity, including when more than one medication is being used.

The EQUETRO™ capsules may be opened and the beads sprinkled over food, such as a teaspoon of applesauce or other similar food products if this method of administration is preferred. EQUETRO™ capsules or their contents should not be crushed or chewed. EQUETRO™ can be taken with or without meals.

HOW SUPPLIED

EQUETRO™ (carbamazepine) extended-release capsules is supplied in three dosage strengths.

100 mg-Two-piece hard gelatin capsule yellow opaque cap with bluish green opaque body printed with the SPD417 on one end, SPD417 and 100 mg on the other in white ink:
Supplied in bottles of 120   NDC 30698-419-12

200 mg-Two-piece hard gelatin capsule yellow opaque cap with blue opaque body printed with the SPD417 on one end and SPD417 and 200 mg on the other in white ink:
Supplied in bottles of 120   NDC 30698-421-12

300 mg-Two-piece hard gelatin capsule yellow opaque cap with blue body printed with the SPD417 on one end and SPD417 and 300 mg on the other in white ink:
Supplied in bottles of 120   NDC 30698-423-12

Store at 25° C (77°F); excursions permitted to 15-30°C (59-86°F) [see USP controlled room temperature].

PROTECT FROM LIGHT AND MOISTURE.

Manufactured for Validus Pharmaceuticals, Inc.,
119 Cherry Hill Road, Suite 310,
Parsippany, NJ 07054, 1-866-9VALIDUS
(1-866-982-5438) info@validuspharma.com
http://www.equetro.com/

By Shire US Inc., 725 Chesterbrook Blvd, Wayne, PA 19087

Made in U.S.A. © 2007 Validus Pharmaceuticals, Inc.

004486 419 1207 XXX (Rev 12/2007)

DRUG INFORMATION CENTERS

ALABAMA

BIRMINGHAM

Drug Information Service
University of Alabama
UAB Hospital Pharmacy
Drug Information-JT1720
619 S. 19th St.
Birmingham, AL 35249-6860
Mon.-Fri. 7 AM-4 PM
205-934-2162
www.health.uab.edu/pharmacy

Global Drug
Information Service
Samford University
McWhorter School
of Pharmacy
800 Lakeshore Dr.
Birmingham, AL 35229-7027
Mon. 8 AM-9 PM
Tues.-Fri. 8 AM-4:30 PM
205-726-2519 or 2891
www.samford.edu/schools/
pharmacy/dic/index.html

HUNTSVILLE

Huntsville Hospital Drug
Information Center
101 Sivley Rd.
Huntsville, AL 35801
Mon.-Fri. 8 AM-4:30 PM
256-265-8284

ARIZONA

TUCSON

Arizona Poison and Drug
Information Center
1259 N. Martin Ave.
Drachman Hall B308
Tucson, AZ 85724
7 days/week, 24 hours
520-626-6016
800-222-1222 **(Emergency)**
www.pharmacy.arizona.edu

ARKANSAS

LITTLE ROCK

Arkansas Drug Information
Center
4301 W. Markham St.
Slot 522-2
Little Rock, AR 72205
Mon.-Fri. 8:30 AM-5 PM
501-686-6161
(Little Rock area only -
for healthcare
professionals only)
888-228-1233
(AR only - **for healthcare**
professionals only)

CALIFORNIA

LOS ANGELES

Los Angeles Regional
Drug Information Center
LAC & USC Medical Center
1200 N. State St.
Trailer 25
Los Angeles, CA 90033
Mon.-Fri. 8 AM-4 PM
Closed 12 PM to 1 PM
323-226-7741

SAN DIEGO

Drug Information Service
University of California
San Diego Medical Center
200 West Arbor Dr.
MC 8925
San Diego, CA 92103-8925
Mon.-Fri. 9 AM-5 PM
619-543-6971
(**for healthcare**
professionals only)

STANFORD

Drug Information Center
University of California
Stanford Hospital and Clinics
300 Pasteur Dr.
Room H-0301
Stanford, CA 94305
Mon.-Fri. 8 AM-4 PM
650-723-6422

COLORADO

DENVER

Rocky Mountain Poison
and Drug Center
990 Bannock St.
(Physical address)
777 Bannock St.
(Mailing address)
Denver, CO 80264
303-739-1100
800-222-1222 **(Emergency)**
www.rmpdc.org

CONNECTICUT

FARMINGTON

Drug Information Service
University of Connecticut
Health Center
263 Farmington Ave.
Farmington, CT 06030
Mon.-Fri. 10 AM-2 PM
860-679-2783

HARTFORD

Drug Information Center
Hartford Hospital
P.O. Box 5037
80 Seymour St.
Hartford, CT 06102
Mon.-Fri. 8:30 AM-5 PM
860-545-2221
860-545-2961(After 5 PM)
www.hartfordhospital.org

NEW HAVEN

Drug Information Center
Yale-New Haven Hospital
20 York St.
New Haven, CT 06540-3202
Mon.-Fri. 9 AM-5 PM
203-688-2248
www.ynhh.org

DISTRICT OF COLUMBIA

Drug Information Service
Howard University Hospital
Room BB06
2041 Georgia Ave. NW
Washington, DC 20060
Mon.-Fri. 8:30 AM-4 PM
202-865-7413
www.huhosp.org/patientpublic/
pharmacy.htm

FLORIDA

FT. LAUDERDALE

Nova Southeastern University
College of Pharmacy
Drug Information Center
3200 S. University Dr.
Ft. Lauderdale, FL 33328
Mon.-Fri. 9 AM-5 PM
954-262-3103
http://pharmacy.nova.edu

GAINESVILLE

Drug Information &
Pharmacy Resource Center
Shands Hospital at
University of Florida
P.O. Box 100316
Gainesville, FL 32610-0316
Mon.-Fri. 9 AM-5 PM
352-265-0408
(**for healthcare**
professionals only)
http://shands.org/professional/
drugs

JACKSONVILLE

Drug Information Service
Shands Jacksonville
655 W. 8th St.
Jacksonville, FL 32209
Mon.-Fri. 8:30 AM-5 PM
904-244-4185
(**for healthcare**
professionals only)
904-244-4700
(**for consumers,**
Mon.-Fri. 9:30 AM-4 PM)
http://jax.shands.org/
education/pharmacy/contact.asp

ORLANDO

Orlando Regional Drug
Information Service
Orlando Regional
Healthcare System
1414 Kuhl Ave., MP 192
Orlando, FL 32806
Mon.-Fri. 8 AM-4 PM
321-841-8717

TALLAHASSEE

Drug Information
Education Center
Florida Agricultural and
Mechanical University
College of Pharmacy and
Pharmaceutical Sciences
Tallahassee, FL 32307
Mon.-Fri. 9 AM-5 PM
850-561-2688

WEST PALM BEACH

Drug Information Center
Nova Southeastern University,
West Palm Beach
3970 RCA Blvd., Suite 7006A
Palm Beach Gardens, FL 33410
Mon.-Fri. 9 AM-5 PM
561-622-0658
(**for healthcare**
professionals only)

GEORGIA

ATLANTA

Emory University Hospital
Dept. of Pharmaceutical
Services-Drug Information
1364 Clifton Rd. NE
Atlanta, GA 30322
Mon.-Fri. 9 AM-4 PM
404-712-4644
(**for healthcare**
professionals only)

Drug Information Service
Northside Hospital
1000 Johnson Ferry Rd. NE
Atlanta, GA 30342
Mon.-Fri. 9 AM-4 PM
404-851-8676 (GA only)

COLUMBUS

**Columbus Regional Drug
Information Center**
710 Center St.
Columbus, GA 31902
Mon.-Fri. 8 AM-5 PM
    706-571-1934
    **(for healthcare
    professionals only)**

IDAHO

POCATELLO

**Drug Information Center
Idaho State University
School of Pharmacy**
970 S. 5th St.
Campus Box 8092
Pocatello, ID 83209
Mon.-Thur. 8:30 AM-5 PM
Fri. 8:30 AM-3 PM
    208-282-4689
    800-334-7139 (ID only)
http://pharmacy.isu.edu

ILLINOIS

CHICAGO

**Drug Information Center
Northwestern Memorial
Hospital**
Feinberg Pavilion, LC 700
251 E. Huron St.
Chicago, IL 60611
Mon.-Fri. 8:30 AM-5 PM
    312-926-7573

**Drug Information Center
University of Illinois at
Chicago**
833 S. Wood St.
MC 886
Chicago, IL 60612-7231
Mon.-Fri. 8 AM-4 PM
    312-996-3681
    **(for healthcare
    professionals only)**
    312-996-5332
    **(for consumers,
    Mon.-Fri. 9 AM-12 PM)**
www.uic.edu/pharmacy/
services/di/index.html

HARVEY

**Drug Information Center
Ingalls Memorial Hospital**
1 Ingalls Dr.
Harvey, IL 60426
Mon.-Fri. 8 AM-7 PM
Sat. 9 AM-3:30 PM
    708-333-4300

HINES

**Drug Information Service
Hines Veterans Administration
Hospital**
Pharmacy Services
MC119
P.O. Box 5000
Hines, IL 60141-5000
Mon.-Fri. 8 AM-4:30 PM
    708-202-8387, ext. 23780

PARK RIDGE

**Drug Information Center
Advocate Lutheran General
Hospital**
1775 Dempster St.
Park Ridge, IL 60068
Mon.-Fri. 7:30 AM-4 PM
    847-723-8128
    **(for healthcare
    professionals only)**

INDIANA

INDIANAPOLIS

**Drug Information Center
St. Vincent Hospital
and Health Services**
2001 W. 86th St.
Indianapolis, IN 46260
Mon.-Fri. 8 AM-4 PM
    317-338-3200
    **(for healthcare
    professionals only)**

**Drug Information Service
Clarian Health Partners**
Pharmacy Department I-65
at 21st St.
Room CG04
Indianapolis, IN 46202
Mon.-Fri. 8 AM-4:30 PM
    317-962-1750

MUNCIE

**Drug Information Center
Ball Memorial Hospital**
2401 University Ave.
Muncie, IN 47303
Mon.-Fri. 8 AM-4:30 PM
    765-747-3033

IOWA

DES MOINES

**Regional Drug
Information Center
Mercy Medical Center-
Des Moines**
1111 Sixth Ave.
Des Moines, IA 50314
Mon.-Fri. 8 AM-4:30 PM
    (regional service; in-house
    service answered 7 days/
    week, 24 hours)
    515-247-3286

IOWA CITY

**Drug Information Center
University of Iowa
Hospitals and Clinics**
200 Hawkins Dr.
Iowa City, IA 52242
Mon.-Fri. 8 AM-4:30 PM
    319-356-2600

KANSAS

KANSAS CITY

**Drug Information Center
University of Kansas
Medical Center**
3901 Rainbow Blvd.
Kansas City, KS 66160
Mon.-Fri. 8:30 AM-4:30 PM
    913-588-2328

KENTUCKY

LEXINGTON

**University of Kentucky
Central Pharmacy
Chandler Medical Center**
800 Rose St., C-114
Lexington, KY 40536-0293
7 days/week, 24 hours
    859-323-5642
    859-323-6289

LOUISIANA

MONROE

**Louisiana Drug and Poison
Information Center
University of Louisiana at
Monroe College of Pharmacy**
Sugar Hall
Monroe, LA 71209-6430
Mon.-Thur. 8 AM-4:30 PM
Fri. 8 AM-11:30 AM
    318-342-1710

NEW ORLEANS

**Xavier University Drug
Information Center
Tulane University
Hospital and Clinic**
1440 Canal St.
Suite 808
New Orleans, LA 70112
Mon.-Fri. 9 AM-5 PM
    504-588-5670

MARYLAND

ANDREWS AFB

Drug Information Services
79 MDSS/SGQP
1050 W. Perimeter Rd.
Suite D1-119
Andrews AFB, MD 20762-6660
Mon.-Fri. 7:30 AM-5 PM
    240-857-4565

BALTIMORE

**Drug Information Service
Johns Hopkins Hospital**
600 N. Wolfe St.
Carnegie 180
Baltimore, MD 21287-6180
Mon.-Fri. 8:30 AM-5 PM
    410-955-6348

**Drug Information Service
University of Maryland
School of Pharmacy**Pharmacy
Hall Room 760
20 North Pine St.
Baltimore, MD 21201
Mon.-Fri. 8:30 AM-5 PM
    410-706-7568
    (consumers only)
    410-706-0898
    **(for healthcare
    professionals only)**
www.pharmacy.umaryland.
edu/umdi

EASTON

**Drug Information
Pharmacy Dept.
Memorial Hospital**
219 S. Washington St.
Easton, MD 21601
7 days/week, 7 AM-5:30 PM
    410-822-1000, ext. 5645

MASSACHUSETTS

BOSTON

**Drug Information Services
Brigham and Women's
Hospital**
75 Francis St.
Boston, MA 02115
Mon.-Fri. 7 AM-3 PM
    617-732-7166

WORCESTER

**Drug Information Pharmacy
UMass Memorial
Medical Center
Healthcare Hospital**
55 Lake Ave. North
Worcester, MA 01655
Mon.-Fri. 8:30 AM-5 PM
    508-856-3456
    508-856-2775 (24-hour)

MICHIGAN

ANN ARBOR

**Drug Information Service
Dept. of Pharmacy Services
University of Michigan
Health System**
1500 East Medical
Center Dr.
UH B2D301
Box 0008
Ann Arbor, MI 48109-0008
Mon.-Fri. 8 AM-5 PM
    734-936-8200

DETROIT

**Drug Information Center
Department of Pharmacy
Services
Detroit Receiving Hospital and
University Health Center**
4201 St. Antoine Blvd.
Detroit, MI 48201
Mon.-Fri. 9 AM-5 PM
    313-745-4556
www.dmcpharmacy.org

LANSING

Drug Information Services
Sparrow Hospital
1215 East Michigan Ave.
Lansing, MI 48912
7 days/week, 24 hours
517-364-2444

PONTIAC

Drug Information Center
St. Joseph Mercy Oakland
44405 Woodward Ave.
Pontiac, MI 48341
Mon.-Fri. 8 AM-4:30 PM
248-858-3055

ROYAL OAK

Drug Information Services
William Beaumont Hospital
3601 West 13 Mile Rd.
Royal Oak, MI 48073-6769
Mon.-Fri. 8 AM-4:30 PM
248-898-4077

SOUTHFIELD

Drug Information Service
Providence Hospital
16001 West 9 Mile Rd.
Southfield, MI 48075
Mon.-Fri. 8 AM-4 PM
248-849-3125

MISSISSIPPI

JACKSON

Drug Information Center
University of Mississippi
Medical Center
2500 N. State St.
Jackson, MS 39216
Mon.-Fri. 8 AM-4:30 PM
601-984-2060

MISSOURI

KANSAS CITY

University of
Missouri-Kansas City
Drug Information Center
2464 Charlotte St., Suite 1220
Kansas City, MO 64108
Mon.-Fri. 9 AM-4 PM
816-235-5490
http://druginfo.umkc.edu/

SPRINGFIELD

Drug Information Center
St. John's Hospital
1235 E. Cherokee St.
Springfield, MO 65804
Mon.-Fri. 8 AM-4:30 PM
417-820-3488

ST. JOSEPH

Regional Medical Center
Pharmacy
5325 Faraon St.
St. Joseph, MO 64506
7 days/week, 24 hours
816-271-6141

MONTANA

MISSOULA

Drug Information Service
University of Montana School
of Pharmacy and Allied Health
Sciences
32 Campus Dr.
1522 Skaggs Bldg.
Missoula, MT 59812-1522
Mon.-Fri. 8 AM-5 PM
406-243-5254
800-501-5491
www.health.umt.edu/dis

NEBRASKA

OMAHA

Drug Informatics Service
School of Pharmacy
Creighton University
2500 California Plaza
Health Science Library
Room 204
Omaha, NE 68178
Mon.-Fri. 8:30 AM-4:30 PM
402-280-5101
http://druginfo.creighton.edu

NEW JERSEY

NEWARK

New Jersey Poison
Information and Education
System
140 Bergen St.
Newark, NJ 07107
Mon.-Fri. 8 AM- 5 PM
973-972-9280
800-222-1222 (Emergency)
www.njpies.org

NEW BRUNSWICK

Drug Information Service
Robert Wood Johnson
University Hospital
Pharmacy Department
1 Robert Wood Johnson Pl.
New Brunswick, NJ 08901
Mon.-Fri. 8:30 AM-4:30 PM
732-937-8842

NEW MEXICO

ALBUQUERQUE

New Mexico Poison Center
University of New Mexico
Health Sciences Center
MSC09 5080
1 University of New Mexico
Albuquerque, NM 87131
7 days/week, 24 hours
505-272-4261
800-222-1222 (Emergency)
http://hsc.unm.edu/pharmacy/
poison

NEW YORK

BROOKLYN

International Drug
Information Center
Long Island University
Arnold & Marie Schwartz
College of Pharmacy &
Health Sciences
75 DeKalb Ave.
RM-HS509
Brooklyn, NY 11201
Mon.-Fri. 9 AM-5 PM
718-488-1064
www.liu.edu

NEW HYDE PARK

Drug Information Center
St. John's University at Long
Island Jewish Medical Center
270-05 76th Ave.
New Hyde Park, NY 11040
Mon.-Fri. 8 AM-3 PM
718-470-DRUG (3784)

NEW YORK CITY

Drug Information Center
Memorial Sloan-Kettering
Cancer Center
1275 York Ave.
RM S-702
New York, NY 10021
Mon.-Fri. 9 AM-5 PM
212-639-7552

Drug Information Center
Mount Sinai Medical Center
1 Gustave Levy Pl.
New York, NY 10029
Mon.-Fri. 9 AM-5 PM
212-241-6619
(for in-house healthcare
professionals only)

ROCHESTER

Finger Lakes
Poison and Drug
Information Center
University of Rochester
601 Elmwood Ave.
Rochester, NY 14642
Mon.-Fri. 8 AM-5 PM
585-275-3718

NORTH CAROLINA

BUIES CREEK

Drug Information Center
School of Pharmacy
Campbell University
P.O. Box 1090
Buies Creek, NC 27506
Mon.-Fri. 8:30 AM-4:30 PM
910-893-1200,
ext. 2701
800-760-9697 (Toll free),
ext. 2701
800-327-5467 (NC only)

CHAPEL HILL

University of North
Carolina Hospitals
Drug Information Center
Dept. of Pharmacy
101 Manning Dr.
Chapel Hill, NC 27514
Mon.-Fri. 8 AM-4:30 PM
919-966-2373

DURHAM

Drug Information Center
Duke University Health
Systems
DUMC Box 3089
Durham, NC 27710
Mon.-Fri. 8 AM-5 PM
919-684-5125

GREENVILLE

Eastern Carolina Drug
Information Center
Pitt County
Memorial Hospital
Dept. of Pharmacy Service
P.O. Box 6028
2100 Stantonsburg Rd.
Greenville, NC 27835
Mon.-Fri. 8 AM-5 PM
252-847-4257

WINSTON-SALEM

Drug Information
Service Center
Wake-Forest University
Baptist Medical Center
Medical Center Blvd.
Winston-Salem, NC 27157
Mon.-Fri. 8 AM-5 PM
336-716-2037
(for healthcare
professionals only)

OHIO

ADA

Drug Information Center
Raabe College of Pharmacy
Ohio Northern University
Ada, OH 45810
Mon.-Thurs. 8:30 AM-5 PM
Fri. 8:30 AM-4 PM
419-772-2307
www.onu.edu/pharmacy/
druginfo

CINCINNATI

Drug and Poison
Information Center
Children's Hospital
Medical Center
3333 Burnet Ave.
Cincinnati, OH 45229
Mon.-Fri. 9 AM-5 PM
513-636-5063
(Administration)
513-636-5111
(7 days/week, 24 hours)

CLEVELAND

Drug Information Service
Cleveland Clinic Foundation
9500 Euclid Ave.
Cleveland, OH 44195
Mon.-Fri. 8:30 AM-4:30 PM
216-444-6456
**(for healthcare
professionals only)**

COLUMBUS

Drug Information Center
Ohio State University Hospital
Dept. of Pharmacy
Doan Hall 368
410 W. 10th Ave.
Columbus, OH 43210-1228
Mon.-Fri. 8 AM-4:30 PM
614-293-8679
**(for in-house healthcare
professionals only)**

Drug Information Center
Riverside Methodist Hospital
3535 Olentangy River Road
Columbus, OH 43214
7 days/week, 24 hours
614-566-5425

TOLEDO

Drug Information Services
St. Vincent Mercy Medical
Center
2213 Cherry St.
Toledo, Ohio 43608-2691
Mon.-Fri. 7 AM-5 PM
419-251-4227
www.rx.medctr.ohio-state.edu

OKLAHOMA

OKLAHOMA CITY

Drug Information Service
Integris Health
3300 Northwest Expressway
Oklahoma City, OK 73112
Mon.-Fri. 8 AM-4:30 PM
405-949-3660

Drug Information Center
OU Medical Center
1200 Everett Dr.
Oklahoma City, OK 73104
Mon.-Fri. 8 AM-4:30 PM
405-271-6226
Fax: 405-271-6281

TULSA

Drug Information Center
Saint Francis Hospital
6161 S. Yale Ave.
Tulsa, OK 74136
Mon.-Fri. 8 AM-4:30 PM
918-494-6339
**(for healthcare
professionals only)**

PENNSYLVANIA

PHILADELPHIA

Drug Information Center
Temple University Hospital
Dept. of Pharmacy
3401 N. Broad St.
Philadelphia, PA 19140
Mon.-Fri. 8 AM-4:30 PM
215-707-4644

Drug Information Service
Dept. of Pharmacy
Thomas Jefferson
University Hospital
111 S. 11th St.
Philadelphia, PA 19107-5089
Mon.-Fri. 8 AM-5 PM
215-955-8877

University of Pennsylvania
Health System Drug
Information Service
Hospital of the University of
Pennsylvania
Department of Pharmacy
3400 Spruce St.
Philadelphia, PA 19104
Mon.-Fri. 8:30 AM-4 PM
215-662-2903

PITTSBURGH

Pharmaceutical
Information Center
Mylan School of Pharmacy
Duquesne University
431 Mellon Hall
Pittsburgh, PA 15282
Mon.-Fri. 8 AM-4 PM
412-396-4600

UPLAND

Drug Information Center
Crozer-Chester Medical Center
Dept. of Pharmacy
1 Medical Center Blvd.
Upland, PA 19013
Mon.-Fri. 8 AM-4:30 PM
610-447-2851
**(for in-house healthcare
professionals only)**

PUERTO RICO

PONCE

Centro Informacion
Medicamentos
Escuela de Medicina de Ponce
P.O. Box 7004
Ponce, PR 00732-7004
Mon.-Fri. 8 AM-4:30 PM
787-840-2575

SAN JUAN

Centro de Informacion de
Medicamentos-CIM
Escuela de Farmacia-RCM
P.O. Box 365067
San Juan, PR 00936-5067
Mon.-Fri. 8 AM-4:30 PM
787-758-2525, ext. 1516

SOUTH CAROLINA

CHARLESTON

Drug Information Service
Medical University of
South Carolina
150 Ashley Ave.
Rutledge Tower Annex
Room 604
P.O. Box 250584
Charleston, SC 29425-0810
Mon.-Fri. 9 AM-5:30 PM
843-792-3896
800-922-5250

SPARTANBURG

Drug Information Center
Spartanburg Regional
Healthcare System
101 E. Wood St.
Spartanburg, SC 29303
Mon.-Fri. 8 AM-4:30 PM
864-560-6910

TENNESSEE

KNOXVILLE

Drug Information Center
University of Tennessee
Medical Center at Knoxville
1924 Alcoa Highway
Knoxville, TN 37920-6999
Mon.-Fri. 8 AM-4:30 PM
865-544-9124

MEMPHIS

South East Regional Drug
Information Center
VA Medical Center
1030 Jefferson Ave.
Memphis, TN 38104
Mon.-Fri. 6:30 AM-4 PM
901-523-8990, ext. 6720

Drug Information Center
University of Tennessee
875 Monroe Ave.
Suite 109
Memphis, TN 38163
Mon.-Fri. 8 AM-5 PM
901-448-5556

TEXAS

AMARILLO

Drug Information Center
Texas Tech Health
Sciences Center
School of Pharmacy
1300 Coulter Rd.
Amarillo, TX 79106
Mon.-Fri. 8 AM-5 PM
806-356-4008

GALVESTON

Drug Information Center
University of Texas
Medical Branch
301 University Blvd.
Galveston, TX 77555-0701
Mon.-Fri. 8 AM-5 PM
409-772-2734

HOUSTON

Drug Information Center
Ben Taub General Hospital
Texas Southern
University/HCHD
1504 Taub Loop
Houston, TX 77030
Mon.-Fri. 8:30 AM-5 PM
713-873-3710

LACKLAND A.F.B.

Drug Information Center
Dept. of Pharmacy
Wilford Hall Medical Center
2200 Bergquist Dr.
Suite 1
Lackland A.F.B., TX 78236
7 days/week, 24 hours
210-292-5414

LUBBOCK

Drug Information and
Consultation Service
Covenant Medical Center
3615 19th St.
Lubbock, TX 79410
7 days/week, 24 hours
806-725-0408

SAN ANTONIO

Drug Information Service
University of Texas
Health Science Center
at San Antonio
Department of Pharmacology
7703 Floyd Curl Drive
San Antonio, TX 78229-3900
Mon.-Fri. 8 AM-4 PM
210-567-4280

TEMPLE

Drug Information Center
Scott and White
Memorial Hospital
2401 S. 31st St.
Temple, TX 76508
Mon.-Fri. 8 AM-5 PM
254-724-4636

UTAH

SALT LAKE CITY
Drug Information Service
University of Utah Hospital
421 Wakara Way
Suite 204
Salt Lake City, UT 84108
Mon.-Fri. 7:30 AM-5 PM
    801-581-2073

VIRGINIA

HAMPTON
Drug Information Center
Hampton University School
of Pharmacy
Hampton Harbors Annex
Hampton, VA 23668
Mon.-Fri. 9 AM-4 PM
    757-728-6693

WEST VIRGINIA

MORGANTOWN
West Virginia Center for
Drug and Health Information
West Virginia University
Robert C. Byrd
Health Sciences Center
1124 HSN, P.O. Box 9520
Morgantown, WV 26506
Mon.-Fri. 8:30 AM-5 PM
    304-293-6640
    800-352-2501 (WV)
www.hsc.wvu.edu/SOP

WYOMING

LARAMIE
Drug Information Center
University of Wyoming
1000 East University Ave.
Dept 3375
Laramie, WY 82071
Mon.-Fri. 8:30 AM-4:30 PM
    307-766-6988

Key to Controlled Substances Categories

Products listed with the symbols shown below are subject to the Controlled Substances Act of 1970. These drugs are categorized according to their potential for abuse. The greater the potential, the more severe the limitations on their prescription.

CATEGORY	INTERPRETATION
℞ II	**HIGH POTENTIAL FOR ABUSE.** Use may lead to severe physical or psychological dependence. Prescriptions must be written in ink, or typewritten and signed by the practitioner. Verbal prescriptions must be confirmed in writing within 72 hours, and may be given only in a genuine emergency. No renewals are permitted.
℞ III	**SOME POTENTIAL FOR ABUSE.** Use may lead to low-to-moderate physical dependence or high psychological dependence. Prescriptions may be oral or written. Up to 5 renewals are permitted within 6 months.
℞ IV	**LOW POTENTIAL FOR ABUSE.** Use may lead to limited physical or psychological dependence. Prescriptions may be oral or written. Up to 5 renewals are permitted within 6 months.
℞ V	**SUBJECT TO STATE AND LOCAL REGULATION.** Abuse potential is low; a prescription may not be required.

Key to FDA Use-in-Pregnancy Ratings

The U.S. Food and Drug Administration's use-in-pregnancy rating system weighs the degree to which available information has ruled out risk to the fetus against the drug's potential benefit to the patient. The ratings, and their interpretation, are as follows:

CATEGORY	INTERPRETATION
A	**CONTROLLED STUDIES SHOW NO RISK.** Adequate, well-controlled studies in pregnant women have failed to demonstrate a risk to the fetus in any trimester of pregnancy.
B	**NO EVIDENCE OF RISK IN HUMANS.** Adequate, well-controlled studies in pregnant women have not shown increased risk of fetal abnormalities despite adverse findings in animals, or, in the absence of adequate human studies, animal studies show no fetal risk. The chance of fetal harm is remote, but remains a possibility.
C	**RISK CANNOT BE RULED OUT.** Adequate, well-controlled human studies are lacking, and animal studies have shown a risk to the fetus or are lacking as well. There is a chance of fetal harm if the drug is administered during pregnancy; but the potential benefits may outweigh the potential risk.
D	**POSITIVE EVIDENCE OF RISK.** Studies in humans, or investigational or post-marketing data, have demonstrated fetal risk. Nevertheless, potential benefits from the use of the drug may outweigh the potential risk. For example, the drug may be acceptable if needed in a life-threatening situation or serious disease for which safer drugs cannot be used or are ineffective.
X	**CONTRAINDICATED IN PREGNANCY.** Studies in animals or humans, or investigational or post-marketing reports, have demonstrated positive evidence of fetal abnormalities or risk which clearly outweighs any possible benefit to the patient.

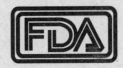

U.S. FOOD AND DRUG ADMINISTRATION

Medical Product Reporting Programs

MedWatch (24-hour service)...800-332-1088
Reporting of problems with drugs, devices, biologics (except vaccines), medical foods, and dietary supplements.

Vaccine Adverse Event Reporting System (24-hour service).............................800-822-7967
Reporting of vaccine-related problems.

Mandatory Medical Device Reporting...240-276-3000
Reporting required from user facilities regarding device-related deaths and serious injuries.

Veterinary Adverse Drug Reaction Program...888-332-8387
Reporting of adverse drug events in animals.

Division of Drug Marketing, Advertising, and Communication (DDMAC)..............301-796-1200
Inquiries from health professionals regarding product promotion.

USP Medication Errors..800-233-7767
Reporting of medication errors or near-errors to help avoid future problems through improvement in product names and packaging.

Information for Health Professionals

Center for Drug Evaluation and Research Drug Information Hotline....................301-827-4573
Information on human drugs including hormones.

Center for Biologics Office of Communications..301-827-2000
Information on biological products including vaccines and blood.

Center for Devices and Radiological Health..301-827-4573
Automated request for information on medical devices and radiation-emitting products.

Emergency Operations...301-443-1240
Emergencies involving FDA-regulated products, tampering reports, and emergency Investigational New Drug requests.

Office of Orphan Products Development...301-827-3666
Information on products for rare diseases.

General Information

General Consumer Inquiries..888-463-6332
Consumer information on regulated products/issues.

Freedom of Information..301-827-6500
Requests for publicly available FDA documents.

Office of Public Affairs..301-827-6250
Interviews/press inquiries on FDA activities.

Center for Food Safety and Applied Nutrition...888-723-3366
Information on food safety, seafood, dietary supplements, women's nutrition, and cosmetics.

Consumer Information Service, Center for Devices and Radiological Health..........800-638-2041
Information on medical devices, mammography facilities, and radiation-emitting products.